Anesthesia Color Codes

PRODUCT	COLOR
Articaine 4% with Epinephrine 1:200,000	
Articaine 4% with Epinephrine 1:100,000	
Bupivacaine 0.5% with Epinephrine 1:200,000	
Lidocaine Plain	
Lidocaine 2% with Epinephrine 1:100,000	
Lidocaine 2% with Epinephrine 1:50,000	
Mepivacaine 2% with Levonordefrin 1:20,000	
Mepivacaine 3% Plain	
Prilocaine 4% Plain	
Prilocaine 4% with Epinephrine 1:200,000	

Anesthesia color code revision. ADA News July 14, 2003; 34(13):12.

MOSBY'S DENTAL DRUG REFERENCE

MOSBY'S DENTAL DRUG REFERENCE

ELEVENTH EDITION

Editor-in-Chief
Arthur H. Jeske, DMD, PhD
Associate Dean for Strategic Planning and Continuing Dental Education
Professor
Department of General Practice and Dental Public Health
The University of Texas School of Dentistry at Houston
Houston, Texas

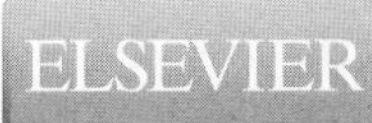

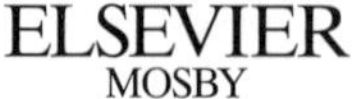

3251 Riverport Lane
St. Louis, Missouri 63043

MOSBY'S DENTAL DRUG REFERENCE, ELEVENTH EDITION

ISBN: 978-0-323-16916-5
ISSN: 2211-5625

Notices

Knowledge and best practice in this field are constantly changing. As new research and experience broaden our understanding, changes in research methods, professional practices, or medical treatment may become necessary.

Practitioners and researchers must always rely on their own experience and knowledge in evaluating and using any information, methods, compounds, or experiments described herein. In using such information or methods they should be mindful of their own safety and the safety of others, including parties for whom they have a professional responsibility.

With respect to any drug or pharmaceutical products identified, readers are advised to check the most current information provided (i) on procedures featured or (ii) by the manufacturer of each product to be administered, to verify the recommended dose or formula, the method and duration of administration, and contraindications. It is the responsibility of practitioners, relying on their own experience and knowledge of their patients, to make diagnoses, to determine dosages and the best treatment for each individual patient, and to take all appropriate safety precautions.

To the fullest extent of the law, neither the Publisher nor the authors, contributors, or editors, assume any liability for any injury and/or damage to persons or property as a matter of products liability, negligence or otherwise, or from any use or operation of any methods, products, instructions, or ideas contained in the material herein.

International Standard Book Number: 978-0-323-16916-5

Vice President and Publisher: Linda Duncan
Executive Content Strategist: Kathy Falk
Content Manager: Kristin Hebberd
Content Development Specialist: Joslyn Dumas
Publishing Services Manager: Pat Joiner
Project Manager: Lisa A.P. Bushey
Design Direction: Maggie Reid

Printed in the United States of America

Last digit is the print number: 9 8 7 6 5 4 3 2

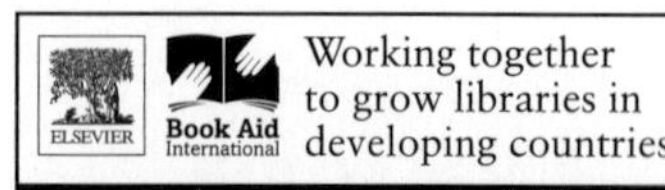

Drug Monograph Content Contributors and Reviewers

Catherine M. Flaitz, DDS, MS
Distinguished Professor
Department of Diagnostic and Biomedical Sciences
Adjunct Professor, Department of Pediatric Dentistry
The University of Texas School of Dentistry at Houston
Houston, Texas

Marshal Shlafer, PhD
Professor of Pharmacology, Medical School
Adjunct Professor of Nursing, School of Nursing
Faculty and Staff, Pharmacology Department
University of Michigan
Ann Arbor, Michigan

Ruth Fearing Tornwall, RDH, MS
Associate Professor
Department of Allied Health Sciences
Lamar Institute of Technology
Beaumont, Texas

Thomas A. Viola, RPh, CCP
Instructor, Writer, and Professional Speaker
Burlington, New Jersey

Preface

This eleventh edition of ***Mosby's Dental Drug Reference*** continues Mosby/Elsevier's tradition of providing comprehensive and current information on prescription drugs and recommendations for the care of the dental patients who take them. As in past editions, new individual drugs, as well as new drug classes, are included in this concise reference book, which is designed to address the need of oral health care practitioners and educators for readily accessible and up-to-date drug information and guidance for the dental management of medically compromised patients. The eleventh edition incorporates many significant improvements, including:

1. *A revised and updated section on the Therapeutic Management of Common Oral Lesions.*
2. *A revised and updated section on Medically Compromised Patients, addressing the most recent antibiotic prophylaxis guidelines for patients at risk of infective endocarditis and for patients with total joint replacements, as well as a summary of monoclonal antibody therapy.*
3. *Revised and updated monographs on cardiovascular drugs.*
4. *Practice-oriented precautions, dental considerations, and recommended medical consultations for every drug entry, and essential drug facts that are placed directly in the context of the dentist's and dental hygienist's care.*
5. *Highlights of serious adverse reactions and contraindications.* In each drug entry, the book calls attention to dangerous or life-threatening reactions so that you can identify them easily and deal with them promptly.
6. *Specialized dental care guidelines, including the most recent recommendations for the prevention of infective endocarditis.* Suggested protocols for the treatment of medically compromised patients and the therapeutic management of common oral lesions are also included.
7. *Combination drug guide.* Detailed index of combination drugs arranged by trade name.
8. *Comprehensive appendices.* Eleven appendices that are now housed on the companion website give you easy access to additional vital drug-related information and detailed sections concerning anesthetics, controlled substances, disorders and conditions, pregnancy and pediatrics, and prevention of medication errors.

Mosby's Dental Drug Reference provides essential drug information in a user-friendly format. The bulk of this handbook contains an alphabetical listing of drug entries by generic name. Drug entries include the following:

Generic and Brand Names. Drug entries begin with the generic drug name, followed by its pronunciation and its U.S., Canadian, and Australian brand names.

Category and Schedule. This section lists the drug's pregnancy risk category and, when appropriate, its controlled substance schedule or over-the-counter (OTC) status.

Mechanism of Action. This section clearly and concisely describes the drug's mechanism of action and therapeutic effects.

Pharmacokinetics. Under this heading, a quick-reference chart outlines the drug's route, onset, peak, and duration, when known. This information is followed by a brief description of the drug's absorption, distribution, metabolism, excretion, and half-life.

Indications and Dosages. Here, you'll find the approved indications and routes, along with age-appropriate dosage information and, for selected agents, dosage adjustments for preexisting conditions, such as liver or kidney disease.

Precautions/Contraindications. Using a practice-oriented format and written specifically for dentistry, this section presents precautions and considerations for each drug entry. Each entry lists conditions in which use of the generic drug is contraindicated.

Interactions. For drugs, herbal supplements, and food, this section supplies vital information about adverse interactions of the medical drug with drugs prescribed in dentistry.

Adverse Effects. Unlike other handbooks that mix more common adverse effects with rare, minor ones in a long, undifferentiated list, this book ranks side effects by frequency of occurrence, indicating expected, frequent, occasional, and rare.

Serious Reactions. Because serious adverse reactions can be life-threatening emergencies that require prompt intervention, this section highlights them separately from other side effects for easy identification.

***Mosby's Dental Drug Reference,* Eleventh Edition**, is an easy-to-use source of current drug information for a wide spectrum of dental care providers. When it comes to providing quality patient care, all members of the dental team can rely on the eleventh edition of *Mosby's Dental Drug Reference* for current, dentally relevant information, presented in an easy-to-use format. As you use the book, please keep in mind the following:

- The majority of the monographs are descriptions of drugs utilized on an outpatient basis and, therefore, more likely to be encountered in dental practice. Vaccines, biologicals, and medications used only intraoperatively in hospitalized patients are generally not included, and the reader is referred to other resources for this information.
- The companion website (www.dentaldrugreference.com) can be consulted for updates and new information pertinent to this text. See more about the companion website in the section titled *About the Companion Website*.
- Several important "Dental Considerations" are relevant to all of the drugs described in the monographs, including:
  1. The use of a prescription medication indicates the presence of a medical condition that is being managed by one or more physicians. The physical status of the patient and his or her ability to tolerate dental treatment must be determined.
  2. In collaboration with the treating physician(s), the physician, not the dentist, should guide all decisions related to changes in the use of prescription drugs for medical conditions.
  3. Vital signs and/or other assessments should be determined at every dental treatment visit, as appropriate and as indicated; many drugs used for systemic conditions result in adverse oral conditions, such as xerostomia. Strict attention must be paid to the prevention of negative outcomes of these conditions, particularly caries and periodontal disease; education of the patient and the patient's family about his or her medications should

be reinforced by the dental team, particularly as it relates to the prevention of oral complications of medication use.

4. This text does not constitute advice about the dental management of specific patients, each of whom must be evaluated individually using all pertinent diagnostic information, and the monographs contained in this book do not constitute full prescribing information for the drugs.

In the production of this book, we have endeavored to make it as current and relevant as possible, while emphasizing the busy oral health care provider's need for rapid access and dentally relevant information. On behalf of the editor-in-chief and Mosby, a sincere debt of gratitude is owed to our reviewers, Catherine M. Flaitz, DDS, MS, The University of Texas School of Dentistry at Houston; Marshal Shlafer, PhD, University of Michigan School of Medicine; and Ruth Fearing Tornwall, RDH, MS, Lamar Institute of Technology, and to our monograph content contributor, Thomas A. Viola, RPh, CCP, for his expertise and contributions. The previous edition of this book was dedicated to Drs. Raymond P. Ahlquist, Gerald O. Carrier, Alfred E. Ciarlone, Louis P. Gangarosa, Sr., James L. Matheny, and Armand M. Karow, and their faculty colleagues at the Medical College of Georgia, who continue to inspire us to be lifelong learners and teachers of pharmacology and its important applications to health care. This edition of the book is respectfully dedicated to dental professionals everywhere, whose quest for knowledge improves patient care and makes this book an important tool and a worthwhile project.

Arthur Jeske, DMD, PhD

Contents

About the Companion Website

The companion website offers a variety of additional learning tools and greatly enhances the text for the user. The companion website offers the following resources:

- Regular updates of drugs removed from the market
- Annual postings of full new monographs with dental-specific information
- Appendices including detailed information on anesthetics, controlled substances, disorders and conditions, pregnancy and pediatrics, and prevention of medication errors
- Color pill atlas that includes a complete listing of the drugs from the book as well as images to correlate with a number of the drugs
- Full, searchable glossary with pronunciations
- Patient teaching guides
- Clinical photos of common oral complications
- Information on Alternative Medicine, Drugs of Abuse, and Drugs Used Short-Term Intravenously
- Medically Compromised Patients
- Therapeutic Management of Common Oral Lesions

To access these resources, please visit www.dentaldrugreference.com.

Therapeutic Management of Common Oral Lesions: Based on Material from the American Academy of Oral Medicine (AAOM) Clinician's Guide to Treatment of Common Oral Conditions

This is a summary of the etiologic factors, clinical description, currently accepted therapeutic management, and patient education for the more common oral conditions. Some of the recommended treatments have been investigated more thoroughly than others, but all have been reported to be of clinical value. Many oral conditions described here have no cure but are managed by a variety of treatment modalities for the purpose of relieving discomfort, shortening their clinical duration and frequency, and minimizing recurrences. The ultimate goal is to provide individuals with some control over the severity of their condition, thereby improving their quality of life.

Clinicians are reminded that an accurate diagnosis is imperative for clinical success. Every effort should be made to determine the diagnosis before initiating treatment. It is critical to confirm that an individual does not have a serious infection, an underlying systemic disease, or a potentially malignant or malignant lesion. When signs, symptoms, microscopic diagnosis, and other laboratory evidence elude a definitive diagnosis, empirical treatment may be initiated and evaluated on a therapeutic, trial basis. Although empiric treatment may be of short-term benefit to the patient, certain drugs may mask or alleviate some of the disease features. Therefore, it is also important to make appropriate and timely referrals in order to obtain a definitive diagnosis when dealing with a persistent oral condition so that the management approach is not masking an underlying condition or to evaluate the individual for drug protocols that are beyond the expertise of the clinician.

In addition to the diagnosis, patient management should be governed by the natural history of the oral condition and whether a palliative, supportive, or curative treatment exists. Referrals of patients should be made when the patients' problems are beyond the scope of the clinician, including the use of more aggressive drug protocols for improved outcome. Furthermore, when healing of a lesion or an anticipated response to treatment is not achieved within an expected period of time, a biopsy or other laboratory studies are recommended.

All drugs require a prescription unless identified as over-the-counter (OTC) drugs. Please note that in recent years, the Food and Drug Administration (FDA) has been active in allowing OTC status for drugs formerly available by prescription only. Be sure to check the dosages of the newly released OTC drugs because they usually are of a different strength than those available by prescription. In addition, these OTC drugs or supplements may contain ingredients, preservatives, and dyes that may cause irritating-to-life-threatening adverse effects, due to relatively minor formulary changes. As with any recommended therapeutic agent, patients should be advised of potential side effects and drug interactions.

SUPPORTIVE CARE

Management of oral mucosal conditions may require topical and systemic interventions. Therapy should address patient nutrition and hydration, oral discomfort, oral hygiene, management of secondary infection, and local control of the disease process. Depending on the extent, severity, and location of oral lesions, consideration should be given to obtaining a consultation from a dentist who specializes in oral medicine, oral and maxillofacial pathology, or oral and maxillofacial surgery. When a question arises involving a medical condition, a physician should be consulted.

Temporary, symptomatic relief of painful conditions can be provided with topical preparations, such as 2% viscous lidocaine hydrochloride or OTC products containing less potent anesthetics in gel, ointment, liquid, spray, and lozenge forms. Topical anesthetics can be used as a rinse in adults to cover a wide surface area but should be applied with a cotton-tipped applicator or other soft applicator in a young child or adult who is unable to expectorate, in order to limit the amount of medication that is swallowed. Swallowing these topical anesthetics is not recommended because it may interfere with the patient's gag reflex and increase the risk for choking, aspiration, and drug toxicity. Symptomatic relief also can be obtained by mixing equal parts of diphenhydramine hydrochloride elixir and magnesium hydroxide/aluminum hydroxide. Children's formula diphenhydramine hydrochloride elixir does not contain alcohol. Sucralfate suspension also can be used before meals. The diphenhydramine mixture and the sucralfate coat the ulcerated lesions and may allow the patient to eat more comfortably. For specific details, refer to "Herpes Simplex, Topical Anesthetics and Coating Agents."

Meticulous oral hygiene is important in patients who have multiple areas of erosion or ulceration. Mucosal lesions contacting bacterial biofilm on the dentition are more likely to become secondarily infected. Patients should be seen by the dentist or dental hygienist for scaling and root planing, under local anesthesia, when necessary, in all cases in which oral hygiene is suboptimal. Patients must be encouraged to brush and floss their teeth after meals in a gentle yet efficient manner. This may be enhanced by placing a soft toothbrush under hot water to further soften the bristles. The use of fluoride toothpaste is strongly encouraged, but some patients with widespread mucosal lesions prefer toothpastes that are not highly flavored and do not contain foaming, whitening, and antitartar agents.

HERPES SIMPLEX INFECTION

Common viral infection causes two types of disease patterns: a primary or acute infection and a secondary or recurrent infection.

Primary Herpetic Gingivostomatitis

Etiology:

A transmissible infection with herpes simplex virus, usually type I or, less commonly, type II.

Clinical description:

Clear-yellowish vesicles develop intraorally and extraorally. These vesicles rupture rapidly and coalesce to form shallow, irregular, painful ulcers. The symptomatic lesions are widespread but the gingivae are affected primarily and are erythematous, enlarged, hemorrhagic, and ulcerated. The patient may have systemic signs and symptoms including anterior cervical lymphadenopathy, fever, anorexia, and malaise. Adults may develop pharyngotonsillitis that is characterized by vesiculo-ulcerative lesions, severe sore throat, and difficulty swallowing. Usually it is self-limiting, with healing in 7–14 days.

Rationale for treatment:
Early treatment to promote healing, relieve symptoms, prevent secondary infection, and support general health is the goal. Supportive therapy includes plenty of fluids, protein, vitamin and mineral food supplements, and rest. Systemic antiviral drugs are most effective when administered in the first 48 hr of onset of symptoms. Topical steroids should be avoided because they tend to permit spread of the viral infection on mucous membranes, particularly ocular membranes. Nutritional liquid supplements and pain and fever control may be needed. Patients should be cautioned to avoid touching the herpetic lesions and then touching the eyes, genitals, or other body areas because of the possibility of self-inoculation.

Topical Anesthetics and Coating Agents

Rx

Diphenhydramine hydrochloride oral solution 12.5 mg/5 ml mixed with aluminum hydroxide, magnesium hydroxide oral suspension. Compound to a 1 : 1 mixture by volume.

Disp. 200 ml

Sig. Rinse with 1–2 teaspoons (5–10 ml) every 2–4 hr for 1 min; swish and spit out.

Although these medications are OTC, it is recommended that a pharmacist compound this oral suspension. Examples of aluminum hydroxide, magnesium hydroxide oral suspensions are Maalox and Mylanta—they are common OTC brands and are available in a number of flavors. Children younger than 6 yr should not swallow this oral suspension.

Rx

Diphenhydramine hydrochloride liquid 12.5 mg/5 ml lidocaine viscous 2% oral solution/aluminum hydroxide, magnesium hydroxide oral suspension. Compound to a 1 : 1 : 1 mixture by volume.

Disp. 200 ml

Sig. Rinse with 1–2 teaspoons (5–10 ml) every 4 hr for 1 min and spit out excess. Shake well before use and store suspension at room temperature.

Compounded by pharmacy and stable for approximately 60 days. Do not use 2% lidocaine hydrochloride in children who cannot expectorate because of potential for aspiration.

Rx

Carafate, generic (sucralfate) suspension 1 g/10 ml

Disp. 200 ml

Sig. Rinse with 1 teaspoon (5 ml) 4 times a day. Rinse for 1 min and spit out excess.

In children younger than 6 yr who cannot expectorate, the amount should be limited to 0.5 g, 4 times a day (2 g/day) in case the suspension is swallowed. Safety and efficacy have not been established in children.

Systemic Antiviral Therapy

Acyclovir and valacyclovir may relieve and decrease the duration of symptoms, but the medications must be initiated at the earliest signs and symptoms for maximum effectiveness.

Rx

Zovirax, generic (acyclovir) capsules 400 mg

Disp. 21 (30) capsules

Sig. Take 1 capsule 3 times a day for 7–10 days or until lesions resolve.

The Centers for Disease Control and Prevention (CDC) recommends this dosage for severe cases of stomatitis or pharyngitis. Current FDA-approved indication is that systemic acyclovir be used to treat oral herpes only in immunocompromised patients.

Rx

Valtrex, generic (valacyclovir) tablet 1 g

Disp. 20 tablets

Sig. Take 1 tablet twice daily for 7–10 days.

The protocol is based on the CDC's recommended dosage for primary genital herpes in the immunocompetent patient. The drug should be taken within the first 48 hr of the initial signs and symptoms.

Recurrent (Orofacial) Herpes Simplex Infection

Etiology:

There is reactivation of the latent virus that resides within the sensory ganglion of the trigeminal nerve. Precipitating factors include fever, stress, exposure to sunlight, trauma, and hormonal alterations.

Clinical description:

Intraoral presentation consists of single or small clusters of vesicles that quickly rupture, forming painful ulcers. The lesions usually occur on the keratinized tissue of the hard palate and attached gingiva.

Labial presentation consists of clusters of vesicles on the vermilion border of the lips or the perioral skin that rupture within hours and then crust.

In immunocompromised patients, recurrent herpetic lesions can occur on any oral mucosal surface and can have an atypical appearance and persistent duration.

Rationale for treatment:

Treatment should be initiated as early as possible in the prodromal stage, with the goal of reducing the duration and symptoms of the lesion. Oral and topical antiviral treatment, prophylactically and therapeutically, can be considered when frequent recurrent herpetic episodes (greater than 6 episodes a year) interfere with daily function and nutrition.

Prevention

If the recurrence on the lips and perioral skin is precipitated by exposure to sunlight, the lesions can be prevented by the repeated application of sunscreen that contains a sun protection factor (SPF) of 30 or higher.

Rx

Suncreen lip balm, SPF 30 (OTC)

Disp. 1 tube

Sig. Apply to susceptible area 1 hr before sun exposure and every hour thereafter.

There are several lip balms or gels that are available that contain an SPF of 30 or higher. Several of these agents contain sensitizers that may result in irritation of the lips and surrounding skin. For maximum protection, concurrent use of a sunscreen on the face and other sun-exposed areas is recommended. A wide-brimmed hat or visor is also recommended when excessive sunlight exposure is a triggering factor. Sharing of these lipsticks should be strongly discouraged because of the potential risk of infection in a susceptible individual.

Topical Antiviral Agents

Topical antiviral medications are most effective when initiated in the early stages of lesion formation. Patients should be instructed to gently apply the medication to the affected site or where the prodromal symptoms are noted. Aggressively rubbing the affected site is not recommended because it can cause tissue trauma and the spread of the infection. To prevent autoinoculation of the virus to the fingers or other sites, the topical agent should be placed on the lesion using a cotton-tipped applicator, and hands should be thoroughly washed. Besides topical antiviral agents, there are many OTC topical anesthetics and coating agents with a variety of ingredients that may provide a protective covering or barrier over the lesion and decrease local discomfort. If these are recommended, the patients should be given the same instructions as noted above.

Rx

Denavir (penciclovir) cream 1%

Disp. 2-g tube

Sig. Dab on lesion every 2 hr while awake, for 4 days, beginning when symptoms first occur.

Rx

Zovirax (acyclovir) cream 5%

Disp. 2- or 5-g tube

Sig. Dab on lesion 5 times a day during waking hours for 4 days, beginning when symptoms first occur.

Rx

Xerese (acyclovir 5%; hydrocortisone 1%) cream

Disp. 5-g tube

Sig. Dab on lesion 5 times a day during waking hours for 5 days, beginning when symptoms first occur.

This topical agent reduces the likelihood of ulcerative lesions developing.

Rx

Abreva (docosanol) cream 10% (OTC)

Disp. 2-g tube

Sig. Dab on lesion 5 times a day during waking hours for 4 days, beginning when symptoms first occur.

Systemic Antiviral Therapy

Systemic antiviral medications are most effective when initiated in the prodromal or early stages of lesion development. The duration of treatment is convenient because the medication is usually taken for 1 day. These medications are used for a longer duration if the patient is immunocompromised. Studies have evaluated the effectiveness of systemic antiviral medications for herpes labialis, but not intraoral lesions.

Rx

Valtrex, generic (valacyclovir) tablets 1 g

Disp. 4 tablets

Sig. Take 2 tablets twice daily, 12 hr apart, when symptoms first occur.

The CDC recommends 1 g PO every 12 hr for 5–10 days for immunocompromised individuals.

To prevent herpetic recurrences from the trauma of dental treatment, some patients may benefit from taking valacyclovir tablets, 2-g dose before dental treatment and 2-g dose in the evening, followed on the next day with 1-g dose in the morning and 1-g dose in the evening.

Rx

Famvir, generic (famciclovir) tablets 500 mg

Disp. 3 tablets

Sig. Take 3 tablets as a single dose at the first sign or symptom of the infection.

The CDC recommends 500 mg PO twice daily for 5–10 days for immunocompromised individuals.

Rx

Zovirax, generic (acyclovir) capsules 400 mg

Disp. 15 (30) capsules

Sig. Take 1 capsule 3 times a day for 5–10 days.

The CDC recommends this dosing schedule for HIV-positive individuals.

HERPES ZOSTER (SHINGLES)

Etiology:

Herpes zoster represents the reactivation of latent varicella-zoster virus following a previous infection with varicella (chickenpox). Precipitating factors include immunosuppressive and cytotoxic drugs, therapeutic radiation, old age, alcohol abuse, malignancies, and trauma, including dental treatment.

Clinical description:

The classic signs and symptoms include painful segmental eruption of small vesicles that later rupture to form punctate or confluent ulcers or crusts. Fever, headache, lymphadenopathy, and referred pain may precede or accompany the lesions. When the head and neck area is involved, one or more of the branches of the trigeminal nerve are affected. It is rare in children, but the risk significantly increases after the age of 50 yr.

Rationale for treatment:

Prompt initiation of antiviral therapy is recommended to reduce duration and symptoms of the lesions. Patients older than 60 yr are especially prone to developing postherpetic neuralgia. Systemic antiviral medications are most effective if initiated within 48 hr of lesion formation. The treatment of acute herpes zoster with famciclovir significantly decreases the incidence and duration of postherpetic neuralgia. Recently, the herpes zoster virus vaccine, Zostavax, a live, attenuated vaccine, has been developed for the prevention of this infection in adults who are 50 yr or older. Length of treatment with these antiviral agents increases when herpes zoster develops in HIV-infected individuals.

Rx

Famvir, generic (famciclovir) tablets 500 mg

Disp. 21 tablets

Sig. Take 1 tablet every 8 hr for 7 days.

Rx

Zovirax, generic (acyclovir) tablets 800 mg

Disp. 50 capsules

Sig. Take 1 tablet every 4 hr, 5 times a day for 7–10 days.

Rx

Valtrex, generic (valacyclovir) tablets 1 g

Disp. 21 tablets

Sig. Take 1 tablet 3 times a day for 7 days.

RECURRENT APHTHOUS STOMATITIS

Etiology:

An altered local immune response is the predisposing factor. Patients with frequent recurrences should be screened for diseases such as anemia, allergies, vitamin deficiency, inflammatory bowel disease, and immunosuppression. Precipitating factors include stress, trauma, salivary gland hypofunction, certain medications, allergies, endocrine alterations, smoking cessation, dietary components, including cheese, chocolate, cow's milk, gluten, nuts, strawberries, and acidic foods and juices. Inspect the oral cavity closely for sources of trauma.

Clinical description:

Minor aphthous ulcerations (canker sores) are the most common clinical variation. These lesions are smaller than 1 cm, shallow, round to oval, and painful. They are covered by a cream-colored membrane and surrounded by an erythematous halo. They usually occur on nonkeratinized (movable) oral mucosa and usually heal in 7–14 days without scarring.

Major aphthous ulcerations are larger lesions that range from 1–3 cm in size and are very painful. These ulcerations are not only larger in size but may be deep with irregular borders. They are often multiple and persistent, taking 2–6 wk and longer to heal. Mucosal scarring may be extensive. These ulcerations may mimic other persistent diseases, such as deep mycotic infection, granulomatous diseases, or malignant lesions.

Herpetiform aphthous ulcerations appear as crops of small, shallow, painful lesions. They usually occur on nonkeratinized oral mucosa, but any mucosal surface may be involved. These ulcerations typically heal within 7–10 days, but closely spaced recurrences are common. Because multiple small ulcers develop suddenly, these lesions resemble recurrent intraoral herpes simplex, clinically.

Rationale for treatment:

Treatment options involve mucosal barriers, topical anesthetics, cauterization, laser therapy, topical or systemic corticosteroids, and immunosuppressant or combination therapy, when indicated. Treatment should be initiated as early as possible in the course of lesions. Identification and elimination of precipitating factors may minimize recurrent episodes. Medications such as mycophenolate mofetil, pentoxifylline, colchicine, thalidomide, and others are used to treat patients with severe, persistent, recurrent aphthous ulcers but should not be routinely used. Placing a dissolvable or bioerodible mucosal patch over a topical steroid may prolong tissue contact of the medication and make the patient more comfortable. Multiple topical over-the-counter anesthetics or protective bioadhesive agents are available for patient comfort.

Topical Steroids

Prolonged use of topical steroids (longer than 2 wk of continuous use) may result in mucosal atrophy and secondary candidiasis and may increase the potential for systemic absorption. It may be necessary to prescribe antifungal therapy with steroids use in some patients.

For Mild-to-Moderate Cases:

Rx

Triamcinolone acetonide in dental paste 0.1%

Disp. 5-g tube

Sig. Coat the lesion with a thin film after each meal and at bedtime.

Rx
Dexamethasone oral solution or elixir 0.5 mg/5 ml
Disp. 240 ml
Sig. Rinse with 1 teaspoon (5 ml) for 2 min 4 times a day and expectorate. Do not eat or drink for 30 min after rinsing.
Rx
Celestone (betamethasone) oral syrup 0.6 mg/5 ml
Disp. 200 ml
Sig. Rinse with 1 teaspoon (5 ml) for 2 min 4 times a day, after meals and before bed and expectorate.
Rx
Fluocinonide 0.05% gel
Disp. 15-g tube
Sig. Apply a thin layer to the ulcer after meals and at bedtime.

Discontinue use of topical steroids when lesions become asymptomatic. If the ulcer does not resolve or significantly improve within 14 days, a biopsy of the lesion is recommended.

Other topical steroid preparations (cream, gel, rinse, ointment) are available. In general, creams are not used intraorally because of very poor mucosal adherence. Many topical steroids come with a warning that they are for external use only. However, several of these agents have been used successfully for managing recurrent aphthous ulcerations. Examples of some of the topical steroid medications are listed below according to potency.

Super-High Potency:
- Betamethasone dipropionate (augmented) 0.05%, gel, ointment
- Clobetasol propionate 0.05%, gel, ointment
- Halobetasol propionate 0.05%, ointment

High Potency:
- Betamethasone dipropionate 0.05%, gel, ointment
- Fluocinonide 0.05%, gel, ointment
- Dexamethasone 0.5 mg/5 ml oral solution, elixir
- Desoximetasone 0.05%, gel; 0.25% ointment

Medium Potency:
- Betamethasone valerate 0.1%, ointment
- Triamcinolone acetonide 0.1%, ointment

Low Potency:
- Alclometasone dipropionate 0.05%, ointment
- Hydrocortisone acetate 1%, gel, ointment
- Desonide 0.05%, gel, ointment

Oral candidiasis may develop from topical steroid use, and, therefore, periodic monitoring for a candidal infection is recommended. Prophylactic antifungal therapy should be initiated in patients with a history of fungal infections during previous steroid administration (see "Candidiasis").

Systemic Steroids and Immunosuppressants for Severe Cases

Rx
Dexamethasone (Decadron) elixir 0.5 mg/5 ml
Disp. 320 ml
Sig. As directed in writing, not to exceed 2 continuous wk.

Directions for using dexamethasone oral solution:
Rinse for 1 min, 4 times daily, after meals and before bedtime. Do not drink or eat for 30 min after rinsing.

1. For 3 days, rinse with 1 tablespoon (15 ml) 4 times a day and swallow. Then,
2. For 3 days, rinse with 1 teaspoonful (5 ml) 4 times a day and swallow. Then,
3. For 3 days, rinse with 1 teaspoonful (5 ml) 4 times a day and swallow every other time. Then,
4. Rinse with 1 teaspoonful (5 ml) 4 times a day and expectorate. Discontinue medication when mouth becomes comfortable.

Rx
Prednisone tablets 5 mg
Disp. 40 tablets
Sig. Take 5 tablets in the morning for 5 days, then 5 tablets in the morning every other day until complete.
For Very Severe Cases
Rx
Prednisone tablets 10 mg
Disp. 26 tablets
Sig. Take 4 tablets in the morning for 5 days, then decrease by 1 tablet on each successive day until complete.

Therapy with medications, such as systemic steroids, immunosuppressants, and immunomodulators is presented to inform the clinician that such modalities have been reported effective for patients suffering from severe, persistent, recurrent aphthous stomatitis. Medications such as azathioprine, pentoxifylline, levamisole, colchicine, dapsone, and thalidomide are used to treat patients with severe, persistent, recurrent aphthous stomatitis but should not be routinely used because of the potential for serious adverse effects. Close collaboration with the patient's physician is recommended when these medications are prescribed.

CANDIDIASIS

Etiology:
Candida albicans and other species are opportunistic fungal organisms that tend to proliferate with the use of broad-spectrum antibiotics, corticosteroids, medications that reduce salivary output, and cytotoxic agents. Conditions that contribute to candidiasis include xerostomia, poorly controlled diabetes mellitus, anemia, poor oral hygiene, prolonged use of prosthetic appliances, and suppression of the immune system (i.e., AIDS or the side effects of some medications). It is important to determine the predisposing factors prior to initiating therapy.
Clinical description:
The disease is characterized by soft, white, slightly elevated plaques that usually can be wiped away, leaving an erythematous area (pseudomembranous form). Candidiasis also may appear as generalized erythematous, sensitive areas (atrophic or erythematous form) or as confluent white areas that are adherent (hyperplastic form). Angular cheilitis, which is also described in this chapter, is frequently associated with this oral disease (see "Angular Cheilitis").

Rationale for treatment:
The goal of treatment is to reestablish a normal balance of oral flora and improve oral hygiene. The disinfection of all removable prostheses with antifungal denture-soaking solutions and the application of antifungal agents on the tissue-contacting surfaces are necessary to eliminate a potential source of fungal infection. Medication for the management of oral candidal infection should be continued for 48 hr after the disappearance of clinical signs to prevent immediate recurrence. For this reason, treating oral candidiasis for 14 days is often recommended. It is also important that salivary flow be evaluated and managed to prevent recurrences (see "Xerostomia").

Topical Antifungal Agents

Rx
Nystatin oral suspension 100,000 units/ml
Disp. 280 ml
Sig. Rinse with 1 teaspoon (5 ml) 4 times a day. Rinse for 2 min and expectorate or swallow.

Nystatin suspension has a high sugar content; therefore, good oral hygiene should be reinforced. A few drops of nystatin oral suspension can be added to the water used for soaking acrylic prostheses.

Rx
Oravig (miconazole) buccal tablets 50 mg
Disp. 14 tablets
Sig. Place 1 tablet above the upper front teeth once daily for 14 days. Alternate sides that you place the tablet.

Rx
Clotrimazole lozenge 10 mg
Disp. 70 lozenges
Sig. Let 1 troche dissolve in mouth 4–5 times a day for 14 days.

In general, lozenges may not be well tolerated when a patient has a dry mouth because of the inability to dissolve this dosage form. Consider a course of systemic antifungal therapy in these cases.

Rx
Nystatin ointment 100,000 units/g
Disp. 15-g tube
Sig. Apply a thin coat to inner surface of prosthesis and to the affected area after each meal.

Rx
Ketoconazole topical cream 2%
Disp. 15-g tube
Sig. Apply a thin coat to inner surface of prosthesis and to the affected area after each meal.

Rx
Clotrimazole topical cream 1%
Disp. 15-g tube
Sig. Apply a thin coat to inner surface of prosthesis and to the affected area after each meal.

This product may be obtained over the counter.

Rx
Miconazole nitrate cream 2%

Disp. 15-g tube
Sig. Apply a thin coat to inner surface of prosthesis and to the affected area after each meal.

This product may be obtained over the counter.

Systemic Antifungal Agents

When topical therapy is not practical or is ineffective, ketoconazole, fluconazole, and itraconazole are effective, well-tolerated, systemic drugs for mucocutaneous candidiasis. They should be used with caution in patients with impaired liver function (i.e., with history of alcoholism or hepatitis) and in patients taking drugs metabolized by the cytochrome P450 isoenzyme. Liver function tests should be performed periodically and/or monitored by the patient's physician when ketoconazole is prescribed for an extended period of time. Diminishing response over time with fluconazole may indicate the development of fungal resistance or the need to temporarily increase the medication dosage.

Several important drug interactions have been reported with these systemic antifungal agents because they are potent inhibitors of cytochrome P450 isoenzymes. For this reason, these antifungals can significantly inhibit the hepatic metabolism of medications such as certain antihistamines, cholesterol-lowering medications, antihypertensive drugs, warfarin compounds, and antiasthmatic agents. Some of these drug interactions may be toxic, so careful review of the patient's medications is recommended before prescribing systemic antifungals. For severely immunocompromised patients, medications in the Echinocardin class such as caspofungin, micafungin, and anidulafungin are available for intravenous administration.

Rx

Ketoconazole tablets 200 mg
Disp. 14 tablets
Sig. Take 1 tablet a day with a meal or orange juice. Do not take with buffered medications or with gastric acid blockers.

Rx

Fluconazole tablets 100 mg
Disp. 15 tablets
Sig. Take 2 tablets stat, then 1 tablet a day until complete.

Systemic Antifungal Agents for Refractory Oropharyngeal Candidiasis

Rx

Itraconazole oral solution 10 mg/1 ml
Disp. 150 ml
Sig. Rinse and swallow 2 teaspoons (10 ml) 2 times a day for 2–4 weeks.

This antifungal medication and dosage is for those patients who are unresponsive or refractory to fluconazole tablets.

ANGULAR CHEILITIS

Etiology:

Fissured lesions in the corners of the mouth are caused by a mixed infection of the microorganisms *Candida albicans, Staphylococcus,* and *Streptococcus.* Predisposing factors include excessive licking, drooling, a decrease in intermaxillary space, anemia, vitamin deficiency, immunosuppression, and an extension of oral infections.

Clinical description:
The commissures may appear wrinkled, red, fissured, cracked, or crusted. Scarring and pigmentation problems may develop in persistent cases. Recurrences are common if the underlying problem is not managed.
Rationale for treatment:
Identification and correction of predisposing factors, elimination of the primary and secondary infections, and decrease of inflammation are the management approaches. Recurrences are common.
Rx
Nystatin/triamcinolone acetonide ointment 100,000 units/g 0.1%
Disp. 15-g tube
Sig. Apply to lips after each meal and at bedtime. Use for no longer than 2 wk and then reevaluate.

This is the preferred topical agent when secondary candidal infection is suspected. Concomitant intraoral antifungal treatment may be indicated.
Rx
Ketoconazole cream 2%
Disp. 15-g tube
Sig. Apply a small dab to corners of mouth after meals and before bedtime. Use for 2 wk and reevaluate.

This topical agent is used when secondary candidal infection is suspected. Concomitant intraoral antifungal treatment may be indicated.
Rx
Hydrocortisone-iodoquinol 1%-1% cream
Disp. 15-g tube
Sig. Apply small dab to the corners of mouth after meals and before bedtime. Use for 2 wk and reevaluate.

This topical agent is used when secondary bacterial and candidal infections are suspected.
Rx
Clotrimazole cream 1%
Disp. 1 tube
Sig. Apply small dab to corner of mouth after meals and before bedtime. Use for 2 wk and reevaluate.

This product may be obtained over the counter.
Rx
Miconazole nitrate antifungal cream 2%
Disp. 1 tube
Sig. Apply small dab to corner of mouth after meals and before bedtime. Use for 2 wk and reevaluate.

This product may be obtained over the counter.
Rx
Bacitracin zinc 500 U; Polymyxin B 10,000 U ointment 2% (OTC)
Disp. 1 tube
Sig. Apply small dab to corner of mouth after meals and before bedtime. Use for 1 wk and reevaluate.

This OTC topical antibacterial agent may be associated with allergic reactions because of its frequent use for skin irritation.

ACTINIC (SOLAR) CHEILITIS

Etiology:

This precancerous lesion is caused by prolonged exposure to sunlight that results in irreversible degenerative changes in the vermilion of the lips, especially the lower lip.

Clinical description:

The normal red translucent appearance of the vermilion border with regular vertical fissuring is replaced by a white plaque or an irregular scaly surface that may exhibit periodic erythema and ulceration. There is often an indistinct margin between the perioral skin and lip vermilion.

Rationale for treatment:

Prevention of the solar-induced changes is recommended. For maximum protection, use sunscreen concurrently on the face and other sun-exposed areas. If exposure to the ultraviolet light in the sun's rays is allowed to continue, the degenerative changes may progress to a malignancy. Sunscreens with an SPF of 30 or higher and protection from both UVA and UVB should be recommended.

Rx

Several OTC sunscreen preparations for the lips are available. For those patients who are allergic to paraaminobenzoic acid (PABA), PABA-free sunscreens should be recommended. For patients with a history of lip cancer, a zinc oxide product should be used. Regular and repeated use of these products is critical for sun protection.

When a lesion on the lip persists, a biopsy is required to exclude epithelial dysplasia or squamous cell carcinoma.

GEOGRAPHIC TONGUE (BENIGN MIGRATORY GLOSSITIS; ERYTHEMA MIGRANS)

Etiology:

Although a common condition, the etiology of geographic tongue is unknown. Although not supported by large epidemiologic studies, this tongue condition has been associated with atopic conditions and pustular psoriasis.

Clinical description:

Geographic tongue is a benign inflammatory condition caused by desquamation of superficial keratin and filiform papillae. It is characterized by both red, denuded, oval to irregularly shaped patches that are surrounded by a slightly raised white border. The primary site of involvement is the dorsal and ventrolateral tongue, but other oral mucosal sites may be affected. The pattern of these lesions frequently changes and ranges from solitary to multiple affected areas.

Rationale for treatment:

Generally, no treatment is necessary because most patients are asymptomatic. When symptoms are present, they may be associated with acidic or spicy foods and beverages. In addition, tender lesions may be associated with secondary candidal infection. Although there is no well-documented treatment for this condition, symptoms can be improved temporally with topical anesthetics or coating agents. For persistent and tender lesions, topical steroids, especially in combination with topical antifungal agents, are the treatment of choice. Patients should be informed that this condition does not suggest a more serious disease and is not contagious. In most cases, a biopsy is not indicated because of the pathognomonic clinical appearance. However, solitary lesions of the lateral tongue that do not resolve should be biopsied to exclude epithelial dysplasia or squamous cell carcinoma.

Rx

Nystatin/triamcinolone acetonide ointment 100,000 units/g 0.1%

Disp. 15-g tube

Sig. Apply to affected area after each meal and at bedtime.

Rx

Lotrisone, generic (clotrimazole/betamethasone dipropionate) cream 1%–0.05%

Disp. 15-g tube

Sig. Apply to affected area after each meal and at bedtime.

Rx

Fluocinonide ointment, gel 0.05%

Disp. 15-g tube

Sig. Apply to affected areas after meals and at bedtime.

If there is a secondary candidal infection, the symptoms may worsen if a topical steroid is used as a single agent.

Rx

Betamethasone valerate ointment 0.1%

Disp. 15-g tube

Sig. Apply to affected areas after meals and at bedtime.

If there is a secondary candidal infection, the symptoms may worsen if a topical steroid is used as a single agent.

XEROSTOMIA (REDUCED SALIVARY FLOW AND DRY MOUTH)

Etiology:

Acute or chronic salivary flow alterations or xerostomia may result from drug therapy, mechanical blockage, dehydration, emotional stress, bacterial infection of the salivary glands, local surgery, avitaminosis, diabetes, anemia, connective tissue diseases, Sjögren's syndrome, radiation therapy, viral infections, and certain congenital disorders.

Clinical description:

The saliva may be ropey with a film forming over the teeth. The tissues may be dry, pale or red, and atrophic. The tongue may be devoid of papillae, atrophic, fissured, and inflamed. Multiple carious lesions may be present, especially at the gingival margin and on exposed root surfaces. The quantity and quality of saliva may be altered.

Rationale for treatment:

Salivary stimulation or replacement therapy is important to keep the mouth moistened and comfortable and for the prevention of caries, candidal infection, and traumatically induced mucosal lesions. For patients with removable prosthetic appliances, the application of an artificial saliva or oral lubricant gel to the tissue contact surface of the prosthesis reduces frictional trauma.

Saliva Substitutes

Rx

Sodium carboxymethylcellulose 0.5% aqueous solution (OTC)

Disp. 8 fl oz

Sig. Use as a rinse as frequently as needed. Solution may be prepared by the pharmacist.

Sipping on plain water or crushed ice is often used with some success in patients with dry mouth.

There are several OTC saliva substitutes and oral moisturizing gels that are commercially available and patients may need to evaluate which product best meets their specific needs and preferences. Relief from oral dryness and accompanying discomfort can be achieved conservatively by the following:

- Sipping water frequently all day long
- Letting ice melt in the mouth
- Restricting caffeine intake
- Avoiding mouth rinses, drinks, and medications containing alcohol
- Avoiding tobacco products
- Humidifying the sleeping area
- Coating the lips (see "Chapped/Cracked Lips")

Saliva Stimulants

The use of sugar-free gum, candy, or mints is a conservative method to temporarily stimulate salivary flow in patients with medication-induced xerostomia or with salivary gland dysfunction. Patients should be cautioned against using products that contain sucrose or other fermentable sugars or have a low pH. Using products that are sweetened with xylitol may decrease the risk for dental caries.

Rx

Salagen, generic (pilocarpine HCl) tablets 5 mg
Disp. 90 tablets
Sig. Take 1 tablet 3 times a day, 30 min prior to meals.

Dosage may be titrated to 2 tablets (10 mg) 3 times a day. An alternative is 1 tablet (5 mg) 4 times a day.

Rx

Evoxac, generic (cevimeline HCl) capsules 30 mg
Disp. 90 capsules
Sig. Take 1 capsule 3 times a day.

Rx

Urecholine, generic (bethanechol chloride) tablets 25 mg
Disp. 90 tablets
Sig. Take 1 tablet 3–5 times a day.

Not FDA-approved for this indication.

Cholinergic drugs should be prescribed in consultation with the patient's physician because of the side effects. The pilocarpine and cevimeline dosage should be adjusted to increase saliva while minimizing the adverse side effects (sweating, stomach upset, etc.). Patients should be warned that there is a wide range of sensitivity and that the adverse side effects may outweigh the benefit of increased salivation. If this occurs, then the cholinergic drug should be discontinued.

Recent alternatives to these systemic medications for xerostomia are supersaturated calcium phosphate rinses such as NeutraSal Solution and Caphosol Solution.

Caries Prevention

Rx

Neutral NaF 1.1% gel
Disp. 1 tube

Sig. Place 1-inch ribbon on a toothbrush; brush teeth for 2 min daily and expectorate. Avoid rinsing or eating for 30 min following application.

As an alternative, place a 1-inch ribbon in a custom tray; apply for 5–10 min daily.

Rx

Stannous fluoride 0.4% gel

Disp. 1 tube

Sig. Place 1-inch ribbon on a toothbrush; brush teeth for 2 min daily and expectorate. Avoid rinsing or eating for 30 min following application.

As an alternative, place a 1-inch ribbon in a custom tray; apply for 5–10 min daily.

Rx

Neutral NaF 1.1% dental cream

Disp. 1 tube

Sig. Place 1-inch ribbon on a toothbrush; brush teeth for 2 min twice daily and expectorate. Avoid rinsing or eating for 30 min following application.

In general, the use of stannous fluoride gels is not recommended because of the high acidity and lower fluoride concentration of 1000 ppm, in contrast to the sodium fluoride gels that have a neutral pH and contain 5000 ppm. Also, stannous fluoride gels may etch ceramic and glass ionomer restorations and cause extrinsic tooth staining.

Note that FDA regulations have limited the size of bottles of fluoride because of toxicity, if ingested by infants. Because most preparations do not come in childproof bottles, the sizes of topical fluoride preparations vary; 24 ml is approximately a 2-wk supply for application to a full dentition in custom carriers.

Recently, bioavailable calcium phosphate with fluoride dentifrices and pastes are available that may be beneficial for remineralization of the teeth and as desensitizing agents in individuals at high risk for caries.

Reduced salivary flow provides an excellent environment for overgrowth of *C. albicans*. The patient is likely to require treatment for candidiasis, along with treatment for dry mouth (see “Candidiasis”). In a dry oral environment, plaque control becomes more difficult. Scrupulous oral hygiene is essential to prevent dental and periodontal disease.

LICHEN PLANUS

Etiology:

Lichen planus is an immunologically mediated, chronic, mucocutaneous disorder. Although many cases develop without a known cause, some lesions are triggered by emotional stress, hypersensitivity to drugs, dental products, foods, and a genetic predilection.

Clinical description:

Lichen planus varies in clinical appearance. Oral forms of this disorder include lacy white lines representing Wickham’s striae (reticular), an erythematous form (atrophic), and an ulcerating form that often is accompanied by striae peripheral to the ulceration (erosive). The lesions are commonly found on the buccal mucosa, gingiva, and tongue, but they can be found on the lips and palate. Lichen planus lesions are chronic and also may affect the skin. The dental and medical literature remains controversial as to whether lichen planus undergoes malignant transformation. Therefore, any persistent or refractory lesion should be biopsied to establish a diagnosis and to rule out a malignancy.

Rationale for treatment:

Since this is a chronic disease, management of the disease focuses on providing oral comfort if the lesions are symptomatic. Systemic and local relief with antiinflammatory and immunosuppressant agents is indicated. Identification of any dietary component, dental product, or medication (lichenoid drug reaction) should be undertaken to ensure against a hypersensitivity reaction. Treatment or prevention of a secondary fungal infection with a systemic antifungal agent also should be considered.

Therapies with steroids and immunomodulating drugs are presented to inform the clinician that such modalities are available. Because of the potential for side effects, close collaboration with the patient's physician is recommended when these medications are prescribed. These modalities may be beyond the scope of the clinical experience of general dentists, and referral to a dental specialist or to an appropriate physician may be necessary.

Topical Steroids

Prolonged use of topical steroids (for a period longer than 2 wk of continuous use) may result in mucosal atrophy and secondary candidiasis and may increase the potential for systemic absorption. The prescribing of antifungal therapy with steroids may be necessary. Therapy with topical steroids, once the lichen planus is under control, should be tapered to alternate-day therapy or less depending on control of the disease and the tendency for recurrence.

Rx

Fluocinonide gel 0.05%

Disp. 30-g tube

Sig. Coat the lesion with a thin film after each meal and at bedtime.

Once the lesions are asymptomatic, decrease to once-daily application, alternate-day use, or less frequently. When there is a flare-up of the oral lesions, increase the use of the topical steroids to 2–4 times a day if needed to decrease the signs and symptoms.

Rx

Dexamethasone elixir, solution 0.5 mg/5 ml

Disp. 240 ml

Sig. Rinse with 1 teaspoon (5 ml) for 2 min 4 times a day and expectorate. Discontinue when lesions become asymptomatic.

Other topical steroid preparations (cream, gel, rinse, ointment) are available. In general, creams are not used intraorally because of very poor mucosal adherence. These topical steroids come with a warning that they are for external use only. However, several of these agents have been used successfully for managing lichen planus. Examples of some of the topical steroid medications are listed below according to potency. Except when lichen planus occurs on the lips, low-potency topical steroids are generally not effective for intraoral lesions.

Super-High Potency:
Betamethasone dipropionate (augmented) 0.05%, gel, ointment
Clobetasol propionate 0.05%, gel, ointment
Halobetasol propionate 0.05%, ointment

High Potency:
Betamethasone dipropionate 0.05%, gel, ointment
Fluocinonide 0.05%, gel, ointment
Dexamethasone 0.5 mg/5 ml oral solution, elixir
Desoximetasone 0.05% gel; – 0.05% ointment

Medium Potency:
Betamethasone valerate 0.1%, ointment
Triamcinolone acetonide 0.1%, ointment

Low Potency:
Alclometasone dipropionate 0.05%, ointment
Desonide 0.05%, cream
Hydrocortisone acetate 1%, gel, ointment

Mixing any of the above steroid ointments with equal parts of benzocaine oral paste promotes adhesion, prolongs tissue contact, and provides temporary pain relief. Prolonged use of topical steroids may result in mucosal atrophy and secondary candidiasis and increase the potential for systemic absorption. It may be necessary to prescribe antifungal therapy with topical steroids. The oral cavity should be monitored for emergence of fungal infection in patients who are placed on therapy. Prophylactic antifungal therapy should be initiated in patients with a history of fungal infection with previous steroid administration (see "Candidiasis"). Therapy with topical steroids, once the lichen planus is under control, should be tapered to alternate-day therapy or less depending on disease control and tendency to recur.

Systemic Steroids and Immunosuppressants for Severe Cases

Rx

Dexamethasone elixir or solution 0.5 mg/5 ml
Disp. 320 ml
Sig. As directed in writing, not to exceed 2 continuous wk.

1. For 3 days, rinse with 1 tablespoonful (15 ml) 4 times a day and swallow. Then,
2. For 3 days, rinse with 1 teaspoonful (5 ml) 4 times a day and swallow. Then,
3. For 3 days, rinse with 1 teaspoonful (5 ml) 4 times a day and swallow every other time. Then,
4. Rinse with 1 teaspoonful (5 ml) 4 times a day and expectorate.

Rx

Prednisone tablets 10 mg
Disp. 26 tablets
Sig. Take 4 tablets in the morning for 5 days, then decrease by 1 tablet on each successive day.

Rx

Prednisone tablets 5 mg
Disp. 40 tablets
Sig. Take 5 tablets in the morning for 5 days, then 5 tablets in the morning every other day until gone.

If oral discomfort recurs, the patient should return to the clinician for reevaluation.

Rx

Protopic (tacrolimus) ointment 0.1%

Disp. 30-g tube

Sig. Apply to the affected sites twice daily. Use for 2 wk and reevaluate.

Rx

Protopic (tacrolimus) ointment 0.03%

Disp. 30-g tube

Sig. Apply to the affected sites twice daily. Use for 2 wk and reevaluate.

Many studies suggest that oral lichen planus has an intrinsic property predisposing to malignant transformation. However, the etiology is complex, with interaction among genetic, infectious agents, environmental, and lifestyle factors. Prospective studies have demonstrated that lichen planus patients have a slightly increased risk to develop oral squamous cell carcinoma. All patients exhibiting lichen planus, intraorally, particularly those who have had the ulcerative form, should receive periodic follow-up.

Therapy with medications such as systemic steroids, immunosuppressants, and immunomodulators is presented to inform the clinician that such modalities have been reported effective for patients suffering from erosive lichen planus. Medications such as azathioprine, mycophenolate mofetil, tacrolimus hydroxychloroquine sulfate, acitretin, and cyclosporine are used to treat patients with severe persistent erosive lichen planus but should not be routinely used because of the potential for side effects. Close collaboration with the patient's physician is recommended when these medications are prescribed.

Topical tacrolimus has been associated with neoplastic disease, such as lymphoma and skin cancers and, therefore, should not be used indiscriminately for long periods of time. This medication is indicated for patients who cannot tolerate or are refractory to topical or systemic steroid therapy.

In addition, periodic scaling and professional dental cleanings every 3–4 mo are important for controlling this chronic disease when the gingival tissues are affected. Patients with gingival involvement are at increased risk for gingival recession and periodontitis. Root sensitivity and root caries may develop due to gingival recession. Meticulous oral hygiene should be reinforced and supplemental topical fluoride may be beneficial (see "Caries Prevention" under "Xerostomia").

PEMPHIGUS VULGARIS AND MUCOUS MEMBRANE PEMPHIGOID

Pemphigus vulgaris and mucous membrane pemphigoid are relatively uncommon lesions. They should be suspected when chronic, multiple oral ulcerations and a history of oral and skin blisters exist. Often, they may occur only in the mouth. Diagnosis is based on history and on microscopic and immunofluorescence studies of a biopsied sample adjacent to a lesion.

Etiology:

Both of these chronic mucocutaneous diseases are autoimmune disorders with autoantibodies against antigens appearing in different areas of the surface epithelium or lining mucosa. In pemphigus vulgaris, the antigens are within the epithelium (desmosomes), whereas in pemphigoid, the antigens are located at the base of the epithelium in the hemidesmosomes.

Clinical description:
In pemphigus vulgaris, the lesion may stay in one location for a long period of time with small placid bullae. The bullae may rupture, leaving areas of ulceration. Approximately 80%–90% of patients have oral lesions. The oral manifestations are the first signs of the disease in approximately two-thirds of patients. All parts of the mouth may be involved. The bullae rupture almost immediately in the mouth but may stay intact for some time on the skin. One of the classic signs, the Nikolsky sign (blister formation induced with gentle rubbing of an affected mucosal site), is positive in pemphigus but is not pathognomonic because it is also positive in other disorders. Because the vesicles or bullae are intraepithelial, they often are filled with clear fluid. Microscopically, Tzanck cells or acantholytic cells are observed within the spinous cell layer of the epithelium.

In pemphigoid, the cleavage or split is beneath the epithelium, resulting in bullae that are often blood filled. Mucous membrane pemphigoid is usually limited to the oral cavity, but some patients have ocular lesions (symblepharon) that must be evaluated by an ophthalmologist. The gingiva is the most common oral site involved. Pemphigoid may appear clinically as red, nonulcerated or ulcerated gingival lesions with a positive Nikolsky sign. Patients should be questioned regarding the signs and symptoms of ocular and pharyngeal involvement.

Rationale for treatment:
Because both pemphigus and pemphigoid are autoimmune disorders, the primary treatment is topical or systemic steroids or other immunomodulating drugs. Pemphigus requires the use of systemic medications. Custom trays can be used to localize topical steroid medications on the gingival tissues (occlusive therapy). Because they can resemble other ulcerative-bullous diseases, a biopsy is necessary for a definitive diagnosis. Specimens should be submitted for light microscopic and immunofluorescence studies, and immunologic testing. Because of the potentially serious nature of these diseases, referral to a specialist in oral medicine, dermatology, and ophthalmology must be considered. When eye lesions are present, an ophthalmologist must be consulted immediately to prevent blindness.

Therapy with medications such as systemic steroids, immunosuppressants, and immunomodulators is presented to inform the clinician that such modalities have been reported effective for patients suffering from vesiculobullous disorders such as pemphigus vulgaris and mucous membrane pemphigoid. Therapies such as dapsone, methotrexate, mycophenolate mofetil, cyclosporine, niacinamide with tetracycline, and plasmapheresis are used to treat patients with vesiculobullous disorders such as pemphigus vulgaris and mucous membrane pemphigoid, but they should not be routinely used because of the potential for serious adverse effects. Close collaboration with the patient's physician is recommended when these medications are prescribed.

Rx
Topical and Systemic Steroids (See Lichen Planus)

ORAL ERYTHEMA MULTIFORME

Etiology:
Oral erythema multiforme is a blistering and ulcerative mucocutaneous disease that is immunologically mediated. It can occur at any age. Drug reactions to

medications such as penicillin and sulfonamides may play a role in some cases. In a few patients who develop oral erythema multiforme, a herpetic infection occurs immediately before the onset of clinical signs. Other infectious diseases have also been implicated.

Clinical description:

Signs of oral erythema multiforme include "blood-crusted" lips, "targetoid" or "bull's-eye" skin lesions, and a nonspecific mucosal erythema, ulceration, and necrosis. The name multiforme is used because its appearance may take different forms. Erythema multiforme, as a skin disease, occurs most frequently because of an allergic reaction. Besides having an acute onset from a specific triggering agent, this condition may also have a chronic or cyclical pattern.

Rationale for treatment:

Treatment is primarily directed at patient comfort, using topical anesthetics and coating agents. Because of the possible relationship of oral erythema multiforme with herpes simplex virus, suppressive antiviral therapy may be indicated to prevent lesion recurrences. Patients should be questioned carefully about a previous history of recurrent herpetic infections and prodromal symptoms that might have preceded the onset of erythema multiforme. It is also important to take a thorough drug history to determine if that is the cause. The use of systemic steroids is controversial and if prescribed should be done so in consultation with the patient's physician. Because some forms of erythema multiforme are very serious, most suspected cases should be referred to appropriate dental or medical specialists for management and identification of the cause.

Topical Anesthetics and Coating Agents

Rx

Diphenhydramine hydrochloride oral solution 12.5 mg/5 ml mixed with aluminum hydroxide, magnesium hydroxide oral suspension

Compound to a 1 : 1 mixture by volume

Disp. 200 ml

Sig. Rinse with 1–2 teaspoons (5–10 ml) every 2–4 hr for 1 min; swish and spit out.

Although these medications are OTC, it is recommended that a pharmacist compound this oral suspension. Examples of aluminum hydroxide, magnesium hydroxide oral suspensions are Maalox and Mylanta—they are common OTC brands and are available in a number of flavors. Children younger than 6 yr should not swallow this oral suspension.

Rx

Diphenhydramine hydrochloride liquid 12.5 mg/5 ml/lidocaine viscous 2% oral solution/aluminum hydroxide, magnesium hydroxide oral suspension

Compound to a 1 : 1 : 1 mixture by volume.

Disp. 200 ml

Sig. Shake well before use. Rinse with 1–2 teaspoons (5–10 ml) every 3–4 hr for 1 min and spit out excess. Store suspension at room temperature.

It is compounded by pharmacy and stable for approximately 60 days. Do not use 2% lidocaine hydrochloride in children who cannot expectorate because of potential for aspiration or swallowing.

Rx

Carafate, generic (sucralfate) suspension 1 g/10 ml

Disp. 200 ml

Sig. Rinse with 1 teaspoon (5 ml) 4 times a day. Rinse for 1 min and spit out excess.

In children younger than 6 yr who cannot expectorate, the amount should be limited to 0.5 g, 4 times a day (2 g/day) in case the suspension is swallowed. Safety and efficacy have not been established in children.

Rx

Sucrets (dyclonine HCl) throat lozenges (OTC)

Disp. 1 package

Sig. Slowly dissolve 1 lozenge in mouth every 2 hr as needed for pain. Do not take more than 10 lozenges a day.

The strength of dyclonine HCl ranges from 3 mg (maximum strength) to 1.2 mg for children's formula.

Suppressive Antiviral Therapy

Rx

Zovirax, generic (acyclovir) tablets 400 mg

Disp. 60 tablets

Sig. Take 1 tablet 2 times daily. Take drug for up to 12 mo and reevaluate.

Rx

Valtrex, generic (valacyclovir) tablets 500 mg

Disp. 60 tablets

Sig. Take 1–2 tablets a day. Take drug for up to 12 mo and reevaluate.

Because of the long-term use of these antiviral agents, patients may be best monitored by a dental specialist or physician.

DENTURE SORE MOUTH

Etiology:

Discomfort under oral prosthetic appliances may result from combinations of candidal infections, bacterial colonization, poor denture hygiene, an occlusal syndrome, overextension, or excessive movement of the appliance. This condition may be erroneously attributed to an allergy to denture material, which is a rare occurrence. This condition may represent a pressure neuropathy due to advanced atrophy of the alveolar bone and trauma to the nerves emanating from the mental foramen and the incisive foramen. The retention and fit of the denture should be evaluated, and mechanical irritation should be ruled out.

Clinical description:

The tissue covered by the appliance, especially if the appliance is made of acrylic, is erythematous and smooth or granular. It may be either asymptomatic or associated with a burning sensation.

Rationale for treatment:

Therapy is directed toward controlling all possible causes and improving oral comfort. If therapy is ineffective, consider underlying systemic conditions such as diabetes mellitus and poor nutrition.

Treatment:

1. Institute appropriate antifungal medication (see "Candidiasis").
2. Improve oral and appliance hygiene. The patient may have to leave the appliance out for extended periods of time and should be instructed to leave the denture out overnight. The appliance should be soaked in a commercially available denture cleanser or soaked in a 1% sodium hypochlorite solution (1 teaspoon of sodium hypochlorite in a denture cup

of water) for 15 min and thoroughly rinsed for at least 2 min under running water. Dentures may be cleaned and soaked in other denture cleansing agents and antibacterial mouth rinses.

3. Reline, rebase, or construct a new appliance.
4. Apply an artificial saliva or oral lubricant gel to the tissue contact surface of the denture to reduce frictional trauma.

If all the above actions fail to control symptoms, a biopsy or short trial of topical steroid therapy can be used to rule out contact mucositis (an allergic reaction to denture materials). If a therapeutic trial fails to resolve the condition, a biopsy should be performed to establish the diagnosis. Furthermore, if the differential diagnosis includes a condition that may be potentially malignant or malignant, a biopsy should be performed immediately to determine a definitive diagnosis.

BURNING MOUTH SYNDROME

Etiology:

Burning mouth syndrome is a common dysesthesia that has been associated with a variety of local and systemic factors. Current literature supports neurogenic, vascular, and psychological causes. However, other conditions, such as xerostomia, candidiasis, referred pain from the tongue musculature, chronic infections, gastrointestinal reflux disease, medications, blood dyscrasias, nutritional deficiencies, hormonal imbalances, and allergic and inflammatory disorders, need to be considered.

Clinical description:

Burning mouth syndrome is characterized by persistent tenderness of usually the tongue, followed by the lips and anterior hard palate, in the absence of clinical signs.

Rationale for treatment:

If an underlying local or systemic cause is not identified, then treatment approaches focus on reducing discomfort.

Treatment:

It is important to reassure the patient that this disorder is not infectious or contagious and does not progress to a malignant condition. On the basis of the history, physical evaluation, and specific laboratory studies, it is important to exclude all local and systemic causes. Minimal blood studies should include complete blood count and differential; fasting glucose, iron, ferritin, folic acid, and vitamin B_{12} levels; and thyroid profile (TSH, T3, T4).

Topical Anesthetics and Coating Agents

Rx

Diphenhydramine hydrochloride oral solution 12.5 mg/5 ml mixed with aluminum hydroxide, magnesium hydroxide oral suspension

Compound to a 1 : 1 mixture by volume

Disp. 200 ml

Sig. Rinse with 1–2 teaspoons (5–10 ml) every 2–4 hr for 1 min; swish and spit out.

Although these medications are OTC, it is recommended that a pharmacist compound this oral suspension. Examples of aluminum hydroxide, magnesium hydroxide oral suspensions are Maalox and Mylanta—they are common OTC brands and are available in a number of flavors.

Rx
Diphenhydramine hydrochloride liquid 12.5 mg/5 ml/lidocaine viscous 2% oral solution/aluminum hydroxide, magnesium hydroxide oral suspension
Compound to a 1 : 1 : 1 mixture by volume.
Disp. 200 ml
Sig. Shake well before use. Rinse with 1–2 teaspoons (5–10 ml) every 3–4 hr for 1 min and spit out excess. Store suspension at room temperature.

It is compounded by pharmacy and stable for approximately 60 days. Do not use 2% lidocaine hydrochloride in adults who cannot expectorate because of potential for aspiration or swallowing.

Rx
Benadryl Children's Allergy (diphenhydramine) solution 12.5 mg/5 ml (OTC)
Disp. 1 bottle
Sig. Rinse with 1–2 teaspoons (5–10 ml) for 2 min before each meal and spit out.

When the burning mouth is considered psychogenic or idiopathic, a tricyclic antidepressant or benzodiazepine in low doses exhibits the properties of analgesia and sedation and frequently is successful in reducing or eliminating the symptoms after several weeks or months. The dosage is adjusted according to patient response and clinical symptoms. The following systemic therapies for burning mouth disorder are best managed by appropriate specialists or the patient's physician, due to the protracted nature of this therapy.

Rx
Clonazepam orally disintegrating tablets 0.25 mg
Disp. 60 tablets
Sig. Take 1 tablet nightly, then adjust dose after 7 days.

This therapy probably is best managed by an appropriate specialist or the patient's physician at this time. Due to the sedative effects, patients may wish to take this medication only at night and increase the dosage to 2 tablets (0.50 mg). Other patients experience more improvement when they take 1–2 tablets 3 times a day.

Rx
Amitriptyline tablets 25 mg
Disp. 50 tablets
Sig. Take 1 tablet at bedtime for 1 wk, then increase to 2 tablets every night for the next week. Increase to 3 tablets every night after 2 wk and maintain at that dosage or titrate as appropriate.

Rx
Chlordiazepoxide capsules 5 mg
Disp. 50 capsules
Sig. Take 1 capsule 3 times a day, then adjust after 1 wk to 2 capsules 3 times a day as appropriate.

Rx
Xanax, generic (alprazolam) tablets 0.25 mg
Disp. 50 tablets
Sig. Take 1 tablet 3 times a day.

The rationale for use of tricyclic antidepressants and other psychotropic drugs should be thoroughly explained to the patient, and the patient's physician should be consulted. These medications have a potential for addiction and dependence.

Rx

Tabasco sauce (capsaicin) (OTC)

Disp. 1 bottle

Sig. Place 1 part Tabasco sauce in 2–4 parts of water. Rinse with 1 teaspoon (5 ml) 4 times a day and expectorate.

Rx

Zostrix, generic (capsaicin) cream 0.025% (OTC)

Disp. 1 tube

Sig. Apply sparingly to affected site(s) 4 times a day.

Wash hands after each application and do not use near the eyes.

Topical capsaicin may produce a burning sensation in some individuals. An increase in discomfort for a 2- to 3-wk period should be anticipated.

Other palliative treatments, along with these medications, include chewing a mildly flavored sugarless gum, slowly dissolving sugarless candy, and sucking on crushed ice.

CHAPPED OR CRACKED LIPS (EXFOLIATIVE CHEILITIS)

Etiology:

Chapped lips are due to alternate wetting and drying of the lip surface that results in inflammation and possible secondary infection. Repeatedly licking, picking, and biting the lips are aggravating factors. Other causes include eczema, contact allergies, xerostomia, and secondary candidal infection.

Clinical description:

The surface of the vermilion is rough, scaly, and peeling and may be ulcerated with bleeding and crusting. In severe and chronic cases, the lips are tender and slightly swollen, and deep fissures and scarring may be detected.

Rationale for treatment:

An interrupted and chronically inflamed surface is at increased risk for scarring and secondary infection. Eliminating the cause, especially if the chapped lips are due to a factitial habit or contact allergy, is important. A protective lip emollient, a topical antiinflammatory agent with or without antimicrobial agents, aids in the healing of the lips, but recurrences are common.

Rx

Aquaphor Healing Ointment, others (OTC)

Disp. 1 tube

Sig. Apply to lips after each meal and at bedtime.

Avoid flavored products because they tend to promote increased licking of the lips. Although medicated products may be soothing initially, they should not be used because they can cause increased drying of the lips. Some patients respond better to lanolin cream or ointment than petroleum-based products.

Rx

Nystatin/triamcinolone acetonide ointment 100,000 units/g 0.1%

Disp. 15-g tube

Sig. Apply to lips after each meal and at bedtime. Use for no longer than 2 wk.

This ointment is best used if a secondary candidal infection is suspected.

Rx
Triamcinolone acetonide ointment 0.1%
Disp. 15-g tube
Sig. Apply to lips after each meal and at bedtime. Use for no longer than 2 wk.
Rx
Aclovate (alclometasone dipropionate) ointment 0.05%
Disp. 15-g tube
Sig. Apply to lips after each meal and at bedtime. Use for no longer than 2 wk.
Rx
Desonide ointment 0.05%
Disp. 15-g tube
Sig. Apply to lips after each meal and at bedtime. Use for no longer than 2 wk.

Pediatric Significance: This is a low-potency topical steroid for short-term use only and is approved for use on the face. Prolonged use of corticosteroids can result in thinning of the tissue, so their use should be closely monitored and for a limited period of time. For maintenance, the frequent application of lip care products that are hypoallergenic should be suggested. Avoid products with desiccants, such as phenols and alcohols, and those with flavoring agents. If the lip lesions do not resolve with treatment, a biopsy may be indicated to rule out other conditions including premalignant and malignant changes associated with actinic changes.

DRUG-INDUCED GINGIVAL OVERGROWTH

Etiology:
Certain drugs, such as phenytoin sodium, calcium channel blocking agents (nifedipine, diltiazem, verapamil, amlodipine, and others), and cyclosporine therapy are known to predispose some individuals to persistent gingival enlargement. Chronic hyperplastic gingivitis, gingival fibromatosis, and granulomatous gingivitis should be ruled out by clinical history, family history, biopsy, and other indicated laboratory tests.

Clinical description:
The gingival tissues, especially in the anterior region, are firm, stippled, nontender, and enlarged. Depending on the degree of inflammation, the gingival tissues vary from normal in color to dark red and hemorrhagic. Especially in drug-induced examples, the enlargements originate in the interdental papillae.

Rationale for treatment:
Local factors, such as plaque and calculus accumulation, contribute to secondary inflammation and the hyperplastic process. This further interferes with plaque control. Specific drugs tend to deplete serum folic acid levels, which result in compromised tissue integrity.

Treatment:
Management approaches consists of (1) meticulous plaque control; (2) gingivectomy or other gingival surgery when indicated; (3) when possible, replacement of the causative drug with an equivalent substitute; and (4) testing for serum folate level and supplement folic acid, if necessary. Use of folic acid rinse, topical antimicrobial mouth rinse, and systemic antibiotics may be effective in some cases.

Rx
Folic acid oral rinse 1 mg/ml
Disp. 16 oz

Sig. Rinse with 1 tablespoonful (10 ml) for 2 min twice a day and expectorate.

Rx

Peridex, PerioGard, generic (chlorhexidine gluconate) oral rinse 0.12%

Disp. 473 ml (16 oz)

Sig. Rinse with 15 ml twice daily for 30 sec and expectorate. Rinse after breakfast and before bedtime.

TASTE DISORDERS

Etiology:

Taste acuity may be affected by medications and by neurologic and physiologic changes. Clinical examination and diagnostic procedures may identify potential causes such as nasal and sinus disease, viral infection, oral candidiasis, neoplasia, malnutrition, metabolic disorders, trauma, illicit drug use, autoimmune diseases affecting salivary glands, and radiation sequelae. A number of medications can result in taste alterations. In addition, individuals with anxiety disorders and depression may complain about changes in taste. Laboratory tests for trace elements may be necessary to identify any existing deficiencies.

Rationale for treatment:

A reduction in salivary flow may concentrate the electrolytes in the saliva, resulting in a salty or metallic taste (see "Xerostomia"). Numerous medications have dysgeusia as a reported side effect. Antibiotics, antihypertensives, antifungals, and antiretrovirals are examples of classes of drugs that have been implicated. Rarely, a deficiency of zinc has been associated with a loss of taste and smell sensation. To prevent deficiency, the current recommended dietary allowance for zinc is 10 mg for men and 12 mg for women. Additional zinc supplementation should be reserved for individuals with true deficiency states and in consultation with the physician.

To Ensure Dietary Allowance for Zinc

Rx

Z-BEC tablets (OTC)

Disp. 60 tablets

Sig. Take 1 tablet daily with food or after meals.

This supplement also contains vitamin B complex, vitamin C, and vitamin E, along with zinc.

Rx

Zinc gluconate lozenges (OTC)

Disp. 48 lozenges

Sig. Dissolve by mouth, 1–2 lozenges daily.

MANAGEMENT OF PATIENTS RECEIVING ANTINEOPLASTIC AGENTS AND RADIATION THERAPY

Etiology:

Cancer chemotherapy and radiation to the head and neck cause direct and indirect effects on the oral tissues. Head and neck radiation treatment for oral cancer can reduce saliva volume and composition when a major salivary gland is in the primary radiation field. This treatment results in a decrease in multiple antimicrobial and other important components of saliva that are needed to maintain oral mucosal health. Due to qualitative and quantitative changes in saliva, patients are at increased risk for extensive dental caries, periodontal disease, chronic candidal infection, and difficulty in eating and swallowing. Advances in care, including salivary gland protection during radiation treatment with amifostine and saliva stimulant intervention, have reduced the morbidity associated with long-term salivary gland hypofunction in this group of patients.

Cytotoxic cancer therapy can also impair normal rapidly dividing cells, including the oral mucosa. Chemotherapy results in direct cytotoxic effects that may lead to painful mucositis and ulceration of the mucosa. To decrease the severity of mucositis, the drug palifermin is available for patients with hematologic malignancies who are receiving a bone marrow transplant. In addition, there are indirect effects of myelosuppression resulting in anemia, thrombocytopenia, and leucopenia. Both local and disseminated infection may develop including fungal, viral, and bacterial infections. Besides odontogenic and periodontal infections, candidal and recurrent herpes simplex infections are among the most common infections in the mouth. Bleeding problems, especially due to decreased platelets, may result in mucosal and gingival bleeding. The use of intravenous bisphosphonates may increase the risk for osteonecrosis of the jaw. The effects of radiation treatment directly affect the targeted tissues. When the head and neck is the targeted site, mucositis, taste alterations, salivary gland hypofunction, dysphagia, osteoradionecrosis, trismus, periodontal disease, and dental caries are potential complications.

The information listed below is intended to assist the practicing dentist in the management of oncology patients who are in the outpatient setting.

Clinical description:

Due to the wide range of potential complications, the oral findings are diverse in appearance. The more common findings include red, inflamed, and/or ulcerated mucosa and chapped lips. The saliva may be viscous or absent.

Rationale for treatment:

The treatment of these patients is symptomatic and supportive. It should be aimed at patient comfort and education, maintenance of proper nutrition and oral hygiene, and prevention of opportunistic infection. Frequent monitoring and close cooperation with the patient's physician are important. To prevent potentially serious oral complication, all patients who undergo chemotherapy and/or radiation therapy should have a thorough oral evaluation to eliminate any source of infection. In patients who will receive radiation treatment to the head and neck region, oral surgical procedures should be performed 14 days prior to the treatment for optimal healing. Oral hygiene is of paramount importance prior to, during, and after radiation treatment.

The oral discomfort may be relieved by periodically using neutral or saline mouth rinses and topical anesthetics and coating agents. Artificial saliva, mouth moisturizing gels, and supersaturated calcium phosphate rinses aid in reducing oral dryness and irritation. Antifungal and antiviral agents are needed to manage specific infections. The use of fluorides and bioavailable calcium phosphate is recommended for caries control and root sensitivity. In some patients, chlorhexidine rinses help control plaque when oral hygiene is poor.

Mouth Rinses (See "Xerostomia")

Rx

Alkaline saline (salt/bicarbonate) mouth rinse

Disp. Mix ½ teaspoon each of salt and baking soda in 16 oz glass of water.
Sig. Rinse for 1 min with copious amounts at least 5 times a day and spit out.

If too irritating, may switch to ½ teaspoon baking soda in 16 oz of water.

Rx

Caphosol (supersaturated calcium phosphate) solution

Disp. 60 ampules

Sig. Mix 2 ampules in a clean glass and swirl contents of glass to mix. Rinse and gargle with half of the solution for 1 min and expectorate. Repeat with the remaining solution. Do not eat or drink for 15 min after use. Use up to 4 times a day.

This solution may be helpful for patients with both dry mouth and mucositis.

Rx

NeutraSal (supersaturated calcium phosphate) rinse

Disp. 30 packets (1 box)

Sig. Dissolve one packet in a clean glass of 30 ml of water. Swish the solution in the mouth thoroughly for 1 min with half of the solution and spit out excess. Repeat with the remaining half of the solution and spit out excess. Use 4–10 times a day or PRN.

This is another supersaturated calcium phosphate rinse that may be beneficial for patients who experience dry mouth and mucositis.

Gingivitis Control

Rx

Peridex, PerioGard, generic (chlorhexidine gluconate) rinse 0.12%

Disp. 473 ml (16 oz)

Sig. Rinse with 0.5 oz (15 ml) twice a day for 30 sec and spit out. Avoid rinsing or eating for 30 min following treatment. Rinse after breakfast and at bedtime.

In xerostomic patients, chlorhexidine rinse should be used concurrently with artificial saliva to provide the needed protein-binding agent for efficacy and substantivity. Because of the alcohol content, this rinse may be too irritating to use. A pharmacy can compound an alcohol-free, 2% aqueous solution. It is important to note that both toothpaste and nystatin reduce the effectiveness of chlorhexidine rinse, so it is important to allow 30 min before using these agents.

Caries Control (See "Xerostomia")

Rx

Neutral NaF gel 1.1%

Disp. 24 ml

Sig. Place a thin ribbon in custom trays. After inserting trays in the mouth, bite on them to create a pumping action. Keep in the mouth for 5–10 min and spit out excess. Avoid rinsing or eating for 30 min after treatment.

An alternative is to brush on NaF gel twice daily for 2 min and spit out excess. Both of these techniques should be supplemented with conventional 1100-ppm sodium fluoride toothpaste twice daily.

The use of SnF2 gels may be substituted, but this agent has high acidity and lower fluoride concentration of 1000 ppm, in contrast to the NaF gels that have a neutral pH and contain 5000 ppm.

Topical Anesthetics

Rx

Lidocaine hydrochloride viscous solution 2%

Disp. 200 ml

Sig. Rinse with 2–3 teaspoons (10–15 ml) every 3–4 hr for 1 min; swish and spit out.

Do not use 2% lidocaine hydrochloride in children or adults who cannot expectorate because of potential for aspiration or swallowing.

Rx

Diphenhydramine hydrochloride oral solution 12.5 mg/5 ml mixed with aluminum hydroxide, magnesium hydroxide oral suspension

Compound to a 1 : 1 mixture by volume

Disp. 200 ml

Sig. Rinse with 1–2 teaspoons (5–10 ml) every 2–4 hr for 1 min; swish and spit out.

Although these medications are OTC, it is recommended that a pharmacist compound this oral suspension.

Rx

Diphenhydramine hydrochloride liquid 12.5 mg/5 ml/lidocaine viscous 2% oral solution/aluminum hydroxide, magnesium hydroxide oral suspension

Compound to a 1 : 1 : 1 mixture by volume

Disp. 200 ml

Sig. Shake well before use. Rinse with 1–2 teaspoons (5–10 ml) every 4 hr for 1 min and spit out excess. Store suspension at room temperature.

It is compounded by pharmacy and is stable for approximately 60 days. Do not use 2% lidocaine hydrochloride in children or adults who cannot expectorate because of potential for aspiration or swallowing.

Rx

Children's Benadryl Allergy Liquid, others (diphenhydramine hydrochloride) oral solution 12.5 mg/5 ml (OTC)

Disp. 4 oz bottle

Sig. Rinse with 1–2 teaspoons (5–10 ml) for 2 min every 2–4 hr and spit out excess.

If swallowed, for adolescents and adults, the maximum amount is 300 mg in 24 hr. For children 6–12 yr, the maximum is 150 mg in 24 hr. Children younger than 6 yr should not swallow this drug.

Rx

Sucrets (dyclonine HCl) throat lozenges (OTC)

Disp. 1 package

Sig. Slowly dissolve 1 lozenge in mouth every 2 hr as needed for pain. Do not take more than 10 lozenges a day.

The strength of dyclonine HCl ranges from 3 mg (maximum strength) to 1.2 mg for children's formula.

In general, when topical anesthetics are used, patients should be warned about a reduced gag reflex and the need for caution while eating and drinking to avoid possible airway compromise. Allergies are rare but may occur.

Antifungal Agents

(See "Candidiasis")

Saliva Stimulants

(See "Xerostomia")

BIBLIOGRAPHY

Neville BW, Damm DD, Allen CM, Bouquot JE, editors: *Oral and maxillofacial pathology*, ed 3, St. Louis, 2009, Saunders, Elsevier.

Rankin KV, Jones DL, Redding SW, editors: *Oral health in cancer therapy. A guide for health care professionals*, ed 3, Dallas, TX, 2008, Dental Oncology Education Program.

Siegel MA, Silverman S Jr, Sollecito TP, editors: *American Academy of Oral Medicine. Clinician's guide to treatment of common oral conditions*, ed 7, Edmonds, WA, 2009, American Academy of Oral Medicine.

Medically Compromised Patients

PREVENTION OF INFECTIVE ENDOCARDITIS

In 2007, the American Heart Association (AHA) updated its recommendations for antibiotic prophylaxis prior to dental procedures to prevent infective endocarditis (Wilson et al., 2007). These guidelines recommend antibiotic prophylaxis only in patients with cardiac conditions that are associated with the highest risk of adverse outcomes from infective endocarditis, including (1) patients with a **prosthetic heart valve,** (2) patients who have **previously had infective endocarditis,** (3) patients with **congenital heart disease** (unrepaired cyanotic heart disease; completely repaired congenital heart defects with prosthetic material or device, whether placed by surgery or catheter intervention, during the first 6 mo after the procedure; or repaired congenital heart disease with residual defects at the site or adjacent to the site of a prosthetic patch or prosthetic device), and (4) **cardiac transplant recipients** who develop cardiac **valvulopathy.** The list of dental procedures for which prophylaxis is recommended includes *all dental procedures* that involve manipulation of gingival tissue or the periapical region of teeth or perforation of the oral mucosa (except for routine anesthetic injections through noninfected tissue, taking dental radiographs, placement of removable prosthodontic or orthodontic appliances, adjustment of orthodontic appliances, placement of orthodontic brackets, shedding of deciduous teeth, and bleeding from trauma to the lips or oral mucosa).

The antibiotic regimens recommended for prophylaxis in patients at risk of adverse outcomes of infective endocarditis are to be administered as a *single dose* and 30 *min to 1 hr before the dental procedure*:

Oral: Amoxicillin 2 g (children 50 mg/kg)

Patients unable to take/absorb oral medications:

- Ampicillin 2 g IM or IV (children 50 mg/kg IM or IV) OR
- Cefazolin or Ceftriaxone 1 g IM or IV (children 50 mg/kg IM or IV)

Patients allergic to penicillins or ampicillin—oral:

- Cephalexin 2 g (children 50 mg/kg) OR
- Clindamycin 600 mg orally (children 20 mg/kg) OR
- Azithromycin or clarithromycin 500 mg (children 15 mg/kg)

Patients allergic to penicillins or ampicillin and unable to take/absorb oral medications:

- Cefazolin or Ceftriaxone 1 g IM or IV (children 50 mg/kg IM or IV) OR
- Clindamycin 600 mg IM or IV (children 20 mg/kg IM or IV)

If the antibiotic was *inadvertently* not administered prior to the procedure, the antibiotic dosage should be administered within 2 hr after the procedure. Practitioners should be cautious of coincidental infective endocarditis in patients at risk who present with a fever or other signs and symptoms of a systemic infection. Patients should also be monitored following the dental procedure for such signs and symptoms, which may be the initial indicators of infective endocarditis. In patients receiving anticoagulant therapy, intramuscular (IM) injections should be avoided and preference given to the oral route of administration if possible.

NONVALVULAR CARDIOVASCULAR DEVICE-RELATED INFECTIONS

In 2011, the AHA updated guidelines regarding the use of antibiotic prophylaxis for patients with cardiovascular implantable electronic devices undergoing dental, respiratory, GI, or GU procedures. A previous (2003) statement addressed devices such as pacemakers, defibrillators, total artificial hearts, ventriculoatrial shunts, patent ductus arteriosus occlusion devices (plugs, umbrellas, buttons, discs, embolization coils), atrial septal defect and ventricular septal defect closure devices (Bard clamshell occluders, discs, buttons, double umbrellas), conduits, patches, peripheral vascular stents, vascular grafts (including hemodialysis), coronary artery stents, and vena caval filters.

Other Surgically Implanted Prosthetic Devices

At this time, there are no guidelines formally promulgated by any professional organizations for antibiotic prophylaxis prior to dental procedures in patients with noncardiac, nonorthopedic implanted devices, such as breast implants. The dental practitioner should consult the patient's physician in cases involving such devices in whom implant infection may be a concern as a result of dental procedures and, with the informed consent of the patient, make a decision regarding the use of antibiotic prophylaxis.

ORTHOPEDIC DEVICES: SCREWS, PLATES, PINS, AND PROSTHETIC JOINTS

In 2012, the American Academy of Orthopaedic Surgeons (AAOS), in collaboration with the American Dental Association (ADA), revised its advisory statement on antibiotic prophylaxis for dental patients with total joint replacements.

The guidelines are now based upon critical assessment of scientific evidence pertaining to the relationship between dental procedures and infection of prosthetic joints. Following are three key recommendations:

1. Based on limited evidence, practitioners should consider changing their long-standing practice of prescribing prophylactic antibiotics who undergo dental procedures, and limited evidence shows that dental procedures are unrelated to prosthetic joint infections.
2. There is no direct evidence that the use of topical oral antimicrobials before dental procedures will prevent prosthetic joint infections.
3. By consensus of the AAOS and ADA, good oral hygiene is recommended in patients with prosthetic joints. The complete guideline and supporting documentation can be found at http://www.aaos.org/guidelines.

Note that these guidelines do not constitute treatment advice for specific patients and caution that "The decision regarding any specific procedure or treatment must be made in light of all circumstances presented by the patients, the needs and resources particular to the locality or institution, and the clinical judgment of the provider."

ADRENAL INSUFFICIENCY (PRIMARY AND SECONDARY): PREVENTION OF ADRENAL CRISIS

Patients with primary (Addison's disease) or secondary (exogenous corticosteroid induced) adrenal insufficiency may be at risk for adrenal crisis during or following surgical procedures performed in dentistry. Adrenal crisis is a medical emergency that requires prompt intervention to save the patient's life. To prevent adrenal crisis, supplemental steroids in rather large doses have been recommended since the mid-1950s for patients with adrenal insufficiency.

Adrenal crisis is a rare event in dentistry, especially in patients with secondary adrenal insufficiency. Four factors appear to be associated with the risk for adrenal crisis: (1) magnitude of surgery, (2) general anesthesia, (3) health status and stability of the patient, and (4) degree of pain control.

The most significant acute adverse outcome of adrenal insufficiency is adrenal crisis. This event can occur when a patient with adrenal insufficiency, most commonly Addison's disease, is challenged by stress (e.g., illness, infection, or surgery) and in response is unable to synthesize adequate amounts of cortisol and aldosterone. This potentially life-threatening emergency usually evolves slowly over a few hours and then is manifested by severe exacerbation of the condition, including profuse sweating, hypotension, weak pulse, cyanosis, nausea, vomiting, weakness, headache, dehydration, fever, sunken eyes, dyspnea, myalgias, arthralgia, hyponatremia, and eosinophilia. If not treated rapidly, the patient may develop hypothermia, severe hypotension, hypoglycemia, confusion, and circulatory collapse that can culminate in death.

Four factors appear to contribute to the risk of adrenal crisis during the perioperative period of oral surgery: (1) magnitude of surgery, (2) general anesthesia, (3) overall health of the patient (e.g., stable vs. ongoing infection), and (4) degree of pain control.

Negligible Risk: Nonsurgical Dental Procedures

The vast majority of patients with adrenal insufficiency can undergo routine, nonsurgical dental treatment *without* the need for supplemental glucocorticoids. This is supported by the fact that routine, nonsurgical dental procedures do not stimulate cortisol production at levels comparable to those occurring during oral surgery, and local anesthesia blocks neural stress pathways required for adrenocorticotropic hormone (ACTH) secretion. This guideline does not advocate dental treatment on patients whose adrenal insufficiency is uncontrolled or undiagnosed. However, stable patients with adrenal insufficiency and those with a history of steroid use in whom glucocorticoid medication was discontinued prior to surgery have withstood general surgical procedures without developing adrenal crisis.

Low-Risk Regimen

For minor oral and periodontal surgery (e.g., a few simple extractions, soft tissue surgery), evidence suggests that adrenal insufficiency is prevented when circulating levels of glucocorticoids are approximately 25 mg hydrocortisone equivalent per day. This is equivalent to a dose of approximately 5 mg prednisone. The clinician should confirm that the patient has taken the recommended amount of steroid within 2 hr of the surgical procedure and schedule the surgery in the morning when normal cortisol levels are highest. Stress-reduction measures should be implemented. Benefits can be gained from use of (1) oral, inhalation, or intravenous sedation, which provides stress reduction; (2) intravenous fluids (i.e., 5% dextrose), which can prevent hypovolemia and hypoglycemia; (3) long-acting local anesthetics; and (4) adequate postoperative analgesics.

Moderate-Risk to Major-Risk Regimen

Patients with adrenocortical suppression undergoing major oral surgery are at increased risk for adrenal crisis when compared with minor surgery. Major surgical procedures are more stressful than minor surgical procedures. They increase the demand for cortisol because of postoperative pain. Blood loss is greater, thus increasing the risk for hypovolemia and hypotension.

For major oral surgical stress (multiple extractions, quadrant periodontal surgery, extraction of bony impactions, osseous surgery, osteotomy, bone resections, cancer surgery), surgical procedures involving use of general anesthesia, procedures lasting more than 1 hr, or procedures associated with significant blood loss, the glucocorticoid target is approximately 50–100 mg/day hydrocortisone equivalent for the day of surgery and at least 1 postoperative day. Higher doses may be necessary if excessive bleeding or complications are encountered. Patients should take their normal steroid dose prior to the procedure and be provided supplemental intravenous hydrocortisone intraoperatively to achieve a total of 100 mg. Hospitalization should be considered for these patients because blood pressure can be more closely monitored postoperatively in this setting. Hydrocortisone 25 mg usually is prescribed every 8 hr following surgery for 24–48 hr, depending on the procedure and anticipated level of postoperative pain.

Following the recommendations listed will further minimize the risk of adrenal crisis associated with surgical stress in adrenally insufficient individuals:

- Define the risk for adrenal insufficiency with a thorough medical history and clinical examination. Patients with a past or present history of tuberculosis or HIV infection are at increased risk for adrenal insufficiency because opportunistic infectious agents can attack the adrenal glands.
- Ensure that adrenally insufficient patients take their glucocorticoid prior to a stressful surgery.
- Schedule surgery in the morning when cortisol levels normally are highest.
- Provide proper stress reduction because anxiety can increase cortisol demand.
- Minor surgeries require minimal steroid coverage. The patient's customary daily dose usually is sufficient.
- Major surgeries and those procedures lasting more than 1 hr or requiring use of general anesthesia should be performed in a hospital with steroid supplementation.
- Use of nitrous oxide-oxygen or intravenous or oral benzodiazepine sedation is helpful, as plasma cortisol levels are not reduced by these agents.
- Avoid outpatient general anesthesia, as general anesthesia increases glucocorticoid demand. Also, avoid use of barbiturates, which increase the metabolism of cortisol and reduce blood levels of cortisol.

SUMMARY OF NEED FOR SUPPLEMENTATION

Negligible-Risk Category

Nonsurgical dental procedures

Regimen: No supplementation required

Low-Risk Category

Minor oral surgery

Few simple extractions, biopsy

Minor periodontal surgery

Regimen: Target 25 mg hydrocortisone equivalent (5 *mg prednisone), day of surgery*

Moderate-Risk to Major-Risk Category
Major oral surgery
Multiple extractions
Quadrant periodontal surgery
Extraction of bony impactions
Osseous surgery
Osteotomy
Bone resections
Cancer surgery
Surgical procedures involving use of general anesthesia
Procedures lasting more than 1 hr
Procedures associated with significant blood loss

Regimen: Target glucocorticoid is approximately 50–100 mg/day hydrocortisone equivalent, day of surgery and at least 1 postoperative day

CONTROL OF BLEEDING IN PATIENTS ON ANTICOAGULANT THERAPY

Oral Anticoagulants

In patients taking oral anticoagulant drugs (e.g., warfarin, Coumadin) to prevent thromboembolic complications (e.g., stroke), the dentist should consult the patient's physician regarding the patient's reason for taking the drug and determine the level of anticoagulation reported as the international normalized ratio (INR). In most patients, the therapeutic range of the INR is approximately 2.5–3.5, whereas some patients may be maintained at higher levels (e.g., up to 4.5). The AMA and the ADA suggest an INR value of 2–3 before a surgical procedure is attempted. Local measures should be used to control bleeding if it occurs.

In patients with INR >3.5, the dentist should consult with the patient's physician regarding possible reduction of the anticoagulant dosage before surgery. Minor surgery usually can be performed safely in patients with an INR up to 3.5.

In general, treating these patients without reducing the anticoagulant dose poses a less significant risk than stopping the anticoagulant. The current literature does not support stopping or reducing the dose of the drug, which would increase the risk for thrombotic events. If the physician recommends an alteration of anticoagulant dosage, he or she should manage the adjustment of anticoagulant dosage. At least 3–4 days must pass before the effect of the reduced dosage will be reflected in a decreased INR. The INR value should be checked on the scheduled day of surgery to be certain that the desired reduction of anticoagulation effect has occurred.

If acute infection is present, surgery should be delayed until the infection has been treated. When the patient is free of acute infection and the INR is 3.5 or lower, routine surgery can be performed. The procedure should be done with as little trauma as possible. If excessive postoperative bleeding (slow blood flow and oozing) occurs, one or more of the following measures can be used to control it:

Use a splint constructed before surgery (in cases with multiple extractions)
Pressure using gauze pack
Absorbable gelatin sponge (Gelfoam)

Dental packing blocks:

20 × 20 × 7 mm, can be cut to fit and applied to bleeding site.
Powder: Apply to bleeding site.

Gelfoam with thrombin

Thrombogen: Powder with isotonic saline diluent (5000-unit container with isotonic saline). For bleeding from skin or mucosa, use solution of 100 units/ml. Do not use with Oxycel, Surgicel, or microfibrillar collagen because they inactivate the thrombin.

Oxidized cellulose (Oxycel)

Pad: 3 × 3 inch; pledget: 2 × 1 × 1 inch; strip: 18 × 2, 5 × ½, 36 × ½ inch. Cut to appropriate size and apply dry.

Tranexamic acid (Cyklokapron)

Solution: 100 mg/ml in 10-ml vials; tablets: 500 mg, after surgery 25 mg/kg orally 3 times a day.

Oxidized regenerated cellulose (Surgicel absorbable hemostat)

Surgicel sheets: 2 × 14, 4 × 8, 2 × 3, ½ × 2 inch; Surgicel Nu-Knit sheets: 1 × 1, 3 × 4, 6 × 9 inch. Pick appropriate size and lay over extraction site to control bleeding.

Microfibrillar collagen hemostat (Avitene, CollaTape, Instat MCH)

Avitene sheets: 35 × 35, 70 × 35, 70 × 70 mm; CollaTape: 1 × 3, ¾ × 1½, ⅜ × ¾ inch.

Instat MCH: Coherent fibers packaged in 0.5- and 1.0-g containers. Apply topically, and it adheres firmly to bleeding surfaces.

Collagen hemostat

Pads: 1 × 2, 3 × 4 inch. Apply directly to bleeding surface with pressure. It is more effective when applied dry.

Antiplatelet Therapy

Patients with drug-eluting stents for treatment of coronary artery disease take a combination of aspirin and another antiplatelet drug from the thienopyridine group (clopidogrel, Plavix; ticlopidine, Ticlid) for at least 1 yr following placement of the stent. Abrupt discontinuation of this dual antiplatelet therapy in patients prior to routine dental procedures is not recommended. In 2007, the AHA issued an advisory statement that strongly advised against the common practice of discontinuing these agents, which included references to very high mortality rates in at-risk patients who develop thromboemboli.

MANAGEMENT OF ANXIETY IN THE DENTAL PATIENT

Anxiety

The dentist may detect anxiety in a patient on the basis of his or her physical appearance, speech, dress, and presence of certain signs and symptoms. The anxious person looks overalert, displayed in ways such as sitting forward in a chair; moving fingers, arms, or legs; getting up and moving; pacing around the room; checking certain parts of clothing; and straightening ties or scarves.

On the other hand, sloppy dress habits and other signs, just the opposite of a concern with perfection, may also be seen. An anxious person may show signs of being watchful of possessions, always trying to keep them in sight.

The anxious person may speak mechanically and rapidly and at times may seem to block out or not connect thoughts together. The anxious person may respond to questions quickly, often not allowing the dentist to finish a question.

Signs of sweating, tension in muscles, increased breathing, and rapid heart rate may be seen. The patient may complain of an inability to sleep, may wake at an early hour, and may not be able to go back to sleep. Attacks of diarrhea and increased frequency of urination may occur. In general, anxious persons are overalert and tense, feel apprehensive, and have a sense of impending disaster that has no apparent cause. Insomnia, tension, and apprehension lead to fatigue, which makes it even more difficult for the individual to deal with anxiety.

The dentist should talk with the patient and show personal interest. Verbal and nonverbal communication must be consistent. The dentist should confront the patient with the observation that the patient appears anxious, then ask if the individual would like to talk about feelings, which may include the person's attitude toward the dentist. During these discussions, tension-free pauses should be allowed to develop between ideas, as a temporary state of regression will help the patient return to a more anxiety-free state. Some patients may respond well to this approach without ever indicating why they were anxious.

If the patient remains anxious in the dental situation, the dentist can plan to use hypnosis, oral or parenteral sedation agents or nitrous oxide, and oxygen to better manage the dental treatment.

Patients with uncontrolled hyperthyroidism may have associated anxiety. Epinephrine must not be used in these patients, including even the small amounts that are used in local anesthetics. Patients with signs and symptoms of hyperthyroidism should be referred for medical evaluation and treatment.

Dental Management of the Anxious Patient

1. Preoperative

   A. *Behavioral*

      Establish effective communication with the patient; provide instructions

      Be open and honest; let the patient see who you are

      Consistent verbal and nonverbal communication

      Explain procedures and answer any questions

      Explain possible discomfort associated with a procedure

      Explain what you will do to make procedures "pain free"

      Possibly confront patient who appears anxious: "You seem tense today. Would you like to talk about it?"

   B. *Pharmacologic*

      Oral sedation: benzodiazepines

      Night before appointment: hypnotic benzodiazepine to aid patient in getting a good night's sleep

      Day of appointment: reduce anxiety prior to appointment

      Select a drug with an onset of 1 hr or less and at the lowest dosage that will be effective

   C. *Informed Consent*

      Use a written and verbal informed consent process to ensure that the patient and the patient's perioperative caretaker understand all aspects of the planned sedative and dental procedures

2. Operative

   A. *Behavioral*

      Allow patient to ask questions

Let patient know if any discomfort will be felt
Reassure patient

B. Pharmacologic

Effective local anesthesia
Oral sedation*: benzodiazepines
Inhalation sedation*: nitrous oxide
Intramuscular sedation*
Intravenous sedation*

3. Postoperative

A. Behavioral

Explain to patient and patient's caretaker what usually occurs after the procedure
Explain to patient and patient's caretaker what the patient needs to do
Explain to patient and patient's caretaker what the patient needs to avoid
Describe to patient and patient's caretaker what complications can occur and what steps to take to manage them:
Pain
Bleeding
Infection
Allergic reaction to medication
Tell patient and patient's caretaker to inform you if any complications develop

B. Pharmacologic

Effective postoperative pain control is essential
Select the most appropriate medication for pain control
Analgesics: nonsteroidal antiinflammatory drugs (NSAIDs) or acetaminophen (in patients who cannot take aspirin/NSAIDs) with codeine, hydrocodone, or oxycodone
Adjunctive medications: antidepressants, muscle relaxants, steroids, anticonvulsants, antibiotics

Specific Drugs and Dosage for Anxiety Control (Dosage for Older Adults and Children Must Be Reduced)*

Nitrous oxide, inhalation, titrated to 20%–50%
Diazepam (Valium), oral (2-, 5-, or 10-mg tablets)
Triazolam (Halcion), oral (0.125- or 0.25-mg tablets)
Lorazepam (Ativan), oral (1- or 3-mg tablets)

Other benzodiazepines or nonbenzodiazepines according to practitioner preference and needs of patient (e.g., oxazepam, alprazolam, diphenhydramine, zolpidem)

DEPRESSION IN DENTAL PATIENTS

Signs of low-grade chronic depression include fatigue (even after adequate sleep); difficulty getting up in the morning; restlessness; loss of interest in

*NOTE: Many states require that dentists have special permits for the use of various sedation modalities; appropriate emergency and monitoring equipment is recommended whenever sedative agents are employed.

family, work, and sex; inability to make decisions; anger and resentment; chronic complaining; self-criticism; feelings of inferiority; and excessive day-dreaming. Signs of more severe depression include excessive crying, change in sleeping habits, thoughts of food making one sick, weight loss without dieting, strong feelings of guilt, nightmares, thoughts about suicide, feeling unreal or in a "fog," and an inability to concentrate.

Patients with major depression are depressed most of the day, show a marked decrease in interest or pleasure in most activities, have a marked gain or loss in weight, and manifest insomnia or hypersomnia. These symptoms must be present for at least 2 wk before major depression can be diagnosed.

Dental Management

Significant impairment of all personal hygiene may occur during the depth of a depressive episode, including a total lack of oral hygiene. Salivary flow may be reduced, and patients may complain of xerostomia (dry mouth), an increased rate of dental caries, and periodontal disease. The xerostomia may be compounded by the side effects of the medications used to treat depression. Complaints of glossodynia and various facial pain syndromes are common.

The dentist should provide an aggressive preventive dental education program for depressed patients, including the use of artificial salivary products, antiseptic mouthwash, and daily fluoride mouth rinses. Xerostomia provides an excellent environment for overgrowth of *Candida albicans*; as a result, patients are likely to require treatment for candidiasis along with treatment for dry mouth.

Small amounts of epinephrine (0.04 mg or 2 cartridges of a 1 : 100,000 concentration) can be used in patients taking tricyclic or heterocyclic antidepressants. Excessive amounts of epinephrine can result in hypertension. A lower dosage of sedative medications may be necessary to avoid excessive CNS depression (Table 1).

Patients taking tricyclic or heterocyclic antidepressant drugs may be prone to orthostatic hypotension. Dentists should avoid rapid changes in chair position for these patients and provide support when patients first get out of the dental chair. Atropine should be used with care because increased intraocular pressure can result. Acetaminophen should be used with care because it can decrease the metabolic rate of the heterocyclics, which could lead to toxic levels of the tricyclic antidepressant. Phenobarbital increases the metabolism of tricyclic antidepressants, which can attenuate their antidepressant effects.

Patients with signs and symptoms of severe depression must be referred for medical evaluation and treatment. If the patient is not responsive to this recommendation, the problem should be shared with a family member and every attempt made to get the individual to medical attention. During severe depression, suicide is always a possibility; however, medical treatment currently is able to reduce this possibility.

Suicidal Patients

Studies have shown that questions about suicide do not prompt these patients to act. The dentist should ask the very depressed patient if he or she has had any thoughts about suicide. Patients who state they have had these thoughts must be referred for immediate medical care; members of the family need to be involved if possible.

TABLE 1
Adverse Drug Interactions of Significance to Dentistry

Dental Drug	Interacting Drug	Medical Condition/ Situation	Effect
Antibiotics			
β-lactams (penicillins, cephalosporins)	Allopurinol (Lopurin, Zyloprim)	Gout	Incidence of minor allergic reactions to ampicillin is increased. Other penicillins have not been implicated. **Recommendation:** Avoid ampicillin.
	β-blockers (Tenormin, Lopressor, Inderal, Corgard)	Hypertension	Serum levels of atenolol are reduced after prolonged use of ampicillin. Anaphylactic reactions to penicillins or other drugs may be more severe in patients taking β-blockers because of increased mediator release from mast cells. **Recommendation:** Use ampicillin cautiously, advise patient of potential reaction.
	Tetracyclines and other bacteriostatic antibiotics	Infection, acne, periodontal disease	Effectiveness of penicillins and cephalosporins may be reduced by bacteriostatic agents. **Recommendation:** Avoid interaction.
Tetracyclines	Antacids	Dyspepsia, gastroesophageal reflux, peptic ulcer	Antacids, dairy products, and other agents containing divalent and trivalent cations will chelate tetracyclines and limit their absorption in the gut. Doxycycline is least influenced by this interaction. **Recommendation:** Avoid interaction.
	Insulin	Diabetes mellitus	Doxycycline and oxytetracycline have been documented as enhancing the hypoglycemic effects of exogenously administered insulin. **Recommendation:** Select different antibiotic or increase carbohydrate intake.

Metronidazole	Ethanol	Alcohol use or abuse	Severe disulfiramlike reactions are well documented. **Recommendation:** Avoid interaction.
	Lithium	Manic depression	Inhibits renal excretion of lithium, leading to elevated/toxic levels of lithium. Lithium toxicity produces confusion, ataxia, and kidney damage. **Recommendation:** Avoid interaction.
	Benzodiazepines	Anxiety	Delayed metabolism of benzodiazepine, increasing the pharmacologic effects can result in excessive sedation and irrational behavior. **Recommendation:** Reduce dose of benzodiazepine.
	Carbamazepine (Tegretol)	Seizure disorder	Increased blood levels of carbamazepine leading to toxicity (symptoms include drowsiness, dizziness, nausea, headache, and blurred vision). Hospitalization has been required. **Recommendation:** Avoid interaction.
	Cyclosporine	Organ transplant	Enhanced immunosuppression and nephrotoxicity. **Recommendation:** Avoid interaction, monitor patient.
	Lovastatin, pravastatin, simvastatin, other statins	Hyperlipidemia	Muscle (eosinophilia) myalgia and rhabdomyolysis. **Recommendation:** Avoid interaction.
	Prednisone, methylprednisolone	Autoimmune disorders, organ transplant	Increased risk of Cushing's syndrome and immunosuppression. **Recommendation:** Monitor patient, shorten duration of antibiotic administration if possible.
	Theophylline (Theo-Dur)	Asthma	Some macrolide antibiotics (erythromycin, clarithromycin) inhibit metabolism of theophylline, leading to toxic serum levels (symptoms of toxicity: headache, nausea, vomiting, confusion, thirst, cardiac arrhythmias, convulsions). Conversely, theophylline reduces serum levels of erythromycin. **Recommendation:** Avoid prescribing these antibiotics in such patients.

(Continued)

TABLE 1
Adverse Drug Interactions of Significance to Dentistry—cont'd

Dental Drug	Interacting Drug	Medical Condition/ Situation	Effect
Antibiotics (especially erythromycin and tetracycline)	Digoxin (Lanoxin)	Congestive heart failure	Alters gastrointestinal flora and retards metabolism of digoxin in approximately 10% of patients, resulting in dangerously high digoxin serum levels that may persist for several weeks after discontinuation of antibiotic. Strongest documentation for erythromycin and tetracycline. Patients should be cautioned to report any signs of digitalis toxicity (salivation, visual disturbances, arrhythmias) during antibiotic therapy. **Recommendation:** Avoid interaction by using noninteractive antibiotic.
Antibiotics (cephalosporins, erythromycin, clarithromycin, metronidazole)	Warfarin (Coumadin)	Atrial fibrillation, MI, post major surgery, stroke prevention	Anticoagulant effect of warfarin may be increased by several antibiotic classes. Reduced synthesis of vitamin K by gut flora is a putative mechanism, but several antibiotics have antiplatelet and anticoagulant activity. Most convincing documentation for cephalosporins, macrolide antibiotics, and metronidazole. **Recommendation:** Penicillins, tetracyclines, and clindamycin are preferred choices but must be used cautiously.
Macrolide antibiotics (erythromycin, clarithromycin)	Benzodiazepines with high oral bioavailability (triazolam, midazolam)	Infection	Reduced hepatic first-pass metabolism of benzodiazepine with increased blood level and unpredictably increased levels of CNS depression. **Recommendation:** Avoid interaction with alternative sedative or reduce dose of interacting benzodiazepine.

Azole antifungal agents (e.g., ketoconazole, Nizoral)	Benzodiazepines	Systemic fungal infection	Reduced hepatic metabolism (CYP3A4 inhibition) of benzodiazepine results in unpredictably increased CNS depression. **Recommendation:** Avoid interaction with alternative sedative agent or reduce dose of interacting benzodiazepine.
Analgesics			
Acetaminophen	Alcohol	Alcohol use and abuse	Increased risk of liver toxicity, especially during fasting state or over 4 g/day acetaminophen, exacerbated by abrupt discontinuation of alcohol use. **Recommendation:** Use lower dose of acetaminophen, allow patient to continue alcohol use. (NOTE: alcohol-related liver damage may absolutely contraindicate use of acetaminophen.)
Aspirin	Oral hypoglycemics (sulfonylureas: glyburide, chlorpropamide, acetohexamide)	Diabetes type 2	Increased hypoglycemic effects. **Recommendation:** Avoid interaction.
Aspirin, NSAIDs	Anticoagulants (warfarin, Coumadin)	Atrial fibrillation, myocardial infarction, postsurgery	Increased risk of gastrointestinal bleeding. **Recommendation:** Avoid interaction.
Aspirin, NSAIDs	Alcohol	Alcohol use and abuse	Increases risk of GI bleeding. **Recommendation:** Lower dose, encourage discontinuation of alcohol use.

(Continued)

TABLE 1
Adverse Drug Interactions of Significance to Dentistry—cont'd

Dental Drug	Interacting Drug	Medical Condition/ Situation	Effect
NSAIDs	β-blocker angiotensin-converting enzyme inhibitor	Hypertension, postmyocardial infarction	Decreased antihypertensive effect. **Recommendation:** Limit duration of NSAID dosage to approximately 4 days.
NSAIDs	Lithium	Manic depression	Produces symptoms of lithium toxicity, including nausea, vomiting, slurred speech, and mental confusion. **Recommendation:** NSAIDs should not be prescribed to patients with manic depression who take lithium. It can result in toxic levels of lithium.
NSAIDs	Methotrexate (MTX)	Connective tissue disease, cancer therapy	Toxic levels of MTX may accumulate. **Recommendation:** Avoid interaction if patient on high-dose MTX for cancer therapy. Low-dose MTX for arthritis is not a concern.
SSRI	Antidepressants	Depressive disease	Increased risk of GI irritation
Anesthetics, local			
All agents	Other local anesthetics		Additive effect of two local anesthetics increases risk. **Recommendation:** Limit dose of each.
	Opioids, sedatives		Sedation with opioids may increase risk of local anesthetic toxicity, especially in children. **Recommendation:** Reduce anesthetic dose.

Sedatives			
Barbiturates	Digoxin, theophylline, corticosteroids, oral anticoagulants	CHF, asthma, autoimmune disease, atrial fibrillation	Barbiturates bind cytochrome P450 system in liver, enhance metabolism of many drugs. **Recommendation:** Limit dose, observe for adverse effects.
	Benzodiazepines, alcohol, antihistamines	Anxiety, alcohol use and abuse, seasonal allergies	Additive effects for sedation and respiratory depression. **Recommendation:** Reduce dose, administer combination of sedatives with extreme caution.
Benzodiazepines (BZ; e.g., alprazolam, chlordiazepoxide, diazepam)	Cimetidine, oral contraceptives, fluoxetine, isoniazid (INH), alcohol	Peptic ulcer disease, depression, tuberculosis, alcohol use and abuse	Delayed metabolism of BZDP, increasing pharmacologic effects can result in excessive sedation and irrational behavior. **Recommendation:** Reduce dose of BZDP. Delayed metabolism of BZDP, increasing pharmacologic effects can result in excessive sedation and irrational behavior. **Recommendation:** Reduce dose of BZDP.
	Digoxin (Lanoxin), phenytoin, theophylline (Theo-Dur)	CHF, epilepsy, asthma	Serum concentrations of digoxin, phenytoin may be increased, resulting in toxicity. Antagonize sedative effects of BZDP. **Recommendation:** Avoid interaction.
	Protease inhibitors (Indinavir, Nelfinavir)	HIV, AIDS	Increased bioavailability and effects of BZDP, especially triazolam and oral midazolam. **Recommendation:** Avoid interaction.
Vasoconstrictor			
Epinephrine and levonordefrin (Neo-Cobefrin)	Nonselective β-blockers: propranolol (Inderal), nadolol (Corgard), penbutolol (Levatol), pindolol (Visken), sotalol (Betapace), timolol (Blocadren)	Angina pectoris, hypertension, glaucoma, migraine, headache, hyperthyroidism, panic syndromes	Unopposed effects: increased B/P with secondary bradycardia. **Recommendation:** Limit or avoid epinephrine, aspirate to avoid intravascular injection, inject slowly. Avoid epinephrine-containing retraction cord and higher concentrations of epinephrine in the dental anesthetic.

(Continued)

TABLE 1
Adverse Drug Interactions of Significance to Dentistry—cont'd

Dental Drug	Interacting Drug	Medical Condition/ Situation	Effect
	Cocaine	Illicit use, topical anesthetic for mucous membrane procedures	Blocks reuptake of norepinephrine and intensifies postsynaptic response to epinephrine-like drugs. This potentiates the adrenergic effects on the heart, with potential for a heart attack. **Recommendation:** Recognize signs and symptoms of cocaine abuse. Avoid use of vasoconstrictors in these patients until cocaine has been withheld for at least 24 hr.
	Halothane	General anesthetic for surgical procedures	Sensitization of sympathetic receptors to epinephrine resulting in arrhythmia at doses greater than 2 g/kg. **Recommendation:** Limit dose to remain below 2 g/kg threshold, aspirate to avoid intravascular injection. Monitor vital signs. Avoid epinephrine-containing retraction cord and concentrations of epinephrine greater than 1 : 100,000.
	Tricyclic antidepressants (amitriptyline [Elavil], doxepin [Sinequan], imipramine [Tofranil])	Depression, severe anxiety, neuropathic pain, attention deficit disorder	Blocks reuptake of norepinephrine resulting in unopposed effects (increased B/P, increased heart rate), potential cardiac arrhythmias; effect is greater with levonordefrin. **Recommendation:** Limit dose or avoid vasoconstrictors, aspirate to avoid intravascular injection. Monitor vital signs. Avoid epinephrine-containing retraction cord and higher concentrations of epinephrine in the dental anesthetic.

	Peripheral adrenergic antagonists (reserpine [Serpasil], guanethidine [Ismelin], guanadrel [Hylorel])	Hypertension	Potential for increased sensitivity of adrenergic receptors to epinephrine and levonordefrin. **Recommendation:** Administer cautiously. Monitor vital signs during and following administration of first cartridge. Limit dose or avoid epinephrine. Aspirate to avoid intravascular injection. Avoid epinephrine-containing retraction cord and higher concentrations of epinephrine in the dental anesthetic.
	Catechol-O-methyltransferase inhibitors (tolcapone [Tasmar], entacapone [Comtan])	Parkinson's disease	Potential for increased sensitivity of adrenergic receptors to epinephrine and levonordefrin, resulting in increased heart rate and B/P and arrhythmias. **Recommendation:** Administer cautiously. Monitor vital signs during and after administration of first cartridge. Limit dose or avoid epinephrine. Aspirate to avoid intravascular injection. Avoid epinephrine-containing retraction cord and higher concentrations of epinephrine in the dental anesthetic.

Bisphosphonate-Associated Osteonecrosis of the Jaw (Osteochemonecrosis)

With the increased frequency of bisphosphonate use for the treatment of osteoporosis (e.g., alendronate, Fosamax), dentists have been alerted to the possibility of osteonecrosis of the jaw related to these drugs. These medications are also used in other resorptive bone diseases, including breast and prostate cancer metastatic to the bones, Paget's disease, and cases of bone fragility related to chronic renal failure. This group of drugs currently includes aminobisphosphonates (alendronate, Fosamax; ibandronate, Boniva; pamidronate, Aredia; risedronate, Actonel; and zoledronate, Zometa) and nonaminobisphosphonates (clodronate, Bonefos; etidronate, Didronel; and tiludronate, Skelid). These agents are used both orally and intravenously, with the intravenous agents appearing to place the patient at a much higher risk for osteonecrosis of the jaw. There are no prospective, randomized scientific studies on which to base dental management algorithms for these patients, but guidelines presently exist, based on retrospective studies and case reports.

Clinically, osteonecrosis of the jaw usually presents as exposed bone in the maxillofacial area, reportedly more frequently in the mandible, spontaneously or following oral surgery, that does not heal within 6 wk (confirmed when other possible causes have been ruled out [e.g., osteoradionecrosis]). Signs and symptoms may include one or more of the following: mucosal ulceration with exposed bone; infection (with or without purulence); pain or swelling in the affected jaw, and/or paresthesia (numbness, tingling) or other sensory alterations (e.g., "heavy jaw"); delayed or incomplete healing; or a sudden deterioration of periodontal health. Additional risk factors include patients in poor health or with a compromised immune system (e.g., long-term corticosteroid therapy) and bony exostoses (e.g., tori). Currently, there are no blood tests that are predictive of the disorder. Endodontically treated teeth in patients with risk factors for bisphosphonate-related osteonecrosis of the jaw must be followed carefully because low-level, residual infection and inflammation may, over time, result in the condition.

This condition occurs only rarely in patients taking oral bisphosphonates, but a higher risk has been determined for the intravenous agents in this group. The dental management of patients at risk for osteonecrosis includes identification of at-risk patients and the following:

- Patients should have a comprehensive dental exam prior to starting bisphosphonate therapy and should be reevaluated every 6 mo or more frequently, as appropriate.
- Oral surgical and other invasive dental procedures should be completed before starting bisphosphonate therapy.
- The dental team should emphasize excellent oral hygiene for patients on bisphosphonate therapy.
- If dental treatment is necessary after bisphosphonate therapy has been started, the least invasive (nonsurgical) technique is recommended, although routine restorative and dental hygiene procedures may be performed.
- The risks and potential benefits of withholding bisphosphonate therapy should be discussed with the patient and the patient's treating physician(s) prior to tooth extraction or other oral surgical procedures. The American

Association of Oral and Maxillofacial Surgeons (AAOMS) has recommended that consideration be given to suspending the use of a bisphosphonate prior to oral and maxillofacial surgery procedures to reduce the risk of bisphosphonate-related osteonecrosis of the jaw, but this measure is not based on randomized, prospective studies and should not be undertaken without consideration of the potential medical consequences (e.g., fractures) and without the input from the physician prescribing the bisphosphonate.

- In patients with oral osteonecrosis, conservative management is recommended and includes the use of antibiotics, antibacterial mouth rinses, limited debridement of the site, and analgesic medications to control pain associated with the osteonecrosis. Steroid drugs may increase the risk for development of osteonecrosis.
- The dental management of patients at risk for bisphosphonate-related osteonecrosis should include appropriate informed consent prior to the performance of actual dental procedures.

ADVERSE DRUG INTERACTIONS

Table 1 provides a summary of adverse drug interactions for commonly used dental drugs. Monographs should be referred to for more specific information.

COMPLEMENTARY MEDICINES, NUTRITIONAL/HERBAL SUPPLEMENTS, AND DENTISTRY

The term alternative medicine is used to describe practices that are used instead of mainstream medical practice. Complementary medicine refers to practices that are used as adjuncts to conventional medicine. These systems are divided into five major categories: alternative medical systems (traditional Chinese medicine, Ayurveda medicine of India, and Native American healing approaches), biologically based therapies (natural products), manipulative and body-based methods (chiropractic and osteopathic manipulation), mind–body interventions (hypnosis, cognitive therapies, and biofeedback), and energy therapies (use of magnets and acupuncture). Both of these systems use treatments that often have no established efficacy. An estimated 42% of Americans use alternative and complementary medicine therapies.

Complementary medicines are defined as herbal medicines, homeopathic remedies, and essential oils. The basic principle of homeopathy is selection of a remedy that, if given to a healthy individual, will produce a range of symptoms similar to those observed in the ill patient (like cures like). Only minute amounts are given to avoid toxicity. Only one remedy is used at any one time. Dilute tinctures are used rather than concentrated ones. In homeopathic practice, medication in tablet form is commonly used.

The standard tinctures used in Western tradition herbal medicine are very different from those used in homeopathy. Alcohol is used to dissolve the plant, and the final product is not diluted. Thus, these remedies are concentrated, highly potent preparations and usually are taken as the unmodified liquid tincture. Other preparations used in herbal remedies include lotions and creams for topical application. Tablet form of medication is not used very often (less than 5%).

Efficacy of Herbal Medicines

Many herbal remedies have been used for hundreds of years. However, traditional use is not a good indication of efficacy. The gold standard for testing efficacy is the randomized clinical trial (RCT). This standard should apply as much to herbal medicines as to conventional medicines. A number of RCTs of herbal medical products have been conducted. However, many of these studies differ with regard to how they were conducted and in their findings. Ernst suggests that the best way to evaluate a number of RCTs on the efficacy of a specific herbal medicine is to do a systematic review or meta-analysis of all RCTs for that product.

Herbal medicines with proven efficacy:
Several herbal remedies have been repeatedly tested in placebo-controlled RCTs. Systematic reviews of these studies have shown that some herbal medicines are effective for certain conditions. For example, ginkgo biloba has been shown to be effective for symptomatic treatment of dementia and intermittent claudication. Table 2 lists the more commonly used herbal medicines that have proved to be effective for the condition(s) listed.

Herbal medicines with doubtful or no efficacy:
Asian ginseng, one of the most popular herbal medicines in the United States, showed no convincing evidence for efficacy as a general tonic or in enhancing mental and physical performance. A review of studies regarding the use of valerian as a hypnotic agent was inconclusive because of flaws in the study designs. A systematic review of RCTs found no evidence that evening primrose was effective for treatment of premenstrual syndrome in women. Garlic was not found to be effective as a cholesterol-lowering drug. *For more information on the efficacy of herbal medicines, see on the companion website Table 3—Claims for Herbal Actions Unsupported by Clinical Trials.*

Side Effects and Adverse Reactions

Recent increased use of herbal remedies seems to come from the public's view that natural products are harmless or at least have fewer side effects than regular drugs. The assumption that phytomedicines (herbal medicines) have only beneficial effects has proved to be incorrect.

Toxicity can be associated with use of herbal remedies. These reactions can be caused by accidental or deliberate contamination of the product. For example, lead, mercury, cadmium, pesticides, microorganisms, and fumigants have been found to contaminate some herbal products. Substitution of animal substances such as enzymes, hormones, or organ extracts and synthetic drugs has accounted for some of the toxic reactions to herbal products. Adulteration by accidental or deliberate substitution of the original plant material by other plant species has been reported to be a source of toxic reactions to herbal products.

Other sources of adverse reactions to herbal products are intrinsic or plant associated. In some cases, the manufacturer ignored the known toxicity of a plant or constituent in the herbal product. In other cases, the product contains plants for which no or insufficient data regarding safety are available. If a highly concentrated or specifically processed extract is used, toxic reactions may occur. If a plant contains constituents known to affect the bioavailability and/or pharmacokinetics of other drugs, serious drug interactions can occur.

TABLE 2
Claims for Herbal Actions Supported by Clinical Trials

Herb	Claimed Action	Effectiveness Supported by Clinical Trials
Kava	Used to treat anxiety.	Clinical trials have shown it reduces anxiety significantly more than placebo.
Artichoke	Used to lower the lipid levels in blood.	Only one randomized clinical study shows it moderately lowers elevated total cholesterol levels when given orally for several weeks.
Feverfew	Used for women's ailments and inflammatory diseases. Recently has been suggested for headache and migraine.	Three studies showed greater effect than placebo in alleviating symptoms of headache or migraine.
Garlic	Used to reduce blood pressure and lower blood lipid levels.	Data show a small but statistically significant reduction in systolic and diastolic blood pressures. No data support claims for lipid-lowering properties of garlic.
Ginger	Used to treat nausea and vomiting.	Several studies support the antiemetic use for ginger. Used to treat or prevent nausea or vomiting.
Ginkgo biloba	Used to treat cerebral insufficiency, prevent loss of cognitive function, and tinnitus.	Studies have shown it is effective in the treatment of cerebral insufficiency when given for 4–6 wk. Data show that regular oral intake of ginkgo biloba slows the loss of cognitive function in patients with dementia.
Hawthorn	Used to treat heart failure.	Various studies show it is effective for the early signs of congestive heart failure.
Horse chestnut	Used to treat venous congestion.	Studies have shown it is effective in reducing signs and symptoms of chronic venous insufficiency.
Saw palmetto	Used in Europe to treat prostate enlargement.	Clinical trials support its use for symptoms of benign prostatic hypertrophy.
St. John's wort	Used to treat depression.	Studies show that it is effective for treating mild to moderate depression. The question of its effectiveness for severe depression remains to be answered.

Long-term users, consumers of large amounts of phytomedicines, or people who use many different medicinal products may be prone to side effects. Pregnant or nursing women, babies, and the elderly, sick, and undernourished are at higher risk for side effects. Some of the more common side effects associated with herbal remedies include bleeding with ginkgo biloba; upset stomach, fatigue, dizziness, confusion, dry mouth, and photosensitivity with St. John's wort; high blood pressure, arrhythmias, nervousness, headaches, heart attack, or stroke with ephedra; and sleepiness, rash, and motor dysfunction of skeletal muscles with kava kava. *For more information on serious adverse reactions from the use of natural products, see on the companion website Table 4—Selected Herbal Medicines with Potentially Serious Adverse Effects.*

Medical Problems

Certain medical problems can make consumption of herbal medicines unsafe. Individuals with high blood pressure, thyroid disease, psychiatric disorders, Parkinson's disease, enlarged prostate gland, diabetes mellitus, heart disease, epilepsy, glaucoma, blood clotting problems, and a history of stroke should check with their physician before taking any herbal remedies. Patients with a history of aspirin allergy can be at risk if they take an herb containing willow bark.

Drug Interactions

For more information on drug interactions, see on the companion website Table 5—Selected Natural Medicines That Potentiate or Interfere with Approved Prescription and Over-the-Counter Drugs. Important drug interactions can occur between certain herbal products and conventional medications. The most common drug involved with drug–herb interactions is warfarin. The most common herb involved with these interactions is St. John's wort. Long-term administration of St. John's wort may result in diminished clinical effectiveness or increased dosage requirements for all CYP3A4 substrates, which represent approximately 50% of all prescription medications. Garlic extracts alter the disposition of coadministered medications metabolized by the CYP3A4 pathway.

Patients taking aspirin, warfarin, ticlopidine, clopidogrel, or dipyridamole should not take ginkgo biloba because bleeding may occur. Patients taking an antidepressant should not take St. John's wort. Patients taking a decongestant, a stimulant drug, or who drink caffeinated beverages should not take ephedra. Individuals taking a benzodiazepine, a barbiturate, an antipsychotic medication, or any medicine used to treat Parkinson's disease should not take kava kava products. It is important that patients notify their general practitioner if they are taking phytomedicines concurrently with conventional drugs, especially those with cardiac, diuretic, sedative, hypotensive, or other properties. Individuals taking a prescription medicine should check with their physician before taking any herbal health product.

Dental Implications

A limited number of papers describe the use of complementary and alternative medical systems for dental problems. Dentists should accept and encompass science-based advances and reject unproved or disproved methods. Selected unconventional treatments can be incorporated into conventional dentistry in certain patients for specific purposes that will be beneficial to the patient.

Information for Dentists

Herbal remedies have the potential to affect the safety of invasive or prolonged dental procedures. Excessive bleeding can occur with some of these medications. Other herbal medicines may affect the cardiovascular system and render the patient more susceptible to cardiac arrhythmias and other cardiovascular complications. Ginseng may cause hypoglycemia. Chinese cancer patients undergoing chemotherapy who were users of Chinese herbal medicine were found to have higher scores of mucositis. It is important for the dentist to include a section in the patient's medical history on the consumption of herbal medications and over-the-counter drugs. Because most U.S. dental schools teach very little on the use, side effects, toxicity, and drug interactions associated with herbal remedies, the dentist must find a way to become informed regarding these issues.

Dentists should use only treatment procedures that have been established to be effective and with minimal risks involved. As clinical trials demonstrate certain alternative and complementary treatments to be effective and safe, they can be incorporated into conventional medicine and dentistry. The dentist may find a medically compromised patient is taking an herbal remedy that is potentially harmful. This should be discussed with the patient and the patient referred to his or her physician for evaluation and management.

MONOCLONAL ANTIBODY THERAPY

Monoclonal antibodies are antibodies that are produced to specifically bind to cells that underlie disease processes (e.g., cancer cells and inflammatory cells involved in autoimmune diseases). They may be produced using viruses, yeasts, or transgenic mice. Monoclonal antibodies that specifically bind to certain substances can also be manufactured and can be used to test for the presence of specific substances within cells, which function as the antigen. Monoclonal antibodies have been produced to treat cancer, cardiovascular disease, inflammatory diseases, macular degeneration, transplant rejection, multiple sclerosis, and viral infections. Dental patients who have received monoclonal antibodies or are in monoclonal antibody therapy have serious systemic medical conditions and should be treated only in consultation with the treating physician(s). Categories of therapeutic monoclonal antibodies include the following specific agents (most named with the suffix "mab" to denote their status as a "Monoclonal Antibody"):

- Antiinflammatory: infliximab, adalimumab, etanercept, basiliximab, daclizumab, omlizumab
- Anticancer: alemtuzumab, bevacizumab, cetuximab, gemtuzumab, nimotuzumab, rituximab, trastuzumab
- Other: palivizumab, abciximab

BIBLIOGRAPHY

ADA: *ADA/PDR Guide to Dental Therapeutics*, ed 5, Chicago, 2006, ADA/Thomson PDR.

American Academy of Oral and Maxillofacial Surgeons. Position paper on bisphosphonate-related osteonecrosis of the jaw—2009 update. www.AAOS.org, 2009.

American Academy of Orthopaedic Surgeons: Antibiotic prophylaxis for bacteremia in patients undergoing dental procedures, 2012. http://www.aaos.org/guidelines

American Heart Association Science Advisory: Prevention of premature discontinuation of dual antiplatelet therapy in patients with coronary artery stents, *Circulation* 115(6):813–818, 2007.

Baddour LM et al: A summary of the update on cardiovascular implantable electronic device infections and their management: A scientific statement from the American Heart Association, *JADA* 142(2):159–165, 2011.

Jeske AH, Suchko GD: Lack of a scientific basis for routine discontinuation of anticoagulant therapy prior to dental therapy, *JADA* 134:1492–1497, 2003.

Little JW: Behavioral and psychiatric disorders. In Little JW, Falace DA, Miller CS, Rhodus NL, editors: *Dental management of the medically compromised patient*, ed 6, St. Louis, 2002, Mosby.

Little JW: Anxiety disorders: dental implications, *J Gen Dent* 51:562–570, 2003.

Little JW: Dental implication of mood disorders, *J Gen Dent* 52:442, 2004.

Little JW: Complementary and alternative medicine: impact on dentistry, *Oral Surg Oral Med Oral Path Oral Radiol Endod* 98:137, 2004.

Little JW: Drugs, drugs, and more drugs: their impact on dentistry, *J Northwest Dent* July–August:23, 2005.

Little JW, et al: Antithrombotic agents: implications in dentistry, *Oral Surg Oral Med Oral Path Oral Radiol Endod* 93:544, 2002.

Miller CS: Drug interactions of significance to dentistry. In Little JW, Falace DA, Miller CS, Rhodus NL, editors: *Dental management of the medically compromised patient*, ed 6, St. Louis, 2002, Mosby.

Miller CS, Little JW, Falace DA: Need of supplemental corticosteroids for dental patients with adrenal insufficiency: reconsideration of the problem, *JADA* 132:1570, 2001.

Rhodus NL: Therapeutic management of common oral lesions. In Little JW, Falace DA, Miller CS, Rhodus NL, editors: *Dental management of the medically compromised patient*, ed 6, St. Louis, 2002, Mosby.

Ruggiero S, Gralow J, Marx RE, et al: Practice guidelines for the prevention, diagnosis and treatment of osteonecrosis of the jaw in patients with cancer, *J Oncol Prac* 2(1):7–14, 2006.

Siegel MA, Silverman S, Sollecato TP, editors: American Academy of Oral Medicine: clinician's guide to treatment of common oral conditions, ed 6, Baltimore, 2005, B.C. Decker.

Wilson W, Taubert KA, Gewitz M, et al: Prevention of infective endocarditis. Guidelines from the American Heart Association, *JADA* 138:739–760, 2007.

abacavir

ah-**bah**′-cah-veer
(Ziagen)

CATEGORY AND SCHEDULE

Pregnancy Risk Category: C

Drug Class: Antiviral, nucleoside analogue

MECHANISM OF ACTION

An antiretroviral that inhibits the activity of HIV-1 reverse transcriptase by competing with the natural substrate deoxyguanosine-5′-triphosphate (dGTP) and by its incorporation into viral DNA.
Therapeutic Effect: Inhibits viral DNA growth.

USES

Used in combination with other antiviral drugs for treatment of HIV-1 infection

PHARMACOKINETICS

Rapidly and extensively absorbed after PO administration. Protein binding: 50%. Widely distributed, including to CSF and erythrocytes. Metabolized in the liver to inactive metabolites. Primarily excreted in urine. Unknown if removed by hemodialysis. ***Half-life:*** 1.5 hr.

INDICATIONS AND DOSAGES

▸ **HIV Infection (in combination with other antiretrovirals)**

PO

Adults. 300 mg twice a day.
Children (3 mo–16 yr). 8 mg/kg twice a day. Maximum: 300 mg twice a day.

▸ **Dosage in Hepatic Impairment**

Mild Impairment. 200 mg twice a day.
Moderate to Severe Impairment. Not recommended.

SIDE EFFECTS/ADVERSE REACTIONS

Adults

Frequent
Nausea, nausea with vomiting, diarrhea, decreased appetite
Occasional
Insomnia

Children

Frequent
Nausea with vomiting, fever, headache, diarrhea, rash
Occasional
Decreased appetite

PRECAUTIONS AND CONTRAINDICATIONS

Hypersensitivity to abacavir or its components
Caution:
Breast-feeding, bone marrow depression, renal or hepatic impairment, use with other antivirals to avoid emergence of resistant viruses, avoid alcohol use

DRUG INTERACTIONS OF CONCERN TO DENTISTRY

- None reported

SERIOUS REACTIONS

! A hypersensitivity reaction may be life threatening. Signs and symptoms include fever, rash, fatigue, intractable nausea and vomiting, severe diarrhea, abdominal pain, cough, pharyngitis, and dyspnea.
! Life-threatening hypotension may occur.
! Lactic acidosis and severe hepatomegaly may occur.

DENTAL CONSIDERATIONS

General:

- Examine for oral manifestation of opportunistic infection.
- Patient on chronic drug therapy may rarely have symptoms of blood dyscrasias, which include infection, bleeding, and poor healing.
- Avoid dental light in patient's eyes; offer dark glasses for patient comfort.
- Place on frequent recall because of oral side effects.
- Consider semisupine chair position for patient comfort if GI side effects occur.

Consultations:

- In a patient with symptoms of blood dyscrasias, request a medical consultation for blood studies and postpone treatment until normal values are reestablished.
- Medical consultation may be required to assess disease control.

Teach Patient/Family to:

- Encourage effective oral hygiene to prevent soft tissue inflammation.
- Prevent trauma when using oral hygiene aids.
- Be alert for the possibility of secondary oral infection and the need to see dentist immediately if signs of infection occur.

abarelix

ah-**bar′**-eh-lix
(Plenaxis)

CATEGORY AND SCHEDULE

Pregnancy Risk Category: X

Drug Class: Antineoplastic

MECHANISM OF ACTION

A luteinizing hormone-releasing hormone (LHRH) antagonist that inhibits gonadotropin and androgen production by blocking gonadotropin releasing-hormone receptors in the pituitary.

Therapeutic Effect: Suppresses luteinizing hormone, follicle-stimulating hormone secretion, reducing the secretion of testosterone by the testes.

USES

Treatment of breast cancer, endometrium, and prostate

PHARMACOKINETICS

Slowly absorbed following intramuscular administration. Distributed extensively. Protein binding: 96%–99%. ***Half-life:*** 13.2 days.

INDICATIONS AND DOSAGES

▸ Prostate Cancer

IM

Adults, Elderly. 100 mg on days 1, 15, and 29 and every 4 wk thereafter. Treatment failure can be detected by obtaining serum testosterone concentration prior to abarelix administration, day 19 and every 8 wk thereafter.

SIDE EFFECTS/ADVERSE REACTIONS

Frequent

Hot flashes, sleep disturbances, breast enlargement

Occasional

Breast pain, nipple tenderness, back pain, constipation, peripheral edema, dizziness, upper respiratory tract infection, diarrhea

Rare

Fatigue, nausea, dysuria, micturition frequency, urinary retention, UTI

PRECAUTIONS AND CONTRAINDICATIONS

This drug should not be used in women and children.

DRUG INTERACTIONS OF CONCERN TO DENTISTRY

- None reported.

SERIOUS REACTIONS

! Immediate-onset systemic allergic reaction characterized by hypotension, urticaria, pruritus, periorbital and/or circumoral edema, shortness of breath, wheezing, and syncope may occur.
! Prolongation of the QT interval may occur. Tightening of throat, tongue swelling, wheezing, shortness of breath, and low blood pressure occur rarely.

DENTAL CONSIDERATIONS

General:

- If additional analgesia is required for dental pain, consider alternative analgesics (NSAIDs) in patients taking opioids for acute or chronic pain.
- This drug may be used in the hospital or on an outpatient basis. Confirm the patient's disease and treatment status.

Consultations:

- Medical consultation may be required to assess disease control and patient's ability to tolerate stress.

Teach Patient/Family to:

- Encourage effective oral hygiene to prevent soft tissue inflammation.
- Prevent trauma when using oral hygiene aids.
- Update health and medication history if physician makes any changes in evaluation or drug regimens; include OTC, herbal, and nonherbal remedies in the update.

abatacept

ah-**bat′**-ah-cept
(Orencia)

CATEGORY AND SCHEDULE

Pregnancy Risk Category: C

Drug Class: Antirheumatic, disease modifying

MECHANISM OF ACTION

Selective costimulation modulator; inhibits T-cell activation by binding to CD80 and CD86 on antigen presenting cells, thus blocking the required CD28 interaction and inhibiting autoimmune T-cell activation.

USES

Rheumatoid arthritis (RA), second-line reduction of signs and symptoms of moderate-to-severe active RA, monotherapy or in combination with other disease-modifying antirheumatic drugs (DMARDs) (e.g., methotrexate). Juvenile idiopathic arthritis, moderate-to-severe active.

PHARMACOKINETICS

Absorbed completely following parenteral administration. Distribution: 0.02–0.13 L/kg. *Half-life*: 13 days (8–25 days).

INDICATIONS AND DOSAGES

▸ **Rheumatoid Arthritis (moderate to severe) in patients who have had an inadequate response to one or more disease-modifying antirheumatic drugs**

IV
Adults. Dose is according to body weight. Administer over a 30-min infusion. Repeat dose at 2 and 4 wk after initial dose, and every 4 wk thereafter:
• <60 kg: 500 mg
• 60–100 kg: 750 mg
• >100 kg: 1000 mg
Children. Juvenile idiopathic arthritis (moderate to severe), active, polyarticular.
IV Infusion
Children (6 yr and older; weighing less than 75 kg). 10 mg/kg given by IV infusion over 30 min; repeat doses at 2 and 4 wk after first infusion and every 4 wk thereafter.

▸ Juvenile Idiopathic Arthritis (moderate to severe), active, polyarticular
IV Infusion
Children (6 yr and older; weighing 75–100 kg). 750 mg given by IV infusion over 30 min; repeat doses at 2 and 4 wk after first infusion and every 4 wk thereafter (MAX dose, 1000 mg).

▸ Juvenile Idiopathic Arthritis (moderate to severe), active, polyarticular
IV Infusion
Children (6 yr and older; weighing more than 100 kg). 1000 mg given by IV infusion over 30 min; repeat doses at 2 and 4 wk after first infusion and every 4 wk thereafter (MAX dose, 1000 mg).
Safety and efficacy not established in children less than 6 yr of age.
Screen for tuberculosis (TB) and hepatitis before initiating therapy.

SIDE EFFECTS/ADVERSE REACTIONS

Frequent
Infection, antibody formation, headache, dizziness, nasopharyngitis

Occasional
Nausea, hypertension, fever, urinary tract infection, cough, back pain

PRECAUTIONS AND CONTRAINDICATIONS

Hypersensitivity to abatacept or any component of the formulation.
Tuberculosis (TB), active or latent; initiate treatment for TB prior to initiating abatacept therapy.
Hepatitis B reactivation has been associated with abatacept therapy; screen for viral hepatitis before initiating abatacept therapy.
Use with caution in patients with chronic obstructive pulmonary disease (COPD) because of worsening of breathing, COPD exacerbations, cough, and dyspnea.

DRUG INTERACTIONS OF CONCERN TO DENTISTRY

• None reported

SERIOUS REACTIONS

! Infections: should be cautious when considering the use of abatacept in patients with a history of recurrent infection, underlying conditions that may increase risks of infections, or chronic, localized infections. These patients should be monitored closely. If a patient develops a serious infection, the treatment should be discontinued.
! Anaphylaxis/hypersensitivity reaction may occur.

DENTAL CONSIDERATIONS

General:
• Examine for oral manifestation of opportunistic infection.
• Monitor vital signs at every appointment because of cardiovascular side effects.
• Consider semisupine chair position for patients with respiratory disease.

Consultations:

• Consult physician to assess disease control and ability of patient to tolerate dental treatment.

Teach Patient/Family to:

• Encourage effective atraumatic oral hygiene measures to prevent soft-tissue inflammation.

• Use soft tooth brush to reduce risk of bleeding.

• Immediately report any sign of infection to the dentist.

abciximab

ab-**six′**-ih-mab
(c7E3 Fab, ReoPro)

CATEGORY AND SCHEDULE

Pregnancy Risk Category: C

Drug Class: Glycoprotein IIb/IIIa receptor inhibitor

MECHANISM OF ACTION

A glycoprotein IIb/IIIa receptor inhibitor that rapidly inhibits platelet aggregation by preventing the binding of fibrinogen to GP IIb/IIIa receptor sites on platelets.

Therapeutic Effect: Prevents closure of treated coronary arteries. Prevents acute cardiac ischemic complications.

USES

Adjunct to aspirin and heparin therapy to prevent cardiac ischemic complications in patients undergoing percutaneous coronary intervention and those with unstable angina not responding to conventional medical therapy.

PHARMACOKINETICS

Rapidly cleared from plasma. Initial-phase half-life is less than 10 min; second-phase half-life is 30 min. Platelet function generally returns within 48 hr.

INDICATIONS AND DOSAGES

▸ **Percutaneous Coronary Intervention (PCI)**

IV Bolus

Adults. 0.25 mg/kg 10–60 min before angioplasty or atherectomy, then 12-hr IV infusion of 0.125 mcg/kg/min. Maximum: 10 mcg/min.

▸ **PCI (unstable angina)**

IV Bolus

Adults. 0.25 mg/kg, followed by 18- to 24-hr infusion of 10 mcg/min, ending 1 hr after procedure.

SIDE EFFECTS/ADVERSE REACTIONS

Frequent

Nausea, hypotension

Occasional

Vomiting

Rare

Bradycardia, confusion, dizziness, pain, peripheral edema, UTI

PRECAUTIONS AND CONTRAINDICATIONS

Active internal bleeding, arteriovenous malformation or aneurysm, cerebrovascular accident (CVA) with residual neurologic defect, history of CVA (within the past 2 yr) or oral anticoagulant use within the past 7 days unless PT is less than 1.2 times control, history of vasculitis, intracranial neoplasm, prior IV dextran use before or during PTCA, recent surgery or trauma (within the past 6 wk), recent (within the past 6 wk or less) GI or GU bleeding, thrombocytopenia (less than 100,000 cells/mcl), and severe uncontrolled hypertension.

DRUG INTERACTIONS OF CONCERN TO DENTISTRY

• Increased risk of bleeding: drugs that interfere with coagulation or platelet function, such as NSAIDs and aspirin.

SERIOUS REACTIONS

! Major bleeding complications may occur. If complications occur, stop the infusion immediately.
! Hypersensitivity reaction may occur.
! Atrial fibrillation or flutter, pulmonary edema, and complete atrioventricular block occur occasionally.

DENTAL CONSIDERATIONS

General:
• Monitor vital signs at every appointment because of cardiovascular side effects.
• For use in hospitals or emergency rooms.
• Review patient's medical and drug history.
• Provide palliative emergency dental care only during drug use.
• Patients may be at risk of bleeding; check for oral signs.
Consultations:
• Medical consultation may be required to assess disease control and patient's ability to tolerate stress.
• Medical consultation should include routine blood counts including platelet counts and bleeding time.
• Avoid products that affect platelet function, such as aspirin and NSAIDs.
Teach Patient/Family to:
• Encourage effective oral hygiene to prevent soft tissue inflammation.
• Prevent trauma when using oral hygiene aids.
• Report oral lesions, soreness, or bleeding to dentist.
• Update health and medication history if physician makes any changes in evaluation or drug regimens; include OTC, herbal, and nonherbal remedies in the update.
• Use soft tooth brush to reduce risk of bleeding.

absorbable gelatin sponge

(Gelfoam)

CATEGORY AND SCHEDULE

Hemostatic

Drug Class: Hemostatic, purified gelatin sponge

MECHANISM OF ACTION

Absorbs blood, provides area for clot formation

USES

Hemostasis adjunct in dental surgery

PHARMACOKINETICS

IMPLANT: Absorbed in 4–6 wk

INDICATIONS AND DOSAGES

▸ **Dental Use**

Adult. Top can be applied dry or moistened with normal saline solution; blot on sterile gauze to remove excess solution, shape to fit with light finger compression; hold pressure until dry. Apply to bleeding surfaces. Material may be cut to appropriate size or secured in extraction sites with sutures.

SIDE EFFECTS/ADVERSE REACTIONS

None reported

PRECAUTIONS AND CONTRAINDICATIONS

Hypersensitivity, frank infection

Caution:

Avoid use in presence of infection, potential nidus of infection, do not resterilize product.

DENTAL CONSIDERATIONS

Teach Patient/Family to:

• Immediately report any sign of infection to the dentist.

acamprosate calcium

ah-kam′-**proe**-sate

(Campral)

CATEGORY AND SCHEDULE

Pregnancy Risk Category: C

Drug Class: Alcohol-abuse deterrent

MECHANISM OF ACTIONS

Actual mechanism unknown; may facilitate balance between GABA and glutamate neurotransmitter systems in the CNS to decrease alcohol craving.

USES

Alcohol-abuse deterrent

PHARMACOKINETICS

Partially absorbed from GI tract, steady-state levels reached within 5 days of dosing. Protein binding negligible. ***Half-life:*** 20–33 hr. Does not undergo metabolism; excreted unchanged in urine.

INDICATIONS AND DOSAGES

▸ Maintenance of Alcohol Abstinence

PO

Adult. 666 mg 3 times a day with or without food.

SIDE EFFECTS/ADVERSE REACTIONS

Oral: Dry mouth

CNS: Headache, somnolence, decreased libido, amnesia, abnormal thinking, tremor

CV: Palpitation, syncope, vasodilation, changes in B/P

GI: Vomiting, dyspepsia, constipation, increased appetite

RESP: Rhinitis, cough, dyspnea, pharyngitis, bronchitis

GU: Impotence

EENT: Abnormal vision, taste alterations

INTEG: Rash

MS: Myalgia, arthralgia

SYST: Back pain, infection, flu syndrome, chest pain, chills, attempts at suicide (see Precautions)

PRECAUTIONS AND CONTRAINDICATIONS

Hypersensitivity, severe renal impairment

Caution:

Renal impairment, depression/suicidal tendency

DRUG INTERACTIONS OF CONCERN TO DENTISTRY

• None reported

DENTAL CONSIDERATIONS

General:

• Assess salivary flow as a factor in caries, periodontal disease, and candidiasis.

• After supine positioning, allow patient to sit upright for 2 min to avoid orthostatic hypotension.

• Avoid alcohol-containing products (elixirs, mouth rinses) to assist maintenance of alcohol abstinence.

Consultations:

• Consult physician to assess disease control.

Teach Patient/Family to:

• Encourage effective oral hygiene to prevent caries and periodontal disease.

• Use sugarless gum, frequent sips of water, and saliva substitutes if dry mouth occurs.

• Use home fluoride products for anticaries effect.

• Avoid mouth rinses with high alcohol content because of drying effects.

acarbose

ah-**car′**-bose

(Glucobay[AUS], Prandase[CAN], Precose)

Do not confuse Precose with PreCare.

CATEGORY AND SCHEDULE

Pregnancy Risk Category: B

Drug Class: Oral antidiabetic

MECHANISM OF ACTION

An alpha-glucosidase inhibitor that delays glucose absorption and digestion of carbohydrates, resulting in a smaller rise in blood glucose concentration after meals.

Therapeutic Effect: Lowers postprandial hyperglycemia.

USES

Use as single drug or in combination with insulin or oral hypoglycemics (sulfonylureas, metformin) in type 2 diabetes (non–insulin-dependent diabetes mellitus [NIDDM]) when diet control is ineffective in controlling blood glucose levels.

PHARMACOKINETICS

PO

Limited oral absorption, absorbed dose excreted in urine, metabolized in the GI tract, and major portion of dose excreted in feces.

INDICATIONS AND DOSAGES

▸ **Diabetes Mellitus**

PO

Adults, Elderly. Initially, 25 mg 3 times a day with first bite of each main meal. Increase at 4- to 8-wk intervals. Maximum: For patients weighing more than 60 kg, 100 mg 3 times a day; for patients weighing 60 kg or less, 50 mg 3 times a day.

SIDE EFFECTS/ADVERSE REACTIONS

Side effects diminish in frequency and intensity over time.

Frequent

Transient GI disturbances: flatulence, diarrhea, abdominal pain

PRECAUTIONS AND CONTRAINDICATIONS

Chronic intestinal diseases associated with marked disorders of digestion or absorption, cirrhosis, colonic ulceration, conditions that may deteriorate as a result of increased gas formation in the intestine, diabetic ketoacidosis, hypersensitivity to acarbose, inflammatory bowel disease, partial intestinal obstruction or predisposition to intestinal obstruction, significant renal dysfunction (serum creatinine level greater than 2 mg/dl)

Caution:

Use glucose for hypoglycemia, monitor blood glucose levels,

pregnancy category B, avoid use in lactation, children.

DRUG INTERACTIONS OF CONCERN TO DENTISTRY

• None reported

SERIOUS REACTIONS

! None known

DENTAL CONSIDERATIONS

General:

• Ensure that patient is following prescribed diet and takes medication regularly.

• Type 2 patients may also be using insulin. If symptomatic hypoglycemia occurs while taking this drug, use dextrose rather than sucrose because of interference with sucrose metabolism.

• Place on frequent recall to evaluate healing response.

• Patients with diabetes may be more susceptible to infection and have delayed wound healing.

• Question the patient about self-monitoring the drug's antidiabetic effect.

• Consider semisupine chair position for patient comfort if GI side effects occur.

Consultations:

• Medical consultation may be required to assess disease control and patient's ability to tolerate stress.

Teach Patient/Family to:

• Encourage effective oral hygiene to prevent soft tissue inflammation.

acebutolol

a-se-**byoo**-toe-lole

(Sectral)

Do not confused Sectral with Factrel, Septra, or Seconal.

CATEGORY AND SCHEDULE

Pregnancy Risk Category: B (D if used in second or third trimester)

Drug Class: Beta-adrenergic blocker (cardioselective); antiarrhythmics, class II

MECHANISM OF ACTION

A $beta_1$-adrenergic blocker that competitively blocks β_1-adrenergic receptors in cardiac tissue; high doses may competitively block both β_1- and β_2-adrenergic receptors. Reduces the rate of spontaneous firing of the sinus pacemaker and delays AV conduction. Exhibits mild intrinsic sympathomimetic activity (ISA) (partial beta-agonist activity). ***Therapeutic Effect:*** Slows heart rate, decreases cardiac output, decreases B/P, and exhibits antiarrhythmic activity.

USES

Mild-to-moderate hypertension
Ventricular arrhythmias

PHARMACOKINETICS

Route	Onset	Peak	Duration
PO (hypertension)	1–1.5 hr	2–8 hr	24 hr
PO (antiarrhythmic)	1 hr	4–6 hr	10 hr

Well absorbed from the GI tract. Bioavailability: approximately 40%. Protein binding: 26%. Undergoes extensive first-pass metabolism to active metabolite. Eliminated via bile and excretion into GI tract through intestinal wall, as well as partly excreted in urine. Removed by hemodialysis. ***Half-life:*** 3–4 hr (parent drug); 8–13 hr (metabolite).

INDICATIONS AND DOSAGES

▸ Mild-to-Moderate Hypertension

PO

Adults. Initially, 400 mg/day in 2 divided doses. Maintenance 400–800 mg/day. Maximum: 1200 mg/day in 2 divided doses.

▸ Ventricular Arrhythmias

PO

Adults. Initially, 200 mg twice a day. Increase gradually to 600–1200 mg/day in 2 divided doses.

Elderly. Initially, 200–400 mg/day. Maximum: 800 mg/day.

▸ Dosage in Renal Impairment

Dosage is modified based on creatinine clearance.

Creatinine Clearance	% of Usual Dosage
Less than 50 ml/min	50
Less than 25 ml/min	25

SIDE EFFECTS/ADVERSE REACTIONS

Frequent

Hypotension manifested as dizziness, nausea, diaphoresis, headache, cold extremities, fatigue, constipation, or diarrhea

Occasional

Insomnia, urinary frequency, impotence or decreased libido

Rare

Rash, arthralgia, myalgia, confusion (especially in the elderly), altered taste

PRECAUTIONS AND CONTRAINDICATIONS

Hypersensitivity to acebutolol or any component of the formulation

Caution:

Cardiogenic shock

Heart block greater than first degree

Overt heart failure

Severe bradycardia

Caution use in patients with bronchospastic disease, diabetes, hyperthyroidism, impaired renal or hepatic function, inadequate cardiac function, or peripheral vascular disease.

DRUG INTERACTIONS OF CONCERN TO DENTISTRY

- Diuretics, other antihypertensives: May increase hypotensive effect of acebutolol.
- Sympathomimetics, xanthines: May antagonize the effects and reduce bronchodilation.
- Oral hypoglycemics and insulin: May mask symptoms of hypoglycemia and prolong hypoglycemic effect of insulin and oral hypoglycemics.
- Catecholamine-depleting drugs (e.g., reserpine): May have additive effect. Monitor for bradycardia or hypotension.
- NSAIDs: May reduce the antihypertensive effect of acebutolol.
- Digoxin: May cause serious bradycardia.
- Calcium channel blockers (verapamil, diltiazem): May cause hypotension and bradycardia.
- Class I antiarrhythmic drugs: May increase atrial conduction time and negative inotropic effects.

SERIOUS REACTIONS

! Overdose may produce profound bradycardia and hypotension.

! Abrupt withdrawal may result in diaphoresis, palpitations, headache, rebound hypertension, and tremors.
! Acebutolol administration may precipitate CHF or MI in patients with heart disease; thyroid storm in those with thyrotoxicosis; or peripheral ischemia in those with existing peripheral vascular disease.
! Hypoglycemia may occur in patients with previously controlled diabetes.
! Signs of thrombocytopenia, such as unusual bleeding or bruising, occur rarely.

DENTAL CONSIDERATIONS

General:

- Monitor vital signs at every appointment because of cardiovascular side effects.
- After supine positioning, have patient sit upright for at least 2 min before standing to avoid orthostatic hypotension.
- Assess salivary flow as a factor in caries, periodontal disease, and candidiasis.
- Limit use of sodium-containing products, such as saline IV fluids, for those patients with dietary salt restriction.
- Stress from dental procedures may compromise cardiovascular function; determine patient risk.

Consultations:

- Medical consultation may be required to assess disease control.

Teach Patient/Family to:

Report oral lesions, soreness, or bleeding to dentist.

When chronic dry mouth occurs, advise patient to:

Avoid mouth rinses with high alcohol content because of drying effects.

Use daily home fluoride products for anticaries effect.

Use sugarless gum, frequent sips of water, or saliva substitutes.

acetaminophen

ah-seet-ah-**min**′-oh-fen
(Abenol[CAN], Apo-Acetaminophen[CAN], Atasol[CAN], Dymadon[AUS], Feverall, Panadol[AUS], Panamax[AUS], Paralgin[AUS], Setamol[AUS], Tempra, Tylenol)
Do not confuse with Fiorinal, Hycodan, Indocin, Percodan, or Tuinal.

CATEGORY AND SCHEDULE

Pregnancy Risk Category: B

Drug Class: Nonnarcotic analgesic

MECHANISM OF ACTION

A central analgesic whose exact mechanism is unknown but appears to inhibit prostaglandin synthesis in the CNS and, to a lesser extent, block pain impulses through peripheral action. Acetaminophen acts centrally on hypothalamic heat-regulating center, producing peripheral vasodilation (heat loss, skin erythema, sweating).
Therapeutic Effect: Results in antipyresis. Produces analgesic effect.

USES

Mild-to-moderate pain, fever; also used in combination with other ingredients, including opioids.

PHARMACOKINETICS

Route	Onset	Peak	Duration
PO	15–30 min	1.5 hr	4–6 hr

Rapidly, completely absorbed from GI tract; rectal absorption variable. Protein binding: 20%–50%. Widely distributed to most body tissues. Metabolized in liver; excreted in urine. Removed by hemodialysis. ***Half-life:*** 1–4 hr (half-life is increased in those with liver disease, elderly, neonates; decreased in children).

INDICATIONS AND DOSAGES

▸ Analgesia and Antipyresis

PO

Adults, Elderly. 325–650 mg q4–6h or 1 g 3–4 times a day. Maximum: 4 g/day.

Children. 10–15 mg/kg/dose q4–6h as needed. Maximum: 5 doses/24 hr.

Neonates. 10–15 mg/kg/dose q6–8h as needed.

Rectal

Adults. 650 mg q4–6h. Maximum: 6 doses/24 hr.

Children. 10–20 mg/kg/dose q4–6h as needed.

Neonates. 10–15 mg/kg/dose q6–8h as needed.

▸ Dosage in Renal Impairment

Creatinine Clearance	Frequency
10–15 ml/min	q6h
Less than 10 ml/min	q8h

SIDE EFFECTS/ADVERSE REACTIONS

Rare

Hypersensitivity reaction

PRECAUTIONS AND CONTRAINDICATIONS

Active alcoholism, liver disease, or viral hepatitis, all of which increase the risk of hepatotoxicity

Caution:

Anemia, hepatic disease, renal disease, chronic alcoholism

DRUG INTERACTIONS OF CONCERN TO DENTISTRY

- Decreased effects: barbiturates, loop diuretics
- Nephrotoxicity: NSAIDs, salicylates (chronic, high-dose, concurrent use)
- Liver toxicity: chronic use of hydantoins, chronic alcohol use, high-dose carbamazepine
- Possible increased effects of zidovudine
- Possible increased effects of acetaminophen: β-blockers, probenecid
- Increased bleeding: warfarin
- Risk of acetaminophen toxicity when used in combination with OTC products

SERIOUS REACTIONS

! Acetaminophen toxicity is the primary serious reaction.

! Early signs and symptoms of acetaminophen toxicity include anorexia, nausea, diaphoresis, and generalized weakness within the first 12–24 hr.

! Later signs of acetaminophen toxicity include vomiting, right upper quadrant tenderness, and elevated liver function tests within 48–72 hr after ingestion.

! The antidote to acetaminophen toxicity is acetylcysteine (Mucomyst), but it should be administered as soon as possible following toxic dose.

DENTAL CONSIDERATIONS

General:

- Reports regarding the concomitant use of acetaminophen and warfarin seem to suggest a possible increase in anticoagulant effects, especially in patients with other diseases or contributing factors, diarrhea, age, debilitation, etc. Patients taking

warfarin should be questioned about recent use of acetaminophen and current international normalized ratio (INR) values. Acetaminophen has been shown to increase the INR depending on the amount and duration of acetaminophen use. A new PT or INR value may be required if surgical procedures are planned. Data from one study (*JAMA* 279:657–662, 1998) indicated that use of four regular-strength acetaminophen tablets (325 mg) qd for 1 wk can increase the INR values. It is important to closely monitor INR values with use of acetaminophen over a long duration and in higher doses.
• Avoid prolonged use with aspirin-containing products or NSAIDs.
• Determine why the patient is taking the drug.
• Patients on chronic drug therapy may rarely have symptoms of blood dyscrasias, which can include infection, bleeding, and poor healing.
• Question patient about the use of other drug products, including OTC products, that contain acetaminophen because of risk of acetaminophen overdose.
• Severe liver injury can occur when more than 4 g of all products that include acetaminophen are taken in a 24-hr period. Warn patient of detrimental effects.

Consultations:
• For a patient with symptoms of blood dyscrasias, request a medical consult for blood studies and postpone dental treatment until normal values are reestablished.

Teach Patient/Family to:
• Question patient concerning other drugs being taken that include acetaminophen. Caution patient to be aware of products that might include acetaminophen.
• Emphasize the potential risks to liver when consuming alcohol and taking acetaminophen.

acetazolamide

ah-seet-ah-**zole**′-ah-mide
(Apo-Acetazolamide[CAN], Dazamide, Diamox, Diamox Sequels)
Do not confuse with acetohexamide.

CATEGORY AND SCHEDULE

Pregnancy Risk Category: C

Drug Class: Diuretic, carbonic anhydrase inhibitor

MECHANISM OF ACTION

A carbonic anhydrase inhibitor that reduces formation of hydrogen and bicarbonate ions from carbon dioxide and water by inhibiting, in proximal renal tubule, the enzyme carbonic anhydrase, thereby promoting renal excretion of sodium, potassium, bicarbonate, water. Ocular: Reduces rate of aqueous humor formation, lowers intraocular pressure.
Therapeutic Effect: Produces anticonvulsant activity.

USES

Treatment of open-angle glaucoma, narrow-angle glaucoma (preoperatively, if surgery delayed), epilepsy (petit mal, grand mal, mixed), edema in CHF, drug-induced edema, acute mountain sickness in climbers, drug-induced edema

PHARMACOKINETICS

Rapidly absorbed. Protein binding: 95%. Widely distributed throughout body tissues including erythrocytes, kidneys, and blood-brain barrier. Not metabolized. Excreted unchanged in urine. Removed by hemodialysis. ***Half-life:*** 2.4–5.8 hr.

INDICATIONS AND DOSAGES

▸ Glaucoma

PO

Adults. 250 mg 1–4 times a day. Extended-Release: 500 mg 1–2 times a day usually given in morning and evening.

▸ Secondary Glaucoma, Preoperative Treatment of Acute Congestive Glaucoma

PO/IV

Adults. 250 mg q4h, 250 mg q12h; or 500 mg, then 125–250 mg q4h.

PO

Children. 10–15 mg/kg/day in divided doses.

IV

Children. 5–10 mg/kg q6h.

▸ Edema

IV

Adults. 25–375 mg once daily.
Children. 5 mg/kg or 150 mg/m^2 once daily.

▸ Epilepsy

PO

Adults, Children. 375–1000 mg/day in 1–4 divided doses.

▸ Acute Mountain Sickness

PO

Adults. 500–1000 mg/day in divided doses. If possible, begin 24–48 hr before ascent; continue at least 48 hr at high altitude.

▸ Usual Elderly Dosage

PO

Initially, 250 mg 2 times a day; use lowest effective dose.

▸ Dosage in Renal Impairment

Creatinine Clearance	Dosage Interval
10–50 ml/min	q12h
Less than 10 ml/min	Avoid use

SIDE EFFECTS/ADVERSE REACTIONS

Frequent

Unusually tired/weak, diarrhea, increased urination/frequency, decreased appetite/weight, altered taste (metallic), nausea, vomiting, numbness in extremities, lips, mouth

Occasional

Depression, drowsiness

Rare

Headache, photosensitivity, confusion, tinnitus, severe muscle weakness, loss of taste

PRECAUTIONS AND CONTRAINDICATIONS

Severe renal disease, adrenal insufficiency, hypochloremic acidosis, hypersensitivity to acetazolamide, to any component of the formulation, or to sulfonamides

Caution:

Hypercalciuria, chronic use of oral sulfonylureas has been associated with increased risk of cardiovascular mortality; risk is controversial.

DRUG INTERACTIONS OF CONCERN TO DENTISTRY

- Toxicity: salicylates (large doses)
- Hypokalemia: corticosteroids (systemic use)
- Crystalluria: ciprofloxacin

SERIOUS REACTIONS

! Long-term therapy may result in acidotic state.

! Nephrotoxicity/hepatotoxicity occurs occasionally, manifested as dark urine/stools, pain in lower back, jaundice, dysuria, crystalluria, renal colic/calculi.

! Bone marrow depression may be manifested as aplastic anemia, thrombocytopenia, thrombocytopenic purpura, leukopenia, agranulocytosis, hemolytic anemia.

DENTAL CONSIDERATIONS

General:

- Patients on chronic drug therapy may rarely have symptoms of blood dyscrasias, which can include infection, bleeding, and poor healing.
- Assess salivary flow as a factor in caries, periodontal disease, and candidiasis.
- Avoid drugs that may exacerbate glaucoma (e.g., anticholinergics).

Consultations:

- In a patient with symptoms of blood dyscrasias, request a medical consultation for blood studies and postpone dental treatment until normal values are reestablished.
- Consultation may be required to assess disease control.

Teach Patient/Family to:

- Encourage effective oral hygiene to prevent soft tissue inflammation.
- Prevent injury when using oral hygiene aids.
- When chronic dry mouth occurs, advise patient to:
  - Avoid mouth rinses with high alcohol content because of drying effects.
  - Use daily home fluoride products for anticaries effect.
  - Use sugarless gum, frequent sips of water, or saliva substitutes.

acetohexamide

ah-seet-oh-**hex′**-ah-mide

(Dymelor)

Do not confuse with acetazolamide.

CATEGORY AND SCHEDULE

Pregnancy Risk Category: D

Drug Class: Sulfonylurea (first generation), antidiabetic

MECHANISM OF ACTION

An intermediate-acting sulfonylurea that promotes the release of insulin from beta cells of pancreas, increases insulin sensitivity at peripheral sites.

Therapeutic Effect: Lowers blood glucose concentration.

USES

Treatment of stable adult-onset diabetes mellitus (type 2)

PHARMACOKINETICS

Well absorbed from the GI tract. Protein binding: 65%–90%. Metabolized in liver. Excreted in urine. Not removed by hemodialysis. ***Half-life:*** 1.3 hr.

INDICATIONS AND DOSAGES

▸ Diabetes Mellitus

PO

Adults, Elderly. Initially, 250 mg/day. Adjust dosage in 250- to 500-mg increments at intervals of 5–7 days. Maximum daily dose: 1.5 g. Elderly patients may be more sensitive and should be started at a lower dosage initially.

SIDE EFFECTS/ADVERSE REACTIONS

Frequent

Altered taste sensation, dizziness, drowsiness, weight gain, constipation, diarrhea, heartburn, nausea, vomiting, stomach fullness, headache

Occasional

Increased sensitivity of skin to sunlight, peeling of skin, itching, rash

PRECAUTIONS AND CONTRAINDICATIONS

Diabetic ketoacidosis with or without coma, type 1 diabetes mellitus, hypersensitivity to acetohexamide or any component of the formulation

Caution:

Elderly, cardiac disease, renal disease, hepatic disease, thyroid disease, severe hypoglycemic reactions

DRUG INTERACTIONS OF CONCERN TO DENTISTRY

- Increased hypoglycemic effects: salicylates (large doses)
- Decreased action: corticosteroids
- Disulfiram-like reaction: alcohol

SERIOUS REACTIONS

! Hypoglycemia may occur because of overdosage or insufficient food intake, especially with increased glucose demands.

! GI hemorrhage, cholestatic hepatic jaundice, leukopenia, thrombocytopenia, pancytopenia, agranulocytosis, aplastic or hemolytic anemia occurs rarely.

DENTAL CONSIDERATIONS

General:

- Monitor vital signs at every appointment because of cardiovascular effects of diabetes.
- Patients on chronic drug therapy may rarely have symptoms of blood dyscrasias, which can include infection, bleeding, and poor healing.
- Place on frequent recall to evaluate healing response.
- Ensure that patient is following prescribed diet and takes medication regularly.
- Question patient about self-monitoring of drug's antidiabetic effect, including self-monitored blood glucose (SMBG) values or finger-stick records.
- Avoid prescribing aspirin-containing products.
- Early-morning appointments and a stress reduction protocol may be required for anxious patients.
- Patients with diabetes may be more susceptible to infection and have delayed wound healing.

Consultations:

- In a patient with symptoms of blood dyscrasias, request a medical consultation for blood studies and postpone dental treatment until normal values are reestablished.
- Medical consultation may include data from patient's blood glucose monitoring, including glycosylated hemoglobin or hemoglobin A1c (HbA1c) testing.

Teach Patient/Family to:

- Encourage effective oral hygiene to prevent soft tissue inflammation.
- Prevent injury when using oral hygiene aids.
- Avoid mouth rinses with high alcohol content.

acetylcholine chloride

ah-seh-teel-**koe′**-leen
(Miochol-E, Miochol-E/ Steri-Tags, Miochol-E System Pak)

CATEGORY AND SCHEDULE

Pregnancy Risk Category: C

Drug Class: Cholinergic

MECHANISM OF ACTION

A cholinergic agonist that causes contraction of the sphincter muscles of the iris.
Therapeutic Effect: Results in miosis and contraction of ciliary muscle, leading to accommodation spasm.

USES

To produce miosis for selected types of eye surgery

PHARMACOKINETICS

Rapid miosis of short duration

INDICATIONS AND DOSAGES

▸ Production of Miosis
Intraocular
Adults, Elderly. 0.5–2 ml instilled into anterior chamber before or after securing one or more sutures.

SIDE EFFECTS/ADVERSE REACTIONS

Rare
Corneal clouding, corneal decompensation

PRECAUTIONS AND CONTRAINDICATIONS

Acute iritis and acute inflammatory disease of the anterior chamber, hypersensitivity to acetylcholine chloride or any component of the formulation

DRUG INTERACTIONS OF CONCERN TO DENTISTRY

- None reported

SERIOUS REACTIONS

! Systemic effects rarely occur. These effects include bradycardia, hypotension, flushing, breathing difficulties, and sweating.

DENTAL CONSIDERATIONS

General:
- Acute-use drug in selected types of eye surgery.
- Avoid dental light in patient's eyes; offer dark glasses for patient comfort.

acetylcysteine

ah-see-til-**sis′**-tay-een
(Acetadote, Mucomyst, Parvolex[CAN])
Do not confuse acetylcysteine with acetylcholine.

CATEGORY AND SCHEDULE

Pregnancy Risk Category: B

Drug Class: Antidotes, mucolytics

MECHANISM OF ACTION

An intratracheal respiratory inhalant that splits the linkage of mucoproteins, reducing the viscosity of pulmonary secretions.
Therapeutic Effect: Facilitates the removal of pulmonary secretions by coughing, postural drainage, mechanical means. Protects against acetaminophen overdose-induced hepatotoxicity.

USES

Adjuvant therapy for patients with abnormal, viscid, or inspissated mucus secretions

PHARMACOKINETICS

INH/INSTILL: Onset 1 min, duration 5–10 min, metabolized by liver, excreted in urine. ***Half-life:*** 5.6 hr (adult); 11 hr (newborn).

INDICATIONS AND DOSAGES

▸ Adjunctive Treatment of Viscid Mucus Secretions from Chronic Bronchopulmonary Disease and for Pulmonary Complications of Cystic Fibrosis

Nebulization

Adults, Elderly, Children. 3–5 ml (20% solution) 3–4 times a day or 6–10 ml (10% solution) 3–4 times a day. Range: 1–10 ml (20% solution) q2–6h or 2–20 ml (10% solution) q2–6h.

Infants. 1–2 ml (20%) or 2–4 ml (10%) 3–4 times a day.

▸ Treatment of Viscid Mucus Secretions in Patients with a Tracheostomy

Intratracheal

Adults, Children. 1–2 ml of 10% or 20% solution instilled into tracheostomy q1–4h.

▸ Acetaminophen Overdose

PO (Oral Solution 5%)

Adults, Elderly, Children. Loading dose of 140 mg/kg, followed in 4 hr by maintenance dose of 70 mg/kg q4h for 17 additional doses (unless acetaminophen assay reveals nontoxic level).

IV

Adults, Elderly, Children.

150 mg/kg infused over 15 min, then 50 mg/kg infused over 4 hr, then 100 mg/kg infused over 16 hr. See administration and handling. Repeat dose if emesis occurs within 1 hr of administration. Continue until all doses are given, even if acetaminophen plasma level drops below toxic range.

▸ Prevention of Renal Damage from Dyes Used During Certain Diagnostic Tests

PO (Oral Solution 5%)

Adults, Elderly. 600 mg twice a day for 4 doses starting the day before the procedure.

SIDE EFFECTS/ADVERSE REACTIONS

Frequent

Inhalation: Stickiness on face, transient unpleasant odor

Occasional

Inhalation: Increased bronchial secretions, throat irritation, nausea, vomiting, rhinorrhea

Rare

Inhalation: Rash

PRECAUTIONS AND CONTRAINDICATIONS

None known

DRUG INTERACTIONS OF CONCERN TO DENTISTRY

- None reported

SERIOUS REACTIONS

! Large doses may produce severe nausea and vomiting.

DENTAL CONSIDERATIONS

General:

- Be aware that aspirin and/or sulfite preservatives in vasoconstrictor-containing products may exacerbate asthma.
- Acute asthmatic episodes may be precipitated in the dental office. A rapid-acting sympathomimetic inhalant (rescue inhaler) should be available for emergency use. Many patients may already have prescribed

rescue inhalers they normally use for acute asthmatic events.
• Consider semisupine chair position for patients with respiratory disease.
• Determine dose and duration of glucocorticoid therapy to assess for risk of stress tolerance and immunosuppression. Patients on chronic glucocorticoid therapy may require supplemental doses for dental treatment.
• Examine for oral manifestation of opportunistic infection.
• Evaluate respiration characteristics and rate.
• Short appointments and a stress reduction protocol may be required for anxious patients.
• Inquire about other drugs patients are using for respiratory disease.

Consultations:
• Consultation with physician may be necessary if sedation or general anesthesia is required.
• Consultation may be required to confirm glucocorticoid dose and duration of use.
• Medical consultation may be required to assess disease control and patient's ability to tolerate stress.

Teach Patient/Family to:
• Encourage effective oral hygiene to prevent soft tissue inflammation.
• Update health and medication history if physician makes any changes in evaluation or drug regimens; include OTC, herbal, and nonherbal remedies in the update.
• Gargle, rinse mouth with water, and expectorate after each aerosol dose.

acitretin

ah-sih-**tre′**-tin
(Soriatane)

CATEGORY AND SCHEDULE

Pregnancy Risk Category: X

Drug Class: Systemic retinoid

MECHANISM OF ACTION

A second-generation retinoid that adjusts factors influencing epidermal proliferation, RNA/DNA synthesis, controls glycoprotein, and governs immune response.
Therapeutic Effect: Regulates keratinocyte growth and differentiation.

USES

Severe psoriasis; unlabeled uses: nonpsoriatic dermatoses, keratinization disorders, palmoplantar keratoses, lichen planus, Darier's disease, Sjögren-Larsson syndrome; should be prescribed only by physicians knowledgeable in the use of systemic retinoids.

PHARMACOKINETICS

Well absorbed from the GI tract. Food increases rate of absorption. Protein binding: greater than 99%. Metabolized in liver. Excreted in bile and urine. Not removed by hemodialysis. ***Half-life:*** 49 hr.

INDICATIONS AND DOSAGES

▸ **Psoriasis**

PO

Adults, Elderly. 25–50 mg/day as a single dose with main meal. May increase to 75 mg/day if necessary and dose tolerated. Maintenance: 25–50 mg/day after the initial response is noted. Continue until lesions have resolved.

SIDE EFFECTS/ADVERSE REACTIONS

Frequent
Lip inflammation, alopecia, skin peeling, shakiness, dry eyes, rash, hyperesthesia, paresthesia, sticky skin, dry mouth, epistaxis, dryness/thickening of conjunctiva
Occasional
Eye irritation, brow and lash loss, sweating, chills, sensation of cold, flushing, edema, blurred vision, diarrhea, nausea, thirst

PRECAUTIONS AND CONTRAINDICATIONS

Women who are pregnant or those who intend to become pregnant within 3 yr following discontinuation of therapy; severely impaired liver or kidney function; chronic abnormal elevated lipid levels; concomitant use of methotrexate or tetracyclines; ingestion of alcohol (in females of reproductive potential); hypersensitivity to acitretin, etretinate, or other retinoids; sensitivity to parabenz (used as preservative in gelatin capsule)
Caution:
Women are advised to use effective contraception during use and for 3 yr after use, renal impairment, lactation, hyperlipidemia, cardiovascular disease

DRUG INTERACTIONS OF CONCERN TO DENTISTRY

- Avoid vitamin preparations containing vitamin A.
- Avoid tetracyclines and other drugs that cause photosensitivity.

SERIOUS REACTIONS

! Benign intracranial hypertension (pseudotumor cerebri) occurs rarely.

DENTAL CONSIDERATIONS

General:
- Determine why patient is taking the drug.
- Apply lubricant to dry lips for patient comfort before dental procedures.
- Assess salivary flow as factor in caries, periodontal disease, and candidiasis.
- Palliative medication may be required for management of oral side effects.
- Place on frequent recall because of oral side effects.
- Consider semisupine chair position for patient comfort if GI side effects occur.
- Avoid dental light in patient's eyes; offer dark glasses for patient comfort.

Consultations:
- Medical consultation may be required to assess disease control.

Teach Patient/Family to:
- Encourage effective oral hygiene to prevent soft tissue inflammation.
- Prevent trauma when using oral hygiene aids.
- Report oral lesions, soreness, or bleeding to dentist.
- When chronic dry mouth occurs, advise patient to:

Avoid mouth rinses with high alcohol content because of drying effects.
Use daily home fluoride products for anticaries effect.
Use sugarless gum, frequent sips of water, or saliva substitutes.

acyclovir

ay-**sye**′-kloe-ver
(Aciclovir-BC IV[AUS], Acihexal[AUS], Acyclo-V[AUS], Avirax[CAN], Lovir[AUS], Zovirax, Zyclir[AUS])
Do not confuse with Zostrix, Zyvox.

CATEGORY AND SCHEDULE

Pregnancy Risk Category: B

Drug Class: Antiviral

MECHANISM OF ACTION

A synthetic nucleoside that converts to acyclovir triphosphate, becoming part of the DNA chain.
Therapeutic Effect: Interferes with DNA synthesis and viral replication. Virustatic.

USES

Management of initial genital herpes and in limited non-life-threatening mucocutaneous herpes simplex infection in immunocompromised patients

PHARMACOKINETICS

Poorly absorbed from the GI tract; minimal absorption following topical application. Protein binding: 9%–36%. Widely distributed. Partially metabolized in liver. Excreted primarily in urine. Removed by hemodialysis. ***Half-life:*** 2.5 hr (increased in impaired renal function).

INDICATIONS AND DOSAGES

▸ **Genital Herpes (initial episode)**
IV
Adults, Elderly, Children 12 yr and older. 5 mg/kg q8h for 5 days.
PO
Adults, Elderly, Children 12 yr and older. 200 mg q4h 5 times a day.

▸ **Genital Herpes (recurrent) fewer than 6 episodes per year**
PO
Adults, Elderly, Children 12 yr and older. 200 mg q4h 5 times a day for 5 days.

▸ **Genital Herpes (recurrent) 6 episodes or more per year**
PO
Adults, Elderly, Children 12 yr and older. 400 mg 2 times a day or 200 mg 3–5 times a day for up to 12 mo.

▸ **Herpes Simplex Mucocutaneous**
IV
Adults, Elderly, Children 12 yr and older. 5 mg/kg/dose q8h for 7 days.
Children younger than 12 yr. 10 mg/kg q8h for 7 days.

▸ **Herpes Simplex Neonatal**
IV
Children younger than 4 mo. 10 mg/kg q8h for 10 days.

▸ **Herpes Simplex Encephalitis**
IV
Adults, Elderly, Children 12 yr and older. 10 mg/kg q8h for 10 days.
Children younger than 12 yr. 20 mg/kg q8h for 10 days.

▸ **Herpes Zoster (Caused by Varicella)**
IV
Adults, Elderly, Children 12 yr and older. 10 mg/kg q8h for 7 days.
Children younger than 12 yr. 20 mg/kg q8h for 7 days.

▸ **Herpes Zoster (Shingles)**
PO
Adults, Elderly, Children 12 yr and older. 800 mg q4h 5 times a day for 7–10 days.
Topical
Adults, Elderly. Apply to affected area 3–6 times a day for 7 days.

▸ **Varicella (chickenpox)**
PO
Adults, Elderly, Children older than 12 yr or Children 2–12 yr, weighing 40 kg or more. 800 mg 4 times a day for 5 days.
Children 2–12 yr, weighing less than 40 kg. 20 mg/kg 4 times a day for 5 days. Maximum: 800 mg/dose.
Children younger than 2 yr. 80 mg/kg/day.

▸ **Dosage in Renal Impairment**
Dosage and frequency are modified on the basis of severity of infection and degree of renal impairment.
PO
For creatinine clearance of 10 ml/min or less, dosage is 200 mg q12h.
IV

Creatinine Clearance	Dosage Percent	Dosage Interval
Greater 50 ml/min	100	8 hr
25–50 ml/min	100	12 hr
10–25 ml/min	100	24 hr
Less than 10 ml/min	50	24 hr

SIDE EFFECTS/ADVERSE REACTIONS

Frequent
Parenteral: Phlebitis or inflammation at IV site, nausea, vomiting
Topical: Burning, stinging
Occasional
Parenteral: Pruritus, rash, urticaria
Oral: Malaise, nausea
Topical: Pruritus
Rare
Oral: Vomiting, rash, diarrhea, headache
Parenteral: Confusion, hallucinations, seizures, tremors
Topical: Rash

PRECAUTIONS AND CONTRAINDICATIONS

Use in neonates when acyclovir is reconstituted with bacteriostatic water containing benzyl alcohol.
Caution:
Modify dose with acute or chronic renal impairment, safety of oral doses in pediatric patients less than 2 yr old not established, lactation, hepatic disease, renal disease, electrolyte imbalance, dehydration.

SERIOUS REACTIONS

! Rapid parenteral administration, excessively high doses, or fluid and electrolyte imbalance may produce renal failure exhibited by such signs and symptoms as abdominal pain, decreased urination, decreased appetite, increased thirst, nausea, and vomiting.
! Toxicity has not been reported with oral or topical use.

DENTAL CONSIDERATIONS

General:
• Postpone dental treatment when oral herpetic lesions are present.
Teach Patient/Family to:
• Dispose of tooth brush or other contaminated oral hygiene devices used during period of infection to prevent reinoculation of herpetic infection.
• Apply with a finger cot or latex glove to prevent herpes infection on fingers.
• Avoid mouth rinses with high alcohol content because of irritating effects.

adalimumab

ah-dah-**lim**′-mu-mab
(Humira)

CATEGORY AND SCHEDULE

Pregnancy Risk Category: B

Drug Class: Monoclonal antibody, antiinflammatory, immunosuppressant

MECHANISM OF ACTION

A monoclonal antibody that binds specifically to tumor necrosis factor (TNF) alpha, blocking its interaction with cell surface TNF receptors.
Therapeutic Effect: Reduces inflammation, tenderness, and swelling of joints; slows or prevents progressive destruction of joints in rheumatoid arthritis.

USES

Treatment of signs and symptoms and inhibition of structural damage in moderately to severely active rheumatoid arthritis in adults who have an inadequate response to one or more disease-modifying antirheumatic drugs (DMARDs)

PHARMACOKINETICS

Half-life: 10–20 days.

INDICATIONS AND DOSAGES

▸ **Rheumatoid Arthritis**

Subcutaneous

Adults, Elderly. 40 mg every other wk. Dose may be increased to 40 mg/wk in those not taking methotrexate.

SIDE EFFECTS/ADVERSE REACTIONS

Frequent

Injection site, erythema, pruritus, pain, and swelling

Occasional

Headache, rash, sinusitis, nausea

Rare

Abdominal or back pain, hypertension

PRECAUTIONS AND CONTRAINDICATIONS

Active infections

Caution:

Appearance of new infection with use; risk of exacerbation of demyelinating diseases; risk of malignancies; risk of TB reactivation; lactation; elderly; safety and effectiveness in children not established.

DRUG INTERACTIONS OF CONCERN TO DENTISTRY

- None reported

SERIOUS REACTIONS

! Rare reactions include hypersensitivity reactions, malignancies, respiratory tract infections, bronchitis, UTIs, and more serious infections (such as pneumonia, tuberculosis, cellulitis, pyelonephritis, and septic arthritis).

DENTAL CONSIDERATIONS

General:

- Patient may need assistance in getting into and out of dental chair.
- Adjust chair position for patient comfort.
- Determine why patient is taking the drug.
- Question patient about other drugs being taken.
- Examine for oral manifestation of opportunistic infection.
- Report oral infections to patient's physician; treat infections aggressively.

• Consider semisupine chair position for patient comfort if GI side effects occur.

Consultations:

• Medical consultation may be required to assess disease control and patient's ability to tolerate stress.

Teach Patient/Family to:

• Encourage effective oral hygiene to prevent soft tissue inflammation.

• Immediately report any signs or symptoms of oral infection.

adapalene

a-**dap**′-ah-leen

(Differin)

CATEGORY AND SCHEDULE

Pregnancy Risk Category: C

Drug Class: Dermatologics, retinoids

MECHANISM OF ACTION

Binds to retinoic acid receptors in cell nuclei modulating cell differentiation, keratinization. Possesses antiinflammatory properties.

Therapeutic Effect: Normalizes differentiation of follicular epithelial cells.

USES

Treatment of acne

PHARMACOKINETICS

Absorption through the skin is low. Trace amount found in plasma following topical application. Excreted primarily by biliary route.

INDICATIONS AND DOSAGES

▸ **Acne Vulgaris**

Topical

Adults, Elderly, Children older than 12 yr. Apply to affected area once daily at bedtime after washing.

SIDE EFFECTS/ADVERSE REACTIONS

Frequent

Erythema, scaling, dryness, pruritus, burning (likely to occur first 2–4 wk, lessens with continued use)

Occasional

Skin irritation, stinging, sunburn, acne flares, erythema, photosensitivity, pruritus, xerosis

PRECAUTIONS AND CONTRAINDICATIONS

Hypersensitivity to adapalene, vitamin A or any one of its components

DRUG INTERACTIONS OF CONCERN TO DENTISTRY

• Avoid use of topical antiinfectives on same skin application site.

SERIOUS REACTIONS

! Concurrent use of other potentially irritating topical products (soaps, cleansers, aftershave, cosmetics) may produce severe topical irritation.

DENTAL CONSIDERATIONS

General:

• Advise patient if dental drugs prescribed have a potential for photosensitivity.

• Apply lubricant to dry lips for patient comfort prior to dental procedures.

• Limit systemic vitamin A doses to no more than the RDA.

Teach Patient/Family to:
• Avoid getting in eyes or mouth, or on other mucous membranes.

adefovir

ah-**deff′**-oh-veer
(Hepsera)

CATEGORY AND SCHEDULE

Pregnancy Risk Category: C

Drug Class: Antiviral

MECHANISM OF ACTION

An antiviral that inhibits the enzyme DNA polymerase, causing DNA chain termination after its incorporation into viral DNA.
Therapeutic Effect: Prevents cell replication of viral DNA.

USES

Treatment of chronic hepatitis B in adults showing evidence of active viral replication and with persistent elevations of ALT or AST or histologically active disease

PHARMACOKINETICS

Binds to proteins after PO administration. Excreted in urine.
Half-life: 7 hr (increased in impaired renal function).

INDICATIONS AND DOSAGES

▸ **Chronic Hepatitis B in Patients with Normal Renal Function**
PO
Adults, Elderly. 10 mg once a day.
▸ **Chronic Hepatitis B in Patients with Impaired Renal Function**
PO
Adults, Elderly with creatinine clearance. 20–49 ml/min. 10 mg q48h.
Adults, Elderly with creatinine clearance. 10–19 ml/min. 10 mg q72h.
Adults, Elderly on hemodialysis. 10 mg every 7 days following dialysis.

SIDE EFFECTS/ADVERSE REACTIONS

Frequent
Asthenia
Occasional
Headache, abdominal pain, nausea, flatulence
Rare
Diarrhea, dyspepsia

PRECAUTIONS AND CONTRAINDICATIONS

Hypersensitivity
Caution:
Severe acute exacerbations of hepatitis in patients who have discontinued drug, renal dysfunction with chronic use, HIV resistance, lactic acidosis, severe hepatomegaly with steatosis, monitor renal and hepatic function, safety and effectiveness in children and lactation not established

DRUG INTERACTIONS OF CONCERN TO DENTISTRY

• None reported

SERIOUS REACTIONS

! Nephrotoxicity (characterized by increased serum creatinine and decreased serum phosphorus levels) is a treatment-limiting toxicity of adefovir therapy.
! Lactic acidosis and severe hepatomegaly occur rarely, particularly in female patients.

DENTAL CONSIDERATIONS

General:

• Examine for oral manifestation of opportunistic infection.
• Determine why patient is taking the drug.
• Consider semisupine chair position for patient comfort if GI side effects occur.
• Do not provide treatment if clinician does not have seroconversion to protective antibodies to hepatitis B.

Consultations:

• Medical consultation may be required to assess disease control and patient's ability to tolerate stress.
• Patients who report feeling symptoms of lactic acidosis, such as weakness, malaise, with unusual muscle pain, difficulty breathing, stomach pain with nausea, cold feeling in arms or legs, dizziness or light-headedness, and irregular heartbeat, should be immediately referred to their physicians.

Teach Patient/Family to:

• Encourage effective oral hygiene to prevent soft tissue inflammation.
• Prevent trauma when using oral hygiene aids.
• Update health and drug history if physician makes any changes in evaluation or drug regimens.

aflibercept

a **flib′** er sept
(Eylea)

CATEGORY AND SCHEDULE

Pregnancy Risk Category: C

Drug Class: Ophthalmic agent, vascular endothelial growth factor (VEGF) inhibitor

MECHANISM OF ACTION

A recombinant fusion protein that prevents VEGF-A and PIGF from binding and activating endothelial cell receptors, thereby suppressing neovascularization and slowing vision loss.
Therapeutic Effect: Inhibits progression of age-related macular degeneration.

USES

Treatment of neovascular (wet) age-related macular degeneration (AMD); treatment of macular edema following central retinal vein occlusion (CRVO)

PHARMACOKINETICS

Low levels are detected in the plasma following intravitreal injection. ***Half-life:*** 5–6 days.

INDICATIONS AND DOSAGES

▸ Age-Related Macular Degeneration (AMD)

Intravitreal injection
Adults. 2 mg (0.05 ml) every 4 wk for 3 mo then every 8 wk thereafter.

▸ Macular Edema Following Central Retinal Vein Occlusion (CRVO)

Intravitreal injection
Adults. 2 mg (0.05 ml) every 4 wk.

SIDE EFFECTS/ADVERSE REACTIONS

Frequent

Conjunctival hemorrhage, eye pain, cataract, vitreous detachment, vitreous floaters

Occasional

Corneal edema, blurred vision, increased lacrimation, increased intraocular pressure

PRECAUTIONS AND CONTRAINDICATIONS

Hypersensitivity to aflibercept or any component of the formulation. Current ocular infection; active ocular inflammation. Intravitreous injections may be associated with endophthalmitis and retinal detachments. Hypersensitivity may present as severe intraocular inflammation; instruct patients to report intraocular inflammation that increases in severity. Following intravitreal injection, intraocular pressure may increase.

DRUG INTERACTIONS OF CONCERN TO DENTISTRY

• None reported

SERIOUS REACTIONS

! Risk of thromboembolic events may be increased following intravitreal administration of VEGF inhibitors.

DENTAL CONSIDERATIONS

General:

• Protect patient's eyes at all times due to increased risk of eye infections.

• Note potentially elevated antinuclear antibody (ANA) levels if diagnosing Sjögren's syndrome.

Consultations:

• Medical consultation may be needed prior to dental procedures to determine disease status and ability of patient to tolerate dental procedures.

Teach Patient/Family to:

• Encourage effective oral hygiene to prevent soft tissue inflammation and oral infection.

• Avoid contamination of eye with mouth fluids.

albendazole

all-**ben′**-dah-zole
(Albenza)

CATEGORY AND SCHEDULE

Pregnancy Risk Category: C

Drug Class: Anthelmintic, systemic

MECHANISM OF ACTION

A benzimidazole carbamate anthelmintic that degrades parasite cytoplasmic microtubules, irreversibly blocks cholinesterase secretion, glucose uptake in helminth and larvae (depletes glycogen, decreases ATP production, depletes energy). Vermicidal.
Therapeutic Effect: Immobilizes and kills worms.

USES

Treatment of infections caused by worms

PHARMACOKINETICS

Poorly and variably absorbed in GI tract. Widely distributed, cyst fluid and including CSF. Protein binding: 70%. Extensively metabolized in liver. Primarily excreted in urine and bile. Not removed by hemodialysis.
Half-life: 8–12 hr.

INDICATIONS AND DOSAGES

▸ **Neurocysticercosis**

PO

Adults, Elderly weighing more than 60 kg. 400 mg 2 times a day. Continue for 28 days, rest 14 days, repeat cycle 3 times.

Adults, Elderly weighing less than 60 kg. 15 mg/kg/day. Continue for 28 days, rest 14 days, repeat cycle 3 times.

▸ **Cystic Hydatid**
PO
Adults, Elderly weighing more than 60 kg. 400 mg 2 times a day. Continue for 8–30 days.
Adults, Elderly weighing less than 60 kg. 15 mg/kg/day. Continue for 8–30 days.

SIDE EFFECTS/ADVERSE REACTIONS

Frequent
Neurocysticercosis: Nausea, vomiting, headache
Hydatid: Abnormal liver function tests, abdominal pain, nausea, vomiting
Occasional
Neurocysticercosis: Increased intracranial pressure, meningeal signs
Hydatid: Headache, dizziness, alopecia, fever

PRECAUTIONS AND CONTRAINDICATIONS

Hypersensitivity to albendazole or any component of the formulation, pregnancy

DRUG INTERACTIONS OF CONCERN TO DENTISTRY

• Possible increase in blood levels: glucocorticoids, cimetidine

SERIOUS REACTIONS

! Pancytopenia occurs rarely.
! In presence of cysticercosis, drug may produce retinal damage in presence of retinal lesions.

DENTAL CONSIDERATIONS

General:
• Determine why patient is taking the drug.
• Patient on chronic drug therapy may rarely present with symptoms of blood dyscrasias, which can include infection, bleeding, and poor healing. If dyscrasia is present, caution patient to prevent oral tissue trauma when using oral hygiene aids.
• Question patients about other drugs they may be taking.
Consultations:
• In a patient with symptoms of blood dyscrasias, request a medical consultation for blood studies and postpone treatment until normal values are reestablished.

albuterol

al-**byoo′**-ter-ole
(AccuNeb, Airomir[AUS], Asmol CFC-Free[AUS], Epaq Inhaler[AUS], Novosalmol[CAN], Proventil, Proventil Repetabs, Respax[AUS], Ventolin, Ventolin CFC-Free[AUS], Volmax, Vospire ER)
Do not confuse albuterol with Albutein or atenolol, or Proventil with Prinivil.

CATEGORY AND SCHEDULE

Pregnancy Risk Category: C

Drug Class: Adrenergic β_2-agonist

MECHANISM OF ACTION

A sympathomimetic that stimulates β_2-adrenergic receptors in the lungs, resulting in relaxation of bronchial smooth muscle.
Therapeutic Effect: Relieves bronchospasm and reduces airway resistance.

USES

Prevention and relief of bronchospasm in reversible obstructive airway disease, exercise-induced bronchospasm;

unlabeled use acute, serious hyperkalemia in hemodialysis patients

PHARMACOKINETICS

Route	Onset	Peak	Duration
PO	15–30 min	2–3 hr	4–6 hr
PO (extended-release)	30 min	2–4 hr	12 hr
Inhalation	5–15 min	0.5–2 hr	2–5 hr

Rapidly, well absorbed from the GI tract; gradually absorbed from the bronchi after inhalation. Metabolized in the liver. Primarily excreted in urine. ***Half-life:*** 2.7–5 hr (PO); 3.8 hr (inhalation).

INDICATIONS AND DOSAGES

▸ **Bronchospasm**

PO

Adults, Children older than 12 yr. 2–4 mg 3–4 times a day. Maximum: 8 mg 4 times a day.

Elderly. 2 mg 3–4 times a day. Maximum: 8 mg 4 times a day.

Children 6–12 yr. 2 mg 3–4 times a day. Maximum: 24 mg/day.

PO (Extended-Release)

Adults, Children older than 12 yr. 4–8 mg q12h.

Inhalation

Adults, Elderly, Children older than 12 yr. 1–2 puffs by metered dose inhaler q4–6h as needed.

Children 4–12 yr. 1–2 puffs 4 times a day.

Nebulization

Adults, Elderly, Children older than 12 yr. 2.5 mg 3–4 times a day.

Children 2–12 yr. 0.63–1.25 mg 3–4 times a day.

▸ **Exercise-Induced Bronchospasm**

Inhalation

Adults, Elderly, Children 4 yr and older. 2 puffs 15–30 min before exercise.

SIDE EFFECTS/ADVERSE REACTIONS

Frequent

Headache; restlessness, nervousness, tremors; nausea; dizziness; throat dryness and irritation, pharyngitis; B/P changes, including hypertension; heartburn; transient wheezing

Occasional

Insomnia, asthenia, altered taste

Inhalation: Dry, irritated mouth or throat; cough; bronchial irritation

Rare

Somnolence, diarrhea, dry mouth, flushing, diaphoresis, anorexia

PRECAUTIONS AND CONTRAINDICATIONS

History of hypersensitivity to sympathomimetics

Caution:

Lactation, cardiac disorders, hyperthyroidism, diabetes mellitus, hypertension, prostatic hypertrophy, narrow-angle glaucoma, seizures, paradoxic bronchospasm

DRUG INTERACTIONS OF CONCERN TO DENTISTRY

• None reported

SERIOUS REACTIONS

! Excessive sympathomimetic stimulation may produce palpitations, extrasystole, tachycardia, chest pain, a slight increase in B/P followed by a substantial decrease, chills, diaphoresis, and blanching of skin.

! Too-frequent or excessive use may lead to decreased bronchodilating effectiveness and severe, paradoxical bronchoconstriction.

DENTAL CONSIDERATIONS

General:

• Monitor vital signs at every appointment because of

cardiovascular and respiratory side effects.
• Assess salivary flow as a factor in caries, periodontal disease, and candidiasis.
• Consider semisupine chair position for patients with respiratory disease.
• Midday appointments and a stress reduction protocol may be required for anxious patients.
• Be aware that aspirin or sulfite preservatives in vasoconstrictor-containing products can exacerbate asthma.
• Acute asthmatic episodes may be precipitated in the dental office. Sympathomimetic inhalants should be available for emergency use.

Consultations:
• Medical consultation may be required to assess disease control and patient's ability to tolerate stress.

Teach Patient/Family to:
• Rinse mouth with water after each dose to prevent dryness (for inhalation dosage forms).
• When chronic dry mouth occurs, advise patient to:
  • Avoid mouth rinses with high alcohol content because of drying effects.
  • Use daily home fluoride products for anticaries effect.
  • To use sugarless gum, frequent sips of water, or saliva substitutes.

alclometasone

al-kloe-**met′**-ah-sone
(Aclovate)

CATEGORY AND SCHEDULE
Pregnancy Risk Category: C

Drug Class: Antiinflammatory, steroidal

MECHANISM OF ACTION
Topical corticosteroids exhibit antiinflammatory, antipruritic, and vasoconstrictive properties. Clinically, these actions correspond to decreased edema, erythema, pruritus, plaque formation, and scaling of the affected skin.

USES
Provide relief of inflammation/pruritus associated with contact dermatitis, eczema, insect bite reactions.

PHARMACOKINETICS
Approximately 3% is absorbed during an 8-hr period. Metabolized in the liver. Excreted in urine.

INDICATIONS AND DOSAGES
▸ **Atopic Dermatitis, Contact Dermatitis, Dermatitis, Discoid Lupus Erythematosus, Eczema, Exfoliative Dermatitis, Granuloma Annulare, Lichen Planus, Lichen Simplex, Polymorphous Light Eruption, Pruritus, Psoriasis, Rhus Dermatitis, Seborrheic Dermatitis, Xerosis**

Topical

Adults, Adolescents, Children 1 yr and older. Apply a thin film to the affected area 2–3 times a day.

SIDE EFFECTS/ADVERSE REACTIONS
Frequent

Burning, erythema, maculopapular rash, pruritus, skin irritation, xerosis

Occasional

Acneiform rash, contact dermatitis, folliculitis, glycosuria, growth inhibition, headache, hyperglycemia, infection, miliaria, papilledema, skin atrophy, skin hypopigmentation, skin ulcer, striae, telangiectasia

Rare

Adrenalcortical insufficiency, increased intracranial pressure, pseudotumor cerebri, impaired wound healing, Cushing's syndrome, hypothalamic-pituitary-adrenal (HPA) suppression, skin ulcers, tolerance, withdrawal, visual impairment, ocular hypertension, cataracts

PRECAUTIONS AND CONTRAINDICATIONS

Hypersensitivity to alclometasone, other corticosteroids, or any of its components

DRUG INTERACTIONS OF CONCERN TO DENTISTRY

- None reported

SERIOUS REACTIONS

! None listed

DENTAL CONSIDERATIONS

General:

- Determine why patient is taking the drug.

Teach Patient/Family to:

- Avoid use on herpetic lesions.

interleukin-2 (aldesleukin)

in-tur-**lew′**-kin

(IL-2, Proleukin)

Do not confuse interleukin-2 with interferon 2.

CATEGORY AND SCHEDULE

Pregnancy Risk Category: C

Drug Class: Antineoplastic

MECHANISM OF ACTION

A biological response modifier that acts like human recombinant interleukin-2, promoting proliferation, differentiation, and recruitment of T and B cells, lymphokine-activated and natural cells, and thymocytes.

Therapeutic Effect: Enhances cytolytic activity in lymphocytes.

USES

Treatment of metastatic renal cell cancer

PHARMACOKINETICS

Primarily distributed into plasma, lymphocytes, lungs, liver, kidney, and spleen. Metabolized to amino acids in the cells lining the kidneys. ***Half-life:*** 85 min.

INDICATIONS AND DOSAGES

▸ **Metastatic Melanoma, Metastatic Renal Cell Carcinoma**

IV

Adults 18 yr and older. 600,000 units/kg q8h for 14 doses; followed by 9 days of rest, then another 14 doses for a total of 28 doses per course. Course may be repeated after rest period of at least 7 wk from date of hospital discharge.

SIDE EFFECTS/ADVERSE REACTIONS

Side effects are generally self-limiting and reversible within 2–3 days after discontinuing therapy.

Frequent

Fever, chills, nausea, vomiting, hypotension, diarrhea, oliguria or anuria, mental status changes, irritability, confusion, depression, sinus tachycardia, pain (abdominal, chest, back), fatigue, dyspnea, pruritus

Occasional

Edema, erythema, rash, stomatitis, anorexia, weight gain, infection (UTI, injection site, catheter tip), dizziness

Rare

Dry skin, sensory disorders (vision, speech, taste), dermatitis, headache, arthralgia, myalgia, weight loss, hematuria, conjunctivitis, proteinuria

PRECAUTIONS AND CONTRAINDICATIONS

Abnormal pulmonary function or thallium stress test results, bowel ischemia or perforation, coma or toxic psychosis lasting longer than 48 hr, GI bleeding requiring surgery, intubation lasting more than 72 hr, organ allografts, pericardial tamponade, renal dysfunction requiring dialysis for longer than 72 hr, repetitive or difficult-to-control seizures; retreatment in those who experience any of the following toxicities: angina, MI, recurrent chest pain with EKG changes, sustained ventricular tachycardia, uncontrolled or unresponsive cardiac rhythm disturbances

DRUG INTERACTIONS OF CONCERN TO DENTISTRY

- Possible reduction in antitumor efficacy: glucocorticoids

SERIOUS REACTIONS

! Anemia, thrombocytopenia, and leukopenia occur commonly.
! GI bleeding and pulmonary edema occur occasionally.
! Capillary leak syndrome results in hypotension (systolic pressure less than 90 mm Hg or a 20-mm Hg drop from baseline systolic pressure), extravasation of plasma proteins and fluid into extravascular space, and loss of vascular tone. It may result in cardiac arrhythmias, angina, MI, and respiratory insufficiency.
! Other rare reactions include fatal malignant hyperthermia, cardiac arrest, CVA, pulmonary emboli, bowel perforation, gangrene, and severe depression leading to suicide.

DENTAL CONSIDERATIONS

General:

- Monitor vital signs at every appointment because of cardiovascular side effects.
- If additional analgesia is required for dental pain, consider alternative analgesics (NSAIDs) in patients taking narcotics for acute or chronic pain.
- Examine for oral manifestation of opportunistic infection.
- Avoid products that affect platelet function, such as aspirin and NSAIDs.
- Chlorhexidine mouth rinse prior to and during chemotherapy may reduce severity of mucositis.
- Patient on chronic drug therapy may rarely present with symptoms of blood dyscrasias, which can include infection, bleeding, and poor healing. If dyscrasia is present, caution patient to prevent oral tissue trauma when using oral hygiene aids.
- Palliative medication may be required for management of oral side effects.
- Short appointments and a stress-reduction protocol may be required for anxious patients.
- Provide emergency dental care only during drug use.
- Patients may be at risk of bleeding; check for oral signs.
- Oral infections should be eliminated and/or treated aggressively.

Consultations:

- Medical consultation should include routine blood counts including platelet counts and bleeding time.
- Consult physician; prophylactic or therapeutic antiinfectives may be indicated if surgery or periodontal treatment is required.

• Medical consultation may be required to assess immunologic status during cancer chemotherapy and determine safety risk, if any, posed by the required dental treatment.
• Medical consultation may be required to assess disease control and patient's ability to tolerate stress.

Teach Patient/Family to:
• See dentist immediately if secondary oral infection occurs.
• Be aware of oral side effects.
• Encourage effective oral hygiene to prevent soft tissue inflammation.
• Report oral lesions, soreness, or bleeding to dentist.
• Prevent trauma when using oral hygiene aids.
• Update health and medication history if physician makes any changes in evaluation or drug regimens; include OTC, herbal, and nonherbal remedies in the update.

alefacept

ah-**leh**′-fa-cept
(Amevive)

CATEGORY AND SCHEDULE

Pregnancy Risk Category: B

Drug Class: Biologic response modifier, immunosuppressant

MECHANISM OF ACTION

An immunologic agent that interferes with the activation of T lymphocytes by binding to the lymphocyte antigen, thus reducing the number of circulating T lymphocytes.
Therapeutic Effect: Prevents T cells from becoming overactive, which may help reduce symptoms of chronic plaque psoriasis.

USES

Treatment of moderate to severe chronic plaque psoriasis in adults who are candidates for systemic therapy or phototherapy

PHARMACOKINETICS

Half-life: 270 hr.

INDICATIONS AND DOSAGES

▸ Plaque Psoriasis

IV
Adults, Elderly. 7.5 mg once weekly for 12 wk.
IM
Adults, Elderly. 15 mg once weekly for 12 wk.

SIDE EFFECTS/ADVERSE REACTIONS

Frequent
Injection site pain and inflammation (with IM administration)
Occasional
Chills
Rare
Pharyngitis, dizziness, cough, nausea, myalgia

PRECAUTIONS AND CONTRAINDICATIONS

History of systemic malignancy, concurrent use of immunosuppressive agents or phototherapy
Caution:
Live or live-attenuated vaccines require regular monitoring of lymphocyte counts; lactation data not available (caution), elderly, safety and efficacy in pediatric patients not known

DRUG INTERACTIONS OF CONCERN TO DENTISTRY

• None reported

SERIOUS REACTIONS

! Rare reactions include hypersensitivity reactions, lymphopenia, malignancies, and serious infections requiring hospitalization (such as abscess, pneumonia, and postoperative wound infection).
! Coronary artery disease and MI occur in less than 1% of patients.

DENTAL CONSIDERATIONS

- None reported

alemtuzumab

al-em-**two′**-zoo-mab
(Campath)

CATEGORY AND SCHEDULE

Pregnancy Risk Category: C

Drug Class: Antineoplastic

MECHANISM OF ACTION

Binds to CD52, a cell surface glycoprotein, found on the surface of all B and T lymphocytes, most monocytes, macrophages, natural killer cells, and granulocytes.
Therapeutic Effect: Produces cytotoxicity reducing tumor size.

USES

Treatment of B-cell chronic lymphocytic leukemia in patients who have been treated with alkylating agents and who have failed fludarabine therapy

PHARMACOKINETICS

Half-life: About 12 days. Peak and trough levels rise during first few weeks of therapy and approach steady state by about week 6.

INDICATIONS AND DOSAGES

▸ **Chronic Lymphocytic Leukemia**

IV

Adults, Elderly. Initially, 3 mg/day as a 2-hr infusion. When the 3-mg daily dose is tolerated (with only low-grade or no infusion-related toxicities), increase daily dose to 10 mg. When the 10 mg/day dose is tolerated, maintenance dose may be initiated. Maintenance: 30 mg/day 3 times a week on alternate days (such as Monday, Wednesday, and Friday or Tuesday, Thursday, and Saturday) for up to 12 wk. The increase to 30 mg/day is usually achieved in 3–7 days.

SIDE EFFECTS/ADVERSE REACTIONS

Frequent

Rigors, tremors, fever, nausea, vomiting, rash, fatigue, hypotension, urticaria, pruritus, skeletal pain, headache, diarrhea, anorexia

Occasional

Myalgia, dizziness, abdominal pain, throat irritation, vomiting, neutropenia, rhinitis, bronchospasm, urticaria

PRECAUTIONS AND CONTRAINDICATIONS

Active systemic infections, history of hypersensitivity or anaphylactic reaction to the drug, immunosuppression

DRUG INTERACTIONS OF CONCERN TO DENTISTRY

- None reported

SERIOUS REACTIONS

! Neutropenia occurs in 85% of patients, anemia occurs in 80% of patients, and thrombocytopenia occurs in 72% of patients.
! A rash occurs in 40% of patients.

! Respiratory toxicity, manifested as dyspnea, cough, bronchitis, pneumonitis, and pneumonia, occurs in 16%–26% of patients.

DENTAL CONSIDERATIONS

General:

- Monitor vital signs at every appointment because of cardiovascular side effects.
- Examine for oral manifestation of opportunistic infection.
- Avoid products that affect platelet function, such as aspirin and NSAIDs.
- This drug may be used in the hospital or on an outpatient basis. Confirm the patient's disease and treatment status.
- Chlorhexidine mouth rinse prior to and during chemotherapy may reduce severity of mucositis.
- Patient on chronic drug therapy may rarely present with symptoms of blood dyscrasias, which can include infection, bleeding, and poor healing. If dyscrasia is present, caution patient to prevent oral tissue trauma when using oral hygiene aids.
- Palliative medication may be required for management of oral side effects.
- Short appointments and a stress reduction protocol may be required for anxious patients.
- Patients may be taking a prophylactic antiinfective.
- Patients are at risk of bleeding; check for oral signs.
- Place on frequent recall because of oral side effects.

Consultations:

- Medical consultation should include routine blood counts including platelet counts and bleeding time.
- Consult physician; prophylactic or therapeutic antiinfectives may be indicated if surgery or periodontal treatment is required.
- Medical consultation may be required to assess immunologic status during cancer chemotherapy and determine safety risk, if any, posed by the required dental treatment.
- Medical consultation may be required to assess disease control and patient's ability to tolerate stress.

Teach Patient/Family to:

- Inform dentist of unusual bleeding episodes following dental treatment.
- See dentist immediately if secondary oral infection occurs.
- Be aware of oral side effects.
- Encourage effective oral hygiene to prevent soft tissue inflammation.
- Report oral lesions, soreness, or bleeding to dentist.
- Prevent trauma when using oral hygiene aids.
- Update health and medication history if physician makes any changes in evaluation or drug regimens; include OTC, herbal, and nonherbal remedies in the update.

alendronate sodium

ah-**len**′-dro-nate
(Fosamax)
Do not confuse Fosamax with Flomax.

CATEGORY AND SCHEDULE

Pregnancy Risk Category: C

Drug Class: Amino bisphosphonate

MECHANISM OF ACTION

A bisphosphonate that inhibits normal and abnormal bone resorption, without retarding mineralization.

Therapeutic Effect: Leads to significantly increased bone mineral density; reverses the progression of osteoporosis.

USES

Osteoporosis treatment and prevention in men and postmenopausal women, glucocorticoid-induced osteoporosis in men and women receiving glucocorticoids at daily dose of 7.5 mg prednisone, Paget's disease of bone

PHARMACOKINETICS

Poorly absorbed after oral administration. Protein binding: 78%. After oral administration, rapidly taken into bone, with uptake greatest at sites of active bone turnover. Excreted in urine.
Terminal Half-life: Greater than 10 yr (reflects release from skeleton as bone is resorbed).

INDICATIONS AND DOSAGES

▸ Osteoporosis (in Men)

PO

Adults, Elderly. 10 mg once a day in the morning.

▸ Glucocorticoid-Induced Osteoporosis

PO

Adults, Elderly. 5 mg once a day in the morning.

Postmenopausal women not receiving estrogen. 10 mg once a day in the morning.

▸ Postmenopausal Osteoporosis

PO (Treatment)

Adults, Elderly. 10 mg once a day in the morning or 70 mg weekly.

PO (Prevention)

Adults, Elderly. 5 mg once a day in the morning or 35 mg weekly.

▸ Paget's Disease

PO

Adults, Elderly. 40 mg once a day in the morning.

SIDE EFFECTS/ADVERSE REACTIONS

Frequent

Back pain, abdominal pain

Occasional

Nausea, abdominal distention, constipation, diarrhea, flatulence

Rare

Rash

PRECAUTIONS AND CONTRAINDICATIONS

GI disease, including dysphagia, frequent heartburn, GI reflux disease, hiatal hernia, and ulcers, inability to stand or sit upright for at least 30 min; renal impairment; sensitivity to alendronate. Carefully evaluate patients when considering the use of dental implants. Osteonecrosis of the jaw has been reported in patients following oral surgical procedures and who are also taking bisphosphonates.

Caution:

Renal insufficiency, active upper GI disease, may see decrease in serum calcium/phosphate, ensure adequate calcium and vitamin D intake, lactation

DRUG INTERACTIONS OF CONCERN TO DENTISTRY

• Increased risk of GI side effects in doses greater than 10 mg/day: Use NSAIDs, aspirin with caution.

• After administration, must wait at least 30 min before taking any other drug.

SERIOUS REACTIONS

! Overdose causes hypocalcemia, hypophosphatemia, and significant GI disturbances.

! Esophageal irritation occurs if alendronate is not given with 6–8 oz of plain water or if the patient lies down within 30 min of drug administration.

DENTAL CONSIDERATIONS

• Bisphosphonate therapy may increase the risk of osteonecrosis of the jaw following dental procedures (see section on Medically Compromised Patients for Management Considerations).

General:

• Be aware of oral manifestations of Paget's disease (macrognathia, alveolar pain).

• Consider semisupine chair position for patient comfort because of pain experienced in osteoporosis and GI side effects of drug.

• Consider short appointments for patient comfort.

Consultations:

• Medical consultation may be required to assess disease control and patient's ability to tolerate stress.

Teach Patient/Family to:

• Observe regular recall schedule and use effective oral hygiene measures to minimize risk of osteonecrosis of the jaw.

alfuzosin

al-**fue′**-zoe-sin

(Uroxatral, Xatral[CAN])

CATEGORY AND SCHEDULE

Pregnancy Risk Category: B

Drug Class: α_1-adrenergic receptor blocker

MECHANISM OF ACTION

An α_1 antagonist that targets receptors around the bladder base, prostate, prostatic urethra, and prostatic capsule and prostate capsule.

Therapeutic Effect: Relaxes smooth muscle and improves urinary flow and symptoms of prostatic hyperplasia.

USES

Benign prostatic hyperplasia (BPH)

PHARMACOKINETICS

Rapidly absorbed and widely distributed. Food reduces absorption. Protein binding: 90%. Extensively metabolized in the liver via CYP3A4 to inactive metabolites. Primarily excreted in feces (69%) and urine (24%). ***Half-life:*** 10 hr.

INDICATIONS AND DOSAGES

▸ BPH

PO

Adults. 10 mg once a day, immediately after same meal each day.

SIDE EFFECTS/ADVERSE REACTIONS

Frequent

Dizziness, headache, malaise, upper respiratory tract infections (bronchitis, sinusitis, pharyngitis)

Occasional

Dry mouth, pain, abdominal pain, constipation, dyspepsia, nausea, impotence, dizziness

Rare

Diarrhea, orthostatic hypotension, tachycardia, drowsiness, priapism, angioedema, chest pain, flushing

PRECAUTIONS AND CONTRAINDICATIONS

Hypersensitivity to alfuzosin or any component of the formulation

Liver disease (moderate or severe)

Concomitant use of cytochrome P450 3A4 inhibitors (e.g., ketoconazole, itraconazole, ritonavir)

Caution:

May increase angina pectoris symptoms

Severe renal impairment, renal failure, renal disease

Known history of QT-interval prolongation

Drugs that prolong QT-interval
Not for use in women and children
Coronary artery disease
Ocular surgery (particularly cataract surgery)

DRUG INTERACTIONS OF CONCERN TO DENTISTRY

• Cimetidine: May increase alfuzosin blood concentration; CYP3A4 inhibitor.
• Cytochrome P450 3A4 inhibitors (e.g., ketoconazole, itraconazole, clarithromycin, ritonavir): May increase alfuzosin blood levels; contraindicated with ketoconazole and itraconazole.
• Antihypertensive agents, other alpha blockers (such as doxazosin, prazosin, tamsulosin, and terazosin): May increase the alpha-blockade effects of both drugs; potential for hypotension.
• Opioids, anticholinergic drugs: May enhance urinary retention in BPH.

SERIOUS REACTIONS

! Priapism has been reported.
! Ischemia-related chest pain may occur rarely.
! Intraoperative floppy iris syndrome (IFIS) has been reported.

DENTAL CONSIDERATIONS

General:
• Monitor vital signs at every appointment because of cardiovascular side effects.
• After supine positioning, have patient sit upright for at least 2 min before standing to avoid orthostatic hypotension.
• Consider semisupine chair position for patient if GI side effects occur.
Consultations:
• Medical consultation may be required to assess disease control.
Teach Patient/Family to:
• Report oral lesions, soreness, or bleeding to dentist.
• When chronic dry mouth occurs, advise patient to:
  Avoid mouth rinses with high alcohol content because of drying effects.
  Use daily home fluoride products for anticaries effect.
  Use sugarless gum, frequent sips of water or saliva substitutes.

alglucosidase alfa

al-gloo-ko-**sy′**-dase **al′**-fa
(Myozyme)

CATEGORY AND SCHEDULE

Pregnancy Risk Category: B

Drug Class: Enzyme

MECHANISM OF ACTION

Alglucosidase alfa is a recombinant form of the enzyme acid alpha-glucosidase (GAA), produced in a Chinese hamster ovary cell line. Alglucosidase alfa binds to mannose-6-phosphate receptors on the cell surface and is internalized and transported to lysosomes, resulting in increased enzymatic activity and glycogen cleavage.
Therapeutic Effect: Provides an exogenous source of GAA, which is the enzyme deficient or absent in Pompe disease.

USES

Used as replacement therapy for Pompe disease (GAA deficiency).

PHARMACOKINETICS

Half-life: 2.3 hr.

INDICATIONS AND DOSAGES

▸ **Replacement Therapy for Pompe Disease**

IV Infusion

Adults. 20 mg/kg over 4 hr, every 2 wk.

Children (1 mo–3.5 yr. at first infusion). 20 mg/kg over 4 hr, every 2 wk.

SIDE EFFECTS/ADVERSE REACTIONS

Frequent

Fever, diarrhea, rash, infusion reaction, vomiting, cough, pneumonia, upper respiratory tract infection, otitis media, oxygen saturation decreased, gastroenteritis, diaper dermatitis, pharyngitis, respiratory distress, oral candidiasis, anemia, respiratory failure, catheter-related infections, pain (postprocedural), gastroesophageal reflux, rhinorrhea, constipation, tachycardia, bronchiolitis, nasopharyngitis, tachypnea, bradycardia, flushing, urticaria. Less frequent adverse effects were not mentioned.

PRECAUTIONS AND CONTRAINDICATIONS

Hypersensitivity to alglucosidase alfa or its components

Caution:

Cardiovascular disease, respiratory impairment, acute underlying illness (increased risk of infusion reactions)

DRUG INTERACTIONS OF CONCERN TO DENTISTRY

• None reported

SERIOUS REACTIONS

! Severe hypersensitivity reactions, including anaphylactic reactions and anaphylactic shock, have been reported during infusion. Infusion-related reactions are common-discontinue immediately for severe hypersensitivity or anaphylactic reaction.

! Cardiac arrhythmia, including ventricular fibrillation, ventricular tachycardia, and bradycardia, resulting in cardiac arrest or death, has been reported.

DENTAL CONSIDERATIONS

General:

• Monitor vital signs at every appointment because of cardiovascular side effects.

• Evaluate carefully for drug-related candidiasis and treat in consultation with patient's physician.

• Place patient on frequent recall and use multiple preventive measures to assist with patient's oral hygiene.

• Consult physician to determine disease control and ability of patient to tolerate dental procedures.

Teach Patient/Family to:

• Use atraumatic, effective oral hygiene measures and assist patient with oral care.

aliskiren

ah-lis-**keer′**-in

(Tekturna)

CATEGORY AND SCHEDULE

Pregnancy Risk Category: C (first trimester), D (second and third trimesters)

Drug Class: Antihypertensive, direct renin inhibitor

MECHANISM OF ACTION

Directly inhibits renin, decreasing plasma renin activity and inhibiting the conversion of angiotensinogen to angiotensin I.

Therapeutic Effect: Reduces blood pressure by blocking renin-mediated production of angiotensin (vasoconstriction) and aldosterone (salt and water retention).

USES

Hypertension, as monotherapy or in combination with a diuretic

PHARMACOKINETICS

Poorly absorbed after oral administration.
Metabolized primarily in the liver (CYP 3A4); 25% excreted in urine in unmetabolized form, also excreted in feces.

INDICATIONS AND DOSAGES

▸ Hypertension (Monotherapy)

Adults. PO 150 mg once daily (antihypertensive effect achieved in 2 wk).
(Daily dose may be increased to 300 mg/day).

SIDE EFFECTS/ADVERSE REACTIONS

Frequent

Diarrhea

Occasional

Dose-related GI disturbances, including abdominal pain, dyspepsia and gastroesophageal reflux; cough

Rare

Rash, elevated uric acid, gout, renal stones

PRECAUTIONS AND CONTRAINDICATIONS

Impaired renal function, hyperkalemia
Hypersensitivity (angioedema), pregnancy
Severe renal dysfunction
Hyperkalemia (especially with an ACE inhibitor in diabetic patients)
Safety during lactation and in pediatric patients not established

DRUG INTERACTIONS OF CONCERN TO DENTISTRY

• CYP3A4 inhibitors: increased blood levels of aliskiren (e.g., azole antifungals, macrolide antibiotics)

SERIOUS REACTIONS

! Head and neck angioedema
! Hypotension

DENTAL CONSIDERATIONS

General:

• Monitor vital signs at every appointment because of underlying disease and cardiovascular side effects of drug.
• Assess salivary flow as a factor in caries, periodontal disease, and candidiasis.
• Early-morning appointments and stress-reduction protocol may be needed for anxious patients.
• Use vasoconstrictors with caution, at low doses and with careful aspiration.
• After supine positioning, allow patient to sit upright for 2 min to avoid occurrence of dizziness.

Consultations:

• Consult with physician to determine disease control and ability to tolerate dental procedures.

Teach patient/family to:

• Update medical history when changes in dosage or disease status occur.

alitretinoin

ah-lee-**tret′**-ih-noyn
(Panretin)

CATEGORY AND SCHEDULE

Pregnancy Risk Category: D

Drug Class: Topical retinoid

MECHANISM OF ACTION

Binds to and activates all known retinoid receptors. Once activated, receptors act as transcription factors, regulating genes that control cellular differentiation and proliferation.
Therapeutic Effect: Inhibits growth of Kaposi's sarcoma (KS) cells.

USES

Topical treatment of cutaneous lesions in patients with AIDS-related KS

PHARMACOKINETICS

Minimally absorbed following topical administration.

INDICATIONS AND DOSAGES

▸ KS Skin Lesions

Topical
Adults. Initially, apply 2 times a day to lesions. May increase to 3–4 times a day.

SIDE EFFECTS/ADVERSE REACTIONS

Frequent
Rash (erythema, scaling, irritation, redness, dermatitis), itching, exfoliative dermatitis (flaking, peeling, desquamation, exfoliation), stinging, tingling, edema skin disorders (scabbing, crusting, drainage)

PRECAUTIONS AND CONTRAINDICATIONS

When systemic therapy is required (more than 10 new KS lesions in previous month, symptomatic pulmonary KS, symptomatic visceral involvement, symptomatic lymphedema, hypersensitivity to retinoids or alitretinoin ingredients)
Caution:
Avoid pregnancy, discontinue breast-feeding when used, safety in children unknown, patients older than 65 yr, occlusive dressings; do not use products containing DEET

DRUG INTERACTIONS OF CONCERN TO DENTISTRY

- Risk of photosensitivity reaction: tetracyclines, fluoroquinolones, other photosensitizing drugs

SERIOUS REACTIONS

! Severe local skin reaction (intense erythema, edema, vesiculation) may limit treatment.

DENTAL CONSIDERATIONS

General:
- Patients will be taking antiviral drugs; note which drugs are being used because some have potential for significant drug interactions.
- Take a complete medical history, including a current drug history with doses and duration of therapy.

allopurinol

al-oh-**pure′**-ih-nole
(Aloprim, Allohexal[AUS], Allosig[AUS], Apo-Allopurinol[CAN], Capurate[AUS], Progout[AUS], Purinol[CAN], Zyloprim)
Do not confuse Zyloprim with ZORprin.

CATEGORY AND SCHEDULE

Pregnancy Risk Category: C

Drug Class: Antigout drug, antihyperuricemic

MECHANISM OF ACTION

A xanthine oxidase inhibitor that decreases uric acid production by inhibiting xanthine oxidase, an enzyme.

Therapeutic Effect: Reduces uric acid concentrations in both serum and urine.

USES

Chronic gout, hyperuricemia associated with malignancies, recurrent calcium oxalate calculi, uric acid nephropathy

PHARMACOKINETICS

Route	Onset	Peak	Duration
PO/IV	2–3 days	1–3 wk	1–2 wk

Well absorbed from the GI tract. Widely distributed. Metabolized in the liver to active metabolite. Excreted primarily in urine. Removed by hemodialysis. ***Half-life:*** 1–3 hr; metabolite, 12–30 hr.

INDICATIONS AND DOSAGES

▸ Chronic Gouty Arthritis

PO

Adults, Children older than 10 yr. Initially, 100 mg/day; may increase by 100 mg/day at weekly intervals. Maximum: 800 mg/day. Maintenance: 100–200 mg 2–3 times a day or 300 mg/day.

▸ To Prevent Uric Acid Nephropathy During Chemotherapy

PO

Adults. Initially, 600–800 mg/day starting 2–3 days before initiation of chemotherapy or radiation therapy.
Children 6–10 yr. 100 mg 3 times a day or 300 mg once a day.
Children younger than 6 yr. 50 mg 3 times a day.

IV

Adults. 200–400 mg/m^2 day beginning 24–48 hr before initiation of chemotherapy.
Children. 200 mg/m^2 day. Maximum: 600 mg/day.

▸ Prevention of Uric Acid Calculi

PO

Adults. 100–200 mg 1–4 times a day or 300 mg once a day.

▸ Recurrent Calcium Oxalate Calculi

PO

Adults. 200–300 mg/day.
Elderly. Initially, 100 mg/day, gradually increased until optimal uric acid level is reached.

▸ Dosage in Renal Impairment

Dosage is modified on the basis of creatinine clearance.

Creatinine Clearance	Dosage Adjustment
10–20 ml/min	200 mg/day
3–9 ml/min	100 mg/day
Less than 3 ml/min	100 mg at extended intervals

SIDE EFFECTS/ADVERSE REACTIONS

Occasional

Oral: Somnolence, unusual hair loss
IV: Rash, nausea, vomiting

Rare

Diarrhea, headache

PRECAUTIONS AND CONTRAINDICATIONS

Asymptomatic hyperuricemia

Caution:

Lactation, renal disease, hepatic disease, children

DRUG INTERACTIONS OF CONCERN TO DENTISTRY

- Increased risk of rash: ampicillin, amoxicillin, bacampicillin, hetacillin

SERIOUS REACTIONS

! Pruritic maculopapular rash possibly accompanied by malaise, fever, chills, joint pain, nausea, and vomiting should be considered a toxic reaction.

! Severe hypersensitivity may follow appearance of rash.
! Bone marrow depression, hepatic toxicity, peripheral neuritis, and acute renal failure occur rarely.

DENTAL CONSIDERATIONS

General:
• Patients on chronic drug therapy may rarely have symptoms of blood dyscrasias, which can include infection, bleeding, and poor healing.
Consultations:
• In a patient with symptoms of blood dyscrasias, request a medical consultation for blood studies and postpone dental treatment until normal values are reestablished.
• Medical consultation may be required to assess disease control.
Teach Patient/Family to:
• Encourage effective oral hygiene to prevent soft tissue inflammation.
• Avoid mouth rinses with high alcohol content because of drying effects.

almotriptan malate

al-moe-**trip**′-tan mal′-ate
(Axert)
Do not confuse Axert with Antivert.

CATEGORY AND SCHEDULE

Pregnancy Risk Category: C

Drug Class: Selective serotonin agonist

MECHANISM OF ACTION

A serotonin receptor agonist that binds selectively to vascular receptors, producing a vasoconstrictive effect on cranial blood vessels.

Therapeutic Effect: Produces relief of migraine headache.

USES

Acute treatment of migraine with or without aura in adults

PHARMACOKINETICS

Well absorbed after PO administration. Metabolized by the liver, excreted in urine. ***Half-life:*** 3–4 hr.

INDICATIONS AND DOSAGES

▸ **Migraine Headache**
PO
Adults, Elderly. 6.25–12.5 mg. If headache improves but then returns, dose may be repeated after 2 hr. Maximum: 2 doses/24 hr.
▸ **Dosage in Renal Impairment**
For adult and elderly patients, recommended initial dose is 6.25 mg, and maximum daily dose is 12.5 mg.

SIDE EFFECTS/ADVERSE REACTIONS

Frequent
Nausea, dry mouth, paresthesia, flushing
Occasional
Changes in temperature sensation, asthenia, dizziness

PRECAUTIONS AND CONTRAINDICATIONS

Arrhythmias associated with conduction disorders, hemiplegic or basilar migraine, ischemic heart disease (including angina pectoris, history of MI, silent ischemia, and Prinzmetal's angina), uncontrolled hypertension, use within 24 hr of ergotamine-containing preparation or another serotonin receptor antagonist, use within 14 days of MAOIs, Wolff-Parkinson-White syndrome

Caution:
Hypertension, diabetes, hepatitis, renal impairment, elevated cholesterol, obesity, smoking, postmenopause, men older than 40 yr, preexisting heart disease, elderly, lactation, safety/efficacy for pediatric patients not evaluated

DRUG INTERACTIONS OF CONCERN TO DENTISTRY

• Avoid concurrent use of ketoconazole, itraconazole, erythromycin

SERIOUS REACTIONS

! Excessive dosage may produce tremor, red extremities, reduced respirations, cyanosis, seizures, and chest pain.
! Serious arrhythmias occur rarely, particularly in patients with hypertension or diabetes, obese patients, smokers, and those with a strong family history of coronary artery disease.

DENTAL CONSIDERATIONS

General:
• This is an acute-use drug; it is doubtful that patients will undergo dental treatment during acute migraine attacks.
• Be aware of patient's disease, its severity, and frequency.
Consultations:
• If treating chronic orofacial pain, consult with physician of record.
• Medical consultation may be required to assess disease control and patient's ability to tolerate stress.
Teach Patient/Family to:
• Avoid mouth rinses with high alcohol content because of drying effects.
• Update health and drug history if physician makes any changes in evaluation or drug regimens.

alosetron

al-**ohs**′-eh-tron
(Lotronex)
Do not confuse Lotronex with Lovenox.

CATEGORY AND SCHEDULE

Pregnancy Risk Category: B

Drug Class: Selective serotonin antagonist, neuroenteric modulator

MECHANISM OF ACTION

A serotonin (5-HT3) receptor antagonist that mediates abdominal pain, bloating, nausea, vomiting, peristalsis, and secretory reflexes.
Therapeutic Effect: Alleviates diarrhea, reduces gastric pain.

USES

Treatment of women with diarrhea-predominant irritable bowel syndrome (IBS) failing to respond to conventional therapy

PHARMACOKINETICS

Rapidly absorbed after PO administration. Extensively metabolized in liver. Excreted primarily in urine and, to a lesser extent, in feces. ***Half-life:*** 1.5 hr.

INDICATIONS AND DOSAGES

▸ **IBS**
PO
Adults (women older than 18 yr).
1 mg twice a day. Maximum: 2 mg/day.

SIDE EFFECTS/ADVERSE REACTIONS

Frequent
Constipation
Occasional
Nausea, GI or abdominal discomfort or pain, dyspepsia, flatulence, hypertension, clinical depression
Rare
Sedation, abnormal dreams, anxiety

PRECAUTIONS AND CONTRAINDICATIONS

Breast-feeding; constipation; diverticulitis (active or history of); GI bleeding, obstruction, or perforation; history of ischemic colitis, ulcerative colitis, or Crohn's disease; thrombophlebitis
Caution:
Food retards absorption, elderly, reduced hepatic or renal function, notify physician immediately if severe constipation or worse occurs, lactation, children; physicians prescribing this drug must be enrolled in the manufacturer's prescribing program

DRUG INTERACTIONS OF CONCERN TO DENTISTRY

- Does not appear to induce CYP450 isoenzymes; no interactions are documented.
- Avoid use of drugs (opioids) that could lead to increased risk of constipation.
- Use NSAIDs or acetaminophen for mild-to-moderate dental pain.

SERIOUS REACTIONS

! Acute ischemic colitis and serious complications of constipation have resulted in the need for blood transfusions and surgery.

DENTAL CONSIDERATIONS

General:
- Short appointments and a stress-reduction protocol may be required for anxious patients.
- Consider semisupine chair position for patient comfort because of GI side effects of disease.
- Avoid drugs with anticholinergic activity, such as antihistamines, opioids, benzodiazepines, propantheline, atropine, and scopolamine.
- Question patient about tolerance of NSAIDs or aspirin related to GI disease.

Consultations:
- Consider consulting with physician before prescribing drugs that can cause constipation (opioids).
- Consultation with physician may be necessary if sedation or general anesthesia is required.
- Medical consultation may be required to assess disease control and patient's ability to tolerate stress.

Teach Patient/Family:
- Importance of updating health and drug history if physician makes any changes in evaluation or drug regimens.

alprazolam

al′-teh-place
(Apo-Alpraz[CAN], Kalma[AUS], Niravam, Novo-Alprazol[CAN], Xanax, Xanax XR)
Do not confuse alprazolam with lorazepam, or Xanax with Tenex or Zantac.

CATEGORY AND SCHEDULE

Pregnancy Risk Category: D
Controlled Substance: Schedule IV

Drug Class: Benzodiazepine

MECHANISM OF ACTION

A benzodiazepine that enhances the action of the inhibitory neurotransmitter gamma-aminobutyric acid in the brain. ***Therapeutic Effect:*** Produces anxiolytic effect from its CNS depressant action.

USES

Treatment of generalized anxiety disorder, panic disorders, anxiety with depressive symptoms; off-label: agoraphobia

PHARMACOKINETICS

Well absorbed from GI tract. Protein binding: 80%. Metabolized in the liver. Primarily excreted in urine. Minimal removal by hemodialysis. ***Half-life:*** 11–16 hr.

INDICATIONS AND DOSAGES

▸ Anxiety Disorders

PO (Immediate-Release)

Adults. Initially, 0.25–0.5 mg 3 times a day. May titrate q3–4 days. Maximum: 4 mg/day in divided doses.

Elderly, debilitated patients, patients with hepatic disease or low serum albumin. Initially, 0.25 mg 2–3 times a day. Gradually increase to optimum therapeutic response.

PO (Orally Disintegrating)

Adults. 0.25–0.5 mg 3 times a day. Maximum: 4 mg/day in divided doses.

▸ Anxiety with Depression

PO

Adults. 2.5–3 mg/day in divided doses.

▸ Panic Disorder

PO (Immediate-Release)

Adults. Initially, 0.5 mg 3 times a day. May increase at 3- to 4-day intervals. Range: 5–6 mg/day. Maximum: 10 mg/day.

Elderly. Initially, 0.125–0.25 mg twice a day. May increase in 0.125-mg increments until desired effect attained.

PO (Extended-Release)

▸ Alert

To switch from immediate-release to extended-release form, give total daily dose (immediate release) as a single daily dose of extended-release form.

Adults. Initially, 0.5–1 mg once a day. May titrate at 3- to 4-day intervals. Range: 3–6 mg/day. Maximum: 10 mg/day.

Elderly. Initially, 0.5 mg once a day.

PO (Orally Disintegrating)

Adults. Initially, 0.5 mg 3 times a day. May increase at 3- to 4-day intervals. Range: 5–6 mg/day. Maximum: 10 mg/day.

▸ Premenstrual Syndrome

PO

Adults. 0.25 mg 3 times a day.

SIDE EFFECTS/ADVERSE REACTIONS

Frequent

Ataxia; light-headedness; transient, mild somnolence; slurred speech (particularly in elderly or debilitated patients)

Occasional

Confusion, depression, blurred vision, constipation, diarrhea, dry mouth, headache, nausea

Rare

Behavioral problems such as anger, impaired memory, paradoxical reactions such as insomnia, nervousness, or irritability

PRECAUTIONS AND CONTRAINDICATIONS

Acute alcohol intoxication with depressed vital signs, acute angle-closure glaucoma, concurrent use of itraconazole or ketoconazole, myasthenia gravis, severe COPD

Caution:
Elderly, debilitated, hepatic disease, renal disease; dependence, potential for abuse; avoid in lactation, safety and efficacy in patients younger than 18 yr not established

DRUG INTERACTIONS OF CONCERN TO DENTISTRY

• Increased CNS depression: alcohol, other CNS depressants, clarithromycin, erythromycin, fluconazole, miconazole, fluoxetine, isoniazid, fluvoxamine, nefazodone, rifamycin; St. John's wort (herb), kava (herb)
• Contraindicated with ketoconazole, itraconazole, ritonavir, indinavir, saquinavir

SERIOUS REACTIONS

! Abrupt or too-rapid withdrawal may result in pronounced restlessness, irritability, insomnia, hand tremors, abdominal and muscle cramps, diaphoresis, vomiting, and seizures.
! Overdose results in somnolence, confusion, diminished reflexes, and coma.
! Blood dyscrasias have been reported rarely.

DENTAL CONSIDERATIONS

General:
• Monitor vital signs at every appointment because of cardiovascular side effects.
• After supine positioning, have patient sit upright for at least 2 min to avoid orthostatic hypotension.
• Assess salivary flow as a factor in caries, periodontal disease, and candidiasis.
• Psychologic and physical dependence may occur with chronic administration.

Consultations:
• Medical consultation may be required to assess disease control.

Teach Patient/Family:
• When chronic dry mouth occurs, advise patient to:
  • Avoid mouth rinses with high alcohol content because of drying effects.
  • Use daily home fluoride products for anticaries effect.
  • Use sugarless gum, frequent sips of water, or saliva substitutes.

alprostadil (prostaglandin e1, pge1)

al-**pros**′-ta-dil
(Caverject, Edex, Muse, Prostin VR Pediatric)

CATEGORY AND SCHEDULE

Pregnancy Risk Category: C
Naturally occurring prostaglandin (E1, PGE1)

MECHANISM OF ACTION

A prostaglandin that directly affects vascular and ductus arteriosus smooth muscle and relaxes trabecular smooth muscle.
Therapeutic Effect: Causes vasodilation; dilates cavernosal arteries, allowing blood flow to and entrapment in the lacunar spaces of the penis.

USES

Treatment of erectile dysfunction because of neurogenic, vasculogenic, psychogenic, or mixed causes

PHARMACOKINETICS

Rapidly metabolized and cleared from body by urinary excretion

INDICATIONS AND DOSAGES

▸ Maintain Patency of Ductus Arteriosus

IV Infusion

Neonates. Initially, 0.05–0.1 mcg/kg/min. Maintenance: 0.01–0.4 mcg/kg/min. Maximum: 0.4 mcg/kg/min.

▸ Impotence

Pellet, Intracavernosal

Adults. Dosage is individualized.

SIDE EFFECTS/ADVERSE REACTIONS

Frequent

Intracavernosal: Penile pain, prolonged erection, hypertension, localized pain, penile fibrosis, injection site hematoma or ecchymosis, headache, respiratory infection, flu-like symptoms

Intraurethral: Penile pain, urethral pain or burning, testicular pain, urethral bleeding, headache, dizziness, respiratory infection, flu-like symptoms

Systemic: Fever, seizures, flushing, bradycardia, hypotension, tachycardia, apnea, diarrhea, sepsis

Occasional

Intracavernosal: Hypotension, pelvic pain, back pain, dizziness, cough, nasal congestion

Intraurethral: Fainting, sinusitis, back and pelvic pain

Systemic: Anxiety, lethargy, myalgia, arrhythmias, respiratory depression, anemia, bleeding, thrombocytopenia, hematuria

PRECAUTIONS AND CONTRAINDICATIONS

Conditions predisposing to anatomic deformation of penis, hyaline membrane disease, penile implants, priapism, respiratory distress syndrome

Caution:

Patients on anticoagulant therapy, use of sterile technique, care of syringe, physician instruction in use required, sexually transmitted disease

DRUG INTERACTIONS OF CONCERN TO DENTISTRY

- None reported

SERIOUS REACTIONS

! Overdose is manifested as apnea, flushing of the face and arms, and bradycardia.

! Cardiac arrest and sepsis occur rarely.

DENTAL CONSIDERATIONS

- None reported

alteplase, recombinant

al′-teh-place

(Activase, Actilyse[AUS], Cathflo Activase)

Do not confuse alteplase or Activase with Altace.

CATEGORY AND SCHEDULE

Pregnancy Risk Category: C

Drug Class: Tissue plasminogen activator

MECHANISM OF ACTION

A tissue plasminogen activator that acts as a thrombolytic by binding to the fibrin in a thrombus and converting entrapped plasminogen to plasmin. This process initiates fibrinolysis.

Therapeutic Effect: Degrades fibrin clots, fibrinogen, and other plasma proteins.

USES
Treatment of acute MI, acute ischemic stroke, acute massive pulmonary embolism; treatment of occluded central venous catheters

PHARMACOKINETICS
Rapidly metabolized in the liver. Primarily excreted in urine.
Half-life: 35 min.

INDICATIONS AND DOSAGES
▸ Acute MI
IV Infusion
Adults weighing greater than 67 kg. 100 mg over 90 min, starting with 15-mg bolus over 1–2 min, then 50 mg over 30 min, then 35 mg over 60 min. Or a 3-hr infusion, giving 60 mg over first hr (6–10 mg as bolus over 1–2 min), 20 mg over second hr, and 20 mg over third hr.
Adults weighing 67 kg or less. 100 mg over 90 min, starting with 15-mg bolus, then 0.75 mg/kg over 30 min (maximum: 50 mg), then 0.5 mg/kg over 60 min (maximum: 35 mg). Or 3-hr infusion of 1.25 mg/kg giving 60% of dose over first hr (6%–10% as 1- to 2-min bolus), 20% over second hr, and 20% over third hr.
▸ Acute Pulmonary Emboli
IV Infusion
Adults. 100 mg over 2 hr. Institute or reinstitute heparin near end or immediately after infusion when aPTT or TT returns to twice normal or less.
▸ Acute Ischemic Stroke
IV Infusion
Adults. 0.9 mg/kg over 60 min (10% total dose as initial IV bolus over 1 min).
▸ Central Venous Catheter Clearance
IV
Adults, Elderly. 2 mg; may repeat after 2 hr.

SIDE EFFECTS/ADVERSE REACTIONS
Frequent
Superficial bleeding at puncture sites, decreased B/P
Occasional
Allergic reaction, such as rash or wheezing; bruising

PRECAUTIONS AND CONTRAINDICATIONS
Active internal bleeding, AV malformation or aneurysm, bleeding diathesis, intracranial neoplasm, intracranial or intraspinal surgery or trauma, recent (within past 2 mo) cerebrovascular accident, severe uncontrolled hypertension

DRUG INTERACTIONS OF CONCERN TO DENTISTRY
• Increased risk of bleeding: drugs that interfere with coagulation or platelet function, such as NSAIDs and aspirin

SERIOUS REACTIONS
! Severe internal hemorrhage may occur.
! Lysis of coronary thrombi may produce atrial or ventricular arrhythmias or stroke.

DENTAL CONSIDERATIONS
General:
• An acute-use drug for use in hospitals or emergency rooms.
• Patients are at risk of bleeding; check for oral signs.
• Avoid products that affect platelet function, such as aspirin and NSAIDs.
• Monitor vital signs every appointment because of cardiovascular side effects.
• Patients who have been treated with drug may present with cardiovascular disease or stroke; review medical and drug history.

Consultations:

- Consultation should include data on coagulation status.
- Medical consultation should include routine blood counts including platelet counts and aggregation.
- In a patient with symptoms of blood dyscrasias, request a medical consultation for blood studies and postpone treatment until normal values are reestablished.
- Medical consultation may be required to assess disease control and patient's ability to tolerate stress.

Teach Patient/Family to:

- Use soft tooth brush to reduce risk of bleeding.
- Encourage effective oral hygiene to prevent soft tissue inflammation.
- Report oral lesions, soreness, or bleeding to dentist.
- Prevent trauma when using oral hygiene aids.
- Update health and medication history if physician makes any changes in evaluation/drug regimens; include OTC, herbal, and nonherbal remedies in the update.

alvimopan

al-**vim**′-oh-pan
(Entereg)

CATEGORY AND SCHEDULE

Pregnancy Risk Category: B

Drug Class: Opioid antagonist

MECHANISM OF ACTION

Peripherally acting mu opioid receptor antagonist (PAM-OR). ***Therapeutic Effect:*** Blocks the adverse side effects of opioid analgesics in the GI tract without interfering with their beneficial CNS effect (analgesia), accelerates time to upper and lower GI recovery following bowel surgery.

USES

Short-term, inpatient control of postoperative ileus (to accelerate recovery following bowel surgery) as an adjunct to opioid pain control (for hospital use only)

PHARMACOKINETICS

Poorly absorbed (absolute bioavailability approximately 6%). Protein binding: 80%. No significant hepatic metabolism, excreted primarily in bile, also in urine (35%). ***Half-life:*** 10–17 hr.

INDICATIONS AND DOSAGES

▸ Postoperative Control of Ileus

Adult. PO 12 mg capsule administered 30 min to 5 hr prior to surgery, followed by 12 mg twice daily beginning the day after surgery for a maximum of 7 days or until discharge. Maximum number of doses: 15.

SIDE EFFECTS/ADVERSE REACTIONS

Frequent

Constipation, flatulence, dyspepsia

Occasional

Anemia, back pain, urinary retention, hypokalemia

PRECAUTIONS AND CONTRAINDICATIONS

May be administered only under the Entereg Access Support and Education program.
Myocardial infarction
Recent use of opioids (increased GI adverse effects)

DRUG INTERACTIONS OF CONCERN TO DENTISTRY

• None reported

SERIOUS REACTIONS

! Hypersensitivity, severe diarrhea, bowel cramping

DENTAL CONSIDERATIONS

General:

• Know status of patient GI disease and surgical recovery.

Consultations:

• Consult with physician to determine disease status of patient and ability to tolerate dental procedures.

Teach patient/family to:

• Update medical history as surgical recovery and GI disease status occur.

amantadine hydrochloride

ah-**man′**-ta-deen hi-droh-**klor′**-ide (Endantadine[CAN], PMS-Amantadine[CAN], Symmetrel)

CATEGORY AND SCHEDULE

Pregnancy Risk Category: C

Drug Class: Antiviral, antiparkinsonian agent

MECHANISM OF ACTION

A dopaminergic agonist that blocks the uncoating of influenza A virus, preventing penetration into the host and inhibiting M2 protein in the assembly of progeny virions. Amantadine also blocks the reuptake of dopamine into presynaptic neurons and causes direct stimulation of postsynaptic receptors.

Therapeutic Effect: Antiviral and antiparkinsonian activity.

USES

Prophylaxis or treatment of respiratory tract illness caused by influenza type A; drug-induced extrapyramidal reactions; parkinsonism

PHARMACOKINETICS

Rapidly and completely absorbed from the GI tract. Protein binding: 67%. Widely distributed. Primarily excreted in urine. Minimally removed by hemodialysis. ***Half-life:*** 11–15 hr (increased in the elderly, decreased in impaired renal function).

INDICATIONS AND DOSAGES

▸ **Prevention and Symptomatic Treatment of Respiratory Illness Caused by Influenza A Virus**

PO

Adults older than 64 yr. 100 mg/day.
Adults 13–64 yr. 200 mg/day.
Children 10–12 yr. 5 mg/kg/day up to 200 mg/day.
Children 1–9 yr. 5 mg/kg/day (up to 150 mg/day).

▸ **Parkinson's Disease, Extrapyramidal Symptoms**

PO

Adults, Elderly. 100 mg twice a day. May increase up to 300 mg/day in divided doses.

▸ **Dosage in Renal Impairment**

Dose and frequency are modified on the basis of creatinine clearance.

Creatinine Clearance	Dosage
30–50 ml/min	200 mg first day; 100 mg/day thereafter
15–29 ml/min	200 mg

SIDE EFFECTS/ADVERSE REACTIONS

Frequent
Nausea, dizziness, poor concentration, insomnia, nervousness

Occasional
Orthostatic hypotension, anorexia, headache, livedo reticularis (reddish blue, netlike blotching of skin), blurred vision, urine retention, dry mouth or nose

Rare
Vomiting, depression, irritation or swelling of eyes, rash

PRECAUTIONS AND CONTRAINDICATIONS

Hypersensitivity, lactation, child younger than 1 yr

Caution:
Epilepsy, CHF, orthostatic hypotension, psychiatric disorders, hepatic disease, renal disease (necessitates dose adjustment)

DRUG INTERACTIONS OF CONCERN TO DENTISTRY

- Increased anticholinergic response: anticholinergic drugs
- Increased CNS depression: alcohol, other CNS depressants

SERIOUS REACTIONS

! CHF, leukopenia, and neutropenia occur rarely.
! Hyperexcitability, seizures, and ventricular arrhythmias may occur.

DENTAL CONSIDERATIONS

General:

- Monitor vital signs at every appointment because of cardiovascular side effects.
- Assess salivary flow as a factor in caries, periodontal disease, and candidiasis.
- After supine positioning, have patient sit upright for at least 2 min to avoid orthostatic hypotension.
- Avoid dental light in patient's eyes; offer dark glasses for patient comfort.
- Short appointments and stress-reduction protocol may be required for anxious patients.
- Consider semisupine chair position for patients with respiratory distress.

Teach Patient/Family to:

- Avoid mouth rinses with high alcohol content because of drying effects.
- Use powered tooth brush if patient has difficulty holding conventional device.

ambenonium

am-be-**noe**′-nee-um
(Mytelase)

CATEGORY AND SCHEDULE

Pregnancy Risk Category: C

Drug Class: Cholinesterase inhibitor

MECHANISM OF ACTION

A cholinesterase inhibitor that enhances and prolongs cholinergic function by increasing the concentration of acetylcholine through inhibition of the hydrolysis of acetylcholine.
Therapeutic Effect: Increases muscle strength in myasthenia gravis.

USES

Treatment of myasthenia gravis, when other drugs cannot be used

PHARMACOKINETICS

Poorly absorbed after PO administration.

INDICATIONS AND DOSAGES

▸ **Myasthenia Gravis**

PO

Adults. 5–25 mg 3 or 4 times a day. If well tolerated, after 1 or 2 days, may increase to 50–75 mg 3 times a day. Range: 5–200 mg/day in divided doses.

SIDE EFFECTS/ADVERSE REACTIONS

Frequent

Abdominal pain, diarrhea, increased salivation, miosis, sweating, and vomiting

Occasional

Anxiety, blurred vision, and urinary urgency

Rare

Trembling, difficulty moving or controlling movement of the tongue, neck, or arms

PRECAUTIONS AND CONTRAINDICATIONS

Not recommended in patients receiving routine administration of atropine or other belladonna derivatives. Not recommended in patients receiving mecamylamine.

Caution:

Seizure disorders, bronchial asthma, coronary occlusion, hyperthyroidism, dysrhythmias, peptic ulcer, megacolon, poor GI motility, bradycardia, hypotension, lactation, children

DRUG INTERACTIONS OF CONCERN TO DENTISTRY

- Avoid drugs with anticholinergic activity and neuromuscular blocking agents.
- Avoid systemic use of ester-type local anesthetics because of reduced plasma cholinesterase activity.
- Use glucocorticoids with caution.

SERIOUS REACTIONS

! Overdosage may result in cholinergic crisis, characterized by severe nausea, vomiting, diarrhea, increased salivation, diaphoresis, bradycardia, hypotension, flushed skin, stomach pain, respiratory depression, seizures, and paralysis of muscles.

! Increasing muscle weakness of myasthenia gravis may occur. Antidote: 0.5–1 mg IV atropine sulfate with other supportive treatment.

DENTAL CONSIDERATIONS

General:

- Control excessive salivary flow with rubber dam and suction.
- Avoid drugs that reduce salivary flow because they will antagonize this drug.
- Patient may be unable to keep mouth open for long periods because of disease; short appointments may be necessary.
- Monitor vital signs at every appointment because of cardiovascular side effects.
- Evaluate respiration characteristics and rate.
- Consider semisupine chair position for patient comfort if GI side effects occur.
- After supine positioning, have patient sit upright for at least 2 min to avoid orthostatic hypotension.

Consultations:

- Consultation with physician may be necessary if sedation or general anesthesia is required.
- Medical consultation may be required to assess disease control and patient's ability to tolerate stress.

Teach Patient/Family to:
• Use powered tooth brush if patient has difficulty holding conventional devices.
• Update health and drug history, reporting changes in health status, drug regimen changes, or disease/treatment status.

ambrisentan

am-bri-**sin**′-tan
(Letairis [U.S.], Volibris [E.U.])

CATEGORY AND SCHEDULE

Pregnancy Risk Category: X

Drug Class: Endothelin receptor antagonist

MECHANISM OF ACTION

Blocks type A endothelin receptor. ***Therapeutic Effect:*** Blocks effects of endothelin on vascular smooth muscle, produces vasodilation.

USES

Treatment of pulmonary arterial hypertension to improve exercise capacity and delay clinical worsening

PHARMACOKINETICS

Well absorbed after oral administration. Protein binding: 99%.
Metabolized primarily in the liver (CYP 3A4, 2C19, UGTs); metabolites excreted primarily by non-renal pathways.

INDICATIONS AND DOSAGES

▸ **Pulmonary Arterial Hypertension**
Adult. PO 5 mg once daily, with or without food, may be increased to 10 mg.

SIDE EFFECTS/ADVERSE REACTIONS

Frequent
Reduced red blood cell count, peripheral edema, nasal congestion, sinusitis, flushing, palpitations, pharyngitis, constipation, dyspnea, headache
Occasional
Hepatic injury

PRECAUTIONS AND CONTRAINDICATIONS

May be administered only under the Letairis Education and Access Program.
Women of childbearing potential (Pregnancy Category X)
Pre-existing hepatic disease (see "SERIOUS REACTIONS")

DRUG INTERACTIONS OF CONCERN TO DENTISTRY

• Increased blood levels: CYP3A4 inhibitors, e.g., azole antifungals and macrolide antibiotics (erythromycin, clarithromycin)

SERIOUS REACTIONS

! Potential liver injury (manifested as elevations of aminotransferases)

DENTAL CONSIDERATIONS

General:
• Monitor vital signs at every appointment because of underlying disease and cardiovascular side effects of drug.
• Position patient for comfort because of underlying respiratory disease.
Consultations:
• Consult with physician to determine disease control and ability to tolerate dental procedures.
Teach patient/family to:
• Update medical history as disease and medication status change.

amcinonide

am-**sin**′-oh-nide
(Cylocort)

CATEGORY AND SCHEDULE

Pregnancy Risk Category: C

Drug Class: Antiinflammatory steroidal, topical

MECHANISM OF ACTION

Topical corticosteroids have antiinflammatory, antipruritic, and vasoconstrictive properties. The exact mechanism of the antiinflammatory process is unclear.
Therapeutic Effect: Reduces or prevents tissue response to inflammatory process.

USES

Relief of redness, swelling, itching, and discomfort of many skin problems

PHARMACOKINETICS

Well absorbed systemically. Large variation in absorption among sites: forearm 1%; scalp 4%, forehead 7%, scrotum 36%. Greatest penetration occurs at groin, axillae, and face. Protein binding in varying degrees. Metabolized in liver. Primarily excreted in urine.

INDICATIONS AND DOSAGES

▸ **Dermatoses**

Topical

Adults, Elderly. Apply sparingly 2–3 times a day.

SIDE EFFECTS/ADVERSE REACTIONS

Frequent

Itching, redness, irritation, burning

Occasional

Dryness, folliculitis, hypertrichosis, acneiform eruptions, hypopigmentation, perioral dermatitis

Rare

Allergic contact dermatitis, maceration of the skin, secondary infection, skin atrophy

Systemic: Absorption more likely with occlusive dressings or extensive application in young children

PRECAUTIONS AND CONTRAINDICATIONS

History of hypersensitivity to amcinonide or other corticosteroids

DRUG INTERACTIONS OF CONCERN TO DENTISTRY

- None reported

SERIOUS REACTIONS

! The serious reactions of long-term therapy and the addition of occlusive dressings are reversible hypothalamic-pituitary-adrenal (HPA) axis suppression, manifestations of Cushing's syndrome, hyperglycemia and glucosuria.

! Abruptly withdrawing the drug after long-term therapy may require supplemental systemic corticosteroids.

DENTAL CONSIDERATIONS

General:

- Determine why patient is taking the drug.
- Side effects include a variety of skin lesions.

Teach Patient/Family to:

- Avoid use on oral herpetic ulcerations.

amifostine

am-ih-**fos′**-teen
(Ethyol)
Do not confuse Ethyol with ethanol.

CATEGORY AND SCHEDULE

Pregnancy Risk Category: C

Drug Class: Cytoprotective, radioprotective

MECHANISM OF ACTION

An antineoplastic adjunct and cytoprotective agent that is converted to an active metabolite by alkaline phosphatase in tissues. The active metabolite binds to and detoxifies metabolites of cisplatin. These actions occur more readily in normal tissues than in tumor tissue. ***Therapeutic Effect:*** Reduces the toxic effect of the chemotherapeutic agent cisplatin.

USES

(1) Reduction of moderate to severe xerostomia in patients undergoing postoperative head and neck radiation for cancer where the radiation port includes a substantial part of the parotid gland; (2) reduction of cumulative renal toxicity associated with repeated cisplatin use in patients with advanced ovarian or non-small cell lung cancers

PHARMACOKINETICS

Rapidly cleared from plasma. Converted in tissue to active free thiol metabolite. Tissue uptake highest in bone marrow, skin, GI mucosa, salivary glands. ***Half-life:*** less than 1 min. Less than 10% remains in plasma 6 min after drug administration.

INDICATIONS AND DOSAGES

▸ To Reduce Cumulative Renal Toxicity from Repeated Administration of Cisplatin in Patients with Advanced Ovarian Cancer

IV

Adults. 910 mg/m^2 once a day as 15-min infusion, beginning 30 min before chemotherapy. A 15-min infusion is better tolerated than extended infusions. If the full dose cannot be administered, dose for subsequent cycles should be 740 mg/m^2.

▸ Treatment of Postoperative Radiation-Induced Xerostomia in Patients with Head and Neck Cancer

IV

Adults. 200 mg/m^2 once a day as 3-min infusion, starting 15–30 min before radiation therapy.

Subcutaneous

Adults. 500 mg/day during radiation therapy.

SIDE EFFECTS/ADVERSE REACTIONS

Frequent

Transient reduction in B/P (usually starts 14 min into infusion, lasts about 6 min and returns to normal in 5–15 min); severe nausea, vomiting

Occasional

Flushing or feeling of warmth or chills or feeling of coldness; dizziness, hiccups, sneezing, somnolence

Rare

Clinically relevant hypocalcemia, mild rash

PRECAUTIONS AND CONTRAINDICATIONS

Sensitivity to aminothiol compounds or mannitol

Caution:
Patients should be well hydrated, monitor blood pressure, safety not established in CV disease; elderly, cerebrovascular disease, lactation, children

DRUG INTERACTIONS OF CONCERN TO DENTISTRY

- None reported

SERIOUS REACTIONS

! A pronounced drop in B/P may require temporary cessation of amifostine and fluid resuscitation.

DENTAL CONSIDERATIONS

General:

- This is an in-hospital or outpatient chemotherapy drug. Confirm the patient's disease and treatment status.
- Dental treatment may be provided if necessary during treatment.
- Monitor vital signs at every appointment because of cardiovascular side effects.
- Consider semisupine chair position for patient comfort if GI side effects occur.
- Patients taking opioids for acute or chronic pain should be given alternative analgesics for dental pain.
- Short appointments and a stress-reduction protocol may be required for anxious patients.
- Palliative medication may be required for management of oral side effects caused by chemotherapeutic drugs.
- Assess salivary flow as a factor in caries, periodontal disease, and candidiasis.
- Chlorhexidine mouth rinse before and during chemotherapy may reduce severity of mucositis.
- Apply lubricant to dry lips for patient comfort before dental procedures.
- Examine for oral manifestation of opportunistic infection.

Consultations:

- Medical consultation may be required to assess immunologic status during cancer therapy and determine safety risks posed by dental treatment.
- Consultation with physician may be necessary if sedation or general anesthesia is required.

Teach Patient/Family to:

- Prevent trauma when using oral hygiene aids.
- Encourage effective oral hygiene to prevent soft tissue inflammation, infection.
- Report oral lesions, soreness, or bleeding to dentist.
- When chronic dry mouth occurs, advise patient to:
  - Avoid mouth rinses with high alcohol content because of drying effects.
  - Use daily home fluoride products for anticaries effect.
  - Use sugarless gum, frequent sips of water, or saliva substitutes.
- Update health and drug history, reporting changes in health status, drug regimen changes, or disease/treatment status.

amiloride hydrochloride

a-**mill′**-oh-ride hi-droh-**klor′**-ide
(Kaluril[AUS], Midamor)
Do not confuse amiloride with amiodarone or amlodipine.

CATEGORY AND SCHEDULE

Pregnancy Risk Category: B (D if used in pregnancy-induced hypertension)

Drug Class: Potassium-sparing diuretic

MECHANISM OF ACTION

A guanidine derivative that acts as a potassium-sparing diuretic, antihypertensive, and antihypokalemic by directly interfering with sodium reabsorption in the distal tubule.
Therapeutic Effect: Increases sodium and water excretion and decreases potassium excretion.

USES

Edema in CHF in combination with other diuretics, for hypertension as an adjunct with other diuretics to maintain potassium

PHARMACOKINETICS

Route	Onset	Peak	Duration
PO	2 hr	6–10 hr	24 hr

Partially absorbed from the GI tract. Protein binding: Minimal. Primarily excreted in urine; partially eliminated in feces. ***Half-life:*** 6–9 hr.

INDICATIONS AND DOSAGES

▸ **To Counteract Potassium Loss Induced by Other Diuretics**

PO

Adults, Children weighing more than 20 kg. 5–10 mg/day up to 20 mg.
Elderly. Initially, 5 mg/day or every other day.
Children weighing 6–20 kg. 0.625 mg/kg/day. Maximum: 10 mg/day.

▸ **Dosage in Renal Impairment**

Creatinine Clearance	Dosage
10–50 ml/min 50% of normal	Less than 10 ml/min Avoid

SIDE EFFECTS/ADVERSE REACTIONS

Frequent
Headache, nausea, diarrhea, vomiting, decreased appetite
Occasional
Dizziness, constipation, abdominal pain, weakness, fatigue, cough, impotence
Rare
Tremors, vertigo, confusion, nervousness, insomnia, thirst, dry mouth, heartburn, shortness of breath, increased urination, hypotension, rash

PRECAUTIONS AND CONTRAINDICATIONS

Acute or chronic renal insufficiency, anuria, diabetic nephropathy, patients on other potassium-sparing diuretics, serum potassium greater than 5.5 mEq/L
Caution:
Dehydration, diabetes, acidosis, lactation

DRUG INTERACTIONS OF CONCERN TO DENTISTRY

• Decreased effects: corticosteroids, NSAIDs, indomethacin

SERIOUS REACTIONS

! Severe hyperkalemia may produce irritability; anxiety; a feeling of heaviness in the legs; paresthesia of hands, face, and lips; hypotension; bradycardia; tented T waves; widening of QRS, and ST depression.

DENTAL CONSIDERATIONS

General:

• Monitor vital signs at every appointment because of cardiovascular side effects.
• Assess salivary flow as a factor in caries, periodontal disease, and candidiasis.
• After supine positioning, have patient sit upright for at least 2 min to avoid orthostatic hypotension.
• Patients on chronic drug therapy may rarely have symptoms of blood dyscrasias, which can include infection, bleeding, and poor healing.
• Limit use of sodium-containing products, such as saline IV fluids, for those patients with a dietary salt restriction.

Consultations:

• Medical consultation may be required to assess patient's ability to tolerate stress.
• Medical consultation may be required to assess disease control.
• In a patient with symptoms of blood dyscrasias, request a medical consultation for blood studies and postpone dental treatment until normal values are reestablished.

Teach Patient/Family to:

• Encourage effective oral hygiene to prevent soft tissue inflammation.
• Prevent injury when using oral hygiene aids.
• When chronic dry mouth occurs, advise patient to:
  - Avoid mouth rinses with high alcohol content because of drying effects.
  - Use daily home fluoride products for anticaries effect.
  - Use sugarless gum, frequent sips of water, or saliva substitutes.

aminoglutethimide

ah-mee-noe-gloo-**teth′**-ih-mide
(Cytadren)

CATEGORY AND SCHEDULE

Pregnancy Risk Category: D

Drug Class: Antineoplastic, antiadrenal

MECHANISM OF ACTION

An antiadrenal agent that partially inhibits the conversion of cholesterol to pregnenolone in the adrenal glands and blocks the conversion of androstenedione to estrone and estradiol in peripheral tissues.
Therapeutic Effect: Suppresses adrenal function.

USES

Treatment of some kinds of tumors that affect the adrenal cortex

PHARMACOKINETICS

Rapidly and completely absorbed from the GI tract. Protein binding: Low (20%–25%). Metabolized in the liver by acetylation. Primarily excreted in urine. ***Half-life:*** 12.5 hr.

INDICATIONS AND DOSAGES

▸ **Cushing's Syndrome**

PO

Adults. Initially, 250 mg q6h. May increase by 250 mg daily every 1–2 wk. Maximum: 2 g/day.

SIDE EFFECTS/ADVERSE REACTIONS

Frequent

Drowsiness, rash, loss of appetite, nausea

Occasional

Dizziness, headache, fever, myalgia, hypotension, tachycardia, pruritus, depression

Rare

Neck tenderness, swelling, increased hair growth in females

PRECAUTIONS AND CONTRAINDICATIONS

Hypersensitivity to glutethimide or aminoglutethimide

DRUG INTERACTIONS OF CONCERN TO DENTISTRY

• None reported

SERIOUS REACTIONS

! Adrenal insufficiency, agranulocytosis, leukopenia, neutropenia, and pancytopenia may occur.

DENTAL CONSIDERATIONS

General:

• Determine why patient is taking the drug.

• Monitor vital signs at every appointment because of cardiovascular side effects.

• Determine dose and duration of glucocorticoid therapy to assess for risk of stress tolerance and immunosuppression. Patients on chronic glucocorticoid therapy may require supplemental doses for dental treatment.

• Precaution if dental surgery is anticipated or general anesthesia is required.

• Patient on chronic drug therapy may rarely present with symptoms of blood dyscrasias, which can include infection, bleeding, and poor healing. If dyscrasia is present, caution patient to prevent oral tissue trauma when using oral hygiene aids.

• After supine positioning, have patient sit upright for at least 2 min before standing to avoid orthostatic hypotension.

• Patient may need assistance in getting into and out of dental chair. Adjust chair position for patient comfort.

• Examine for oral manifestation of opportunistic infection.

• Caution: use of additional CNS depressants.

• If cancer is present, evaluate surgical, radiation, and chemotherapy history.

Consultations:

• Consultation may be required to confirm glucocorticoid dose and duration of use.

• Medical consultation may be required to assess disease control and patient's ability to tolerate stress.

• In a patient with symptoms of blood dyscrasias, request a medical consultation for blood studies and postpone treatment until normal values are reestablished.

Teach Patient/Family to:

• Update health and medication history if physician makes any changes in evaluation or drug regimens; include OTC, herbal, and nonherbal remedies in the update.

• Report oral lesions, soreness, or bleeding to dentist.

• Avoid driving or performing other tasks requiring mental alertness while taking aminoglutethimide.
• Encourage effective oral hygiene to prevent soft tissue inflammation.
• Prevent trauma when using oral hygiene aids.

aminophylline/ theophylline

am-in-**off'**-ih-lin
(aminophylline) Phyllocontin, (theophylline) Elixophyllin, Quibron-T, Quibron-T/SR, Nuelin[AUS], Nuelin SR[AUS], Slo-Bid Gyrocaps, Theo-24, Thoechron, Theodur, Theolair, T-Phyl, Uniphyl
Do not confuse aminophylline with amitriptyline or ampicillin, or Slo-Bid with Dolobid.

CATEGORY AND SCHEDULE

Pregnancy Risk Category: C

Drug Class: Xanthine

MECHANISM OF ACTION

A xanthine derivative that acts as a bronchodilator by directly relaxing smooth muscle of the bronchial airways and pulmonary blood vessels.
Therapeutic Effect: Relieves bronchospasm and increases vital capacity.

USES

Treatment of bronchial asthma, bronchospasm, Cheyne-Stokes respirations

PHARMACOKINETICS

PO: Peak 1 hr; metabolized in liver; excreted in urine, breast milk; crosses placenta.

INDICATIONS AND DOSAGES

▸ Chronic Bronchospasm

PO

Adults, Elderly, Children. 16 mg/kg or 400 mg/day (whichever is less) in 3–4 divided doses (8-hr intervals); may increase by 25% every 2–3 days. Maximum: 13 mg/kg/day (children 13–16 yr); 18 mg/kg/day (children 9–12 yr); 20 mg/kg/day (children 1–8 yr). Maximum dosages are based on serum theophylline concentrations, clinical condition, and presence of toxicity.

▸ Acute Bronchospasm in Patients Not Currently Taking Theophylline

PO

Adults, Children older than 1 yr. Initially, loading dose of 5 mg/kg (theophylline); then maintenance dosage of theophylline based on patient group (shown below).

Patient Group	Maintenance Theophylline Dosage
Healthy, nonsmoking adults	3 mg/kg q8h
Elderly patients, patients with cor pulmonale	2 mg/kg q8h
Patients with CHF or hepatic disease	1–2 mg/kg q12h
Children 9–16 yr, young adult smokers	3 mg/kg q6h
Children 1–8 yr	4 mg/kg q6h

IV

Adults, Children older than 1 yr. Initially, loading dose of 6 mg/kg (aminophylline); maintenance dosage of aminophylline based on patient group (shown below).

Patient Group	Maintenance Aminophylline Dosage
Healthy, nonsmoking adults	0.7 mg/kg/hr
Elderly patients, patients with cor pulmonale, CHF, or hepatic impairment	0.25 mg/kg/hr
Children 13–16 yr	0.7 mg/kg/hr
Children 9–12 yr, young adult smokers	0.9 mg/kg/hr
Children 1–8 yr	1–1.2 mg/kg/hr
Children 6 mo–1 yr	0.6–0.7 mg/kg/hr
Children 6 wk–6 mo	0.5 mg/kg/hr
Neonates	5 mg/kg q12h

▸ **Acute Bronchospasm In Patients Currently Taking Theophylline**

PO, IV

Adults, Children older than 1 yr. Obtain serum theophylline level. If not possible and patient is in respiratory distress and not experiencing toxic effects, may give 2.5 mg/kg dose. Maintenance: Dosage based on peak serum theophylline concentration, clinical condition, and presence of toxicity.

SIDE EFFECTS/ADVERSE REACTIONS

Frequent

Altered smell (during IV administration), restlessness, tachycardia, tremor

Occasional

Heartburn, vomiting, headache, mild diuresis, insomnia, nausea

PRECAUTIONS AND CONTRAINDICATIONS

History of hypersensitivity to caffeine or xanthine

Caution:

Elderly, CHF, cor pulmonale, hepatic disease, active peptic ulcer disease, diabetes mellitus, hyperthyroidism, hypertension, children, glaucoma, prostatic hypertrophy

DRUG INTERACTIONS OF CONCERN TO DENTISTRY

- Increased action: erythromycin (macrolides), ciprofloxacin
- Cardiac dysrhythmia: CNS stimulants, hydrocarbon inhalation anesthetics
- Decreased effects: barbiturates, carbamazepine
- Decreased effects of benzodiazepines

SERIOUS REACTIONS

! Too-rapid IV administration may produce marked hypotension with accompanying faintness, light-headedness, palpitations, tachycardia, hyperventilation, nausea, vomiting, angina-like pain, seizures, ventricular fibrillation, and cardiac standstill.

DENTAL CONSIDERATIONS

General:

- Monitor vital signs at every appointment because of cardiovascular and respiratory side effects.
- Consider semisupine chair position for patient comfort because of respiratory disease and GI side effects of drug.
- Midday appointments and a stress reduction protocol may be required for anxious patients.
- Be aware that aspirin or sulfite preservatives in vasoconstrictor-containing products can exacerbate asthma.
- Acute asthmatic episodes may be precipitated in the dental office. Sympathomimetic inhalants should be available for emergency use.

Consultations:

• Medical consultation may be required to assess disease control.

aminosalicylic acid

ah-**mee**′-noe-sal-ih-sil-ik as′-id
(Nemasol[CAN], Paser)

CATEGORY AND SCHEDULE

Pregnancy Risk Category: C

Drug Class: Antitubercular antiinfective

MECHANISM OF ACTION

An antitubercular agent active against *M. tuberculosis.* Thought to exhibit competitive antagonism of folic acid synthesis.
Therapeutic Effect: Bacteriostatic activity in susceptible microorganisms.

USES

Tuberculosis, in combination with other *M. tuberculosis* antiinfectives

PHARMACOKINETICS

Readily absorbed from the GI tract. Protein binding: 50%–60%. Widely distributed (including CSF). Metabolized in liver. Primarily excreted in urine. Removed by hemodialysis. ***Half-life:*** 1.1–1.62 hr.

INDICATIONS AND DOSAGES

▸ **Tuberculosis**

PO

Adults, Elderly. 4 g in divided doses 3 times a day.
Children. 150 mg/kg/day in divided doses 3 times a day. Maximum: 12 g/day.

SIDE EFFECTS/ADVERSE REACTIONS

Occasional

Abdominal pain, diarrhea, nausea, vomiting

Rare

Hypersensitivity reactions, hepatotoxicity, thrombocytopenia

PRECAUTIONS AND CONTRAINDICATIONS

End-stage renal disease, hypersensitivity to aminosalicylic acid products

Caution:

Hepatic dysfunction, refrigeration required for storage, malabsorption of vitamin B_{12}, no data on safe use in children or lactation

DRUG INTERACTIONS OF CONCERN TO DENTISTRY

• None reported

SERIOUS REACTIONS

! Liver toxicity and hepatitis, blood dyscrasias occur rarely.
! Agranulocytosis, methemoglobinemia, thrombocytopenia have been reported.

DENTAL CONSIDERATIONS

General:

• Determine that noninfectious status exists by ensuring that:
  • Anti-tuberculosis (TB) drugs have been taken for more than 3 wk.
  • Culture confirmed TB susceptibility to antiinfectives.
  • Patient has had three consecutive negative sputum smears.
  • Patient is not in the coughing stage.

• Determine why patient is taking drug (i.e., for prophylaxis or active therapy).
• Explain importance of taking medication for full length of regimen to ensure effectiveness of treatment and to prevent the emergence of resistant strains.
• Patients on chronic drug therapy may rarely have symptoms of blood dyscrasias, which can include infection, bleeding, and poor healing.
• Consider semisupine chair position for patient comfort if GI side effects occur.

Consultations:

• Medical consultation may be required to assess disease control and patient's ability to tolerate stress.
• In a patient with symptoms of blood dyscrasias, request a medical consultation for blood studies and postpone treatment until normal values are reestablished.

Teach Patient/Family to:

• Update health and drug history if physician makes any changes in evaluation or drug regimens.
• Prevent trauma when using oral hygiene aids.

amiodarone hydrochloride

a-mi-**oh′**-da-rone
hi-droh-**klor′**-ide
(Aratac[AUS], Cordarone, Cordarone X[AUS], Pacerone)
Do not confuse amiodarone with amiloride or Cordarone with Cardura.

CATEGORY AND SCHEDULE

Pregnancy Risk Category: D

Drug Class: Antidysrhythmic (class III)

MECHANISM OF ACTION

A cardiac agent that prolongs duration of myocardial cell action potential and refractory period by acting directly on all cardiac tissue. Decreases AV and SN function. ***Therapeutic Effect:*** Suppresses arrhythmias.

USES

Documented life-threatening ventricular tachycardia; unapproved: ventricular fibrillation not controlled by first-line agents

PHARMACOKINETICS

Route	Onset	Peak	Duration
PO	3 days–1 wk	1 wk–5 mo	7–50 days after discontinuation

Slowly, variably absorbed from GI tract. Protein binding: 96%. Extensively metabolized in the liver to active metabolite. Excreted via bile; not removed by hemodialysis. ***Half-life:*** 26–107 days; metabolite, 61 days.

INDICATIONS AND DOSAGES

▸ Life-Threatening Recurrent Ventricular Fibrillation or Hemodynamically Unstable Ventricular Tachycardia

PO

Adults, Elderly. Initially, 800–1600 mg/day in 2–4 divided doses for 1–3 wk. After arrhythmia is controlled or side effects occur, reduce to 600–800 mg/day for about 4 wk. Maintenance: 200–600 mg/day.

Children. Initially, 10–15 mg/kg/day for 4–14 days, then 5 mg/kg/day for several wk. Maintenance: 2.5 mg/kg or lowest effective maintenance dose for 5 of 7 days/wk.

IV Infusion
Adults. Initially, 1050 mg over 24 hr; 150 mg over 10 min, then 360 mg over 6 hr; then 540 mg over 18 hr. May continue at 0.5 mg/min for up to 2–3 wk regardless of age or renal or left ventricular function.

SIDE EFFECTS/ADVERSE REACTIONS

Expected
Corneal microdeposits are noted in almost all patients treated for more than 6 mo (can lead to blurry vision).
Frequent
Parenteral: Hypotension, nausea, fever, bradycardia
Oral: Constipation, headache, decreased appetite, nausea, vomiting, paresthesias, photosensitivity, muscular incoordination
Occasional
Oral: Bitter or metallic taste; decreased libido; dizziness; facial flushing; blue-gray coloring of skin (face, arms, and neck); blurred vision; bradycardia; asymptomatic corneal deposits
Rare
Oral: Rash, vision loss, blindness

PRECAUTIONS AND CONTRAINDICATIONS

Bradycardia-induced syncope (except in the presence of a pacemaker), second- and third-degree AV block, severe hepatic disease, severe SN dysfunction
Caution:
Goiter, Hashimoto's thyroiditis, SN dysfunction, second- or third-degree AV block, electrolyte imbalances, bradycardia; lactation, not recommended for children

DRUG INTERACTIONS OF CONCERN TO DENTISTRY

- Bradycardia, hypotension: inhalation anesthetics, lidocaine, anticholinergics, vasoconstrictors
- Increased photosensitization: tetracyclines
- Do not use with grapefruit juice, gatifloxacin, moxifloxacin, or sparfloxacin.
- Amiodarone is both a substrate and an inhibitor of CYP3A4; potential interactions with strong inhibitors of CYP3A4 isoenzymes.

SERIOUS REACTIONS

! Serious, potentially fatal pulmonary toxicity (alveolitis, pulmonary fibrosis, pneumonitis, acute respiratory distress syndrome) may begin with progressive dyspnea and cough with crackles, decreased breath sounds, pleurisy, CHF, or hepatotoxicity.
! Amiodarone may worsen existing arrhythmias or produce new arrhythmias (called proarrhythmias).

DENTAL CONSIDERATIONS

General:
- Monitor vital signs at every appointment because of cardiovascular and respiratory side effects.
- Assess salivary flow as a factor in caries, periodontal disease, and candidiasis.
- Avoid dental light in patient's eyes; offer dark glasses for patient comfort.
- After supine positioning, have patient sit upright for at least 2 min before standing to avoid orthostatic hypotension.
- Use vasoconstrictors with caution, in low doses, and with careful aspiration. Avoid gingival retraction cord with epinephrine.

• Stress from dental procedures may compromise cardiovascular function; determine patient risk.
• Delay or avoid dental treatment if patient shows signs of cardiac symptoms or respiratory distress.
Consultations:
• Medical consultation may be required to assess patient's ability to tolerate stress.
• Medical consultation may be required to assess disease control.
Teach Patient/Family to:
• Update health and drug history, reporting changes in health status, drug regimen changes, or disease/treatment status.
• When chronic dry mouth occurs, advise patient to:
  • Avoid mouth rinses with high alcohol content because of drying effects.
  • Use daily home fluoride products for anticaries effect.
  • Use sugarless gum, frequent sips of water, or saliva substitutes.

amitriptyline hydrochloride

ah-mee-**trip′**-ti-leen
hi-droh-**klor′**-ide
(Apo-Amitriptyline[CAN], Elavil, Endep[AUS], Levate[CAN], Novo-Triptyn[CAN], Tryptanol[AUS])
Do not confuse amitriptyline with aminophylline or nortriptyline, or Elavil with Equanil or Mellaril.

CATEGORY AND SCHEDULE

Pregnancy Risk Category: C

Drug Class:
Antidepressant-tricyclic

MECHANISM OF ACTION

A tricyclic antidepressant that blocks the reuptake of neurotransmitters, including norepinephrine and serotonin, at presynaptic membranes, thus increasing their availability at postsynaptic receptor sites. Also has strong anticholinergic activity.
Therapeutic Effect: Relieves depression.

USES

Treatment of major depression; unapproved: treatment of enuresis and neurogenic pain

PHARMACOKINETICS

Rapidly and well absorbed from the GI tract. Protein binding: 90%. Undergoes first-pass metabolism in the liver. Primarily excreted in urine. Minimal removal by hemodialysis. ***Half-life:*** 10–26 hr.

INDICATIONS AND DOSAGES

▸ **Depression**
PO
Adults. 30–100 mg/day as a single dose at bedtime or in divided doses. May gradually increase up to 300 mg/day. Titrate to lowest effective dosage.
Elderly. Initially, 10–25 mg at bedtime. May increase by 10–25 mg at weekly intervals. Range: 25–150 mg/day.
Children 6–12 yr. 1–5 mg/kg/day in 2 divided doses.
IM
Adults. 20–30 mg 4 times a day.
▸ **Pain Management**
PO
Adults, Elderly. 25–100 mg at bedtime.

SIDE EFFECTS/ADVERSE REACTIONS

Frequent

Dizziness, somnolence, dry mouth, orthostatic hypotension, headache, increased appetite, weight gain, nausea, unusual fatigue, unpleasant taste

Occasional

Blurred vision, confusion, constipation, hallucinations, delayed micturition, eye pain, arrhythmias, fine muscle tremors, parkinsonian syndrome, anxiety, diarrhea, diaphoresis, heartburn, insomnia

Rare

Hypersensitivity, alopecia, tinnitus, breast enlargement, photosensitivity

PRECAUTIONS AND CONTRAINDICATIONS

Acute recovery period after MI, use within 14 days of MAOIs.

Caution:

Suicidal patients, convulsive disorders, prostatic hypertrophy, asthma, schizophrenia, psychotic disorders, severe depression, increased intraocular pressure, narrow-angle glaucoma, urinary retention, cardiac disease, hepatic disease, renal disease, hyperthyroidism, electroshock therapy, elective surgery, children younger than 12 yr, elderly, MAOIs, St. John's wort

DRUG INTERACTIONS OF CONCERN TO DENTISTRY

- Increased anticholinergic effects: muscarinic blockers, antihistamines, phenothiazines
- Increased effects of direct-acting sympathomimetics (epinephrine, levonordefrin)
- Possible risk of increased CNS depression: alcohol, barbiturates, benzodiazepines, CNS depressants, antidepressants
- Possible increase in serum levels: fluconazole, ketoconazole, bupropion, fluvoxamine, paroxetine, sertraline
- Decreased antihypertensive effect: clonidine, guanadrel, guanethidine
- Possible decrease in serum levels: barbiturates, St. John's wort (herb)

SERIOUS REACTIONS

! Overdose may produce confusion, seizures, severe somnolence, arrhythmias, fever, hallucinations, agitation, dyspnea, vomiting, and unusual fatigue or weakness.

! Abrupt discontinuation after prolonged therapy may produce headache, malaise, nausea, vomiting, and vivid dreams.

! Blood dyscrasias and cholestatic jaundice occur rarely.

DENTAL CONSIDERATIONS

General:

- Take vital signs every appointment because of cardiovascular side effects.
- Assess salivary flow as a factor in caries, periodontal disease, and candidiasis.
- Patients on chronic drug therapy may rarely have symptoms of blood dyscrasias, which can include infection, bleeding, and poor healing.
- After supine positioning, have patient sit upright for at least 2 min to avoid orthostatic hypotension.
- Use vasoconstrictors with caution, in low doses, and with careful aspiration. Avoid use of gingival retraction cord with epinephrine.
- Place on frequent recall because of oral side effects.

Consultations:

- In a patient with symptoms of blood dyscrasias, request a medical consultation for blood studies and

postpone dental treatment until normal values are reestablished.
• Medical consultation may be required to assess disease control.
• Physician should be informed if significant xerostomic side effects occur (e.g., increased caries, sore tongue, problems eating or swallowing, difficulty wearing prosthesis) so that a medication change can be considered.

Teach Patient/Family to:
• Encourage effective oral hygiene to prevent soft tissue inflammation.
• Prevent injury when using oral hygiene aids.
• When chronic dry mouth occurs, advise patient to:
  Avoid mouth rinses with high alcohol content because of drying effects.
  Use daily home fluoride products for anticaries effect.
  Use sugarless gum, frequent sips of water, or saliva substitutes.

amlexanox

am-**lecks**′-ah-knocks
(Aphthasol)
Do not confuse with Ambesol.

CATEGORY AND SCHEDULE

Pregnancy Risk Category: B

Drug Class: Topical antiinflammatory

MECHANISM OF ACTION

A mouth agent that has antiallergic and antiinflammatory properties. Appears to inhibit formation and/or release of inflammatory mediators (e.g., histamine) from mast cells, neutrophils, mononuclear cells.

Therapeutic Effect: Alleviates signs and symptoms of aphthous ulcers.

USES

Treatment of aphthous ulcers in patients with normal immune systems

PHARMACOKINETICS

After topical application, most systemic absorption occurs from the GI tract. Metabolized to inactive metabolite. Excreted in urine. ***Half-life:*** 3.5 hr.

INDICATIONS AND DOSAGES

▸ Aphthous Ulcers

Topical

Adults, Elderly. Administer ¼ inch directly to ulcers 4 times a day (after meals and at bedtime) following oral hygiene.

SIDE EFFECTS/ADVERSE REACTIONS

Rare

Stinging, burning at administration site, transient pain, rash

PRECAUTIONS AND CONTRAINDICATIONS

Hypersensitivity

Caution:

Wash hands immediately before and after each use; discontinue if mucositis appears, lactation, children

DRUG INTERACTIONS OF CONCERN TO DENTISTRY

• None reported

SERIOUS REACTIONS

! Ingestion of a full tube would result in nausea, vomiting, and diarrhea.

DENTAL CONSIDERATIONS

General:

• Recurrent aphthous ulcers may be associated with systemic conditions; evaluate as needed if healing has not occurred after 10 days.

Teach Patient/Family to:

• Apply paste as directed and wash hands immediately before and after each use.

• Report oral lesions or soreness to dentist.

amlodipine

am-**loh**′-dip-een

(Norvasc)

CATEGORY AND SCHEDULE

Pregnancy Risk Category: C

Drug Class: Calcium channel antagonist, dihydropyridine class

MECHANISM OF ACTION

Antianginal and antihypertensive agent that inhibits calcium ion movement across cell members, depressing contraction of cardiac and vascular smooth muscle.
Therapeutic Effect: Decreases myocardial oxygen demand, decreases systemic vascular resistance and blood pressure.

USES

Essential hypertension, chronic stable angina, vasospastic angina (Prinzmetal's or variant angina)

PHARMACOKINETICS

64%–90% bioavailable after oral administration. Protein binding: 93%. Primarily metabolized in the liver (90%), primarily excreted in urine. ***Half-life:*** 30–50 hr.

INDICATIONS AND DOSAGES

▸ Essential Hypertension, Stable Angina and Vasospastic Angina

Adult. PO 5 mg once daily, titrated over 7–14 days up to 10 mg daily maximum.

Child (6–17 yr). PO 2.5 to 5 mg once daily.

SIDE EFFECTS/ADVERSE REACTIONS

Frequent

Peripheral edema, headache, flushing, dizziness, palpitation

Occasional

Headache, fatigue, nausea, abdominal pain, somnolence

Rare

Arrhythmias (ventricular tachycardia, atrial fibrillation), bradycardia, chest pain, hypotension, peripheral ischemia, syncope, tachycardia, postural hypotension, vasculitis

Hypoesthesia, peripheral neuropathy, paresthesia, tremor, vertigo

Anorexia, constipation, dyspepsia, dysgeusia, diarrhea, flatulence, pancreatitis, vomiting, gingival enlargement, dry mouth, hyperglycemia, thirst

Allergy, back pain, arthralgia, myalgia, pruritus, rash

Angioedema, erythema multiforme, leukopenia, thrombocytopenia

PRECAUTIONS AND CONTRAINDICATIONS

Advanced aortic stenosis, severe hypotension

CHF, hypotension, hepatic disease, lactation, children under the age of 6, hepatic disease, beta-blocker withdrawal

DRUG INTERACTIONS OF CONCERN TO DENTISTRY

• Decreased effect: NSAIDs (antagonize antihypertensive effect)

• Increased hypotension: sedatives, opioids with hypotensive actions

SERIOUS REACTIONS

! Amlodipine may precipitate CHF and MI in patients with chronic cardiac disease and peripheral ischemia.
! Overdose produces nausea, somnolence, confusion, and slurred speech.

DENTAL CONSIDERATIONS

General:
• Monitor vital signs at every appointment because of underlying disease and possible cardiovascular side effects.
• After supine positioning, have patient sit upright for at least 2 min before standing to avoid orthostatic hypotension.
• Use stress-reduction protocol.
• Use vasoconstrictors with caution, in low doses, and with careful aspiration.
• Place on frequent recall to monitor gingival condition for possible gingival enlargement.
Consultations:
• Consult with physician to determine disease control and ability of patient to tolerate dental treatment.
• Consult with physician if gingival enlargement occurs, to discuss use of alternative medical drug, or to emphasize need for frequent monitoring of gingival condition.
Teach Patient/Family to:
• Encourage effective oral hygiene to minimize gingivitis and gingival enlargement.
• Schedule frequent oral hygiene recall visits to control gingivitis and gingival enlargement.
• When chronic dry mouth occurs, advise patient to:
• Avoid mouth rinses with high alcohol content because of drying effects.
• Use daily home fluoride products for anticaries effect.
• Use sugarless gum, frequent sips of water, or saliva substitutes.

amoxapine

ah-**moks**′-ah-peen
(Ascendin)
Do not confuse amoxapine with atomoxetine or atropine.

CATEGORY AND SCHEDULE

Pregnancy Risk Category: C

Drug Class: Antidepressant, tricyclic

MECHANISM OF ACTION

A tricyclic antidepressant that blocks the reuptake of neurotransmitters, such as norepinephrine and serotonin, at CNS presynaptic membranes, increasing their availability at postsynaptic receptor sites. The metabolite 7-OH-amoxapine has significant dopamine receptor blocking activity similar to haloperidol.
Therapeutic Effect: Produces antidepressant effects.

USES

Treatment of depression

PHARMACOKINETICS

Rapidly, well absorbed from the GI tract. Protein binding: 90%. Metabolized in liver. Excreted in urine and feces. ***Half-life:*** 8 hr.

INDICATIONS AND DOSAGES

▸ Depression

PO

Adults. 25 mg 2–3 times a day. May increase to 100 mg 2–3 times a day.

Adolescents. Initially, 25–50 mg/day as single or divided doses. May increase to 100 mg/day.

Elderly. Initially, 25 mg at bedtime. May increase by 25 mg/day q3–7 days. Maximum: 400 mg/day (outpatient), 600 mg/day (inpatient).

SIDE EFFECTS/ADVERSE REACTIONS

Frequent

Drowsiness, fatigue, xerostomia, constipation, weight gain

Occasional

Nausea, dizziness, headache, confusion, nervousness, restlessness, insomnia, edema, tremor, blurred vision, aggressiveness, muscle weakness

Rare

Paradoxical reactions (agitation, restlessness, nightmares, insomnia, extrapyramidal symptoms, particularly fine hand tremor), laryngitis, seizures

PRECAUTIONS AND CONTRAINDICATIONS

Acute recovery period following MI, within 14 days of MAOI ingestion, hypersensitivity to dibenzoxazepine compounds

Caution:

Suicidal patients, severe depression, increased intraocular pressure, narrow-angle glaucoma, urinary retention, cardiac disease, hepatic disease, hyperthyroidism, electroshock therapy, elective surgery, elderly, MAOIs

DRUG INTERACTIONS OF CONCERN TO DENTISTRY

- Increased anticholinergic effects: muscarinic blockers, antihistamines, phenothiazines
- Increased effects of direct-acting sympathomimetics (epinephrine, levonordefrin)
- Potential risk of increased CNS depression: alcohol, barbiturates, benzodiazepines, CNS depressants
- Decreased antihypertensive effect: clonidine, guanadrel, guanethidine

SERIOUS REACTIONS

! High dosage may produce cardiovascular effects, including severe postural hypotension, dizziness, tachycardia, palpitations, arrhythmias, and seizures. High dosage may also result in altered temperature regulation, such as hyperpyrexia or hypothermia.

! Abrupt withdrawal from prolonged therapy may produce headache, malaise, nausea, vomiting, and vivid dreams.

DENTAL CONSIDERATIONS

General:

- Take vital signs every appointment because of cardiovascular side effects.
- Assess salivary flow as a factor in caries, periodontal disease, and candidiasis.
- Patients on chronic drug therapy may rarely have symptoms of blood dyscrasias, which can include infection, bleeding, and poor healing.
- After supine positioning, have patient sit upright for at least 2 min to avoid orthostatic hypotension.
- Use vasoconstrictors with caution, in low doses, and with careful aspiration. Avoid use of gingival retraction cord with epinephrine.

• Place on frequent recall because of oral side effects.

Consultations:

• In a patient with symptoms of blood dyscrasias, request a medical consultation for blood studies and postpone dental treatment until normal values are reestablished.

• Medical consultation may be required to assess disease control.

• Physician should be informed if significant xerostomic side effects occur (e.g., increased caries, sore tongue, problems eating or swallowing, difficulty wearing prosthesis) so that a medication change can be considered.

Teach Patient/Family to:

• Encourage effective oral hygiene to prevent soft tissue inflammation.

• Prevent injury when using oral hygiene aids.

• When chronic dry mouth occurs, advise patient to:

  • Avoid mouth rinses with high alcohol content because of drying effects.
  • Use daily home fluoride products for anticaries effect.
  • Use sugarless gum, frequent sips of water, or saliva substitutes.

amoxicillin

ah-mox-eh-**sill′**-in

(Amoxil, Moxage, others)

CATEGORY AND SCHEDULE

Pregnancy Risk Category: B

Drug Class: Antibacterial aminopenicillin, extended spectrum

MECHANISM OF ACTION

Inhibits bacterial cell wall synthesis, resulting in death of susceptible bacteria (bactericidal).

Therapeutic Effect: Bactericidal effect on susceptible microorganisms, reduces severity of or eliminates infection.

USES

For treatment of infections caused by susceptible bacterial species in the orofacial region, upper and lower respiratory tract (including pneumonia), sinuses, pharyngeal/tonsillar region, middle ear, genitourinary tract, skin structures, and in otitis media and sinusitis. Used as a single dose for prophylaxis in patients at high risk of infective endocarditis and to prevent infections of artificial joints in susceptible patients (see section on “Medically Compromised Patients”). Also used in combination therapy of *H. pylori*–related GI disease.

PHARMACOKINETICS

Well absorbed after oral administration. Protein binding: 20%. Widely distributed, does not cross blood-brain barrier except in the presence of inflamed meninges. Partially metabolized in the liver, primarily excreted unchanged in urine. ***Half-life:*** 1–1.5 hr.

INDICATIONS AND DOSAGES

▸ **Ear, Nose, and Throat Infections**

Adult. PO 250 mg q8h or 500 mg q12h (mild to moderate).
PO 500 mg q8h or 875 mg q12h (severe).

Child. PO 20 mg/kg/day in divided doses q8h or 25 mg/kg/day in divided doses q12h (mild to moderate).

PO 40 mg/kg/day in divided doses q8h or 45 mg/kg/day in divided doses q12h (severe).

▸ Lower Respiratory Tract

Adult. PO 500 mg q8h or 875 mg q12h (mild, moderate or severe).

Child. PO 40 mg/kg/day in divided doses q8h or 45 mg/kg/day in divided doses q12h (mild, moderate or severe).

▸ Skin/Skin Structure

Adult. PO 250 mg q8h or 500 mg q12h (mild to moderate).

PO 500 mg q8h or 875 mg q12h (severe).

Child. PO 20 mg/kg/day in divided doses q8h or 25 mg/kg/day in divided doses q12h (mild to moderate).

PO 40 mg/kg/day in divided doses q8h or 45 mg/kg/day in divided doses q12h (severe).

▸ Genitourinary Tract

Adult. PO 250 mg q8h or 500 mg q12h (mild to moderate).

PO 500 mg q8h or 875 mg q1h (severe).

Child. 20 mg/kg/day in divided doses q8h or 25 mg/kg/day in divided doses q12h (mild to moderate).

40 mg/kg/day in divided doses q8h or 45 mg/kg/day in divided doses q12h (severe).

SIDE EFFECTS/ADVERSE REACTIONS

Frequent

Mild GI disturbances (nausea, vomiting, mild diarrhea), headache, oral or vaginal candidiasis

Occasional

Generalized rash, urticaria

Rare

Severe allergic reactions, fatal anaphylaxis

PRECAUTIONS AND CONTRAINDICATIONS

Hypersensitivity to penicillins and cross-sensitivity to cephalosporins, including fatal anaphylaxis

Superinfections

Phenylketonuria (chewable tablets contain phenylalanine)

False-positive urinary glucose tests (if amoxicillin reaches high concentration in urine)

DRUG INTERACTIONS OF CONCERN TO DENTISTRY

• Decreased antimicrobial effectiveness: tetracyclines, macrolide antibiotics, lincosamide antibiotics

SERIOUS REACTIONS

! Antibiotic-associated colitis and other superinfections may result from altered bacterial flora.

! Severe hypersensitivity reactions, including anaphylaxis and acute interstitial nephritis

DENTAL CONSIDERATIONS

General:

• Take precautions regarding allergy to medications.

• If medically prescribed, determine why patient is taking drug.

• If used for prophylaxis, determine that patient has taken drug prior to dental procedure.

• Amoxicillin may be considered among first-choice antibiotics for odontogenic infections, and may be taken with food and liquid if needed.

• May be associated with brown, yellow, or gray tooth staining in pediatric patients (can be removed with brushing or prophylaxis paste).

Consultations:
- Consult with physician to determine disease control and ability of patient to tolerate dental procedures.

Teach Patient/Family to:
- When used for dental infection, advise patient to take at prescribed intervals and complete dosage regimen.
- Discontinue taking drug and immediately notify dentist if signs/ symptoms of allergy or diarrhea occur.
- Immediately notify dentist if signs/ symptoms of infection are not relieved or increase.

amoxicillin/ clavulanate potassium

ah-**mox′**-ih-sill-in /clav-u-**lan′**-ate poh-**tass′**-ee-um
(Augmentin, Augmentin ES 600, Augmentin XR, Ausclay[AUS], Ausclay Duo Forte[AUS], Ausclay Duo 400[AUS], Clamoxyl[AUS], Clamoxyl Duo 400[AUS], Clamoxyl Duo Forte[AUS], Clavulin[CAN], Clavulin Duo Forte[AUS])
Do not confuse amoxicillin with amoxapine.

CATEGORY AND SCHEDULE

Pregnancy Risk Category: B

Drug Class: Aminopenicillin with a β-lactamase inhibitor

MECHANISM OF ACTION

Amoxicillin inhibits bacterial cell wall synthesis, while clavulanate inhibits bacterial β-lactamase.

Therapeutic Effect: Amoxicillin is bactericidal in susceptible microorganisms. Clavulanate protects amoxicillin from enzymatic degradation.

USES

For treatment of infections caused by susceptible ß-lactamase-producing strains of microorganisms as listed: lower respiratory tract infections, otitis media, and sinusitis caused by *H. influenzae, M. catarrhalis;* skin and skin structure infections caused by *S. aureus, E. coli, Klebsiella* species; UTIs caused by *E. coli, Klebsiella, Enterobacter* species; Augmentin ES-600: treatment of recurrent or persistent otitis media, *S. pneumoniae,* and β-lactamase-producing strains of *H. influenzae* or *M. catarrhalis*

PHARMACOKINETICS

Well absorbed from the GI tract. Protein binding: 20%. Partially metabolized in the liver. Primarily excreted in urine. Removed by hemodialysis. ***Half-life:*** 1–1.3 hr (increased in impaired renal function).

INDICATIONS AND DOSAGES

▸ **Mild-to-Moderate Infections**
PO
Adults, Elderly. 500 mg q12h or 250 mg q8h.

▸ **Severe Infections, Respiratory Tract Infections**
PO
Adults, Elderly. 875 mg q12h or 500 mg q8h.

▸ **Community-Acquired Pneumonia, Sinusitis**
PO
Adults, Elderly. 2 g (extended-release tablets) q12h for 7–10 days.

▸ **Usual Pediatric Dosage**
PO
Children weighing 40 kg and less. 25–45 mg/kg/day (200 or 400 mg/5 ml powder or 200 or 400 mg chewable tablets) in 2 divided doses or 20–40 mg/kg/day (125 or 250 mg/5 ml powder or 125 or 250 mg chewable tablets) in 3 divided doses.

▸ **Otitis Media**
PO
Children. 90 mg/kg/day (600 mg/5 ml suspension) in divided doses q12h for 10 days.

▸ **Usual Neonate Dosage**
PO
Neonates, Children younger than 3 mo. 30 mg/kg/day (125 mg/5 ml suspension) in divided doses q12h.

▸ **Dosage in Renal Impairment**
Dosage and frequency are modified on the basis of creatinine clearance.
Creatinine clearance 10–30 ml/min. 250–500 mg q12h. Creatinine clearance less than 10 ml/min. 250–500 mg q24h.

SIDE EFFECTS/ADVERSE REACTIONS

Frequent
GI disturbances (mild diarrhea, nausea, vomiting), headache, oral or vaginal candidiasis
Occasional
Generalized rash, urticaria

PRECAUTIONS AND CONTRAINDICATIONS

Hypersensitivity to any penicillins, infectious mononucleosis
Caution:
Hypersensitivity to cephalosporins, hepatic function impairment

DRUG INTERACTIONS OF CONCERN TO DENTISTRY

- Decreased antimicrobial effectiveness: tetracyclines, erythromycins, lincomycins
- Increased amoxicillin concentrations: probenecid
- Increased risk of skin rashes: allopurinol

SERIOUS REACTIONS

! Antibiotic-associated colitis and other superinfections may result from altered bacterial balance.
! Severe hypersensitivity reactions including anaphylaxis and acute interstitial nephritis occur rarely.

DENTAL CONSIDERATIONS

General:
- Take precautions regarding allergy to medication.
- Determine why the patient is taking the drug.

Consultations:
- Medical consultation may be required to assess disease control.

Teach Patient/Family:
- Importance of good oral hygiene to prevent soft tissue inflammation.
- Caution to prevent injury when using oral hygiene aids.
- When used for dental infection, advise patient:
  - To report sore throat, oral burning sensation, fever, and fatigue, any of which could indicate superinfection.
  - To take at prescribed intervals and complete dosage regimen.
  - To immediately notify the dentist if signs or symptoms of infection increase.

amphetamine

am-**fet′**-ah-meen

CATEGORY AND SCHEDULE

Pregnancy Risk Category: C
Controlled substance: Schedule II

Drug Class: Amphetamine

MECHANISM OF ACTION

A sympathomimetic amine that produces CNS and respiratory stimulation, mydriasis, bronchodilation, a pressor response, and contraction of the urinary sphincter. Directly affects α and β receptor sites in peripheral system. Enhances release of norepinephrine by blocking reuptake.
Therapeutic Effect: Increases motor activity, mental alertness; decreases drowsiness, fatigue.

USES

Narcolepsy, attention deficit/hyperactivity disorder (ADHD)

PHARMACOKINETICS

Well absorbed from the GI tract. Protein binding: 20%. Widely distributed (including CSF). Metabolized in liver. Excreted in urine. Unknown if removed by hemodialysis. ***Half-life:*** 7–31 hr.

INDICATIONS AND DOSAGES

▸ **ADHD**

PO

Adults. 5–20 mg 1–3 times a day.
Adults, Children older than 12 yr. Initially, 5 mg twice a day. Increase by 10 mg at weekly intervals until therapeutic response achieved.
Children 6–12 yr. Initially, 2.5 mg twice a day. Increase by 5 mg/day at weekly intervals until therapeutic response achieved.
Children 3–6 yr. Initially, 2.5 mg twice a day. Increase by 2.5 mg/day at weekly intervals until therapeutic response achieved.

▸ **Narcolepsy**

PO

Adults. 5–20 mg 1–3 times a day.
Adults, Children older than 12 yr. Initially, 5 mg twice a day. Increase by 10 mg at weekly intervals until therapeutic response achieved.
Children 6–12 yr. Initially, 2.5 mg twice a day. Increase by 5 mg/day at weekly intervals until therapeutic response achieved.

SIDE EFFECTS/ADVERSE REACTIONS

Frequent

Irregular pulse, increased motor activity, talkativeness, nervousness, mild euphoria, insomnia

Occasional

Headache, chills, dry mouth, GI distress, worsening depression in patients who are clinically depressed, tachycardia, palpitations, chest pain

PRECAUTIONS AND CONTRAINDICATIONS

Advanced arteriosclerosis, agitated states, glaucoma, history of drug abuse, history of hypersensitivity to sympathomimetic amines, hyperthyroidism, moderate to severe hypertension, symptomatic cardiovascular disease, within 14 days following discontinuation of an MAOI

Caution:

Gilles de la Tourette's syndrome, lactation, children younger than 3 yr

DRUG INTERACTIONS OF CONCERN TO DENTISTRY

• Increased sensitivity to effects of sympathomimetics; increased risk of serotonin syndrome with selective serotonin reuptake inhibitors (SSRIs)
• Increased pressor response: tricyclic antidepressants

SERIOUS REACTIONS

! Overdose may produce skin pallor or flushing, arrhythmias, and psychosis.
! Abrupt withdrawal following prolonged administration of high dosage may produce lethargy (may last for weeks).
! Prolonged administration to children with ADHD may produce a temporary suppression of normal weight and height patterns.

DENTAL CONSIDERATIONS

General:
• Monitor vital signs at every appointment because of cardiovascular side effects.
• Assess salivary flow as a factor in caries, periodontal disease, and candidiasis.
• Psychologic and physical dependence may occur with chronic use.
• Consider short appointments, frequent recall if patient becomes restless during a dental appointment.
Consultations:
• Medical consultation may be required to assess disease control and patient's ability to tolerate stress.
Teach Patient/Family to:
• Update health and drug history, reporting changes in health status, drug regimen changes, or disease/treatment status.
• Encourage effective oral hygiene to prevent soft tissue inflammation, infection.
• Prevent trauma when using oral hygiene aids.
• When chronic dry mouth occurs, advise patient to:
  • Avoid mouth rinses with high alcohol content because of drying effects.
  • Use daily home fluoride products for anticaries effect.
  • Use sugarless gum, frequent sips of water, or saliva substitutes.

amphotericin b

am-foe-**ter**′-ih-sin bee
(Abelcet, AmBisome, Amphocin, Amphotec, Fungizone)

CATEGORY AND SCHEDULE

Pregnancy Risk Category: B

Drug Class: Polyene antifungal

MECHANISM OF ACTION

An antifungal and antiprotozoal that is generally fungistatic but may become fungicidal with high dosages or very susceptible microorganisms. This drug binds to sterols in the fungal cell membrane.
Therapeutic Effect: Increases fungal cell-membrane permeability, allowing loss of potassium and other cellular components.

USES

Oral mucocutaneous infections caused by *Candida* species

PHARMACOKINETICS

Protein binding: 90%. Widely distributed. Metabolic fate unknown.

Cleared by nonrenal pathways. Minimal removal by hemodialysis. Amphotec and Abelcet are not dialyzable. ***Half-life:*** Fungizone, 24 hr (increased in neonates and children); Amphotec, 26–28 hr; Abelcet, 7.2 days; AmBisome, 100–153 hr.

INDICATIONS AND DOSAGES

▸ Cryptococcosis; Blastomycosis; Systemic Candidiasis; Disseminated Forms of Moniliasis, Coccidioidomycosis, and Histoplasmosis; Zygomycosis; Sporotrichosis; Aspergillosis

IV Infusion (Fungizone)

Adults, Elderly. Dosage based on patient tolerance and severity of infection. Initially, 1-mg test dose is given over 20–30 min. If test dose is tolerated, 5-mg dose may be given the same day. Subsequently, dosage is increased by 5 mg q12–24h until desired daily dose is reached. Alternatively, if test dose is tolerated, 0.25 mg/kg is given on same day and 0.5 mg/kg on second day; then dosage is increased until desired daily dose reached. Total daily dose: 1 mg/kg/day up to 1.5 mg/kg every other day. Maximum: 1.5 mg/kg/day.

Children. Test dose of 0.1 mg/kg/dose (maximum 1 mg) is infused over 20–60 min. If test dose is tolerated, initial dose of 0.4 mg/kg may be given on same day; dosage is then increased in 0.25-mg/kg increments as needed. Maintenance dose: 0.25–1 mg/kg/day.

▸ Invasive Fungal Infections Unresponsive to or Intolerant of Fungizone

IV Infusion (Abelcet)

Adults, Children. 5 mg/kg at rate of 2.5 mg/kg/hr.

▸ Empiric Treatment of Fungal Infections in Patients with Febrile Neutropenia; Aspergillosis, Candidiasis, or Cryptococcosis in Patients with Renal Impairment and Those Who Have Experienced Toxicity or Treatment Failure with Fungizone

IV Infusion (Ambisome)

Adults, Children. 3–5 mg/kg over 1 hr.

▸ Invasive Aspergillosis in Patients with Renal Impairment and Those Who Have Experienced Toxicity or Treatment Failure with Fungizone

IV Infusion (Amphotec)

Adults, Children. 3–4 mg/kg over 2–4 hr.

▸ Cutaneous and Mucocutaneous Infections Caused by *Candida albicans,* such as Paronychia, Oral Thrush, Perléche, Diaper Rash, and Intertriginous Candidiasis

Topical

Adults, Elderly, Children. Apply liberally to affected area and rub in 2–4 times a day.

SIDE EFFECTS/ADVERSE REACTIONS

Frequent

Chills, fever, increased serum creatinine level, multiple organ failure

Hypokalemia, hypomagnesemia, hyperglycemia, hypocalcemia, edema, abdominal pain, back pain, chills, chest pain, hypotension, diarrhea, nausea, vomiting, headache, rigors, insomnia, dyspnea, epistaxis, altered hepatic or renal function, hypotension, tachycardia, hypokalemia, bilirubinemia, headache, anemia, hypokalemia, anorexia, malaise

Topical: Local irritation, dry skin
Rare
Topical: Rash

PRECAUTIONS AND CONTRAINDICATIONS

Hypersensitivity to amphotericin B or sulfites
Caution:
Lactation; not for systemic fungal infections

DRUG INTERACTIONS OF CONCERN TO DENTISTRY

- None reported

SERIOUS REACTIONS

! Cardiovascular toxicity (as evidenced by hypotension, ventricular fibrillation, and anaphylaxis) occurs rarely.
! Altered vision and hearing, seizures, hepatic failure, coagulation defects, multiple organ failure, and sepsis may be noted.

DENTAL CONSIDERATIONS

General:

- Determine why the patient is taking the drug.
- Broad-spectrum antibiotics may contribute to oral *Candida* infections.

Teach Patient/Family to:

- Complete entire course of medication.
- Not use commercial mouthwashes for mouth infection unless prescribed by dentist.
- Soak removable appliance in antifungal agent overnight.
- Prevent reinoculation of *Candida* infection by disposing of tooth brush or other contaminated oral hygiene devices used during period of infection.

amphotericin b, lipid-based

am-foe-**ter**′-ih-sin bee
(Abelcet, Amphotec, AmBisome)

CATEGORY AND SCHEDULE

Pregnancy Risk Category: B

Drug Class: Antifungal

MECHANISM OF ACTION

An antifungal and antiprotozoal that is generally fungistatic but may become fungicidal with high dosages or very susceptible microorganisms. This drug binds to sterols in the fungal cell membrane.
Therapeutic Effect: Increases fungal cell-membrane permeability, allowing loss of potassium and loss of other cellular components.

USES

Treatment of infections caused by fungus

PHARMACOKINETICS

Protein binding: 90%. Widely distributed. Metabolic fate unknown. Cleared by nonrenal pathways. Minimal removal by hemodialysis. Not dialyzable. ***Half-life:*** 7.2 days.

INDICATIONS AND DOSAGES

▸ Invasive Fungal Infections Unresponsive to, or Intolerant of, Fungizone.
IV Infusion
Adults, Children. 5 mg/kg at rate of 2.5 mg/kg/hr.

SIDE EFFECTS/ADVERSE REACTIONS

Frequent
Chills, fever, increased serum creatinine, multiple organ failure

Occasional
Nausea, hypotension, vomiting, dyspnea, diarrhea, headache, hypokalemia, abdominal pain, rash

PRECAUTIONS AND CONTRAINDICATIONS

Hypersensitivity to amphotericin B or sulfites

DRUG INTERACTIONS OF CONCERN TO DENTISTRY

• Risk of hypokalemia: glucocorticoids and mineralocorticoids

SERIOUS REACTIONS

! Cardiovascular toxicity (as evidenced by hypotension, ventricular fibrillation, and anaphylaxis) occurs rarely.
! Altered vision and hearing, seizures, hepatic failure, coagulation defects, multiple organ failure, and sepsis may be noted.

DENTAL CONSIDERATIONS

General:
• Intended for serious systemic fungal infections; palliative emergency dental care only.
• Determine why patient is taking the drug.
• Patient on chronic drug therapy may rarely present with symptoms of blood dyscrasias, which can include infection, bleeding, and poor healing. If dyscrasia is present, caution patient to prevent oral tissue trauma when using oral hygiene aids.
• Monitor vital signs at every appointment because of cardiovascular side effects.
• Avoid prescribing aspirin-containing products.

Consultations:
• In a patient with symptoms of blood dyscrasias, request a medical consultation for blood studies and postpone treatment until normal values are reestablished.
• Medical consultation may be required to assess disease control and patient's ability to tolerate stress.

Teach Patient/Family to:
• Encourage effective oral hygiene to prevent soft tissue inflammation.
• Report oral lesions, soreness, or bleeding to dentist.
• Prevent trauma when using oral hygiene aids.

ampicillin

am′-pi-sill-in
(Alpovex[AUS], Amficot, Apo-Ampi[CAN], Novo-Ampicillin[CAN], Nu-Ampi[CAN], Omnipen, Omnipen-N, Polycillin, Polycillin-N, Principen, Totacillin, Totacillin-N)
Do not confuse with aminophylline, Imipenem, or Unipen.

CATEGORY AND SCHEDULE

Pregnancy Risk Category: B

Drug Class: Aminopenicillin

MECHANISM OF ACTION

A penicillin that inhibits cell wall synthesis in susceptible microorganisms.
Therapeutic Effect: Produces bactericidal effect.

USES

Treatment of sinus infections, pneumonia, otitis media, skin infections, UTIs; effective for susceptible strains of β-lactamase negative *E. coli, P. mirabilis, H. influenzae, S. faecalis, S. pneumoniae, S. typhosa, N. gonorrhoeae, N. meningitidis, L. monocytogenes,* shigella, enterococci

PHARMACOKINETICS

Moderately absorbed from the GI tract. Protein binding: 28%. Widely distributed. Partially metabolized in liver. Primarily excreted in urine. Removed by hemodialysis. ***Half-life:*** 1–1.9 hr (half-life increased in impaired renal function).

INDICATIONS AND DOSAGES

▸ **Respiratory Tract, Skin/Skin-Structure Infections**

PO

Adults, Elderly, Children weighing more than 20 kg. 250–500 mg q6h.

Children weighing less than 20 kg. 50 mg/kg/day in divided doses q6h.

IM/IV

Adults, Elderly, Children weighing more than 40 kg. 250–500 mg q6h.

Children weighing less than 40 kg. 25–50 mg/kg/day in divided doses q6–8h.

▸ **Bacterial Meningitis, Septicemia**

IM/IV

Adults, Elderly. 2 g q4h or 3 g q6h.

Children. 100–200 mg/kg/day in divided doses q4h.

▸ **Gonococcal Infections**

PO

Adults. 3.5 g one time with 1 g probenecid.

▸ **Perioperative Prophylaxis**

IM/IV

Adults, Elderly. 2 g 30 min before procedure. May repeat in 8 hr.

Children. 50 mg/kg using same dosage regimen.

▸ **Usual Neonate Dosage**

IM/IV

Neonates 7–28 days old. 75 mg/kg/day in divided doses q8h up to 200 mg/kg/day in divided doses q6h.

Neonates 0–7 days old. 50 mg/kg/day in divided doses q12h up to 150 mg/kg/day in divided doses q8h.

SIDE EFFECTS/ADVERSE REACTIONS

Frequent

Pain at IM injection site, GI disturbances, including mild diarrhea, nausea, or vomiting, oral or vaginal candidiasis

Occasional

Generalized rash, urticaria, phlebitis, thrombophlebitis with IV administration, headache

Rare

Dizziness, seizures, especially with IV therapy

PRECAUTIONS AND CONTRAINDICATIONS

Hypersensitivity to any penicillin, infectious mononucleosis

DRUG INTERACTIONS OF CONCERN TO DENTISTRY

- Decreased antimicrobial effectiveness: tetracyclines, erythromycins, lincomycins
- Increased ampicillin concentrations: probenecid
- Increased skin rash: allopurinol
- Decreased effects of atenolol
- Suspected increased risk of methotrexate toxicity

SERIOUS REACTIONS

! Altered bacterial balance may result in potentially fatal superinfections and antibiotic-associated colitis as evidenced by abdominal cramps, watery or severe diarrhea, and fever.
! Severe hypersensitivity reactions including anaphylaxis and acute interstitial nephritis occur rarely.

DENTAL CONSIDERATIONS

General:
- Take precautions regarding allergy to medication.
- Determine why the patient is taking the drug.

Consultations:
- Medical consultation may be required to assess disease control.

Teach Patient/Family to:
- Encourage effective oral hygiene to prevent soft tissue inflammation.
- Prevent injury when using oral hygiene aids.
- When used for dental infection, advise patient to:
  - Report sore throat, oral burning sensation, fever, and fatigue, any of which could indicate superinfection.
  - Take at prescribed intervals and complete dosage regimen.
  - Immediately notify the dentist if signs or symptoms of infection increase.

ampicillin sodium

am-pi-**sill′**-in **soe′**-dee-um
(Alphacin[AUS], Apo-Ampi[CAN], Novo-Ampicillin[CAN], Nu-Ampi[CAN], Polycillin, Principen)
Do not confuse ampicillin with aminophylline, Imipenem, or Unipen.

CATEGORY AND SCHEDULE

Pregnancy Risk Category: B

Drug Class: Aminopenicillin

MECHANISM OF ACTION

A penicillin that inhibits cell wall synthesis in susceptible microorganisms.
Therapeutic Effect: Bactericidal.

USES

Sinus infections, pneumonia, otitis media, skin infections, UTIs; effective for susceptible strains of β-lactamase negative) *E. coli, P. mirabilis, H. influenzae, S. faecalis, S. pneumoniae, S. typhosa, N. gonorrhoeae, N. meningitidis, L. monocytogenes,* shigella, enterococci

PHARMACOKINETICS

Moderately absorbed from the GI tract. Protein binding: 28%. Widely distributed. Partially metabolized in the liver. Primarily excreted in urine. Removed by hemodialysis. ***Half-life:*** 1–1.5 hr (increased in impaired renal function).

INDICATIONS AND DOSAGES

▸ Respiratory Tract, Skin and Skin-Structure Infections
PO
Adults, Elderly. 250–500 mg q6h.

Children. 50–100 mg/kg/day in divided doses q6h. Maximum: 3 g/day.
IV, IM
Adults, Elderly. 500 mg to 3 g q6h. Maximum: 14 g/day.
Children. 100–200 mg/kg/day in divided doses q6h.
Neonates. 50–100 mg/kg/day in divided doses q6–12h.

▸ Meningitis
IV
Children. 200–400 mg/kg/day in divided doses q6h. Maximum: 12 g/day.
Neonates. 100–200 mg/kg/day in divided doses q6–12h.

▸ Gonococcal Infections
PO
Adults. 3.5 g one time with 1 g probenecid.

▸ Perioperative Prophylaxis
IV, IM
Adults, Elderly. 2 g 30 min before procedure. May repeat in 8 hr.
Children. 50 mg/kg 30 min before procedure. May repeat in 8 hr.

▸ Dosage in Renal Impairment

Creatinine Clearance	% of Normal Dosage
10–30 ml/min	Give q6–12h
Less than 10 ml/min	Give q12h

SIDE EFFECTS/ADVERSE REACTIONS

Frequent
Pain at IM injection site, GI disturbances (mild diarrhea, nausea, vomiting), oral or vaginal candidiasis

Occasional
Generalized rash, urticaria, phlebitis or thrombophlebitis (with IV administration), headache

Rare
Dizziness, seizures (especially with IV therapy)

PRECAUTIONS AND CONTRAINDICATIONS

Hypersensitivity to any penicillin, infectious mononucleosis

DRUG INTERACTIONS OF CONCERN TO DENTISTRY

- Decreased antimicrobial effectiveness: tetracyclines, erythromycins, lincomycins
- Increased ampicillin concentrations: probenecid
- Increased skin rash: allopurinol
- Decreased effects of atenolol
- Suspected increased risk of methotrexate toxicity

SERIOUS REACTIONS

! Antibiotic-associated colitis and other superinfections may result from altered bacterial balance.

! Severe hypersensitivity reactions, including anaphylaxis and acute interstitial nephritis, occur rarely.

DENTAL CONSIDERATIONS

General:
- Take precautions regarding allergy to medication.
- Determine why the patient is taking the drug.

Consultations:
- Medical consultation may be required to assess disease control.

Teach Patient/Family to:
- Encourage effective oral hygiene to prevent soft tissue inflammation.
- Prevent injury when using oral hygiene aids.
- When used for dental infection, advise patient to:
    - Report sore throat, oral burning sensation, fever, and

fatigue, any of which could indicate superinfection.

- Take at prescribed intervals and complete dosage regimen.
- Immediately notify the dentist if signs or symptoms of infection increase.

ampicillin/sulbactam sodium

am′-pi-sill-in/sul-**bac′**-tam **so′**-dee-um
(Unasyn)

CATEGORY AND SCHEDULE

Pregnancy Risk Category: B

Drug Class: Aminopenicillin

MECHANISM OF ACTION

Ampicillin inhibits bacterial cell wall synthesis, while sulbactam inhibits bacterial β-lactamase. ***Therapeutic Effect:*** Ampicillin is bactericidal in susceptible microorganisms. Sulbactam protects ampicillin from enzymatic degradation.

USES

Elimination of bacteria

PHARMACOKINETICS

Protein binding: 28%–38%. Widely distributed. Partially metabolized in the liver. Primarily excreted in urine. Removed by hemodialysis. ***Half-life:*** 1 hr (increased in impaired renal function).

INDICATIONS AND DOSAGES

▸ **Skin and Skin-Structure, Intraabdominal, and Gynecologic Infections**

IV, IM

Adults, Elderly. 1.5 g (1 g ampicillin/500 mg sulbactam) to 3 g (2 g ampicillin/1 g sulbactam) q6h.

▸ **Dosage in Renal Impairment**

Dosage and frequency are modified based on creatinine clearance and the severity of the infection.

Creatinine Clearance	Dosage
Greater than 30 ml/min	0.5–3 g q6–8h
15–29 ml/min	1.5–3 g q12h
5–14 ml/min	1.5–3 g q24h
Less than 5 ml/min	Not recommended

SIDE EFFECTS/ADVERSE REACTIONS

Frequent

Diarrhea and rash (most common), urticaria, pain at IM injection site, thrombophlebitis with IV administration, oral or vaginal candidiasis

Occasional

Nausea, vomiting, headache, malaise, urine retention

PRECAUTIONS AND CONTRAINDICATIONS

Hypersensitivity to any penicillin, infectious mononucleosis

DRUG INTERACTIONS OF CONCERN TO DENTISTRY

- Decreased antimicrobial effectiveness: tetracyclines, erythromycins, lincomycins
- Increased ampicillin concentration: probenecid
- Increased skin rash: allopurinol
- Decreased effects of atenolol
- Suspected increased risk of methotrexate toxicity

• Increased risk of bleeding with anticoagulants: large IV doses of penicillins

SERIOUS REACTIONS

! Severe hypersensitivity reactions including anaphylaxis, acute interstitial nephritis, and blood dyscrasias may occur.
! Antibiotic-associated colitis and other superinfections may result from altered bacterial balance.
! Overdose may produce seizures.

DENTAL CONSIDERATIONS

General:
• For selected infections in the hospital setting, provide emergency dental treatment only.
• Caution regarding allergy to medication.
• Examine for oral manifestation of opportunistic infection.
• Determine why patient is taking the drug.
Consultations:
• Medical consultation may be required to assess disease control.
• Consult patient's physician if an acute dental infection occurs and another antiinfective is required.
Teach Patient/Family to:
• Encourage effective oral hygiene to prevent soft tissue inflammation.
• Report oral lesions, soreness, or bleeding to dentist.
• Prevent trauma when using oral hygiene aids.
• See dentist immediately if secondary oral infection occurs.
• When used for dental infection, advise patient to:
• Report sore throat, oral burning sensation, fever, or fatigue, any of which could indicate superinfection.
• Take at prescribed intervals and complete dosage regimen.
• Immediately notify the dentist if signs or symptoms of infection increase.

amprenavir

am-**pren**′-eh-veer
(Agenerase)
Do not confuse Agenerase with asparaginase.

CATEGORY AND SCHEDULE

Pregnancy Risk Category: C

Drug Class: Antiviral

MECHANISM OF ACTION

An antiretroviral that inhibits HIV-1 protease by binding to the enzyme's active site, thus preventing processing of viral precursors and resulting in the formation of immature, noninfectious viral particles.
Therapeutic Effect: Impairs HIV replication and proliferation.

USES

HIV-1 infection, in combination with other antiretroviral agents

PHARMACOKINETICS

Rapidly absorbed after PO administration. Protein binding: 90%. Metabolized in the liver. Primarily excreted in feces.
Half-life: 7.1–10.6 hr.

INDICATIONS AND DOSAGES

▸ HIV-1 Infection (in combination with other antiretrovirals)

PO

Adults, Children 13–16 yr. 1200 mg capsules twice a day.

Children 4–12 yr, and children 13–16 yr weighing less than 50 kg. 20 mg/kg twice a day or 15 mg/kg 3 times a day. Maximum: 2400 mg/day.

Oral Solution

Adults. 1400 mg 2 times/day.

Children 4–12 yr, and children 13–16 yr weighing less than 50 kg. 22.5 mg/kg/day (1.5 ml/kg) oral solution twice a day or 17 mg/kg/day (1.1 ml/kg) 3 times a day. Maximum: 2800 mg/day.

▸ Dosage in Hepatic Impairment

Dosage and frequency are modified on the basis of the Child-Pugh score.

Child-Pugh Scores	Capsules	Oral Solution
5–8	450 mg bid	513 mg bid
9–12	300 mg bid	342 mg bid

SIDE EFFECTS/ADVERSE REACTIONS

Frequent

Diarrhea or loose stools, nausea, oral paresthesia, rash, vomiting

Occasional

Peripheral paresthesia, depression

PRECAUTIONS AND CONTRAINDICATIONS

Concurrent use with midazolam, triazolam, bepridil, disulfiram, metronidazole, pimozide, and ergot-like drugs; hypersensitivity; serious reactions could occur with lidocaine (systemic) or other antiarrhythmics and tricyclic antidepressants; avoid use of drugs metabolized by CYP3A4 enzymes; lactation

Caution:

Exacerbation of diabetes, hyperglycemia, use of additional vitamin E, hemophilia, viral resistance, risk of cross allergy with sulfonamides, fat redistribution, hepatic disease, patients on oral contraceptives, sildenafil; oral solution contains propylene glycol with risk of toxicity to children younger than 4 yr

DRUG INTERACTIONS OF CONCERN TO DENTISTRY

- Contraindicated with midazolam, triazolam, tricyclic antidepressants
- Increased plasma levels of erythromycin, clarithromycin, itraconazole, alprazolam, clorazepate, diazepam, carbamazepine, loratadine, flurazepam, ketoconazole, itraconazole; lidocaine (systemic use for cardiac arrhythmias)
- Decreased effectiveness: dexamethasone, St. John's wort (herb)
- Use with caution: sildenafil, vardenafil, todalafil

SERIOUS REACTIONS

! Severe hypersensitivity reactions or Stevens-Johnson syndrome as evidenced by blisters, peeling of the skin, loosening of skin and mucous membranes, and fever may occur.

DENTAL CONSIDERATIONS

General:

- Palliative medication may be required for management of oral side effects.
- Examine for oral manifestation of opportunistic infection.

• Patients on chronic drug therapy may rarely have symptoms of blood dyscrasias, which can include infection, bleeding, and poor healing.
• Consider semisupine chair position for patient comfort if GI side effects occur.

Consultations:

• In a patient with symptoms of blood dyscrasias, request a medical consultation for blood studies and postpone treatment until normal values are reestablished.
• Medical consultation may be required to assess disease control and patient's ability to tolerate stress.

Teach Patient/Family to:

• Encourage effective oral hygiene to prevent soft tissue inflammation.
• Prevent trauma when using oral hygiene aids.
• Update health and drug history if physician makes any changes in evaluation or drug regimens.
• See dentist immediately if secondary oral infection occurs.

amyl nitrite

am′-il **nye′**-trite
(Amyl Nitrite)
Do not confuse with Nicobid, Nicoderm, Nilstat, nitroprusside, Nizoral, or Nystatin.

CATEGORY AND SCHEDULE

Pregnancy Risk Category: C

Drug Class: Antianginal

MECHANISM OF ACTION

A nitrite vasodilator that relaxes smooth muscles. Reduces afterload and improves vascular supply to the myocardium.
Therapeutic Effect: Dilates coronary arteries, improves blood flow to ischemic areas within myocardium, systemic vasodilation reduces workload on heart.

USES

Pain relief of anginal attacks

PHARMACOKINETICS

The vapors are absorbed rapidly through the pulmonary alveoli and metabolized rapidly. Partially excreted in the urine.

INDICATIONS AND DOSAGES

▸ **Acute Relief of Angina Pectoris**

Nasal Inhalation
Adults, Elderly. Place crushed capsule to nostrils for 0.18–0.3 ml inhalation of vapors. Repeat at 5–10 min intervals. No more than 3 doses in a 15–30 min period.

SIDE EFFECTS/ADVERSE REACTIONS

Frequent

Headache (may be severe) occurs mostly in early therapy, diminishes rapidly in intensity, usually disappears during continued treatment; transient flushing of face and neck; dizziness (especially if patient is standing immobile or is in a warm environment); weakness; postural hypotension

Occasional

Nausea, rash, vomiting

Rare

Involuntary passage of urine and feces, restlessness, weakness

PRECAUTIONS AND CONTRAINDICATIONS

Closed-angle glaucoma, severe anemia, head injury, postural

hypotension, pregnancy, hypersensitivity to nitrates

DRUG INTERACTIONS OF CONCERN TO DENTISTRY

• None reported

SERIOUS REACTIONS

! Large doses may produce hemolytic anemia or methemoglobinemia.
! Severe postural hypotension manifested by fainting, pulselessness, cold or clammy skin, and profuse sweating may occur.
! Tolerance may occur with repeated, prolonged therapy.
! High dose tends to produce severe headache.

DENTAL CONSIDERATIONS

General:

• For emergency relief of acute angina; if angina is not relieved, call 911 for transfer of patient to a medical emergency facility.
• Prior to treatment, inquire about disease control and frequency of angina episodes.
• Ensure that patient's rescue antianginal drug is available for use.
• Monitor vital signs at every appointment because of cardiovascular side effects.
• Postpone elective dental treatment if patient shows signs of cardiac symptoms or respiratory distress.
• After supine positioning, have patient sit upright for at least 2 min before standing to avoid orthostatic hypotension.

Consultations:

• Medical consultation may be required to assess disease control and patient's ability to tolerate stress.

Teach Patient/Family to:

• Report angina symptoms to physician.
• Update health and medication history if physician makes any changes in evaluation or drug regimens; include OTC, herbal, and nonherbal remedies in the update.
• Encourage effective oral hygiene to prevent soft tissue inflammation.

anagrelide

ah-**na**′-greh-lide
(Agrylin)

CATEGORY AND SCHEDULE

Pregnancy Risk Category: C

Drug Class: Platelet count-reducing agent

MECHANISM OF ACTION

A hematologic agent that reduces platelet production and prevents platelet shape changes caused by platelet aggregating substances. ***Therapeutic Effect:*** Inhibits platelet aggregation.

USES

Decreases the risk of blood clots in patients who have too many platelet cells

PHARMACOKINETICS

After oral administration, plasma concentration peak within 1 hr. Extensively metabolized. Primarily excreted in urine. ***Half-life:*** About 3 days.

INDICATIONS AND DOSAGES

▸ **Thrombocythemia**

PO

Adults, Elderly. Initially, 0.5 mg 4 times a day or 1 mg twice a day. Adjust to lowest effective dosage, increasing by up to 0.5 mg/day or less in any 1 wk. Maximum: 10 mg/day or 2.5 mg/dose.

SIDE EFFECTS/ADVERSE REACTIONS

Frequent

Headache, palpitations, diarrhea, abdominal pain, nausea, flatulence, bloating, asthenia, pain, dizziness

Occasional

Tachycardia, chest pain, vomiting, paresthesia, peripheral edema, anorexia, dyspepsia, rash

Rare

Confusion, insomnia

PRECAUTIONS AND CONTRAINDICATIONS

Caution:

Cardiac disease, renal impairment, hepatic impairment, monitor reduction in platelets, risk of thrombocytopenia especially while correct dose is being found, sudden discontinuance of use, lactation, children younger than 16 yr

DRUG INTERACTIONS OF CONCERN TO DENTISTRY

• Possible risk of hemorrhage: NSAIDs, aspirin

SERIOUS REACTIONS

! Angina, heart failure, and arrhythmias occur rarely.

DENTAL CONSIDERATIONS

General:

• Laboratory studies should include routine complete blood counts (CBCs).

• Patients have risk of thrombohemorrhagic complications; prolonged bleeding time, anemia, or splenomegaly may occur in some patients with this disease. However, thrombosis may also occur in some patients.

• Mucosal bleeding can be a symptom of disease.

• Patients with severe symptoms may be taking chemotherapy.

• Monitor vital signs at every appointment because of cardiovascular side effects.

• Consider semisupine chair position for patient comfort if GI side effects occur.

Consultations:

• Medical consultation with hematologist or physician directing therapy is essential before dental treatment.

Teach Patient/Family to:

• Inform dentist of unusual bleeding episodes following dental treatment.

• Update health and drug history if physician makes any changes in evaluation or drug regimens.

anakinra

an-ah-**kin**′-ra

(Kineret)

CATEGORY AND SCHEDULE

Pregnancy Risk Category: B

Drug Class: Antirheumatic

MECHANISM OF ACTION

An interleukin-1 (IL-1) receptor antagonist that blocks the binding of IL-1, a protein that is a major mediator of joint disease and is present in excess amounts in patients with rheumatoid arthritis.

Therapeutic Effect: Inhibits the inflammatory response.

USES

Treatment of moderate to severe symptoms of rheumatoid arthritis

PHARMACOKINETICS

No accumulation of anakinra in tissues or organs was observed after daily subcutaneous doses. Excreted in urine. ***Half-life:*** 4–6 hr.

INDICATIONS AND DOSAGES

▸ Rheumatoid Arthritis

Subcutaneous

Adults, Children older than 18 yr, Elderly. 100 mg/day, given at same time each day.

SIDE EFFECTS/ADVERSE REACTIONS

Occasional

Injection site ecchymosis, erythema, and inflammation

Rare

Headache, nausea, diarrhea, abdominal pain

PRECAUTIONS AND CONTRAINDICATIONS

Known hypersensitivity to *Escherichia coli*-derived proteins, serious infection

DRUG INTERACTIONS OF CONCERN TO DENTISTRY

- None reported

SERIOUS REACTIONS

! Infections, including upper respiratory tract infection, sinusitis, flu-like symptoms, and cellulitis, have been noted.

! Neutropenia may occur, particularly when anakinra is used in combination with tumor necrosis factor-blocking agents.

DENTAL CONSIDERATIONS

General:

- Question patient about other drugs or products he or she may be taking for arthritis.
- Patient may be at risk for infection.
- Oral infections should be eliminated and/or treated aggressively.
- Evaluate efficacy of oral hygiene home care; preventive instruction appointment may be necessary.
- Patient on chronic drug therapy may rarely present with symptoms of blood dyscrasias, which can include infection, bleeding, and poor healing. If dyscrasia is present, caution patient to prevent oral tissue trauma when using oral hygiene aids.
- Patient may need assistance in getting into and out of dental chair. Adjust chair position for patient comfort.

Consultations:

- Medical consultation may be required to assess disease control.
- In a patient with symptoms of blood dyscrasias, request a medical consultation for blood studies and postpone treatment until normal values are reestablished.

Teach Patient/Family to:

- Use powered tooth brush if patient has difficulty holding conventional devices.
- Prevent trauma when using oral hygiene aids.
- Encourage effective oral hygiene to prevent soft tissue inflammation.
- Update health and medication history if physician makes any changes in evaluation or drug regimens; include OTC, herbal, and nonherbal remedies in the update.

anastrozole

ah-**nas**′-trow-zole
(Arimidex)
Do not confuse Arimidex with Imitrex.

CATEGORY AND SCHEDULE

Pregnancy Risk Category: D

Drug Class: Antineoplastic

MECHANISM OF ACTION

Decreases the circulating estrogen level by inhibiting aromatase, the enzyme that catalyzes the final step in estrogen production.
Therapeutic Effect: Inhibits the growth of breast cancers that are stimulated by estrogens.

USES

Treatment of breast cancer

PHARMACOKINETICS

Well absorbed into systemic circulation (absorption not affected by food). Protein binding: 40%. Extensively metabolized in the liver. Eliminated by biliary system and, to a lesser extent, kidneys. ***Mean Half-life:*** 50 hr in postmenopausal women. Steady-state plasma levels reached in about 7 days.

INDICATIONS AND DOSAGES

▸ **Breast Cancer**

PO

Adults, Elderly. 1 mg once a day.

SIDE EFFECTS/ADVERSE REACTIONS

Frequent

Asthenia, nausea, headache, hot flashes, back pain, vomiting, cough, diarrhea

Occasional

Constipation, abdominal pain, anorexia, bone pain, pharyngitis, dizziness, rash, dry mouth, peripheral edema, pelvic pain, depression, chest pain, paresthesia

Rare

Weight gain, diaphoresis

PRECAUTIONS AND CONTRAINDICATIONS

None known

DRUG INTERACTIONS OF CONCERN TO DENTISTRY

- None reported

SERIOUS REACTIONS

! Thrombophlebitis, anemia, leukopenia, and vaginal hemorrhage occur rarely.

! Vaginal hemorrhage occurs rarely (2%).

DENTAL CONSIDERATIONS

General:

- Monitor vital signs at every appointment because of cardiovascular side effects.
- If additional analgesia is required for dental pain, consider alternative analgesics (NSAIDs) in patients taking narcotics for acute or chronic pain.
- Avoid products that affect platelet function, such as aspirin and NSAIDs.
- Consider semisupine chair position for patient comfort if GI side effects occur.
- Examine for oral manifestation of opportunistic infection.
- Patient on chronic drug therapy may rarely present with symptoms of blood dyscrasias, which can include infection, bleeding, and poor healing. If dyscrasia is present, caution patient to prevent oral tissue

trauma when using oral hygiene aids.

• Assess salivary flow as a factor in caries, periodontal disease, and candidiasis.

Consultations:

• Consider consulting with physician before prescribing drugs that may cause constipation (narcotics).

• Consultation with physician may be necessary if sedation or general anesthesia is required.

• In a patient with symptoms of blood dyscrasias, request a medical consultation for blood studies and postpone treatment until normal values are reestablished.

• Medical consultation may be required to assess disease control and patient's ability to tolerate stress.

Teach Patient/Family to:

• Encourage effective oral hygiene to prevent soft tissue inflammation.

• Prevent trauma when using oral hygiene aids.

• Update health and medication history if physician makes any changes in evaluation or drug regimens; include OTC, herbal, and nonherbal remedies in the update.

• When chronic dry mouth occurs, advise patient to:

  • Avoid mouth rinses with high alcohol content because of drying effects.

  • Use daily home fluoride products for anticaries effect.

  • Use sugarless gum, frequent sips of water, or saliva substitutes.

anidulafungin

ann-id-yoo-la-**fun**′-jin

(Eraxis)

CATEGORY AND SCHEDULE

Pregnancy Risk Category: C

Drug Class: Antifungal

MECHANISM OF ACTION

An antifungal that inhibits the synthesis of 1,3-β-D-glucan, an essential component of the fungal cell wall.

Therapeutic Effect: Fungistatic.

USES

Treatment of fungal infections including candidemia and esophageal candidiasis.

PHARMACOKINETICS

Protein binding: 84%. Metabolism in the liver has not been observed. Approximately 30% eliminated in feces; less than 1% excreted in the urine. ***Half-life:*** 26.5 hr.

INDICATIONS AND DOSAGES

▸ Candidemia

IV

Adults. 200 mg loading dose on day 1, followed by 100 mg daily thereafter. Continue for at least 14 days after the last positive culture.

▸ Esophageal Candidiasis

IV

Adult. 100 mg loading dose on day 1, followed by 50 mg daily for a minimum of 14 days and for at least 7 days following resolution of symptoms.

Children. Safety and efficacy have not been established.

SIDE EFFECTS/ADVERSE REACTIONS

Rare

Diarrhea, hypokalemia, abnormal liver function, rash, urticaria, flushing, pruritus, dyspnea, hypotension, deep vein thrombosis

PRECAUTIONS AND CONTRAINDICATIONS

Hypersensitivity to anidulafungin or its components

Caution:

Do not breast-feed, hepatic impairment

DRUG INTERACTIONS OF CONCERN TO DENTISTRY

• None reported

SERIOUS REACTIONS

! Histamine-mediated symptoms including rash, urticaria, flushing, pruritus, dyspnea, and hypotension have been reported.

DENTAL CONSIDERATIONS

General:

• Determine why the patient is taking the drug.
• Examine oral mucous membranes for signs of residual fungal infection.
• Monitor vital signs at each appointment because of cardiovascular side effects.
• Consult physician to determine control of disease.
• Consider removable prostheses as residual source of candidal organisms.

Teach Patient/Family to:

• Soak full or partial dentures in an antifungal solution at night until lesions are absent; prolonged infections may require fabrication of new prosthesis.
• Dispose of tooth brush used during oral infection after oral lesions are absent to prevent reinoculation.
• Comply with antifungal therapy completely to eliminate infection and complete entire course of medication.

anthralin

anth-**rah′**-lin

(A-Fil, Anthra-Derm, Anthraforte[CAN], Anthranol[CAN], Anthrascalp[CAN], Dithrocream[AUS], Drithocreme, Dritho-Scalp, Micanol, Psoriatec)

(capsules, tablets, chewable tablets, syrup, elixir, cream, spray)

Do not confuse with Antagon, Antabuse, or Andriol.

CATEGORY AND SCHEDULE

Pregnancy Risk Category: C

Drug Class: Antipsoriatic

MECHANISM OF ACTION

A topical agent that binds DNA, inhibiting synthesis of nucleic protein, and reduces mitotic activity.

Therapeutic Effect: Results in damage to DNA sugar and enhances membrane lipid peroxidation, which may play a critical role in the antipsoriatic action.

USES

Treatment of psoriasis

PHARMACOKINETICS

Poorly absorbed systemically, but excellent epidermal absorption. Auto-oxidized to inactive metabolites-danthrone and dianthrone. Rapid urinary excretion, so significant levels do not accumulate in the blood or other tissues. ***Half-life:*** 6 hr.

INDICATIONS AND DOSAGES

▸ **Psoriasis**

Topical

Adults, Elderly. Apply in a thin layer to affected areas q12h or q24h.

SIDE EFFECTS/ADVERSE REACTIONS

Frequent

Irritation

Rare

Neutrophilia, proteinuria, staining of the skin

PRECAUTIONS AND CONTRAINDICATIONS

Acute psoriasis where inflammation is present, erythroderma, hypersensitivity to anthralin

DRUG INTERACTIONS OF CONCERN TO DENTISTRY

• None reported

SERIOUS REACTIONS

! Patients with renal disease should have routine urine tests for albuminuria.

! Hypersensitivity reaction, such as burning, erythema, and dermatitis, may occur.

DENTAL CONSIDERATIONS

General:

• Determine why patient is taking the drug.

• Arthritic symptoms may occur in some patients; inquire about use of other medications.

apomorphine

ah-poe-**more′**-feen

(Apokyn)

CATEGORY AND SCHEDULE

Pregnancy Risk Category: C

Drug Class: Anti-Parkinson's agent

MECHANISM OF ACTION

Stimulation of postsynaptic dopamine receptors in the brain, counteracting the excess cholinergic activity responsible for striatal excitation and involuntary movements.

USES

Control of acute loss of control of body movements in advanced Parkinson's disease

PHARMACOKINETICS

Rapidly absorbed after subcutaneous injection. Protein binding: 99.9%. Widely distributed. ***Half-life:*** 45 min; rapidly metabolized, not detectable in urine or bodily secretions in unchanged form.

INDICATIONS AND DOSAGES

▸ **Acute, Intermittent Treatment of Hypomobility ("Off Episodes") Associated with Advanced Parkinson's Disease**

Injection Pen for Subcutaneous Administration

Adult, Elderly. Subcutaneous, 0.2 ml (2 mg) initially; may be increased in 0.1-ml (1-mg) increments every few days, up to a maximum of 0.6 ml (6 mg).

SIDE EFFECTS/ADVERSE REACTIONS

ORAL: Stomatitis, taste alterations

CNS: Somnolence, dizziness, headache, depression, hallucinations (rare)
CV: Chest pain, tachycardia, shortness of breath
GI: Nausea, vomiting
RESP: Respiratory depression, tachypnea
INTEG: Injection site discomfort
MS: May exacerbate preexisting dyskinesias

PRECAUTIONS AND CONTRAINDICATIONS

Hypersensitivity, irritable bowel or antiemetic therapy with 5-HT3 antagonists (e.g., ondansetron). Do not administer with antiemetics other than 5-HT3 antagonists. Use with caution in patients with cardiac decompensation or impaired hepatic or renal function. Do not use if solution is cloudy, contains particulates, or is discolored.

DRUG INTERACTIONS OF CONCERN TO DENTISTRY

• CNS depressants may intensify adverse effects of therapy (e.g., dizziness).
• Phenothiazines may reduce effectiveness of apomorphine.

DENTAL CONSIDERATIONS

General:
• Monitor vital signs because of possible cardiovascular and respiratory effects.
• Understand limitations of Parkinson's disease on dental treatment.
• After supine positioning, have patient sit upright for 2 min before standing to avoid orthostatic hypotension.
• Assist patient with ambulation if dizziness or loss of coordination occurs.
• Differentiate taste alterations because of drug from those associated with restorative materials.

Consultations:
• Consult physician to determine degree of disease control and patient's ability to tolerate dental treatment.

Teach Patient/Family to:
• Encourage effective oral hygiene measures to prevent soft tissue inflammation.
• Help patient with effective dental home care to minimize oral diseases if patient lacks adequate motor coordination.

apraclonidine hydrochloride

ap-ra-**kloe**′-ni-deen
hi-droh-**klor**′-ide
(Iopidine)
Do not confuse with Cetapred, clomiphene, Klonopin, or quinidine.

CATEGORY AND SCHEDULE

Pregnancy Risk Category: C

Drug Class: Selective α_2-adrenergic agonist

MECHANISM OF ACTION

An ocular α-adrenergic agent that is relatively selective for α_2 receptor agonist.
Therapeutic Effect: Reduces intraocular pressure.

USES

Control or prevention of increases in intraocular pressure related to laser surgery of eye; short-term control of increased intraocular pressure as an adjunctive drug

PHARMACOKINETICS

Onset of action occurs within 1 hr. The duration of a single dose is about 12 hr. ***Half-life:*** 8 hr.

INDICATIONS AND DOSAGES

▸ Glaucoma

Ophthalmic

Adults, Elderly. Instill 1 drop of 0.5% solution to affected eye(s) 3 times a day.

▸ Intraocular Hypertension, Post Laser Surgery

Ophthalmic

Adults, Elderly. Instill 1 drop of 1% solution in operative eye(s) 1 hr before surgery and 1 drop postoperatively.

SIDE EFFECTS/ADVERSE REACTIONS

Frequent

Eye discomfort, dry mouth

Occasional

Headache, constipation, redness around eye, conjunctivitis, changes in visual acuity, mydriasis, ocular inflammation

Rare

Nasal decongestion

PRECAUTIONS AND CONTRAINDICATIONS

Hypersensitivity to apraclonidine or clonidine or any component of the formulation

Caution:

Tachyphylaxis, impaired renal or liver function, depression, lactation, children, cardiovascular disease, cardiovascular drugs

DRUG INTERACTIONS OF CONCERN TO DENTISTRY

- No drug interactions have been reported; this is a new drug and data are lacking.
- Avoid using drugs that can exacerbate glaucoma: anticholinergic drugs.

SERIOUS REACTIONS

! Allergic reaction occurs rarely.

! Peripheral edema and arrhythmias have been reported.

DENTAL CONSIDERATIONS

General:

- Protect patient's eyes from accidental spatter during dental treatment.
- Avoid dental light in patient's eyes; offer dark glasses for patient comfort.
- Determine why the patient is taking the drug.
- Assess salivary flow as a factor in caries, periodontal disease, and candidiasis.

Consultations:

- Medical consultation may be required to assess disease control.

Teach Patient/Family to:

- When chronic dry mouth occurs, advise patient to:
  - Avoid mouth rinses with high alcohol content because of drying effects.
  - Use daily home fluoride to prevent caries.
  - Use sugarless gum, frequent sips of water, or saliva substitutes.

aprepitant

ah-**prep**′-ih-tant

(Emend)

CATEGORY AND SCHEDULE

Pregnancy Risk Category: B

Drug Class: Antiemetic

MECHANISM OF ACTION

A selective human substance P and neurokinin-1 (NK1) receptor antagonist that inhibits chemotherapy-induced nausea and vomiting centrally in the chemoreceptor trigger zone.
Therapeutic Effect: Prevents the acute and delayed phases of chemotherapy-induced emesis, including vomiting caused by high-dose cisplatin.

USES

Prevention of acute and delayed nausea/vomiting associated with cancer chemotherapy, including high-dose cisplatin; for acute use only

PHARMACOKINETICS

Crosses the blood-brain barrier. Extensively metabolized in the liver. Eliminated primarily by liver metabolism (not excreted renally).
Half-life: 9–13 hr.

INDICATIONS AND DOSAGES

▸ Prevention of Chemotherapy-Induced Nausea and Vomiting

PO

Adults, Elderly. 125 mg 1 hr before chemotherapy on day 1 and 80 mg once a day in the morning on days 2 and 3.

SIDE EFFECTS/ADVERSE REACTIONS

Frequent

Fatigue, nausea, hiccups, diarrhea, constipation, anorexia

Occasional

Headache, vomiting, dizziness, dehydration, heartburn

Rare

Abdominal pain, epigastric discomfort, gastritis, tinnitus, insomnia

PRECAUTIONS AND CONTRAINDICATIONS

Breast-feeding, concurrent use of pimozide (Orap)

Caution:

Patients taking drugs metabolized by CYP3A4 enzymes; not for chronic use; acts as a moderate inhibitor of CYP3A4 and an inducer of CYP3A4 and CYP2C9; use with caution in lactation, safety and efficacy in pediatric patients not established

DRUG INTERACTIONS OF CONCERN TO DENTISTRY

- Increased plasma concentrations of midazolam and other benzodiazepines metabolized by CYP3A4
- Increased plasma levels: concurrent use of drugs that inhibit CYP3A4 enzymes (fluconazole, itraconazole, ketoconazole, erythromycin, and clarithromycin)
- Decreased plasma levels: concurrent use of drugs that induce CYP3A4 enzymes (carbamazepine)

SERIOUS REACTIONS

! Neutropenia and mucous membrane disorders occur rarely.

DENTAL CONSIDERATIONS

General:

- Patients using this drug are also undergoing or have recently undergone cancer chemotherapy; take a complete health history.
- Chemotherapy patients may show stomatitis and ulceration; palliative therapy may be required.
- Consider semisupine chair position for patient comfort if GI side effects occur.
- Examine for oral manifestation of opportunistic infection.

• Short appointments and a stress-reduction protocol may be required for anxious patients.
• Patients taking opioids for acute or chronic pain should be given alternative analgesics for dental pain.
• Patients on chronic drug therapy may rarely have symptoms of blood dyscrasias, which can include infection, bleeding, and poor healing.
• Consult physician; prophylactic or therapeutic antibiotics may be indicated to prevent or treat infection if surgery or periodontal debridement is required for patients undergoing chemotherapy.

Consultations:

• Medical consultation may be required to assess immunologic status during cancer therapy and determine safety risks posed by dental treatment.
• Consultation with physician may be necessary if sedation or general anesthesia is required.
• Medical consultation may be required to assess disease control and patient's ability to tolerate stress.

Teach Patient/Family to:

• Encourage effective oral hygiene to prevent soft tissue inflammation.
• Prevent trauma when using oral hygiene aids.
• Importance of updating health and drug history if physician makes any changes in evaluation or drug regimens.

arformoterol tartrate

ar-for-**moe′**-ter-ole **tar′**-trate
(Brovana)

CATEGORY AND SCHEDULE

Pregnancy Risk Category: C

Drug Class: β_2 agonist

MECHANISM OF ACTION

A long-acting β_2 agonist that stimulates adrenergic receptors in bronchial smooth muscle causing relaxation of smooth muscle.
Therapeutic Effect: Produces bronchodilation.

USES

Used for chronic obstructive pulmonary disease (COPD).

PHARMACOKINETICS

Primarily absorbed by the pulmonary system following inhalation. Protein binding: 52%–65%. Primarily metabolized by glucuronidation. Primarily excreted in urine; partial elimination in feces. ***Half-life:*** 26 hr.

INDICATIONS AND DOSAGES

▸ COPD

Oral Inhalation
Adults. 15 mcg (2 ml) twice a day by nebulization.
Children. Safety and efficacy have not been established in children.

SIDE EFFECTS/ADVERSE REACTIONS

Occasional

Pain, chest pain, back pain, sinusitis, rash, leg cramps, dyspnea, peripheral edema

Rare

Oral candidiasis, pulmonary congestion

PRECAUTIONS AND CONTRAINDICATIONS

Hypersensitivity to arformoterol or its components

Caution:

Acutely deteriorating COPD, cardiovascular disorders, convulsive disorders, diabetes mellitus, thyrotoxicosis, coadministration with other long-acting β_2 agonists

DRUG INTERACTIONS OF CONCERN TO DENTISTRY

- Methylxanthines (e.g., aminophylline, theophylline), steroids, diuretics: may potentiate hypokalemic effects.
- Tricyclic antidepressants, drugs that prolong QT interval: may potentiate cardiovascular effects.

SERIOUS REACTIONS

! May increase the risk of asthma-related death.

! May exacerbate cardiovascular conditions including arrhythmias and hypertension.

! Hypersensitivity reactions including urticaria, angioedema, rash, bronchospasm, and anaphylaxis may occur.

DENTAL CONSIDERATIONS

General:

- Monitor vital signs at every appointment because of cardiovascular and respiratory side effects.
- Evaluate oral mucous membranes for signs of candidiasis.
- Consider semisupine chair position for patients with respiratory disease.
- Midday appointments and stress-reduction protocol may be required for anxious patients.
- Aspirin, NSAIDs, and bisulfites in local anesthetics may exacerbate asthma.
- Acute asthmatic episodes may be precipitated in the dental office. Sympathomimetic/bronchodilator inhalants should be available for emergency use.

Consultations:

- Consult physician to determine control of disease and ability of patient to tolerate dental procedures.

Teach Patient/Family to:

- Rinse mouth with water after each dose of drug to prevent dryness.

argatroban

ar-**gat**′-tro-ban

(Acova)

Do not confuse argatroban with Aggrestat or Orgaran.

CATEGORY AND SCHEDULE

Pregnancy Risk Category: B

Drug Class: Anticoagulant

MECHANISM OF ACTION

A direct thrombin inhibitor that reversibly binds to thrombin-active sites. Inhibits thrombin-catalyzed or thrombin-induced reactions, including fibrin formation, activation of coagulant factors V, VIII, and XIII; also inhibits protein C formation and platelet aggregation. ***Therapeutic Effect:*** Produces anticoagulation.

USES

An anticoagulant for prophylaxis or treatment of thrombosis in patients with heparin-induced thrombocytopenia

PHARMACOKINETICS

Following IV administration, distributed primarily in extracellular fluid. Protein binding: 54%.

Metabolized in the liver. Primarily excreted in the feces, presumably through biliary secretion. ***Half-life:*** 39–51 min.

INDICATIONS AND DOSAGES

▸ To Prevent and Treat Heparin-Induced Thrombocytopenia

IV Infusion

Adults, Elderly. Initially, 2 mcg/kg/min administered as a continuous infusion. After initial infusion, dose may be adjusted until steady state aPTT is 1.5–3 times initial baseline value, not to exceed 100 sec.

▸ Percutaneous Coronary Intervention

IV Infusion

Adults, Elderly. Initially, 25 mcg/kg/min and administer bolus of 350 mcg/kg over 3–5 min. ACT (activated clotting time) checked in 5–10 min following bolus. If ACT is less than 300 sec, give additional bolus 150 mcg/kg, increase infusion to 30 mcg/kg/min. If ACT is greater than 450 sec, decrease infusion to 15 mcg/kg/min. Once ACT of 300–450 sec achieved, proceed with procedure.

▸ Dosage in Hepatic Impairment

Adults, Elderly. Initially, 0.5 mcg/kg/min.

SIDE EFFECTS/ADVERSE REACTIONS

Frequent

Dyspnea, hypotension, fever, diarrhea, nausea, pain, vomiting, infection, cough

PRECAUTIONS AND CONTRAINDICATIONS

Overt major bleeding

DRUG INTERACTIONS OF CONCERN TO DENTISTRY

• Increased risk of bleeding: drugs that interfere with coagulation or platelet function, such as NSAIDs and aspirin

SERIOUS REACTIONS

! Ventricular tachycardia and atrial fibrillation occur occasionally.

! Major bleeding and sepsis occur rarely.

DENTAL CONSIDERATIONS

General:

• Patients are at risk of bleeding; check for oral signs.

• Delay elective dental treatment until patient completes parenteral anticoagulant therapy.

• Determine why patient is taking the drug.

• Avoid products that affect platelet function, such as aspirin and NSAIDs.

• Consider local hemostasis measures to prevent excessive bleeding.

Consultations:

• Medical consultation should include partial prothrombin time, prothrombin time, or INR.

• Medical consultation should include routine blood counts including platelet counts and aggregation.

Teach Patient/Family to:

• Use soft tooth brush to reduce risk of bleeding.

• Encourage effective oral hygiene to prevent soft tissue inflammation.

• Report oral lesions, soreness, or bleeding to dentist.

• Prevent trauma when using oral hygiene aids.

• Update health and medication history if physician makes any changes in evaluation or drug regimens; include OTC, herbal, and nonherbal remedies in the update.

• Inform dentist of unusual bleeding episodes following dental treatment.

aripiprazole

ar-ah-**pip**′-rah-zole
(Abilify)

CATEGORY AND SCHEDULE

Pregnancy Risk Category: C

Drug Class: Antipsychotic

MECHANISM OF ACTION

An antipsychotic agent that provides partial agonist activity at dopamine and serotonin (5-HT1A) receptors and antagonist activity at serotonin (5-HT2A) receptors.
Therapeutic Effect: Diminishes schizophrenic behavior.

USES

Treatment of schizophrenia

PHARMACOKINETICS

Well absorbed through the GI tract. Protein binding: 99% (primarily albumin). Reaches steady levels in 2 wk. Metabolized in the liver. Eliminated primarily in feces and, to a lesser extent, in urine. Not removed by hemodialysis. ***Half-life:*** 75 hr.

INDICATIONS AND DOSAGES

▸ **Schizophrenia, Bipolar Disorder**

PO

Adults, Elderly. Initially, 10–15 mg once a day. May increase up to 30 mg/day.

SIDE EFFECTS/ADVERSE REACTIONS

Frequent

Weight gain, headache, insomnia, vomiting

Occasional

Light-headedness, nausea, akathisia, somnolence

Rare

Blurred vision, constipation, asthenia or loss of energy and strength, anxiety, fever, rash, cough, rhinitis, orthostatic hypotension

PRECAUTIONS AND CONTRAINDICATIONS

Hypersensitivity

Caution:

Known cardiovascular diseases, cerebrovascular disease, or other conditions predisposing the patient to hypotension; seizures, may impair judgment or motor skills, elevated body temperature, suicide, dysphagia, dehydration, severe renal or hepatic impairment, avoid breast-feeding and use in children

DRUG INTERACTIONS OF CONCERN TO DENTISTRY

- Possible lowering of blood levels: carbamazepine and other inducers of CYP3A4 isoenzymes
- Increased blood levels: ketoconazole and other inhibitors of CYP3A4 or CYP2D6 isoenzymes
- Caution with CNS depressants and alcohol

SERIOUS REACTIONS

! Extrapyramidal symptoms and neuroleptic malignant syndrome occur rarely.

DENTAL CONSIDERATIONS

General:

- Assess for presence of extrapyramidal motor symptoms, such as tardive dyskinesia and akathisia. Extrapyramidal motor activity may complicate dental treatment.
- Consider semisupine chair position for patient comfort if GI side effects occur.

Consultations:

• Consultation with physician may be necessary if sedation or general anesthesia is required.

• Medical consultation may be required to assess disease control and patient's ability to tolerate stress.

Teach Patient/Family to:

• Consult physician if signs of tardive dyskinesia or akathisia are present.

• Encourage effective oral hygiene to prevent soft tissue inflammation.

• Use powered tooth brush if patient has difficulty holding conventional devices.

• Update health and drug history if physician makes any changes in evaluation or drug regimens.

armodafinil

ar-moe-**daf'**-i-nil

(Nuvigil)

CATEGORY AND SCHEDULE

Pregnancy Risk Category: C

Controlled Substance: Schedule IV

Drug Class: CNS stimulant

MECHANISM OF ACTION

Alpha-1 agonist and the R-enantiomer of modafinil. The exact mechanism of action is unknown. Binds to dopamine transporter and inhibits dopamine reuptake.

USES

Narcolepsy; obstructive sleep apnea/hypopnea syndrome (OSAHS); shift-work sleep disorder (SWSD)

PHARMACOKINETICS

Readily absorbed after oral administration. Food may delay absorption. Protein binding: 60%. Widely distributed. Metabolized in liver to R-modafinil acid and modafinil sulfone. Excreted primarily in urine (80%, and <10% unchanged drug). ***Half-life*:** 15 hr.

INDICATIONS AND DOSAGES

▸ **Narcolepsy, Improve Wakefulness in Patients with Excessive Sleepiness; Obstructive Sleep Apnea**

PO

Adults. 150 mg or 250 mg as a single dose in the morning.

▸ **Shift-Work Sleep Disorder**

PO

Adults. 150 mg daily approximately 1 hr before to the start of work shift.

Pediatric. Not approved for use in children.

Dose adjustments. Severe hepatic impairment: dose should be reduced by half.

Renal impairment: Inadequate data to determine safety and efficacy.

SIDE EFFECTS/ADVERSE REACTIONS

Frequent

Neurologic: dizziness, headache (dose-related), insomnia

Gastrointestinal: diarrhea, nausea, xerostomia

Occasional

Rash, indigestion, increased heart rate, anxiety

Rare

Stevens-Johnson syndrome, anaphylaxis, angioedema, dyspnea

PRECAUTIONS AND CONTRAINDICATIONS

Contraindications: hypersensitivity to modafinil, armodafinil, or any component of the formulation.

Serious and life-threatening rashes, including Stevens-Johnson syndrome, and rare cases of multi-organ hypersensitivity reactions have occurred with armodafinil use.
Use with caution in patients with cardiovascular diseases (increased risk of cardiac adverse events), hepatic impairment, psychiatric disorder (increased risk of psychiatric adverse effects), renal impairment (drug clearance may be reduced); and excessive sleepiness. Avoid or limit alcohol.

DRUG INTERACTIONS OF CONCERN TO DENTISTRY

- CYP3A4 substrates: Armodafinil may decrease the levels and effects of CYP3A4 substrates (e.g., lidocaine).
- CYP3A4 inhibitors: May increase the concentrations of armodafinil.

SERIOUS REACTIONS

! Serious and life-threatening rashes, including Stevens-Johnson syndrome. Patients should be advised to discontinue drug at first sign of rash.
! Rare cases of angioedema reactions have been reported with the use of armodafinil.

DENTAL CONSIDERATIONS

General:

- Xerostomia may complicate dental treatment and oral hygiene.
- Monitor vital signs at every appointment because of cardiovascular effects.
- Consider semisupine chair position for patient comfort if GI side effects occur.
- Use vasoconstrictors with caution, at low doses, and with careful aspiration.

Teach Patient/Family to:

- Encourage effective oral hygiene to prevent soft tissue inflammation.
- Prevent injury when using oral hygiene aids.
- When chronic dry mouth (xerostomia) occurs, advise patient to:
  - Avoid mouth rinses with high alcohol content because of drying effects.
  - Use daily home fluoride products for anticaries effect.
  - Use sugarless gum, frequent sips of water, or saliva substitutes.

artemether/ lumefantrine

ar-**tem**′-e-ther / **loo**-me-**fan**′-treen
(Coartem)

CATEGORY AND SCHEDULE

Pregnancy Risk Category: C

Drug Class: Antimalarial

MECHANISM OF ACTION

A semisynthetic derivative of artemisinin that destroys the malarial pathogen *Plasmodium falciparum*. Artemether is rapidly metabolized into an active metabolite dihydroartemisinin (DHA). The antimalarial activity of artemether and DHA has been attributed to endoperoxide moiety. Both artemether and lumefantrine were shown to inhibit nucleic acid and protein synthesis.
Therapeutic Effect: Inhibits parasite growth.

USES

Malaria due to *Plasmodium falciparum*

PHARMACOKINETICS

Well absorbed after PO administration. Protein binding: 95.4% (artemether); 99.7% (lumefantrine). Binds to α_1-acid glycoprotein and erythrocytes. Rapidly and extensively metabolized in liver. Food enhances absorption. ***Half-life:*** 1–7 hr (artemether); 130 hr (lumefantrine).

INDICATIONS AND DOSAGES

▸ **Malaria due to *Plasmodium falciparum***

PO

Adults, 16 yr and older (who weigh 35 kg or greater). Four tablets of oral combination of artemether (20 mg) and lumefantrine (120 mg) as an initial dose; 4 more tablets 8 hr later; 4 tablets in the morning and 4 tablets in the evening for the next 2 days (total course of 24 tablets).

Children younger than 16 yr old who weigh 25 to less than 35 kg. Three tablets as an initial dose; take 3 more tablets 8 hr later; 3 tablets in the morning and 3 tablets in the evening for the next 2 days.

Children younger than 16 yr old who weigh 15 to less than 25 kg. Two tablets as an initial dose; 2 more tablets 8 hr later; 2 tablets in the morning and 2 tablets in the evening for the next 2 days.

Children younger than 16 yr old who weigh 5 to less than 15 kg. One tablet as an initial dose; second tablet 8 hr later. One tablet in the morning and 1 tablet in the evening for the next 2 days.

SIDE EFFECTS/ADVERSE REACTIONS

Frequent

Adults: Headache, anorexia, dizziness, asthenia, arthralgia, myalgia, nausea, vomiting, abdominal pain, sleep disorder, palpitations, fatigue, fever, shivering

Children: Pyrexia, cough, vomiting, anorexia, headache

Occasional

Adults: diarrhea, insomnia, hepatomegaly, splenomegaly, headache

Children: abdominal pain, diarrhea, splenomegaly, anemia, hepatomegaly

Rare

Adults: Anemia, cough, pruritus, rash, vertigo, nasopharyngitis

Children: Chills, asthenia, fatigue, nausea, rhinitis, dizziness, aspartate aminotransferase increased, arthralgia, myalgia, rash

PRECAUTIONS AND CONTRAINDICATIONS

Hypersensitivity to artemether, lumefantrine, or its components

Caution:

Hypokalemia

Hypomagnesemia

Drugs that prolong the QT interval (e.g. quinine, quinidine)

Cardiovascular disease

Hepatic impairment

Renal insufficiency

Halofantrine (within one month of Coartem therapy)

CYP450 3A4 substrates, inhibitors, inducers

Food aversion: increased risk of recrudescence due to reduced drug absorption

DRUG INTERACTIONS OF CONCERN TO DENTISTRY

- Antiretroviral agents: May increase the risk of QT prolongation, loss of antiviral efficacy, or loss of Coartem efficacy.
- Aurothioglucose: May increase risk of blood dyscrasias.
- CYP3A4 inhibitors (ketoconazole, itraconazole): May increase Coartem

levels; increase risk of QT prolongation.
• CYP450 2D6: May increase the risk of adverse effects and QT prolongation.
• Clarithromycin, telithromycin: May increase Coartem concentrations; increase risk of QT prolongation.
• Drugs that prolong the QT interval: May increase the risk of QT prolongation.
• Halofantrine: May cause additive effects and increase the risk of QT prolongation.
• Hormonal contraceptives: May reduce hormone contraceptive concentrations.
• Mefloquine: May decrease efficacy of Coartem.
• Grapefruit juice: This can increase concentrations of artemether/lumefantrine and increase risk of QT interval prolongation; avoid.

SERIOUS REACTIONS

! QTc prolongation may occur.
! Ototoxicity has been reported.
! Angioedema may occur.
! Hepatomegaly and splenomegaly have been reported.

DENTAL CONSIDERATIONS

General:
• QTc prolongation has been reported.
• Use caution with coadministration of CYP3A4 substrates, inducers, or inhibitors.
• Examine for oral manifestation of opportunistic infection.
• Patient on chronic drug therapy may rarely have symptoms of blood dyscrasias, which include infection, bleeding, and poor healing.
• Avoid dental light in patient's eyes; offer dark glasses for patient comfort.
• Place on frequent recall because of oral side effects.
• Consider semisupine chair position for patient comfort if GI side effects occur.

Consultations:
• In a patient with symptoms of blood dyscrasias, request a medical consultation for blood studies and postpone treatment until normal values are reestablished.
• Medical consultation may be required to assess disease control.

Teach Patient/Family to:
• Encourage effective oral hygiene to prevent soft tissue inflammation.
• Prevent trauma when using oral hygiene aids.
• Be alert for the possibility of secondary oral infection and the need to see dentist immediately if signs of infection occur.
• Recommend using an additional non-hormonal method of birth control.
• Instruct patient to take drug with food.
• Advise patient to avoid drinking grapefruit juice while taking this drug.

articaine hydrochloride

ar′-ti-kane hi-droh-**klor**′-ide
(Astracaine[CAN], Astracaine Forte[CAN], Septocaine, Zorcaine)

CATEGORY AND SCHEDULE

Pregnancy Risk Category: C

Drug Class: Amide local anesthetic with vasoconstrictor (epinephrine)

MECHANISM OF ACTION

An amide anesthetic that inhibits conduction of nerve impulses. ***Therapeutic Effect:*** Causes temporary loss of feeling and sensation.

USES

Local, infiltrative, or conductive anesthesia in both simple and complex dental and periodontal procedures

PHARMACOKINETICS

Onset of action occurs within 1–6 min depending on route of administration. Complete anesthesia lasts approximately 1 hr. Well absorbed. Protein binding: 60%–80%. Rapidly metabolized by plasma carboxyesterase to its primary metabolite, articainic acid, which is inactive. Excreted in urine. ***Half-life:*** 20–120 min.

INDICATIONS AND DOSAGES

These recommended doses serve only as a guide to the amount of anesthetic required for most routine procedures. The actual volumes to be used depend on a number of factors, such as type and extent of surgical procedure, depth of anesthesia, degree of muscular relaxation, and condition of the patient.

▸ **Local, Infiltrative, or Conductive Anesthesia in Both Simple and Complex Dental or Periodontal Procedures**

Infiltration

Adults, Elderly, Children older than 4 yr. 0.5–2.5 ml of a 4% solution, which corresponds to 20–100 mg. Maximum dose administered should not exceed 7 mg/kg (0.175 ml/kg) or 3.2 mg/lb (0.0795 ml/lb) of body weight (up to 500 mg).

SIDE EFFECTS/ADVERSE REACTIONS

Rare

Drowsiness, dizziness, disorientation, light-headedness, tremors, blurred or double vision, nausea, sensation of heat, cold, numbness

PRECAUTIONS AND CONTRAINDICATIONS

History of hypersensitivity to local anesthetics of the amide type or sodium metabisulfite

Caution:

Accidental intravascular injections may be associated with convulsions, CNS depression, or cardiorespiratory depression; reduce dose for elderly, debilitated, or pediatric patients; exaggerated response to intravascular epinephrine, severe hepatic impairment, lactation

DRUG INTERACTIONS OF CONCERN TO DENTISTRY

- CNS depressants: increased risk of CNS depression with all CNS depressants, especially in children and when larger doses are used.
- Avoid placing dental cartridges in disinfectant solutions with heavy metals or surface-active agents; may see release of metal ions into local anesthetic solutions with tissue irritation following injection.
- Risk of cardiovascular side effects; rapid intravascular administration of local anesthetic containing vasoconstrictor, either alone or in patients taking tricyclic antidepressants, MAOIs, digitalis drugs, cocaine, phenothiazines, β-blockers, and in presence of halogenated hydrocarbon general anesthetics; use smallest effective vasoconstrictor dose and careful aspiration technique.

• Avoid use of vasoconstrictors in patients with uncontrolled hyperthyroidism, diabetes, angina, or hypertension; refer these patients for medical treatment before elective dental procedures.

SERIOUS REACTIONS

! Tachycardia or bradycardia, B/P changes, syncope, cardiac arrest, and seizures have been observed in some patients during dental procedures.

DENTAL CONSIDERATIONS

General:

• Monitor vital signs at every appointment because of cardiovascular side effects.
• Apply lubricant to dry lips for patient comfort before dental procedures.
• Use vasoconstrictor with caution, in low doses, and with careful aspiration.

Teach Patient/Family to:

• Use care to prevent injury while numbness exists and to not chew gum or eat following dental anesthesia.
• Report any signs of infection, muscle pain, or fever to dentist when feeling returns.
• Report any unusual soft tissue reactions.

ascorbic acid (vitamin c)

ah-**skor**′-bic **as**′-id
(Apo-C[CAN], Cecon, Cenolate, Pro-C[AUS], Redoxon[CAN])

CATEGORY AND SCHEDULE

Pregnancy Risk Category: C
OTC

Drug Class: Vitamin C, water-soluble vitamin

MECHANISM OF ACTION

Assists in collagen formation and tissue repair and is involved in oxidation reduction reactions and other metabolic reactions.
Therapeutic Effect: Involved in carbohydrate use and metabolism, as well as synthesis of carnitine, lipids, and proteins. Preserves blood vessel integrity.

USES

Vitamin C deficiency, scurvy, urine acidification, and supplemental use in a variety of debilitated patients with poor vitamin C intake

PHARMACOKINETICS

Readily absorbed from the GI tract. Protein binding: 25%. Metabolized in the liver. Excreted in urine. Removed by hemodialysis.

INDICATIONS AND DOSAGES

▸ **Dietary Supplement**

PO

Adults, Elderly. 50–200 mg/day.
Children. 35–100 mg/day.

▸ **Acidification of Urine**

PO

Adults, Elderly. 4–12 g/day in 3–4 divided doses.
Children. 500 mg q6–8h.

▸ Scurvy
PO
Adults, Elderly. 100–250 mg 1–2 times a day.
Children. 100–300 mg/day in divided doses.

▸ Prevention and Reduction of Severity of Colds
PO
Adults, Elderly. 1–3 g/day in divided doses.

SIDE EFFECTS/ADVERSE REACTIONS

Rare
Abdominal cramps, nausea, vomiting, diarrhea, increased urination with doses exceeding 1 g
Parenteral: Flushing, headache, dizziness, sleepiness or insomnia, soreness at injection site

PRECAUTIONS AND CONTRAINDICATIONS

Caution:
Gout

DRUG INTERACTIONS OF CONCERN TO DENTISTRY

- Increased urinary excretion: salicylates, barbiturates

SERIOUS REACTIONS

! Ascorbic acid may acidify urine, leading to crystalluria.
! Large doses of IV ascorbic acid may lead to deep vein thrombosis.
! Abrupt discontinuation after prolonged use of large doses may produce rebound ascorbic acid deficiency.

DENTAL CONSIDERATIONS

General:
- An increased incidence of caries and soft tissue injury has been reported with excessive use of chewable ascorbic acid tablets.

asenapine

a-sen′ a-peen
(Saphris)
Do not confuse asenapine with amoxapine (Asendin).

CATEGORY AND SCHEDULE

Pregnancy Risk Category: C

Drug Class: Antimanic agent, atypical antipsychotic agent

MECHANISM OF ACTION

Asenapine is an atypical antipsychotic with mixed serotonin-dopamine antagonist activity. The addition of serotonin antagonism to dopamine antagonism is thought to improve symptoms of psychoses and reduce extrapyramidal side effects as compared to typical antipsychotics.
Therapeutic Effect: Diminishes manifestations of psychotic symptoms.

USES

Acute and maintenance treatment of schizophrenia; treatment of acute mania or mixed episodes associated with bipolar I disorder (as monotherapy or in combination with lithium or valproate)

PHARMACOKINETICS

Rapidly absorbed following sublingual administration; bioavailability is decreased if swallowed or administered with food or liquid. Peak plasma concentrations reached in 0.5–1.5 hr. 95% plasma protein bound. Undergoes hepatic metabolism.

Excreted via urine and feces.
Half-life: 24 hr.

INDICATIONS AND DOSAGES

▸ Schizophrenia

PO

Adults. SL acute treatment: Initially, 5 mg twice daily. Daily doses >20 mg/day in clinical trials did not appear to offer any additional benefits and increased risk of adverse effects.

Maintenance treatment: Initially, 5 mg twice daily; may increase to 10 mg twice daily after 1 wk based on tolerability. Sublingual tablets should be placed under the tongue and allowed to disintegrate. Do not crush, chew, or swallow. Advise patients to avoid eating or drinking for at least 10 min after administration.

▸ Bipolar Disorder

PO

Adults. SL monotherapy: Initially, 10 mg twice daily; decrease to 5 mg twice daily if dose not tolerated. Combination therapy (with lithium or valproate): 5 mg twice daily; may increase to 10 mg twice daily if tolerated.

SIDE EFFECTS/ADVERSE REACTIONS

Frequent

Somnolence, insomnia, extrapyramidal symptoms, headache, akathisia, dizziness, hypertriglyceridemia, impaired temperature regulation, weight gain

Occasional

Arthralgia, peripheral edema, hypertension, fatigue, anxiety, depression, hyperglycemia, constipation, vomiting, dyspepsia, xerostomia and increase in salivation, abnormal taste, toothache, edema of the tongue

PRECAUTIONS AND CONTRAINDICATIONS

Hypersensitivity to asenapine or any component of the formulation.

Hepatic impairment, blood dyscrasias, cerebrovascular incidents, dyslipidemia, esophageal dysmotility, extrapyramidal symptoms, hyperglycemia, neuroleptic malignant syndrome, orthostatic hypotension, suicidal tendencies

DRUG INTERACTIONS OF CONCERN TO DENTISTRY

- Increased risk of seizures: tramadol (e.g., Ultram), opioid analgesics, cyclobenazaprine, phenothiazines, cholinergics (e.g., Salagen), buproprion (e.g., Zyban), dextromethorphan
- Cardiac dysrhythmias: increased risk of tachycardia with fluoroquinolone antibiotics (e.g., moxifloxacin), opioids, benzodiazepine sedatives, epinephrine

SERIOUS REACTIONS

! Elderly patients with dementia-related psychosis treated with antipsychotic drugs are at an increased risk of death compared to those treated with a placebo.

DENTAL CONSIDERATIONS

General:

- Avoid conditions that lower seizure threshold (e.g., hypoxia).
- Monitor vital signs for possible cardiovascular adverse effects.
- Assess salivary flow as a factor in caries, periodontal disease, and candidiasis.
- Avoid or limit doses of epinephrine in local anesthetic.
- After supine positioning, have patient sit upright for at least 2 min

before standing to avoid orthostatic hypotension.
• Beware of possible drug-related hyperglycemia and symptoms of diabetes mellitus.
• Drug therapy may cause dysgeusia and numbness in lips and oral cavity.

Consultations:
• Consult physician to determine control of disease and ability of patient to tolerate dental procedures.

Teach Patient/Family to:
• Use effective oral hygiene regimen to reduce adverse effects of dry mouth.
• Avoid mouth rinses with high alcohol content because of drying effect.
• Use home fluoride products for anticaries effect.
• Use sugarless/xylitol gum, frequent sips of water, or saliva substitutes if dry mouth occurs.

aspirin/ acetylsalicylic acid

as′-pir-in/ah-**seet′**-il-sill-ic **as′**-id
(Ascriptin, Aspro[AUS], Bayer, Bex[AUS], Bufferin, Disprin[AUS], Ecotrin, Entrophen[CAN], Halfprin, Novasen[CAN], Solprin[AUS], Spren[AUS])
Do not confuse aspirin or Ascriptin with Aricept, Afrin, or Asendin, or Ecotrin with Edecrin.

CATEGORY AND SCHEDULE

Pregnancy Risk Category: D
OTC

Drug Class: Nonnarcotic analgesic salicylate

MECHANISM OF ACTION

A nonsteroidal salicylate that inhibits prostaglandin synthesis, acts on the hypothalamus heat-regulating center, and interferes with the production of thromboxane A_2, a substance that stimulates platelet aggregation.
Therapeutic Effect: Reduces inflammatory response and intensity of pain; decreases fever; inhibits platelet aggregation.

USES

Treatment of mild-to-moderate pain or fever, including arthritis, thromboembolic disorders, transient ischemic attacks in men, rheumatic fever, post-MI

PHARMACOKINETICS

Route	Onset	Peak	Duration
PO	1 hr	2–4 hr	24 hr

Rapidly and completely absorbed from GI tract; enteric-coated absorption delayed; rectal absorption delayed and incomplete. Protein binding: High. Widely distributed. Rapidly hydrolyzed to salicylate.
Half-life: 15–20 min (aspirin); 2–3 hr (salicylate at low dose); more than 20 hr (salicylate at high dose).

INDICATIONS AND DOSAGES

▸ **Analgesia, Fever**
PO, Rectal
Adults, Elderly. 325–1000 mg q4–6h. Maximum: 4 g/day.
Children. 10–15 mg/kg/dose q4–6h.

▸ **Antiinflammatory**
PO
Adults, Elderly. Initially, 2.4–3.6 g/day in divided doses; then 3.6–5.4 g/day.

Children. Initially, 60–90 mg/kg/day in divided doses; then 80–100 mg/kg/day.

▸ **Suspected MI**

PO

Adults, Elderly. 162 mg as soon as the MI is suspected, then daily for 30 days after the MI.

▸ **Prevention of MI**

PO

Adults, Elderly. 75–325 mg/day.

▸ **Prevention of Stroke After Transient Ischemic Attack**

PO

Adults, Elderly. 50–325 mg/day.

▸ **Kawasaki Disease**

PO

Children. 80–100 mg/kg/day in divided doses.

SIDE EFFECTS/ADVERSE REACTIONS

Occasional

GI distress (including abdominal distention, cramping, heartburn, and mild nausea); allergic reaction (including bronchospasm, pruritus, and urticaria)

PRECAUTIONS AND CONTRAINDICATIONS

Allergy to tartrazine dye, bleeding disorders, chickenpox or flu in children and teenagers, GI bleeding or ulceration, hepatic impairment, history of hypersensitivity to aspirin or NSAIDs

Caution:

Anemia, hepatic disease, renal disease, Hodgkin's disease, preoperative, postoperative

DRUG INTERACTIONS OF CONCERN TO DENTISTRY

- Increased risk of GI complaints and occult blood loss: alcohol, NSAIDs, corticosteroids
- Buffered aspirin: Decreased absorption of tetracycline
- Recent report indicated ibuprofen may block clot-preventing effects of aspirin
- Interactions when used as a dental drug:
  - Increased risk of bleeding: oral anticoagulants, valproic acid, dipyridamole
  - Increased risk of hypoglycemia: sulfonylureas
  - Increased risk of toxicity: methotrexate, lithium, zidovudine
  - Decreased effects of probenecid, sulfinpyrazone
  - Avoid prolonged or concurrent use with NSAIDs, corticosteroids, acetaminophen
  - Suspected reduction in antihypertensives and vasodilator effects of angiotensin-converting enzyme (ACE) inhibitors; monitor blood pressure if used concurrently

SERIOUS REACTIONS

! High doses of aspirin may produce GI bleeding and gastric mucosal lesions.

! Dehydrated, febrile children may experience aspirin toxicity quickly. Reye's syndrome may occur in children with the chickenpox or the flu.

! Low-grade toxicity is characterized by tinnitus, generalized pruritus (possibly severe), headache, dizziness, flushing, tachycardia, hyperventilation, diaphoresis, and thirst.

! Marked toxicity is characterized by hyperthermia, restlessness, seizures, abnormal breathing patterns, respiratory failure, and coma.

DENTAL CONSIDERATIONS

General:

- Patients on chronic drug therapy may rarely have symptoms of blood

dyscrasias, which can include infection, bleeding, and poor healing.

• Avoid prescribing buffered aspirin-containing products if patient is on a sodium-restricted diet.

• Chewable forms of aspirin should not be used for 7 days following oral surgery because of possible soft tissue injury.

• Evaluate allergic reactions: rash, urticaria; patients with allergy to salicylates may not be able to take NSAIDs; drug may need to be discontinued.

• Severe stomach bleeding may occur in patients who regularly use NSAIDs in recommended doses, when the patient is also taking another NSAID, a blood thinning or steroid drug, if the patient has GI or peptic ulcer disease, if they are 60 yr or older, or when NSAIDs are taken longer than directed. Warn patients of the potential for severe stomach bleeding.

Consultations:

• In a patient with symptoms of blood dyscrasias, request a medical consultation for blood studies and postpone dental treatment until normal values are reestablished.

• Take precautions if dental surgery is anticipated because of risk of increased bleeding; avoid prescribing aspirin before dental surgery.

• Tinnitus, ringing, roaring in ears after high-dose and long-term therapy necessitates referral for salicylism.

Teach Patient/Family to:

• Not place aspirin or buffered aspirin tablets directly on a tooth or mucosal surface because of the risk of chemical burn.

• Read label on other OTC drugs; may contain aspirin.

• Avoid alcohol ingestion; GI bleeding may occur.

• Warn patient of potential risks of NSAIDs.

atazanavir sulfate

ah-tah-**zan′**-ah-veer **sul′**-fate

(Reyataz)

Do not confuse Reyataz with Retavase.

CATEGORY AND SCHEDULE

Pregnancy Risk Category: B

Drug Class: Antiviral, HIV-1 protease inhibitor

MECHANISM OF ACTION

An antiviral that acts as an HIV-1 protease inhibitor, selectively preventing the processing of viral precursors found in cells infected with HIV-1.

Therapeutic Effect: Prevents the formation of mature HIV cells.

USES

HIV-1 infection in combination with other antiretroviral medications

PHARMACOKINETICS

Rapidly absorbed after PO administration. Protein binding: 86%. Extensively metabolized in the liver. Excreted primarily in urine and, to a lesser extent, in feces.

Half-life: 5–8 hr.

INDICATIONS AND DOSAGES

▸ **HIV-1 Infection**

PO

Adults, Elderly (antiretroviral-naive). 400 mg (2 capsules) once a day with food.

Adults, Elderly (antiretroviral-experienced). 300 mg and ritonavir (Norvir) 100 mg once a day.

▸ **HIV-1 Infection (concurrent therapy with efavirenz)**
PO
Adults, Elderly. 300 mg atazanavir, 100 mg ritonavir, and 600 mg efavirenz as a single daily dose with food.
▸ **HIV-1 Infection (concurrent therapy with didanosine)**
PO
Adults, Elderly. Give atazanavir with food 2 hr before or 1 hr after didanosine.
▸ **HIV-1 Infection (concurrent therapy with tenofovir)**
PO
Adults, Elderly. 300 mg atazanavir and 100 mg ritonavir and 300 mg tenofovir given as a single daily dose with food.
▸ **HIV-1 Infection in Patients with Mild-to-Moderate Hepatic Impairment**
PO
Adults, Elderly. 300 mg once a day with food.

SIDE EFFECTS/ADVERSE REACTIONS

Frequent
Nausea, headache
Occasional
Rash, vomiting, depression, diarrhea, abdominal pain, fever
Rare
Dizziness, insomnia, cough, fatigue, back pain

PRECAUTIONS AND CONTRAINDICATIONS

Concurrent use with ergot derivatives, midazolam, pimozide, or triazolam; severe hepatic insufficiency
Caution:
Prolongs PR interval, use with caution in preexisting conduction disorders; diabetes mellitus, hyperglycemia, hepatic impairment; monitor liver function, HBV infection, redistribution of body fat, do not breast-feed infants, safety and efficacy in children not established

DRUG INTERACTIONS OF CONCERN TO DENTISTRY

- Avoid drugs metabolized by CYP3A4 isoenzymes; however, the package insert notes that significant drug interactions are not expected with azithromycin, erythromycin, itraconazole, or ketoconazole; use with caution and monitor.

SERIOUS REACTIONS

! A severe hypersensitivity reaction (marked by angioedema and chest pain) and jaundice may occur.

DENTAL CONSIDERATIONS

General:
- Short appointments and a stress-reduction protocol may be required for anxious patients.
- Use precaution if sedation or general anesthesia is required; risk of hypotensive episode.
- Consider semisupine chair position for patient comfort if GI side effects occur.
- Patient history should include all medications and herbal or nonherbal remedies taken by the patient.
- Assess salivary flow as a factor in caries, periodontal disease, and candidiasis.
- Examine for oral manifestation of opportunistic infection.
- Palliative medication may be required for management of oral side effects.
- Advise patient if dental drugs prescribed have a potential for photosensitivity.

• Take precautions if dental surgery is anticipated and general anesthesia required.
• Patients on chronic drug therapy may rarely have symptoms of blood dyscrasias, which can include infection, bleeding, and poor healing.

Consultations:

• Consultation with physician may be necessary if sedation or general anesthesia is required.
• Medical consultation may be required to assess disease control and patient's ability to tolerate stress.

Teach Patient/Family to:

• Be aware of oral side effects and potential sequelae.
• Update health and drug history, reporting changes in health status, drug regimen changes, or disease/treatment status.
• Encourage effective oral hygiene to prevent soft tissue inflammation, infection.
• Prevent trauma when using oral hygiene aids.

atenolol

ah-**ten**′-oh-lol
(Apo-Atenol[CAN], AteHexal[AUS], Noten[AUS], Tenolin[CAN], Tenormin, Tensig[AUS])
Do not confuse atenolol with albuterol or timolol.

CATEGORY AND SCHEDULE

Pregnancy Risk Category: D

Drug Class: Antihypertensive, selective β_1-blocker

MECHANISM OF ACTION

A β_1-adrenergic blocker that acts as an antianginal, antiarrhythmic, and antihypertensive agent by blocking β1-adrenergic receptors in cardiac tissue.
Therapeutic Effect: Slows SN heart rate, decreasing cardiac output and B/P. Decreases myocardial oxygen demand.

USES

Treatment of mild-to-moderate hypertension, treatment and prophylaxis of angina pectoris, arrhythmia, adjunct therapy in hypertrophic cardiomyopathy, MI therapy and prophylaxis, adjunct therapy in pheochromocytoma, prophylaxis for vascular headache, adjunct therapy in thyrotoxicosis, mitral valve prolapse syndrome, mild-to-moderate heart failure

PHARMACOKINETICS

Route	Onset	Peak	Duration
PO	1 hr	2–4 hr	24 hr

Incompletely absorbed from the GI tract. Protein binding: 6%–16%. Minimal liver metabolism. Primarily excreted unchanged in urine. Removed by hemodialysis. ***Half-life:*** 6–7 hr (increased in impaired renal function).

INDICATIONS AND DOSAGES

▸ **Hypertension**

PO

Adults. Initially, 25–50 mg once a day. May increase dose up to 100 mg once a day.
Elderly. Usual initial dose, 25 mg a day.
Children. Initially, 0.8–1 mg/kg/dose given once a day. Range: 0.8–1.5 mg/kg/day. Maximum: 2 mg/kg/day or 100 mg/day.

▸ **Angina Pectoris**
PO
Adults. Initially, 50 mg once a day. May increase dose up to 200 mg once a day.
Elderly. Usual initial dose, 25 mg a day.
▸ **Acute MI**
IV
Adults. Give 5 mg over 5 min; may repeat in 10 min. In those who tolerate full 10-mg IV dose, begin 50-mg tablets 10 min after last IV dose followed by another 50-mg oral dose 12 hr later. Thereafter, give 100 mg once a day or 50 mg twice a day for 6–9 days. Or, for those who do not tolerate full IV dose, give 50 mg orally twice a day or 100 mg once a day for at least 7 days.
▸ **Dosage in Renal Impairment**
Dosage interval is modified on the basis of creatinine clearance.

Creatinine Clearance	Dosage Interval
15–35 ml/min	50 mg a day
Less than 15 ml/min	50 mg every other day

SIDE EFFECTS/ADVERSE REACTIONS

Atenolol is generally well tolerated, with mild and transient side effects.
Frequent
Hypotension manifested as cold extremities, constipation or diarrhea, diaphoresis, dizziness, fatigue, headache, and nausea
Occasional
Insomnia, flatulence, urinary frequency, impotence or decreased libido, depression
Rare
Rash, arthralgia, myalgia, confusion (especially in the elderly), altered taste

PRECAUTIONS AND CONTRAINDICATIONS

Cardiogenic shock, overt heart failure, second- or third-degree heart block, severe bradycardia
Caution:
Major surgery, lactation, diabetes mellitus, severe renal disease, thyroid disease, COPD, asthma, well-compensated heart failure

DRUG INTERACTIONS OF CONCERN TO DENTISTRY

- Decreased antihypertensive effects: NSAIDs, indomethacin, salicylates
- May slow metabolism of lidocaine
- Decreased β-blocking effects (or decreased β-adrenergic effects) of epinephrine, levonordefrin, isoproterenol, and other sympathomimetics
- Reduced bioavailability suspected with ampicillin

SERIOUS REACTIONS

! Overdose may produce profound bradycardia and hypotension.
! Abrupt atenolol withdrawal may result in diaphoresis, palpitations, headache, and tremors.
! Atenolol administration may precipitate CHF or MI in patients with cardiac disease; thyroid storm in those with thyrotoxicosis; and peripheral ischemia in those with existing peripheral vascular disease.
! Hypoglycemia may occur in patients with previously controlled diabetes.
! Thrombocytopenia, manifested as unusual bruising or bleeding, occurs rarely.

DENTAL CONSIDERATIONS

General:
- Monitor vital signs at every appointment because of cardiovascular and respiratory side effects.

- After supine positioning, have patient sit upright for at least 2 min before standing to avoid orthostatic hypotension.
- Patients on chronic drug therapy may rarely have symptoms of blood dyscrasias, which can include infection, bleeding, and poor healing.
- Assess salivary flow as a factor in caries, periodontal disease, and candidiasis.
- Stress from dental procedures may compromise cardiovascular function; determine patient risk.
- Short appointments and a stress-reduction protocol may be required for anxious patients.
- Use vasoconstrictors with caution, in low doses, and with careful aspiration. Avoid use of gingival retraction cord with epinephrine.
- Patient should never abruptly discontinue.

Consultations:

- In a patient with symptoms of blood dyscrasias, request a medical consultation for blood studies and postpone dental treatment until normal values are reestablished.
- Medical consultation may be required to assess disease control and stress tolerance of patient.
- Use precautions if general anesthesia is required for dental surgery.

Teach Patient/Family to:

- Encourage effective oral hygiene to prevent soft tissue inflammation.
- Use caution to prevent injury when using oral hygiene aids.
- When chronic dry mouth occurs, advise patient to:
  - Avoid mouth rinses with high alcohol content because of drying effects.
  - Use daily home fluoride products for anticaries effect.
  - Use sugarless gum, frequent sips of water, or saliva substitutes.

atomoxetine

ah-toh-**mox′**-eh-teen
(Strattera)

CATEGORY AND SCHEDULE

Pregnancy Risk Category: C

Drug Class: Selective norepinephrine reuptake inhibitor

MECHANISM OF ACTION

A norepinephrine reuptake inhibitor that enhances noradrenergic function by selective inhibition of the presynaptic norepinephrine transporter.

Therapeutic Effect: Improves symptoms of attention deficit/hyperactivity disorder (ADHD).

USES

Treatment of ADHD

PHARMACOKINETICS

Rapidly absorbed after PO administration. Protein binding: 98% (primarily to albumin). Eliminated primarily in urine and, to a lesser extent, in feces. Not removed by hemodialysis. ***Half-life:*** 4–5 hr in general population, 22 hr in 7% of Caucasians and 2% of African-Americans (increased in moderate to severe hepatic insufficiency).

INDICATIONS AND DOSAGES

▸ **ADHD**

PO

Adults, Children weighing 70 kg and more. 40 mg once a day. May increase after at least 3 days to 80 mg as a single daily dose or in divided doses. Maximum: 100 mg.
Children weighing less than 70 kg. Initially, 0.5 mg/kg/day. May increase after at least 3 days to

1.2 mg/kg/day. Maximum: 1.4 mg/kg/day or 100 mg.

▸ **Dosage in Hepatic Impairment**

Expect to administer 50% of normal atomoxetine dosage to patients with moderate hepatic impairment and 25% of normal dosage to those with severe hepatic impairment.

SIDE EFFECTS/ADVERSE REACTIONS

Frequent

Headache, dyspepsia, nausea, vomiting, fatigue, decreased appetite, dizziness, altered mood

Occasional

Tachycardia, hypertension, weight loss, delayed growth in children, irritability

Rare

Insomnia, sexual dysfunction in adults, fever

PRECAUTIONS AND CONTRAINDICATIONS

Angle-closure glaucoma, use within 14 days of MAOIs

Caution:

Hypertension, tachycardia, CV disease, urinary retention, nursing, use of herbs, poor metabolizers of CYP2D6 drugs, hepatic impairment, monitor weight and growth changes, use in geriatric patients not established

DRUG INTERACTIONS OF CONCERN TO DENTISTRY

- No dental drug interactions reported; however, drugs that inhibit CYP2D6 enzymes (paroxetine, fluoxetine) can increase plasma levels.
- Albuterol and other β_2-agonists should be used with caution because of potential effects on the cardiovascular system.

SERIOUS REACTIONS

! Urine retention or urinary hesitance may occur.

! In overdose, gastric emptying and repeated use of activated charcoal may prevent systemic absorption.

DENTAL CONSIDERATIONS

General:

- Assess salivary flow as a factor in caries, periodontal disease, and candidiasis.
- Monitor vital signs at every appointment because of cardiovascular side effects.
- Consider semisupine chair position for patient comfort if GI side effects occur.
- Use vasoconstrictor with caution, in low doses, and with careful aspiration.

Consultations:

- Medical consultation may be required to assess disease control and patient's ability to tolerate stress.

Teach Patient/Family to:

- Encourage effective oral hygiene to prevent soft tissue inflammation, infection.
- When chronic dry mouth occurs, advise patient to:
    - **Avoid mouth rinses with high alcohol content because of drying effects.**
    - Use daily home fluoride products for anticaries effect.
    - Use sugarless gum, frequent sips of water, or saliva substitutes.

atorvastatin

ah-**tore**-vah′-stah-tin
(Lipitor)
Do not confuse Lipitor with Levatol.

CATEGORY AND SCHEDULE

Pregnancy Risk Category: X

Drug Class: Cholesterol-lowering agent

MECHANISM OF ACTION

An antihyperlipidemic that inhibits HMG-CoA reductase, the enzyme that catalyzes the early step in cholesterol synthesis.
Therapeutic Effect: Decreases LDL and VLDL cholesterol, and plasma triglyceride levels; increases HDL cholesterol concentration.

USES

An adjunct in homozygous familial hypercholesterolemia, mixed lipidemia, elevated serum triglyceride levels, and type IV hyperproteinemia; also reduces total cholesterol, LDL-C, apo B, and triglyceride levels; patient should first be placed on cholesterol-lowering diet; familial hypercholesterolemia age 10–17 yr

PHARMACOKINETICS

Poorly absorbed from the GI tract. Protein binding: greater than 98%. Metabolized in the liver. Minimally eliminated in urine. Plasma levels are markedly increased in chronic alcoholic hepatic disease but are unaffected by renal disease.
Half-life: 14 hr.

INDICATIONS AND DOSAGES

▸ **Hyperlipidemia, Reduction of Risk of MI, Angina Revascularization Procedures**
PO
Adults, Elderly. Initially, 10–40 mg a day given as a single dose. Dose range: Increase at 2- to 4-wk intervals to maximum of 80 mg/day.
Children 10–17 yr. Initially, 10 mg/day, may increase to 20 mg/day.
▸ **Familial Hypercholesterolemia**
PO
Children 10–17 yr. Initially, 10 mg/day. May increase to 20 mg/day.

SIDE EFFECTS/ADVERSE REACTIONS

Atorvastatin is generally well tolerated. Side effects are usually mild and transient.
Frequent
Headache
Occasional
Myalgia, rash or pruritus, allergy
Rare
Flatulence, dyspepsia

PRECAUTIONS AND CONTRAINDICATIONS

Active hepatic disease, lactation, pregnancy, unexplained elevated hepatic function test results
Caution:
Chronic alcohol liver disease, pregnancy risk category X, monitor liver function and lipid levels

DRUG INTERACTIONS OF CONCERN TO DENTISTRY

• Severe myopathy or rhabdomyolysis: erythromycin, niacin, itraconazole, ketoconazole
• Increase in plasma levels: erythromycin, itraconazole, alcohol, ketoconazole
• Suspected increase in midazolam effects when used in general anesthesia (*Anesthesia* 58:899–904, 2003)

SERIOUS REACTIONS

! Cataracts may develop, and photosensitivity may occur.

DENTAL CONSIDERATIONS

General:

- Consider semisupine chair position for patient comfort if GI side effects occur.

atropine sulfate

a′-troe-peen

(Atropine Sulfate, Sal-Tropine Atropt[AUS])

Do not confuse atropine sulfate with Akarpine or Aplisol.

CATEGORY AND SCHEDULE

Pregnancy Risk Category: C

Drug Class: Anticholinergic

MECHANISM OF ACTION

An acetylcholine antagonist that inhibits the action of acetylcholine by competing with acetylcholine for common binding sites on muscarinic receptors, which are located on exocrine glands, cardiac and smooth-muscle ganglia, and intramural neurons. This action blocks all muscarinic effects.

Therapeutic Effect: Decreases GI motility and secretory activity, and GU muscle tone (ureter, bladder); produces ophthalmic cycloplegia and mydriasis.

USES

Reduction of salivary and bronchial secretions

PHARMACOKINETICS

Onset 0.5–1 hr, moderate protein binding, duration of action 4–6 hr, renal excretion

INDICATIONS AND DOSAGES

▸ **Asystole, Slow, Pulseless Electrical Activity**

IV

Adults, Elderly. 1 mg; may repeat q3–5 min up to total dose of 0.04 mg/kg.

▸ **Preanesthetic**

IV/IM/Subcutaneous

Adults, Elderly. 0.4–0.6 mg 30–60 min preoperatively.

Children weighing 5 kg and more. 0.01–0.02 mg/kg/dose to maximum of 0.4 mg/dose.

Children weighing less than 5 kg. 0.02 mg/kg/dose 30–60 min pre-op.

▸ **Bradycardia**

IV

Adults, Elderly. 0.5–1 mg q5min not to exceed 2 mg or 0.04 mg/kg.

Children. 0.02 mg/kg with a minimum of 0.1 mg to a maximum of 0.5 mg in children and 1 mg in adolescents. May repeat in 5 min. Maximum total dose: 1 mg in children, 2 mg in adolescents.

SIDE EFFECTS/ADVERSE REACTIONS

Frequent

Dry mouth, nose, and throat that may be severe; decreased sweating, constipation, irritation at subcutaneous or IM injection site

Occasional

Swallowing difficulty, blurred vision, bloated feeling, impotence, urinary hesitancy

Rare

Allergic reaction, including rash and urticaria; mental confusion or excitement, particularly in children, fatigue

PRECAUTIONS AND CONTRAINDICATIONS

Bladder neck obstruction because of prostatic hypertrophy, cardiospasm, intestinal atony, myasthenia gravis in those not treated with neostigmine, narrow-angle glaucoma, obstructive disease of the GI tract, paralytic ileus, severe ulcerative colitis, tachycardia secondary to cardiac insufficiency or thyrotoxicosis, toxic megacolon, unstable cardiovascular status in acute hemorrhage

DRUG INTERACTIONS OF CONCERN TO DENTISTRY

• Increased anticholinergic effects: tricyclic antidepressants, antihistamines, opioid analgesics, antipsychotic medications, or other drugs with anticholinergic activity
• Decreased absorption of ketoconazole

SERIOUS REACTIONS

! Overdosage may produce tachycardia, palpitations, hot, dry or flushed skin, absence of bowel sounds, increased respiratory rate, nausea, vomiting, confusion, somnolence, slurred speech, dizziness, and CNS stimulation.
! Overdosage may also produce psychosis as evidenced by agitation, restlessness, rambling speech, visual hallucinations, paranoid behavior, and delusions, followed by depression.

DENTAL CONSIDERATIONS

General:
• Give PO dose 30–60 min before drying effects are required for dental procedures.
• Request that patient remove contact lenses before using drug because of possible drying effects in the eyes.
• Caution patients that they may feel a dry, burning sensation in the throat and experience blurred vision.
• This drug is intended for acute use, usually in single doses only; therefore, chronic dry mouth should not be a concern.
• Avoid dental light in patient's eyes; offer dark glasses for patient comfort.
• Patient should avoid heat and exercise while taking due to reduced sweat production.
Consultations:
• Medical consultation is advisable before using this drug in patients with a history of GI disease, cardiac disease, or glaucoma.

aurothioglucose/ gold sodium thiomalate

ȯr-o-thī-o-**glu**′-kos
(Gold-50[AUS], Solganal);
(Myochrysine, Myocrisin[AUS])

CATEGORY AND SCHEDULE

Pregnancy Risk Category: C

Drug Class: Antiinflammatory gold compound

MECHANISM OF ACTION

Aurothioglucose: A gold compound that alters cellular mechanisms, collagen biosynthesis, enzyme systems, and immune responses.
Therapeutic Effect: Suppresses synovitis of the active stage of rheumatoid arthritis.
Gold sodium thiomalate: A gold compound whose mechanism of action is unknown. May decrease prostaglandin synthesis or alter cellular mechanisms by inhibiting sulfhydryl groups.
Therapeutic Effect: Decreases synovial inflammation, retards cartilage and bone destruction, suppresses or prevents but does not cure, arthritis, synovitis.

USES

Treatment of rheumatoid arthritis; juvenile arthritis; unapproved: psoriatic arthritis, Felty's syndrome

PHARMACOKINETICS

Aurothioglucose (50% gold): Slow, erratic absorption after IM administration. Protein binding: 95%–99%. Primarily excreted in urine. ***Half-life:*** 3–27 days (half-life increased with increased number of doses).
Gold sodium thiomalate: Well absorbed. Protein binding: 95%. Widely distributed. Metabolized in liver. Excreted in urine and feces. Not removed by hemodialysis. ***Half-life:*** 5 days.

INDICATIONS AND DOSAGES

▸ Rheumatoid Arthritis (Aurothioglucose)

IM
Adults, Elderly. Initially, 10 mg, then 25 mg for 2 doses, then 50 mg weekly thereafter until total dose of 0.8–1 g given. If patient is improved and there are no signs of toxicity, may give 50 mg at 3- to 4-wk intervals for many months.
Children. 0.25 mg/kg, may increase by 0.25 mg/kg each week. Maintenance: 0.75–1 mg/kg/dose. Maximum: 25-mg dose for total of 20 doses, then q2–4wk.

▸ Rheumatoid Arthritis (Gold Sodium Thiomalate)

IM
Adults, Elderly. Initially, 10 mg, then 25 mg for second dose. Follow with 25–50 mg/wk until improvement noted or total of 1 g administered. Maintenance: 25–50 mg q2wk for 2–20 wk; if stable, may increase to q3–4wk intervals.
Children. Initially, 10 mg, then 1 mg/kg/wk. Maximum single dose: 50 mg. Maintenance: 1 mg/kg/dose at 2- to 4-wk intervals.

▸ Dosage in Renal Impairment

Creatinine Clearance	Dosage
50–80 ml/min	50% of usual dosage
Less than 50 ml/min	Not recommended

SIDE EFFECTS/ADVERSE REACTIONS

Frequent
Aurothioglucose: Rash, stomatitis, diarrhea
Gold sodium thiomalate: Pruritic dermatitis, stomatitis, marked by erythema, redness, shallow ulcers of oral mucous membranes, sore throat, and difficulty swallowing, diarrhea or loose stools, abdominal pain, nausea
Occasional
Aurothioglucose: Nausea, vomiting, anorexia, abdominal cramps
Gold sodium thiomalate: Vomiting, anorexia, flatulence, dyspepsia, conjunctivitis, photosensitivity
Rare
Gold sodium thiomalate: Constipation, urticaria, rash

PRECAUTIONS AND CONTRAINDICATIONS

Aurothioglucose: Bone marrow aplasia, history of gold-induced pathologies, including blood dyscrasias, exfoliative dermatitis, necrotizing enterocolitis, and pulmonary fibrosis, serious adverse effects with previous gold therapy, severe blood dyscrasias
Gold sodium thiomalate: Colitis, concurrent use of antimalarials, immunosuppressive agents, penicillamine, or phenylbutazone, CHF, exfoliative dermatitis, history of blood dyscrasias, severe liver or renal impairment, systemic lupus erythematosus

DRUG INTERACTIONS OF CONCERN TO DENTISTRY

• None reported

SERIOUS REACTIONS

! Gold toxicity is the primary serious reaction. Signs and symptoms of gold toxicity include decreased hemoglobin, leukopenia (WBC count less than 4000/mm^3), reduced granulocyte counts (less than 150,000/mm^3), proteinuria, hematuria, stomatitis (sores, ulcers, and white spots in the mouth and throat), blood dyscrasias (anemia, leukopenia, thrombocytopenia, and eosinophilia), glomerulonephritis, nephritic syndrome, and cholestatic jaundice.

DENTAL CONSIDERATIONS

General:

• Patients on chronic drug therapy may rarely have symptoms of blood dyscrasias, which can include infection, bleeding, and poor healing.

• Palliative medication may be required for management of oral side effects.

• Consider semisupine chair position for patient comfort because of arthritic disease.

Consultations:

• Medical consultation may be required to assess disease control and patient's ability to tolerate stress.

• In a patient with symptoms of blood dyscrasias, request a medical consultation for blood studies and postpone dental treatment until normal values are reestablished.

Teach Patient/Family to:

• Encourage effective oral hygiene to prevent soft tissue inflammation.

• Be aware of the possibility of secondary oral infection and the need to see dentist immediately if infection occurs.

• Report oral lesions, soreness, or bleeding to dentist.

• Avoid mouth rinses with high alcohol content because of drying effects.

avanafil

a-**van**′-a-fil

(Stendra)

Do not confuse with sildenafil, tadalafil, or vardenafil.

CATEGORY AND SCHEDULE

Pregnancy Risk Category: C

Drug Class: Phosphodiesterase type 5 enzyme inhibitor

MECHANISM OF ACTION

An erectile dysfunction agent that inhibits phosphodiesterase type 5, the enzyme responsible for degrading cyclic guanosine monophosphate in the corpus cavernosum of the penis, resulting in smooth muscle relaxation and increased blood flow.

Therapeutic Effect: Facilitates erection in male erectile dysfunction

USES

Treatment of male erectile dysfunction (ED)

PHARMACOKINETICS

Rapidly absorbed following oral administration. Peak plasma concentrations reached in 30–45 min. 99% plasma protein bound. Undergoes hepatic metabolism and forms active and inactive metabolites. Excreted 62% via feces and 21% via urine. Drug has no effect on penile blood flow

without sexual stimulation.
Half-life: 5 hr.

INDICATIONS AND DOSAGES

▸ **Erectile Dysfunction**

PO

Adults. Initially, 100 mg 30 min prior to sexual activity; to be given as one single dose and not given more than once daily; dosing range: 50–200 mg once daily. May be administered with or without food. Avoid grapefruit juice.

SIDE EFFECTS/ADVERSE REACTIONS

Frequent

Headache, dizziness, flushing

Occasional

Back pain, nasal congestion, nasopharyngitis, color vision change

PRECAUTIONS AND CONTRAINDICATIONS

Hypersensitivity to avanafil or any component of the formulation. Concurrent use of nitrates in any form. May cause auditory and visual disturbances, including hearing and vision loss. Not recommended for use in patients with severe cardiovascular disease (hypotension, uncontrolled hypertension, angina, arrhythmias, stroke) and bleeding disorders.

DRUG INTERACTIONS OF CONCERN TO DENTISTRY

• CYP3A4 inhibitors: increase likelihood of adverse effects if taken with macrolide antibiotics (e.g., clarithromycin, erythromycin), azole antifungals (e.g., ketoconazole)
• Nitrates (e.g., nitroglycerin): potentially serious reductions in blood pressure
• Alpha blockers (e.g., phentolamine mesylate, Oraverse): potentially significant hypotension

SERIOUS REACTIONS

! Prolonged erections (lasting longer than 4 hr) and priapism (painful erections lasting longer than 6 hr) occur rarely. Instruct patients to seek immediate medical attention if erection persists for more than 4 hr.

DENTAL CONSIDERATIONS

General:

• Avoid postural hypotension, especially if patient has taken drug during period overlapping with dental appointment.
• Monitor vital signs for possible cardiovascular adverse effects.

Teach Patient/Family to:

• Inform dentist if taking drug overlaps with dental appointment or if drug dosage is changed.

axitinib

ax-i-**ti**′-nib
(Inlyta)
Do not confuse axitinib with gefitinib, imatinib, pazopanib, sorafenib, sunitinib, vandetanib, or vemurafenib.

CATEGORY AND SCHEDULE

Pregnancy Risk Category: D

Drug Class: Antineoplastic agent, tyrosine kinase inhibitor, vascular endothelial growth factor (VEGF) inhibitor

MECHANISM OF ACTION

An antineoplastic that binds to and inhibits VEGF, a protein that plays a major role in the formation of new blood vessels to tumors.
Therapeutic Effect: Inhibits tumor growth by inhibiting angiogenesis.

USES

Treatment of advanced renal cell cancer (RCC) after failure of one prior treatment

PHARMACOKINETICS

Rapidly absorbed following oral administration. Peak plasma concentrations reached in 2.5–4 hr. 99% plasma protein bound. Undergoes hepatic metabolism. Excreted 41% via feces (12% unchanged) and 23% via urine (metabolites). ***Half-life:*** 2.5–6 hr.

INDICATIONS AND DOSAGES

▸ Renal Cell Cancer, Advanced

PO

Adults. Initially, 5 mg twice daily (approximately every 12 hr). If dose is tolerated for at least 2 consecutive wk, may increase the dose to 7 mg twice daily, and then further increase to 10 mg twice daily. If dose is not tolerated, reduce dose from 5 mg twice daily to 3 mg twice daily; further reduce to 2 mg twice daily if intolerance persists. Tablet should be swallowed whole with a glass of water. May be taken with or without food. Do not make up missed or vomited doses. Avoid grapefruit juice.

SIDE EFFECTS/ADVERSE REACTIONS

Frequent

Hypertension, fatigue, dysphonia, headache, rash, hypocalcemia, hyperglycemia, hypoglycemia, hypothyroidism, hyperkalemia, diarrhea, inappetence, nausea, vomiting, weight loss, anemia, thrombocytopenia, leukopenia, weakness, arthralgia, cough, dyspnea

Occasional

Epistaxis, dry skin, alopecia, erythema, dyspepsia, myalgia, tinnitus, dizziness, oral mucosal inflammation, stomatitis, and taste alteration

PRECAUTIONS AND CONTRAINDICATIONS

Hypersensitivity to axitinib or any component of the formulation. May cause gastrointestinal events such as perforation and fistulas, hemorrhagic events, hypertension and hypertensive crisis, proteinuria, thyroid dysfunction, and wound healing complications. Not recommended for use in patients with severe hepatic impairment.

DRUG INTERACTIONS OF CONCERN TO DENTISTRY

• Increased adverse effects: CYP3A4 inhibitors (e.g., macrolide antibiotics, azole antifungals)
• Reduced effectiveness: CYP3A4 inducers (e.g., barbiturates, corticosteroids, St. John's wort)

SERIOUS REACTIONS

! Arterial thrombotic events (cerebrovascular accident, MI, transient ischemic attack) and venous thrombotic events (pulmonary embolism, deep vein thrombosis) have been observed with fatalities. Use with caution in patients with a history of risks for arterial or venous thrombotic events.

DENTAL CONSIDERATIONS

General:

• Adverse drug effects include increased bleeding; consult physician for preoperative management of drug therapy and plan for hemostasis during invasive procedures.
• Increased incidence of oral ulcerations, stomatitis.
• Dysgeusia may alter patient's response to preventive and restorative materials.

• Take precautions when seating and dismissing patient due to possible arm or leg numbness, confusion, dizziness, loss of balance or coordination, loss of vision.

Consultations:

• Consult physician to determine patient's ability to tolerate dental procedures and to adjust drug regimen prior to invasive procedures due to risk of bleeding.

Teach Patient/Family to:

• Avoid mouth rinses with high alcohol content because of drying effect.

• Use home fluoride products for anticaries effect.

• See section "Therapeutic Management of Common Oral Lesions" to determine appropriate therapy for oral ulcers, oral inflammation, and taste alterations associated with antineoplastic drugs.

azatadine maleate

ah-**za**′-ta-deen **mal**′-ee-ate

(Optimine)

Do not confuse with azelastine or azacitidine.

CATEGORY AND SCHEDULE

Pregnancy Risk Category: B

Drug Class: Antihistamine, H1-receptor antagonist

MECHANISM OF ACTION

A piperazine-derivative antihistamine that has both anticholinergic and antiserotonin activity. Inhibits mediator release from mast cells and prevents calcium entry into mast cells through voltage-dependent calcium channels.

Therapeutic Effect: Relieves allergic conditions, including urticaria and pruritus. Anticholinergic effects cause drying of nasal mucosa.

USES

Allergy symptoms, rhinitis, chronic urticaria, pruritus

PHARMACOKINETICS

Rapidly and extensively absorbed from the GI tract. Protein binding: minimal. Metabolized in liver. Excreted in urine. ***Half-life:*** 8.7 hr.

INDICATIONS AND DOSAGES

▸ **Allergic Rhinitis**

PO

Adults, Elderly, Children 12 yr or older. 1–2 mg 2 times a day.

SIDE EFFECTS/ADVERSE REACTIONS

Frequent

Slight to moderate drowsiness, thickening of bronchial secretions

Rare

Headache, fatigue, nervousness, dizziness, appetite increase, weight gain, nausea, diarrhea, abdominal pain, dry mouth, arthralgia, pharyngitis

PRECAUTIONS AND CONTRAINDICATIONS

History of hypersensitivity to azatadine, antihistamines, or any other component of the formulation or to other related antihistamines including cyproheptadine, concomitant use of MAOIs

DRUG INTERACTIONS OF CONCERN TO DENTISTRY

• Increased CNS depression: all CNS depressants, alcohol

• Increased anticholinergic effect: anticholinergics

SERIOUS REACTIONS

! Hepatitis, bronchospasm, and epistaxis have been reported.

DENTAL CONSIDERATIONS

General:

• Assess salivary flow as a factor in caries, periodontal disease, and candidiasis.

• Patients on chronic drug therapy may rarely have symptoms of blood dyscrasias, which can include infection, bleeding, and poor healing.

• Consider semisupine chair position for patient comfort because of respiratory disease.

• Monitor vital signs at every appointment because of cardiovascular side effects.

Consultations:

• In a patient with symptoms of blood dyscrasia, request a medical consultation for blood studies and postpone dental treatment until normal values are reestablished.

Teach Patient/Family to:

• Encourage effective oral hygiene to prevent soft tissue inflammation.

• Prevent injury when using oral hygiene aids.

• When chronic dry mouth occurs, advise patient to:

  • **Avoid mouth rinses with high alcohol content because of drying effects.**

  • Use daily home fluoride products for anticaries effect.

  • Use sugarless gum, frequent sips of water, or saliva substitutes.

azathioprine

ay-za-**thye**′-oh-preen
(Alti-Azathioprine[CAN], Azasan, Imuran, Thioprine[AUS])
Do not confuse azathioprine with Azulfidine or azatadine, or Imuran with Elmiron or Imferon.

CATEGORY AND SCHEDULE

Pregnancy Risk Category: D

Drug Class: Immunosuppressant

MECHANISM OF ACTION

An immunologic agent that antagonizes purine metabolism and inhibits DNA, protein, and RNA synthesis.
Therapeutic Effect: Suppresses cell-mediated hypersensitivities; alters antibody production and immune response in transplant recipients; reduces the severity of arthritis symptoms.

USES

Renal transplants to prevent graft rejection, refractory rheumatoid arthritis; unapproved use in refractory ITP, glomerulonephritis, nephrotic syndrome, bone marrow transplant; unapproved: pemphigoid and pemphigus, chronic ulcerative colitis, Behçet's syndrome, Crohn's disease

PHARMACOKINETICS

Metabolized in liver; excreted in urine (active metabolite); crosses placenta.

INDICATIONS AND DOSAGES

▸ **Adjunct in Prevention of Renal Allograft Rejection**

PO, IV

Adults, Elderly, Children. 2–5 mg/kg/day on day of transplant, then 1–3 mg/kg/day as maintenance dose.

▸ **Rheumatoid Arthritis**
PO
Adults. Initially, 1 mg/kg/day as a single dose or in 2 divided doses. May increase by 0.5 mg/kg/day after 6–8 wk at 4-wk intervals up to maximum of 2.5 mg/kg/day. Maintenance: Lowest effective dosage. May decrease dose by 0.5 mg/kg or 25 mg/day q4wk (while other therapies, such as rest, physiotherapy, and salicylates, are maintained).
Elderly. Initially, 1 mg/kg/day (50–100 mg); may increase by 25 mg/day until response or toxicity.
▸ **Dosage in Renal Impairment**
Dosage is modified on the basis of creatinine clearance.

Creatinine Clearance	Dose
10–50 ml/min	75% of usual dose
Less than 10 ml/min	50% of usual dose

SIDE EFFECTS/ADVERSE REACTIONS

Frequent
Nausea, vomiting, anorexia (particularly during early treatment and with large doses)
Occasional
Rash
Rare
Severe nausea and vomiting with diarrhea, abdominal pain, hypersensitivity reaction

PRECAUTIONS AND CONTRAINDICATIONS

Pregnant patients with rheumatoid arthritis

DRUG INTERACTIONS OF CONCERN TO DENTISTRY

• Increased blood dyscrasias: NSAIDs, especially phenylbutazone, dapsone, phenothiazines
• Increased immunosuppression, risk of infection: corticosteroids

SERIOUS REACTIONS

! Azathioprine use increases the risk of developing neoplasia (new abnormal-growth tumors).
! Significant leukopenia and thrombocytopenia may occur, particularly in those undergoing kidney transplant rejection.
! Hepatotoxicity occurs rarely.

DENTAL CONSIDERATIONS

General:
• Patients on chronic drug therapy may rarely have symptoms of blood dyscrasias, which can include infection, bleeding, and poor healing.
• To prevent infection if surgery or deep scaling is planned, prophylactic antibiotics may be indicated in patients who develop neutropenia.
• Determine why the patient is taking the drug.
• Alert the patient to the possibility of secondary oral infection; must see dentist immediately if infection occurs.
Consultations:
• In a patient with symptoms of blood dyscrasias, request a medical consultation for blood studies and postpone dental treatment until normal values are reestablished.
• Medical consultation may be required to assess disease control and patient's ability to tolerate stress.
Teach Patient/Family to:
• Encourage effective oral hygiene to prevent soft tissue inflammation.
• Use caution to prevent injury when using oral hygiene aids.
• Avoid mouth rinses with high alcohol content because of drying effects and irritation of mucous membranes.

azelaic acid

aye-zeh-**lay**′-ick **as**′-id
(Azelex, Finacea, Finevin)

CATEGORY AND SCHEDULE

Pregnancy Risk Category: B

Drug Class: Topical antimicrobial, antiacne

MECHANISM OF ACTION

The exact mechanism of action of azelaic acid is not known. Possesses antimicrobial activity against *Propionibacterium acnes* and *Staphylococcus epidermidis*. ***Therapeutic Effect:*** Inhibits microbial cellular protein synthesis.

USES

Topical therapy of mild-to-moderate inflammatory acne vulgaris; unapproved: melasma

PHARMACOKINETICS

Minimal absorption after topical administration. Metabolized in liver. Excreted in urine as unchanged drug. ***Half-life:*** 12 hr.

INDICATIONS AND DOSAGES

▸ Mild-to-Moderate Acne

Topical

Adults, Adolescents. Apply cream or gel to affected area twice daily (morning and evening).

SIDE EFFECTS/ADVERSE REACTIONS

Occasional

Pruritus, stinging, burning, tingling, erythema, dryness, rash, peeling, irritation, contact dermatitis

Rare

Worsening of asthma, vitiligo depigmentation, small depigmented spots, hypertrichosis, reddening (signs of keratosis pilaris), exacerbation of recurrent cold sore, fever blister, or oral herpes simplex

PRECAUTIONS AND CONTRAINDICATIONS

Hypersensitivity to azelaic acid or any component of the formulation

DRUG INTERACTIONS OF CONCERN TO DENTISTRY

- None reported

SERIOUS REACTIONS

! None reported

DENTAL CONSIDERATIONS

General:

- Topical use rarely causes exacerbation of recurrent herpes labialis.
- Keep away from mouth and other mucous membranes; wash eyes if cream comes in contact; irritation can occur.

azelastine

ah-**zel**′-ah-steen
(Astelin, Optivar)
Do not confuse Optivar with Optiray.

CATEGORY AND SCHEDULE

Pregnancy Risk Category: C

Drug Class: Antihistamine

MECHANISM OF ACTION

An antihistamine that competes with histamine for histamine receptor sites on cells in the blood vessels, GI tract, and respiratory tract. ***Therapeutic Effect:*** Relieves symptoms associated with seasonal allergic rhinitis such as increased mucus production and sneezing, and symptoms associated with allergic conjunctivitis, such as redness, itching, and excessive tearing.

USES

Temporary relief of signs and symptoms of allergic conjunctivitis. Control of symptoms associated with seasonal allergic rhinitis, nonallergic vasomotor rhinitis, nasal pruritus.

PHARMACOKINETICS

Route	Onset	Peak	Duration
Nasal spray	0.5–1 hr	2–3 hr	12 hr
Ophthalmic	N/A	3 min	8 hr

Well absorbed through nasal mucosa. Primarily excreted in feces. ***Half-life:*** 22 hr.

INDICATIONS AND DOSAGES

▸ **Allergic Rhinitis**

Nasal

Adults, Elderly, Children 12 yr and older. 2 sprays in each nostril twice a day.

Children 5–11 yr. 1 spray in each nostril twice a day.

▸ **Allergic Conjunctivitis**

Ophthalmic

Adults, Elderly, Children 3 yr or older. 1 drop into affected eye twice a day.

SIDE EFFECTS/ADVERSE REACTIONS

Frequent

Headache, bitter taste

Rare

Nasal burning, paroxysmal sneezing

Ophthalmic: Transient eye burning or stinging, bitter taste, headache

PRECAUTIONS AND CONTRAINDICATIONS

Breast-feeding women, history of hypersensitivity to antihistamines, neonates or premature infants, third trimester of pregnancy

DRUG INTERACTIONS OF CONCERN TO DENTISTRY

- Increased risk of anticholinergic effects: anticholinergics
- Possible additive sedation: alcohol, anxiolytics, opioid analgesics

SERIOUS REACTIONS

! Epistaxis occurs rarely.

DENTAL CONSIDERATIONS

General:

- Protect patient's eyes from accidental spatter during dental treatment.
- Assess salivary flow as factor in caries, periodontal disease, and candidiasis.

Teach Patient/Family:

- When chronic dry mouth occurs, advise patient to:
  - Avoid mouth rinses with high alcohol content because of drying effects.
  - Use daily home fluoride products for anticaries effect.
  - Use sugarless gum, frequent sips of water, or saliva substitutes.

azilsartan medoxomil

a-zil-**sar**′-tan mee-dox′-o-mil

ay zil sar tan

(Edarbi)

CATEGORY AND SCHEDULE

Pregnancy Risk Category: D

Drug Class: Angiotensin II receptor antagonist, antihypertensive

MECHANISM OF ACTION

An angiotensin II receptor, type AT1, antagonist that blocks the vasoconstrictor and aldosterone-secreting effects of angiotensin II, inhibiting the binding of angiotensin II to the AT1 receptors.
Therapeutic Effect: Causes vasodilation, decreases peripheral resistance and decreases blood pressure.

USES

Treatment of hypertension, as a single drug or in combination with other antihypertensives

PHARMACOKINETICS

Rapidly absorbed following oral administration. Peak plasma concentrations reached in 1.5–3 hr. 99% plasma protein bound. Azilsartan medoxomil is a prodrug, hydrolyzed to active form via hepatic metabolism and then further via the CYP2C9 enzyme system to inactive metabolites. Excreted 55% via feces and 42% via urine (15% as unchanged drug). ***Half-life:*** 11 hr.

INDICATIONS AND DOSAGES

▸ Hypertension

PO

Adults. 80 mg once daily; consider initial dose of 40 mg once daily in patients taking diuretics. May be taken with or without food.

SIDE EFFECTS/ADVERSE REACTIONS

Frequent

Hypotension, orthostatic hypotension, dizziness, fatigue, diarrhea, nausea

Occasional

Hematologic changes (leukopenia, thrombocytopenia), muscle spasm and weakness, cough

PRECAUTIONS AND CONTRAINDICATIONS

Hypersensitivity to azilsartan or any component of the formulation. May cause hyperkalemia, hypotension, and renal function deterioration. Use with caution in patients with renal artery stenosis and renal impairment. Contraindicated in concomitant use with aliskiren in patients with diabetes mellitus.

DRUG INTERACTIONS OF CONCERN TO DENTISTRY

- Risk of decreased renal function, potential renal failure: NSAIDs (e.g., ibuprofen, naproxen).
- Potential for increased hypotensive effects with other hypotensive drugs and sedatives.
- Diarrhea associated with azilsartan may be worsened by antibiotic therapy.

SERIOUS REACTIONS

! Drugs that act on the renin-angiotensin system can cause injury and death to the developing fetus. Discontinue as soon as possible once pregnancy is detected.

DENTAL CONSIDERATIONS

General:

- Monitor vital signs at every appointment because of cardiovascular effects.
- After supine positioning, have patient sit upright for at least 2 min before standing to avoid orthostatic hypotension.
- Stress from dental procedures may compromise cardiovascular function; determine patient risk and use a stress-reduction protocol for anxious patients.
- Assess salivary flow as a factor in caries, periodontal disease, and candidiasis.

• Limit use of sodium-containing products, such as saline IV fluids, for patients with a dietary salt restriction.
• Short appointments and a stress-reduction protocol may be required for anxious patients.

Consultations:

• Medical consultation may be required to assess disease control and patient's ability to tolerate dental procedures.

Teach Patient/Family to:

• Avoid mouth rinses with high alcohol content because of drying effect.
• Use home fluoride products for anticaries effect.
• Use sugarless/xylitol gum, frequent sips of water, or saliva substitutes if dry mouth occurs.

azithromycin

ah-zi-thro-**mye'**-sin
(Zithromax, Zithromax TRI-PAK, Zithromax Z-PAK, Zmax)
Do not confuse azithromycin with erythromycin.

CATEGORY AND SCHEDULE

Pregnancy Risk Category: B

Drug Class: Macrolide antibiotic

MECHANISM OF ACTION

A macrolide antibiotic that binds to ribosomal receptor sites of susceptible organisms, inhibiting RNA-dependent protein synthesis. ***Therapeutic Effect:*** Bacteriostatic or bactericidal, depending on the drug dosage.

USES

Treatment of mild-to-moderate infections of the upper or lower respiratory tract; COPD exacerbations caused by *H. influenzae, M. catarrhalis,* or *S. pneumoniae;* gonorrhea, chancroid, uncomplicated skin and skin structure infections caused by *M. catarrhalis, S. pneumoniae, S. pyogenes, S. aureus, S. agalactiae, H. influenzae, Clostridium,* or *L. pneumophila;* nongonococcal urethritis; cervicitis caused by *C. trachomatis;* otitis media caused by *H. influenzae, S. pneumoniae,* or *M. catarrhalis;* chlamydia; *Mycobacterium avium* complex (MAC) in HIV infection

PHARMACOKINETICS

Rapidly absorbed from the GI tract. Protein binding: 7%–50%. Widely distributed. Eliminated primarily unchanged by biliary excretion. ***Half-life:*** 68 hr.

INDICATIONS AND DOSAGES

▸ Respiratory Tract, Skin, and Skin-Structure Infections

PO

Adults, Elderly. 500 mg once, then 250 mg/day for 4 days.
Children 6 mo and older. 10 mg/kg once (maximum 500 mg) then 5 mg/kg/day for 4 days (maximum 250 mg).

▸ Acute Bacterial Exacerbations of COPD

PO

Adults. 500 mg/day for 3 days.

▸ Otitis Media

PO

Children 6 mo and older. 10 mg/kg once (maximum 500 mg) then 5 mg/kg/day for 4 days (maximum 250 mg). Single dose: 30 mg/kg. Maximum: 1500 mg. Three-day regimen: 10 mg/kg/day as single daily dose. Maximum: 500 mg/day.

▸ **Pharyngitis, Tonsillitis**
PO
Children older than 2 yr. 12 mg/kg/day (maximum 500 mg) for 5 days.
▸ **Chancroid**
PO
Adults, Elderly. 1 g as single dose.
Children. 20 mg/kg as single dose. Maximum: 1 g.
▸ **Treatment of MAC**
PO
Adults, Elderly. 500 mg/day in combination.
Children. 5 mg/kg/day (maximum 250 mg) in combination.
▸ **Prevention of MAC**
PO
Adults, Elderly. 1200 mg/wk alone or with rifabutin.
Children. 5 mg/kg/day (maximum 250 mg) or 20 mg/kg/wk (maximum 1200 mg) alone or with rifabutin.
▸ **Nongonococcal Urethritis and Cervicitis Caused by *Chlamydia trachomatis***
PO
Adults. 1 g as a single dose.
▸ **Usual Pediatric Dosage**
PO
Children older than 6 mo. 10 mg/kg once (maximum: 500 mg) then 5 mg/kg/day for 4 days (maximum 250 mg).
▸ **Usual Parenteral Dosage (Community-Acquired Pneumonia, PID)**
IV
Adults. 500 mg/day, followed by oral therapy.

SIDE EFFECTS/ADVERSE REACTIONS

Occasional
Nausea, vomiting, diarrhea, abdominal pain
Rare
Headache, dizziness, allergic reaction

PRECAUTIONS AND CONTRAINDICATIONS

Hypersensitivity to azithromycin or other macrolide antibiotics

DRUG INTERACTIONS OF CONCERN TO DENTISTRY

- Risk of severe myopathy, rhabdomyolysis: hydroxymethylglutaryl coenzyme A (HMG-CoA) reductase inhibitors (statins)
- Decreased action of clindamycin, penicillin, lincomycin
- Possible increase in anticoagulant effect: warfarin
- Increased serum levels of theophylline

SERIOUS REACTIONS

! Antibiotic-associated colitis and other superinfections may result from altered bacterial balance.
! Acute interstitial nephritis and hepatotoxicity occur rarely.

DENTAL CONSIDERATIONS

General:
- An alternative drug of choice for mild infection caused by susceptible organisms in patients allergic to penicillin.
- Determine why the patient is taking the drug.
- Consider semisupine chair position for patient comfort if GI side effects occur.

Teach Patient/Family:
- When used for dental infection, advise patient to:
  - Report sore throat, oral burning sensation, fever, and fatigue, any of which could indicate superinfection.
  - Take at prescribed intervals and complete dosage regimen.

• Immediately notify the dentist if signs or symptoms of infection increase.

aztreonam

az-**tree**′-oo-nam
(Azactam)

CATEGORY AND SCHEDULE

Pregnancy Risk Category: B

Drug Class: Antibacterial

MECHANISM OF ACTION

A monobactam antibiotic that inhibits bacterial cell wall synthesis. ***Therapeutic Effect:*** Bactericidal.

USES

Treatment of infections caused by bacteria

PHARMACOKINETICS

Completely absorbed after IM administration. Protein binding: 56%–60%. Partially metabolized by hydrolysis. Primarily excreted unchanged in urine. Removed by hemodialysis. ***Half-life:*** 1.4–2.2 hr (increased in impaired renal or hepatic function).

INDICATIONS AND DOSAGES

▸ **UTIs**

IV, IM

Adults, Elderly. 500 mg–1 g q8–12h.

▸ **Moderate to Severe Systemic Infections**

IV, IM

Adults, Elderly. 1–2 g q8–12h.

▸ **Severe or Life-Threatening Infections**

IV

Adults, Elderly. 2 g q6–8h.

▸ **Cystic Fibrosis**

IV

Children. 50 mg/kg/dose q6–8h up to 200 mg/kg/day. Maximum: 8 g/day.

▸ **Mild to Severe Infections in Children**

IV

Children. 30 mg/kg q6–8h. Maximum: 120 mg/kg/day.
Neonates. 60–120 mg/kg/day q6–12h.

▸ **Dosage in Renal Impairment**

Dosage and frequency are modified on the basis of creatinine clearance and the severity of the infection.

Creatinine Clearance	Dosage
10–30 ml/min	1–2 g initially, then usual dose at usual intervals
Less than 10 ml/min	1–2 g initially, then usual dose at usual intervals

SIDE EFFECTS/ADVERSE REACTIONS

Occasional

Discomfort and swelling at IM injection site, nausea, vomiting, diarrhea, rash

Rare

Phlebitis or thrombophlebitis at IV injection site, abdominal cramps, headache, hypotension

PRECAUTIONS AND CONTRAINDICATIONS

None known

DRUG INTERACTIONS OF CONCERN TO DENTISTRY

• None reported

SERIOUS REACTIONS

! Antibiotic-associated colitis and other superinfections may result from altered bacterial balance.

! Severe hypersensitivity reactions, including anaphylaxis, occur rarely.

DENTAL CONSIDERATIONS

General:

- For selected infections in the hospital setting.
- Provide palliative dental care for dental emergencies only.
- Caution regarding allergy to medication.
- Examine for oral manifestation of opportunistic infection.
- Determine why patient is taking the drug.

Consultations:

- Medical consultation may be required to assess disease control.
- Consult patient's physician if an acute dental infection occurs and another antiinfective is required.

Teach Patient/Family to:

- Encourage effective oral hygiene to prevent soft tissue inflammation.
- Report oral lesions, soreness, or bleeding to dentist.
- Prevent trauma when using oral hygiene aids.

bacitracin

bass-ih-**tray′**-sin
(Baciguent, Baci-IM, Bacitracin)
Do not confuse bacitracin with Bactrim or Bactroban.

CATEGORY AND SCHEDULE

Pregnancy Risk Category: C
OTC

Drug Class: Antiinfective, antibiotic

MECHANISM OF ACTION

An antibiotic that interferes with plasma membrane permeability and inhibits bacterial cell wall synthesis in susceptible bacteria.
Therapeutic Effect: Bacteriostatic.

USES

Treatment of superficial ocular infections (conjunctivitis, keratitis, corneal ulcers, blepharitis). Minor skin abrasions, superficial infections. Treatment, prophylaxis of surgical procedures.

INDICATIONS AND DOSAGES

▸ **Superficial Ocular Infections**
Ophthalmic
Adults. ½-inch ribbon in conjunctival sac q3–4h.

▸ **Skin Abrasions, Superficial Skin Infections**
Topical
Adults, Children. Apply to affected area 1–5 times a day.

▸ **Surgical Treatment and Prophylaxis**
Irrigation
Adults, Elderly. 50,000–150,000 units, as needed.

SIDE EFFECTS/ADVERSE REACTIONS

Rare
Ophthalmic: Burning, itching, redness, swelling, pain
Topical: Hypersensitivity reaction (allergic contact dermatitis, burning, inflammation, pruritus)

PRECAUTIONS AND CONTRAINDICATIONS

None known

DRUG INTERACTIONS OF CONCERN TO DENTISTRY

- None reported

SERIOUS REACTIONS

! Severe hypersensitivity reactions, including apnea and hypotension, occur rarely.

DENTAL CONSIDERATIONS

General:
- Use protective glove or finger cot to apply.
- Determine why patient is taking the drug.

Teach Patient/Family to:
- Report burning, itching, or rash.

baclofen

bak′-loe-fen
(Apo-Baclofen[CAN], Baclo[AUS], Clofen[AUS], Lioresal, Liotec[CAN], Novo-Baclofen[CAN], Nu-Baclofen[CAN], Stelax[AUS])
Do not confuse baclofen with Bactroban or Beclovent.

CATEGORY AND SCHEDULE

Pregnancy Risk Category: C

Drug Class: Skeletal muscle relaxant, central acting

MECHANISM OF ACTION

A direct-acting skeletal muscle relaxant that inhibits transmission of reflexes at the spinal cord level. ***Therapeutic Effect:*** Relieves muscle spasticity.

USES

Treatment of skeletal muscle spasticity in multiple sclerosis, spinal cord injury, children with cerebral palsy; intrathecal dose form for severe spasticity in spinal cord injury or those not responsive to oral dose form; unapproved: trigeminal neuralgia

PHARMACOKINETICS

Well absorbed from the GI tract. Protein binding: 30%. Partially metabolized in the liver. Primarily excreted in urine. ***Half-life:*** 2.5–4 hr; intrathecal: 1.5 hr.

INDICATIONS AND DOSAGES

▸ Spasticity

PO

Adults. Initially, 5 mg 3 times a day. May increase by 15 mg/day at 3-day intervals. Range: 40–80 mg/day. Maximum: 80 mg/day.

Elderly. Initially, 5 mg 2–3 times a day. May gradually increase dosage.

Children. Initially, 10–15 mg/day in divided doses q8h. May increase by 5–15 mg/day at 3-day intervals. Maximum: 40 mg/day (children 2–7 yr); 60 mg/day (children 8 yr and older).

Usual Intrathecal Dosage

Adults, Elderly, Children older than 12 yr. 300–800 mcg/day.

Children 12 yr and younger. 100–300 mcg/day.

SIDE EFFECTS/ADVERSE REACTIONS

Frequent

Transient somnolence, asthenia, dizziness, light-headedness, nausea, vomiting

Occasional

Headache, paresthesia, constipation, anorexia, hypotension, confusion, nasal congestion

Rare

Paradoxical CNS excitement or restlessness, slurred speech, tremor, dry mouth, diarrhea, nocturia, impotence

PRECAUTIONS AND CONTRAINDICATIONS

Skeletal muscle spasm due to cerebral palsy, Parkinson's disease, rheumatic disorders, CVA, cough, intractable hiccups, neuropathic pain

DRUG INTERACTIONS OF CONCERN TO DENTISTRY

- Increased CNS depression: alcohol, all CNS depressants
- Muscle hypertonia: tricyclic antidepressants
- Warn patient of sedative effects while taking medication

SERIOUS REACTIONS

! Abrupt discontinuation of baclofen may produce hallucinations and seizures.

! Overdose results in blurred vision, seizures, myosis, mydriasis, severe muscle weakness, strabismus, respiratory depression, and vomiting.

DENTAL CONSIDERATIONS

General:

- Monitor vital signs at every appointment because of cardiovascular side effects.

• Assess salivary flow as a factor in caries, periodontal disease, and candidiasis.
• After supine positioning, have patient sit upright for at least 2 min to avoid orthostatic hypotension.

Teach Patient/Family:

• When chronic dry mouth occurs, advise patient to:
  • Avoid mouth rinses with high alcohol content because of drying effects.
  • Use daily home fluoride products for anticaries effect.
  • Use sugarless gum, frequent sips of water, or saliva substitutes.

balsalazide

ball-**sal′**-ah-zide
(Colazal)

CATEGORY AND SCHEDULE

Pregnancy Risk Category: B

Drug Class: Antiinflammatory

MECHANISM OF ACTION

A 5-aminosalicylic acid derivative that changes intestinal microflora, altering prostaglandin production and inhibiting function of natural killer cells, mast cells, neutrophils, and macrophages.
Therapeutic Effect: Diminishes inflammatory effect in colon.

USES

Treatment of mild to moderately active ulcerative colitis

PHARMACOKINETICS

PO: Drug reaches colon intact; bacterial azoreductases release 5-aminobenzyl-B-analine and mesalamine (active metabolite); low, variable systemic absorption; peak concentration 1–2 hr, protein binding ≈99%; less than 1% renal excretion; most excreted in feces (65%).

INDICATIONS AND DOSAGES

▸ **Ulcerative Colitis**

PO
Adults, Elderly. Three 750-mg capsules 3 times a day for 8 wk.

SIDE EFFECTS/ADVERSE REACTIONS

Frequent
Headache, abdominal pain, nausea, diarrhea
Occasional
Vomiting, arthralgia, rhinitis, insomnia, fatigue, flatulence, coughing, dyspepsia

PRECAUTIONS AND CONTRAINDICATIONS

Hypersensitivity, including hypersensitivity to mesalamine or salicylates

DRUG INTERACTIONS OF CONCERN TO DENTISTRY

• None reported

SERIOUS REACTIONS

! Liver toxicity occurs rarely.

DENTAL CONSIDERATIONS

General:

• Consider semisupine chair position for patient comfort because of GI side effects of disease.

Consultations:

• To reduce any potential risk of antibiotic-associated pseudomembranous colitis, a consultation is recommended before selecting an antibiotic for a dental infection.

B

becaplermin

beh-**kap′**-lear-min
(Regranex)

CATEGORY AND SCHEDULE

Pregnancy Risk Category: C

Drug Class: Topical wound repair

MECHANISM OF ACTION

A platelet-derived growth factor that heals open wounds.
Therapeutic Effect: Stimulates body to grow new tissue.

USES

An adjunct to good ulcer care practices in lower extremity diabetic, neuropathic ulcers that extend into subcutaneous tissues or beyond and have adequate blood supply

PHARMACOKINETICS

None reported

INDICATIONS AND DOSAGES

▸ **Ulcers**

Topical

Adults, Elderly. Apply once daily (spread evenly; cover with saline-moistened gauze dressing). After 12 hr, rinse ulcer, re-cover with saline gauze.

SIDE EFFECTS/ADVERSE REACTIONS

Occasional

Local rash near ulcer

Precautions and Contraindications

Hypersensitivity, neoplasms at the site of application, ulcers caused by vascular insufficiency

Caution:

Nonsterile, low-bioburden product that is not for use in ulcers that heal by primary intention, lactation, children younger than 16 yr, external use only, do not apply with fingers

DRUG INTERACTIONS OF CONCERN TO DENTISTRY

• Unknown

SERIOUS REACTIONS

! None reported

DENTAL CONSIDERATIONS

General:

• Patients requiring use of this medication probably will be limited in activities or bedridden.

• Determine why patient is taking the drug.

• Diabetes: question patient about self-monitoring of blood glucose values or finger-stick records.

• Diabetics may be more susceptible to infection and have delayed wound healing.

• Examine for oral manifestation of opportunistic infection.

• Patients with advanced diabetes should be questioned about any limitations in activities or stress tolerance. Some will also be receiving dialysis treatment if renal function is compromised. Dental treatment usually can be performed the day after dialysis.

Consultations:

• Medical consultation may be required to assess disease control and patient's ability to tolerate stress.

• Medical consultation may include data from patient's blood glucose monitoring, including glycosylated hemoglobin or HbA1c testing.

• Patients in dialysis may require antibiotic prophylaxis; determine need.

Teach Patient/Family to:

• Encourage effective oral hygiene to prevent soft tissue inflammation.

- Prevent trauma when using oral hygiene aids.
- Update health and drug history if physician makes any changes in evaluation or drug regimens.

beclomethasone dipropionate/ beclomethasone dipropionate hfa

be-kloe-**meth′**-ah-sone di-**pro′**-pi-o-nate

Oral inhalation: Qvar

Nasal inhalation: Beconase, Beconase AQ Nasal, Vancenase AQ 84 mcg, Vancenase Pockethaler

CATEGORY AND SCHEDULE

Pregnancy Risk Category: C

Drug Class: Corticosteroid, synthetic

MECHANISM OF ACTION

Glucocorticoids have multiple actions that include antiinflammatory and immunosuppressant effects. They inhibit phospholipase A_2, interfering with or reducing the synthesis of prostaglandins and leukotrienes. They also bind to cytoplasmic glucocorticoid receptors (GRs) and enter the cell nucleus to bind with DNA. This results in the synthesis of various enzymes such as collagenase, elastase, and cytokines that play important roles in inflammation control and immunosuppression. They also suppress the production of lymphocytes, monocytes, and eosinophils.

USES

Treatment of chronic asthma, prevention of recurrent nasal polyps, allergic and nonallergic rhinitis

PHARMACOKINETICS

Inhalation: Onset 10 min, half-life 3–15 hr; crosses placenta; metabolized in lungs, liver, GI system; excreted in feces (metabolites).

INDICATIONS AND DOSAGES

Oral Inhalation (QVAR only)

Adults, Adolescents. 40–160 mcg bid; limit to 320 mcg bid.

Children 5–11 yr. 40 mcg bid; limit 80 mcg bid.

Nasal Inhalation

Adults, Children older than 12 yr. 1–2 sprays in each nostril bid-qid; 84 mcg double strength: use once daily.

Children 6–12 yr. 1 spray in each nostril once daily.

Pockethaler

Adults, Children older than 12 yr. 1 spray in each nostril bid–qid.

SIDE EFFECTS/ADVERSE REACTIONS

Occasional

Dry mouth, candidiasis

Rare

Bronchospasm, hoarseness, sore throat

PRECAUTIONS AND CONTRAINDICATIONS

Hypersensitivity; status asthmaticus (primary treatment); nonasthmatic bronchial disease; bacterial, fungal, or viral infections of mouth, throat, or lungs; children younger than 3 yr

Caution:

Nasal disease/surgery

DRUG INTERACTIONS OF CONCERN TO DENTISTRY

- None reported

SERIOUS REACTIONS

! Potential acute adrenal insufficiency if used to replace systemic corticosteroid use
! Signs and symptoms of hypercorticism

DENTAL CONSIDERATIONS

General:

- Evaluate respiration characteristics and rate.
- Assess salivary flow as a factor in caries, periodontal disease, and candidiasis.
- Place on frequent recall because of oral side effects.
- Be aware that aspirin or sulfite preservatives in vasoconstrictor-containing products can exacerbate asthma.
- Acute asthmatic episodes may be precipitated in the dental office. Sympathomimetic inhalants should be available for emergency use.
- Morning appointments and a stress-reduction protocol may be required for anxious patients.

Consultations:

- Medical consultation may be required to assess patient's ability to tolerate stress.

Teach Patient/Family:

- Gargling and rinsing with water after each dose helps prevent candidiasis.
- When chronic dry mouth occurs, advise patient to:
  - Avoid mouth rinses with high alcohol content because of drying effects.
  - Use daily home fluoride products for anticaries effect.
  - Use sugarless gum, frequent sips of water, or saliva substitutes.

benazepril

be-**naze′**-ah-pril
(Lotensin)
Do not confuse benazepril with Benadryl, or Lotensin with Loniten or lovastatin.

CATEGORY AND SCHEDULE

Pregnancy Risk Category: C (D if used in second or third trimester)

Drug Class: Angiotensin-converting enzyme (ACE) inhibitor

MECHANISM OF ACTION

An ACE inhibitor that decreases the rate of conversion of angiotensin I to angiotensin II, a potent vasoconstrictor. Reduces peripheral arterial resistance.
Therapeutic Effect: Lowers B/P.

USES

Treatment of hypertension, alone or in combination with thiazide diuretics

PHARMACOKINETICS

Route	Onset	Peak	Duration
PO	1 hr	2–4 hr	24 hr

Partially absorbed from the GI tract. Protein binding: 97%. Metabolized in the liver to active metabolite. Primarily excreted in urine. Minimal removal by hemodialysis. ***Half-life:*** 35 min; metabolite 10–11 hr.

INDICATIONS AND DOSAGES

▸ **Hypertension (monotherapy)**

PO

Adults. Initially, 10 mg/day. Maintenance: 20–40 mg/day as

single or in 2 divided doses. Maximum: 80 mg/day.
Elderly. Initially, 5–10 mg/day. Range: 20–40 mg/day.

▸ **Hypertension (combination therapy)**
PO
Adults. Discontinue diuretic 2–3 days prior to initiating benazepril, then dose as noted above. If unable to discontinue diuretic, begin benazepril at 5 mg/day.

▸ **Dosage in Renal Impairment**
For adult patients with creatinine clearance less than 30 ml/min, initially, 5 mg/day titrated up to maximum of 40 mg/day.

SIDE EFFECTS/ADVERSE REACTIONS

Frequent
Cough, headache, dizziness
Occasional
Fatigue, somnolence or drowsiness, nausea
Rare
Rash, fever, myalgia, diarrhea, loss of taste

PRECAUTIONS AND CONTRAINDICATIONS

History of angioedema from previous treatment with ACE inhibitors
Caution:
Impaired renal or liver function, dialysis patients, hypovolemia, blood dyscrasias, CHF, chronic obstructive pulmonary disease (COPD), asthma, elderly

DRUG INTERACTIONS OF CONCERN TO DENTISTRY

- Increased hypotension: alcohol, phenothiazines
- Decreased hypotensive effects: indomethacin and possibly other NSAIDs, sympathomimetics
- Suspected reduction in the antihypertensive and vasodilator effects by salicylates; monitor blood pressure if used concurrently

SERIOUS REACTIONS

! Excessive hypotension ("first-dose syncope") may occur in patients with CHF and in those who are severely salt or volume depleted.
! Angioedema (swelling of the face and lips) and hyperkalemia occur rarely.
! Agranulocytosis and neutropenia may be noted in those with collagen vascular disease, including scleroderma and systemic lupus erythematosus, and impaired renal function.
! Nephrotic syndrome may be noted in patients with history of renal disease.

DENTAL CONSIDERATIONS

General:
- Monitor vital signs at every appointment because of cardiovascular and respiratory side effects.
- After supine positioning, have patient sit upright for at least 2 min to avoid orthostatic hypotension.
- Patients on chronic drug therapy may rarely have symptoms of blood dyscrasias, which can include infection, bleeding, and poor healing.
- Assess salivary flow as a factor in caries, periodontal disease, and candidiasis.
- Limit use of sodium-containing products, such as saline IV fluids, for those patients with a dietary salt restriction.
- Use vasoconstrictors with caution, in low doses, and with careful aspiration.

B

• Stress from dental procedures may compromise cardiovascular function; determine patient risk.
• Short appointments and a stress-reduction protocol may be required for anxious patients.

Consultations:
• Medical consultation may be required to assess disease control and patient's ability to tolerate stress.
• In a patient with symptoms of blood dyscrasias, request a medical consultation for blood studies and postpone dental treatment until normal values are reestablished.
• Take precautions if dental surgery is anticipated and sedation or general anesthesia is required; risk of hypotensive episode.

Teach Patient/Family to:
• Use effective oral hygiene to prevent soft tissue inflammation.
• Use caution to prevent injury when using oral hygiene aids.
• When chronic dry mouth occurs, advise patient to:
  • Avoid mouth rinses with high alcohol content because of drying effects.
  • Use daily home fluoride products for anticaries effect.
  • Use sugarless gum, frequent sips of water, or saliva substitutes.

bendamustine

ben-da-**mus′**-teen
(Treanda)

CATEGORY AND SCHEDULE

Pregnancy Risk Category: D

Drug Class: Antineoplastic agent, alkylating agent

MECHANISM OF ACTION

The exact mechanism of action of bendamustine is unknown. Bendamustine is an alkylating drug and (PARP) modulator. Dissociates into electrophilic alkyl groups, forms covalent bonds with electron-rich nucleophilic moieties, which results in tumor cell death through different pathways.

USES

Chronic lymphocytic leukemia (CLL)

PHARMACOKINETICS

Protein binding: 94%–96%. Metabolism occurs in liver primarily by hydrolysis; active minor metabolites formed primarily by CYP1A2. Excreted primarily in the feces (90%). ***Half-life***: 40 min.

INDICATIONS AND DOSAGES

IV
Adult. CLL: 100 mg/m^2 on days 1 and 2 of a 28-day treatment cycle (maximum: 6 cycles).
Allopurinol may be given to prevent tumor lysis syndrome. Prophylactic antibiotics may be considered.
Pediatric Dosing. Safety and efficacy has not been established.
Dose Adjustments. Renal impairment: Creatinine clearance less than 40 ml/min: DO NOT USE.
Hematologic toxicity, grade 3 or higher: reduce dose to 50 mg/m^2 on days 1 and 2 of each 28-day cycle. For recurrent hematologic toxicity, grade 3 or higher: reduce dose to 25 mg/m^2 on days 1 and 2 of each 28-day cycle.
Delay treatment for hematologic toxicity of grade 4 or high until ANC = 1000/mm^3, platelets = 75,000/mm^3.

For nonhematologic toxicity, grade 2 or higher: delay treatment until resolves to grade 1 or higher.
Hepatic impairment: Moderate (AST or ALT 2.5–10 times ULN and total bilirubin 1.5–3 times ULN) or severe (total bilirubin >3 times ULN): DO NOT USE.

SIDE EFFECTS/ADVERSE REACTIONS

Frequent
Fever, nausea and vomiting, anemia, bilirubin increased, myelosuppression, neutropenia, pyrexia, thrombocytopenia, and leukopenia

Occasional
Hypertension, fatigue, chills, rash, diarrhea, weight loss, cough

PRECAUTIONS AND CONTRAINDICATIONS

Hypersensitivity to bendamustine, mannitol, or any component of the formulation.
May cause fetal harm if administered to a woman during pregnancy.
Use appropriate precautions for handling and disposal.
Do not administer to children.
Hepatic impairment, moderate to severe: not recommended.
Smoking tobacco may decrease the levels and effects of bendamustine. May increase the levels and effects of the active metabolites of bendamustine.

DRUG INTERACTIONS OF CONCERN TO DENTISTRY

- CYP1A2 inhibitors (e.g., ciprofloxacin): May increase the levels and effects of bendamustine. May decrease the levels and effects of the active metabolites of bendamustine.

SERIOUS REACTIONS

! Bone marrow suppression has occurred.
! Dermatologic toxicity including hypersensitivity/infusion reaction (chills, fever, pruritus, and rash) may occur.
! Infection such as pneumonia and sepsis have been reported.
! Tumor lysis syndrome occurring in the first treatment cycle. May lead to life-threatening acute renal failure.

DENTAL CONSIDERATIONS

General:
- Monitor vital signs at every appointment because of cardiovascular side effects.
- Patients on chronic drug therapy may have symptoms of blood dyscrasias, which can include infection, bleeding, and poor healing.
- Examine for oral manifestation of opportunistic infection.
- Consider semisupine chair position for patient comfort if GI side effects occur.
- Evaluate allergic reactions: rash, urticaria.
- Stomatitis and xerostomia may complicate dental treatment and oral hygiene.

Consultations:
- Medical consultation may be required to assess disease control and ability of patient to tolerate dental treatment.

Teach Patient/Family to:
- Use effective atraumatic oral hygiene measures to prevent soft tissue inflammation.
- Report oral lesions, soreness, or bleeding to dentist.
- Be alert for the possibility of stomatitis and xerostomia and the need to see dentist immediately if signs of inflammation.

B

- If dry mouth occurs:
  - Avoid mouth rinse with high alcohol content because of dryness effects.
  - Use sugarless gum, frequent sips of water, or saliva substitutes.

bendroflumethiazide

ben-droe-floo-meth-**eye′**-ah-zide
(Naturetin-5)

CATEGORY AND SCHEDULE

Pregnancy Risk Category: C

Drug Class: Antidiuretic, central and nephrogenic diabetes insipidus; antihypertensive; antiurolithic, calcium calculi; diuretic

MECHANISM OF ACTION

A benzothiadiazine derivative that acts as a thiazide diuretic and antihypertensive. As a diuretic blocks reabsorption of water, sodium, and potassium at cortical diluting segment of distal tubule. As an antihypertensive reduces plasma, extracellular fluid volume, peripheral vascular resistance by direct effect on blood vessels.
Therapeutic Effect: Promotes diuresis, reduces B/P.

USES

Commonly used to treat high B/P. May also be used to help reduce the amount of water in the body by increasing the flow of urine.

PHARMACOKINETICS

Route	Onset	Peak	Duration
PO	2 hr	4 hr	6–12 hr

Variably absorbed from the GI tract. Primarily excreted unchanged in urine. Not removed by hemodialysis.
Half-life: 5.6–14.8 hr.

INDICATIONS AND DOSAGES

▸ **Edema**

PO

Adults. 5 mg/day, preferably given in the morning. To initiate therapy, doses up to 20 mg may be given once a day or divided into 2 doses.

▸ **Hypertension**

PO

Adults. 5–20 mg/day, preferably given in the morning. Maintenance: 2.5–15 mg/day.

SIDE EFFECTS/ADVERSE REACTIONS

Expected

Increase in urine frequency and volume

Frequent

Potassium depletion

Occasional

Postural hypotension, headache, GI disturbances, photosensitivity reaction

PRECAUTIONS AND CONTRAINDICATIONS

Anuria, history of hypersensitivity to sulfonamides or thiazide diuretics

DRUG INTERACTIONS OF CONCERN TO DENTISTRY

- Decreased hypotensive response: NSAIDs, especially indomethacin

SERIOUS REACTIONS

! Vigorous diuresis may lead to profound water and electrolyte depletion, resulting in hypokalemia, hyponatremia, and dehydration.
! Acute hypotensive episodes may occur.

! Hyperglycemia may be noted during prolonged therapy.
! Pancreatitis, blood dyscrasias, pulmonary edema, allergic pneumonitis, and dermatologic reactions occur rarely.
! Overdose can lead to lethargy and coma without changes in electrolytes or hydration.

DENTAL CONSIDERATIONS

General:

• Monitor vital signs at every appointment due to cardiovascular side effects.
• Patient on chronic drug therapy may rarely present with symptoms of blood dyscrasias, which can include infection, bleeding, and poor healing. If dyscrasia is present, caution patient to prevent oral tissue trauma when using oral hygiene aids.
• After supine positioning, have patient sit upright for at least 2 min before standing to avoid orthostatic hypotension.
• Limit use of sodium-containing products, such as saline IV fluids, for patients with a dietary salt restriction.
• Stress from dental procedures may compromise cardiovascular function; determine patient risk.
• Short appointments and a stress-reduction protocol may be required for anxious patients.
• Advise patient if dental drugs prescribed have a potential for photosensitivity.
• Patients taking diuretics should be monitored for serum K levels.

Consultations:

• In a patient with symptoms of blood dyscrasias, request a medical consultation for blood studies and postpone treatment until normal values are reestablished.
• Medical consultation may be required to assess disease control and patient's ability to tolerate stress.

Teach Patient/Family to:

• Use effective oral hygiene to prevent soft tissue inflammation.
• Prevent trauma when using oral hygiene aids.
• Update health and medication history if physician makes any changes in evaluation or drug regimens; include OTC, herbal, and nonherbal remedies in the update.

benzocaine

ben′-zoe-kane

(Americaine Anesthetic Lubricant, Americaine Otic, Anbesol, Anbesol Baby Gel, Anbesol Maximum Strength, Babee Teething, Benzodent, Cepacol, Cetacaine, Chiggerex, Chigger-Tox, Cylex, Dermoplast, Detaine, Foille, Foille Medicated First Aid, Foille Plus, HDA Toothache, Hurricaine, Lanacaine, Mycinettes, Omedia, Orabase-B, Orajel, Orajel Baby, Orajel Baby Nighttime, Orajel Maximum Strength, Orasol, Otricaine, Otocain, Retre-Gel, Solarcaine, Topicaine[AUS], Trocaine, Zilactin, Zilactin Baby Topicale)

CATEGORY AND SCHEDULE

Pregnancy Risk Category: C

Drug Class: Topical ester, local anesthetic. Action: Inhibits conduction of nerve impulses from sensory nerves

B

MECHANISM OF ACTION

A local anesthetic that blocks nerve conduction in the autonomic, sensory, and motor nerve fibers. Reduces permeability of resting nerves to potassium and sodium ions.

Therapeutic Effect: Produces local analgesic effect.

USES

Treatment of oral irritation, toothache, cold sore, canker sore, pain, teething pain, pain caused by dental prostheses or orthodontic appliances

PHARMACOKINETICS

Poorly absorbed by topical administration. Well absorbed from mucous membranes and traumatized skin. Metabolized in liver and by hydrolysis with cholinesterase. Minimal excretion in urine.

INDICATIONS AND DOSAGES

▸ Canker Sores

Topical

Adults, Elderly, Children older than 2 yr. Apply gel, liquid, or ointment to affected area. Maximum: 4 times a day.

▸ Denture Irritation

Topical

Adults, Elderly. Apply thin layer of gel to affected area up to 4 times a day or until pain is relieved.

▸ General Lubrication

Topical

Adults, Elderly, Children older than 2 yr. Apply gel to exterior of tube or instrument prior to use.

▸ Otitis Externa, Otitis Media

Otic

Adults, Elderly, Children older than 1 yr. Instill 4–5 drops into external ear canal of affected ears. Repeat q1–2h as needed.

▸ Pain and Itching Associated with Sunburn, Insect Bites, Minor Cuts, Scrapes, Minor Burns, Minor Skin Irritations

Topical

Adults, Elderly, Children older than 2 yr. Apply to affected area 3–4 times a day.

▸ Pharyngitis

PO

Adults, Elderly. 1 lozenge q2h. Maximum 8 lozenges a day.

▸ Toothache/Teething Pain

Topical

Adults, Elderly, Children older than 2 yr. Apply gel, liquid, or ointment to affected areas. Maximum: 4 times a day.

▸ Anesthesia

Topical

Adults, Elderly. Apply aerosol, gel, ointment, liquid q4–12h as needed.

SIDE EFFECTS/ADVERSE REACTIONS

Occasional

Burning, stinging, angioedema, contact dermatitis, taste disorders

Rare

Allergic ulceration of oral mucosa

PRECAUTIONS AND CONTRAINDICATIONS

Hypersensitivity to benzocaine or ester-type local anesthetics, perforated tympanic membrane or ear discharge (otic preparations)

DRUG INTERACTIONS OF CONCERN TO DENTISTRY

- None reported

SERIOUS REACTIONS

! Methemoglobinemia occurs rarely in infants and young children.

DENTAL CONSIDERATIONS

General:

- Do not use for topical anesthesia if medical history reveals allergy to procaine, PABA, parabens, or other ester-type local anesthetics.
- Use smallest effective amount in infants and children.
- Avoid applying to large denuded areas of mucosa to prevent excessive systemic absorption and potential toxicity.

benzonatate

ben-**zoe′**-na-tate
(Tessalon Perles)

CATEGORY AND SCHEDULE

Pregnancy Risk Category: C

Drug Class: Antitussive, non-narcotic

MECHANISM OF ACTION

A non-narcotic antitussive that anesthetizes stretch receptors in respiratory passages, lungs, and pleura.
Therapeutic Effect: Reduces cough.

USES

Relief of nonproductive cough

PHARMACOKINETICS

PO: Onset 15–20 min, duration 3–8 hr; metabolized by liver; excreted in urine.

INDICATIONS AND DOSAGES

▸ **Antitussive**

PO

Adults, Elderly, Children older than 10 yr: 100 mg 3 times a day or every 4 hr up to 600 mg/day.

SIDE EFFECTS/ADVERSE REACTIONS

Occasional

Mild somnolence, mild dizziness, constipation, GI upset, skin eruptions, nasal congestion

PRECAUTIONS AND CONTRAINDICATIONS

Hypersensitivity

Caution:

Lactation

DRUG INTERACTIONS OF CONCERN TO DENTISTRY

- Increased CNS depression: slight risk of increased sedation with other CNS depressants

SERIOUS REACTIONS

! A paradoxical reaction, including restlessness, insomnia, euphoria, nervousness, and tremor, has been noted.

DENTAL CONSIDERATIONS

General:

- Elective dental treatment may not be possible with significant coughing episodes.

B

benzoyl peroxide

ben′-zoe-ill per-**ox′**-ide

(Acetoxyl[CAN], Benoxyl[CAN], Benzac, Benzac AC, Benzac AC Wash, Benzac W, Benzac W Wash, Benzagel, Benzagel Wash, Benzashave, Brevoxyl, Brevoxyl Cleansing, Brevoxyl Wash, Clearplex, Clinac BPO, Del Aqua, Desquam-E, Desquam-X, Exact Acne Medication, Fostex 10% BPO, Loroxide, Neutrogena Acne Mask, Neutrogena On the Spot Acne Treatment, Oxy[AUS], Oxy 10 Balanced Medicated Face Wash, Oxy 10 Balance Spot Treatment, Palmer's Skin Success Acne, Oxyderm[CAN], PanOxyl, PanOxyl-AQ, PanOxyl Aqua Gel, PanOxyl Bar, Seba-Gel, Solugel[CAN], Triaz, Triaz Cleanser, Zapzyt)

CATEGORY AND SCHEDULE

Pregnancy Risk Category: C
OTC

Drug Class: Antiacne agent, topical; keratolytic, topical

MECHANISM OF ACTION

A keratolytic agent that releases free-radical oxygen, which oxidizes bacterial proteins in the sebaceous follicles, decreasing the number of anaerobic bacteria and decreasing irritating-type free fatty acids.
Therapeutic Effect: Bactericidal action against *Propionibacterium acnes* and *Staphylococcus epidermidis.*

USES

Treatment of acne

PHARMACOKINETICS

Minimal absorption through skin. Gel is more penetrating than cream. Metabolized to benzoic acid in skin. Excreted in urine as benzoate.

INDICATIONS AND DOSAGES

▸ **Acne**

Topical

Adults. Apply 2.5%–10% concentration 1–2 times a day.

SIDE EFFECTS/ADVERSE REACTIONS

Occasional

Irritation, dryness, burning, peeling, stinging, contact dermatitis, bleaching of hair

PRECAUTIONS AND CONTRAINDICATIONS

Hypersensitivity to benzoyl peroxide or any component of the formulation

DRUG INTERACTIONS OF CONCERN TO DENTISTRY

• None reported

SERIOUS REACTIONS

! Hypersensitivity reactions have been reported with benzoyl peroxide use.

DENTAL CONSIDERATIONS

General:

• Determine why patient is taking the drug.
• Advise patient if dental drugs prescribed have a potential for photosensitivity.
• Inquire about other drugs the patient may be using for acne.

Teach Patient/Family to:

• Avoid application to eyes, nose, mouth, and mucous membranes.
• Update health and medication history if physician makes any

changes in evaluation or drug regimens; include OTC, herbal, and nonherbal remedies in the update.

benzthiazide

benz-**thigh′**-ah-zide
(Exna)

CATEGORY AND SCHEDULE

Pregnancy Risk Category: C

Drug Class: Diuretic, thiazide

MECHANISM OF ACTION

Thiazide diuretic and antihypertensive. As a diuretic, blocks reabsorption of water, sodium, and potassium at cortical diluting segment of distal tubule. As an antihypertensive, reduces plasma and extracellular fluid volume and reduces peripheral vascular resistance by direct effect on blood vessels.
Therapeutic Effect: Promotes diuresis, reduces B/P.

USES

Treatment of high B/P

PHARMACOKINETICS

Route	Onset	Peak	Duration
PO	2 hr	4 hr	6–12 hr

Variably absorbed from the GI tract. Primarily excreted unchanged in urine. Not removed by hemodialysis. ***Half-life:*** Unknown.

INDICATIONS AND DOSAGES

▸ **Edema**

PO

Adults. Initially, 50–200 mg/day. Maintenance: 50–150 mg/day.

▸ **Hypertension**

PO

Adults. Initially, 50–100 mg/day. Dosage should be adjusted according to the patient response, either upward to as much as 50 mg 4 times a day or downward to the minimal effective dosage level.

SIDE EFFECTS/ADVERSE REACTIONS

Expected

Increase in urine frequency and volume

Frequent

Potassium depletion

Occasional

Postural hypotension, headache, GI disturbances, photosensitivity reaction

PRECAUTIONS AND CONTRAINDICATIONS

Anuria, history of hypersensitivity to sulfonamide-derived drugs or thiazide diuretics

DRUG INTERACTIONS OF CONCERN TO DENTISTRY

- Decreased hypotensive response: NSAIDs

SERIOUS REACTIONS

! Vigorous diuresis may lead to profound water and electrolyte depletion, resulting in hypokalemia, hyponatremia, and dehydration.
! Acute hypotensive episodes may occur.
! Hyperglycemia may be noted during prolonged therapy.
! Pancreatitis, blood dyscrasias, pulmonary edema, allergic pneumonitis, and dermatologic reactions occur rarely.
! Overdose can lead to lethargy and coma without changes in electrolytes or hydration.

DENTAL CONSIDERATIONS

General:

• Monitor vital signs at every appointment due to cardiovascular side effects.

• Patient on chronic drug therapy may rarely present with symptoms of blood dyscrasias, which can include infection, bleeding, and poor healing. If dyscrasia is present, caution patient to prevent oral tissue trauma when using oral hygiene aids.

• Observe appropriate limitations of vasoconstrictor doses.

• After supine positioning, have patient sit upright for at least 2 min before standing to avoid orthostatic hypotension.

• Limit use of sodium-containing products, such as saline IV fluids, for patients with a dietary salt restriction.

• Stress from dental procedures may compromise cardiovascular function; determine patient risk.

• Short appointments and a stress-reduction protocol may be required for anxious patients.

• Advise patient if dental drugs prescribed have a potential for photosensitivity.

• Patients taking diuretics should be monitored for serum K levels.

Consultations:

• In a patient with symptoms of blood dyscrasias, request a medical consultation for blood studies and postpone treatment until normal values are reestablished.

• Medical consultation may be required to assess disease control and patient's ability to tolerate stress.

Teach Patient/Family to:

• Use effective oral hygiene to prevent soft tissue inflammation.

• Prevent trauma when using oral hygiene aids.

• Update health and medication history if physician makes any changes in evaluation or drug regimens; include OTC, herbal, and nonherbal remedies in the update.

benztropine mesylate

benz′-troe-peen **mess′**-ah-late
(Apo-Benztropine[CAN], Bentrop[AUS], Cogentin)
Do not confuse benztropine with bromocriptine.

CATEGORY AND SCHEDULE

Pregnancy Risk Category: C

Drug Class: Anticholinergic, antidyskinetic

MECHANISM OF ACTION

An antiparkinson agent that selectively blocks central cholinergic receptors, helping to balance cholinergic and dopaminergic activity.

Therapeutic Effect: Reduces the incidence and severity of akinesia, rigidity, and tremor.

USES

Treatment of Parkinson symptoms, extrapyramidal symptoms associated with neuroleptic drugs

PHARMACOKINETICS

IM/IV: Onset 15 min, duration 6–10 hr. **PO:** Onset 1 hr, duration 6–10 hr.

INDICATIONS AND DOSAGES

▸ **Parkinsonism**

PO

Adults. 0.5–6 mg/day as a single dose or in 2 divided doses. Titrate by 0.5 mg at 5–6 day intervals.
Elderly. Initially, 0.5 mg once or twice a day. Titrate by 0.5 mg at 5–6 day intervals. Maximum: 4 mg/day.

▸ **Drug-Induced Extrapyramidal Symptoms**

PO, IM

Adults. 1–4 mg once or twice a day.
Children older than 3 yr. 0.02–0.05 mg/kg/dose once or twice a day.

▸ **Acute Dystonic Reactions**

IV, IM

Adults. Initially, 1–2 mg; then 1–2 mg PO twice a day to prevent recurrence.

SIDE EFFECTS/ADVERSE REACTIONS

Frequent

Somnolence, dry mouth, blurred vision, constipation, decreased sweating or urination, GI upset, photosensitivity

Occasional

Headache, memory loss, muscle cramps, anxiety, peripheral paresthesia, orthostatic hypotension, abdominal cramps

Rare

Rash, confusion, eye pain

PRECAUTIONS AND CONTRAINDICATIONS

Angle-closure glaucoma, benign prostatic hyperplasia, children younger than 3 yr, GI obstruction, intestinal atony, megacolon, myasthenia gravis, paralytic ileus, severe ulcerative colitis

Caution:

Elderly, lactation, tachycardia, prostatic hypertrophy, liver or kidney disease, drug abuse history, dysrhythmias, hypotension, hypertension, psychiatric patients

DRUG INTERACTIONS OF CONCERN TO DENTISTRY

- Increased anticholinergic effect: antihistamines, anticholinergics, and meperidine
- Decreased effects of phenothiazines

SERIOUS REACTIONS

! Overdose may produce severe anticholinergic effects, such as unsteadiness, somnolence, tachycardia, dyspnea, skin flushing, and severe dryness of the mouth, nose, or throat.

! Severe paradoxical reactions, marked by hallucinations, tremor, seizures, and toxic psychosis, may occur.

DENTAL CONSIDERATIONS

General:

- Monitor vital signs at every appointment because of cardiovascular side effects.
- Assess salivary flow as a factor in caries, periodontal disease, and candidiasis.
- After supine positioning, have patient sit upright for at least 2 min to avoid orthostatic hypotension.
- Avoid dental light in patient's eyes; offer dark glasses for patient comfort.
- Do not use ingestible sodium bicarbonate products, such as the Prophy-Jet air polishing system, within 1 hr of taking benztropine.
- Place on frequent recall because of oral side effects.

Consultations:

- Medical consultation may be required to assess disease control and patient's ability to tolerate stress.

B

Teach Patient/Family to:
• Use effective oral hygiene to prevent soft tissue inflammation.
• Use a powered tooth brush if patient has difficulty holding conventional devices.
• When chronic dry mouth occurs, advise patient to:
  • Avoid mouth rinses with high alcohol content because of drying effects.
  • Use daily home fluoride products for anticaries effect.
  • Use sugarless gum, frequent sips of water, or saliva substitutes.

bepotastine

bep ′ oh-tas ′ teen
(Bepreve)

CATEGORY AND SCHEDULE

Pregnancy Risk Category: C

Drug Class: Histamine H_1 antagonist (second generation)

MECHANISM OF ACTION

An ophthalmic H_1 receptor antagonist that inhibits the release of histamine from the mast cell. ***Therapeutic Effect:*** Prevents pruritus associated with allergic conjunctivitis.

USES

Treatment of itching associated with allergic conjunctivitis

PHARMACOKINETICS

Minimal systemic absorption following ocular administration. Peak plasma concentrations reached in 1–2 hr. 55% plasma protein bound. Onset of action is within 3 min with duration of action up to 8 hr. Excreted via urine (75%–90% as unchanged drug). ***Half-life:*** Not reported.

INDICATIONS AND DOSAGES

▸ **Allergic Conjunctivitis**

Ophthalmic

Adults, Elderly, Children 2 yr and older. Instill 1 drop into the affected eye(s) twice daily.

SIDE EFFECTS/ADVERSE REACTIONS

Frequent

Taste abnormality

Occasional

Headache, ocular irritation, nasopharyngitis

PRECAUTIONS AND CONTRAINDICATIONS

Hypersensitivity to bepotastine or any component of the formulation. Not for the treatment of contact lens irritation. Do not wear contact lens if the eye is red; otherwise, contact may be placed in eye 10 min after dosing; use in nursing and in children younger than 2 yr has not been established.

DRUG INTERACTIONS OF CONCERN TO DENTISTRY

• None reported

SERIOUS REACTIONS

! None known

DENTAL CONSIDERATIONS

General:
• Protect patient's eyes at all times due to underlying eye disease.
• Drug use may result in transient dysgeusia following application and may alter patient's response to preventive and restorative materials.

bepridil

beh'-prih-dill
(Bapadin, Vascor)

CATEGORY AND SCHEDULE

Pregnancy Risk Category: C

Drug Class: Calcium channel blocker

MECHANISM OF ACTION

A calcium channel blocker that inhibits calcium ion entry across cell membranes of cardiac and vascular smooth muscle; decreases heart rate, myocardial contractility, slows SA and AV conduction.
Therapeutic Effect: Dilates coronary arteries, peripheral arteries/arterioles.

USES

Treatment of stable angina, used alone or in combination with propranolol

PHARMACOKINETICS

Rapidly, completely absorbed from GI tract. Undergoes first-pass metabolism in liver to active metabolite. Primarily excreted in urine. Not removed by hemodialysis.
Half-life: less than 24 hr.

INDICATIONS AND DOSAGES

▸ **Chronic Stable Angina**

PO

Adults, Elderly. Initially, 200 mg/day; after 10 days, dosage may be adjusted. Maintenance: 200–400 mg/day.

SIDE EFFECTS/ADVERSE REACTIONS

Frequent

Dizziness, light-headedness, nervousness, headache, asthenia (loss of strength), hand tremor, nausea, diarrhea

Occasional

Drowsiness, insomnia, tinnitus, abdominal discomfort, palpitations, dry mouth, shortness of breath, wheezing, anorexia, constipation

Rare

Peripheral edema, anxiety, flatulence, nasal congestion, paresthesia

PRECAUTIONS AND CONTRAINDICATIONS

Sick sinus syndrome/second- or third-degree AV block (except in presence of pacemaker), severe hypotension (90 mm Hg, systolic), history of serious ventricular arrhythmias, uncompensated cardiac insufficiency, congenital QT interval prolongation, use with other drugs prolonging QT interval

Caution:

CHF, hypotension, hepatic injury, lactation, children, renal disease, may induce new arrhythmias, prolongs QT interval with risk of torsades de pointes

DRUG INTERACTIONS OF CONCERN TO DENTISTRY

- Decreased effect: NSAIDs, phenobarbital
- Increased effect: parenteral and inhalational general anesthetics or other drugs with hypotensive actions
- Increased effects of carbamazepine

B

SERIOUS REACTIONS

! CHF, second- and third-degree AV block occur rarely.
! Serious arrhythmias can be induced.
! Overdosage produces nausea, drowsiness, confusion, slurred speech, profound bradycardia.

DENTAL CONSIDERATIONS

General:

- Monitor cardiac status; take vital signs at every appointment because of cardiovascular side effects.
- Consider a stress-reduction protocol to prevent stress-induced angina during the dental appointment.
- Observe appropriate limitations of vasoconstrictor doses.
- After supine positioning, have patient sit upright for at least 2 min to avoid orthostatic hypotension.
- Limit use of sodium-containing products, such as saline IV fluids, for those patients with a dietary salt restriction.
- Assess salivary flow as a factor in caries, periodontal disease, and candidiasis.

Consultations:

- Medical consultation may be required to assess disease control and stress tolerance of patient.

Teach Patient/Family to:

- Schedule frequent oral prophylaxis if gingival overgrowth occurs.
- When chronic dry mouth occurs, advise patient to:
  - Avoid mouth rinses with high alcohol content because of drying effects.
  - Use daily home fluoride products for anticaries effect.
  - Use sugarless gum, frequent sips of water, or saliva substitutes.

besifloxacin

bess-ih-**flox′**-ah-sin
(Besivance)

CATEGORY AND SCHEDULE

Pregnancy Risk Category: C

Drug Class: Antibacterial, ophthalmic

MECHANISM OF ACTION

A bactericidal, broad-spectrum fluoroquinolone that inhibits bacterial DNA gyrase and topoisomerase.

USES

Bacterial conjunctivitis

PHARMACOKINETICS

Following single topical application to the eye, tear concentration averages 610 mcg/ml. Peak plasma concentrations less than 1.3 ng/ml. Distribution not reported. Protein binding: 39%–44%. Does not undergo hepatic metabolism. ***Half-life:*** 7 hr. Primarily excreted unchanged in feces (73%) and urine (23%).

INDICATIONS AND DOSAGES

▸ **Conjunctivitis**

Adults, Children over 1 yr: Shake bottle, instill 1 drop in the affected eye every 8 hr for 7 days.

SIDE EFFECTS/ADVERSE REACTIONS

Frequent

Conjunctival redness

Occasional

Blurred vision, eye pain, eye irritation, itching eyes, headache

PRECAUTIONS AND CONTRAINDICATIONS

Hypersensitivity to besifloxacin or any of its ingredients

DRUG INTERACTIONS OF CONCERN TO DENTISTRY

- None reported

SERIOUS REACTIONS

! Increased risk of congestive circulatory failure in patients at risk for peripheral edema

DENTAL CONSIDERATIONS

General:

Protect patient's eyes from irritants (splatter, excessive gas flow from nitrous oxide nasal hood).

betamethasone

bay-ta-**meth′**-ah-sone

(Alphatrex, Betaderm[CAN], Betatrex, Beta-Val, Betnesol[CAN], Celestone, Diprolene, Luxiq, Maxivate)

CATEGORY AND SCHEDULE

Pregnancy Risk Category: C (D if used in first trimester)

Drug Class: Antiinflammatory

MECHANISM OF ACTION

An adrenocortical steroid that controls the rate of protein synthesis, depresses the migration of polymorphonuclear leukocytes and fibroblasts, reduces capillary permeability, and prevents or controls inflammation.

Therapeutic Effect: Decreases tissue response to inflammatory process.

USES

Treatment of psoriasis, eczema, contact dermatitis, pruritus, oral ulcerative inflammatory lesions, mild-to-moderate ulcerative colitis. Also used to relieve swelling, itching, and discomfort of some other rectal problems, including hemorrhoids and inflammation of the rectum caused by radiation therapy.

PHARMACOKINETICS

PO: Onset 1–2 hr, peak 1 hr, duration 3 days.

IM/IV: Onset 10 min, peak 4–8 hr, duration 1–1.5 days.

Metabolized in liver, excreted in urine as steroids, crosses placenta.

INDICATIONS AND DOSAGES

▸ **Antiinflammation, Immunosuppression, Corticosteroid Replacement Therapy**

PO

Adults, Elderly. 0.6–7.2 mg/day.

Children. 0.063–0.25 mg/kg/day in 3–4 divided doses.

▸ **Relief of Inflamed and Pruritic Dermatoses**

Topical

Adults, Elderly. 1–3 times a day.

Foam: Apply twice a day.

B

SIDE EFFECTS/ADVERSE REACTIONS

Frequent

Systemic: Increased appetite, abdominal distention, nervousness, insomnia, false sense of well-being

Topical: Burning, stinging, pruritus

Occasional

Systemic: Dizziness, facial flushing, diaphoresis, decreased or blurred vision, mood swings

Topical: Allergic contact dermatitis, purpura or blood-containing blisters, thinning of skin with easy bruising, telangiectases, or raised dark red spots on skin

PRECAUTIONS AND CONTRAINDICATIONS

Hypersensitivity to betamethasone, systemic fungal infections

DRUG INTERACTIONS OF CONCERN TO DENTISTRY

- Decreased action: barbiturates
- Increased GI side effects: alcohol, salicylates, and other NSAIDs
- Increased action: ketoconazole, macrolide antibiotics

SERIOUS REACTIONS

! Overdose may cause systemic hypercorticism and adrenal suppression.

DENTAL CONSIDERATIONS

General:

- Monitor vital signs at every appointment because of cardiovascular side effects.
- Patients on chronic drug therapy may rarely have symptoms of blood dyscrasias, which can include infection, bleeding, and poor healing.
- Symptoms of oral infections may be masked.
- Determine dose and duration of steroid therapy for each patient to assess risk for stress tolerance and immunosuppression.
- Avoid prescribing aspirin-containing products.
- Place on frequent recall to evaluate healing response.
- Prophylactic antibiotics may be indicated to prevent infection if surgery or deep scaling is planned.
- Patients who have been or are currently on chronic steroid therapy (longer than 2 wk) may require supplemental steroids for dental treatment.

Consultations:

- In a patient with symptoms of blood dyscrasias, request a medical consultation for blood studies and postpone dental treatment until normal values are reestablished.
- Medical consultation may be required to assess disease control.
- Consultation may be required to confirm steroid dose and duration of use.

Teach Patient/Family to:

- Use effective oral hygiene to prevent soft tissue inflammation.
- Use caution to prevent injury when using oral hygiene aids.

betaxolol

bee-**tax′**-oh-lol

(Betoptic[AUS], Betoptic-S, Betoquin[AUS], Kerlone)

Do not confuse betaxolol with bethanechol.

CATEGORY AND SCHEDULE

Pregnancy Risk Category: C (D if used in second or third trimester)

Drug Class: Antihypertensive, selective β_1-blocker

MECHANISM OF ACTION

An antihypertensive and antiglaucoma agent that blocks β_1-adrenergic receptors in cardiac tissue. Reduces aqueous humor production.

Therapeutic Effect: Slows sinus heart rate, decreases B/P, and reduces intraocular pressure (IOP).

USES

Treatment of hypertension, alone or in combination with other antihypertensive drugs, especially thiazide diuretics

PHARMACOKINETICS

PO: Peak 3–4 hr. ***Half-life:*** 14–22 hr; protein binding 50%; some hepatic metabolism; excreted in urine mostly unchanged.

INDICATIONS AND DOSAGES

▸ Hypertension

PO

Adults. Initially, 5–10 mg/day. May increase to 20 mg/day after 7–14 days.

Elderly. Initially, 5 mg/day.

▸ Chronic Open-Angle Glaucoma and Ocular Hypertension

Ophthalmic (Eye Drops)

Adults, Elderly. 1 drop twice a day.

▸ Dosage in Renal Impairment

For adult and elderly patients who are on dialysis, initially give 5 mg/day; increase by 5 mg/day q2wk. Maximum: 20 mg/day.

SIDE EFFECTS/ADVERSE REACTIONS

Betaxolol is generally well tolerated, with mild and transient side effects.

Frequent

Systemic: Hypotension manifested as dizziness, nausea, diaphoresis, headache, fatigue, constipation or diarrhea, dyspnea

Ophthalmic: Eye irritation, visual disturbances

Occasional

Systemic: Insomnia, flatulence, urinary frequency, impotence or decreased libido

Ophthalmic: Increased light sensitivity, watering of eye

Rare

Systemic: Rash, arrhythmias, arthralgia, myalgia, confusion, altered taste, increased urination

Ophthalmic: Dry eye, conjunctivitis, eye pain

PRECAUTIONS AND CONTRAINDICATIONS

Cardiogenic shock, overt cardiac failure, second- or third-degree heart block, sinus bradycardia

Caution:

Major surgery, lactation, diabetes mellitus, renal disease, thyroid disease, COPD, asthma, well-compensated heart failure, aortic or mitral valve disease

DRUG INTERACTIONS OF CONCERN TO DENTISTRY

- Decreased antihypertensive effects: NSAIDs, indomethacin
- May slow metabolism of lidocaine
- Decreased β-blocking effects (or decreased β-adrenergic effects) of epinephrine, levonordefrin, isoproterenol, and other sympathomimetics

SERIOUS REACTIONS

! Overdose may produce profound bradycardia, hypotension, and bronchospasm.

! Abrupt withdrawal may result in diaphoresis, palpitations, headache, and tremors.

! Betaxolol administration may precipitate CHF or MI in patients with cardiac disease; thyroid storm in those with thyrotoxicosis; and peripheral ischemia in those with existing peripheral vascular disease.

! Hypoglycemia may occur in patients with previously controlled diabetes.

! Ophthalmic overdose may produce bradycardia, hypotension, bronchospasm, and acute cardiac failure.

DENTAL CONSIDERATIONS

General:

- Monitor vital signs at every appointment because of cardiovascular and respiratory side effects.
- After supine positioning, have patient sit upright for at least 2 min to avoid orthostatic hypotension.
- Assess salivary flow as a factor in caries, periodontal disease, and candidiasis.
- Stress from dental procedures may compromise cardiovascular function; determine patient risk.
- Short appointments and a stress-reduction protocol may be required for anxious patients.
- Use vasoconstrictors with caution, in low doses, and with careful aspiration. Avoid use of gingival retraction cord with epinephrine.

Consultations:

- Medical consultation may be required to assess disease control and stress tolerance of patient.
- Use precautions if general anesthesia is required for dental surgery.

Teach Patient/Family to:

- Use effective oral hygiene to prevent soft tissue inflammation.
- Use caution to prevent injury when using oral hygiene aids.
- When chronic dry mouth occurs, advise patient to:
  - Avoid mouth rinses with high alcohol content because of drying effects.
  - Use daily home fluoride products for anticaries effect.
  - Use sugarless gum, frequent sips of water, or saliva substitutes.

bethanechol chloride

beh-**than′**-eh-kole
(Duvoid[CAN], Myotonachol[CAN], Urecholine, Urocarb[AUS])
Do not confuse bethanechol with betaxolol.

CATEGORY AND SCHEDULE

Pregnancy Risk Category: C

Drug Class: Cholinergic stimulant

MECHANISM OF ACTION

A cholinergic that acts directly at cholinergic receptors in the smooth muscle of the urinary bladder and GI tract. Increases detrusor muscle tone.

Therapeutic Effect: May initiate micturition and bladder emptying. Improves gastric and intestinal motility.

USES

Treatment of urinary retention (postoperative, postpartum), neurogenic atony of bladder with retention; unapproved: gastric atony

PHARMACOKINETICS

PO: Onset 30–90 min, duration 6 hr. **SC:** Onset 5–15 min, duration 2 hr; excreted by kidneys.

B

INDICATIONS AND DOSAGES

▸ **Postoperative and Postpartum Urine Retention, Atony of Bladder**

PO

Adults, Elderly. 10–50 mg 3–4 times a day. Minimum effective dose determined by giving 5–10 mg initially, then repeating same amount at 1-hr intervals until desired response is achieved, or maximum of 50 mg is reached.

Children. 0.6 mg/kg/day in 3–4 divided doses.

SIDE EFFECTS/ADVERSE REACTIONS

Occasional

Belching, blurred or changed vision, diarrhea, urinary urgency

PRECAUTIONS AND CONTRAINDICATIONS

Active or latent bronchial asthma, acute inflammatory GI tract conditions, anastomosis, bladder wall instability, cardiac or coronary artery disease, epilepsy, hypertension, hyperthyroidism, hypotension, GI or urinary tract obstruction, parkinsonism, peptic ulcer, pronounced bradycardia, recent GI resection, vasomotor instability

Caution:

Hypertension, lactation, children younger than 8 yr, urinary retention

DRUG INTERACTIONS OF CONCERN TO DENTISTRY

- Decreased effects: anticholinergics

SERIOUS REACTIONS

! Overdosage produces CNS stimulation (including insomnia, anxiety, and orthostatic hypotension), and cholinergic stimulation (such as headache, increased salivation diaphoresis, nausea, vomiting, flushed skin, abdominal pain, and seizures).

DENTAL CONSIDERATIONS

General:

- Monitor vital signs at every appointment because of cardiovascular and respiratory side effects.
- After supine positioning, have patient sit upright for at least 2 min to avoid orthostatic hypotension.

Consultations:

- For excessive, troublesome salivation, reassure patient that treatment duration usually is limited to a few days; otherwise, consult to lower bethanechol dose.

bevacizumab

beh-vah-**siz′**-you-mab

(Avastin)

CATEGORY AND SCHEDULE

Pregnancy Risk Category: C

Drug Class: Antineoplastic monoclonal antibody; vascular endothelial growth factor (VEGF) inhibitor

MECHANISM OF ACTION

An antineoplastic that binds to and inhibits VEGF, a protein that plays a major role in the formation of new blood vessels to tumors.

Therapeutic Effect: Inhibits metastatic disease progression.

USES

Prevents the growth of certain types of blood vessels to cancer cells by starving the cells of nutrients needed to grow

PHARMACOKINETICS

Clearance varies by body weight, gender, and tumor burden. ***Half-life:*** 20 days (range, 11–50 days).

INDICATIONS AND DOSAGES

▸ First-Line Treatment of Metastatic Carcinoma of the Colon or Rectum in Combination with 5-Fluorouracil (5-FU)

IV

Adults, Elderly. 5 mg/kg once every 14 days.

SIDE EFFECTS/ADVERSE REACTIONS

Frequent

Asthenia, vomiting, anorexia, hypertension, epistaxis, stomatitis, constipation, headache, dyspnea

Occasional

Altered taste, dry skin, exfoliative dermatitis, dizziness, flatulence, excessive lacrimation, skin discoloration, weight loss, myalgia

Rare

Nail disorder, skin ulcer, alopecia, confusion, abnormal gait, dry mouth

PRECAUTIONS AND CONTRAINDICATIONS

GI perforation, hypertensive crisis, nephrotic syndrome, recent hemoptysis, serious bleeding, wound dehiscence requiring medical intervention

DRUG INTERACTIONS OF CONCERN TO DENTISTRY

• None reported

SERIOUS REACTIONS

! UTIs, manifested as urinary frequency or urgency and proteinuria, occur frequently.

! CHF, deep vein thrombosis, GI perforation, hypertensive crisis, nephrotic syndrome, and severe hemorrhage are the most serious reactions that occur.

! Anemia, neutropenia, and thrombocytopenia occur occasionally.

! Hypersensitivity reactions occur rarely.

DENTAL CONSIDERATIONS

General:

• Assess salivary flow as a factor in caries, periodontal disease, and candidiasis.

• If additional analgesia is required for dental pain, consider alternative analgesics (NSAIDs) in patients taking opioids for acute or chronic pain.

• Avoid products that affect platelet function, such as aspirin and NSAIDs.

• This drug may be used in the hospital or on an outpatient basis. Confirm the patient's disease and treatment status.

• Consider semisupine chair position for patient comfort if GI side effects occur.

• Chlorhexidine mouth rinse prior to and during chemotherapy may reduce severity of mucositis.

• Patient on chronic drug therapy may rarely present with symptoms of blood dyscrasias, which can include infection, bleeding, and poor healing. If dyscrasia is present, caution patient to prevent oral tissue trauma when using oral hygiene aids.

• Palliative medication may be required for management of oral side effects.

• Short appointments and a stress-reduction protocol may be required for anxious patients.

• Monitor vital signs at every appointment for cardiovascular side effects.

- Patients may have received other chemotherapy or radiation; confirm medical and drug history.
- Patients may be taking a prophylactic antiinfective.
- Patients may be at risk of bleeding; check for oral signs.
- Oral infections should be eliminated and/or treated aggressively.
- Place on frequent recall due to oral side effects.

Consultations:

- Medical consultation should include routine blood counts including platelet counts and bleeding time.
- Consult physician; prophylactic or therapeutic antiinfectives may be indicated if surgery or periodontal treatment is required.
- Medical consultation may be required to assess immunologic status during cancer chemotherapy and determine safety risk, if any, posed by the required dental treatment.
- Medical consultation may be required to assess disease control and patient's ability to tolerate stress.

Teach Patient/Family to:

- Inform dentist of unusual bleeding episodes following dental treatment.
- Be aware of oral side effects.
- Use effective oral hygiene to prevent soft tissue inflammation.
- Report oral lesions, soreness, or bleeding to dentist.
- Prevent trauma when using oral hygiene aids.
- Update health and medication history if physician makes any changes in evaluation or drug regimens; include OTC, herbal, and nonherbal remedies in the update.
- If abdominal pain associated with constipation and/or vomiting occur, advise patient to consult physician immediately.
- When chronic dry mouth occurs advise patient to:
  - Avoid mouth rinses with high alcohol content due to drying effects.
  - Use daily home fluoride products for anticaries effect.
  - Use sugarless gum, frequent sips of water, or saliva substitutes.

bexarotene

becks-**aye′**-row-teen
(Targretin)

CATEGORY AND SCHEDULE

Pregnancy Risk Category: X

Drug Class: Antineoplastic

MECHANISM OF ACTION

Retinoid antineoplastic agent that binds to and activates retinoid X receptor subtypes, which regulate the genes that control cellular differentiation and proliferation.
Therapeutic Effect: Inhibits growth of tumor cell lines of hematopoietic and squamous cell origin and induces tumor regression.

USES

Treatment of a form of cancer called cutaneous T-cell lymphoma (CTCL)

PHARMACOKINETICS

Moderately absorbed from the GI tract. Protein binding: greater than 99%. Metabolized in the liver. Primarily eliminated through the hepatobiliary system. ***Half-life:*** 7 hr.

INDICATIONS AND DOSAGES

▸ **Cutaneous T-Cell Lymphoma Refractory to at Least One Prior Systemic Therapy**

PO

Adults. 300 mg/m²/day. If no response and initial dose is well tolerated, may be increased to 400 mg/m²/day. If not tolerated, may decrease to 200 mg/m²/day, then to 100 mg/m²/day.

Topical

Adults. Initially, apply once every other day. May increase at weekly intervals up to 4 times a day.

SIDE EFFECTS/ADVERSE REACTIONS

Frequent

Hyperlipidemia, headache, hypothyroidism, asthenia

Occasional

Rash, nausea, peripheral edema, dry skin, abdominal pain, chills, exfoliative dermatitis, diarrhea

PRECAUTIONS AND CONTRAINDICATIONS

Hypersensitivity to bexarotene or any component of the formulation

DRUG INTERACTIONS OF CONCERN TO DENTISTRY

- Erythromycin, itraconazole

SERIOUS REACTIONS

! Pancreatitis, hepatic failure, and pneumonia occur rarely.

DENTAL CONSIDERATIONS

General:

- Consult patient for ability to tolerate dental procedure and to determine why patient is taking drug.

bicalutamide

by-kal-**yew′**-tah-myd
(Casodex, Cosudex[AUS])

CATEGORY AND SCHEDULE

Pregnancy Risk Category: X

Drug Class: Nonsteroidal antiandrogen, antineoplastic

MECHANISM OF ACTION

An antiandrogen antineoplastic agent that competitively inhibits androgen action by binding to androgen receptors in target tissue.

Therapeutic Effect: Decreases growth of prostatic carcinoma.

USES

Combination therapy with a luteinizing hormone-releasing hormone (LHRH) analogue for advanced prostate cancer

PHARMACOKINETICS

Well absorbed from the GI tract. Protein binding: 96%. Metabolized in the liver to inactive metabolite. Excreted in urine and feces. Not removed by hemodialysis. ***Half-life:*** 5.8 days.

INDICATIONS AND DOSAGES

▸ **Prostatic Carcinoma**

PO

Adults, Elderly. 50–100 mg once a day in morning or evening, given concurrently with a LHRH analogue or after surgical castration.

SIDE EFFECTS/ADVERSE REACTIONS

Frequent

Hot flashes, breast pain, muscle pain, constipation, asthenia, nausea, diarrhea

Occasional
Nocturia, abdominal pain, peripheral edema
Rare
Vomiting, weight loss, dizziness, insomnia, rash, impotence, gynecomastia

PRECAUTIONS AND CONTRAINDICATIONS
Hypersensitivity, women who may become pregnant, pregnancy category X
Caution:
Hepatic impairment, lactation, children

DRUG INTERACTIONS OF CONCERN TO DENTISTRY
- Avoid drugs that could exacerbate urinary retention, such as anticholinergics.

SERIOUS REACTIONS
! Sepsis, CHF, hypertension, and iron deficiency anemia may occur.

DENTAL CONSIDERATIONS
General:
- Patients taking opioids for acute or chronic pain should be given alternative analgesics for dental pain.
- Palliative medication may be required for management of oral side effects.
- Assess salivary flow as a factor in caries, periodontal disease, and candidiasis.
- Monitor vital signs at every appointment because of cardiovascular and respiratory side effects.
- Short appointments may be required for patient comfort.
- Consider semisupine chair position for patient comfort because of disease and drug side effects.
- Place on frequent recall because of oral side effects.

Consultations:
- Medical consultation may be required to assess disease control and patient's ability to tolerate stress.

Teach Patient/Family to:
- Update medical/drug record if physician makes any changes in evaluation or drug regimens.
- When chronic dry mouth occurs, advise patient to:
  - Avoid mouth rinses with high alcohol content because of drying effects.
  - Use daily home fluoride products for anticaries effect.
  - Use sugarless gum, frequent sips of water, or saliva substitutes.

bimatoprost
bye-**mat′**-oh-prost
(Lumigan)

CATEGORY AND SCHEDULE
Pregnancy Risk Category: C

Drug Class: A prostamide (synthetic structural analogue of prostaglandin)

MECHANISM OF ACTION
A synthetic analogue of prostaglandin with ocular hypotensive activity.
Therapeutic Effect: Reduces intraocular pressure (IOP) by increasing the outflow of aqueous humor.

USES
Reduction of elevated IOP in patients with open-angle glaucoma or ocular hypertension who are intolerant of, or insufficiently

B

responsive to, other IOP-lowering drugs

PHARMACOKINETICS

Absorbed through the cornea and hydrolyzed to the active free acid form. Protein binding: 88%. Moderately distributed into body tissues. Metabolized in liver. Primarily excreted in urine; some elimination in feces. ***Half-life:*** 45 min.

INDICATIONS AND DOSAGES

▸ Glaucoma, Ocular Hypertension

Ophthalmic

Adults, Elderly. 1 drop in affected eye(s) once daily, in the evening.

SIDE EFFECTS/ADVERSE REACTIONS

Frequent

Conjunctival hyperemia, growth of eyelashes, and ocular pruritus

Occasional

Ocular dryness, visual disturbance, ocular burning, foreign body sensation, eye pain, pigmentation of the periocular skin, blepharitis, cataract, superficial punctate keratitis, eyelid erythema, ocular irritation, and eyelash darkening

Rare

Intraocular inflammation (iritis)

PRECAUTIONS AND CONTRAINDICATIONS

Hypersensitivity to bimatoprost or any other component of the formulation

Caution:

Increased pigmentation in iris and eyelid, change in eye color, changes in eyelashes (color, length, shape); uveitis, macular edema; renal or hepatic impairment, lactation, pediatric use, remove contact lenses to apply

DRUG INTERACTIONS OF CONCERN TO DENTISTRY

- None reported

SERIOUS REACTIONS

! Systemic adverse events, including infections (colds and upper respiratory tract infections), headaches, asthenia, and hirsutism, have been reported.

DENTAL CONSIDERATIONS

General:

- Avoid drugs with anticholinergic activity, such as antihistamines, opioids, benzodiazepines, propantheline, atropine, and scopolamine.
- Protect patient's eyes from accidental spatter during dental treatment.
- Avoid dental light in patient's eyes; offer dark glasses for patient comfort.

Consultations:

- Medical consultation may be required to assess disease control.

Teach Patient/Family to:

- Update health and drug history if physician makes any changes in evaluation or drug regimens.

biperiden

bye-**per′**-ih-den

(Akineton HCl)

CATEGORY AND SCHEDULE

Pregnancy Risk Category: C

Drug Class: Anticholinergic

MECHANISM OF ACTION

A weak anticholinergic that exhibits competitive antagonism of acetylcholine at cholinergic

receptors in the corpus striatum, which restores balance.
Therapeutic Effect: Antiparkinson activity.

USES

Treatment of Parkinson symptoms, extrapyramidal symptoms secondary to neuroleptic drug therapy

PHARMACOKINETICS

Well absorbed from GI tract. Protein binding: 23%–33%. Widely distributed. ***Half-life:*** 18–24 hr.

INDICATIONS AND DOSAGES

▸ **Extrapyramidal Symptoms**

PO

Adults, Elderly. 2 mg 3–4 times a day. Dosage in renal impairment.

▸ **Parkinsonism**

PO

Adults, Elderly. 2 mg 1–3 times a day.

SIDE EFFECTS/ADVERSE REACTIONS

Frequent

Orthostatic hypotension, anorexia, headache, blurred vision, urinary retention, dry mouth or nose

Occasional

Insomnia, agitation, euphoria

Rare

Vomiting, depression, irritation or swelling of eyes, rash

PRECAUTIONS AND CONTRAINDICATIONS

Hypersensitivity, narrow-angle glaucoma, myasthenia gravis, GI/GU obstruction, megacolon, stenosing peptic ulcers

Caution:

Elderly, lactation, tachycardia, prostatic hypertrophy, dysrhythmias, liver or kidney disease, drug abuse, hypotension, hypertension, psychiatric patients, children

DRUG INTERACTIONS OF CONCERN TO DENTISTRY

- Increased anticholinergic effect: antihistamines, anticholinergic-acting drugs, meperidine
- Increased CNS depression: alcohol, CNS depressants
- Decreased effects of phenothiazines

SERIOUS REACTIONS

! Overdosage may vary from severe anticholinergic effects, such as unsteadiness, severe drowsiness, dryness of mouth, nose, or throat, tachycardia, shortness of breath, and skin flushing.

! Also produces severe paradoxical reaction, marked by hallucinations, tremor, seizures, and toxic psychosis.

DENTAL CONSIDERATIONS

General:

- Monitor vital signs at every appointment because of cardiovascular side effects.
- After supine positioning, have patient sit upright for at least 2 min to avoid orthostatic hypotension.
- Assess salivary flow as a factor in caries, periodontal disease, and candidiasis.
- Avoid dental light in patient's eyes; offer dark glasses for patient comfort.

Consultations:

- Medical consultation may be required to assess disease control and patient's ability to tolerate stress.

Teach Patient/Family to:

- Use powered tooth brush if patient has difficulty holding conventional devices.
- Use effective hygiene to prevent soft tissue inflammation.

B

- When chronic dry mouth occurs, advise patient to:
  - Avoid mouth rinses with high alcohol content because of drying effects.
  - Use daily home fluoride products for anticaries effect.
  - Use sugarless gum, frequent sips of water, or saliva substitutes.

bisacodyl

bis-ah-**koe′**-dill

(Alophen, Apo-Bisacodyl[CAN], Bisa-Lax[AUS], Dulcolax, Femilax, Gentlax, Modane, Veracolate)

Do not confuse Veracolate with Accolate, or Modane with Mudrane.

CATEGORY AND SCHEDULE

Pregnancy Risk Category: C

OTC

Drug Class: Laxative, carbon dioxide-releasing; hyperosmotic; laxative, hyperosmotic, saline; laxative, lubricant; laxative, stimulant (contact); laxative, stool softener (emollient)

MECHANISM OF ACTION

A GI stimulant that has a direct effect on colonic smooth musculature by stimulating the intramural nerve plexus.

Therapeutic Effect: Promotes fluid and ion accumulation in the colon, increasing peristalsis and producing a laxative effect.

USES

As enemas or suppositories to produce bowel movements in a short time

PHARMACOKINETICS

Route	Onset	Peak	Duration
PO	6–12 hr	N/A	N/A
Rectal	15–30 min	N/A	N/A

Minimal absorption following oral and rectal administration. Absorbed drug is excreted in urine; remainder is eliminated in feces.

INDICATIONS AND DOSAGES

▸Treatment of Constipation

PO

Adults, Children older than 12 yr. 5–15 mg as needed. Maximum: 30 mg.

Children 3–12 yr. 5–10 mg or 0.3 mg/kg at bedtime or after breakfast.

Elderly. Initially, 5 mg/day.

Rectal

Adults, Children 12 yr and older. 10 mg to induce bowel movement.

Children 2–11 yr. 5–10 mg as a single dose.

Children younger than 2 yr. 5 mg.

Elderly. 5–10 mg/day.

SIDE EFFECTS/ADVERSE REACTIONS

Frequent

Some degree of abdominal discomfort, nausea, mild cramps, faintness

Occasional

Rectal administration: burning of rectal mucosa, mild proctitis

PRECAUTIONS AND CONTRAINDICATIONS

Abdominal pain, appendicitis, intestinal obstruction, nausea, undiagnosed rectal bleeding, vomiting

DRUG INTERACTIONS OF CONCERN TO DENTISTRY

• None reported; however, a delayed absorption time may be expected for orally administered drugs.

SERIOUS REACTIONS

! Long-term use may result in laxative dependence, chronic constipation, and loss of normal bowel function.
! Prolonged use or overdose may result in electrolyte or metabolic disturbances (such as hypokalemia, hypocalcemia, and metabolic acidosis or alkalosis), as well as persistent diarrhea, vomiting, muscle weakness, malabsorption, and weight loss.

DENTAL CONSIDERATIONS

General:
• Determine why patient is taking the drug.
• Consider semisupine chair position for patient comfort if GI side effects occur.
• Avoid the use of drugs that may exacerbate constipation, e.g., opioids.

bismuth subsalicylate

bis′-muth sub-sal-**ih′**-sah-late
(Bismed[CAN], Colo-Fresh, Devrom, Kaopectate, Pepto-Bismol)

CATEGORY AND SCHEDULE

Pregnancy Risk Category: C
OTC

Drug Class: Antidiarrheal

MECHANISM OF ACTION

An antinauseant and antiulcer agent that absorbs water and toxins in the large intestine and forms a protective coating in the intestinal mucosa. Also possesses antisecretory and antimicrobial effects.
Therapeutic Effect: Prevents diarrhea. Helps treat *Helicobacter pylori*-associated peptic ulcer disease.

USES

Treatment of diarrhea (cause undetermined), prevention of diarrhea when traveling

PHARMACOKINETICS

PO: Onset 1 hr, peak 2 hr, duration 4 hr.

INDICATIONS AND DOSAGES

▸ Diarrhea, Gastric Distress

PO
Adults, Elderly. 2 tablets (30 ml) q30–60 min. Maximum: 8 doses in 24 hr.
Children 9–12 yr. 1 tablet or 15 ml q30–60 min. Maximum: 8 doses in 24 hr.
Children 6–8 yr. Two-thirds of a tablet or 10 ml q30–60 min. Maximum: 8 doses in 24 hr.
Children 3–5 yr. One-third of a tablet or 5 ml q30–60 min. Maximum: 8 doses in 24 hr.

▸ *H. pylori*-Associated Duodenal Ulcer, Gastritis

PO
Adults, Elderly. 525 mg 4 times a day, with 500 mg amoxicillin and 500 mg metronidazole, 3 times a day after meals, for 7–14 days.

B

▸ **Chronic Infant Diarrhea**
PO
Children 2–24 mo. 2.5 ml q4h.

SIDE EFFECTS/ADVERSE REACTIONS

Frequent
Grayish-black stools
Rare
Constipation

PRECAUTIONS AND CONTRAINDICATIONS

Bleeding ulcers, gout, hemophilia, hemorrhagic states, renal impairment
Caution:
Anticoagulant therapy

DRUG INTERACTIONS OF CONCERN TO DENTISTRY

- Salicylate toxicity: other salicylates
- Decreased absorption of tetracyclines, other antibiotics
- Suspected reduction in antihypertensives and vasodilator effects of ACE inhibitors; monitor blood pressure if used concurrently

SERIOUS REACTIONS

! Debilitated patients and infants may develop impaction.

DENTAL CONSIDERATIONS

General:
- Avoid prescribing aspirin-containing products for analgesia.

bisoprolol fumarate

bis-**ope′**-pro-lal foo′-mar-ate
(Bicor[AUS], Zebeta)
Do not confuse Zebeta with DiaBeta.

CATEGORY AND SCHEDULE

Pregnancy Risk Category: C (D if used in second or third trimester)

Drug Class: Antihypertensive, selective β_1-blocker

MECHANISM OF ACTION

An antihypertensive that blocks β_1-adrenergic receptors in cardiac tissue.
Therapeutic Effect: Slows sinus heart rate and decreases B/P.

USES

Treatment of hypertension as a single agent or in combination with other antihypertensives, mild to moderate heart failure

PHARMACOKINETICS

Well absorbed from the GI tract. Protein binding: 26%–33%. Metabolized in the liver. Primarily excreted in urine. Not removed by hemodialysis. ***Half-life:*** 9–12 hr (increased in impaired renal function).

INDICATIONS AND DOSAGES

▸ **Hypertension**
PO
Adults. Initially, 5 mg/day. May increase up to 20 mg/day.
Elderly. Initially, 2.5–5 mg/day. May increase by 2.5–5 mg/day. Maximum: 20 mg/day.
▸ **Dosage in Hepatic Impairment**
For adults and elderly patients with cirrhosis or hepatitis whose

creatinine clearance is less than 40 ml/min, initially give 2.5 mg.

SIDE EFFECTS/ADVERSE REACTIONS

Frequent

Hypotension manifested as dizziness, nausea, diaphoresis, headache, cold extremities, fatigue, constipation, or diarrhea

Occasional

Insomnia, flatulence, urinary frequency, impotence, or decreased libido

Rare

Rash, arthralgia, myalgia, confusion (especially in the elderly), altered taste

PRECAUTIONS AND CONTRAINDICATIONS

Cardiogenic shock, overt cardiac failure, second- or third-degree heart block

Caution:

Major surgery, lactation, diabetes mellitus, renal disease, thyroid disease, COPD, heart failure, CAD, nonallergic bronchospasm, hepatic disease

DRUG INTERACTIONS OF CONCERN TO DENTISTRY

- Decreased antihypertensive effects: NSAIDs, indomethacin, sympathomimetics
- May slow metabolism of lidocaine
- Decreased β-blocking effects (or decreased β-adrenergic effects) of epinephrine, levonordefrin, isoproterenol, and other sympathomimetics

SERIOUS REACTIONS

! Overdose may produce profound bradycardia and hypotension.

! Abrupt withdrawal may result in diaphoresis, palpitations, headache, and tremulousness.

! Bisoprolol administration may precipitate CHF and MI in patients with heart disease, thyroid storm in those with thyrotoxicosis, and peripheral ischemia in those with existing peripheral vascular disease.

! Hypoglycemia may occur in patients with previously controlled diabetes.

! Thrombocytopenia, including unusual bruising and bleeding, occurs rarely.

DENTAL CONSIDERATIONS

General:

- Monitor vital signs at every appointment because of cardiovascular side effects.
- After supine positioning, have patient sit upright for at least 2 min to avoid orthostatic hypotension.
- Patients on chronic drug therapy may rarely have symptoms of blood dyscrasias, which can include infection, bleeding, and poor healing.
- Patient should never abruptly discontinue.
- Assess salivary flow as a factor in caries, periodontal disease, and candidiasis.
- Stress from dental procedures may compromise cardiovascular function; determine patient risk.
- Short appointments and a stress-reduction protocol may be required for anxious patients.
- Use vasoconstrictors with caution, in low doses, and with careful aspiration. Avoid use of gingival retraction cord with epinephrine.

Consultations:

- In a patient with symptoms of blood dyscrasias, request a medical consultation for blood studies and postpone dental treatment until normal values are reestablished.

B

• Medical consultation may be required to assess disease control and patient's ability to tolerate stress.
• Take precautions if general anesthesia is required for dental surgery.

Teach Patient/Family to:
• When chronic dry mouth occurs, advise patient to:
  • Avoid mouth rinses with high alcohol content because of drying effects.
  • Use daily home fluoride products for anticaries effect.
  • Use sugarless gum, frequent sips of water, or saliva substitutes.

bivalirudin

bye-va-**leer′**-uh-din
(Angiomax)

CATEGORY AND SCHEDULE

Pregnancy Risk Category: B

Drug Class: Anticoagulants, thrombin inhibitors

MECHANISM OF ACTION

An anticoagulant that specifically and reversibly inhibits thrombin by binding to its receptor sites.
Therapeutic Effect: Decreases acute ischemic complications in patients with unstable angina pectoris.

USES

Treatment of unstable angina in patients undergoing percutaneous transluminal coronary angioplasty

PHARMACOKINETICS

Route	Onset	Peak	Duration
IV	Immediate	N/A	1 hr

Primarily eliminated by kidneys. Twenty-five percent removed by hemodialysis. ***Half-life:*** 25 min (increased in moderate to severe renal impairment).

INDICATIONS AND DOSAGES

▸Anticoagulant in Patients with Unstable Angina Who Are Undergoing Percutaneous Transluminal Coronary Angioplasty (PTCA) in Conjunction with Aspirin

IV

Adults, Elderly. 1 mg/kg as IV bolus followed by 4-hr IV infusion at rate of 2.5 mg/kg/hr. After initial 4-hr infusion is completed, give additional IV infusion at rate of 0.2 mg/kg/hr for 20 hr or less, if necessary.

Dosage in Renal Impairment

GFR	Dosage Reduced By
30–59 ml/min	20%
10–29 ml/min	60%
Dialysis	90%

SIDE EFFECTS/ADVERSE REACTIONS

Frequent
Back pain
Occasional
Nausea, headache, hypotension, generalized pain
Rare
Injection site pain, insomnia, hypertension, anxiety, vomiting, pelvic or abdominal pain, bradycardia, nervousness, dyspepsia, fever, urine retention

PRECAUTIONS AND CONTRAINDICATIONS

Active major bleeding

DRUG INTERACTIONS OF CONCERN TO DENTISTRY

- Increased risk of bleeding: anticoagulants, antiplatelet agents, thrombolytics, ginkgo biloba (herb)

SERIOUS REACTIONS

! A hemorrhagic event occurs rarely and is characterized by a fall in B/P or HCT.

DENTAL CONSIDERATIONS

General:

- Intended for use in hospitals or emergency rooms.
- Patients are at risk of bleeding; check for oral signs.
- Provide palliative dental care for dental emergencies only.

Consultations:

- Medical consultation should include routine blood counts including coagulation platelet counts and aggregation.
- In a patient with symptoms of blood dyscrasias, request a medical consultation for blood studies and postpone treatment until normal values are reestablished.

Teach Patient/Family to:

- Use soft tooth brush to reduce risk of bleeding.
- Use effective oral hygiene to prevent soft tissue inflammation.
- Report oral lesions, soreness, or bleeding to dentist.
- Prevent trauma when using oral hygiene aids.
- Update health and medication history if physician makes any changes in evaluation or drug regimens; include OTC, herbal, and nonherbal remedies in the update.

bleomycin sulfate

blee-oh-**my′**-sin **sull′**-fate
(Blenamax[AUS], Blenoxane)

CATEGORY AND SCHEDULE

Pregnancy Risk Category: D

Drug Class: Antineoplastic

MECHANISM OF ACTION

A glycopeptide antibiotic whose mechanism of action is unknown. Is most effective in the G2 phase of cell division.

Therapeutic Effect: Appears to inhibit DNA synthesis and, to a lesser extent, RNA and protein synthesis.

USES

Treatment of cancer of head, neck, penis, cervix, vulva of squamous cell origin, Hodgkin's and non-Hodgkin's disease, lymphosarcoma, reticulum cell sarcoma, testicular carcinoma, as a sclerosing agent for malignant pleural effusion

PHARMACOKINETICS

Half-life: 2 hr; when creatinine clearance is greater than 35 ml/min, half-life is increased in lower clearance; metabolized in liver, 50% excreted in urine (unchanged).

INDICATIONS AND DOSAGES

▸ **As Monotherapy to Treat Testicular Carcinoma; Lymphomas (Including Hodgkin's Disease, Choriocarcinoma, Reticulum Cell Sarcoma, and Lymphosarcoma); and Squamous Cell Carcinomas of the**

Head and Neck (Including Mouth, Tongue, Tonsil, Nasopharynx, Oropharynx, Sinus, Palate, Lip, Buccal Mucosa, Gingiva, Epiglottis, and Larynx)
IV, IM, Subcutaneous
Adults, Elderly. 10–20 units/m^2 (0.25–0.5 units/kg) 1–2 times/wk.
IV (Continuous)
Adults, Elderly. 15 units/m^2 over 24 hr for 4 days.

▸ **In Combination Therapy to Treat Testicular Carcinoma; Lymphomas (Including Hodgkin's Disease, Choriocarcinoma, Reticulum Cell Sarcoma, and Lymphosarcoma); and Squamous Cell Carcinomas of the Head and Neck (Including Mouth, Tongue, Tonsil, Nasopharynx, Oropharynx, Sinus, Palate, Lip, Buccal Mucosa, Gingiva, Epiglottis, and Larynx)**
IV, IM
Adults, Elderly. 3–4 units/m^2.

▸ **As a Sclerosing Agent to Treat Malignant Pleural Effusions and Prevent Recurrent Pleural Effusions**
Intrapleural
Adults, Elderly. 60–240 units as a single injection.

SIDE EFFECTS/ADVERSE REACTIONS

Frequent
Anorexia, weight loss, erythematous skin swelling, urticaria, rash, striae, vesiculation, hyperpigmentation (particularly at areas of pressure, skin folds, cuticles, IM injection sites, and scars), stomatitis (usually evident 1–3 wk after initial therapy); may also be accompanied by decreased skin sensitivity followed by skin hypersensitivity, nausea, vomiting, alopecia, and—with parenteral form—fever or chills (typically occurring a few hours after large single dose and lasting 4–12 hr)

PRECAUTIONS AND CONTRAINDICATIONS

Previous allergic reaction

DRUG INTERACTIONS OF CONCERN TO DENTISTRY

- None reported

SERIOUS REACTIONS

! Interstitial pneumonitis occurs in 10% of patients and occasionally progresses to pulmonary fibrosis. This condition appears to be dose or age related, occurring more often in patients receiving a total dose greater than 400 units and those older than 70 yr.

! Nephrotoxicity and hepatotoxicity occur infrequently.

DENTAL CONSIDERATIONS

General:

- Monitor vital signs at every appointment due to cardiovascular side effects.
- Examine for oral manifestation of opportunistic infection.
- This drug may be used in the hospital or on an outpatient basis. Confirm the patient's disease and treatment status.
- Chlorhexidine mouth rinse prior to and during chemotherapy may reduce severity of mucositis.
- Patient on chronic drug therapy may rarely present with symptoms of blood dyscrasias, which can include infection, bleeding, and poor healing. If dyscrasia is present, caution patient to prevent oral tissue trauma when using oral hygiene aids.
- Palliative medication may be required for management of oral side effects.
- Patients may have received other chemotherapy or radiation; confirm medical and drug history.

• Patients may be taking a prophylactic antiinfective.
• Place on frequent recall due to oral side effects.

Consultations:

• Consult physician; prophylactic or therapeutic antiinfectives may be indicated if surgery or periodontal treatment is required.
• Medical consultation may be required to assess immunologic status during cancer chemotherapy and determine safety risk, if any, posed by the required dental treatment.
• Medical consultation may be required to assess disease control and patient's ability to tolerate stress.

Teach Patient/Family to:

• Be aware of oral side effects.
• Use effective oral hygiene to prevent soft tissue inflammation.
• Report oral lesions, soreness, or bleeding to dentist.
• Prevent trauma when using oral hygiene aids.
• Update health and medication history if physician makes any changes in evaluation or drug regimens; include OTC, herbal, and nonherbal remedies in the update.

boceprevir

boe-**se**′-pre-vir
(Victrelis)

CATEGORY AND SCHEDULE

Pregnancy Risk Category: B / X (in combination with ribavirin)

Drug Class: Antiviral agent, protease inhibitor

MECHANISM OF ACTION

Binds reversibly to nonstructural protein 3 serine protease and inhibits replication of the hepatitis C virus.

Therapeutic Effect: Inhibits replication of hepatitis C virus, slowing progression of or improving the clinical status of hepatitis infection.

USES

Treatment of chronic hepatitis C (in combination with peginterferon alfa and ribavirin) in adult patients with compensated liver disease who were previously untreated or have failed prior therapy with peginterferon alfa and ribavirin

PHARMACOKINETICS

Following oral administration, food enhances absorption up to 65%. Peak plasma concentrations reached in 2 hr. 75% plasma protein bound. Hepatic metabolism via aldo-ketoreductase and CYP3A4/5 pathways to inactive metabolites. Excreted 79% via feces and 9% via urine. ***Half-life:*** 3 hr.

INDICATIONS AND DOSAGES

▸ Treatment of Chronic Hepatitis C (CHC)

PO

Adults. 800 mg 3 times/day (in combination with peginterferon alfa and ribavirin). Administer with food. Doses should be taken approximately every 7–9 hr. Should not be used as monotherapy; administer concurrently with peginterferon alfa and ribavirin.

SIDE EFFECTS/ADVERSE REACTIONS

Frequent

Fatigue, chills, insomnia, irritability, dizziness, headache, alopecia, dry skin, rash, nausea, abnormal taste, inappetence, diarrhea, vomiting, xerostomia, arthralgia, weakness, dyspnea

Occasional

Thrombocytopenia, thromboembolic events

B

PRECAUTIONS AND CONTRAINDICATIONS

Hypersensitivity to boceprevir or any component of the formulation; contraindicated during pregnancy and in male partners of pregnant women

DRUG INTERACTIONS OF CONCERN TO DENTISTRY

• Increased risk adverse effects: CYP3A4 inhibitors, e.g., macrolide antibiotics (clarithromycin), azole antifungals (e.g., ketoconazole)
• Increased blood levels and CNS depressant effects of some benzodiazepines (midazolam, triazolam)
• Decreased therapeutic effect of boceprevir: CYP3A4 inducers (e.g., carbamazepine, phenobarbital, St. John's wort)

SERIOUS REACTIONS

! Addition of boceprevir may result in higher incidence of neutropenia and anemia (resulting from ribavirin/peginterferon alfa therapy) and may require use of erythropoietic-stimulating agents, dose reduction, or termination of therapy

DENTAL CONSIDERATIONS

General:
• Dysgeusia may alter patient's response to preventive and restorative materials.
• After supine positioning, have patient sit upright for at least 2 min to avoid orthostatic hypotension.

Consultations:
• Consult patient's physician to assess disease control and ability to tolerate dental procedures.

Teach Patient/Family to:
• Avoid mouth rinses with high alcohol content because of drying effect.
• Report changes in disease status and medication regimen.

bosentan

bo′-sen-tan
(Tracleer)
Do not confuse with TriCor.

CATEGORY AND SCHEDULE

Pregnancy Risk Category: X

Drug Class: Antihypertensive

MECHANISM OF ACTION

An endothelin receptor antagonist that blocks endothelin-1, the neurohormone that constricts pulmonary arteries.
Therapeutic Effect: Improves exercise ability and slows clinical worsening of pulmonary arterial hypertension (PAH).

USES

Treatment of pulmonary arterial hypertension in patients with World Health Organization (WHO) class III and IV symptoms

PHARMACOKINETICS

Highly bound to plasma proteins, mainly albumin. Metabolized in the liver. Eliminated by biliary excretion. ***Half-life:*** Approximately 5 hr.

INDICATIONS AND DOSAGES

▸ PAH in Those with WHO Class III or IV Symptoms

PO

Adults, Elderly. 62.5 mg twice a day for 4 wk; then increase to maintenance dosage of 125 mg twice a day.
Children weighing less than 40 kg. 62.5 mg twice a day.

SIDE EFFECTS/ADVERSE REACTIONS

Occasional
Headache, nasopharyngitis, flushing

Rare
Dyspepsia (heartburn, epigastric distress), fatigue, pruritus, hypotension

PRECAUTIONS AND CONTRAINDICATIONS

Administration with cyclosporine or glyburide, pregnancy
Caution:
Hepatic impairment, pregnancy category X, use during lactation or in children has not been determined, necessitates monthly tests for pregnancy during use

DRUG INTERACTIONS OF CONCERN TO DENTISTRY

- Increased plasma concentrations: ketoconazole and possibly other drugs that inhibit or induce CYP450 enzymes involved with metabolism
- See contraindications for other drugs

SERIOUS REACTIONS

! Abnormal hepatic function, lower extremity edema, and palpitations occur rarely.

DENTAL CONSIDERATIONS

General:
- Acute PAH rarely occurs and is a major medical problem. Patients are at high risk.
- Chronic PAH also occurs. Patients may be taking a variety of antihypertensive medications. It is advisable to consult with the physician of record to determine quality of disease control, patient's ability to tolerate stress, and, with this particular drug, liver function.

Teach Patient/Family to:
- Use effective oral hygiene to prevent tissue inflammation and dental caries.
- Update health and drug history if physician makes any changes in evaluation or drug regimens; include OTC, herbal, and nonherbal drugs in the update.

brimonidine

bry-**mo′**-nih-deen
(Alphagan P)
Do not confuse with bromocriptine.

CATEGORY AND SCHEDULE

Pregnancy Risk Category: B

Drug Class: α-adrenergic receptor agonist

MECHANISM OF ACTION

An ophthalmic agent that is a selective α_2-adrenergic agonist.
Therapeutic Effect: Reduces intraocular pressure (IOP).

USES

Lowering of intraocular pressure in open-angle glaucoma or ocular hypertension; prevention of postoperative intraocular pressure elevation after argon laser trabeculoplasty

PHARMACOKINETICS

Plasma concentrations peak within 0.5–2.5 hr after ocular administration. Distributed into aqueous humor. Metabolized in liver. Primarily excreted in urine. ***Half-life:*** 3 hr.

INDICATIONS AND DOSAGES

▸ **Glaucoma, Ocular Hypertension**
Ophthalmic
Adults, Elderly, Children 2 yr and older. 1 drop in affected eye(s) 3 times a day.

B

SIDE EFFECTS/ADVERSE REACTIONS

Occasional

Allergic conjunctivitis, conjunctival hyperemia, eye pruritus, burning sensation, conjunctival folliculosis, oral dryness, visual disturbances

PRECAUTIONS AND CONTRAINDICATIONS

Concurrent use of MAOI therapy, hypersensitivity to brimonidine tartrate or any other component of the formulation

Caution:

Wait 15 min after using before inserting contact lens; tricyclic antidepressants, β-blockers, CNS depressants; severe CV disease, hepatic or renal impairment, depression, cerebral or coronary insufficiency, Raynaud's phenomenon, orthostatic hypotension, thromboangiitis obliterans, lactation, children younger than 2 yr

DRUG INTERACTIONS OF CONCERN TO DENTISTRY

- Drug interactions have not been studied; however, the following possibilities exist:
  - Increased CNS depression: opioids, sedatives, alcohol, and general anesthetics
  - Possible risk of interference with lowering intraocular pressure: anticholinergic drugs or drugs with anticholinergic actions; tricyclic antidepressants; benzodiazepines

SERIOUS REACTIONS

! Bradycardia, hypotension, iritis, miosis, skin reactions, including erythema, eyelid, pruritus, rash, vasodilation, and tachycardia have been reported.

DENTAL CONSIDERATIONS

General:

- Assess salivary flow as factor in caries, periodontal disease, and candidiasis.
- Avoid dental light in patient's eyes; offer dark glasses for patient comfort.
- Question patient about compliance with prescribed drug regimen for glaucoma.
- Avoid drugs with anticholinergic activity, such as antihistamines, opioids, benzodiazepines, propantheline, atropine, and scopolamine.
- Monitor vital signs at every appointment because of cardiovascular side effects.

Consultations:

- Consultation with physician may be necessary if sedation or general anesthesia is required.

Teach Patient/Family to:

- Update health and drug history if physician makes any changes in evaluation or drug regimens.
- When chronic dry mouth occurs, advise patient to:
  - Avoid mouth rinses with high alcohol content because of drying effects.
  - Use daily home fluoride products for anticaries effect.
  - Use sugarless gum, frequent sips of water, or saliva substitutes.

brinzolamide

brin-**zol'**-ah-mide

(Azopt)

CATEGORY AND SCHEDULE

Pregnancy Risk Category: C

Drug Class: Carbonic anhydrase inhibitor

MECHANISM OF ACTION
An ophthalmic agent that inhibits carbonic anhydrase. Decreases aqueous humor secretion.
Therapeutic Effect: Reduces intraocular pressure (IOP).

USES
Treatment of ocular hypertension, open-angle glaucoma

PHARMACOKINETICS
Systemically absorbed to some degree. Protein binding: 60%. Distributed extensively in red blood cells. Site of metabolism has not been established. Metabolized to active and inactive metabolites. Primarily excreted unchanged in urine.

INDICATIONS AND DOSAGES
▸ **Glaucoma, Ocular Hypertension**
Ophthalmic
Adults, Elderly. Instill 1 drop in affected eye(s) 3 times a day.

SIDE EFFECTS/ADVERSE REACTIONS
Occasional
Blurred vision, bitter taste, dry eye, ocular discharge, ocular discomfort and pain, ocular pruritus, headache, rhinitis
Rare
Allergic reactions, alopecia, chest pain, conjunctivitis, diarrhea, diplopia, dizziness, dry mouth, dyspnea, dyspepsia, eye fatigue, hypertonia, keratoconjunctivitis, keratopathy, kidney pain, lid margin crusting or sticky sensation, nausea, pharyngitis, tearing, urticaria

PRECAUTIONS AND CONTRAINDICATIONS
Hypersensitivity to brinzolamide or any other component of the formulation
Caution:
Lactation, no data for pediatric use

DRUG INTERACTIONS OF CONCERN TO DENTISTRY
• Avoid drugs that can exacerbate glaucoma (e.g., anticholinergics).

SERIOUS REACTIONS
! Electrolyte imbalance, development of an acidotic state, and possible CNS effects may occur.

DENTAL CONSIDERATIONS
General:
• Avoid dental light in patient's eyes; offer dark glasses for patient comfort.
• Question patient about compliance with prescribed drug regimen for glaucoma.
Consultations:
• Medical consult may be required to assess disease control.

bromocriptine mesylate
broe-moe-**krip′**-teen **mess′**-ah-late
(Apo-Bromocriptine[CAN], Bromohexal[AUS], Kripton[AUS], Parlodel)
Do not confuse bromocriptine with benztropine, or Parlodel with pindolol.

CATEGORY AND SCHEDULE
Pregnancy Risk Category: C

Drug Class: Dopamine receptor agonist, ovulation stimulant

MECHANISM OF ACTION

A dopamine agonist that directly stimulates dopamine receptors in the corpus striatum and inhibits prolactin secretion. Also suppresses secretion of growth hormone. ***Therapeutic Effect:*** Improves symptoms of parkinsonism, suppresses galactorrhea, and reduces serum growth hormone concentrations in acromegaly.

USES

Treatment of female infertility, Parkinson's disease, prevention of postpartum lactation, amenorrhea caused by hyperprolactinemia, acromegaly

PHARMACOKINETICS

Indication	Onset	Peak	Duration
Prolactin lowering	2 hr	8 hr	24 hr
Antiparkinson	0.5–1.5 hr	2 hr	N/A
Growth hormone suppressant	1–2 hr	4–8 wk	4–8 hr

Minimally absorbed from the GI tract. Protein binding: 90%–96%. Metabolized in the liver. Excreted in feces by biliary secretion. ***Half-life:*** 15 hr.

INDICATIONS AND DOSAGES

▸ Hyperprolactinemia

PO

Adults, Elderly. Initially, 1.25–2.5 mg/day. May increase by 2.5 mg/day at 3- to 7-day intervals. Range: 2.5 mg 2–3 times a day.

▸ Parkinson's Disease

PO

Adults, Elderly. Initially, 1.25 mg twice a day. May increase by 2.5 mg/day every 14–28 days. Range: 30–90 mg/day.

▸ Acromegaly

PO

Adults, Elderly. Initially, 1.25–2.5 mg. May increase at 3- to 7-day intervals. Usual dose 20–30 mg/day.

SIDE EFFECTS/ADVERSE REACTIONS

Frequent

Nausea, headache, dizziness

Occasional

Fatigue, light-headedness, vomiting, abdominal cramps, diarrhea, constipation, nasal congestion, somnolence, dry mouth

Rare

Muscle cramps, urinary hesitancy

PRECAUTIONS AND CONTRAINDICATIONS

Hypersensitivity to ergot alkaloids, peripheral vascular disease, pregnancy, severe ischemic heart disease, uncontrolled hypertension

Caution:

Lactation, hepatic disease, renal disease, children

DRUG INTERACTIONS OF CONCERN TO DENTISTRY

- None reported

SERIOUS REACTIONS

! Visual or auditory hallucinations have been noted in patients with Parkinson's disease.

! Long-term, high-dose therapy may produce continuing rhinorrhea, syncope, GI hemorrhage, peptic ulcer, and severe abdominal pain.

DENTAL CONSIDERATIONS

General:

- Monitor vital signs at every appointment because of cardiovascular side effects.

• After supine positioning, have patient sit upright for at least 2 min to avoid orthostatic hypotension.
• Assess salivary flow as a factor in caries, periodontal disease, and candidiasis.
• Short appointments may be required because of disease effects on musculature.

Consultations:

• Medical consultation may be required to assess disease control.

Teach Patient/Family to:

• Avoid mouth rinses with high alcohol content because of drying effects.

brompheniramine

brome-fen-**ir′**-ah-meen
(BroveX, BroveX CT, Codimal A, Colhist, Dimetane, Dimetane Extentabs, Dimetapp, Lodrane 12 Hour, Nasahist B, ND Stat)

CATEGORY AND SCHEDULE

Pregnancy Risk Category: B
OTC (tablets, elixir)

Drug Class: Antihistamine, H_1-receptor antagonist

MECHANISM OF ACTION

An alkylamine that competes with histamine at histaminic receptor (H_1) sites. Inhibits central acetylcholine.
Therapeutic Effect: Results in anticholinergic, antipruritic, antitussive, antiemetic effects. Produces antidyskinetic, sedative effect.

USES

Allergy symptoms, rhinitis, hay fever

PHARMACOKINETICS

Rapidly absorbed after PO administration. Widely distributed. Metabolized in liver. Primarily excreted in urine. ***Half-life:*** 25 hr.

INDICATIONS AND DOSAGES

▸ **Allergic Rhinitis, Anaphylaxis, Urticarial Transfusion Reactions, Urticaria**

PO

Adults, Elderly, Children 12 yr and older. 4 mg q4–6h or 8–12 mg extended/timed-release q12h.
Children younger than 12 yr. 1–2 mg q4–6h.

▸ **Amelioration of Allergic Reactions to Blood or Plasma, Anaphylaxis as an Adjunct to Epinephrine and Other Standard Measures After the Acute Symptoms Have Been Controlled, Other Uncomplicated Allergic Conditions of the Immediate Type When Oral Therapy Is Impossible or Contraindicated**

IM/IV/SC

Adults, Elderly, Children 12 yr and older. 5–20 mg/day in 2 divided doses. Maximum: 40 mg/day.
Children younger than 12 yr. 0.125 mg/kg/day or 3.75 mg/m^2 in 3–4 divided doses.

SIDE EFFECTS/ADVERSE REACTIONS

Frequent

Drowsiness; dizziness; dry mouth, nose, or throat; urinary retention; thickening of bronchial secretions
Elderly. Sedation, dizziness, hypotension

Occasional

Epigastric distress, flushing, blurred vision, tinnitus, paresthesia, sweating, chills

B

PRECAUTIONS AND CONTRAINDICATIONS

Concurrent MAOI therapy, focal CNS lesions, newborn or premature infants, hypersensitivity to brompheniramine or related drugs

Caution:

Increased intraocular pressure, renal disease, cardiac disease, hypertension, bronchial asthma, seizure disorder, stenosed peptic ulcers, hyperthyroidism, prostatic hypertrophy, bladder neck obstruction

DRUG INTERACTIONS OF CONCERN TO DENTISTRY

- Increased CNS depression: alcohol, all CNS depressants
- Additive photosensitization: tetracyclines
- Increased drying effect: anticholinergics
- Hypotension: general anesthetics

SERIOUS REACTIONS

! Children may experience dominant paradoxical reactions, including restlessness, insomnia, euphoria, nervousness, and tremors.

! Overdosage in children may result in hallucinations, seizures, and death.

! Hypersensitivity reaction, such as eczema, pruritus, rash, cardiac disturbances, and photosensitivity, may occur.

DENTAL CONSIDERATIONS

General:

- Assess salivary flow as a factor in caries, periodontal disease, and candidiasis.
- Consider semisupine chair position for patients with respiratory disease.
- Determine why the patient is taking the drug.

Teach Patient/Family to:

- Use effective oral hygiene to prevent soft tissue inflammation.
- Avoid mouth rinses with high alcohol content because of drying effects.

bucindolol

byoo′-sin-doe-lole

(Gencaro)—currently unavailable in the U.S.

Drug Class: β-adrenergic blocker, nonselective

MECHANISM OF ACTION

Nonselective β-blocking activity. Mild vasodilatory activity.

Therapeutic Effect: Decreases B/P, increases left ventricular ejection fraction, reduces plasma rennin activity.

USES

Hypertension

Congestive heart failure

PHARMACOKINETICS

Route	Onset	Peak	Duration
PO (hypertension)	1 hr	2–3 hr	6–12 hr
PO (CHF)	4 hr	3 months	< 24 hr

Well absorbed from the GI tract. Bioavailability: approximately 30%. Undergoes extensive first-pass metabolism to active metabolite. ***Half-life:*** 3.6 hr.

INDICATIONS AND DOSAGES

▸ **Hypertension**

PO

Adults. Initially, 50 mg three times/day, followed by weekly increases until target blood pressure is achieved.

▸ **Congestive Heart Failure**

PO

Adults. Initially, 12.5mg every 12 hr. If tolerated, may increase. Maximum dose: 100 mg twice/day.

SIDE EFFECTS/ADVERSE REACTIONS

Frequent

Drowsiness, nausea, vomiting, abdominal cramps, dyspepsia, hypotension manifested as dizziness, faintness, light-headedness

Occasional

Facial flushing, hypoglycemia, hyperglycemia, arthralgias, myalgias, bronchospasms

Rare

Elevated liver enzymes

PRECAUTIONS AND CONTRAINDICATIONS

Hypersensitivity to bucindolol or any component of the formulation
Cardiogenic shock
Overt cardiac failure
Second- or third-degree AV block
Severe sinus bradycardia or hypotension

Caution:

Anesthesia/surgery
Abrupt withdrawal
Bronchial asthma or related bronchospastic conditions
Cerebrovascular insufficiency
Diabetes mellitus
Hyperthyroidism/thyrotoxicosis
Myasthenic conditions
Peripheral vascular disease
Renal disease

DRUG INTERACTIONS OF CONCERN TO DENTISTRY

- Amiodarone: increased risk of hypotension, bradycardia, or cardiac arrest
- β_2-agonists: decreased effectiveness
- Calcium channel blockers: increase risk of conduction disturbances
- Digoxin: increases concentrations of digoxin
- Diuretics, other antihypertensives: may increase hypotensive effect
- Insulin, oral hypoglycemics: may mask symptoms of hypoglycemia and prolong hypoglycemic effect of these drugs
- NSAIDs: decreased antihypertensive effect
- Epinephrine: may cause reflex tachycardia, hypertension, resistance to epinephrine

SERIOUS REACTIONS

! Overdose may produce profound bradycardia and hypotension.

! Abrupt withdrawal may result in rebound hypertension.

! Bucindolol administration may precipitate CHF or MI in patients with heart disease; thyroid storm in those with thyrotoxicosis; or peripheral ischemia in those with existing peripheral vascular disease.

! Hypoglycemia may occur in patients with previously controlled diabetes.

DENTAL CONSIDERATIONS

General:

- Monitor vital signs at every appointment because of cardiovascular side effects.
- After supine positioning, have patient sit upright for at least 2 min before standing to avoid orthostatic hypotension.

- Assess salivary flow as a factor in caries, periodontal disease, and candidiasis.
- Limit use of sodium-containing products, such as saline IV fluids, for those patients with dietary salt restriction.
- Stress from dental procedures may compromise cardiovascular function; determine patient risk.
- Limit or avoid vasoconstrictors.

Consultations:

- Medical consultation may be required to assess disease control.

Teach Patient/Family to:

- Report oral lesions, soreness, or bleeding to dentist.
- When chronic dry mouth occurs, advise patient to:
  - Avoid mouth rinses with high alcohol content because of drying effects.
  - Use daily home fluoride products for anticaries effect.
  - Use sugarless gum, frequent sips of water, or saliva substitutes.

buclizine hydrochloride

bew′-klih-zeen hi-droh-**klor′**-ide
(Bucladin-S)

CATEGORY AND SCHEDULE

Pregnancy Risk Category: C

Drug Class: Antiemetic

MECHANISM OF ACTION

A centrally acting agent that suppresses nausea and vomiting. Buclizine is an anticholinergic that reduces labyrinth excitability and diminishes vestibular stimulation of labyrinth, affecting chemoreceptor trigger zone (CTZ). Possesses anticholinergic activity.

Therapeutic Effect: Reduces nausea, vomiting, vertigo.

USES

Prophylaxis of nausea, vomiting, and dizziness associated with motion sickness

PHARMACOKINETICS

None reported

INDICATIONS AND DOSAGES

▸ **Motion Sickness**

PO

Adults, Elderly, Children 12 yr and older. 50 mg 30 min before travel. Dose may be repeated every 4–6 hr as needed. Maximum: 150 mg/day.

SIDE EFFECTS/ADVERSE REACTIONS

Frequent

Drowsiness

Occasional

Dryness of mouth, headache, jitteriness

PRECAUTIONS AND CONTRAINDICATIONS

Early pregnancy, hypersensitivity to buclizine or other components of the formulation, including tartrazine

DRUG INTERACTIONS OF CONCERN TO DENTISTRY

- None reported

SERIOUS REACTIONS

! Children may experience dominant paradoxical reaction, including restlessness, insomnia, euphoria, nervousness, and tremors.

! Overdosage in children may result in hallucinations, convulsions, and death.

! Hypersensitivity reaction, marked by eczema, pruritus, rash, cardiac disturbances, and photosensitivity, may occur.

! Overdosage may vary from CNS depression, such as sedation, apnea, cardiovascular collapse, or death, to severe paradoxical reaction, including hallucinations, tremors, or seizures.

DENTAL CONSIDERATIONS

General:

- Symptoms may preclude elective dental treatment.
- Assess salivary flow as a factor in caries, periodontal disease, and candidiasis.
- Consider semisupine chair position for patient comfort because of GI effects of disease.

Teach Patient/Family to:

- Use effective oral hygiene to prevent soft tissue inflammation.
- When chronic dry mouth occurs, advise patient to:
  - Avoid mouth rinses with high alcohol content because of drying effects.
  - Use daily home fluoride products for anticaries effect.
  - Use sugarless gum, frequent sips of water, or saliva substitutes.

budesonide

bu-**dess'**-ah-nide

(Burinex[AUS], Entocort EC, Pulmicort Respules, Pulmicort Turbuhaler, Rhinocort Aqua, Rhinocort Aqueous[AUS], Rhinocort Hayfever[AUS])

CATEGORY AND SCHEDULE

Pregnancy Risk Category: B

Drug Class: Glucocorticoid, long-acting

MECHANISM OF ACTION

A glucocorticoid that inhibits the accumulation of inflammatory cells and decreases and prevents tissues from responding to the inflammatory process.

Therapeutic Effect: Relieves symptoms of allergic rhinitis or Crohn's disease.

USES

Treatment of mild-to-moderate active Crohn's disease of the ileum or ascending colon

PHARMACOKINETICS

Minimally absorbed from nasal tissue; moderately absorbed from inhalation. Protein binding: 88%. Primarily metabolized in the liver. ***Half-life:*** 2–3 hr.

INDICATIONS AND DOSAGES

▸ **Rhinitis**

Intranasal (Rhinocort Aqua)

Adults, Elderly, Children 6 yr and older. 1 spray in each nostril once a day. Maximum: 8 sprays a day for adults and children 12 yr and older; 4 sprays a day for children younger than 12 yr.

▸ **Bronchial Asthma**

Nebulization

Children 6 mo–8 yr. 0.25–1 mg/day titrated to lowest effective dosage.

Inhalation

Adults, Elderly, Children 6 yr and older. Initially, 200–400 mcg twice a day. Maximum: Adults: 800 mcg twice a day. Children: 400 mcg twice a day.

▸ **Crohn's Disease**

PO

Adults, Elderly. 9 mg once a day for up to 8 wk.

B

SIDE EFFECTS/ADVERSE REACTIONS

Frequent
Nasal: Mild nasopharyngeal irritation, burning, stinging, or dryness; headache; cough
Inhalation: Flu-like symptoms, headache, pharyngitis
Occasional
Nasal: Dry mouth, dyspepsia, rebound congestion, rhinorrhea, loss of taste
Inhalation: Back pain, vomiting, altered taste, voice changes, abdominal pain, nausea, dyspepsia

PRECAUTIONS AND CONTRAINDICATIONS

Hypersensitivity to any corticosteroid or its components, persistently positive sputum cultures for *Candida albicans,* primary treatment of status asthmaticus, systemic fungal infections, untreated localized infection involving nasal mucosa
Caution:
Tuberculosis, hypertension, diabetes mellitus, osteoporosis, peptic ulcer, glaucoma, cataracts, suppression of the hypothalamic-pituitary-adrenal (HPA) axis, discontinue use during nursing or discontinue drug, safety in children has not been established, geriatric patients

SERIOUS REACTIONS

! An acute hypersensitivity reaction marked by urticaria, angioedema, and severe bronchospasm; occurs rarely.

DENTAL CONSIDERATIONS

General:
- Evaluate respiration characteristics and rate.
- Assess salivary flow as a factor in caries, periodontal disease, and candidiasis.
- Morning appointments are suggested with stress-reduction protocol for anxious patients.
- Place on frequent recall because of oral side effects.
- Acute asthmatic episodes may be precipitated in the dental office. Rapid-acting sympathomimetic inhalants should be available for emergency use. Budesonide is not a rapid-acting drug and is not intended for use in acute asthmatic attacks.

Consultations:
- Medical consultation may be required to assess disease control.

Teach Patient/Family to:
- Use effective oral hygiene to prevent soft tissue inflammation.
- Gargle and rinse with water after each dose.
- When chronic dry mouth occurs, advise patient to:
  - Avoid mouth rinses with high alcohol content because of drying effects.
  - Use daily home fluoride products for anticaries effect.
  - Use sugarless gum, frequent sips of water, or artificial saliva substitutes.

bumetanide

byoo-**met′**-ah-nide
(Bumex, Burinex[CAN])

CATEGORY AND SCHEDULE

Pregnancy Risk Category: C (D if used in pregnancy-induced hypertension)

Drug Class: Loop diuretic

MECHANISM OF ACTION

A loop diuretic that enhances excretion of sodium, chloride, and, to lesser degree, potassium, by direct action at the ascending limb of the loop of Henle and in the proximal tubule.

Therapeutic Effect: Produces diuresis.

USES

Treatment of edema in CHF, liver disease, renal disease (nephrotic syndrome), pulmonary edema, ascites (nephrotic syndrome), hypertension

PHARMACOKINETICS

Route	Onset	Peak	Duration
PO	30–60 min	60–120 min	60–120 min
IV	Rapid	15–30 min	2–3 hr
IM	40 min	4–6 hr	4–6 hr

Completely absorbed from the GI tract (absorption decreased in CHF and nephrotic syndrome). Protein binding: 94%–96%. Partially metabolized in the liver. Primarily excreted in urine. Not removed by hemodialysis. ***Half-life:*** 1–1.5 hr.

INDICATIONS AND DOSAGES

▸ Edema

PO

Adults, Children older than 18 yr. 0.5–2 mg as a single dose in the morning. May repeat at q4–5 hr.

Elderly. 0.5 mg/day, increased as needed.

IV, IM

Adults, Elderly. 0.5–2 mg/dose; may repeat in 2–3 hr. Or 0.5–1 mg/hr by continuous IV infusion.

▸ Hypertension

PO

Adults, Elderly. Initially, 0.5 mg/day. Range: 1–4 mg/day. Maximum: 5 mg/day. Larger doses may be given 2–3 doses a day.

▸ Usual Pediatric Dosage

PO, IV, IM

Children. 0.015–0.1 mg/kg/dose q6–24h.

SIDE EFFECTS/ADVERSE REACTIONS

Expected

Increased urinary frequency and urine volume

Frequent

Orthostatic hypotension, dizziness

Occasional

Blurred vision, diarrhea, headache, anorexia, premature ejaculation, impotence, dyspepsia

Rare

Rash, urticaria, pruritus, asthenia, muscle cramps, nipple tenderness

PRECAUTIONS AND CONTRAINDICATIONS

Anuria, hepatic coma, severe electrolyte depletion

Caution:

Dehydration, ascites, severe renal disease

DRUG INTERACTIONS OF CONCERN TO DENTISTRY

- Decreased diuretic effect: NSAIDs, indomethacin
- Masked ototoxicity: phenothiazines
- Increased electrolyte imbalance: nondepolarizing skeletal muscle relaxants, corticosteroids

SERIOUS REACTIONS

! Vigorous diuresis may lead to profound water and electrolyte depletion, resulting in hypokalemia, hyponatremia, dehydration, coma, and circulatory collapse.

! Ototoxicity—manifested as deafness, vertigo, or tinnitus—may occur, especially in patients with

B

severe renal impairment and those taking other ototoxic drugs.
! Blood dyscrasias and acute hypotensive episodes have been reported.

DENTAL CONSIDERATIONS

General:

- Monitor vital signs at every appointment because of cardiovascular side effects.
- Patients on chronic drug therapy may rarely have symptoms of blood dyscrasias, which can include infection, bleeding, and poor healing.
- After supine positioning, have patient sit upright for at least 2 min to avoid orthostatic hypotension.
- Assess salivary flow as a factor in caries, periodontal disease, and candidiasis.
- Limit or avoid vasoconstrictors.
- Limit use of sodium-containing products, such as saline IV fluids, for patients with a dietary salt restriction.
- Patients on high-potency diuretics should be monitored for serum K^+ levels.

Consultations:

- In a patient with symptoms of blood dyscrasias, request a medical consultation for blood studies and postpone dental treatment until normal values are reestablished.
- Medical consultation may be required to assess disease control.

Teach Patient/Family to:

- Use effective oral hygiene to prevent soft tissue inflammation.
- Use caution to prevent injury when using oral hygiene aids.
- When chronic dry mouth occurs, advise patient to:
- Avoid mouth rinses with high alcohol content because of drying effects.
- Use daily home fluoride products for anticaries effect.
- Use sugarless gum, frequent sips of water, or saliva substitutes.

bupivacaine

byoo-**piv′**-ah-caine
(Marcaine, Marcaine Spinal, Sensorcaine, Sensorcaine-MPF)

CATEGORY AND SCHEDULE

Pregnancy Risk Category: C

Drug Class: Amide local anesthetic

MECHANISM OF ACTION

An amide-type anesthetic that stabilizes neuronal membranes and prevents initiation and transmission of nerve impulses, thereby effecting local anesthetic actions.
Therapeutic Effect: Produces local analgesia.

USES

Local dental anesthesia, epidural anesthesia, peripheral nerve block, caudal anesthesia

PHARMACOKINETICS

Onset of action occurs within 4–10 min depending on route of administration. Duration is 1.5–8.5 hr, depending on site of administration. Well absorbed. Protein binding: 95%. Metabolized in liver. Excreted in urine. **Half-life:** 1.5–5.5 hr (adults), 8.1 hr (neonates).

INDICATIONS AND DOSAGES

Dose varies with procedure, depth of anesthesia, vascularity of tissues, duration of anesthesia, and condition of patient.

▸ Analgesic, Epidural (partial to moderate motor blockade)

IV

Adults, Elderly. 10–20 ml (25–50 mg) of a 0.25% solution. Repeat once q3h as needed.

Children weighing more than 10 kg. 1–2.5 mg/kg single dose as a 0.125% or 0.25% solution or 0.2–0.4 mg/kg/hr continuous infusion as a 0.1%, 0.125%, or 0.25% solution. Maximum: 0.4 mg/kg/hr.

Children weighing less than 10 kg. 1–1.25 mg/kg single dose as a 0.125% or 0.25% solution or 0.1–0.2 mg/kg/hr continuous infusion as a 0.1%, 0.125%, or 0.25% solution. Maximum: 0.2 mg/kg/hr.

▸ Analgesic, Epidural (moderate to complete motor blockade)

IV

Adults, Elderly. 10–20 ml (50–100 mg) as a 0.5% solution. Repeat once q3h as needed.

Children weighing more than 10 kg. 1–2.5 mg/kg single dose as a 0.125% or 0.25% solution or 0.2–0.4 mg/kg/hr continuous infusion as a 0.1%, 0.125%, or 0.25% solution. Maximum: 0.4 mg/kg/hr.

Children weighing less than 10 kg. 1–1.25 mg/kg single dose as a 0.125% or 0.25% solution or 0.1–0.2 mg/kg/hr continuous infusion as a 0.1%, 0.125%, or 0.25% solution. Maximum: 0.2 mg/kg/hr.

▸ Analgesic, Epidural (complete motor blockade)

IV

Adults. 10–20 ml (75–150 mg) as a 0.75% solution. Repeat once q3h as needed.

Children weighing more than 10 kg. 1–2.5 mg/kg single dose as a 0.125% or 0.25% solution or 0.2–0.4 mg/kg/hr continuous infusion as a 0.1%, 0.125%, or 0.25% solution. Maximum: 0.4 mg/kg/hr.

Children weighing less than 10 kg. 1–1.25 mg/kg single dose as a 0.125% or 0.25% solution or 0.1–0.2 mg/kg/hr continuous infusion as a 0.1%, 0.125%, or 0.25% solution. Maximum: 0.2 mg/kg/hr.

▸ Analgesic, Intrapleural

IV

Adults, Elderly. 10–30 ml bolus of 0.25%, 0.375%, or 0.5% q4–8h or 0.375% solution with epinephrine continuous infusion at 6 ml/hr after 20-ml loading dose.

▸ Analgesic, Caudal (moderate to complete blockade)

IV

Adults, Elderly. 15–30 ml of 0.5% solution (75–150 mg) or 0.25% solution (37.5–75 mg), repeated once every 3 hr as needed.

Children weighing more than 10 kg. 1–2.5 mg/kg single dose as a 0.125% or 0.25% solution or 0.2–0.4 mg/kg/hr continuous infusion as a 0.1%, 0.125%, or 0.25% solution. Maximum: 0.4 mg/kg/hr.

Children weighing less than 10 kg. 1–1.25 mg/kg single dose as a 0.125% or 0.25% solution or 0.1–0.2 mg/kg/hr continuous infusion as a 0.1%, 0.125%, or 0.25% solution. Maximum: 0.2 mg/kg/hr.

▸ Analgesic, Dental
IV
Adults, Elderly. 1.8–3.6 ml of 0.5% solution (9–18 mg) with epinephrine. A second dose of 9 mg may be administered. Maximum: 90 mg total dose.

▸ Analgesic, Peripheral Nerve Block (moderate to complete motor blockade)
IV
Adults, Elderly. 5–37.5 ml (25–175 mg) of 0.5% solution or 5–70 ml (12.5–175 mg) of 0.25% solution. Repeat q3h as needed. Maximum: up to 400 mg/day.
Children 12 yr and older. 0.3–2.5 mg/kg as a 0.25% or 0.5% solution. Maximum: 1 ml/kg of 0.25% solution or 0.5 ml/kg of 0.5% solution.

▸ Analgesic, Retrobulbar (complete motor blockade)
IV
Adults, Elderly. 2–4 ml (15–30 mg) of 0.75% solution.

▸ Analgesic, Sympathetic Blockade
IV
Adults, Elderly. 20–50 ml (50–125 mg) of 0.25% (no epinephrine) solution. Repeat once q3h as needed.

▸ Analgesic, Hyperbaric Spinal (obstetrical, normal vaginal delivery)
IV
Adults, Elderly. 0.8 ml (6 mg) bupivacaine in dextrose as 0.75% solution.

▸ Analgesic, Hyperbaric Spinal (obstetrical, cesarean section)
IV
Adults, Elderly. 1–1.4 ml (7.5–10.5 mg) bupivacaine in dextrose as 0.75% solution.

▸ Anesthesia, Hyperbaric Spinal (surgical, lower extremity, and perineal procedures)
IV
Adults, Elderly. 1 ml (7.5 mg) bupivacaine in dextrose as 0.75% solution.
Children 12 yr and older. 0.3–0.6 mg/kg bupivacaine in dextrose as a 0.75% solution.

▸ Anesthesia, Spinal (surgical, lower abdominal procedures)
IV
Adults, Elderly. 1.6 ml (12 mg) bupivacaine in dextrose as 0.75% solution.
Children 12 yr and older. 0.3–0.6 mg/kg bupivacaine in dextrose as a 0.75% solution.

▸ Anesthesia, Spinal (surgical, hyperbaric, upper abdominal procedures)
IV
Adults, Elderly. 2 ml (15 mg) bupivacaine in dextrose administered in horizontal position.
Children 12 yr and older. 0.3–0.6 mg/kg bupivacaine in dextrose as a 0.75% solution.

▸ Analgesic, Local Infiltration
IV
Adults, Elderly. 0.25% solution. Maximum: 225 mg with epinephrine or 175 mg without epinephrine.
Children 12 yr and older. 0.5–2.5 mg/kg as a 0.25% or 0.5% solution. Maximum: 1 ml/kg of 0.25% solution or 0.5 ml/kg of 0.5% solution.

SIDE EFFECTS/ADVERSE REACTIONS

Occasional

Hypotension, bradycardia, palpitations, respiratory depression, dizziness, headache, vomiting, nausea, restlessness, weakness, blurred vision, tinnitus, apnea

PRECAUTIONS AND CONTRAINDICATIONS

Local infection at the site of proposed lumbar puncture (spinal anesthesia), obstetrical paracervical block anesthesia, septicemia (spinal anesthesia), severe hemorrhage, severe hypotension or shock, arrhythmias such as complete heart block, which severely restricts cardiac output (spinal anesthesia), sulfite allergy (epinephrine-containing solutions only), hypersensitivity to bupivacaine products or to other amide-type anesthetics

Caution:

Elderly, severe drug allergies, use in children (risk of local injury because of long duration of anesthesia)

DRUG INTERACTIONS OF CONCERN TO DENTISTRY

- CNS depressants: may see increased risk of CNS depression with all CNS depressants, especially in children and when larger doses are used.
- Avoid placing dental cartridges in disinfectant solutions with heavy metals or surface-active agents; may see release of metal ions into local anesthetic solutions, with tissue irritation following injection.
- Avoid excessive exposure of dental cartridges to light or heat; it hastens deterioration of vasoconstrictors; color change in local anesthetic solution indicates breakdown of vasoconstrictor.
- Risk of cardiovascular side effects: rapid intravascular administration of local anesthetic containing vasoconstrictors, either alone or in patients taking tricyclic antidepressants, MAOIs, digitalis drugs, cocaine, phenothiazines, ß-blockers, and in the presence of halogenated hydrocarbon general anesthetics; always use the smallest effective vasoconstrictor dose and careful aspiration technique.
- Avoid use of vasoconstrictors in patients with uncontrolled hyperthyroidism, diabetes, angina, or hypertension; refer these patients for medical treatment before elective dental procedures.

SERIOUS REACTIONS

! Arterial hypotension, bradycardia, ventricular arrhythmias, central nervous system (CNS) depression and excitation, convulsions, respiratory arrest, tinnitus have been reported.

! Solutions with epinephrine contain metabisulfite, a sulfite that may cause allergic-type reactions, including anaphylaxis.

DENTAL CONSIDERATIONS

General:

- Monitor vital signs at every appointment because of cardiovascular and respiratory side effects.
- Lubricate dry lips before injection or dental treatment as required.

Teach Patient/Family to:

- Use care to prevent injury while numbness exists; do not chew gum or eat following dental anesthesia.
- Remember that numbness with this drug is expected to last for a considerable period.
- Report any signs of infection, muscle pain, or fever to dentist when oral sensations return.
- Report any unusual soft tissue reactions.

B

buprenorphine hydrochloride

byoo-pre-**nor′**-feen
hi-droh-**klor′**-ide
(Buprenex, Subutex, Temgesic[CAN])

CATEGORY AND SCHEDULE

Pregnancy Risk Category: C
Controlled Substance: Schedule III

Drug Class: Opioid agonist-antagonist

MECHANISM OF ACTION

An opioid agonist-antagonist that binds with opioid receptors in the CNS.
Therapeutic Effect: Alters the perception of and emotional response to pain; blocks the effects of heroin and produces minimal opioid withdrawal symptoms.

USES

Relief of moderate to severe pain (injection) and for treatment of opioid dependence (tablets)

PHARMACOKINETICS:

IM: Onset 15–30 min, duration 4–6 hr; absorption 90%–100%; hepatic metabolism; excreted in feces (68%–71%); also renal excretion.

INDICATIONS AND DOSAGES

▸ **Analgesia**
IV, IM
Adults, Children older than 12 yr. 0.3 mg q6–8h as needed. May repeat once in 30–60 min. Range: 0.15–0.6 mg q4–8h as needed.
Children 2–12 yr. 2–6 mcg/kg q4–6h as needed.
Elderly. 0.15 mg q6h as needed.

▸ **Opioid Dependence**
Sublingual
Adults, Elderly, Children older than 16 yr. Initially, 12–16 mg/day, beginning at least 4 hr after last use of heroin or short-acting opioid. Maintenance: 16 mg/day. Range: 4–24 mg/day. Patients should be switched to buprenorphine and naloxone combination, preferred for maintenance treatment.

SIDE EFFECTS/ADVERSE REACTIONS

Frequent
Tablet: Headache, pain, insomnia, anxiety, depression, nausea, abdominal pain, constipation, back pain, weakness, rhinitis, withdrawal syndrome, infection, diaphoresis
Injection (more than 10%): Sedation
Occasional
Injection: Hypotension, respiratory depression, dizziness, headache, vomiting, nausea, vertigo

PRECAUTIONS AND CONTRAINDICATIONS

Hypersensitivity to buprenorphine; hypersensitivity to naloxone for those receiving the fixed combination product containing naloxone (Suboxone)
Caution:
Hepatic impairment, hepatitis, risk of allergic reaction, bile tract disease, impaired respiration (COPD, cor pulmonale, decreased respiratory reserve, hypoxia, hypercapnia, preexisting respiratory depression); naloxone may not be effective as a narcotic reversal agent, head injury, impairment of reaction time, low abuse potential, opioid-dependent patients, debilitated patients, elderly, children younger than 2 yr, use not advised during lactation

DRUG INTERACTIONS OF CONCERN TO DENTISTRY

• Increased risk of respiratory and cardiovascular collapse: benzodiazepines, opioids
• Increased CNS depression: all CNS depressants, concomitant use of other opioids

SERIOUS REACTIONS

! Overdose results in cold and clammy skin, weakness, confusion, severe respiratory depression, cyanosis, pinpoint pupils, and extreme somnolence progressing to seizures, stupor, and coma.

DENTAL CONSIDERATIONS

General:
• Patients taking this drug for opioid dependence; avoid the use of any drug with abuse potential.
• Consider aspirin, acetaminophen, or NSAIDs for the management of dental-related pain.
• Monitor vital signs at every appointment because of cardiovascular side effects.
• After supine positioning, have patient sit upright for at least 2 min to avoid orthostatic hypotension.
• Assess salivary flow as a factor in caries, periodontal disease, and candidiasis.
• Consider semisupine chair position for patient comfort if GI or respiratory side effects occur.
• Take precautions if dental surgery is anticipated and general anesthesia is required.
• If opioid or sedative drugs are required for patient management and comfort, advise current drug abuse care facility or after-care program as appropriate.
Consultations:
• Consultations may be difficult to obtain where treatment confidentiality of drug dependence is followed.
• Medical consultation may be required to assess disease control.
Teach Patient/Family to:
• Use effective oral hygiene to prevent soft tissue inflammation.
• When chronic dry mouth occurs, advise patient to:
  • Avoid mouth rinses with high alcohol content because of drying effects.
  • Use daily home fluoride products for anticaries effect.
  • Use sugarless gum, frequent sips of water, or saliva substitutes.

bupropion

byoo-**proe′**-pee-on
(Wellbutrin, Wellbutrin SR, Wellbutrin XL, Zyban, Zyban sustained release[AUS])
Do not confuse bupropion with buspirone, Wellbutrin with Wellcovorin or Wellferon, or Zyban with Zagam.

CATEGORY AND SCHEDULE

Pregnancy Risk Category: B

Drug Class: Antidepressant

MECHANISM OF ACTION

An aminoketone that blocks the reuptake of neurotransmitters, including serotonin and norepinephrine at CNS presynaptic membranes, increasing their availability at postsynaptic receptor sites. Also reduces the firing rate of noradrenergic neurons.
Therapeutic Effect: Relieves depression and nicotine withdrawal symptoms.

B

USES

Treatment of depression; smoking cessation treatment (Zyban)

PHARMACOKINETICS

Rapidly absorbed from the GI tract. Protein binding: 84%. Crosses the blood-brain barrier. Undergoes extensive first-pass metabolism in the liver to active metabolite. Primarily excreted in urine. ***Half-life:*** 14 hr.

INDICATIONS AND DOSAGES

▸ Depression

PO (Immediate-Release)
Adults. Initially, 100 mg twice a day. May increase to 100 mg 3 times a day no sooner than 3 days after beginning therapy. Maximum: 450 mg/day.
Elderly. 37.5 mg twice a day. May increase by 37.5 mg q3–4 days. Maintenance: Lowest effective dosage.
PO (Sustained-Release)
Adults. Initially, 150 mg/day as a single dose in the morning. May increase to 150 mg twice a day as early as day 4 after beginning therapy. Maximum: 400 mg/day.
Elderly. 50–100 mg/day. May increase by 50–100 mg/day q3–4 days. Maintenance: Lowest effective dosage.
PO (Extended-Release)
Adults. 150 mg once a day. May increase to 300 mg once a day. Maximum: 450 mg a day.

▸ Smoking Cessation

PO
Adults. Initially, 150 mg a day for 3 days; then 150 mg twice a day for 7–12 wk.

SIDE EFFECTS/ADVERSE REACTIONS

Frequent
Constipation, weight gain or loss, nausea, vomiting, anorexia, dry mouth, headache, diaphoresis, tremors, sedation, insomnia, dizziness, agitation
Occasional
Diarrhea, akinesia, blurred vision, tachycardia, confusion, hostility, fatigue

PRECAUTIONS AND CONTRAINDICATIONS

Current or prior diagnosis of anorexia nervosa or bulimia, seizure disorder, use within 14 days of MAOIs
Caution:
Renal and hepatic disease, recent MI, cranial trauma, lactation, children, low abuse potential; increased CNS or psychiatric symptoms may occur with use

DRUG INTERACTIONS OF CONCERN TO DENTISTRY

- Increased adverse reactions (seizures): tricyclic antidepressants, phenothiazines, benzodiazepines, alcohol, haloperidol, and trazodone
- Decreased serum levels with carbamazepine
- Inhibits CYP2D6 isoenzymes; use with caution; other drugs metabolized by this enzyme

SERIOUS REACTIONS

! The risk of seizures increases in patients taking more than 150 mg/dose of bupropion, in patients with a history of bulimia or seizure disorders, and in patients discontinuing drugs that may lower the seizure threshold.

DENTAL CONSIDERATIONS

General:

- Assess salivary flow as a factor in caries, periodontal disease, and candidiasis.
- Short appointments and a stress-reduction protocol may be required for anxious patients.
- See nicotine dose forms for additional smoking cessation considerations.

Consultations:

- Medical consultation may be required to assess disease control and patient's ability to tolerate stress.
- Physician should be informed if significant xerostomic side effects occur (e.g., increased caries, sore tongue, problems eating or swallowing, difficulty wearing prosthesis) so that a medication change can be considered.

Teach Patient/Family:

- When chronic dry mouth occurs, advise patient to:
  - Avoid mouth rinses with high alcohol content because of drying effects.
  - Use daily home fluoride products for anticaries effect.
  - Use sugarless gum, frequent sips of water, or saliva substitutes.

buspirone hydrochloride

byoo-**spir′**-own hi-droh-**klor′**-ide
(BuSpar, Buspirex[CAN], Bustab[CAN])
Do not confuse buspirone with bupropion.

CATEGORY AND SCHEDULE

Pregnancy Risk Category: B

Drug Class: Antianxiety agent

MECHANISM OF ACTION

Although its exact mechanism of action is unknown, this nonbarbiturate is thought to bind to serotonin and dopamine receptors in the CNS. The drug may also increase norepinephrine metabolism in the locus ceruleus.
Therapeutic Effect: Produces anxiolytic effect.

USES

Management and short-term relief of anxiety disorders; unapproved: PMS

PHARMACOKINETICS

Rapidly and completely absorbed from the GI tract. Protein binding: 95%. Undergoes extensive first-pass metabolism. Metabolized in the liver to active metabolite. Primarily excreted in urine. Not removed by hemodialysis. ***Half-life:*** 2–3 hr.

INDICATIONS AND DOSAGES

▸ Short-Term Management (up to 4 wk) of Anxiety Disorders

PO

Adults. 5 mg 2–3 times a day or 7.5 mg twice a day. May increase by 5 mg/day every 2–4 days. Maintenance: 15–30 mg/day in 2–3

B

divided doses. Maximum: 60 mg/day.
Elderly. Initially, 5 mg twice a day. May increase by 5 mg/day every 2–3 days. Maximum: 60 mg/day.
Children. Initially, 5 mg/day. May increase by 5 mg/day at weekly intervals. Maximum: 60 mg/day.

SIDE EFFECTS/ADVERSE REACTIONS

Frequent
Dizziness, somnolence, nausea, headache
Occasional
Nervousness, fatigue, insomnia, dry mouth, light-headedness, mood swings, blurred vision, poor concentration, diarrhea, paresthesia
Rare
Muscle pain and stiffness, nightmares, chest pain, involuntary movements

PRECAUTIONS AND CONTRAINDICATIONS

Concurrent use of MAOIs, severe hepatic or renal impairment
Caution:
Lactation, elderly, impaired hepatic/renal function

DRUG INTERACTIONS OF CONCERN TO DENTISTRY

• Increased sedation: alcohol, all CNS depressants
• Increased plasma levels: fluconazole, ketoconazole, itraconazole, miconazole, erythromycin, clarithromycin, troleandomycin

SERIOUS REACTIONS

! Buspirone does not appear to cause drug tolerance, psychological or physical dependence, or withdrawal syndrome.
! Overdose may produce severe nausea, vomiting, dizziness, drowsiness, abdominal distention, and excessive pupil contraction.

DENTAL CONSIDERATIONS

General:
• Monitor vital signs at every appointment because of cardiovascular side effects.
• Assess salivary flow as a factor in caries, periodontal disease, and candidiasis.
• Short appointments and a stress-reduction protocol may be required for anxious patients.
• Determine why the patient is taking the drug.
Consultations:
• Medical consultation may be required to assess disease control.
Teach Patient/Family:
• When chronic dry mouth occurs, advise patient to:
  • Avoid mouth rinses with high alcohol content because of drying effects.
  • Use daily home fluoride products for anticaries effect.
  • Use sugarless gum, frequent sips of water, or saliva substitutes.

busulfan

byoo-**sull′**-fan
(Busulfex, Myleran)
Do not confuse Myleran with Alkeran, Leukeran, or Mylicon.

CATEGORY AND SCHEDULE

Pregnancy Risk Category: D

Drug Class: Antineoplastic

MECHANISM OF ACTION

An alkylating agent that interferes with DNA replication and RNA synthesis. Cell cycle-phase nonspecific.

Therapeutic Effect: Disrupts nucleic acid function and causes myelosuppression.

USES

Treatment of chronic myelogenous leukemia, orphan drug in preparative therapy for malignancies treated with bone marrow transplant

PHARMACOKINETICS

Completely absorbed from the GI tract. Protein binding: 33%. Metabolized in the liver. Primarily excreted in urine. Minimally removed by hemodialysis. ***Half-life:*** 2.5 hr.

INDICATIONS AND DOSAGES

▸ Remission Induction in Chronic Myelogenous Leukemia (CML)

PO

Adults, Elderly. 4–8 mg/day up to 12 mg/day. Maintenance: 1–4 mg/day to 2 mg/wk. Continue until WBC count is 10,000–20,000/mm^3, resume when WBC count reaches 50,000/mm^3.

Children. 0.06–0.12 mg/kg/day. Maintenance: Titrate to maintain leukocyte count above 40,000/mm^3, reduce dose by 50% if count is 30,000–40,000/mm^3, and discontinue if the count is 20,000/mm^3 or less.

▸ Marrow Ablative Conditioning for Bone Marrow Transplantation

IV

Adults, Elderly, Children weighing more than 12 kg. 0.8 mg/kg/dose q6h for total of 16 doses. (Use IBW or ABW, whichever is lower.)

Children weighing 12 kg or less. 1.1 mg/kg/dose (IBW) q6h for 16 doses.

PO

Adults, Elderly, Children. 1 mg/kg/dose (IBW) q6h for 16 doses.

SIDE EFFECTS/ADVERSE REACTIONS

Expected

Nausea, stomatitis, vomiting, anorexia, insomnia, diarrhea, fever, abdominal pain, anxiety

Frequent

Headache, rash, asthenia, infection, chills, tachycardia, dyspepsia

Occasional

Constipation, dizziness, edema, pruritus, cough, dry mouth, depression, abdominal enlargement, pharyngitis, hiccups, back pain, alopecia, myalgia

Rare

Injection site pain, arthralgia, confusion, hypotension, lethargy

PRECAUTIONS AND CONTRAINDICATIONS

Disease resistance to previous therapy with this drug

Caution:

Women of childbearing age, leukopenia, thrombocytopenia, anemia, hepatotoxicity, renal toxicity

DRUG INTERACTIONS OF CONCERN TO DENTISTRY

- Acetaminophen may reduce clearance if given within 72 hr before busulfan administration.

SERIOUS REACTIONS

! Busulfan's major adverse effect is myelosuppression, resulting in hematologic toxicity, as evidenced by anemia, severe leukopenia, and severe thrombocytopenia.

! Very high busulfan dosages may produce blurred vision, muscle twitching, and tonic-clonic seizures.

! Long-term therapy (more than 4 yr) may produce pulmonary syndrome ("busulfan lung"), characterized by persistent cough, congestion, crackles, and dyspnea.

! Hyperuricemia may produce uric acid nephropathy, renal calculi, and acute renal failure.

DENTAL CONSIDERATIONS

General:

• Patients taking opioids for acute or chronic pain should be given alternative analgesics for dental pain.

• Consider semisupine chair position for patient comfort if GI side effects occur.

• Chlorhexidine mouth rinse (nonalcoholic) before and during chemotherapy may reduce severity of mucositis.

• Patients on chronic drug therapy may rarely have symptoms of blood dyscrasias, which can include infection, bleeding, and poor healing.

• Palliative medication may be required for management of oral side effects.

• Apply lubricant to dry lips for patient comfort before dental procedures.

• Assess salivary flow as factor in caries, periodontal disease, and candidiasis.

• Patients in active chemotherapy treatment should have adequate WBC count before completing dental procedures that may produce a wound. Consultation with the oncologist may be required to determine WBC counts before treatment.

Consultations:

• Medical consultation may be required to assess disease control and patient's ability to tolerate stress.

• In a patient with symptoms of blood dyscrasias, request a medical consultation for blood studies and postpone dental treatment until normal values are reestablished.

• Consult oncologist; prophylactic or therapeutic antibiotics may be indicated to prevent or treat infection if surgery or deep scaling is planned.

Teach Patient/Family to:

• Use effective oral hygiene to prevent soft tissue inflammation.

• Prevent trauma when using oral hygiene aids.

• Report oral lesions, soreness, or bleeding to dentist.

• See dentist immediately if secondary oral infection occurs.

• Update medical/drug record if physician makes any changes in evaluation or drug regimen.

• When chronic dry mouth occurs, advise patient to:

  • Avoid mouth rinses with high alcohol content because of drying effects.
  • Use daily home fluoride products for anticaries effect.
  • Use sugarless gum, frequent sips of water, or artificial saliva substitutes.

butabarbital sodium

byoo-tah-**bar′**-bi-tal
(Butisol)

CATEGORY AND SCHEDULE

Pregnancy Risk Category: D
Controlled Substance: Schedule III

Drug Class: Anticonvulsant; antihyperbilirubinemic; sedative-hypnotic

MECHANISM OF ACTION

A barbiturate and nonselective CNS depressant that binds at GABA receptor complex, enhancing GABA activity.
Therapeutic Effect: Produces hypnotic effect caused by CNS depression.

USES

May be used before surgery to relieve anxiety or tension. In addition, some are used as anticonvulsants to help control seizures in certain disorders or diseases, such as epilepsy.

PHARMACOKINETICS

Widely distributed. Metabolized in liver. Minimally excreted unchanged in urine. ***Half-life:*** 34–100 hr.

INDICATIONS AND DOSAGES

▸ **Insomnia, Short-Term**

PO

Adults. 50–100 mg at bedtime.

▸ **Preoperative Sedation**

PO

Adults. 50–100 mg, 60–90 min before surgery.
Children. 2–6 mg/kg. Maximum: 100 mg.

▸ **Sedation, Daytime**

PO

Adults. 15–30 mg 3–4 times a day.

SIDE EFFECTS/ADVERSE REACTIONS

Occasional
Somnolence
Rare
Confusion, dizziness, agitation, nausea, vomiting, constipation, headache, hypotension, acne

PRECAUTIONS AND CONTRAINDICATIONS

Porphyria, barbiturate sensitivity

DRUG INTERACTIONS OF CONCERN TO DENTISTRY

- Nephrotoxicity and/or hepatotoxicity: halogenated hydrocarbon anesthetics
- Increased CNS depression: alcohol and all other CNS depressants
- Increased metabolism of oral anticoagulants, glucocorticoids, carbamazepine, tricyclic antidepressants

SERIOUS REACTIONS

! Skin eruptions appear as hypersensitivity reaction.
! Blood dyscrasias, liver disease, and hypocalcemia occur rarely.

DENTAL CONSIDERATIONS

General:

- Determine why patient is taking the drug.
- Monitor vital signs at every appointment due to cardiovascular side effects.
- Patient on chronic drug therapy may rarely present with symptoms of blood dyscrasias, which can include infection, bleeding, and poor healing. If dyscrasia is present, caution patient to prevent oral tissue trauma when using oral hygiene aids.
- When used for sedation in dentistry:
  - Have responsible person drive patient to and from dental office when drug used for conscious sedation.
  - After supine positioning, have patient sit upright for at least 2 min before standing to avoid orthostatic hypotension.
  - Geriatric patients are more susceptible to drug effects; use lower dose.
  - Barbiturates induce certain liver enzymes that can alter the

B

metabolism of other drugs (see drug interactions).

Consultations:

• In a patient with symptoms of blood dyscrasias, request a medical consultation for blood studies and postpone treatment until normal values are reestablished.

Teach Patient/Family to:

• Avoid driving or other activities requiring mental alertness.
• Avoid alcohol ingestion or CNS depressants; serious CNS depression may result.
• Avoid OTC preparations that contain CNS depressants (antihistamine, cold remedies).
• Update health and medication history if physician makes any changes in evaluation or drug regimens; include OTC, herbal, and nonherbal remedies in the update.

butenafine

byoo-**ten′**-ah-feen
(Mentax)

CATEGORY AND SCHEDULE

Pregnancy Risk Category: B

Drug Class: Antifungal

MECHANISM OF ACTION

An antifungal agent that blocks biosynthesis of ergosterol, essential for fungal cell membrane. Fungicidal.
Therapeutic Effect: Relieves athlete's foot.

USES

Treatment of tinea pedis caused by *E. floccosum, T. mentagrophytes*, or *T. rubrum;* and tinea versicolor caused by *Malassezia furfur*

PHARMACOKINETICS

Total amount absorbed into systemic circulation has not been determined. Metabolized in liver. Excreted in urine. ***Half-life:*** 35 hr.

INDICATIONS AND DOSAGES

▸ **Tinea Pedis, Tinea Corporis, Tinea Cruris, Tinea Versicolor**

Topical

Adults, Elderly, Children 12 yr and older. Apply to affected area and immediate surrounding skin daily for 4 wk.

SIDE EFFECTS/ADVERSE REACTIONS

Occasional

Contact dermatitis, burning/stinging, worsening of the condition

Rare

Erythema, irritation, pruritus

PRECAUTIONS AND CONTRAINDICATIONS

Hypersensitivity to butenafine or any component of the formulation

Caution:

External use only, lactation, children younger than 12 yr, not for oral use

DRUG INTERACTIONS OF CONCERN TO DENTISTRY

• None reported

SERIOUS REACTIONS

! None known

butoconazole

byoo-toe-**ko′**-na-zole
(Gynazole-1, Femstat One[CAN] Mycelex-32%)

CATEGORY AND SCHEDULE

Pregnancy Risk Category: C

Drug Class: Antifungal

MECHANISM OF ACTION
An antifungal similar to imidazole derivatives that inhibits the steroid synthesis, a vital component of fungal cell formation, thereby damaging the fungal cell membrane. ***Therapeutic Effect:*** Fungistatic.

USES
Treatment of vulvovaginal infections caused by *Candida* spp.

PHARMACOKINETICS
Not known

INDICATIONS AND DOSAGES
▸ **Treatment of Candidiasis**

Topical

Adults, Elderly. Insert 1 full applicator intravaginally at bedtime for up to 6 days.

SIDE EFFECTS/ADVERSE REACTIONS
Occasional

Vaginal itching, burning, irritation

PRECAUTIONS AND CONTRAINDICATIONS
Hypersensitivity to butoconazole or any of its components

Caution:

Lactation

SERIOUS REACTIONS
! Soreness, swelling, pelvic pain, or cramping rarely occurs.

DENTAL CONSIDERATIONS
General:

• Examine oral mucous membranes for signs of yeast infection.

• Broad-spectrum antibiotics for dental infections may cause vaginal yeast infection.

B

butorphanol tartrate
byoo-**tor′**-fa-nole **tar′**-trate

(Stadol, Stadol NS)

Do not confuse butorphanol with butabarbital, or Stadol with Haldol.

CATEGORY AND SCHEDULE
Pregnancy Risk Category: C, D if used for prolonged time, high dose at term

Controlled Substance: Schedule IV

Drug Class: Analgesic; anesthesia adjunct; opioid analgesic; antidiarrheal; antitussive; pulmonary edema therapy adjunct; suppressant, narcotic abstinence syndrome

MECHANISM OF ACTION
An opioid that binds to opiate receptor sites in the CNS. Reduces intensity of pain stimuli incoming from sensory nerve endings. ***Therapeutic Effect:*** Alters pain perception and emotional response to pain.

USES
Pain relief

PHARMACOKINETICS

Route	Onset	Peak	Duration
IM	10–30 min	30–60 min	3–4 hr
IV	Less than 1 min	30 min	2–4 hr
Nasal	15 min	1–2 hr	4–5 hr

Rapidly absorbed after IM injection. Protein binding: 80%. Extensively metabolized in the liver. Primarily excreted in urine. ***Half-life:*** 2.5–4 hr.

INDICATIONS AND DOSAGES

▸ **Analgesia**

IV

Adults. 0.5–2 mg q3–4h as needed.
Elderly. 1 mg q4–6h as needed.

IM

Adults. 1–4 mg q3–4h as needed.
Elderly. 1 mg q4–6h as needed.

▸ **Migraine**

Nasal

Adults. 1 mg or 1 spray in one nostril. May repeat in 60–90 min. May repeat 2-dose sequence q3–4h as needed. Alternatively, 2 mg or 1 spray each nostril if patient remains recumbent, may repeat in 3–4 hr.

SIDE EFFECTS/ADVERSE REACTIONS

Frequent

Parenteral: Somnolence, dizziness
Nasal: Nasal congestion, insomnia

Occasional

Parenteral: Confusion, diaphoresis, clammy skin, lethargy, headache, nausea, vomiting, dry mouth
Nasal: Vasodilation, constipation, unpleasant taste, dyspnea, epistaxis, nasal irritation, upper respiratory tract infection, tinnitus

Rare

Parenteral: Hypotension, pruritus, blurred vision, sensation of heat, CNS stimulation, insomnia
Nasal: Hypertension, tremor, ear pain, paresthesia, depression, sinusitis

PRECAUTIONS AND CONTRAINDICATIONS

CNS disease that affects respirations, physical dependence on other opioid analgesics, preexisting respiratory depression, pulmonary disease

DRUG INTERACTIONS OF CONCERN TO DENTISTRY

- Increased CNS depression: alcohol and all CNS depressants
- Decreased effects of: buprenorphine
- Use caution or avoid use in patients taking MAOIs
- Avoid use in narcotic-dependent persons
- Possible decrease in effects: drugs that induce CYP3A4 isoenzymes (phenobarbital, carbamazepine)
- Possible increase in effects: drugs that inhibit CYP3A4 isoenzymes (ketoconazole, itraconazole, erythromycin, protease inhibitors)

SERIOUS REACTIONS

! Abrupt withdrawal after prolonged use may produce symptoms of narcotic withdrawal, such as abdominal cramping, rhinorrhea, lacrimation, anxiety, increased temperature, and piloerection or goose bumps.

! Overdose results in severe respiratory depression, skeletal muscle flaccidity, cyanosis, and extreme somnolence progressing to seizures, stupor, and coma.

! Tolerance to analgesic effect and physical dependence may occur with chronic use.

DENTAL CONSIDERATIONS

General:

- Monitor vital signs at every appointment due to cardiovascular side effects.
- This is an acute-use drug; it is doubtful that patients will undergo dental treatment during severe migraine attacks.
- After supine positioning, have patient sit upright for at least 2 min before standing to avoid orthostatic hypotension.

• Psychologic and physical dependence may occur with chronic administration.
• Determine why patient is taking the drug.
• If additional analgesia is required for dental pain, consider alternative analgesics (NSAIDs) in patients taking narcotics for acute or chronic pain.

Teach Patient/Family to:

• Avoid driving or other activities requiring mental alertness.
• Avoid alcohol ingestion or CNS depressants; serious CNS depression may result.
• Avoid OTC preparations that contain CNS depressants (antihistamine, cold remedies).
• Update health and medication history if physician makes any changes in evaluation or drug regimens; include OTC, herbal, and nonherbal remedies in the update.

C

cabergoline

ka-**ber**′-goe-leen
(Dostinex)

CATEGORY AND SCHEDULE

Pregnancy Risk Category: B

Drug Class: Dopamine agonist; antihyperprolactinemic

MECHANISM OF ACTION

Agonist at dopamine D_2 receptors, suppressing prolactin secretion.
Therapeutic Effects: Shrinks prolactinomas, restores gonadal function.

USES

Treatment of different types of medical problems that occur when too much of the hormone prolactin is produced. It can be used to treat certain menstrual problems, fertility problems in men and women, and pituitary prolactinomas (tumors of the pituitary gland).

PHARMACOKINETICS

Cabergoline is administered orally and undergoes significant first-pass metabolism following systemic absorption. Extensively metabolized in the liver. Elimination is primarily in the feces. ***Half-life:*** 63-69 hr.

INDICATIONS AND DOSAGES

▸ **Hyperprolactinemia (Idiopathic or Primary Pituitary Adenomas)**

PO

Adults, Elderly. 0.25 mg 2 times a week, titrate by 0.25 mg/dose no more than every 4 wk up to 1 mg 2 times a week.

PV

Adults. 0.5 mg 2 to 5 times a week.

▸ **Parkinson's Disease**

PO

Adults. 0.5 mg/day and titrate to response. Mean effective dose is 3 mg/day and ranges from 0.5 to 6 mg/day.

▸ **Restless Legs Syndrome (RLS)**

PO

Adults. 0.5 mg once daily at bedtime, slowly titrate until symptoms resolve or drug-intolerance limits further adjustment. Mean effective dose is 2 mg/day and ranges from 1 to 4 mg/day.

SIDE EFFECTS/ADVERSE REACTIONS

Frequent

Nausea, orthostatic hypotension, confusion, dyskinesia, hallucinations, peripheral edema

Occasional

Headache, vertigo, dizziness, dyspepsia, postural hypotension, constipation, asthenia, fatigue, abdominal pain, drowsiness

Rare

Vomiting, dry mouth, diarrhea, flatulence, anxiety, depression, dysmenorrhea, dyspepsia, mastalgia, paresthesias, vertigo, visual impairment, pleuropulmonary changes, pleural effusion, pulmonary fibrosis, heart failure, peptic ulcer

PRECAUTIONS AND CONTRAINDICATIONS

Hypersensitivity to cabergoline, ergot alkaloids or any one of its components. Uncontrolled hypertension.

DRUG INTERACTIONS OF CONCERN TO DENTISTRY

- None reported

SERIOUS REACTIONS

! Overdosage may produce nasal congestion, syncope, or hallucinations.

DENTAL CONSIDERATIONS

General:

- Determine why patient is taking the drug.
- Monitor vital signs at every appointment for cardiovascular side effects.
- After supine positioning, have patient sit upright for at least 2 min before standing to avoid orthostatic hypotension.
- Use precaution if sedation or general anesthesia is required; risk of hypotensive episode.
- Assess salivary flow as a factor in caries, periodontal disease, and candidiasis.
- Consider semisupine chair position for patient comfort if GI side effects occur.

Consultations:

- Medical consultation may be required to assess disease control.

Teach Patient/Family:

- When chronic dry mouth occurs, advise patient to:
  - Avoid mouth rinses with high alcohol content because of drying effects.
  - Use daily home fluoride products for anticaries effect.
  - Use sugarless gum, frequent sips of water, or saliva substitutes.
  - Update health and medication history if physician makes any changes in evaluation or drug regimens; include OTC, herbal, and nonherbal remedies in the update.

calcitonin

kal-si-**toe**′-nin
(Calcimar, Caltine[CAN], Cibacalcin, Miacalcin)
Do not confuse calcitonin with calcitriol.

CATEGORY AND SCHEDULE

Pregnancy Risk Category: C

Drug Class: Synthetic polypeptide calcitonins

MECHANISM OF ACTION

A synthetic hormone that decreases osteoclast activity in bones, decreases tubular reabsorption of sodium and calcium in the kidneys, and increases absorption of calcium in the GI tract.
Therapeutic Effect: Regulates serum calcium concentrations.

USES

Treatment of Paget's disease, postmenopausal osteoporosis, hypercalcemia

PHARMACOKINETICS

Injection form rapidly metabolized (primarily in kidneys); primarily excreted in urine. Nasal form rapidly absorbed. ***Half-life:*** 70–90 min (injection); 43 min (nasal).

INDICATIONS AND DOSAGES

▸ **Skin Testing Before Treatment in Patients with Suspected Sensitivity to Calcitonin-Salmon**

Intracutaneous

Adults, Elderly. Prepare a 10-international units/ml dilution; withdraw 0.05 ml from a 200-international units/ml vial in a tuberculin syringe; fill up to 1 ml with 0.9% NaCl. Take 0.1 ml and inject intracutaneously on inner aspect of forearm. Observe after 15 min; a positive response is the appearance of more than mild erythema or wheal.

▸ **Paget's Disease**
IM, Subcutaneous
Adults, Elderly. Initially, 100 international units/day.
Maintenance: 50 international units/day or 50–100 international units every 1–3 days.
Intranasal
Adults, Elderly. 200–400 international units/day.

▸ **Osteoporosis Imperfecta**
IM, Subcutaneous
Adults. 2 international units/kg 3 times a wk.

▸ **Postmenopausal Osteoporosis**
IM, Subcutaneous
Adults, Elderly. 100 international units/day with adequate calcium and vitamin D intake.
Intranasal
Adults, Elderly. 200 international units/day as a single spray, alternating nostrils daily.

▸ **Hypercalcemia**
IM, Subcutaneous
Adults, Elderly. Initially, 4 international units/kg q12h; may increase to 8 international units/kg q12h if no response in 2 days; may further increase to 8 international units/kg q6h if no response in another 2 days.

SIDE EFFECTS/ADVERSE REACTIONS

Frequent
IM, Subcutaneous: Nausea (may occur 30 min after injection, usually diminishes with continued therapy), inflammation at injection site
Nasal: Rhinitis, nasal irritation, redness, sores
Occasional
IM, Subcutaneous: Flushing of face or hands
Nasal: Back pain, arthralgia, epistaxis, headache
Rare
IM, Subcutaneous: Epigastric discomfort, dry mouth, diarrhea, flatulence
Nasal: Itching of earlobes, edema of feet, rash, diaphoresis

PRECAUTIONS AND CONTRAINDICATIONS

Hypersensitivity to gelatin desserts or salmon protein
Caution:
Allergy, hypocalcemic tetany, routine monitoring of urine sediment, osteogenic sarcoma in Paget's disease, lactation, children

DRUG INTERACTIONS OF CONCERN TO DENTISTRY

• Supplemental calcium and vitamin D may already be used; do not use additional amounts.

SERIOUS REACTIONS

! Patients with a protein allergy may develop a hypersensitivity reaction.

DENTAL CONSIDERATIONS

General:
• Consider semisupine chair position for patient comfort because of effects of disease or if GI side effects occur.
• Assess salivary flow as factor in caries, periodontal disease, and candidiasis.

Teach Patient/Family to:
• Encourage effective oral hygiene to prevent soft tissue inflammation.
• When chronic dry mouth occurs, advise patient to:
  • Avoid mouth rinses with high alcohol content because of drying effects.
  • Use daily home fluoride products for anticaries effect.

• Use sugarless gum, frequent sips of water, or saliva substitutes.

calcitriol

kal-si-**trye′**-ole
(Calcijex, Rocaltrol, Vectical)

CATEGORY AND SCHEDULE

Pregnancy Risk Category: C

Drug Class: Fat-soluble vitamin, vitamin D analogue

MECHANISM OF ACTION

A fat-soluble vitamin that is essential for absorption, utilization of calcium and phosphate, and normal calcification of bone. ***Therapeutic Effect:*** Stimulates calcium and phosphate absorption from small intestine, promotes secretion of calcium from bone to blood, promotes renal tubule phosphate resorption, acts on bone cells to stimulate skeletal growth and on parathyroid gland to suppress hormone synthesis and secretion.

USES

Renal failure
Hypoparathyroidism/ pseudohypoparathyroidism
Mild-to-moderate plaque psoriasis
Vitamin D-dependent rickets
Vitamin D-resistant rickets

PHARMACOKINETICS

Rapidly absorbed from small intestine. Extensive metabolism in kidneys. Primarily excreted in feces; minimal excretion in urine. Topical: some systemic absorption. ***Half-life:*** 5–8 hr. Topical: 3–6 hr.

INDICATIONS AND DOSAGES

▸ Renal Failure

PO

Adults, Elderly. 0.25 mcg/day or 0.5–1 mcg every other day. Increases can be made every 4–8 wk, if necessary.

Children. 0.25–2 mcg/day with hemodialysis; 0.014–0.41 mcg/kg/day without hemodialysis.

IV

Adults, Elderly. Initially, 1–2 mcg (0.02 mcg/kg) 3 times/wk. Dose range: 0.5–4 mcg (0.01–0.05 mcg/kg) 3 times/wk. Adjust dose at 2- to 4-wk intervals.

Children. 0.01–0.05 mcg/kg 3 times/wk with hemodialysis.

▸ Hypoparathyroidism/ Pseudohypoparathyroidism

PO

Adults, Elderly. Initially, 0.25 mcg/day. Range: 0.5–2 mcg/day.

Children 6 yr and older. Initially, 0.25 mcg/day. Range: 0.5–2 mcg/day.

Children 1–5 yr. 0.25–0.75 mcg once daily.

Children less than 1 yr. 0.04–0.08 mcg/kg once daily.

▸ Psoriasis, Mild-Moderate Plaque

Topical

Adults. Apply twice/day. Max: 200 g/wk.

▸ Vitamin D-Dependent Rickets

PO

Adults, Elderly, Children. 1 mcg once daily.

▸ Vitamin D-Resistant Rickets

PO

Adults, Elderly, Children. 0.015–0.02 mcg/kg once daily. Maintenance: 0.03–0.06 mcg/kg once daily. Maximum: 2 mcg once daily.

C

SIDE EFFECTS/ADVERSE REACTIONS

Occasional
Oral: Hypercalcemia, headache, irritability, constipation, metallic taste, nausea, polyuria, photophobia, dry mouth, hypercalciuria, nephrolithiasis
Topical: skin discomfort, pruritus, psoriasis (worsening)

PRECAUTIONS AND CONTRAINDICATIONS

Hypersensitivity to calcitriol or other vitamin D products or analogues
Hypercalcemia
Malabsorption syndrome
Vitamin D toxicity

Caution:
Concurrent use with digitalis
Surgery or prolonged immobilization
Ocular exposure
Cardiac disease
Breast-feeding

DRUG INTERACTIONS OF CONCERN TO DENTISTRY

- Aluminum-containing antacid (long-term use): May increase aluminum concentration and aluminum bone toxicity.
- Calcium-containing preparations, thiazide diuretics: May increase the risk of hypercalcemia.
- Didanosine: May alter intestinal phosphate absorption; increased risk of hypermagnesemia.
- Digoxin: May increase risk of arrhythmia.
- Magnesium-containing antacids: May increase magnesium concentration.
- Mineral oil: May cause fat-soluble vitamin malabsorption.
- Vitamin D analogues: Increased risk of hypervitaminosis D, hypercalcemia.

SERIOUS REACTIONS

! Early signs of overdosage are manifested as weakness, headache, somnolence, nausea, vomiting, dry mouth, constipation, muscle and bone pain, and metallic taste sensation.
! Later signs of overdosage are evidenced by polyuria, polydipsia, anorexia, weight loss, nocturia, photophobia, rhinorrhea, pruritus, disorientation, hallucinations, hyperthermia, hypertension, and cardiac arrhythmias.

DENTAL CONSIDERATIONS

General:
- Monitor the patient's BUN, serum alkaline phosphatase, serum calcium, serum creatinine, serum magnesium, serum phosphate, and urinary calcium levels. Know that the therapeutic serum calcium level is 9 to 10 mg/dl.
- Estimate the patient's daily dietary calcium intake.
- Encourage the patient to maintain adequate fluid intake.
- Avoid bright light in the patient's eyes; offer dark glasses for patient comfort.
- Consider semisupine position if the patient experiences GI discomfort.

Consultations:
- Medical consultation may be required to assess disease control.

Teach Patient/Family to:
- Encourage the patient to consume foods rich in vitamin D including eggs, leafy vegetables, margarine, meats, milk, vegetable oils, and vegetable shortening.
- Warn the patient not to take mineral oil during calcitriol therapy.
- Advise the patient receiving chronic renal dialysis not to take

magnesium-containing antacids during calcitriol therapy.
• Encourage the patient to drink plenty of liquids.

candesartan cilexetil

kan-de-**sar′**-tan sill-**ex′**-eh-till
(Atacand)

CATEGORY AND SCHEDULE

Pregnancy Risk Category: C (D if used in second or third trimester)

Drug Class: Angiotensin II (AT1) receptor antagonist, antihypertensive

MECHANISM OF ACTION

An angiotensin II receptor, type AT_1, antagonist that blocks the vasoconstrictor and aldosterone-secreting effects of angiotensin II, inhibiting the binding of angiotensin II to the AT_1 receptors.
Therapeutic Effect: Causes vasodilation, decreases peripheral resistance, and decreases B/P.

USES

Treatment of hypertension, as a single drug or in combination with other antihypertensives

PHARMACOKINETICS

Rapidly, completely absorbed. Protein binding: greater than 99%. Undergoes minor hepatic metabolism to inactive metabolite. Excreted unchanged in urine and in the feces through the biliary system. Not removed by hemodialysis.
Half-life: 9 hr.

INDICATIONS AND DOSAGES

▸ Hypertension Alone or in Combination with Other Antihypertensives

PO

Adults, Elderly, Patients with mildly impaired liver or renal function. Initially, 16 mg once a day in those who are not volume depleted. Can be given once or twice a day with total daily doses of 8–32 mg. Give lower dosage in those treated with diuretics or with severely impaired renal function.

SIDE EFFECTS/ADVERSE REACTIONS

Occasional

Upper respiratory tract infection, dizziness, back and leg pain

Rare

Pharyngitis, rhinitis, headache, fatigue, diarrhea, nausea, dry cough, peripheral edema

PRECAUTIONS AND CONTRAINDICATIONS

Hypersensitivity to candesartan

Caution:

Discontinue drug if pregnancy occurs, risk of fetal and neonatal injury, correct volume depletion if present, renal impairment, pregnancy category C (first trimester) and D (second and third trimesters), lactation

DRUG INTERACTIONS OF CONCERN TO DENTISTRY

• Potential for increased hypotensive effects with other hypotensive and sedative drugs

SERIOUS REACTIONS

! Overdosage may manifest as hypotension and tachycardia. Bradycardia occurs less often.
! Institute supportive measures.

C

DENTAL CONSIDERATIONS

General:

• Monitor vital signs at every appointment in patients with history of hypertension.
• Evaluate respiration characteristics and rate.
• Consider semisupine chair position for patient comfort if GI side effects occur.
• Observe appropriate limitations of vasoconstrictor doses.
• Limit use of sodium-containing products, such as saline IV fluids, for those patients with a dietary salt restriction.
• Stress from dental procedures may compromise cardiovascular function; determine patient risk.
• Short appointments and a stress-reduction protocol may be required for anxious patients.
• Use precaution if sedation or general anesthesia is required; risk of hypotensive episode.

Consultations:

• Medical consultation may be required to assess disease control and patient's ability to tolerate stress.

Teach Patient/Family to:

• Update health and drug history if physician makes any changes in evaluation or drug regimens.

capecitabine

cap-eh-**site'**-ah-bean
(Xeloda)
Do not confuse Xeloda with Xenical.

CATEGORY AND SCHEDULE

Pregnancy Risk Category: D

Drug Class: Antineoplastic

MECHANISM OF ACTION

An antimetabolite that is enzymatically converted to 5-fluorouracil. Inhibits enzymes necessary for synthesis of essential cellular components.
Therapeutic Effect: Interferes with DNA synthesis, RNA processing, and protein synthesis.

USES

First-line treatment of patients with metastatic colorectal cancer and metastatic breast cancer resistant to both paclitaxel and anthracycline-containing chemotherapy regimens; colorectal cancer when treatment with a fluoropyrimidine alone is preferred

PHARMACOKINETICS

Readily absorbed from the GI tract. Protein binding: less than 60%. Metabolized in the liver. Primarily excreted in urine. ***Half-life:*** 45 min.

INDICATIONS AND DOSAGES

▸ Metastatic Breast Cancer, Colon Cancer

PO

Adults, Elderly. Initially, 2500 mg/m^2/day in 2 equally divided doses approximately q12h for 2 wk. Follow with a 1-wk rest period; given in 3-wk cycles.

SIDE EFFECTS/ADVERSE REACTIONS

Frequent

Diarrhea (sometimes severe), nausea, vomiting, stomatitis, hand-and-foot syndrome (painful palmar-plantar swelling with paresthesia, erythema, and blistering), fatigue, anorexia, dermatitis

Occasional
Constipation, dyspepsia, nail disorder, headache, dizziness, insomnia, edema, myalgia

PRECAUTIONS AND CONTRAINDICATIONS

Severe renal impairment
Caution:
Food reduces absorption, renal insufficiency, altered coagulation when taken with Coumadin, patients older than 80 yr, pregnancy category D, hepatic dysfunction because of liver metastases, lactation, children younger than 18 yr, avoid use of folic acid

DRUG INTERACTIONS OF CONCERN TO DENTISTRY

• Dental drug interactions not reported; however, patients taking this drug with coumarin oral anticoagulants have altered coagulation parameters, bleeding, or both; INR or PT should be physician-monitored.

SERIOUS REACTIONS

! Serious reactions may include myelosuppression (evidenced by neutropenia, thrombocytopenia, and anemia), cardiovascular toxicity (marked by angina, cardiomyopathy, and deep vein thrombosis), respiratory toxicity (marked by dyspnea, epistaxis, and pneumonia), and lymphedema.

DENTAL CONSIDERATIONS

General:
• Monitor vital signs at every appointment because of cardiovascular side effects.
• Patients on chronic drug therapy may have symptoms of blood dyscrasias, which can include infection, bleeding, and poor healing.
• Patients taking opioids for acute or chronic pain should be given alternative analgesics for dental pain.
• Short appointments and a stress reduction protocol may be required for anxious patients.
• Consider semisupine chair position for patient comfort if GI side effects occur.
• Question patient about tolerance of NSAIDs or aspirin related to GI side effects of drug.
• Consider local hemostasis measures to control and prevent excessive bleeding.
• Examine for oral manifestation of opportunistic infection.
• Be aware of oral side effects and potential sequelae.
• Palliative medication may be required for management of oral side effects.
• Avoid dental light in patient's eyes; offer dark glasses for patient comfort.
• Prophylactic or therapeutic antibiotics may be indicated to prevent or treat infection if surgery or periodontal debridement is required.
Consultations:
• In a patient with symptoms of blood dyscrasias, request a medical consultation for blood studies and postpone treatment until normal values are reestablished.
• Medical consultation may be required to assess disease control and patient's ability to receive dental treatment.
• Consultation with physician may be necessary if sedation or general anesthesia is required.

C

Teach Patient/Family to:
• Prevent trauma when using oral hygiene aids.
• See dentist immediately if secondary oral infection occurs.
• Encourage effective oral hygiene to prevent soft tissue inflammation.
• Report oral lesions, soreness, or bleeding to dentist.
• Update health and drug history if physician makes any changes in evaluation or drug regimens.

caprylidene

ka-**pril**′-e-dene
(Axona)

CATEGORY AND SCHEDULE

Pregnancy Risk Category: C

Drug Class: Nutritionals, medical food

MECHANISM OF ACTION

Axona is a prescription medical food containing a proprietary formulation of medium chain triglycerides (MCTs) that are metabolized to ketone bodies to induce hyperketonemia, thus providing an alternate glucose substrate and energy source to the brain when its ability to process glucose is impaired. Brain-imaging scans of older adults and those with Alzheimer's disease reveal a dramatically decreased uptake of glucose.
Therapeutic Effect: Dietary management for the treatment of symptoms of Alzheimer's Disease.

USES

Clinical dietary management of metabolic processes associated with mild-to-moderate Alzheimer's disease

PHARMACOKINETICS

Well absorbed after oral administration. Initial metabolism via lipases in the gut to medium chain fatty acids that undergo hepatic oxidation to ketone bodies. ***Half-life:*** Not reported.

INDICATIONS AND DOSAGES

▸ **Dietary Management of Metabolic Processes Associated with Mild-to-Moderate Alzheimer's Disease**

PO
Adults. 40 g (1 packet of powder, containing 20 g MCTs) once daily.

SIDE EFFECTS/ADVERSE REACTIONS

Frequent
Diarrhea, flatulence
Occasional
Dizziness, headache, dyspepsia

PRECAUTIONS AND CONTRAINDICATIONS

Allergy to milk or soy (contains caseinate, whey, and lecithin) and/or hypersensitivity to palm or coconut oil. Use with caution in patients at risk for ketoacidosis (alcoholics, poorly controlled diabetics) and in patients with a history of GI inflammatory conditions (IBS, diverticulitis, chronic gastritis, GERD). May increase serum triglycerides. May increase BUN, uric acid, or serum creatinine.

DRUG INTERACTIONS OF CONCERN TO DENTISTRY

• Antibiotics: possible increased frequency or worsening of diarrhea

SERIOUS REACTIONS

! None known

DENTAL CONSIDERATIONS

General:

• Patients taking caprylidene usually suffer from mild-to-moderate Alzheimer's disease and should be treated according to appropriate protocols (e.g., in-patient settings).

Consultations:

• Medical consultation is advisable to assess status of patient's disease and ability of patient to tolerate dental procedures.

Teach Patient/Family to:

• Report changes in disease status and changes in medication(s).

• Assist patient with oral hygiene methods, as appropriate for the abilities of the patient.

capsaicin

kap-**say**′-sin

(Zostrix)

Do not confuse with Zovirax.

CATEGORY AND SCHEDULE

Pregnancy Risk Category: C

OTC

Drug Class: Topical analgesic

MECHANISM OF ACTION

A topical analgesic that depletes and prevents reaccumulation of the chemomediator of pain impulses (substance P) from peripheral sensory neurons to CNS.

Therapeutic Effect: Relieves pain.

USES

Treatment of neuralgia associated with herpes zoster or diabetic neuropathy; pain of osteoarthritis and rheumatoid arthritis

PHARMACOKINETICS

None reported

INDICATIONS AND DOSAGES

▸ Treatment of Neuralgia, Osteoarthritis, Rheumatoid Arthritis

Topical

Adults, Elderly, Children older than 2 yr. Apply directly to affected area 3–4 times a day. Continue for 14–28 days for optimal clinical response.

SIDE EFFECTS/ADVERSE REACTIONS

Frequent

Burning, stinging, erythema at site of application

PRECAUTIONS AND CONTRAINDICATIONS

Hypersensitivity to capsaicin or any component of the formulation

Caution:

Lactation, avoid use on broken skin

DRUG INTERACTIONS OF CONCERN TO DENTISTRY

• None reported

SERIOUS REACTIONS

! None known

DENTAL CONSIDERATIONS

General:

• Determine why the patient is taking the drug.

• Consider location of lesions and alter dental procedures accordingly.

Teach Patient/Family to:

• Wash hands thoroughly after use and avoid contact with mouth or eyes.

C

captopril

kap′-toe-pril

(Acenorm[AUS], Capoten, Captohexal[AUS], Novo-Captoril[CAN], Topace[AUS])

Do not confuse captopril with Capitrol.

CATEGORY AND SCHEDULE

Pregnancy Risk Category: C (D if used in second or third trimester)

Drug Class: Angiotensin-converting enzyme (ACE) inhibitor

MECHANISM OF ACTION

An ACE inhibitor that suppresses the renin-angiotensin-aldosterone system and prevents conversion of angiotensin I to angiotensin II, a potent vasoconstrictor; may also inhibit angiotensin II at local vascular and renal sites. Decreases plasma angiotensin II, increases plasma renin activity, and decreases aldosterone secretion.

Therapeutic Effect: Reduces peripheral arterial resistance, pulmonary capillary wedge pressure; improves cardiac output and exercise tolerance.

USES

Treatment of hypertension, heart failure not responsive to conventional therapy, left ventricular dysfunction (LVD) after MI, diabetic nephropathy

PHARMACOKINETICS

Rapidly, well absorbed from the GI tract (absorption is decreased in the presence of food). Protein binding: 25%–30%. Metabolized in the liver. Primarily excreted in urine. Removed by hemodialysis.

Half-life: less than 3 hr (increased in those with impaired renal function).

INDICATIONS AND DOSAGES

▸ **Hypertension**

PO

Adults, Elderly. Initially, 12.5–25 mg 2–3 times a day. After 1–2 wk, may increase to 50 mg 2–3 times a day. Diuretic may be added if no response in additional 1–2 wk. If taken in combination with diuretic, may increase to 100–150 mg 2–3 times a day after 1–2 wk. Maintenance: 25–150 mg 2–3 times a day. Maximum: 450 mg/day.

▸ **CHF**

PO

Adults, Elderly. Initially, 6.25–25 mg 3 times a day. Increase to 50 mg 3 times a day. After at least 2 wk, may increase to 50–100 mg 3 times a day. Maximum: 450 mg/day.

▸ **Post-Myocardial Infarction, Impaired Liver Function**

PO

Adults, Elderly. 6.25 mg a day, then 12.5 mg 3 times a day. Increase to 25 mg 3 times a day over several days up to 50 mg 3 times a day over several week.

▸ **Diabetic Nephropathy Prevention of Kidney Failure**

PO

Adults, Elderly. 25 mg 3 times a day.

Children. Initially 0.3–0.5 mg/kg/dose titrated up to a maximum of 6 mg/kg/day in 2–4 divided doses.

Neonates. Initially, 0.05–0.1 mg/kg/dose q8–24h titrated up to 0.5 mg/kg/dose given q6–24 hr.

Dosage in Renal Impairment. Creatinine clearance 10–50 ml/min. 75% of normal dosage. Creatinine clearance less than 10 ml/min. 50% of normal dosage.

SIDE EFFECTS/ADVERSE REACTIONS

Frequent
Rash
Occasional
Pruritus, dysgeusia (altered taste)
Rare
Headache, cough, insomnia, dizziness, fatigue, paresthesia, malaise, nausea, diarrhea or constipation, dry mouth, tachycardia

PRECAUTIONS AND CONTRAINDICATIONS

History of angioedema from previous treatment with ACE inhibitors
Caution:
Dialysis patients, hypovolemia, leukemia, scleroderma, lupus erythematosus, blood dyscrasias, CHF, diabetes mellitus, renal disease, thyroid disease, COPD, asthma, discontinue drug if pregnancy is detected

DRUG INTERACTIONS OF CONCERN TO DENTISTRY

- Increased hypotension: alcohol, phenothiazines
- Decreased hypotensive effects: indomethacin and possibly other NSAIDs, sympathomimetics
- Suspected reduction in the antihypertensive and vasodilator effects by salicylates; monitor blood pressure if used concurrently

SERIOUS REACTIONS

! Excessive hypotension ("first-dose syncope") may occur in patients with CHF and in those who are severely salt and volume depleted.
! Angioedema (swelling of face and lips) and hyperkalemia occur rarely.
! Agranulocytosis and neutropenia may be noted in those with collagen vascular disease, including scleroderma and systemic lupus erythematosus, and impaired renal function.
! Nephrotic syndrome may be noted in those with history of renal disease.

DENTAL CONSIDERATIONS

General:
- Monitor vital signs at every appointment because of cardiovascular side effects.
- Observe appropriate limitations of vasoconstrictor doses.
- After supine positioning, have patient sit upright for at least 2 min before standing to avoid orthostatic hypotension.
- Patients on chronic drug therapy may rarely have symptoms of blood dyscrasias, which can include infection, bleeding, and poor healing.
- Assess salivary flow as a factor in caries, periodontal disease, and candidiasis.
- Limit use of sodium-containing products, such as saline IV fluids, for patients with a dietary salt restriction.
- Stress from dental procedures may compromise cardiovascular function; determine patient risk.
- Short appointments and a stress-reduction protocol may be required for anxious patients.

Consultations:
- Medical consultation may be required to assess patient's ability to tolerate stress.
- In a patient with symptoms of blood dyscrasias, request a medical consultation for blood studies and postpone dental treatment until normal values are reestablished.
- Take precautions if dental surgery is anticipated and sedation or

general anesthesia is required; risk of hypotensive episode.

Teach Patient/Family to:

- Encourage effective oral hygiene to prevent soft tissue inflammation.
- Use caution to prevent injury when using oral hygiene aids.
- When chronic dry mouth occurs, advise patient to:
  - Avoid mouth rinses with high alcohol content because of drying effects.
  - Use daily home fluoride products for anticaries effect.
  - Use sugarless gum, frequent sips of water, or saliva substitutes.

carbachol

kar′-ba-kole

(Caroptic, Isopto Carbachol, Miostat)

CATEGORY AND SCHEDULE

Pregnancy Risk Category: C

Drug Class: Antiglaucoma agent, ophthalmic; Antihypertensive agent, ocular, postsurgical; Miotic

MECHANISM OF ACTION

A direct-acting parasympathomimetic agent that stimulates cholinergic receptors resulting in muscarinic and nicotinic effects. Indirectly promotes release of acetylcholine.

Therapeutic Effect: Produces contraction of the iris sphincter muscle, resulting in miosis, and reduction in intraocular pressure associated with decreased resistance to aqueous humor outflow.

USES

Used in the eye to treat glaucoma

PHARMACOKINETICS

None reported

INDICATIONS AND DOSAGES

▸ Glaucoma

Ophthalmic

Adults, Elderly. Instill 1–2 drops of 0.75%–3% solution in affected eye(s) up to 3 times a day.

▸ Miosis, Ophthalmic Surgery

Ophthalmic

Adults, Elderly. Instill 0.5 ml of 0.01% solution into anterior chamber before or after securing sutures.

SIDE EFFECTS/ADVERSE REACTIONS

Occasional

Blurred vision, burning/irritation of eye, decreased night vision, headache

PRECAUTIONS AND CONTRAINDICATIONS

Acute iritis, hypersensitivity to carbachol or any component of the formulation

DRUG INTERACTIONS OF CONCERN TO DENTISTRY

- None reported

SERIOUS REACTIONS

! None reported

DENTAL CONSIDERATIONS

General:

- Determine why patient is taking the drug.
- Avoid drugs with anticholinergic activity, such as antihistamines, opioids, benzodiazepines, propantheline, atropine, and scopolamine.

• Avoid dental light in patient's eyes; offer dark glasses for patient comfort.
• Protect patient's eyes from accidental spatter during dental treatment.
• Question glaucoma patient about compliance with prescribed drug regimen.

Consultations:

• Medical consultation may be required to assess disease control.

Teach Patient/Family to:

• Update health and medication history if physician makes any changes in evaluation or drug regimens; include OTC, herbal, and nonherbal remedies in the update.

carbamazepine

kar-ba-**maz'**-eh-peen
(Apo-Carbamazepine[CAN], Carbatrol, Epitol, Equetro, Tegretol, Tegretol CR[AUS], Tegretol XR, Teril[AUS])
Do not confuse Tegretol with Cartrol, Toradol, or Trental.

CATEGORY AND SCHEDULE

Pregnancy Risk Category: D

Drug Class: Anticonvulsant

MECHANISM OF ACTION

An iminostilbenes derivative that decreases sodium and calcium ion influx into neuronal membranes, reducing post-tetanic potentiation at synapses.
Therapeutic Effect: Reduces seizure activity.

USES

Treatment of tonic-clonic, complex-partial, and mixed seizures; trigeminal neuralgia; unapproved: neurogenic pain, some psychotic disorders, diabetes insipidus, alcohol withdrawal

PHARMACOKINETICS

Slowly and completely absorbed from the GI tract. Protein binding: 75%. Metabolized in the liver to active metabolite. Primarily excreted in urine. Not removed by hemodialysis. ***Half-life:*** 25–65 hr (decreased with chronic use).

INDICATIONS AND DOSAGES

▸ Seizure Control

PO

Adults, Children older than 12 yr. Initially, 200 mg twice a day. May increase dosage by 200 mg/day at weekly intervals. Range: 400–1200 mg/day in 2–4 divided doses. Maximum: 1.6–2.4 g/day.
Children 6–12 yr. Initially, 100 mg twice a day. May increase by 100 mg/day at weekly intervals. Range: 20–30 mg/kg/day. Maximum: 1000 mg/day.
Children younger than 6 yr. Initially 5 mg/kg/day. May increase at weekly intervals to 10 mg/kg/day up to 20 mg/kg/day.
Elderly. Initially 100 mg 1–2 times a day. May increase by 100 mg/day at weekly intervals. Usual dose 400–1000 mg/day.

▸ Trigeminal Neuralgia, Diabetic Neuropathy

PO

Adults. Initially, 100 mg twice a day. May increase by 100 mg twice a day up to 400–800 mg/day. Maximum: 1200 mg/day.
Elderly. Initially 100 mg 1–2 times a day. May increase by 100 mg/day at weekly intervals. Usual dose 400–1000 mg/day.

SIDE EFFECTS/ADVERSE REACTIONS

Frequent

Drowsiness, dizziness, nausea, vomiting

Occasional

Visual abnormalities (spots before eyes, difficulty focusing, blurred vision), dry mouth or pharynx, tongue irritation, headache, fluid retention, diaphoresis, constipation or diarrhea, behavioral changes in children

PRECAUTIONS AND CONTRAINDICATIONS

Concomitant use of MAOIs, history of myelosuppression, hypersensitivity to tricyclic antidepressants.

Caution:

Glaucoma, hepatic disease, renal disease, cardiac disease, psychosis, lactation, children younger than 6 yr

DRUG INTERACTIONS OF CONCERN TO DENTISTRY

- Decreased metabolism: erythromycin, clarithromycin, propoxyphene, troleandomycin, metronidazole, ketoconazole, fluconazole, itraconazole, or any drug that inhibits CYP450 3A4 enzymes
- Increased serum levels: tricyclic antidepressants, fluoxetine, fluvoxamine, nefazodone, ketoconazole, itraconazole
- Increased CNS depression: haloperidol, phenothiazines
- Decreased half-life: doxycycline
- Potential hepatotoxicity: chronic high doses of carbamazepine with acetaminophen
- Decreased effects of phenobarbital, corticosteroids, benzodiazepines, doxycycline, sertraline

SERIOUS REACTIONS

! Toxic reactions may include blood dyscrasias (such as aplastic anemia, agranulocytosis, thrombocytopenia, leukopenia, leukocytosis, and eosinophilia), cardiovascular disturbances (such as CHF, hypotension or hypertension, thrombophlebitis, and arrhythmias), and dermatologic effects (such as rash, urticaria, pruritus, and photosensitivity).

! Abrupt withdrawal may precipitate status epilepticus.

DENTAL CONSIDERATIONS

General:

- Monitor vital signs at every appointment because of cardiovascular side effects.
- Patients on chronic drug therapy may rarely have symptoms of blood dyscrasias, which can include infection, bleeding, and poor healing.
- Assess salivary flow as a factor in caries, periodontal disease, and candidiasis.
- Short appointments and a stress-reduction protocol may be required for anxious patients.
- Talk with patient about type of epilepsy, seizure frequency, and quality of seizure control.
- Recommend sealants and home fluoride therapy if patient is using the chewable dose form.

Consultations:

- In a patient with symptoms of blood dyscrasias, request a medical consultation for blood studies and postpone dental treatment until normal values are reestablished.
- Medical consultation may be required to assess disease control and patient's ability to tolerate stress.

Teach Patient/Family to:
- Encourage effective oral hygiene to prevent soft tissue inflammation.
- Use caution to prevent injury when using oral hygiene aids.
- Use caution when driving or performing other tasks requiring alertness.
- When chronic dry mouth occurs, advise patient to:
  - Avoid mouth rinses with high alcohol content because of drying effects.
  - Use daily home fluoride products for anticaries effect.
  - Use sugarless gum, frequent sips of water, or saliva substitutes.

carbamide peroxide

kahr′-buh-mide

(Auro Ear Drops, Debrox, E • R • O Ear, Gly-Oxide, Mollifene Ear Wax Removing, Murine Ear Drops, Orajel Perioseptic, Proxigel) (gel, solution)

CATEGORY AND SCHEDULE
Pregnancy Risk Category: C

Drug Class: Ceruminolytic; topical oral antiinflammatory

MECHANISM OF ACTION
A ceruminolytic that releases oxygen on contact with moist mouth tissues to provide cleansing effects, reduce inflammation, relieve pain, and inhibit odor-forming bacteria. In the ear, oxygen is released and hydrogen peroxide is reduced to water, which enables the chemical reaction.

Therapeutic Effect: Relieves inflammation of gums and lips. Emulsifies and disperses ear wax.

USES
Dental whitener

PHARMACOKINETICS
Not known

INDICATIONS AND DOSAGES
▸ **Earwax Removal**

Topical, Solution

Adults, Elderly, Children 12 yr or older. Tilt head and administer 5–10 drops twice a day for up to 4 days.

Children 12 yr or younger. Tilt head and administer 1–5 drops twice a day for up to 4 days.

▸ **Oral Lesions**

Topical, gel

Adults, Elderly, Children. Apply to affected area 4 times a day.

Topical, solution

Adults, Elderly, Children. Apply several drops undiluted on affected area 4 times a day after meals and at bedtime.

SIDE EFFECTS/ADVERSE REACTIONS
Occasional

Oral: Gingival sensitivity

PRECAUTIONS AND CONTRAINDICATIONS
Dizziness, ear discharge or drainage, ear injury, ear pain, irritation, or rash, hypersensitivity to carbamide peroxide or any one of its components

DRUG INTERACTIONS OF CONCERN TO DENTISTRY
- None reported

SERIOUS REACTIONS
! Opportunistic infections caused by organisms like *Candida albicans* are possible with prolonged use.

C

DENTAL CONSIDERATIONS

General:

• For oral ulcers, perform an oral exam to rule out possible local contributing factors such as broken tooth or filling or ill-fitting dentures.

• Question patient about symptom history; onset, duration, and frequency.

• This drug is the principal ingredient in tooth bleaching or whitening agents; avoid excessive use.

Teach Patient/Family:

• To see the dentist if symptoms worsen or do not abate within 7 days.

carbinoxamine maleate

kar-bi-**nox′**-ah-meen **mal′**-ee-ate (Carboxine, Histex CT, Histex I/E, Histex PD, Histex Pd 12, Palgic, Pediatex, Pediox)

CATEGORY AND SCHEDULE

Pregnancy Risk Category: C

Drug Class: Antihistaminic (H_1-receptor)-decongestant

MECHANISM OF ACTION

An antihistamine that exhibits H_1 receptor blocking action.

Therapeutic Effect: Prevents allergic responses mediated by histamine, such as rhinitis.

USES

Treatment of the nasal congestion (stuffy nose), sneezing, and runny nose caused by colds and hay fever

PHARMACOKINETICS

Virtually no intact drug is excreted in urine. ***Half-life:*** 1–20 hr.

INDICATIONS AND DOSAGES

▸ **Allergic Rhinitis**

PO

Adults, Children 6 yr and older. 1 tsp 4 times a day.

Children 18 mo–6 yr. ½ tsp 4 times a day.

Children 9–18 mo. ¼–½ tsp 4 times a day.

SIDE EFFECTS/ADVERSE REACTIONS

Frequent

Somnolence, dizziness, muscle weakness, hypotension, urine retention, thickening of bronchial secretions, dry mouth, nose, throat, or lips; in elderly, sedation, dizziness, hypotension

Occasional

Epigastric distress, vomiting, headache

Rare

Excitability in children

PRECAUTIONS AND CONTRAINDICATIONS

Hypersensitivity or idiosyncrasy to any ingredients, patients taking MAOIs

DRUG INTERACTIONS OF CONCERN TO DENTISTRY

• Increased sedation: alcohol and all CNS depressants

• Prolonged sedative and anticholinergic effects: MAOIs

SERIOUS REACTIONS

! Overdose symptoms may vary from CNS depression, including sedation, apnea, hypotension, cardiovascular collapse, and death, to severe paradoxical reactions, such as hallucinations, tremor, and seizures.

DENTAL CONSIDERATIONS

General:

- Assess salivary flow as a factor in caries, periodontal disease, and candidiasis.
- Determine why patient is taking the drug.

Teach Patient/Family to:

- Encourage effective oral hygiene to prevent soft tissue inflammation.
- Prevent trauma when using oral hygiene aids.
- When chronic dry mouth occurs, advise patient to:
  - Avoid mouth rinses with high alcohol content because of drying effects.
  - Use daily home fluoride products for anticaries effect.
  - Use sugarless gum, frequent sips of water, or saliva substitutes.

carboplatin

kar-bow-**play**′-tin
(Paraplatin)
Do not confuse carboplatin with Cisplatin or Platinol.

CATEGORY AND SCHEDULE

Pregnancy Risk Category: D

Drug Class: Antineoplastic

MECHANISM OF ACTION

A platinum coordination complex that inhibits DNA synthesis by cross-linking with DNA strands, preventing cell division. Cell cycle-phase nonspecific.
Therapeutic Effect: Interferes with DNA function.

USES

Treatment of cancer of the ovaries

PHARMACOKINETICS

Protein binding: Low. Hydrolyzed in solution to active form. Primarily excreted in urine. ***Half-life:*** 2.6–5.9 hr.

INDICATIONS AND DOSAGES

▸ Ovarian Carcinoma (Monotherapy)

IV

Adults. 360 mg/m^2 on day 1, every 4 wk. Do not repeat dose until neutrophil and platelet counts are within acceptable levels. Adjust drug dosage in previously treated patients based on lowest post-treatment platelet or neutrophil count. Increase dosage only once to no more than 125% of starting dose.

▸ Ovarian Carcinoma (Combination Therapy)

IV

Adults. 300 mg/m^2 (with cyclophosphamide) on day 1, every 4 wk. Don't repeat dose until neutrophil and platelet counts are within acceptable levels.
Children. 300–600 mg/m^2 every 4 wk for solid tumor, or 175 mg/m^2 every 4 wk for brain tumor.

▸ Dosage in Renal Impairment

Initial dosage is based on creatinine clearance; subsequent dosages are based on the patient's tolerance and degree of myelosuppression.

Creatinine Clearance	Dosage Day 1
60 ml/min or greater	360 mg/m^2
41–59 ml/min	250 mg/m^2
16–40 ml/min	200 mg/m^2

SIDE EFFECTS/ADVERSE REACTIONS

Frequent

Nausea, vomiting

C

Occasional
Generalized pain, diarrhea or constipation, peripheral neuropathy
Rare
Alopecia, asthenia, hypersensitivity reaction (erythema, pruritus, rash, urticaria)

PRECAUTIONS AND CONTRAINDICATIONS
History of severe allergic reaction to cisplatin, platinum compounds, or mannitol; severe bleeding, severe myelosuppression

DRUG INTERACTIONS OF CONCERN TO DENTISTRY
• None reported

SERIOUS REACTIONS
! Myelosuppression may be severe, resulting in anemia, infection, (sepsis, pneumonia), and bleeding.
! Prolonged treatment may result in peripheral neurotoxicity.

DENTAL CONSIDERATIONS
General:
• Determine why patient is taking the drug.
• If additional analgesia is required for dental pain, consider alternative analgesics (NSAIDs) in patients taking narcotics for acute or chronic pain.
• Examine for oral manifestation of opportunistic infection.
• Avoid prescribing aspirin-containing products.
• This drug may be used in the hospital or on an outpatient basis. Confirm the patient's disease and treatment status.
• Patient on chronic drug therapy may rarely present with symptoms of blood dyscrasias, which can include infection, bleeding, and poor healing. If dyscrasia is present, caution patient to prevent oral tissue trauma when using oral hygiene aids.
• Short appointments and a stress-reduction protocol may be required for anxious patients.
• Patients may have received other chemotherapy or radiation; confirm medical and drug history.
• Patients may be at risk of bleeding; check for oral signs.
• Patients may be at risk of infection.
• Patients may be taking prophylactic antiinfectives.
• Oral infections should be eliminated and/or treated aggressively.
Consultations:
• Medical consultation should include routine blood counts including platelet counts and bleeding time.
• Consult physician; prophylactic or therapeutic antiinfectives may be indicated if surgery or periodontal treatment is required.
• Medical consultation may be required to assess immunologic status during cancer chemotherapy and determine safety risk, if any, posed by the required dental treatment.
• Medical consultation may be required to assess disease control and patient's ability to tolerate stress.
Teach Patient/Family to:
• See dentist immediately if secondary oral infection occurs.
• Encourage effective oral hygiene to prevent soft tissue inflammation.
• Report oral lesions, soreness, or bleeding to dentist.
• Prevent trauma when using oral hygiene aids.
• Updating health and medication history if physician makes any

changes in evaluation or drug regimens; include OTC, herbal, and nonherbal remedies in the update.

carglumic acid

kar-**glu**-mik as′-id
(Carbaglu)

CATEGORY AND SCHEDULE

Pregnancy Risk Category: C

Drug Class: Metabolic alkalosis agent, urea cycle disorder treatment agent

MECHANISM OF ACTION

Carglumic acid is a structural analogue to NAG, a required activator of the hepatic mitochondrial enzyme CPS1, which converts ammonia into urea in the first step of the urea cycle.
Therapeutic Effect: Reduces blood ammonia levels.

USES

Adjunctive treatment of acute hyperammonemia and maintenance therapy of chronic hyperammonemia due to the deficiency of the hepatic enzyme N-acetylglutamate synthase (NAGS)

PHARMACOKINETICS

Peak plasma concentrations reached in 3 hr. Metabolism via intestinal flora to carbon dioxide. Excreted via feces (60% unchanged drug) and urine (9% unchanged drug).
Half-life: 5.6 hr.

INDICATIONS AND DOSAGES

▸ Acute Hyperammonemia

PO

Adults, Children. 100–250 mg/kg/day given in 2 or 4 divided doses; titrate to age-appropriate plasma ammonia levels. Concomitant adjunctive ammonia-lowering therapy recommended. Administer immediately prior to meals. Carglumic acid tablets should not be crushed or swallowed whole. Each 200-mg tablet should be dispersed in at least 2.5 ml of water (no other foods/liquids) and taken immediately. Tablets do not dissolve completely, and some particles may remain; container should be rinsed with water and contents consumed immediately.

▸ Chronic Hyperammonemia

PO

Adults, Children. Less than 100mg/kg/day given in 2 or 4 divided doses; titrate to age-appropriate plasma ammonia levels.

SIDE EFFECTS/ADVERSE REACTIONS

Frequent

Fever, headache, vomiting, abdominal pain, diarrhea, anemia, ear infection, tonsillitis, nasopharyngitis

Occasional

Somnolence hyperhidrosis, rash, anorexia, dysgeusia, weight loss, weakness, pneumonia, influenza

PRECAUTIONS AND CONTRAINDICATIONS

With acute episodes of hyperammonemia, protein restriction and a hypercaloric diet are recommended until normalization of plasma ammonia concentrations.

DRUG INTERACTIONS OF CONCERN TO DENTISTRY

- No studies reported

C

SERIOUS REACTIONS

! Increased risk of respiratory and other infections

DENTAL CONSIDERATIONS

General:

• Possible increase in vomiting and abdominal pain; caution advised when considering use of analgesics (opioids, NSAIDs).

• Differential diagnosis of odontogenic infections may be complicated by adverse effects of carglumic acid (e.g., pyrexia, tonsillitis, nasopharyngitis, headache).

• Carglumic acid provokes diarrhea, which could be worsened by ingestion of antibiotics.

Consultations:

• Consult physician to assess disease status and ability of patient to tolerate dental procedures.

Teach Patient/Family to:

• Report changes in medical status and drug therapy.

• Report indications of blood and lymphatic system disorders (anemia).

carisoprodol

kar-ih-so-**pro′**-dol

(Soma)

CATEGORY AND SCHEDULE

Pregnancy Risk Category: C

Drug Class: Skeletal muscle relaxant, central acting

MECHANISM OF ACTION

A centrally acting skeletal muscle relaxant whose exact mechanism is unknown. Effects may be because of its CNS depressant actions.

Therapeutic Effect: Relieves muscle spasms and pain.

USES

Adjunct for relief of acute, painful musculoskeletal conditions

PHARMACOKINETICS

Onset 2 hr, duration 4–6 hr. ***Half-life:*** 2.5 hr. Metabolized in liver to meprobamate by the CYP 2C19 isoenzyme; excreted by kidneys.

INDICATIONS AND DOSAGES

▸ **Adjunct to Rest, Physical Therapy, Analgesics, and Other Measures for Relief of Discomfort from Acute, Painful Musculoskeletal Conditions**

PO

Adults, Elderly. 350 mg 4 times a day.

SIDE EFFECTS/ADVERSE REACTIONS

Frequent

Somnolence

Occasional

Tachycardia, facial flushing, dizziness, headache, light-headedness, dermatitis, nausea, vomiting, abdominal cramps, dyspnea

PRECAUTIONS AND CONTRAINDICATIONS

Acute intermittent porphyria, sensitivity to meprobamate

Caution:

Renal disease, hepatic disease, addictive personalities, elderly, children younger than 12 yr

DRUG INTERACTIONS OF CONCERN TO DENTISTRY

• Increased CNS depression: alcohol, all CNS depressants

SERIOUS REACTIONS

! Overdose may cause CNS and respiratory depression, shock, and coma.

DENTAL CONSIDERATIONS

General:

• When used in dentistry, may be more effective when used in combination with aspirin or NSAIDs.

Teach Patient/Family to:

• Use powered tooth brush if patient has difficulty holding conventional devices.

carmustine

kar-**muss**′-teen

(BiCNU, Gliadel)

CATEGORY AND SCHEDULE

Pregnancy Risk Category: D

Drug Class: Antineoplastic

MECHANISM OF ACTION

An alkylating agent and nitrosourea that inhibits DNA and RNA synthesis by cross-linking with DNA and RNA strands, preventing cell division. Cell cycle-phase nonspecific.

Therapeutic Effect: Interferes with DNA and RNA function.

USES

Treatment of certain types of brain cancer

PHARMACOKINETICS

Degraded within 15 min; crosses blood-brain barrier; 70% excreted in urine within 96 hr; 10% excreted as CO_2; fate of 20% is unknown.

INDICATIONS AND DOSAGES

▸ **Disseminated Hodgkin's Disease, Non-Hodgkin's Lymphoma, Multiple Myeloma, and Primary and Metastatic Brain Tumors in Previously Untreated Patients (Monotherapy)**

IV (BiCNu)

Adults, Elderly. 150–200 mg/m^2 as a single dose or 75–100 mg/m^2 on 2 successive days.

Children. 200–250 mg/m^2 every 4–6 wk as a single dose.

▸ **Implantation (Gliadel)**

Adults, Elderly, Children. Up to 8 wafers may be placed in resection cavity.

SIDE EFFECTS/ADVERSE REACTIONS

Frequent

Nausea and vomiting within min to 2 hr after administration (may last up to 6 hr)

Occasional

Diarrhea, esophagitis, anorexia, dysphagia

Rare

Thrombophlebitis

PRECAUTIONS AND CONTRAINDICATIONS

None known

DRUG INTERACTIONS OF CONCERN TO DENTISTRY

• None reported

SERIOUS REACTIONS

! Hematologic toxicity because of myelosuppression occurs frequently. Thrombocytopenia occurs about 4 wk after carmustine treatment begins and lasts 1–2 wk.

! Leukopenia is evident 5–6 wk after treatment begins and lasts 1–2 wk. Anemia occurs less frequently and is less severe.

C

! Mild, reversible hepatotoxicity also occurs frequently.
! Prolonged high-dose carmustine therapy may produce impaired renal function and pulmonary toxicity (pulmonary infiltrate or fibrosis).

DENTAL CONSIDERATIONS

General:

- Determine why patient is taking the drug.
- If additional analgesia is required for dental pain, consider alternative analgesics in patients taking narcotics for acute or chronic pain.
- Avoid products that affect platelet function, such as aspirin and NSAIDs.
- This drug may be used in the hospital or on an outpatient basis. Confirm the patient's disease and treatment status.
- Consider semisupine chair position for patient comfort if GI side effects occur.
- Patient on chronic drug therapy may rarely present with symptoms of blood dyscrasias, which can include infection, bleeding, and poor healing. If dyscrasia is present, caution patient to prevent oral tissue trauma when using oral hygiene aids.
- Examine for oral manifestation of opportunistic infection.
- Consider local hemostasis measures to prevent excessive bleeding.
- Monitor vital signs at every appointment because of cardiovascular side effects.
- Use caution with use of potentially hepatotoxic drugs.

Consultations:

- Medical consultation should include routine blood counts including platelet counts and bleeding time.
- Consult physician; prophylactic or therapeutic antiinfectives may be indicated if surgery or periodontal treatment is required.
- In a patient with symptoms of blood dyscrasias, request a medical consultation for blood studies and postpone treatment until normal values are reestablished.
- Medical consultation may be required to assess disease control and patient's ability to tolerate stress.

Teach Patient/Family to:

- Encourage effective oral hygiene to prevent soft tissue inflammation.
- Prevent trauma when using oral hygiene aids.
- Update health and medication history if physician makes any changes in evaluation or drug regimens; include OTC, herbal, and nonherbal remedies in the update.
- Report oral lesions, soreness, or bleeding to dentist.

carteolol

kar-**tee**′-oh-lole
(Cartrol, Ocupress)
Do not confuse carteolol with carvedilol.

CATEGORY AND SCHEDULE

Pregnancy Risk Category: C (D if after first trimester)

Drug Class: β-adrenergic blocker

MECHANISM OF ACTION

An antihypertensive that blocks β_1-adrenergic receptor at normal doses and β_2-adrenergic receptors at large doses. Predominantly blocks β_1-adrenergic receptors in cardiac

tissue. Reduces aqueous humor production.
Therapeutic Effect: Slows sinus heart rate, decreases cardiac output, decreases B/P, increases airway resistance, decreases intraocular pressure.

USES

Treatment of chronic open-angle glaucoma, ocular hypertension

PHARMACOKINETICS

Well absorbed from the GI tract. Protein binding: unknown. Minimally metabolized in liver. Primarily excreted unchanged in urine. Not removed by hemodialysis. ***Half-life:*** 6 hr (increased in decreased renal function).

INDICATIONS AND DOSAGES

▸ **Ocular Hypertension**

PO

Adults, Elderly. Initially, 2.5 mg/day as single dose either alone or in combination with diuretic. May increase gradually to 5–10 mg/day as a single dose. Maintenance: 2.5–5 mg/day.

▸ **Dosage in Renal Impairment**

Creatinine Clearance	Dosage Interval
Greater than 60 ml/min	24 hr
20–60 ml/min	48 hr
Less than 20 ml/min	72 hr

▸ **Open-Angle Glaucoma, Ocular Hypertension**

Ophthalmic

Adults, Elderly. 1 drop 2 times a day.

SIDE EFFECTS/ADVERSE REACTIONS

Frequent

Oral: Hypotension manifested as dizziness, nausea, diaphoresis, headache, cold extremities, fatigue, constipation/diarrhea

Ophthalmic: Redness of eye or inside of eyelids, decreased night vision

Occasional

Oral: Insomnia, flatulence, urinary frequency, impotence or decreased libido

Ophthalmic: Blepharoconjunctivitis, edema, droopy eyelid, staining of cornea, blurred vision, brow ache, increased light sensitivity, burning, stinging

Rare

Rash, arthralgia, myalgia, confusion (especially elderly), taste disturbances

PRECAUTIONS AND CONTRAINDICATIONS

Bronchial asthma, COPD, bronchospasm, overt cardiac failure, cardiogenic shock, heart block greater than first degree, persistently severe bradycardia.

Caution:

Major surgery, lactation, diabetes mellitus, renal disease, thyroid disease, COPD, well-compensated heart failure, coronary artery disease (CAD), nonallergic bronchospasm

DRUG INTERACTIONS OF CONCERN TO DENTISTRY

- Decreased hypotensive effect: indomethacin, NSAIDs
- Increased hypotension, myocardial depression: hydrocarbon inhalation anesthetics
- Hypertension, bradycardia: sympathomimetics (epinephrine, ephedrine)
- Bradycardia: fluoxetine, paroxetine

SERIOUS REACTIONS

! Abrupt withdrawal (particularly in those with CAD) may produce angina or precipitate MI.

C

! May precipitate thyroid crisis in those with thyrotoxicosis.
! β-blockers may mask signs and symptoms of acute hypoglycemia (tachycardia, B/P changes) in diabetic patients.

DENTAL CONSIDERATIONS

General:

- Monitor vital signs at every appointment because of cardiovascular side effects.
- After supine positioning, have patient sit upright for at least 2 min before standing to avoid orthostatic hypotension.
- Assess salivary flow as a factor in caries, periodontal disease, and candidiasis.
- Patients on chronic drug therapy may rarely have symptoms of blood dyscrasias, which can include infection, bleeding, and poor healing.
- Limit use of sodium-containing products, such as saline IV fluids, for those patients with a dietary salt restriction.
- Stress from dental procedures may compromise cardiovascular function; determine patient risk.
- Short appointments and a stress-reduction protocol may be required for anxious patients.

Consultations:

- In a patient with symptoms of blood dyscrasias, request a medical consultation for blood studies and postpone dental treatment until normal values are reestablished.
- Medical consultation may be required to assess disease control and patient's ability to tolerate stress.

Teach Patient/Family to:

- Report oral lesions, soreness, or bleeding to dentist.
- When chronic dry mouth occurs, advise patient to:
  - Avoid mouth rinses with high alcohol content because of drying effects.
  - Use daily home fluoride products for anticaries effect.
  - Use sugarless gum, frequent sips of water, or saliva substitutes.

carvedilol

kar-vea-die-lole
(Coreg, Coreg CR)

CATEGORY AND SCHEDULE

Pregnancy Risk Category: C (D if used in second or third trimester)

Drug Class: β-Adrenergic Blocker with α-Blocking Activity
Do not confuse carvedilol with carteolol or captopril.

MECHANISM OF ACTION

A cardiovascular agent that possesses nonselective β-blocking and α-adrenergic blocking activity. Causes vasodilation.
Therapeutic Effect: Reduces cardiac output, exercise-induced tachycardia, and reflex orthostatic tachycardia; reduces peripheral vascular resistance; inhibits renin release.

USES

Hypertension
Left ventricular dysfunction following myocardial infarction
Heart failure

PHARMACOKINETICS

Rapidly and extensively absorbed from the GI tract following oral administration. Bioavailability: 25%–35% (immediate release formulation); 85% (extended-release). Protein binding: 98%, primarily to albumin. Metabolized in the liver primarily through CYP3A4, 2C19, and 2D6 pathway to active metabolites. Excreted primarily via bile into feces. Minimally removed by hemodialysis. ***Half-life:*** 7–10 hr. Food delays rate of absorption.

INDICATIONS AND DOSAGES

▸ **Hypertension**

PO (Immediate Release)

Adults, Elderly. Initially, 6.25 mg twice a day. May double at 7- to 14-day intervals to highest tolerated dosage. Maximum: 50 mg/day. (25 mg twice a day); if pulse drops below 55 bpm, reduce dose.

PO (Extended Release)

Adults, Elderly. Initially, 20 mg once a day, in the morning with food. May double the dose at 7- to 14-day intervals. Maximum: 80 mg/day. Note: 6.25 mg of immediate release is equivalent to 20 mg of extended release.

▸ **Myocardial Infarction Prophylaxis in Stable Patients with Left Ventricular Dysfunction**

PO (Immediate Release)

Adults, Elderly. Initially, 3.125–6.25 mg twice a day with food. May increase at intervals of 3–10 days up to target dose of 25 mg twice a day. Maximum: 50 mg/day.

PO (Extended Release)

Adults, Elderly. Initially, 20 mg once a day, in the morning with food. Increase at 3- to 10-day intervals to a target dose of 80 mg a day.

SIDE EFFECTS/ADVERSE REACTIONS

Carvedilol is generally well tolerated, with mild and transient side effects.

Adults

Frequent

Fatigue, dizziness, hyperglycemia, diarrhea, weight gain, hypotension, weakness

Occasional

Bradycardia, rhinitis, back pain, syncope, headache, blurred vision, impotence, nausea, vomiting, angina

Rare

Orthostatic hypotension, somnolence, UTI, viral infection, rash, hypercholesterolemia, gout, weight loss

PRECAUTIONS AND CONTRAINDICATIONS

Hypersensitivity to carvedilol or any component of the formulation

Caution:

Bronchial asthma or related bronchospastic conditions
Cardiogenic shock
Pulmonary edema
Second- or third-degree AV block
Severe bradycardia
Hepatic disease
Heart rate below 55 bpm
Caution use in patients undergoing anesthesia and in those with CHF controlled with ACE inhibitor, digoxin or diuretics; diabetes mellitus; hypoglycemia; impaired hepatic function; peripheral vascular disease; and thyrotoxicosis
Avoid abrupt withdrawal

DRUG INTERACTIONS OF CONCERN TO DENTISTRY

- Calcium blockers: Increase risk of conduction disturbances, hypotension, and/or bradycardia.
- Cimetidine: May increase carvedilol blood concentration.
- Digoxin: Increases concentrations of digoxin.
- Diuretics, other antihypertensives: May increase hypotensive effect.

C

• Insulin, oral hypoglycemics: May mask symptoms of hypoglycemia and prolong hypoglycemic effect of these drugs.
• Rifampin: Decreases carvedilol blood concentration.
• CYP450 2D6 inhibitors: May decrease the metabolism of CYP2D6 substrates.
• Cyclosporine: Increases concentrations of cyclosporine.

SERIOUS REACTIONS

! Overdose may produce profound bradycardia and hypotension.
! Abrupt withdrawal may result in diaphoresis, palpitations, headache, and tremors.
! Carvedilol administration may precipitate CHF or MI in patients with heart disease; thyroid storm in those with thyrotoxicosis; or peripheral ischemia in those with existing peripheral vascular disease.
! Hypoglycemia may occur in patients with previously controlled diabetes.
! Signs of thrombocytopenia, such as unusual bleeding or bruising, occur rarely.

DENTAL CONSIDERATIONS

General:
• Monitor vital signs at every appointment because of cardiovascular side effects.
• After supine positioning, have patient sit upright for at least 2 min before standing to avoid orthostatic hypotension.
• Assess salivary flow as a factor in caries, periodontal disease, and candidiasis.
• Limit use of sodium-containing products, such as saline IV fluids, for those patients with dietary salt restriction.
• Stress from dental procedures may compromise cardiovascular function; determine patient risk.

Consultations:
• Medical consultation may be required to assess disease control.

Teach Patient/Family to:
Report oral lesions, soreness, or bleeding to dentist.
• When chronic dry mouth occurs, advise patient to:
  • Avoid mouth rinses with high alcohol content because of drying effects.
  • Use daily home fluoride products for anticaries effect.
  • Use sugarless gum, frequent sips of water, or saliva substitutes.

caspofungin acetate

kas-poe-**fun′**-gin **ass′**-eh-tayte
(Cancidas)

CATEGORY AND SCHEDULE

Pregnancy Risk Category: C

Drug Class: Antifungal, systemic

MECHANISM OF ACTION

An antifungal that inhibits the synthesis of glucan, a vital component of fungal cell formation, thereby damaging the fungal cell membrane.
Therapeutic Effect: Fungistatic.

USES

Help the body overcome serious fungus infections

PHARMACOKINETICS

Distributed in tissue. Extensively bound to albumin. Protein binding: 97%. Slowly metabolized in liver to active metabolite. Excreted primarily in urine and to a lesser extent in feces. Not removed by hemodialysis. ***Half-life:*** 40–50 hr.

INDICATIONS AND DOSAGES

▸ Aspergillosis

IV

Adults, Elderly, Children older than 12 yr. Give single 70-mg loading dose on day 1, followed by 50 mg/day thereafter. For patients with moderate hepatic insufficiency, daily dose reduced to 35 mg.

▸ Invasive Candidiasis

IV

Adults, Elderly. Initially, 70 mg followed by 50 mg daily.

▸ Esophageal Candidiasis

IV

Adults, Elderly. 50 mg a day.

SIDE EFFECTS/ADVERSE REACTIONS

Frequent

Fever

Occasional

Headache, nausea, phlebitis

Rare

Paresthesia, vomiting, diarrhea, abdominal pain, myalgia, chills, tremor, insomnia

PRECAUTIONS AND CONTRAINDICATIONS

None known

DRUG INTERACTIONS OF CONCERN TO DENTISTRY

• Reduction in concentration: dexamethasone, carbamazepine

SERIOUS REACTIONS

! Hypersensitivity reactions (characterized by rash, facial swelling, pruritus, and a sensation of warmth) may occur.

DENTAL CONSIDERATIONS

General:

• For selected infections in the hospital setting.
• Provide palliative dental care for dental emergencies only.
• Patient on chronic drug therapy may rarely present with symptoms of blood dyscrasias, which can include infection, bleeding, and poor healing. If dyscrasia is present, caution patient to prevent oral tissue trauma when using oral hygiene aids.

Consultations:

• In a patient with symptoms of blood dyscrasias, request a medical consultation for blood studies and postpone treatment until normal values are reestablished.
• Medical consultation may be required to assess disease control and patient's ability to tolerate stress.
• Medical consultation should include PPT, PT, or INR.

Teach Patient/Family to:

• Encourage effective oral hygiene to prevent soft tissue inflammation.
• Report oral lesions, soreness, or bleeding to dentist.
• Prevent trauma when using oral hygiene aids.

cefaclor

sef'-ah-klor

(Apo-Cefaclor[CAN], Ceclor, Ceclor CD, Cefkor[AUS], Cefkor CD[AUS], Keflor[AUS])

CATEGORY AND SCHEDULE

Pregnancy Risk Category: B

Drug Class: Antibiotic, cephalosporin (second generation)

MECHANISM OF ACTION

A second-generation cephalosporin that binds to bacterial cell membranes and inhibits cell wall synthesis.
Therapeutic Effect: Bactericidal.

USES

For use in the treatment of the following infections when caused by susceptible strains of named microorganisms: otitis media caused by *S. pneumoniae, H. influenzae,* staphylococci, and *S. pyogenes*; lower respiratory tract infections caused by *S. pneumoniae, H. influenzae,* and *S. pyogenes*; pharyngitis and tonsillitis caused by *S. pyogenes*; UTIs caused by *E. coli, P. mirabilis, Klebsiella* species, and coagulase-negative staphylococci; skin and skin structure infections caused by *S. aureus* and *S. pyogenes*; and in vitro activity against *Peptococcus, Peptostreptococcus,* and *Propionibacterium* (clinical significance unknown)

PHARMACOKINETICS

Well absorbed from the GI tract. Protein binding: 25%. Widely distributed. Primarily excreted unchanged in urine. Moderately removed by hemodialysis. ***Half-life:*** 0.6–0.9 hr (increased in impaired renal function).

INDICATIONS AND DOSAGES

▸ Bronchitis

PO (Extended-Release)
Adults, Elderly. 500 mg q12h for 7 days.

▸ Lower Respiratory Tract Infections

PO
Adults, Elderly. 250–500 mg q8h.

▸ Otitis Media

PO
Children. 20–40 mg/kg/day in 2–3 divided doses. Maximum: 1 g/day.

▸ Pharyngitis, Skin/Skin Structure Infections, Tonsillitis

PO (Extended-Release)
Adults, Elderly. 375 mg q12h.
PO (Regular-Release)
Adults, Elderly. 250–500 mg q8h.
Children. 20–40 mg/kg/day in 2–3 divided doses. Maximum: 1 g/day.

▸ UTIs

PO
Adults, Elderly. 250–500 mg q8h.
Children. 20–40 mg/kg/day in 2–3 divided doses q8h. Maximum: 1 g/day.
PO (Extended-Release)
Adults, Children older than 16 yr. 375–500 mg q12h.

▸ Otitis Media

PO
Children older than 1 mo. 40 mg/kg/day in divided doses q8h. Maximum: 1 g/day.

▸ Dosage in Renal Impairment

Decreased dosage may be necessary in patients with creatinine clearance less than 40 ml/min.

SIDE EFFECTS/ADVERSE REACTIONS

Frequent

Oral candidiasis, mild diarrhea, mild abdominal cramping, vaginal candidiasis

Occasional

Nausea, serum sickness-like reaction (marked by fever and joint pain; usually occurs after the second course of therapy and resolves after the drug is discontinued)

Rare

Allergic reaction (pruritus, rash, and urticaria)

PRECAUTIONS AND CONTRAINDICATIONS
History of anaphylactic reaction to penicillins or hypersensitivity to cephalosporins
Caution:
Hypersensitivity to penicillins, lactation, renal disease

DRUG INTERACTIONS OF CONCERN TO DENTISTRY
- Decreased bactericidal effects: tetracyclines, erythromycins
- Increased and prolonged serum levels: probenecid

SERIOUS REACTIONS
! Antibiotic-associated colitis and other superinfections may result from altered bacterial balance.
! Nephrotoxicity may occur, especially in patients with preexisting renal disease.
! Patients with a history of allergies, especially to penicillin, are at increased risk for developing a severe hypersensitivity reaction, marked by severe pruritus, angioedema, bronchospasm, and anaphylaxis.

DENTAL CONSIDERATIONS
General:
- Take precautions regarding allergy to medication.
- Determine why the patient is taking the drug.

Consultations:
- Medical consultation may be required to assess disease control.

Teach Patient/Family to:
- Encourage effective oral hygiene to prevent soft tissue inflammation.
- When used for dental infection, advise patient to:
- Report sore throat, oral burning sensation, fever, and fatigue, any of which could indicate superinfection.
- Take at prescribed intervals and complete dosage regimen.
- Immediately notify the dentist if signs or symptoms of infection increase.

cefadroxil
sef-ah-**drox′**-ill
(Duricef)

CATEGORY AND SCHEDULE
Pregnancy Risk Category: B

Drug Class: Cephalosporin (first generation)

MECHANISM OF ACTION
A first-generation cephalosporin that binds to bacterial cell membranes and inhibits cell wall synthesis.
Therapeutic Effect: Bactericidal.

USES
Treatment of gram-negative bacilli: *E. coli, P. mirabilis, Klebsiella* (UTI only); gram-positive organisms: *S. pneumoniae, S. pyogenes, S. aureus*; upper/lower respiratory tract, urinary tract, skin infections; otitis media; tonsillitis; particularly for UTI

PHARMACOKINETICS
Well absorbed from the GI tract. Protein binding: 15%–20%. Widely distributed. Primarily excreted unchanged in urine. Removed by hemodialysis. ***Half-life:*** 1.2–1.5 hr

(increased in impaired renal function).

C

INDICATIONS AND DOSAGES

▸ UTIs

PO

Adults, Elderly. 1–2 g/day as a single dose or in 2 divided doses.

Children. 30 mg/kg/day in 2 divided doses. Maximum: 2 g/day.

▸ Skin and Skin-Structure Infections, Group A β-Hemolytic Streptococcal Pharyngitis, Tonsillitis

PO

Adults, Elderly. 1–2 g in 2 divided doses.

Children. 30 mg/kg/day in 2 divided doses. Maximum: 2 g/day.

▸ Impetigo

PO

Children. 30 mg/kg/day as a single or in 2 divided doses. Maximum: 2 g/day.

▸ Dosage in Renal Impairment

After an initial 1-g dose, dosage and frequency are modified on the basis of creatinine clearance and the severity of the infection.

Creatinine Clearance	Dosage Interval
25–50 ml/min	500 mg q12h
10–25 ml/min	500 mg q24h
0–10 ml/min	500 mg q36h

SIDE EFFECTS/ADVERSE REACTIONS

Frequent

Oral candidiasis, mild diarrhea, mild abdominal cramping, vaginal candidiasis

Occasional

Nausea, unusual bruising or bleeding, serum sickness-like reaction (marked by fever and joint pain; usually occurs after the second course of therapy and resolves after the drug is discontinued)

Rare

Allergic reaction (rash, pruritus, urticaria), thrombophlebitis (pain, redness, swelling at injection site)

PRECAUTIONS AND CONTRAINDICATIONS

History of anaphylactic reaction to penicillins or hypersensitivity to cephalosporins

Caution:

Hypersensitivity to penicillins, lactation, renal disease

DRUG INTERACTIONS OF CONCERN TO DENTISTRY

• Decreased bactericidal effects: tetracyclines, erythromycins

• Increased and prolonged serum levels: probenecid

SERIOUS REACTIONS

! Antibiotic-associated colitis and other superinfections may result from altered bacterial balance.

! Nephrotoxicity may occur, especially in patients with preexisting renal disease.

! Patients with a history of allergies, especially to penicillin, are at increased risk for developing a severe hypersensitivity reaction, marked by severe pruritus, angioedema, bronchospasm, and anaphylaxis.

DENTAL CONSIDERATIONS

General:

• Take precautions regarding allergy to medication.

• Determine why the patient is taking the drug.

Consultations:

• Medical consultation may be required to assess disease control.

Teach Patient/Family to:

- Encourage effective oral hygiene to prevent soft tissue inflammation.
- When used for dental infection, advise patient to:
  - Report sore throat, oral burning sensation, fever, and fatigue, any of which could indicate superinfection.
  - Take at prescribed intervals and complete dosage regimen.
  - Immediately notify the dentist if signs or symptoms of infection increase.

cefazolin sodium

sef-**a**′-zoe-lin **so**′-dee-um
(Ancef, Kefzol)
Do not confuse cefazolin with cefprozil or Cefzil.

CATEGORY AND SCHEDULE

Pregnancy Risk Category: B

Drug Class: Cephalosporin (first generation)

MECHANISM OF ACTION

A first-generation cephalosporin that binds to bacterial cell membranes and inhibits cell wall synthesis. ***Therapeutic Effect:*** Bactericidal.

USES

Indicated for use when infection is caused by susceptible microorganisms: respiratory tract infections caused by *S. pneumoniae, Klebsiella* species, *H. influenzae, S. aureus,* and group A β-hemolytic streptococci; UTI infections caused by *E. coli, P. mirabilis, Klebsiella* species, and some Enterobacter and enterococci; skin and skin structure infections caused by *S. aureus,* group A β-hemolytic streptococci; biliary tract infections caused by *E. coli, P. mirabilis, S. aureus, Klebsiella* species, and various strains of streptococci; bone and joint infections caused by *S. aureus*; genital infections caused by *E. coli, P. mirabilis, Klebsiella* species, and some enterococci; septicemia caused by *S. aureus, S. viridans, P. mirabilis, E. coli*, and *Klebsiella* species, group A β-hemolytic streptococci

PHARMACOKINETICS

Widely distributed. Protein binding: 85%. Primarily excreted unchanged in urine. Moderately removed by hemodialysis. ***Half-life:*** 1.4–1.8 hr (increased in impaired renal function).

INDICATIONS AND DOSAGES

▸ **Uncomplicated UTIs**

IV, IM

Adults, Elderly. 1 g q12h.

▸ **Mild to Moderate Infections**

IV, IM

Adults, Elderly. 250–500 mg q8–12h.

▸ **Severe Infections**

IV, IM

Adults, Elderly. 0.5–1 g q6–8h.

▸ **Life-Threatening Infections**

IV, IM

Adults, Elderly. 1–1.5 g q6h. Maximum: 12 g/day.

▸ **Perioperative Prophylaxis**

IV, IM

Adults, Elderly. 1 g 30–60 min before surgery, 0.5–1 g during surgery, and q6–8h for up to 24 hr postoperatively.

▸ **Usual Pediatric Dosage**

Children. 50–100 mg/kg/day in divided doses q8h. Maximum: 6 g/day.

C

Neonates older than 7 days.
40–60 mg/kg/day in divided doses q8–12h.
Neonates 7 days and younger.
40 mg/kg/day in divided doses q12h.

▸ **Dosage in Renal Impairment**

Dosing frequency is modified on the basis of creatinine clearance.

Creatinine Clearance	Dosage Interval
10–30 ml/min	Usual dose q12h
Less than 10 ml/min	Usual dose q24h

SIDE EFFECTS/ADVERSE REACTIONS

Frequent
Discomfort with IM administration, oral candidiasis, mild diarrhea, mild abdominal cramping, vaginal candidiasis
Occasional
Nausea, serum sickness-like reaction (marked by fever and joint pain; usually occurs after the second course of therapy and resolves after the drug is discontinued)
Rare
Allergic reaction (rash, pruritus, urticaria), thrombophlebitis (pain, redness, swelling at injection site)

PRECAUTIONS AND CONTRAINDICATIONS

History of anaphylactic reaction to penicillins or hypersensitivity to cephalosporins
Caution:
Hypersensitivity to penicillins, lactation, renal disease

DRUG INTERACTIONS OF CONCERN TO DENTISTRY

• Decreased bactericidal effects: tetracyclines, erythromycins
• Increased and prolonged serum levels: probenecid

SERIOUS REACTIONS

! Antibiotic-associated colitis and other superinfections may result from altered bacterial balance.
! Nephrotoxicity may occur, especially in patients with preexisting renal disease.
! Patients with a history of allergies, especially to penicillin, are at increased risk for developing a severe hypersensitivity reaction, marked by severe pruritus, angioedema, bronchospasm, and anaphylaxis.

DENTAL CONSIDERATIONS

General:
• Take precautions regarding allergy to medication.
• Determine why the patient is taking the drug.
Consultations:
• Medical consultation may be required to assess disease control.
Teach Patient/Family to:
• Encourage effective oral hygiene to prevent soft tissue inflammation.
• When used for dental infection, advise patient to:
  • Report sore throat, oral burning sensation, fever, and fatigue, any of which could indicate superinfection.
  • Take at prescribed intervals and complete dosage regimen.
  • Immediately notify the dentist if signs or symptoms of infection increase.

cefdinir

sef'-di-neer

(Omnicef)

CATEGORY AND SCHEDULE

Pregnancy Risk Category: B

Drug Class: Cephalosporin (third generation)

MECHANISM OF ACTION

A third-generation cephalosporin that binds to bacterial cell membranes and inhibits cell wall synthesis.

Therapeutic Effect: Bactericidal.

USES

Community-acquired pneumonia, acute exacerbations of chronic bronchitis, acute maxillary sinusitis, pharyngitis/tonsillitis

PHARMACOKINETICS

Moderately absorbed from the GI tract. Protein binding: 60%–70%. Widely distributed. Not appreciably metabolized. Primarily excreted unchanged in urine. Minimally removed by hemodialysis. ***Half-life:*** 1–2 hr (increased in impaired renal function).

INDICATIONS AND DOSAGES

▸ **Community-Acquired Pneumonia**

PO

Adults, Elderly, Children 13 yr and older. 300 mg q12h for 10 days.

▸ **Acute Exacerbation of Chronic Bronchitis**

PO

Adults, Elderly. 300 mg q12h for 5–10 days.

▸ **Acute Maxillary Sinusitis**

PO

Adults, Elderly, Children 13 yr and older. 300 mg q12h or 600 mg q24h for 10 days.

Children 6 mo–12 yr. 7 mg/kg q12h or 14 mg/kg q24h for 10 days.

▸ **Pharyngitis or Tonsillitis**

PO

Adults, Elderly, Children 13 yr and older. 300 mg q12h for 5–10 days or 600 mg q24h for 10 days.

Children 6 mo–12 yr. 7 mg/kg q12h for 5–10 days or 14 mg/kg q24h for 10 days.

▸ **Uncomplicated Skin or Skin-Structure Infections**

PO

Adults, Elderly, Children 13 yr and older. 300 mg q12h for 10 days.

Children 6 mo–12 yr. 7 mg/kg q12h for 10 days.

▸ **Acute Bacterial Otitis Media**

PO (Capsules)

Children 6 mo–12 yr. 7 mg/kg q12h or 14 mg/kg q24h for 10 days.

▸ **Usual Pediatric Dosage for Oral Suspension**

Children weighing 81–95 lb (37–43 kg). 12.5 ml (2.5 tsp) q12h or 25 ml (5 tsp) q24h.

Children weighing 61–80 lb (28–36 kg). 10 ml (2 tsp) q12h or 20 ml (4 tsp) q24h.

Children weighing 41–60 lb (19–27 kg). 7.5 ml (1 tsp) q12h or 15 ml (3 tsp) q24h.

Children weighing 20–40 lb (9–18 kg). 5 ml (1 tsp) q12h or 10 ml (2 tsp) q24h.

Infants weighing less than 20 lb (9 kg). 2.5 ml (1/2 tsp) q12h or 5 ml (1 tsp) q24h.

▸ **Dosage in Renal Impairment**

For patients with creatinine clearance less than 30 ml/min, dosage is 300 mg/day as single daily dose. For hemodialysis patients, dosage is 300 mg or 7 mg/kg/dose every other day.

SIDE EFFECTS/ADVERSE REACTIONS

Frequent

Oral candidiasis, mild diarrhea, mild abdominal cramping, vaginal candidiasis

Occasional

Nausea, serum sickness-like reaction (marked by fever and joint pain; usually occurs after the second course of therapy and resolves after the drug is discontinued)

Rare

Allergic reaction (rash, pruritus, urticaria)

PRECAUTIONS AND CONTRAINDICATIONS

History of anaphylactic reaction to penicillins or hypersensitivity to cephalosporins

Caution:

Hypersensitivity to other cephalosporins, penicillins, or penicillamine; renal impairment (need dose reduction); ulcerative colitis, pseudomembranous colitis, bleeding disorders, renal impairment, hemodialysis, β-lactamase-resistant organisms, not detected in breast milk, children younger than 6 mo

DRUG INTERACTIONS OF CONCERN TO DENTISTRY

- Absorption retarded by iron salts, magnesium, or aluminum antacids: take antiinfective dose at least 2 hr before antacids or iron preparations
- Increased plasma levels: probenecid

SERIOUS REACTIONS

! Antibiotic-associated colitis and other superinfections may result from altered bacterial balance.

! Nephrotoxicity may occur, especially in patients with preexisting renal disease.

! Patients with a history of allergies, especially to penicillin, are at increased risk for developing a severe hypersensitivity reaction, marked by severe pruritus, angioedema, bronchospasm, and anaphylaxis.

DENTAL CONSIDERATIONS

General:

- Use precaution regarding allergy to medication.
- Determine why patient is taking the drug.
- Examine for oral manifestation of opportunistic infection.

Consultations:

- Medical consultation may be required to assess disease control.

Teach Patient/Family to:

- Encourage effective oral hygiene to prevent soft tissue inflammation.

cefditoren pivoxil

seff-di-**tore**′-en

(Spectracef)

CATEGORY AND SCHEDULE

Pregnancy Risk Category: B

Drug Class: Cephalosporin, third generation

MECHANISM OF ACTION

A third-generation cephalosporin that binds to bacterial cell membranes and inhibits cell wall synthesis.

Therapeutic Effect: Bactericidal.

USES

Treatment of mild-to-moderate infections in adults and children older than 12 yr; for susceptible microorganisms causing (1) acute bacterial exacerbation of chronic bronchitis (*H. influenzae, H. parainfluenzae, S. pneumoniae* (penicillin susceptible only), or *M. catarrhalis*); (2) pharyngitis/tonsillitis (*S. pyogenes*); (3) uncomplicated skin and skin-structure infections (*S. aureus* and *S. pyogenes*)

PHARMACOKINETICS

Moderately absorbed from the GI tract. Protein binding: 88%. Not metabolized. Excreted in the urine. Minimally removed by hemodialysis. ***Half-life:*** 1.6 hr (half-life increased with impaired renal function).

INDICATIONS AND DOSAGES

▸ Pharyngitis, Tonsillitis, Skin Infections

PO

Adults, Elderly, Children older than 12 yr: 200 mg twice a day for 10 days.

▸ Acute Exacerbation of Chronic Bronchitis

PO

Adults, Elderly, Children older than 12 yr: 400 mg twice a day for 10 days.

▸ Community-Acquired Pneumonia

PO

Adults, Elderly, Children older than 12 yr: 400 mg 2 twice a day for 14 days.

▸ Dosage in Renal Impairment

Dosage and frequency are modified on the basis of creatinine clearance.

Creatinine Clearance	Dosage Interval
50–80 ml/min	No adjustment necessary
30–49 ml/min	200 mg twice a day
Less than 30 ml/min	200 mg twice a day

SIDE EFFECTS/ADVERSE REACTIONS

Occasional

Diarrhea

Rare

Nausea, headache, abdominal pain, vaginal candidiasis, dyspepsia, vomiting

PRECAUTIONS AND CONTRAINDICATIONS

Carnitine deficiency, inborn errors of metabolism, known allergy to cephalosporins, hypersensitivity to milk protein

Caution:

Penicillin-allergic patients, diarrhea, not for prolonged treatment, risk of resistance emergence, alteration of normal GI flora, decrease in prothrombin activity (long-term use, renal or hepatic impairment, taking anticoagulants), take with meals, lactation, safety and efficiency has not been established in children younger than 12 yr, elderly patients with impaired renal function, reduce dose in severe renal impairment

DRUG INTERACTIONS OF CONCERN TO DENTISTRY

- Reduced absorption: concurrent use with antacids, H2-receptor antagonist
- Increased and prolonged serum levels: probenecid

SERIOUS REACTIONS

! Antibiotic-associated colitis and other superinfections may occur.

! Patients with a history of allergies, especially to penicillin, are at increased risk for developing a severe hypersensitivity reaction, marked by severe pruritus, angioedema, bronchospasm, and anaphylaxis.

DENTAL CONSIDERATIONS

General:

- Caution regarding allergy to medication.
- Assess salivary flow as a factor in caries, periodontal disease, and candidiasis.
- Determine why patient is taking the drug.
- Consider semisupine chair position for patient comfort if GI side effects occur.
- Consult with patient's physician if an acute dental infection occurs and another antiinfective is required.
- Examine for oral manifestation of opportunistic infection.
- Patients on chronic drug therapy may rarely have symptoms of blood dyscrasias, which can include infection, bleeding, and poor healing.

Consultations:

- Medical consultation may be required to assess disease control.
- In a patient with symptoms of blood dyscrasias, request a medical consultation for blood studies and postpone treatment until normal values are reestablished.

Teach Patient/Family to:

- Encourage effective oral hygiene to prevent soft tissue inflammation and infection.
- When chronic dry mouth occurs, advise patient to:
  - Avoid mouth rinses with high alcohol content because of drying effects.
  - Use daily home fluoride products for anticaries effect.
  - Use sugarless gum, frequent sips of water, or saliva substitutes.

cefepime

sef′-eh-peem

(Maxipime)

Do not confuse cefepime with ceftidine.

CATEGORY AND SCHEDULE

Pregnancy Risk Category: B

Drug Class: Cephalosporin (fourth generation)

MECHANISM OF ACTION

A fourth-generation cephalosporin that binds to bacterial cell membranes and inhibits cell wall synthesis.

Therapeutic Effect: Bactericidal.

USES

Treatment of UTIs (uncomplicated and complicated), uncomplicated skin and soft tissue infections, complicated intraabdominal infections (in combination with metronidazole), and pneumonia caused by susceptible strains of microorganisms, including *S. pneumoniae*; febrile neutropenia

PHARMACOKINETICS

Well absorbed after IM administration. Protein binding: 20%. Widely distributed. Primarily excreted unchanged in urine. Removed by hemodialysis.

Half-life: 2–2.3 hr (increased in impaired renal function, and in the elderly).

INDICATIONS AND DOSAGES

▸ **Pneumonia**

IV

Adults, Elderly. 1–2 g q12h for 7–10 days.

Children 2 mo and older. 50 mg/kg q12h. Maximum: 2 g/dose.

▸ **Intraabdominal Infections**

IV

Adults, Elderly. 2 g q12h for 10 days.

▸ **Skin and Skin-Structure Infections**

IV

Adults, Elderly. 2 g q12h for 10 days.

Children 2 mo and older. 50 mg/kg q12h. Maximum: 2 g/dose.

▸ **UTIs**

IV

Adults, Elderly. 0.5–2 g q12h for 7–10 days.

Children 2 mo and older. 50 mg/kg q12h. Maximum: 2 g/dose.

▸ **Febrile Neutropenia**

IV

Adults, Elderly. 2 g q8h.

Children 2 mo and older. 50 mg/kg q8h. Maximum: 2 g/dose.

▸ **Dosage in Renal Impairment**

Dosage and frequency are modified on the basis of creatinine clearance and the severity of the infection.

Creatinine Clearance	Dosage
30–60 ml/min	0.5–2 g q24h
11–29 ml/min	0.5–1 g q24h
10 ml/min or less	0.25–0.5 g q24h

SIDE EFFECTS/ADVERSE REACTIONS

Frequent

Discomfort with IM administration, oral candidiasis, mild diarrhea, mild abdominal cramping, vaginal candidiasis

Occasional

Nausea, serum sickness-like reaction (marked by fever and joint pain; usually occurs after the second course of therapy and resolves after the drug is discontinued)

Rare

Allergic reaction (rash, pruritus, urticaria), thrombophlebitis (pain, redness, swelling at injection site)

PRECAUTIONS AND CONTRAINDICATIONS

History of anaphylactic reaction to penicillins or hypersensitivity to cephalosporins

Caution:

Renal impairment, overgrowth of resistant organisms, colitis, monitor prothrombin, lactation, children younger than 12 yr; renal insufficiency patient at risk for encephalopathy, myoclonus, seizures, renal failure

DRUG INTERACTIONS OF CONCERN TO DENTISTRY

• Increased risk of nephrotoxicity, ototoxicity: aminoglycosides in high doses, furosemide

SERIOUS REACTIONS

! Antibiotic-associated colitis manifested and other superinfections may result from altered bacterial balance.

! Nephrotoxicity may occur, especially in patients with preexisting renal disease.

! Patients with a history of allergies, especially to penicillin, are at increased risk for developing a severe hypersensitivity reaction, marked by severe pruritus, angioedema, bronchospasm, and anaphylaxis.

C

DENTAL CONSIDERATIONS

General:

• Precaution regarding allergy to medication.

• Determine why patient is taking the drug.

Consultation:

• Medical consultation may be required to assess disease control.

Teach Patient/Family to:

• Encourage effective oral hygiene to prevent soft tissue inflammation.

• Report sore throat, oral burning sensation, fever, and fatigue, any of which could indicate presence of a superinfection.

cefixime

sef-**ix**′-zeem

(Suprax)

Do not confuse Suprax with Sporanox, Surbex, or Surfak.

CATEGORY AND SCHEDULE

Pregnancy Risk Category: B

Drug Class: Cephalosporin (third generation)

MECHANISM OF ACTION

A third-generation cephalosporin that binds to bacterial cell membranes and inhibits cell wall synthesis.

Therapeutic Effect: Bactericidal.

USES

Treatment of uncomplicated UTI (*E. coli, P. mirabilis*), pharyngitis and tonsillitis (*S. pyogenes*), otitis media (*H. influenzae, M. catarrhalis*), acute bronchitis, and acute exacerbations of chronic bronchitis (*S. pneumoniae, H. influenzae*)

PHARMACOKINETICS

Moderately absorbed from the GI tract. Protein binding: 65%–70%. Widely distributed. Primarily excreted unchanged in urine. Minimally removed by hemodialysis.

Half-life: 3–4 hr (increased in renal impairment).

INDICATIONS AND DOSAGES

▸ Otitis Media, Acute Bronchitis, Acute Exacerbations of Chronic Bronchitis, Pharyngitis, Tonsillitis, and Uncomplicated UTIs

PO

Adults, Elderly, Children weighing more than 50 kg. 400 mg/day as a single dose or in 2 divided doses.

Children 6 mo–12 yr weighing less than 50 kg. 8 mg/kg/day as a single dose or in 2 divided doses.

Maximum: 400 mg.

▸ Uncomplicated Gonorrhea

PO

Adults. 400 mg as a single dose.

▸ Dosage in Renal Impairment

Dosage is modified on the basis of creatinine clearance.

Creatinine Clearance	% of Usual Dose
21–60 ml/min	75%
20 ml/min or less	50%

SIDE EFFECTS/ADVERSE REACTIONS

Frequent

Oral candidiasis, mild diarrhea, mild abdominal cramping, vaginal candidiasis

Occasional

Nausea, serum sickness-like reaction (marked by arthralgia and fever; usually occurs after second course of therapy and resolves after drug is discontinued)

Rare

Allergic reaction (rash, pruritus, urticaria)

PRECAUTIONS AND CONTRAINDICATIONS

History of anaphylactic reaction to penicillins, hypersensitivity to cephalosporins.
Caution:
Hypersensitivity to penicillins, lactation, renal disease

DRUG INTERACTIONS OF CONCERN TO DENTISTRY

• Decreased antibacterial effects: tetracyclines, erythromycins
• Increased and prolonged serum levels: probenecid

SERIOUS REACTIONS

! Antibiotic-associated colitis and other superinfections may result from altered bacterial balance.
! Nephrotoxicity may occur, especially in patients with preexisting renal disease.
! Patients with a history of allergies, especially to penicillin, are at increased risk for developing a severe hypersensitivity reaction, marked by severe pruritus, angioedema, bronchospasm, and anaphylaxis.

DENTAL CONSIDERATIONS

General:
• Take precautions regarding allergy to medication.
• Determine why the patient is taking the drug.
Consultations:
• Medical consultation may be required to assess disease control.
Teach Patient/Family to:
• Encourage effective oral hygiene to prevent soft tissue inflammation.
• Avoid mouth rinses with high alcohol content because of drying effects and possible drug-drug reaction.
• When used for dental infection, advise patient to:
  • Report sore throat, oral burning sensation, fever, and fatigue, any of which could indicate superinfection.
  • Take at prescribed intervals and complete dosage regimen.
  • Immediately notify the dentist if signs or symptoms of infection increase.

cefonicid sodium

sef-on-**ih′**-sid
(Monocid)
Do not confuse with cefoxitin.

CATEGORY AND SCHEDULE

Pregnancy Risk Category: B

Drug Class: Antibacterial, systemic

MECHANISM OF ACTION

A second-generation cephalosporin that binds to bacterial cell membranes and inhibits cell wall synthesis.
Therapeutic Effect: Bactericidal.

USES

Treatment of infections caused by bacteria

PHARMACOKINETICS

Protein binding: greater than 90%. Widely distributed. Not metabolized. Primarily excreted unchanged in urine. Not removed by hemodialysis. ***Half-life:*** 4.5 hr.

INDICATIONS AND DOSAGES

▸ **UTIs**
IV, IM
Adults, Elderly. 0.5 g q24h.

C

▸ Mild to Moderate Infections
IV, IM
Adults, Elderly. 1 g q24h.
▸ Severe or Life-Threatening Infections
IV, IM
Adults, Elderly. 2 g q24h.
▸ Surgical Prophylaxis
IV
Adults, Elderly. 1 g 60 min before surgery.
▸ Dosage in Renal Impairment
Dosage and frequency are modified on the basis of creatinine clearance and the severity of infection.

Creatinine Clearance	Dosage (mild to moderate infections)
60–79 ml/min	10 mg/kg q24h
59–40 ml/min	8 mg/kg q24h
39–20 ml/min	4 mg/kg q24h
19–10 ml/min	4 mg/kg q48h
9–5 ml/min	4 mg/kg q3–5days
Less than 5 ml/min	3 mg/kg q3–5days

SIDE EFFECTS/ADVERSE REACTIONS

Frequent
Discomfort with IM administration, oral candidiasis, mild diarrhea, mild abdominal cramping, vaginal candidiasis
Occasional
Nausea, unusual bleeding or bruising, serum sickness-like reaction (marked by fever and joint pain)
Rare
Allergic reaction (rash, pruritus, urticaria), thrombophlebitis (pain, redness, swelling at injection site)

PRECAUTIONS AND CONTRAINDICATIONS

History of anaphylactic reaction to penicillins or hypersensitivity to cephalosporins

DRUG INTERACTIONS OF CONCERN TO DENTISTRY

• Increased or prolonged plasma levels: probenecid

SERIOUS REACTIONS

! Antibiotic-associated colitis and other superinfections may result from altered bacterial balance.
! Nephrotoxicity may occur, especially in patients with preexisting renal disease.
! Patients with a history of allergies, especially to penicillin, are at an increased risk for developing a severe hypersensitivity reaction, marked by severe pruritus, angioedema, bronchospasm, and anaphylaxis.

DENTAL CONSIDERATIONS

General:
• For selected infections in the hospital setting; provide palliative emergency dental care only.
• Use with caution in patients with a history of antibiotic-associated colitis.
• Determine why patient is taking the drug.
• Examine for oral manifestation of opportunistic infection.
• Caution regarding allergy to medication.
Consultations:
• Medical consultation may be required to assess disease control and patient's ability to tolerate stress.
Teach Patient/Family to:
• Encourage effective oral hygiene to prevent soft tissue inflammation.
• Report sore throat, oral burning sensation, fever, or fatigue, any of which could indicate presence of a superinfection.

cefoperazone

sef-oh-**per′**-ah-zone
(Cefobid)
Do not confuse with Ceftin, cefotetan, and cefamandole.

CATEGORY AND SCHEDULE

Pregnancy Risk Category: B

Drug Class: Antibacterial, systemic

MECHANISM OF ACTION

A third-generation cephalosporin that binds to bacterial cell membranes.
Therapeutic Effect: Inhibits synthesis of bacterial cell wall. Bactericidal.

USES

Treatment of infections caused by bacteria

PHARMACOKINETICS

Widely distributed, including CSF. Protein binding: 82%–93%. Metabolized and excreted in kidney and urine. Removed by hemodialysis. ***Half-life:*** 1.6–2.4 hr (half-life is increased with impaired renal function).

INDICATIONS AND DOSAGES

▸ Mild to Moderate Infections

IM/IV

Adults, Elderly. 2–4 g/day in 2 divided doses q12h.

▸ Severe or Life-Threatening Infections

IM/IV

Adults, Elderly. Total daily dose and/or frequency may be increased to 6–12 g/day divided into 2, 3, or 4 equal doses of 1.5–4 g per dose.

▸ Dosage in Renal and/or Hepatic Impairment

Do not exceed 4 g/day in those with liver disease and/or biliary obstruction. Modification of dose usually not necessary in those with renal impairment. Dose should not exceed 1–2 g/day in those with both hepatic and substantial renal impairment.

SIDE EFFECTS/ADVERSE REACTIONS

Frequent

Discomfort with IM administration, oral candidiasis, mild diarrhea, mild abdominal cramping, vaginal candidiasis

Occasional

Nausea, unusual bruising/bleeding, serum sickness reaction

Rare

Allergic reaction, rash, pruritus, urticaria, thrombophlebitis (pain, redness, swelling at injection site)

PRECAUTIONS AND CONTRAINDICATIONS

Anaphylactic reaction to penicillins, history of hypersensitivity to cephalosporins or any one of its components

DRUG INTERACTIONS OF CONCERN TO DENTISTRY

- Avoid alcohol, risk of disulfiram-like reaction.
- Increased risk of bleeding: drugs that interfere with platelet action.

SERIOUS REACTIONS

! Antibiotic-associated colitis manifested as severe abdominal pain and tenderness, fever, and watery and severe diarrhea, and other superinfections may result from altered bacterial balance.

C

! Nephrotoxicity may occur, especially in patients with preexisting renal disease. Severe hypersensitivity reaction including severe pruritus, angioedema, bronchospasm, and anaphylaxis, particularly in patients with a history of allergies, especially to penicillins, may occur.

DENTAL CONSIDERATIONS

General:

- For selected infections in the hospital setting; provide palliative emergency dental treatment only.
- Use with caution in patients with a history of antibiotic-associated colitis.
- May interfere with prothrombin levels.
- Examine for oral manifestation of opportunistic infection.
- Determine why patient is taking the drug.
- Caution regarding allergy to medication.

Consultations:

- Medical consultation may be required to assess disease control and patient's ability to tolerate stress.
- Medical consultation should include INR.

Teach Patient/Family to:

- Encourage effective oral hygiene to prevent soft tissue inflammation.
- Report sore throat, oral burning sensation, fever, or fatigue, any of which could indicate presence of a superinfection.

cefotaxime sodium

sef-oh-**taks**′-eem **so**′-dee-um
(Claforan)
Do not confuse cefotaxime with cefoxitin, ceftizoxime, or cefuroxime, or Claforan with Claritin.

CATEGORY AND SCHEDULE

Pregnancy Risk Category: B

Drug Class: Antibacterial, systemic

MECHANISM OF ACTION

A third-generation cephalosporin that binds to bacterial cell membranes and inhibits cell wall synthesis.
Therapeutic Effect: Bactericidal.

USES

Treatment of infections caused by bacteria

PHARMACOKINETICS

Widely distributed, including to CSF. Protein binding: 30%–50%. Partially metabolized in the liver to active metabolite. Primarily excreted in urine. Moderately removed by hemodialysis. ***Half-life:*** 1 hr (increased in impaired renal function).

INDICATIONS AND DOSAGES

▸ **Uncomplicated Infections**
IV, IM
Adults, Elderly. 1 g q12h.

▸ **Mild to Moderate Infections**
IV, IM
Adults, Elderly. 1–2 g q8h.

▸ **Severe Infections**
IV, IM
Adults, Elderly. 2 g q6–8h.

▸ Life-Threatening Infections
IV, IM
Adults, Elderly. 2 g q4h.
Children. 2 g q4h. Maximum: 12 g/day.

▸ Gonorrhea
IM
Adults (Male). 1 g as a single dose.
Adults (Female). 0.5 g as a single dose.

▸ Perioperative Prophylaxis
IV, IM
Adults, Elderly. 1 g 30–90 min before surgery.

▸ Cesarean Section
IV
Adults. 1 g as soon as umbilical cord is clamped, then 1 g 6 and 12 hr after first dose.

▸ Usual Pediatric Dosage
Children weighing 50 kg or more. 1–2 g q6–8h.
Children 1 mo–12 yr weighing less than 50 kg. 100–200 mg/kg/day in divided doses q6–8h.

▸ Dosage in Renal Impairment
For patients with creatinine clearance less than 20 ml/min give half of dose at usual dosing intervals.

SIDE EFFECTS/ADVERSE REACTIONS

Frequent
Discomfort with IM administration, oral candidiasis, mild diarrhea, mild abdominal cramping, vaginal candidiasis

Occasional
Nausea, serum sickness-like reaction (marked by fever and joint pain; usually occurs after the second course of therapy and resolves after the drug is discontinued)

Rare
Allergic reaction (rash, pruritus, urticaria), thrombophlebitis (pain, redness, swelling at injection site)

PRECAUTIONS AND CONTRAINDICATIONS

History of anaphylactic reaction to penicillins or hypersensitivity to cephalosporins

DRUG INTERACTIONS OF CONCERN TO DENTISTRY

• Increased or prolonged plasma levels: probenecid

SERIOUS REACTIONS

! Antibiotic-associated colitis and other superinfections may result from altered bacterial balance.
! Nephrotoxicity may occur, especially in patients with preexisting renal disease.
! Patients with a history of allergies, especially to penicillin, are at increased risk for developing a severe hypersensitivity reaction, marked by severe pruritus, angioedema, bronchospasm, and anaphylaxis.

DENTAL CONSIDERATIONS

General:
• For selected infections in the hospital setting; provide palliative emergency dental treatment only.
• Use caution in patients with a history of antibiotic-associated colitis.
• Examine for oral manifestation of opportunistic infection.
• Determine why patient is taking the drug.
• Caution regarding allergy to medication.

Consultations:
• Medical consultation may be required to assess disease control and patient's ability to tolerate stress.

C

Teach Patient/Family to:
• Encourage effective oral hygiene to prevent soft tissue inflammation.
• Report sore throat, oral burning sensation, fever, or fatigue, any of which could indicate presence of a superinfection.

cefotetan disodium

sef′-oh-tee-tan die-**so′**-dee-um
(Apatef[AUS], Cefotan)
Do not confuse cefotetan with cefoxitin or Ceftin.

CATEGORY AND SCHEDULE

Pregnancy Risk Category: B

Drug Class: Antibacterial, systemic

MECHANISM OF ACTION

A second-generation cephalosporin that binds to bacterial cell membranes and inhibits cell wall synthesis.
Therapeutic Effect: Bactericidal.

USES

Treatment of infections caused by bacteria

PHARMACOKINETICS

Protein binding: 78%–91%. Primarily excreted unchanged in urine. Minimally removed by hemodialysis. ***Half-life:*** 3–4.6 hr (increased in impaired renal function).

INDICATIONS AND DOSAGES

▸ **UTIs**
IV, IM
Adults, Elderly. 1–2 g in divided doses q12–24h.

▸ **Mild to Moderate Infections**
IV, IM
Adults, Elderly. 1–2 g q12h.

▸ **Severe Infections**
IV, IM
Adults, Elderly. 2 g q12h.

▸ **Life-Threatening Infections**
IV, IM
Adults, Elderly. 3 g q12h.

▸ **Perioperative Prophylaxis**
IV
Adults, Elderly. 1–2 g 30–60 min before surgery.

▸ **Cesarean Section**
IV
Adults. 1–2 g as soon as umbilical cord is clamped.

▸ **Usual Pediatric Dosage**
Children. 40–80 mg/kg/day in divided doses q12h. Maximum: 6 g/day.

▸ **Dosage in Renal Impairment**
Dosing frequency is modified on the basis of creatinine clearance and the severity of the infection.

Creatinine Clearance	Dosage Interval
10–30 ml/min	Usual dose q24h
Less than 10 ml/min	Usual dose q48h

SIDE EFFECTS/ADVERSE REACTIONS

Frequent
Discomfort with IM administration, oral candidiasis, mild diarrhea, mild abdominal cramping, vaginal candidiasis
Occasional
Nausea, unusual bleeding or bruising, serum sickness-like reaction (marked by fever and joint pain; usually occurs after the second course of therapy and resolves after the drug is discontinued)

Rare
Allergic reaction (rash, pruritus, urticaria), thrombophlebitis (pain, redness, swelling at injection site)

PRECAUTIONS AND CONTRAINDICATIONS
History of anaphylactic reaction to penicillins or hypersensitivity to cephalosporins

DRUG INTERACTIONS OF CONCERN TO DENTISTRY
- Avoid alcohol, risk of disulfiram-like reaction
- Increased or prolonged plasma levels: probenecid
- Increased risk of bleeding: drugs that interfere with platelet action

SERIOUS REACTIONS
! Antibiotic-associated colitis and other superinfections may result from altered bacterial balance.
! Nephrotoxicity may occur, especially in patients with preexisting renal disease.
! Patients with a history of allergies, especially to penicillin, are at increased risk for developing a severe hypersensitivity reaction, marked by severe pruritus, angioedema, bronchospasm, and anaphylaxis.

DENTAL CONSIDERATIONS
General:
- For selected infections in the hospital setting; provide palliative emergency dental treatment only.
- Use with caution in patients with a history of antibiotic-associated colitis.
- May interfere with prothrombin levels.
- Examine for oral manifestation of opportunistic infection.
- Determine why patient is taking the drug.
- Caution regarding allergy to medication.

Consultations:
- Medical consultation may be required to assess disease control and patient's ability to tolerate stress.
- Medical consultation should include INR.

Teach Patient/Family to:
- Encourage effective oral hygiene to prevent soft tissue inflammation.
- Report sore throat, oral burning sensation, fever, or fatigue, any of which could indicate presence of a superinfection.

cefoxitin sodium
se-**fox**′-ih-tin **so**′-dee-um
(Mefoxin)
Do not confuse cefoxitin with cefotaxime, cefotetan, or Cytoxan.

CATEGORY AND SCHEDULE
Pregnancy Risk Category: B

Drug Class: Antibacterial, systemic

MECHANISM OF ACTION
A second-generation cephalosporin that binds to bacterial cell membranes and inhibits cell wall synthesis.
Therapeutic Effect: Bactericidal.

USES
Treatment of infections caused by bacteria

PHARMACOKINETICS

Peak levels reached within 5 min following IV infusion. ***Half-life:*** 45 m–1 hr; 85% excreted unchanged in urine.

INDICATIONS AND DOSAGES

▸ **Mild to Moderate Infections**
IV, IM
Adults, Elderly. 1–2 g q6–8h.

▸ **Severe Infections**
IV, IM
Adults, Elderly. 1 g q4h or 2 g q6–8h up to 2 g q4h.

▸ **Uncomplicated Gonorrhea**
IM
Adults. 2 g one time with 1 g probenecid.

▸ **Perioperative Prophylaxis**
IV, IM
Adults, Elderly. 2 g 30–60 min before surgery, then q6h for up to 24 hr after surgery.
Children older than 3 mo. 30–40 mg/kg 30–60 min before surgery, then q6h for up to 24 hr after surgery.

▸ **Cesarean Section**
IV
Adults. 2 g as soon as umbilical cord is clamped, then 2 g 4 and 8 hr after first dose, then q6h for up to 24 hr.

▸ **Usual Pediatric Dosage**
Children older than 3 mo. 80–160 mg/kg/day in 4–6 divided doses. Maximum: 12 g/day.
Neonates. 90–100 mg/kg/day in divided doses q6–8h.

▸ **Dosage in Renal Impairment**
After a loading dose of 1–2 g, dosage and frequency are modified on the basis of creatinine clearance and the severity of the infection.

Creatinine Clearance	Dosage
30–50 ml/min	1–2 g q8–12h
10–29 ml/min	1–2 g q12–24h
5–9 ml/min	500 mg–1 g q12–24h
Less than 5 ml/min	500 mg–1 g q24–48h

SIDE EFFECTS/ADVERSE REACTIONS

Frequent
Discomfort with IM administration, oral candidiasis, mild diarrhea, mild abdominal cramping, vaginal candidiasis

Occasional
Nausea, serum sickness-like reaction (marked by fever and joint pain; usually occurs after the second course of therapy and resolves after the drug is discontinued)

Rare
Allergic reaction (pruritus, rash, urticaria), thrombophlebitis (pain, redness, swelling at injection site)

PRECAUTIONS AND CONTRAINDICATIONS

History of anaphylactic reaction to penicillins or hypersensitivity to cephalosporins

DRUG INTERACTIONS OF CONCERN TO DENTISTRY

• Increased or prolonged plasma levels: probenecid

SERIOUS REACTIONS

! Antibiotic-associated colitis and other superinfections may result from altered bacterial balance.
! Nephrotoxicity may occur, especially in patients with preexisting renal disease.
! Patients with a history of allergies, especially to penicillin, are at increased risk for developing a severe hypersensitivity reaction, marked by severe pruritus,

angioedema, bronchospasm, and anaphylaxis.

DENTAL CONSIDERATIONS

General:

- For selected infections in the hospital setting; provide palliative emergency dental treatment only.
- Use with caution in patients with a history of antibiotic-associated colitis.
- Examine for oral manifestation of opportunistic infection.
- Determine why patient is taking the drug.
- Caution regarding allergy to medication.

Consultations:

- Consult patient's physician if an acute dental infection occurs and another antiinfective is required.
- Medical consultation may be required to assess disease control and patient's ability to tolerate stress.

Teach Patient/Family to:

- Encourage effective oral hygiene to prevent soft tissue inflammation.
- Report sore throat, oral burning sensation, fever, or fatigue, any of which could indicate presence of a superinfection.

cefpodoxime proxetil

sef-poe-**dox′**-ime **prox′**-eh-til
(Vantin)
Do not confuse Vantin with Ventolin.

CATEGORY AND SCHEDULE

Pregnancy Risk Category: B

Drug Class: Cephalosporin (third generation)

MECHANISM OF ACTION

A third-generation cephalosporin that binds to bacterial cell membranes and inhibits cell wall synthesis.
Therapeutic Effect: Bactericidal.

USES

Treatment of upper and lower respiratory tract infections, pharyngitis (tonsillitis), gonorrhea, UTI, uncomplicated skin and skin structure infections caused by susceptible organisms, acute otitis media, community-acquired pneumonia, acute bacterial exacerbation of chronic bronchitis, anorectal infections in women

PHARMACOKINETICS

Well absorbed from the GI tract (food increases absorption). Protein binding: 21%–40%. Widely distributed. Primarily excreted unchanged in urine. Partially removed by hemodialysis. ***Half-life:*** 2.3 hr (increased in impaired renal function and elderly patients).

INDICATIONS AND DOSAGES

▸ **Chronic Bronchitis, Pneumonia**

PO

Adults, Elderly, Children older than 13 yr. 200 mg q12h for 10–14 days.

▸ **Gonorrhea, Rectal Gonococcal Infection (Female Patients Only)**

PO

Adults, Children older than 13 yr. 200 mg as a single dose.

▸ **Skin and Skin-Structure Infections**

PO

Adults, Elderly, Children older than 13 yr. 400 mg q12h for 7–14 days.

▸ **Pharyngitis, Tonsillitis**

PO

Adults, Elderly, Children older than 13 yr. 100 mg q12h for 5–10 days.

C

Children 6 mo–13 yr. 5 mg/kg q12h for 5–10 days. Maximum: 100 mg/dose.

▸ **Acute Maxillary Sinusitis**

PO

Adults, Children older than 13 yr. 200 mg twice a day for 10 days.

Children 2 mo–13 yr. 5 mg/kg q12h for 10 days. Maximum: 400 mg/day.

▸ **UTIs**

PO

Adults, Elderly, Children older than 13 yr. 100 mg q12h for 7 days.

▸ **Acute Otitis Media**

PO

Children 6 mo–13 yr. 5 mg/kg q12h for 5 days. Maximum: 400 mg/dose.

▸ **Dosage in Renal Impairment**

For patients with creatinine clearance less than 30 ml/min, usual dose is given q24h. For patients on hemodialysis, usual dose is given 3 times a wk after dialysis.

SIDE EFFECTS/ADVERSE REACTIONS

Frequent

Oral candidiasis, mild diarrhea, mild abdominal cramping, vaginal candidiasis

Occasional

Nausea, serum sickness-like reaction (marked by fever and joint pain; usually occurs after the second course of therapy and resolves after the drug is discontinued)

Rare

Allergic reaction (pruritus, rash, urticaria)

PRECAUTIONS AND CONTRAINDICATIONS

History of anaphylactic reaction to penicillins or hypersensitivity to cephalosporins

Caution:

Hypersensitivity to penicillins, lactation, renal disease, safety and efficacy in infants younger than 5 mo not established

DRUG INTERACTIONS OF CONCERN TO DENTISTRY

- Decreased bactericidal effects: tetracyclines, erythromycins
- Increased and prolonged serum levels: probenecid

SERIOUS REACTIONS

! Antibiotic-associated colitis and other superinfections may result from altered bacterial balance.

! Nephrotoxicity may occur, especially in patients with preexisting renal disease.

! Patients with a history of allergies, especially to penicillin, are at increased risk for developing a severe hypersensitivity reaction, marked by severe pruritus, angioedema, bronchospasm, and anaphylaxis.

DENTAL CONSIDERATIONS

General:

- Take precautions regarding allergy to medication.
- Determine why the patient is taking the drug.

Consultations:

- Medical consultation may be required to assess disease control.

Teach Patient/Family to:

- Encourage effective oral hygiene to prevent soft tissue inflammation.
- Avoid mouth rinses with high alcohol content because of drying effects and possible drug-drug reaction.
- When used for dental infection, advise patient to:

• Report sore throat, oral burning sensation, fever, and fatigue, any of which could indicate superinfection.
• Take at prescribed intervals and complete dosage regimen.
• Immediately notify the dentist if signs or symptoms of infection increase.

cefprozil

sef-**pro′**-zil
(Cefzil)
Do not confuse cefprozil with Cefazolin or Cefzil with Cefol, Ceftin or Kefzol.

CATEGORY AND SCHEDULE

Pregnancy Risk Category: B

Drug Class: Cephalosporin (second generation)

MECHANISM OF ACTION

A second-generation cephalosporin that binds to bacterial cell membranes and inhibits cell wall synthesis.
Therapeutic Effect: Bactericidal.

USES

Treatment of pharyngitis/tonsillitis, otitis media, secondary bacterial infection of acute bronchitis, sinusitis; acute bacterial sinusitis; acute bacterial exacerbation of chronic bronchitis and uncomplicated skin and skin structure infections

PHARMACOKINETICS

Well absorbed from the GI tract. Protein binding: 36%–45%. Widely distributed. Primarily excreted unchanged in urine. Moderately removed by hemodialysis. ***Half-life:*** 1.3 hr (increased in impaired renal function).

INDICATIONS AND DOSAGES

▸ **Pharyngitis, Tonsillitis**
PO
Adults, Elderly. 500 mg q24h for 10 days.
Children 2–12 yr. 7.5 mg/kg q12h for 10 days.

▸ **Acute Bacterial Exacerbation of Chronic Bronchitis, Secondary Bacterial Infection of Acute Bronchitis**
PO
Adults, Elderly. 500 mg q12h for 10 days.

▸ **Skin and Skin-Structure Infections**
PO
Adults, Elderly. 250–500 mg q12h for 10 days.
Children. 20 mg/kg q24h for 10 days.

▸ **Acute Sinusitis**
PO
Adults, Elderly. 250–500 mg q12h for 10 days.
Children 6 mo–12 yr. 7.5–15 mg/kg q12h for 10 days.

▸ **Otitis Media**
PO
Children 6 mo–12 yr. 15 mg/kg q12h for 10 days. Maximum: 1 g/day.

▸ **Dosage in Renal Impairment**
Patients with creatinine clearance less than 30 ml/min receive 50% of usual dose at usual interval.

SIDE EFFECTS/ADVERSE REACTIONS

Frequent
Oral candidiasis, mild diarrhea, mild abdominal cramping, vaginal candidiasis

C

Occasional
Nausea, serum sickness reaction (marked by fever and joint pain; usually occurs after the second course of therapy and resolves after the drug is discontinued)
Rare
Allergic reaction (pruritus, rash, urticaria)

PRECAUTIONS AND CONTRAINDICATIONS

History of anaphylactic reaction to penicillins or hypersensitivity to cephalosporins
Caution:
Lactation, elderly, hypersensitivity to penicillins, renal disease

DRUG INTERACTIONS OF CONCERN TO DENTISTRY

- Decreased bactericidal effects: tetracyclines, erythromycins
- Increased and prolonged serum levels: probenecid

SERIOUS REACTIONS

! Antibiotic-associated colitis and other superinfections may result from altered bacterial balance.
! Nephrotoxicity may occur, especially in patients with preexisting renal disease.
! Patients with a history of allergies, especially to penicillin, are at increased risk for developing a severe hypersensitivity reaction, marked by severe pruritus, angioedema, bronchospasm, and anaphylaxis.

DENTAL CONSIDERATIONS

General:
- Take precautions regarding allergy to medication.
- Determine why the patient is taking the drug.
- Examine for evidence of oral manifestations of blood dyscrasia (infection, bleeding, poor healing) and superinfection.

Consultations:
- Medical consultation may be required to assess disease control.

Teach Patient/Family to:
- Encourage effective oral hygiene to prevent soft tissue inflammation.
- When used for dental infection, advise patient to:
  - Report sore throat, oral burning sensation, fever, and fatigue, any of which could indicate superinfection.
  - Take at prescribed intervals and complete dosage regimen.
  - Immediately notify the dentist if signs or symptoms of infection increase.

ceftaroline fosamil

sef-**tar**′-oh-leen **foe**′-seh-mil
(Teflaro)

CATEGORY AND SCHEDULE

Pregnancy Risk Category: B

Drug Class: Fifth-generation cephalosporin; antibiotic

MECHANISM OF ACTION

A fifth-generation cephalosporin that binds to bacterial cell membranes and inhibits cell wall synthesis.
Therapeutic Effect: Bactericidal

USES
Treatment of acute bacterial skin and skin structure infections and community-acquired pneumonia

PHARMACOKINETICS
Peak plasma concentrations reached in 1 hr. 20% plasma protein bound. Ceftaroline fosamil (a prodrug) is converted to bioactive ceftaroline in plasma by phosphatase enzyme, further hydrolyzed to inactive metabolites. Excreted via feces (6%) and urine (88%). ***Half-life:*** 2.4 hr.

INDICATIONS AND DOSAGES
▸ Pneumonia, Community-Acquired
IV infusion
Adults. 600 mg every 12 hr for 5–7 days (as 60-min infusion).

▸ Skin and Skin Structure Infections, Complicated
IV infusion
Adults. 600 mg every 12 hr for 5–14 days (as 60-min infusion).

▸ Dosage in Renal Impairment
For patients with a creatinine clearance of 31–50 ml/min, administer 400 mg every 12 hr. For patients with a creatinine clearance of 15–30 ml/min, administer 300 mg every 12 hr. For patients with a creatinine clearance of less than 15 ml/min, administer 200 mg every 12 hr.

SIDE EFFECTS/ADVERSE REACTIONS
Frequent
Headache, insomnia, rash, hypokalemia, diarrhea, nausea, vomiting, oral and vaginal candidiasis
Occasional
Abdominal pain, anemia, bradycardia, dizziness, eosinophilia, hyperglycemia, hyperkalemia, neutropenia, palpitation, seizures, renal failure, thrombocytopenia, urticaria

PRECAUTIONS AND CONTRAINDICATIONS
Hypersensitivity to ceftaroline, other cephalosporins, or any component of the formulation. Use with caution in patients with a history of penicillin allergy. Use with caution in patients with renal impairment.

DRUG INTERACTIONS OF CONCERN TO DENTISTRY
• Possible interaction with inhibitors of CYP liver enzymes (e.g., macrolide antibiotics, azole antifungals) or inducers of CYP liver enzymes (e.g., barbiturates)
• Antibiotics: potential reduction of efficacy of ceftaroline by coadministered antibiotics

SERIOUS REACTIONS
! Antibiotic-associated colitis and other superinfections may result from altered bacterial balance. Nephrotoxicity may occur, especially in patients with preexisting renal disease. Patients with a history of allergies, especially to penicillin, are at increased risk for developing a severe hypersensitivity reaction, marked by severe pruritus, angioedema, bronchospasm, and anaphylaxis.

DENTAL CONSIDERATIONS
General:
• Diarrhea associated with ceftaroline can progress to pseudomembranous colitis if unrecognized and untreated.
• Nausea produced by ceftaroline may be worsened by opioid analgesics, NSAIDs.
• Health care personnel treating patients taking ceftaroline may be at risk for exposure to pneumonia.

C

C

ceftazidime

sef-**taz'**-ih-deem

(Ceptaz, Fortaz, Fortum[AUS], Tazicef, Tazidime)

Do not confuse ceftazidime with ceftizoxime.

CATEGORY AND SCHEDULE

Pregnancy Risk Category: B

Drug Class: Third-generation cephalosporin; antibiotic

MECHANISM OF ACTION

A third-generation cephalosporin that binds to bacterial cell membranes and inhibits cell wall synthesis.

Therapeutic Effect: Bactericidal.

USES

Treatment of intraabdominal, biliary tract, respiratory tract, GU tract, skin, bone infections; meningitis; septicemia

PHARMACOKINETICS

Widely distributed (including to CSF). Protein binding: 5%–17%. Primarily excreted unchanged in urine. Removed by hemodialysis. ***Half-life:*** 2 hr (increased in impaired renal function).

INDICATIONS AND DOSAGES

▸ **UTIs**

IV, IM

Adults. 250–500 mg q8–12h.

▸ **Mild-to-Moderate Infections**

IV, IM

Adults. 1 g q8–12h.

▸ **Uncomplicated Pneumonia, Skin and Skin-Structure Infections**

IV, IM

Adults. 0.5–1 g q8h.

▸ **Bone and Joint Infections**

IV, IM

Adults. 2 g q12h.

▸ **Meningitis, Serious Gynecologic and Intraabdominal Infections**

IV, IM

Adults. 2 g q8h.

▸ **Pseudomonal Pulmonary Infections in Patients with Cystic Fibrosis**

IV

Adults. 30–50 mg/kg q8h. Maximum: 6 g/day.

▸ **Usual Elderly Dosage**

Elderly (normal renal function). 500 mg–1 g q12h.

▸ **Usual Pediatric Dosage**

Children 1 mo–12 yr. 100–150 mg/kg/day in divided doses q8h. Maximum: 6 g/day.

Neonates 0–4 wk. 100–150 mg/kg/day in divided doses q8–12h.

▸ **Dosage in Renal Impairment**

After an initial 1-g dose, dosage and frequency are modified on the basis of creatinine clearance and the severity of the infection.

Creatinine Clearance	Dosage
31–50 ml/min	1 g q12h
16–30 ml/min	1 g q24h
6–15 ml/min	500 mg q24h
Less than 5 ml/min	500 mg q48h

SIDE EFFECTS/ADVERSE REACTIONS

Frequent

Discomfort with IM administration, oral candidiasis, mild diarrhea, mild abdominal cramping, vaginal candidiasis

Occasional

Nausea, serum sickness-like reaction (marked by fever and joint pain; usually occurs after the second course of therapy and resolves after the drug is discontinued)

Rare

Allergic reaction (pruritus, rash, urticaria), thrombophlebitis (pain, redness, swelling at injection site)

PRECAUTIONS AND CONTRAINDICATIONS
History of anaphylactic reaction to penicillins or hypersensitivity to cephalosporins

DRUG INTERACTIONS OF CONCERN TO DENTISTRY
- None reported

SERIOUS REACTIONS
! Antibiotic-associated colitis and other superinfections may result from altered bacterial balance.
! Nephrotoxicity may occur, especially in patients with preexisting renal disease.
! Patients with a history of allergies, especially to penicillin, are at increased risk for developing a severe hypersensitivity reaction, marked by severe pruritus, angioedema, bronchospasm, and anaphylaxis.

DENTAL CONSIDERATIONS
General:
- For selected infections in the hospital setting; provide palliative emergency dental treatment only.
- Use with caution in patients with a history of antibiotic-associated colitis.
- Examine for oral manifestation of opportunistic infection.
- Determine why patient is taking the drug.
- Caution regarding allergy to medication.

Consultations:
- Medical consultation may be required to assess disease control and patient's ability to tolerate stress.

Teach Patient/Family to:
- Encourage effective oral hygiene to prevent soft tissue inflammation.
- Report sore throat, oral burning sensation, fever, or fatigue, any of which could indicate presence of a superinfection.

ceftibuten
cef'-te-bute-in
(Cedax)

CATEGORY AND SCHEDULE
Pregnancy Risk Category: B

Drug Class: Cephalosporin (third generation)

MECHANISM OF ACTION
A third-generation cephalosporin that binds to bacterial cell membranes and inhibits cell wall synthesis.
Therapeutic Effect: Bactericidal.

USES
Treatment of acute exacerbations of chronic bronchitis caused by susceptible strains of *H. influenzae, M. catarrhalis,* or *S. pneumoniae*; acute otitis media caused by susceptible strains of *H. influenzae, M. catarrhalis,* or *S. pyogenes*; pharyngitis and tonsillitis caused by *S. pyogenes*

PHARMACOKINETICS
Rapidly absorbed from the GI tract. Excreted primarily in urine.
Half-life: 2–3 hr.

INDICATIONS AND DOSAGES
▸ Chronic Bronchitis
PO
Adults, Elderly. 400 mg/day once a day for 10 days.

▸ Pharyngitis, Tonsillitis
PO
Adults, Elderly. 400 mg once a day for 10 days.

Children older than 6 mo. 9 mg/kg once a day for 10 days. Maximum: 400 mg/day.

▸ **Otitis Media**

PO

Children older than 6 mo. 9 mg/kg once a day for 10 days. Maximum: 400 mg/day.

▸ **Dosage in Renal Impairment**

Dosage is modified on the basis of creatinine clearance.

Creatinine Clearance	Dosage
50 ml/min and higher	400 mg or 9 mg/kg q24h
30–49 ml/min	200 mg or 4.5 mg/kg q24h
Less than 30 ml/min	100 mg or 2.25 mg/kg q24h

SIDE EFFECTS/ADVERSE REACTIONS

Frequent

Oral candidiasis, mild diarrhea (discharge, itching)

Occasional

Nausea, serum sickness-like reaction (marked by fever and joint pain; usually occurs after the second course of therapy and resolves after the drug is discontinued)

Rare

Allergic reaction (rash, pruritus, urticaria)

PRECAUTIONS AND CONTRAINDICATIONS

History of anaphylactic reaction to penicillins or hypersensitivity to cephalosporins

Caution:

Hypersensitivity to penicillins, renal impairment, lactation, infants younger than 6 mo, pseudomembranous colitis, oral suspension contains 1 g sucrose/5 ml

DRUG INTERACTIONS OF CONCERN TO DENTISTRY

- Decreased bactericidal effects: tetracyclines, erythromycins
- Increased and prolonged serum levels: probenecid
- Aminoglycosides increase nephrotoxic potential

SERIOUS REACTIONS

! Antibiotic-associated colitis and other superinfections may result from altered bacterial balance.

! Nephrotoxicity may occur, especially in patients with preexisting renal disease.

! Patients with a history of allergies, especially to penicillin, are at increased risk for developing a severe hypersensitivity reaction, marked by severe pruritus, angioedema, bronchospasm, and anaphylaxis.

DENTAL CONSIDERATIONS

General:

- Take precautions regarding allergy to medication.
- Assess salivary flow as factor in caries, periodontal disease, and candidiasis.
- Oral suspension contains sucrose; patient should rinse mouth after use.
- Determine why the patient is taking the drug.

Consultations:

- Medical consultation may be required to assess disease control.

Teach Patient/Family to:

- Encourage effective oral hygiene to prevent soft tissue inflammation.
- When used for dental infection, advise patient to:
  - Report sore throat, oral burning sensation, fever, and fatigue, any of which could indicate superinfection.
  - Take at prescribed intervals and complete dosage regimen.

• Immediately notify the dentist if signs or symptoms of infection increase.

ceftizoxime sodium

sef-ti-**zox′**-eem **so′**-dee-um

(Cefizox)

Do not confuse ceftizoxime with cefotaxime or ceftazidime.

CATEGORY AND SCHEDULE

Pregnancy Risk Category: B

Drug Class: Cephalosporin (third-generation)

MECHANISM OF ACTION

A third-generation cephalosporin that binds to bacterial cell membranes and inhibits cell wall synthesis.

Therapeutic Effect: Bactericidal.

USES

Treatment of intraabdominal, biliary tract, respiratory tract, GU tract, skin, bone infections; gonorrhea; meningitis; septicemia; pelvic inflammatory disease (PID)

PHARMACOKINETICS

Widely distributed (including to CSF). Protein binding: 30%. Primarily excreted unchanged in urine. Moderately removed by hemodialysis. ***Half-life:*** 1.7 hr (increased in impaired renal function).

INDICATIONS AND DOSAGES

▸ **Uncomplicated UTIs**

IV, IM

Adults, Elderly. 500 mg q12h.

▸ **Mild, Moderate, or Severe Infections of the Biliary, Respiratory, and GU Tracts; Skin, Bone, and Intraabdominal Infections; Meningitis; and Septicemia**

IV, IM

Adults, Elderly. 1–2 g q8–12h.

▸ **Life-Threatening Infections of the Biliary, Respiratory, and GU Tracts; Skin, Bone and Intraabdominal Infections; Meningitis; and Septicemia**

IV

Adults, Elderly. 3–4 g q8h, up to 2 g q4h.

▸ **PID**

IV

Adults. 2 g q4–8h.

▸ **Uncomplicated Gonorrhea**

IM

Adults. 1 g 1 time.

▸ **Usual Pediatric Dosage**

Children older than 6 mo. 50 mg/kg q6–8h. Maximum: 12 g/day.

▸ **Dosage in Renal Impairment**

After a loading dose of 0.5–1 g, dosage and frequency are modified on the basis of creatinine clearance and the severity of the infection.

Creatinine Clearance	Dosage
50–79 ml/min	0.5 g–1.5 g q8h
5–49 ml/min	0.25 g–1 g q12h
Less than 5 ml/min	0.25–0.5 g q24h or 0.5 g–1 g q48h

SIDE EFFECTS/ADVERSE REACTIONS

Frequent

Discomfort with IM administration, oral candidiasis, mild diarrhea, mild abdominal cramping, vaginal candidiasis

C

Occasional
Nausea, serum sickness-like reaction (fever, joint pain; usually occurs after the second course of therapy and resolves after the drug is discontinued)
Rare
Allergic reaction (rash, pruritus, urticaria), thrombophlebitis (pain, redness, swelling at injection site)

PRECAUTIONS AND CONTRAINDICATIONS

History of anaphylactic reaction to penicillins or hypersensitivity to cephalosporins

DRUG INTERACTIONS OF CONCERN TO DENTISTRY

• Increased or prolonged plasma levels: probenecid

SERIOUS REACTIONS

! Antibiotic-associated colitis manifested and other superinfections may result from altered bacterial balance.
! Nephrotoxicity may occur, especially in patients with preexisting renal disease.
! Patients with a history of allergies, especially to penicillin, are at increased risk for developing a severe hypersensitivity reaction, marked by severe pruritus, angioedema, bronchospasm, and anaphylaxis.

DENTAL CONSIDERATIONS

General:
• For selected infections in the hospital setting; provide palliative emergency dental treatment only.
• Use with caution in patients with a history of antibiotic-associated colitis.
• Examine for oral manifestation of opportunistic infection.
• Determine why patient is taking the drug.
• Caution regarding allergy to medication.
Consultations:
• Medical consultation may be required to assess disease control and patient's ability to tolerate stress.
Teach Patient/Family to:
• Encourage effective oral hygiene to prevent soft tissue inflammation.
• Report sore throat, oral burning sensation, fever, or fatigue, any of which could indicate presence of a superinfection.

ceftriaxone sodium

sef-try-**ax**′-one **so**′-dee-um
(Rocephin)

CATEGORY AND SCHEDULE

Pregnancy Risk Category: B

Drug Class: Cephalosporin (third-generation)

MECHANISM OF ACTION

A third-generation cephalosporin that binds to bacterial cell membranes and inhibits cell wall synthesis.
Therapeutic Effect: Bactericidal.

USES

Treatment of respiratory tract, GU tract, skin, bone, intraabdominal, biliary tract infections; septicemia; meningitis; gonorrhea; Lyme disease; acute bacterial otitis media

PHARMACOKINETICS

Widely distributed (including to CSF). Protein binding: 83%–96%. Primarily excreted unchanged in urine. Not removed by hemodialysis. ***Half-life:*** 4.3–4.6 hr IV; 5.8–8.7 hr IM (increased in impaired renal function).

INDICATIONS AND DOSAGES

▸ **Mild to Moderate Infections**
IV, IM
Adults, Elderly. 1–2 g as a single dose or in 2 divided doses.

▸ **Serious Infections**
IV, IM
Adults, Elderly. Up to 4 g/day in 2 divided doses.
Children. 50–75 mg/kg/day in divided doses q12h. Maximum: 2 g/day.

▸ **Skin and Skin-Structure Infections**
IV, IM
Children. 50–75 mg/kg/day as a single dose or in 2 divided doses. Maximum: 2 g/day.

▸ **Meningitis**
IV
Children. Initially, 75 mg/kg, then 100 mg/kg/day as a single dose or in divided doses q12h. Maximum: 4 g/day.

▸ **Lyme Disease**
IV
Adults, Elderly. 2–4 g a day for 10–14 days.

▸ **Acute Bacterial Otitis Media**
IM
Children. 50 mg/kg once a day for 3 days. Maximum: 1 g/day.

▸ **Perioperative Prophylaxis**
IV, IM
Adults, Elderly. 1 g 0.5–2 hr before surgery.

▸ **Uncomplicated Gonorrhea**
IM
Adults. 250 mg plus doxycycline one time.

▸ **Dosage in Renal Impairment**
Dosage modification is usually unnecessary, but liver and renal function test results should be monitored in those with both renal and liver impairment or severe renal impairment.

SIDE EFFECTS/ADVERSE REACTIONS

Frequent
Discomfort with IM administration, oral candidiasis, mild diarrhea, mild abdominal cramping, vaginal candidiasis

Occasional
Nausea, serum sickness-like reaction (marked by fever and joint pain; usually occurs after the second course of therapy and resolves after the drug is discontinued)

Rare
Allergic reaction (rash, pruritus, urticaria), thrombophlebitis (pain, redness, swelling at injection site)

PRECAUTIONS AND CONTRAINDICATIONS

History of anaphylactic reaction to penicillins or hypersensitivity to cephalosporins

Caution:
Hypersensitivity to penicillins, lactation, renal disease

DRUG INTERACTIONS OF CONCERN TO DENTISTRY

- None reported

SERIOUS REACTIONS

! Antibiotic-associated colitis and other superinfections may result from altered bacterial balance.

! Nephrotoxicity may occur, especially in patients with preexisting renal disease.

! Patients with a history of allergies, especially to penicillin, are at increased risk for developing a severe hypersensitivity reaction, marked by severe pruritus, angioedema, bronchospasm, and anaphylaxis.

C

DENTAL CONSIDERATIONS

General:

• For selected infections in the hospital setting; provide palliative emergency dental treatment only.
• Use with caution in patients with a history of antibiotic-associated colitis.
• May interfere with prothrombin levels.
• Examine for oral manifestation of opportunistic infection.
• Determine why patient is taking the drug.
• Caution regarding allergy to medication.

Consultations:

• Medical consultation may be required to assess disease control and patient's ability to tolerate stress.
• Medical consultation should include partial prothrombin time, prothrombin time, or INR.

Teach Patient/Family to:

• Encourage effective oral hygiene to prevent soft tissue inflammation.
• Report sore throat, oral burning sensation, fever, or fatigue, any of which could indicate presence of a superinfection.

cefuroxime axetil/ cefuroxime sodium

sef-yur-**ox′**-ime
(cefuroxime axetil) Ceftin, Zinnat[AUS] (cefuroxime sodium), Kefurox, Zinacef
Do not confuse cefuroxime with cefotaxime or deferoxamine or Ceftin with Cefzil.

CATEGORY AND SCHEDULE

Pregnancy Risk Category: B

Drug Class: Cephalosporin (second generation)

MECHANISM OF ACTION

A second-generation cephalosporin that binds to bacterial cell membranes and inhibits cell wall synthesis.
Therapeutic Effect: Bactericidal.

USES

Gram-negative bacilli (*H. influenzae, E. coli, Neisseria, P. mirabilis, Klebsiella*); gram-positive organisms (*S. pneumoniae, S. pyogenes, S. aureus*); serious lower respiratory tract, urinary tract, skin, gonococcal infections; septicemia; meningitis; early Lyme disease; acute bronchitis, acute bacterial maxillary sinusitis, pharyngitis, tonsillitis, impetigo, bone and joint infections

PHARMACOKINETICS

Rapidly absorbed from the GI tract. Protein binding: 33%–50%. Widely distributed (including to CSF). Primarily excreted unchanged in urine. Moderately removed by hemodialysis. ***Half-life:*** 1.3 hr (increased in impaired renal function).

INDICATIONS AND DOSAGES

▸ **Ampicillin-Resistant Influenza; Bacterial Meningitis; Early Lyme Disease; GU Tract, Gynecologic, Skin and Bone Infections; Septicemia; Gonorrhea and Other Gonococcal Infections**

IV, IM
Adults, Elderly. 750 mg–1.5 g q8h.
Children. 75–100 mg/kg/day divided q8h. Maximum: 8 g/day.
Neonates. 50–100 mg/kg/day divided q12h.
PO
Adults, Elderly. 125–500 mg twice a day, depending on the infection.

▸ **Pharyngitis, Tonsillitis**
PO
Children 3 mo–12 yr. 125 mg (tablets) q12h or 20 mg/kg/day (suspension) in 2 divided doses.

▸ **Acute Otitis Media, Acute Bacterial Maxillary Sinusitis, Impetigo**
PO
Children 3 mo–12 yr. 250 mg (tablets) q12h or 30 mg/kg/day (suspension) in 2 divided doses.

▸ **Bacterial Meningitis**
IV
Children 3 mo–12 yr. 200–240 mg/kg/day in divided doses q6–8h.

▸ **Perioperative Prophylaxis**
IV
Adults, Elderly. 1.5 g 30–60 min before surgery and 750 mg q8h after surgery.

▸ **Usual Neonatal Dosage**
IV, IM
Neonates. 20–100 mg/kg/day in divided doses q12h.

▸ **Dosage in Renal Impairment**
Adult dosage and frequency are modified based on creatinine clearance and the severity of the infection.

SIDE EFFECTS/ADVERSE REACTIONS

Frequent
Discomfort with IM administration, oral candidiasis, mild diarrhea, mild abdominal cramping, vaginal candidiasis

Occasional
Nausea, serum sickness-like reaction (marked by fever and joint pain; usually occurs after the second course of therapy and resolves after the drug is discontinued)

Rare
Allergic reaction (rash, pruritus, urticaria), thrombophlebitis (pain, redness, swelling at injection site)

PRECAUTIONS AND CONTRAINDICATIONS

History of anaphylactic reaction to penicillins or hypersensitivity to cephalosporins

DRUG INTERACTIONS OF CONCERN TO DENTISTRY

- Decreased bactericidal effects: tetracyclines, erythromycins
- Increased and prolonged serum levels: probenecid

SERIOUS REACTIONS

! Antibiotic-associated colitis and other superinfections may result from altered bacterial balance.
! Nephrotoxicity may occur, especially in patients with preexisting renal disease.
! Patients with a history of allergies, especially to penicillin, are at increased risk for developing a severe hypersensitivity reaction, marked by severe pruritus, angioedema, bronchospasm, and anaphylaxis.

DENTAL CONSIDERATIONS

General:
- Take precautions regarding allergy to medication.
- Determine why the patient is taking the drug.

Consultations:
- Medical consultation may be required to assess disease control.

Teach Patient/Family to:
- Encourage effective oral hygiene to prevent soft tissue inflammation.
- When used for dental infection, advise patient to:

- Report sore throat, oral burning sensation, fever, and fatigue, any of which could indicate superinfection.
- Take at prescribed intervals and complete dosage regimen.
- Immediately notify the dentist if signs or symptoms of infection increase.

celecoxib

sel-eh-**kox′**-ib

(Celebrex, DisperDose, Panixine)

Do not confuse Celebrex with Cerebyx or Celexa.

CATEGORY AND SCHEDULE

Pregnancy Risk Category: C (D if used in third trimester or near delivery)

Drug Class: Cox-2-selective nonsteroidal antiinflammatory, analgesic

MECHANISM OF ACTION

An NSAID that inhibits cyclo-oxygenase-2, the enzyme responsible for prostaglandin synthesis. Mechanism of action in treating familial adenomatous polyposis is unknown.
Therapeutic Effect: Reduces inflammation and relieves pain.

USES

Relief of signs and symptoms of osteoarthritis and relief of signs and symptoms of rheumatoid arthritis in adults; also approved for reducing the number of intestinal polyps in patients with familial adenomatous polyposis; acute pain and primary dysmenorrhea

PHARMACOKINETICS

Widely distributed. Protein binding: 97%. Metabolized in the liver. Primarily eliminated in feces.
Half-life: 11.2 hr.

INDICATIONS AND DOSAGES

▸ **Osteoarthritis**

PO

Adults, Elderly. 200 mg/day as a single dose or 100 mg twice a day.

▸ **Rheumatoid Arthritis**

PO

Adults, Elderly. 100–200 mg twice a day.

▸ **Acute Pain**

PO

Adults, Elderly. Initially, 400 mg with additional 200 mg on day 1, if needed. Maintenance: 200 mg twice a day as needed.

▸ **Familial Adenomatous Polyposis**

PO

Adults, Elderly. 400 mg twice daily (with food).

SIDE EFFECTS/ADVERSE REACTIONS

Frequent

Diarrhea, dyspepsia, headache, upper respiratory tract infection

Occasional

Abdominal pain, flatulence, nausea, back pain, peripheral edema, dizziness, rash

PRECAUTIONS AND CONTRAINDICATIONS

NSAIDs may cause an increased risk of serious cardiovascular thrombotic events, including myocardial infarction and stroke, which may be fatal. Patients with cardiovascular disease may be at greater risk.

Hypersensitivity to aspirin, NSAIDs, or sulfonamides

Caution:

Geriatric patients weighing less than 50 kg use lowest dose, children younger than 18 yr, severe hepatic or renal impairment, upper active GI disease, GI bleeding, avoid in late pregnancy (category D after 34 wk), lactation, dehydrated patients, heart failure, hypertension, asthma, patients suspected or known to be poor CYP2C9 isoenzyme metabolizers

DRUG INTERACTIONS OF CONCERN TO DENTISTRY

- Increased plasma levels: fluconazole
- Increased risk of thromboembolism
- Increased risk of GI bleeding: NSAIDs, aspirin, oral glucocorticoids, alcoholism, smoking, older age, generally poor health
- Increased plasma levels of lithium
- Possible risk of increased INR in elderly patients taking warfarin
- Possible reduction in blood pressure control: ACE inhibitors, diuretics
- Users of SSRIs also taking NSAIDs may have a higher risk of GI side effects; until more data are available, it may be advisable to avoid use of NSAIDs in these patients (*Br J Clin Pharmacol* 55:591–595, 2003)

SERIOUS REACTIONS

! None known

DENTAL CONSIDERATIONS

General:

- Patients on chronic drug therapy may rarely have symptoms of blood dyscrasias, which can include infection, bleeding, and poor healing.
- Assess salivary flow as a factor in caries, periodontal disease, and candidiasis.
- Consider semisupine chair position for patient comfort because of effects of disease and GI side effects of drug.
- Severe stomach bleeding may occur in patients who regularly use NSAIDs in recommended doses, when the patient is also taking another NSAID, an antiplatelet or anticoagulant drug, or steroid drug, if the patient has GI or peptic ulcer disease, if they are 60 yr or older, or when NSAIDs are taken longer than directed. Warn patients of the potential for severe stomach bleeding.

Teach Patient/Family to:

- Encourage effective oral hygiene to prevent soft tissue inflammation.
- Update health and drug history if physician makes any changes in evaluation or drug regimens.
- Use powered tooth brush if patient has difficulty holding conventional devices.
- When chronic dry mouth occurs, advise patient to:
  - Avoid mouth rinses with high alcohol content because of drying effects.
  - Use daily home fluoride products for anticaries effect.
  - Use sugarless gum, frequent sips of water, or saliva substitutes.
- Warn patient of potential risks of NSAIDs.

C

cephalexin

sef-ah-**lex′**-in

(Apo-Cephalex[CAN], Biocef, Ceporex[AUS], Ibilex[AUS], Keflex, Keftab, Novolexin[CAN])

CATEGORY AND SCHEDULE

Pregnancy Risk Category: B

Drug Class: Cephalosporin (first generation)

MECHANISM OF ACTION

A first-generation cephalosporin that binds to bacterial cell membranes and inhibits cell wall synthesis. ***Therapeutic Effect:*** Bactericidal.

USES

Treatment of the following infections when caused by susceptible microorganisms: respiratory tract infections caused by *S. pneumoniae* and group A β-hemolytic streptococci; otitis media caused by *S. pneumoniae, H. influenzae, M. catarrhalis,* staphylococci, and streptococci; skin and skin structure infections caused by staphylococci and streptococci; bone infections caused by staphylococci and *P. mirabilis*; and GU tract infections caused by *E. coli, P. mirabilis,* and *K. pneumoniae*

PHARMACOKINETICS

Rapidly absorbed from the GI tract. Protein binding: 10%–15%. Widely distributed. Primarily excreted unchanged in urine. Moderately removed by hemodialysis. ***Half-life:*** 0.9–1.2 hr (increased in impaired renal function).

INDICATIONS AND DOSAGES

▸ Bone Infections, Prophylaxis of Rheumatic Fever, Follow-up to Parenteral Therapy

PO

Adults, Elderly. 250–500 mg q6h up to 4 g/day.

▸ Streptococcal Pharyngitis, Skin and Skin-Structure Infections, Uncomplicated Cystitis

PO

Adults, Elderly. 500 mg q12h.

▸ Usual Pediatric Dosage

Children. 25–100 mg/kg/day in 2–4 divided doses.

▸ Otitis Media

PO

Children. 75–100 mg/kg/day in 4 divided doses.

▸ Dosage in Renal Impairment

After usual initial dose, dosing frequency is modified on the basis of creatinine clearance and the severity of the infection.

Creatinine Clearance	Dosage Interval
10–50 ml/min	250 mg q6h
0–10 ml/min	125 mg q6h

SIDE EFFECTS/ADVERSE REACTIONS

Frequent

Oral candidiasis, mild diarrhea, mild abdominal cramping, vaginal candidiasis

Occasional

Nausea, serum sickness-like reaction (marked by fever and joint pain; usually occurs after the second course of therapy and resolves after the drug is discontinued)

Rare

Allergic reaction (rash, pruritus, urticaria)

PRECAUTIONS AND CONTRAINDICATIONS

History of anaphylactic reaction to penicillins or hypersensitivity to cephalosporins

Caution:

Hypersensitivity to penicillins, lactation, renal disease

DRUG INTERACTIONS OF CONCERN TO DENTISTRY

- Decreased bactericidal effects: tetracyclines, erythromycins
- Increased and prolonged serum levels: probenecid

SERIOUS REACTIONS

! Antibiotic-associated colitis and other superinfections may result from altered bacterial balance.

! Nephrotoxicity may occur, especially in patients with preexisting renal disease.

! Patients with a history of allergies, especially to penicillin, are at increased risk for developing a severe hypersensitivity reaction, marked by severe pruritus, angioedema, bronchospasm, and anaphylaxis.

DENTAL CONSIDERATIONS

General:

- Take precautions regarding allergy to medication.
- Determine why the patient is taking the drug.

Consultations:

- Medical consultation may be required to assess disease control.

Teach Patient/Family to:

- Encourage effective oral hygiene to prevent soft tissue inflammation.
- Avoid mouth rinses with high alcohol content because of drying effects and possible drug-drug reaction.
- When used for dental infection, advise patient to:
  - Report sore throat, oral burning sensation, fever, and fatigue, any of which could indicate superinfection.
  - Take at prescribed intervals and complete dosage regimen.
  - Immediately notify the dentist if signs or symptoms of infection increase.

cephradine

sef'-ra-deen

(Velosef)

CATEGORY AND SCHEDULE

Pregnancy Risk Category: B

Drug Class: Cephalosporin (first generation)

MECHANISM OF ACTION

A first-generation cephalosporin that binds to bacterial cell membranes. Inhibits synthesis of bacterial cell wall.

Therapeutic Effect: Bactericidal.

USES

Treatment of gram-negative bacilli: *H. influenzae, E. coli, P. mirabilis, Klebsiella*; gram-positive organisms: *S. pneumoniae, S. pyogenes, S. aureus*; serious respiratory tract, urinary tract, skin, and skin structure infections; otitis media

PHARMACOKINETICS

Well absorbed from the GI tract. Protein binding: 18%–20%. Widely distributed. Primarily excreted unchanged in urine. Removed by hemodialysis. ***Half-life:*** 1–2 hr (half-life is increased with impaired renal function).

C

INDICATIONS AND DOSAGES

▸ **Mild, Moderate or Severe Infections of the Respiratory and GU Tracts; Bone, Joint and Skin Infections; Prostatitis; Otitis Media**

PO

Adults, Elderly. 250–500 mg q6h. Maximum: 8 g/day.

Children older than 9 mo. 25–50 mg/kg/day in divided doses q6–12h. Maximum: 4 g/day.

▸ **Dosage in Renal Impairment**

Dosage and frequency are based on the degree of renal impairment and the severity of infection. In patients with renal impairment, starting doses of 250 mg are recommended, with longer dosing intervals of up to 12 hr. Consult physician for use in patients on dialysis.

SIDE EFFECTS/ADVERSE REACTIONS

Frequent

Diarrhea, mild abdominal cramping, vaginal candidiasis (discharge, itching)

Occasional

Nausea, headache, unusual bruising or bleeding, serum sickness-like reaction (fever, joint pain)

Rare

Allergic reaction (rash, pruritus, urticaria)

PRECAUTIONS AND CONTRAINDICATIONS

History of hypersensitivity to penicillins and cephalosporins

Caution:

Hypersensitivity to penicillins, lactation, renal disease

DRUG INTERACTIONS OF CONCERN TO DENTISTRY

- Decreased bactericidal effects: tetracyclines, erythromycins
- Increased and prolonged serum levels: probenecid

SERIOUS REACTIONS

! Antibiotic-associated colitis as evidenced by severe abdominal pain and tenderness, fever, and watery and severe diarrhea, and other superinfections may result from altered bacterial balance.

! Nephrotoxicity may occur, especially in patients with preexisting renal disease.

! Severe hypersensitivity reaction including severe pruritus, angioedema, bronchospasm, and anaphylaxis, particularly in patients with history of allergies, especially penicillin, may occur.

DENTAL CONSIDERATIONS

General:

- Take precautions regarding allergy to medication.
- Determine why the patient is taking the drug.

Consultations:

- Medical consultation may be required to assess disease control.

Teach Patient/Family to:

- Encourage effective oral hygiene to prevent soft tissue inflammation.
- When used for dental infection, advise patient to:
  - Report sore throat, oral burning sensation, fever, and fatigue, any of which could indicate superinfection.
  - Take at prescribed intervals and complete dosage regimen.
  - Immediately notify the dentist if signs or symptoms of infection increase.

certolizumab

cer-to-**liz**′-u-mab
(Cimzia)

CATEGORY AND SCHEDULE

Pregnancy Risk Category: B

Drug Class: Antiinflammatory, monoclonal antibody

MECHANISM OF ACTION

Humanized, pegylated tumor necrosis factor alpha (TNF-α) inhibitor. Reduces infiltration of inflammatory cells. Higher binding affinity for TNF-α than adalimumab or infliximab.

USES

Crohn's disease, moderately to severely active disease in patients who have inadequate response to conventional therapy

PHARMACOKINETICS

Approximately 80% bioavailability following SC administration. ***Half-life***: 14 days.

INDICATIONS AND DOSAGES

Adult. Subcutaneous (sc)
Crohn's disease: Initially, 400 mg (as 2 SC injections of 200 mg) once and then repeat at weeks 2 and 4.
Maintenance: 400 mg (as 2 SC injections of 200 mg) once every 4 wk.
Note: Evaluate patients for tuberculosis (TB) risk factors and test for latent TB infection before starting therapy.
Do not start therapy with certolizumab in patients with an active infection.
Evaluate patients at risk for hepatitis B virus infection for signs of prior HBV infection.
Pediatric. Safety and efficacy have not been established.

SIDE EFFECTS/ADVERSE REACTIONS

Frequent
Upper respiratory infection, urinary tract infectious disease, headache, nausea, infection
Occasional
Dizziness, vomiting, abdominal pain, arthralgia, injection site reactions (bleeding, burning, inflammation, pain, rash), cough
Rare
Congestive heart failure, myocardial infarction, bowel obstruction, opportunistic infection, sepsis

PRECAUTIONS AND CONTRAINDICATIONS

There are no contraindications listed within the manufacturer's labeling.
Caution:
Tuberculosis, children and young adults, cytopenias (e.g., leucopenia), heart failure, hepatitis B virus, infection

DRUG INTERACTIONS OF CONCERN TO DENTISTRY

- None reported

SERIOUS REACTIONS

! Sepsis and occasionally serious infections have occurred.
! Heart failure, hypersensitivity reactions, and opportunistic infections have been reported.
! Lupus-like syndrome may occur; discontinue if symptoms occur.

! Immunogenicity: Patients develop antibodies to certolizumab during therapy.

DENTAL CONSIDERATIONS

General:

- Patients on chronic drug therapy may rarely have symptoms of blood dyscrasias, which can include infection, bleeding, and poor healing.
- Aphthous ulcers may require postponement of dental treatment.
- Examine for oral manifestations of opportunistic infection.
- Monitor vital signs at every appointment because of cardiovascular side effects.

Consultations:

- In a patient with symptoms of blood dyscrasias, request a medical consultation for blood studies and postpone treatment until normal values are reestablished.

Teach Patient/Family to:

- Encourage effective oral hygiene to prevent soft tissue inflammation, infection.
- Report oral lesions, soreness, or bleeding to dentist.
- Prevent trauma when using oral hygiene aids.

cetirizine

si-**tear′**-ah-zeen
(Reactine[CAN], Zyrtec)
Do not confuse Zyrtec with Zantac or Zyprexa.

CATEGORY AND SCHEDULE

Pregnancy Risk Category: B

Drug Class: Antihistamine

MECHANISM OF ACTION

A second-generation piperazine that competes with histamine for H_1-receptor sites on effector cells in the GI tract, blood vessels, and respiratory tract.

Therapeutic Effect: Prevents allergic response, produces mild bronchodilation, blocks histamine-induced bronchitis.

USES

Treatment of symptoms of seasonal allergic rhinitis, perennial allergic rhinitis, chronic urticaria

PHARMACOKINETICS

Rapidly and almost completely absorbed from the GI tract (absorption not affected by food). Protein binding: 93%. Undergoes low first-pass metabolism; not extensively metabolized. Primarily excreted in urine (more than 80% as unchanged drug). ***Half-life:*** 6.5–10 hr.

INDICATIONS AND DOSAGES

▸ **Allergic Rhinitis, Urticaria**

PO

Adults, Elderly, Children older than 5 yr. Initially, 5–10 mg/day as a single or in 2 divided doses.
Children 2–5 yr. 2.5 mg/day. May increase up to 5 mg/day as a single or in 2 divided doses.
Children 12–23 mo. Initially, 2.5 mg/day. May increase up to 5 mg/day in 2 divided doses.
Children 6–11 mo. 2.5 mg once a day.

▸ **Dosage in Renal or Hepatic Impairment**

For adult and elderly patients with renal impairment (creatinine clearance of 11–31 ml/min), those receiving hemodialysis (creatinine clearance of 7 ml/min), and those with hepatic impairment, dosage is decreased to 5 mg once a day.

SIDE EFFECTS/ADVERSE REACTIONS

Occasional

Pharyngitis; dry mucous membranes, nose, or throat; nausea and vomiting; abdominal pain; headache; dizziness; fatigue; thickening of mucus; somnolence; photosensitivity; urine retention

PRECAUTIONS AND CONTRAINDICATIONS

Hypersensitivity to cetirizine or hydroxyzine

Caution:

Renal impairment (requires dose reduction), elderly, glaucoma, urinary obstruction, lactation

DRUG INTERACTIONS OF CONCERN TO DENTISTRY

- No drug interactions reported, but should be similar to other antihistamines; anticipate increased sedation with other CNS depressants and increased anticholinergic effects with anticholinergic drugs.

SERIOUS REACTIONS

! Children may experience paradoxical reactions, including restlessness, insomnia, euphoria, nervousness, and tremor.

! Dizziness, sedation, and confusion are more likely to occur in elderly patients.

DENTAL CONSIDERATIONS

General:

- Assess salivary flow as factor in caries, periodontal disease, and candidiasis.

Teach Patient/Family:

- When chronic dry mouth occurs, advise patient to:
  - Avoid mouth rinses with high alcohol content because of drying effects.
  - Use daily home fluoride products for anticaries effect.
  - Use sugarless gum, frequent sips of water, or saliva substitutes.

cetuximab

ceh-**tux′**-ih-mab

(Erbitux)

CATEGORY AND SCHEDULE

Pregnancy Risk Category: C

Drug Class: Monoclonal antibody; antineoplastic

MECHANISM OF ACTION

A monoclonal antibody that binds to the epidermal growth factor receptor (EGFR), a glycoprotein on normal and tumor cells, thus inhibiting cell growth and inducing apoptosis.

Therapeutic Effect: Inhibits the growth and survival of tumor cells that overexpress EGFR.

USES

As a single agent or in combination with irinotecan for treatment of EGFR-expressing, metastatic colorectal carcinoma in patients who are refractory or intolerant to irinotecan-based chemotherapy

PHARMACOKINETICS

Reaches steady state levels by the third weekly infusion. Clearance decreases as dose increases.

Half-life: 114 hr (range, 75–188 hr).

C

INDICATIONS AND DOSAGES

▸ **Metastatic Colorectal Carcinoma**

IV

Adults, Elderly. Initially, 400 mg/m^2 as a loading dose. Maintenance: 250 mg/m^2 infused over 60 min weekly.

SIDE EFFECTS/ADVERSE REACTIONS

Frequent

Acneiform rash, malaise, fever, nausea, diarrhea, constipation, headache, abdominal pain, anorexia, vomiting

Occasional

Nail disorder, back pain, stomatitis, peripheral edema, pruritus, cough, insomnia

Rare

Weight loss, depression, dyspepsia, conjunctivitis, alopecia

PRECAUTIONS AND CONTRAINDICATIONS

None known

DRUG INTERACTIONS OF CONCERN TO DENTISTRY

- None reported

SERIOUS REACTIONS

! Anemia occurs in 10% of patients.

! A severe infusion reaction, characterized by rapid onset of airway obstruction, a precipitous drop in B/P, and severe urticaria, occurs rarely.

! Dermatologic toxicity, pulmonary embolus, leukopenia, and renal failure occur rarely.

DENTAL CONSIDERATIONS

General:

- Monitor vital signs at every appointment because of cardiovascular side effects.
- If additional analgesia is required for dental pain, consider alternative analgesics (NSAIDs) in patients taking narcotics for acute or chronic pain.
- Examine for oral manifestation of opportunistic infection.
- Consider semisupine chair position for patient comfort because of GI effects of disease.
- Patient on chronic drug therapy may rarely present with symptoms of blood dyscrasias, which can include infection, bleeding, and poor healing. If dyscrasia is present, caution patient to prevent oral tissue trauma when using oral hygiene aids.
- Advise patient if dental drugs prescribed have a potential for photosensitivity.
- Patients may be taking a prophylactic antiinfective.
- Use caution in the use of drugs that may cause diarrhea or constipation.
- Patients may have received other chemotherapy or radiation; confirm medical and drug history.

Consultations:

- Consult physician; prophylactic or therapeutic antiinfectives may be indicated if surgery or periodontal treatment is required.
- Medical consultation may be required to assess immunologic status during cancer chemotherapy and determine safety risk, if any, posed by the required dental treatment.
- Medical consultation may be required to assess disease control and patient's ability to tolerate stress.
- Medical consultation should include routine blood counts including platelet counts and bleeding time.

Teach Patient/Family to:

- Encourage effective oral hygiene to prevent soft tissue inflammation.
- Report oral lesions, soreness, or bleeding to dentist.
- Prevent trauma when using oral hygiene aids.
- Update health and medication history if physician makes any changes in evaluation or drug regimens; include OTC, herbal, and nonherbal remedies in the update.

cevimeline

sev-**im**′-el-ine

(Evoxac)

Do not confuse Evoxac with Eurax.

CATEGORY AND SCHEDULE

Pregnancy Risk Category: C

Drug Class: Cholinergic (muscarinic) agonist

MECHANISM OF ACTION

A cholinergic agonist that binds to muscarinic receptors of effector cells, thereby increasing secretion of exocrine glands, such as salivary glands.

Therapeutic Effect: Relieves dry mouth.

USES

Treatment of symptoms of dry mouth associated with Sjögren's syndrome

PHARMACOKINETICS

Rapid absorption after oral administration, peak levels 1.5–2 hr. Protein binding: 20%. Metabolized in liver by CYP 2D6 and CYP 3A4 isoenzymes. ***Half-life:*** 5 hr. 84% excreted in urine within 24 hr.

INDICATIONS AND DOSAGES

▸ **Dry Mouth**

PO

Adults. 30 mg 3 times a day.

SIDE EFFECTS/ADVERSE REACTIONS

Frequent

Diaphoresis, headache, nausea, sinusitis, rhinitis, upper respiratory tract infection, diarrhea

Occasional

Dyspepsia, abdominal pain, cough, UTI, vomiting, back pain, rash, dizziness, fatigue

Rare

Skeletal pain, insomnia, hot flashes, excessive salivation, rigors, anxiety

PRECAUTIONS AND CONTRAINDICATIONS

Acute iritis, angle-closure glaucoma, uncontrolled asthma

Caution:

Has the potential to alter heart rate or cardiac conduction; use with care in cardiovascular disease, asthma, bronchitis, COPD, seizure disorders, Parkinson's disease, urinary tract/bladder obstruction, cholecystitis, cholangitis, biliary obstruction, GI ulcers, lactation, children (no data), history of adverse effects to other cholinergic agonists

DRUG INTERACTIONS OF CONCERN TO DENTISTRY

- Use with caution in patients taking β-adrenergic blockers: possible conduction disturbances.
- There are no specific data on dental drug interactions; however, use caution with other cholinergic agonists.

C

• Possibility that a cholinergic antagonist could interfere with this drug's action.
• Although there are no supporting data, use with caution in patients taking drugs that inhibit cytochrome P-450 (CYP3A3/4 and CYP2D6 isoenzymes).

SERIOUS REACTIONS

! Cevimeline use may result in decreased visual acuity, especially at night, and impaired depth perception.

DENTAL CONSIDERATIONS

General:
• Assess salivary flow as a factor in caries, periodontal disease, and candidiasis.
• Place on frequent recall to assess effectiveness.
• Consider semisupine chair position for patient comfort if GI side effects occur.

Consultations:
• Medical consultation may be required to assess disease control.
• Medical consultation may be necessary before prescribing for those patients with cardiovascular or respiratory disease.

Teach Patient/Family to:
• Be aware that this drug may cause visual disturbances, especially with night driving, which may impair driving safety.
• Drink extra fluids (water) to compensate for excessive sweating.
• When chronic dry mouth occurs, advise patient to:
  • Avoid mouth rinses with high alcohol content because of drying effects.
  • Use daily home fluoride to prevent caries.
  • Use sugarless gum, frequent sips of water, or saliva substitutes.

chloral hydrate

klor′-al **hye′**-drate
(Aquachloral Supprettes, PMS-Chloral Hydrate[CAN], Somnote)

CATEGORY AND SCHEDULE

Pregnancy Risk Category: C
Controlled Substance Schedule IV

Drug Class: Sedative hypnotic, chloral derivative

MECHANISM OF ACTION

A nonbarbiturate chloral derivative that produces CNS depression.
Therapeutic Effect: Induces quiet, deep sleep, with only a slight decrease in respiratory rate and B/P.

USES

Sedation, insomnia

PHARMACOKINETICS

Rapid absorption after oral administration, peak levels 30–45 min. Duration: 2–5 hr. Metabolized to trichloroethanol in liver and other tissues and, to a lesser extent, trichloroacetic acid, in liver. ***Half-life:*** 7–9.5 hr. Glucuronide conjugate excreted in urine.

INDICATIONS AND DOSAGES

▸ **Premedication for Dental or Medical Procedures**

PO, Rectal
Adults. 0.5–1 g.
Children. 75 mg/kg up to 1 g total. (Dosage reduced when combined with other sedatives.)

▸ **Premedication for EEG**
PO, Rectal
Adults. 0.5–1.5 g.
Children. 25–50 mg/kg/dose 30–60 min prior to EEG. May repeat in 30 min. Maximum: 1 g for infants, 2 g for children.

SIDE EFFECTS/ADVERSE REACTIONS

Occasional
Gastric irritation (nausea, vomiting, flatulence, diarrhea), rash, sleepwalking
Rare
Headache, paradoxical CNS hyperactivity or nervousness in children, excitement or restlessness in the elderly (particularly in patients with pain)

PRECAUTIONS AND CONTRAINDICATIONS

Gastritis, marked hepatic or renal impairment, severe cardiac disease
Caution:
Severe cardiac disease, depression, suicidal individuals, asthma, intermittent porphyria, lactation, elderly; no specific reversal agent available, use extreme caution in dose calculation when used in pediatric patients for sedation

DRUG INTERACTIONS OF CONCERN TO DENTISTRY

- Increased action of both drugs: alcohol, all CNS depressants, including nitrous oxide
- Sensitization of myocardium to vasoconstrictors

SERIOUS REACTIONS

! Overdose may produce somnolence, confusion, slurred speech, severe incoordination, respiratory depression, and coma.

DENTAL CONSIDERATIONS

General:
- Consider semisupine chair position for patient comfort because of GI side effects of drug.
- Administer syrup in juice or beverage to mask taste and reduce GI upset.
- Contraindicated for use in patients with GI ulcerative disease.
- Have someone drive patient to and from dental office when drug used for conscious sedation.
- Geriatric patients are more susceptible to drug effects; use lower dose.
- Psychologic and physical dependence may occur with chronic administration.

chlordiazepoxide

klor-dye-az-eh-**pox′**-ide
(Apo-Chlordiazepoxide[CAN], Librium, Novopoxide[CAN])
Do not confuse Librium with Librax.

CATEGORY AND SCHEDULE

Pregnancy Risk Category: D
Controlled Substance Schedule IV

Drug Class: Benzodiazepine antianxiety

MECHANISM OF ACTION

A benzodiazepine that enhances the action of the inhibitory neurotransmitter gamma-aminobutyric acid in the CNS.
Therapeutic Effect: Produces anxiolytic effect.

USES

Short-term management of anxiety, acute alcohol withdrawal, preoperatively for relaxation

PHARMACOKINETICS

Slow onset after oral administration, peak levels 2 hr. Metabolized in liver (active metabolites). ***Half-life:*** 24–48 hr. Metabolites excreted in urine.

INDICATIONS AND DOSAGES

▸ Alcohol Withdrawal Symptoms

PO

Adults, Elderly. 50–100 mg. May repeat q2–4h. Maximum: 300 mg/24 hr.

▸ Anxiety

PO

Adults. 15–100 mg/day in 3–4 divided doses.

Elderly. 5 mg 2–4 times a day.

IV, IM

Adults. Initially, 50–100 mg, then 25–50 mg 3–4 times a day as needed.

SIDE EFFECTS/ADVERSE REACTIONS

Frequent

Pain at IM injection site; somnolence, ataxia, dizziness, confusion with oral dose (particularly in elderly or debilitated patients)

Occasional

Rash, peripheral edema, GI disturbances

Rare

Paradoxical CNS reactions, such as hyperactivity or nervousness in children and excitement or restlessness in the elderly (generally noted during first 2 wk of therapy, particularly in presence of uncontrolled pain)

PRECAUTIONS AND CONTRAINDICATIONS

Acute alcohol intoxication, acute angle-closure glaucoma

Caution:

Elderly, debilitated, hepatic disease, renal disease

DRUG INTERACTIONS OF CONCERN TO DENTISTRY

- Delayed elimination: erythromycin
- Increased CNS depression: CNS depressants, alcohol, disulfiram, nefazodone
- Increased serum levels and prolonged effects of benzodiazepines: ketoconazole, itraconazole, fluconazole, miconazole (systemic), cimetidine, fluvoxamine, omeprazole, rifabutin, rifampin
- Contraindicated with ritonavir, indinavir, saquinavir
- Possible increase in CNS side effects: kava kava (herb)
- Decreased plasma levels: St. John's wort (herb)

SERIOUS REACTIONS

! IV administration may produce pain, swelling, thrombophlebitis, and carpal tunnel syndrome.

! Abrupt or too-rapid withdrawal may result in pronounced restlessness, irritability, insomnia, hand tremors, abdominal or muscle cramps, diaphoresis, vomiting, and seizures.

! Overdose results in somnolence, confusion, diminished reflexes, and coma.

DENTAL CONSIDERATIONS

General:

- After supine positioning, have patient sit upright for at least 2 min to avoid orthostatic hypotension.
- Assess salivary flow as a factor in caries, periodontal disease, and candidiasis.

• Psychologic and physical dependence may occur with chronic administration.
• Geriatric patients are more susceptible to drug effects; use lower dose.
• Have someone drive patient to and from dental office if used for conscious sedation.

Consultations:
• Medical consultation may be required to assess disease control.

Teach Patient/Family to:
• Encourage effective oral hygiene to prevent soft tissue inflammation.
• Avoid mouth rinses with high alcohol content because of drying effects.

chlorhexidine gluconate

klor-**hex'**-ih-deen **gloo'**-ko-nate
(Chlorhexidine Mouthwash[AUS], Chlorhexidine Obstetric Lotion[AUS], Chlorohex Gel[AUS], Chlorohex Gel Forte[AUS], Chlorohex Mouth Rinse[AUS], Peridex, PerioChip, PerioGard, Perisol)

CATEGORY AND SCHEDULE

Pregnancy Risk Category: C

Drug Class: Antiinfective-oral rinse

MECHANISM OF ACTION

An antiseptic and antimicrobial agent that is active against a broad spectrum of microbes. The chlorhexidine molecule, because of its positive charge, reacts with the microbial cell surface, destroys the integrity of the cell membrane, penetrates into the cell, precipitates the cytoplasm, and the cell dies.

Therapeutic Effect: Causes cell death.

USES

Treatment of gingivitis; unlabeled use: acute aphthous ulcers and denture stomatitis

PHARMACOKINETICS

Initially, the chlorhexidine gluconate dental chip releases approximately 40% of the drug within the first 24 hr, then releases the remainder in an almost linear fashion for 7–10 days.
Approximately 30% of the active ingredient, chlorhexidine gluconate, is retained in the oral cavity following oral rinsing. This retained drug is slowly released into the oral fluids. Poorly absorbed from the GI track. Primarily excreted in feces.
Half-life: Unknown.

INDICATIONS AND DOSAGES

▸ **Gingivitis**

Oral Rinse

Adults, Elderly. Swish and spit for 30 sec twice daily.

▸ **Periodontitis**

Oral Insert

Adults, Elderly. One chip is inserted into a periodontal pocket; insert a new chip q3mo; maximum of 8 chips per dental visit.

SIDE EFFECTS/ADVERSE REACTIONS

Occasional

Altered taste, staining of teeth, toothache

PRECAUTIONS AND CONTRAINDICATIONS

Hypersensitivity to chlorhexidine gluconate or any component of the formulation

C

Caution:
Lactation, efficacy not established for children younger than 18 yr, not intended for periodontitis

DRUG INTERACTIONS OF CONCERN TO DENTISTRY

- Disulfiram-like effects resulting from alcohol content: Antabuse, metronidazole

SERIOUS REACTIONS

! Anaphylaxis has been reported.

DENTAL CONSIDERATIONS

General:

- Perform dental examination and prophylaxis/scaling/root planing before starting rinse.
- Place on frequent recall because of oral side effects.
- Use discretion when prescribing to patients with anterior facial restorations with rough surfaces or margins.

Teach Patient/Family to:

- Eat, brush, and floss before using rinse.
- Not rinse with water after using chlorhexidine.
- Not dilute solution; not swallow solution.
- Beware of oral side effects.
- Not brush or use dental floss at site of chip placement.

chlorhexidine gluconate chip

klor-**hex**′-ih-deen **gloo**′-ko-nate
(Perio Chip)

CATEGORY AND SCHEDULE

Pregnancy Risk Category: C

Drug Class: Antiinfective

MECHANISM OF ACTION

Interferes with the integrity of the bacterial cell membrane, causing leakage of the intracellular components; penetrates into the cell, precipitates the cytoplasm, and the cell dies; effective against numerous supragingival and subgingival bacteria.

USES

Adjunct to scaling and root planing for reduction of the subgingival bacterial flora

PHARMACOKINETICS

40% of chlorhexidine released in first 24 hr, remainder released over 7–10 days; no detectable plasma levels.

INDICATIONS AND DOSAGES

Adults. Insert chip into a periodontal pocket with probing depth 5 mm or greater; up to 8 chips may be inserted per single visit; treatment 5 mm in depth; if chip dislodges within 48 hr of placement, replace with new chip; do not replace chips lost after 48 hr, but reevaluate in 3 mo and insert a new chip if pocket depth has not been reduced to less than 5mm; if chip is dislodged 7 days or more after placement, consider this a full course of treatment.

SIDE EFFECTS/ADVERSE REACTIONS

Oral: Localized pain, tenderness, aching, throbbing, toothache
Note: All other side effects reported did not differ from placebo chip

PRECAUTIONS AND CONTRAINDICATIONS

Hypersensitivity
Caution:
Not recommended for acutely abscessed periodontal pocket, use in children not established

DRUG INTERACTIONS OF CONCERN TO DENTISTRY

- None reported

DENTAL CONSIDERATIONS

General:
- Do not brush or use dental floss at site of chip placement.

Teach Patient/Family to:
- Notify dentist immediately if chip is dislodged or if pain, swelling, or other symptoms occur.

chloroquine/ chloroquine phosphate

klor′-oh-kwin/**klor′**-oh-kwin **foss′**-fate
(Aralen hydrochloride, Aralen[CAN]) (Aralen phosphate)

CATEGORY AND SCHEDULE

Pregnancy Risk Category: C

Drug Class: Antimalarial

MECHANISM OF ACTION

An amebacide that concentrates in parasite acid vesicles and may interfere with parasite protein synthesis.
Therapeutic Effect: Increases pH and inhibits parasite growth.

USES

Treatment of malaria caused by *P. vivax, P. malariae, P. ovale, P. falciparum* (some strains); rheumatoid arthritis; amebiasis

PHARMACOKINETICS

Rate of absorption is variable. Chloroquine is almost completely absorbed from the GI tract. Protein binding: 50%–65%. Widely distributed into body tissues such as eyes, heart, kidneys, liver, and lungs. Partially metabolized to active de-ethylated metabolites (principal metabolite is desethylchloroquine). Excreted in urine. Removed by hemodialysis. ***Half-life:*** 1–2 mo.

INDICATIONS AND DOSAGES

Chloroquine Phosphate

▸ **Treatment of Malaria (Acute Attack): Dose (mg Base)**

Dose	Time	Adults	Children
Initial	1 hr	600 mg	10 mg/kg
Second	6 hr later	300 mg	5 mg/kg
Third	Day 2	300 mg	5 mg/kg
Fourth	Day 3	300 mg	5 mg/kg

▸ **Suppression of Malaria**
PO
Adults. 300 mg (base)/wk on same day each week beginning 2 wk before exposure; continue for 6–8 wk after leaving endemic area.
Children. 5 mg (base)/kg/wk.

▸ **Malaria Prophylaxis**
PO
Adults. 600 mg base initially given in 2 divided doses 6 hr apart.
Children. 10 mg base/kg.

C

▸ **Amebiasis**
PO
Adults. 1 g (600 mg base) daily for 2 days; then, 500 mg (300 mg base)/day for at least 2–3 wk.
Chloroquine HCL
▸ **Treatment of Malaria**
IM
Adults. Initially, 160–200 mg base (4–5 ml), repeat in 6 hr. Maximum: 800 mg base in first 24 hr. Begin oral therapy as soon as possible and continue for 3 days until approximately 1.5 g base given.
Children. Initially, 5 mg base/kg, repeat in 6 hr. Do not exceed 10 mg base/kg/24 hr.
▸ **Amebiasis**
IM
Adults. 160–200 mg base (4–5 ml) daily for 10–12 days. Change to oral therapy as soon as possible.

SIDE EFFECTS/ADVERSE REACTIONS

Frequent
Discomfort with IM administration, mild transient headache, anorexia, nausea, vomiting
Occasional
Visual disturbances (blurring, difficulty focusing); nervousness, fatigue, pruritus especially of palms, soles, scalp; bleaching of hair, irritability, personality changes, diarrhea, skin eruptions
Rare
Phlebitis or thrombophlebitis at IV injection site, abdominal cramps, headache, hypotension

PRECAUTIONS AND CONTRAINDICATIONS

Hypersensitivity to 4-aminoquinoline compounds, retinal or visual field changes

DRUG INTERACTIONS OF CONCERN TO DENTISTRY

• Hepatotoxicity: alcohol, hepatotoxic drugs

SERIOUS REACTIONS

! Ocular toxicity and ototoxicity have been reported.
! Prolonged therapy: peripheral neuritis and neuromyopathy, hypotension, ECG changes, agranulocytosis, aplastic anemia, thrombocytopenia, convulsions, psychosis.
! Overdosage includes symptoms of headache, vomiting, visual disturbance, drowsiness, convulsions, hypokalemia followed by cardiovascular collapse, and death.

DENTAL CONSIDERATIONS

General:
• Patients on chronic drug therapy may rarely have symptoms of blood dyscrasias, which can include infection, bleeding, and poor healing.
• Avoid dental light in patient's eyes; offer dark glasses for patient comfort.
• Determine why the patient is taking the drug.
Consultations:
• In a patient with symptoms of blood dyscrasias, request a medical consultation for blood studies and postpone dental treatment until normal values are reestablished.
Teach Patient/Family to:
• Encourage effective oral hygiene to prevent soft tissue inflammation.
• Avoid mouth rinses with high alcohol content because of drying effects.

chlorothiazide

klor-oh-**thye′**-ah-zide
(Diuril, Diuril Sodium)

CATEGORY AND SCHEDULE

Pregnancy Risk Category: C

Drug Class: Thiazide diuretic

MECHANISM OF ACTION

A sulfonamide derivative that acts as a thiazide diuretic and antihypertensive. As a diuretic blocks reabsorption of water, the electrolytes sodium and potassium at cortical diluting segment of distal tubule. As an antihypertensive reduces plasma, extracellular fluid volume, decreases peripheral vascular resistance (PVR) by direct effect on blood vessels.
Therapeutic Effect: Promotes diuresis, reduces B/P.

USES

Treatment of edema, hypertension, diuresis

PHARMACOKINETICS

Poorly absorbed from the GI tract. Not metabolized. Primarily excreted unchanged in urine. Not removed by hemodialysis. ***Half-life:*** 45–120 min.

INDICATIONS AND DOSAGES

▸ **Edema, Hypertension**

PO

Adults. 0.5–1 g 1–2 times a day. May give every other day or 3–5 days a wk.
Children 12 yr and older. 10–20 mg/kg/dose in divided doses q8–12h. Maximum: 2g/day.
Children 2–12 yr. 1 g/day.
Children 6 mo–2 yr. 10–20 mg/kg/day in divided doses q12–24h. Maximum: 375 mg/day.
Children younger than 6 mo. 20–30 mg/kg/day in divided doses q12h. Maximum: 375 mg/day.

▸ **Hypertension**

IV

Adults. 0.5–1 g in divided doses q12–24h.

SIDE EFFECTS/ADVERSE REACTIONS

Expected
Increase in urine frequency and volume
Frequent
Potassium depletion
Occasional
Postural hypotension, headache, GI disturbances, photosensitivity reaction, muscle spasms, alopecia, rash, urticaria

PRECAUTIONS AND CONTRAINDICATIONS

Anuria, history of hypersensitivity to sulfonamides or thiazide diuretics, renal decompensation
Caution:
Hypokalemia, renal disease, hepatic disease, gout, COPD, lupus erythematosus, diabetes mellitus, elderly

DRUG INTERACTIONS OF CONCERN TO DENTISTRY

- Increased photosensitization: tetracyclines
- Decreased hypotensive response, nephrotoxicity: NSAIDs

SERIOUS REACTIONS

! Vigorous diuresis may lead to profound water loss and electrolyte

depletion, resulting in hypokalemia, hyponatremia, and dehydration.
! Acute hypotensive episodes may occur.
! Hyperglycemia may be noted during prolonged therapy.
! GI upset, pancreatitis, dizziness, paresthesias, headache, blood dyscrasias, pulmonary edema, allergic pneumonitis, and dermatologic reactions occur rarely.
! Overdosage can lead to lethargy and coma without changes in electrolytes or hydration.

DENTAL CONSIDERATIONS

General:

- Monitor vital signs at every appointment because of cardiovascular side effects.
- After supine positioning, have patient sit upright for at least 2 min before standing to avoid orthostatic hypotension.
- Patients on chronic drug therapy may rarely have symptoms of blood dyscrasias, which can include infection, bleeding, and poor healing.
- Observe appropriate limitations of vasoconstrictor doses.
- Assess salivary flow as a factor in caries, periodontal disease, and candidiasis.
- Limit use of sodium-containing products, such as saline IV fluids, for patients with a dietary salt restriction.
- Stress from dental procedures may compromise cardiovascular function; determine patient risk.
- Short appointments and a stress-reduction protocol may be required for anxious patients.
- Patients taking diuretics should be monitored for serum K levels.

Consultations:

- In a patient with symptoms of blood dyscrasias, request a medical consultation for blood studies and postpone dental treatment until normal values are reestablished.
- Medical consultation may be required to assess disease control and patient's ability to tolerate stress.
- Physician should be informed if significant xerostomic side effects occur (increased caries, sore tongue, problems eating or swallowing, difficulty wearing prosthesis) so that a medication change can be considered.

Teach Patient/Family to:

- Encourage effective oral hygiene to prevent soft tissue inflammation.
- Use caution to prevent injury when using oral hygiene aids.
- When chronic dry mouth occurs, advise patient to:
  - Avoid mouth rinses with high alcohol content because of drying effects.
  - Use daily home fluoride products for anticaries effect.
  - Use sugarless gum, frequent sips of water, or saliva substitutes.

C

chlorpheniramine

klor-fen-**ir′**-ah-meen
(Aller-Chlor, Chlor-Trimeton, Chlor-Trimeton Allergy, Chlor-Trimeton Allergy 12 Hour, Chlor-Trimeton Allergy 8 Hour, Chlor-Tripolon[CAN], Chlorate, Chlorphen, Diabetic Tussin Allergy Relief)
Do not confuse with chlorpromazine or chlorpropamide.

CATEGORY AND SCHEDULE

Pregnancy Risk Category: C
OTC (tablets, syrup)

Drug Class: Antihistamine, H_1-receptor antagonist

MECHANISM OF ACTION

A propylamine derivative antihistamine that competes with histamine for H_1 histamine receptor sites on cells in the blood vessels, GI tract, and respiratory tract. ***Therapeutic Effect:*** Inhibits symptoms associated with seasonal allergic rhinitis such as increased mucus production and sneezing.

USES

Allergy symptoms, rhinitis

PHARMACOKINETICS

Well absorbed after PO and parenteral administration. Food delays absorption. Widely distributed. Metabolized in liver. Primarily excreted in urine. Not removed by dialysis. ***Half-life:*** 20 hr.

INDICATIONS AND DOSAGES

▸ **Allergic Rhinitis, Common Cold**

PO

Adults, Elderly. 4 mg q6–8h or 8–12 mg (sustained-release) q8–12h. Maximum: 24 mg/day.

Children 12 yr and older. 4 mg q6–8h or 8 mg (sustained-release) q12h. Maximum: 24 mg/day.

Children 6–11 yr. 2 mg q4–6h. Maximum: 12 mg/day.

IM/IV/SC

Adults, Elderly. 5–40 mg as a single dose. Maximum: 40 mg/day.

SC

Children 6 yr and older. 87.5 mcg/kg or 2.5 mg/m^2 4 times a day.

SIDE EFFECTS/ADVERSE REACTIONS

Frequent

Drowsiness, dizziness, muscular weakness, hypotension, dry mouth, nose, throat, and lips, urinary retention, thickening of bronchial secretions

Elderly: Sedation, dizziness, hypotension

Occasional

Epigastric distress, flushing, visual or hearing disturbances, paresthesia, diaphoresis, chills

PRECAUTIONS AND CONTRAINDICATIONS

Hypersensitivity to chlorpheniramine or its components

DRUG INTERACTIONS OF CONCERN TO DENTISTRY

- Increased CNS depression: alcohol, all CNS depressants
- Increased anticholinergic effect: other anticholinergics, phenothiazines, tricyclic antidepressants

C

SERIOUS REACTIONS

! Children may experience dominant paradoxical reactions, including restlessness, insomnia, euphoria, nervousness, and tremors.
! Overdosage in children may result in hallucinations, seizures, and death.
! Hypersensitivity reaction, such as eczema, pruritus, rash, cardiac disturbances, and photosensitivity, may occur.
! Overdosage may vary from CNS depression, including sedation, apnea, hypotension, cardiovascular collapse, or death to severe paradoxical reaction, such as hallucinations, tremors, and seizures.

DENTAL CONSIDERATIONS

General:

- Assess salivary flow as a factor in caries, periodontal disease, and candidiasis.
- Consider semisupine chair position for patients with respiratory disease.
- Determine why the patient is taking the drug.

Teach Patient/Family to:

- Encourage effective oral hygiene to prevent soft tissue inflammation.
- Use caution to prevent injury when using oral hygiene aids.
- When chronic dry mouth occurs, advise patient to:
  - Avoid mouth rinses with high alcohol content because of drying effects.
  - Use daily home fluoride products for anticaries effect.
  - Use sugarless gum, frequent sips of water, or saliva substitutes.

chlorpromazine

klor-**proe**′-ma-zeen
(Chlorpromanyl[CAN], Largactil[CAN], Thorazine)
Do not confuse chlorpromazine with chlorpropamide, clomipramine, or prochlorperazine, or Thorazine with thiamide or thioridazine.

CATEGORY AND SCHEDULE

Pregnancy Risk Category: C

Drug Class: Phenothiazine antipsychotic

MECHANISM OF ACTION

A phenothiazine that blocks dopamine neurotransmission at postsynaptic dopamine receptor sites. Possesses strong anticholinergic, sedative, and antiemetic effects; moderate extrapyramidal effects; and slight antihistamine action.
Therapeutic Effect: Relieves nausea and vomiting; improves psychotic conditions; controls intractable hiccups and porphyria.

USES

Psychotic disorders, mania, schizophrenia, anxiety, intractable hiccups, nausea, vomiting, preoperatively for relaxation, acute intermittent porphyria, behavioral problems in children

PHARMACOKINETICS

Rapidly absorbed after oral or IM administration. Protein binding: 92%–97%. Metabolized in the liver. Excreted in urine. ***Half-life:*** 6 hr.

INDICATIONS AND DOSAGES

▸ Severe Nausea or Vomiting

PO
Adults, Elderly. 10–25 mg q4–6h.
Children. 0.5–1 mg/kg q4–6h.
IV, IM
Adults, Elderly. 25–50 mg q4–6h.
Children. 0.5–1 mg/kg q6–8h.
Rectal
Adults, Elderly. 50–100 mg q6–8h.
Children. 1 mg/kg q6–8h.

▸ Psychotic Disorders

PO
Adults, Elderly. 30–800 mg/day in 1–4 divided doses.
Children older than 6 mo. 0.5–1 mg/kg q4–6h.
IV, IM
Adults, Elderly. Initially, 25 mg; may repeat in 1–4 hr. May gradually increase to 400 mg q4–6h. Maximum: 300–800 mg/day.
Children older than 6 mo. 0.5–1 mg/kg q6–8h. Maximum: 75 mg/day for children 5–12 yr; 40 mg/day for children younger than 5 yr.

▸ Intractable Hiccups

PO, IV, IM
Adults. 25–50 mg 3 times a day.

▸ Porphyria

PO
Adults. 25–50 mg 3–4 times a day.
IM
Adults, Elderly. 25 mg 3–4 times a day.

SIDE EFFECTS/ADVERSE REACTIONS

Frequent
Somnolence, blurred vision, hypotension, color vision or night vision disturbances, dizziness, decreased sweating, constipation, dry mouth, nasal congestion
Occasional
Urinary retention, photosensitivity, rash, decreased sexual function, swelling or pain in breasts, weight gain, nausea, vomiting, abdominal pain, tremors

PRECAUTIONS AND CONTRAINDICATIONS

Comatose states, myelosuppression, severe cardiovascular disease, severe CNS depression, subcortical brain damage
Caution:
Lactation, seizure disorders, hypertension, hepatic disease, cardiac disease, elderly

DRUG INTERACTIONS OF CONCERN TO DENTISTRY

- Increased sedation: other CNS depressants, alcohol, barbiturate anesthetics, opioid analgesics
- Hypotension, tachycardia: epinephrine (systemic)
- Increased extrapyramidal effects: related drugs, such as haloperidol, droperidol, and metoclopramide
- Additive photosensitization: tetracyclines
- Increased anticholinergic effects: anticholinergics

SERIOUS REACTIONS

! Extrapyramidal symptoms appear to be dose related and are divided into three categories: akathisia (including inability to sit still, tapping of feet), parkinsonian symptoms (such as masklike face, tremors, shuffling gait, hypersalivation), and acute dystonias (including torticollis, opisthotonos, and oculogyric crisis). A dystonic reaction may also produce diaphoresis and pallor.
! Tardive dyskinesia, including tongue protrusion, puffing of the cheeks, and puckering of the mouth is a rare reaction that may be irreversible.

C

! Abrupt discontinuation after long-term therapy may precipitate nausea, vomiting, gastritis, dizziness, and tremors.
! Blood dyscrasias, particularly agranulocytosis and mild leukopenia, may occur.
! Chlorpromazine may lower the seizure threshold.

DENTAL CONSIDERATIONS

General:

- Monitor vital signs at every appointment because of cardiovascular side effects.
- Patients on chronic drug therapy may rarely have symptoms of blood dyscrasias, which can include infection, bleeding, and poor healing.
- After supine positioning, have patient sit upright for at least 2 min before standing to avoid orthostatic hypotension.
- Assess salivary flow as a factor in caries, periodontal disease, and candidiasis.
- Avoid dental light in patient's eyes; offer dark glasses for patient comfort.
- Assess for presence of extrapyramidal motor symptoms, such as tardive dyskinesia and akathisia. Extrapyramidal motor activity may complicate dental treatment.
- Geriatric patients are more susceptible to drug effects; use a lower dose.

Consultations:

- In a patient with symptoms of blood dyscrasias, request a medical consultation for blood studies and postpone dental treatment until normal values are reestablished.
- Take precautions if dental surgery is anticipated and anesthesia is required.
- If signs of tardive dyskinesia or akathisia are present, refer to physician.
- Physician should be informed if significant xerostomic side effects occur (increased caries, sore tongue, problems eating or swallowing, difficulty wearing prosthesis) so that a medication change can be considered.

Teach Patient/Family to:

- Encourage effective oral hygiene to prevent soft tissue inflammation.
- Use caution to prevent injury when using oral hygiene aids.
- Use powered tooth brush if patient has difficulty holding conventional devices.
- When chronic dry mouth occurs, advise patient to:
  - Avoid mouth rinses with high alcohol content because of drying effects.
  - Use daily home fluoride products for anticaries effect.
  - Use sugarless gum, frequent sips of water, or saliva substitutes.

chlorpropamide

klor-**pro′**-pa-mide
(Apo-Chlorpropamide[CAN], Diabinese)
Do not confuse with chlorpromazine.

CATEGORY AND SCHEDULE

Pregnancy Risk Category: C

Drug Class: Antidiabetic, sulfonylurea (first generation)

MECHANISM OF ACTION

A first-generation sulfonylurea that promotes release of insulin from beta cells of pancreas.

Therapeutic Effect: Lowers blood glucose concentration.

USES

Treatment of stable adult-onset diabetes mellitus (Type 2)

PHARMACOKINETICS

Rapidly absorbed from the GI tract. Protein binding: 60%–90%. Extensively metabolized in liver. Excreted primarily in urine. Removed by hemodialysis. ***Half-life:*** 30–42 hr.

INDICATIONS AND DOSAGES

▸ Diabetes Mellitus, Combination Therapy

PO

Adults. Initially, 250 mg once a day. Maintenance: 250–500 mg once a day. Maximum: 750 mg/day.

Elderly. Initially, 100–125 mg once a day. Maintenance: 100–250 mg once a day. Increase or decrease by 50–125 mg a day for 3- to 5-day intervals.

▸ Renal Function Impairment

Not recommended.

SIDE EFFECTS/ADVERSE REACTIONS

Frequent

Headache, upper respiratory tract infection

Occasional

Sinusitis, myalgia (muscle aches), pharyngitis, aggravated diabetes mellitus

PRECAUTIONS AND CONTRAINDICATIONS

Diabetic complications, such as ketosis, acidosis, and diabetic coma, severe liver or renal impairment, sole therapy for type 1 diabetes mellitus, or hypersensitivity to sulfonylureas

Caution:

Elderly, cardiac disease, thyroid disease, renal disease, hepatic disease, severe hypoglycemic reactions, avoid use in lactation, use in children not established

DRUG INTERACTIONS OF CONCERN TO DENTISTRY

- Increased hypoglycemic effects: salicylates, NSAIDs, ketoconazole, miconazole
- Decreased action: corticosteroids, sympathomimetics
- Disulfiram-like reaction: alcohol

SERIOUS REACTIONS

! Possible increased risk of cardiovascular mortality with this class of drugs.

! Overdosage can cause severe hypoglycemia prolonged by extended half-life.

DENTAL CONSIDERATIONS

General:

- Patients on chronic drug therapy may rarely have symptoms of blood dyscrasias, which can include infection, bleeding, and poor healing.
- Short appointments and a stress-reduction protocol may be required for anxious patients.
- Question patient about self-monitoring of drug's antidiabetic effect, including blood glucose values or finger-stick records.
- Ensure that patient is following prescribed diet and regularly takes medication.
- Determine if medication controls disease. Patients with diabetes may be more susceptible to infection and have delayed wound healing.
- Avoid prescribing aspirin-containing products.

C

Consultations:
- In a patient with symptoms of blood dyscrasias, request a medical consultation for blood studies and postpone dental treatment until normal values are reestablished.
- Medical consultation may be required to assess disease control.
- Medical consultation may include data from patient's blood glucose monitoring, including glycosylated hemoglobin or HbA1c testing.

Teach Patient/Family to:
- Encourage effective oral hygiene to prevent soft tissue inflammation.
- Use caution to prevent injury when using oral hygiene aids.
- Avoid mouth rinses with high alcohol content because of drying effects.

chlorthalidone

klor-**thal′**-ih-doan
(Apo-Chlorthalidone[CAN], Hygroton[AUS], Thalitone)

CATEGORY AND SCHEDULE

Pregnancy Risk Category: B (D if used in pregnancy-induced hypertension)

Drug Class: Diuretic with thiazide-like effects

MECHANISM OF ACTION

A thiazide diuretic that blocks reabsorption of sodium, potassium, and water at the distal convoluted tubule; also decreases plasma and extracellular fluid volume and peripheral vascular resistance.
Therapeutic Effect: Produces diuresis; lowers B/P.

USES

Treatment of edema, hypertension, diuresis, CHF

PHARMACOKINETICS

Rapidly absorbed from the GI tract. Excreted unchanged in urine.
Half-life: 35–50 hr. Onset of antihypertensive effect: 3–4 days; optimal therapeutic effect: 3–4 wk.

INDICATIONS AND DOSAGES

▸ **Hypertension, Edema**

PO

Adults. 25–100 mg/day or 100 mg 3 times a week.

Elderly. Initially, 12.5–25 mg/day or every other day.

SIDE EFFECTS/ADVERSE REACTIONS

Expected

Increase in urinary frequency and urine volume

Frequent

Potassium depletion (rarely produces symptoms)

Occasional

Anorexia, impotence, diarrhea, orthostatic hypotension, GI disturbances, photosensitivity

Rare

Rash

PRECAUTIONS AND CONTRAINDICATIONS

Anuria, history of hypersensitivity to sulfonamides or thiazide diuretics, renal decompensation

Caution:

Hypokalemia, renal disease, hepatic disease, gout, diabetes mellitus, elderly, lactation

DRUG INTERACTIONS OF CONCERN TO DENTISTRY

- Increased photosensitization: tetracyclines

• Decreased hypotensive response, nephrotoxicity: NSAIDs, indomethacin

SERIOUS REACTIONS

! Vigorous diuresis may lead to profound water and electrolyte depletion, resulting in hypokalemia, hyponatremia, and dehydration.
! Acute hypotensive episodes may occur.
! Hyperglycemia may occur during prolonged therapy.
! Overdose can lead to lethargy and coma without changes in electrolytes or hydration.

DENTAL CONSIDERATIONS

General:
• Monitor vital signs at every appointment because of cardiovascular side effects.
• After supine positioning, have patient sit upright for at least 2 min before standing to avoid orthostatic hypotension.
• Patients on chronic drug therapy may rarely have symptoms of blood dyscrasias, which can include infection, bleeding, and poor healing.
• Assess salivary flow as a factor in caries, periodontal disease, and candidiasis.
• Limit use of sodium-containing products, such as saline IV fluids, for those patients with a dietary salt restriction.
• Short appointments and a stress-reduction protocol may be required for anxious patients.
• Observe appropriate limitations of vasoconstrictor doses.
• Stress from dental procedures may compromise cardiovascular function; determine patient risk.

Consultations:
• In a patient with symptoms of blood dyscrasias, request a medical consultation for blood studies and postpone dental treatment until normal values are reestablished.
• Medical consultation may be required to assess disease control and patient's ability to tolerate stress.

Teach Patient/Family to:
• Encourage effective oral hygiene to prevent soft tissue inflammation.
• Use caution to prevent injury when using oral hygiene aids.
• When chronic dry mouth occurs, advise patient to:
  • Avoid mouth rinses with high alcohol content because of drying effects.
  • Use daily home fluoride products for anticaries effect.
  • Use sugarless gum, frequent sips of water, or saliva substitutes.

chlorzoxazone

klor-zox′-ah-zone
(Parafon Forte DSC, Remular, Remular-S)
Do not confuse with chlorthalidone.

CATEGORY AND SCHEDULE

Pregnancy Risk Category: C

Drug Class: Skeletal muscle relaxant, centrally acting

MECHANISM OF ACTION

A skeletal muscle relaxant that inhibits transmission of reflexes at the spinal cord level.
Therapeutic Effect: Relieves muscle spasticity.

C

USES
Adjunct for relief of muscle spasm in musculoskeletal conditions

PHARMACOKINETICS
Readily absorbed from the GI tract. Metabolized in liver. Primarily excreted in urine. ***Half-life:*** 1.1 hr.

INDICATIONS AND DOSAGES
▸ **Musculoskeletal Pain**
PO
Adults, Elderly. 250–500 mg 3–4 times a day. Maximum: 750 mg 3–4 day.
Children. 20 mg/kg/day in 3–4 divided doses.

SIDE EFFECTS/ADVERSE REACTIONS
Frequent
Drowsiness, fever, headache
Occasional
Nausea, vomiting, stomach cramps, rash

PRECAUTIONS AND CONTRAINDICATIONS
Hypersensitivity to chlorzoxazone or any one of its components
Caution:
Lactation, hepatic disease, elderly

DRUG INTERACTIONS OF CONCERN TO DENTISTRY
- Increased CNS depression: alcohol, narcotics, barbiturates, sedatives, hypnotics

SERIOUS REACTIONS
! Overdosage results in nausea, vomiting, diarrhea, and hypotension.

DENTAL CONSIDERATIONS
General:
- Determine why the patient is taking the drug.
- Consider semisupine chair position if back is involved.
- When used for dental-related problems, consider aspirin or NSAIDs to improve response.

cholestyramine resin
koe-less-**tir′**-ah-meen
(Novo-Cholamine[CAN], Prevalite, Questran[CAN], Questran Lite[AUS])
Do not confuse Questran with Quarzan.

CATEGORY AND SCHEDULE
Pregnancy Risk Category: B

Drug Class: Antihyperlipidemic

MECHANISM OF ACTION
An antihyperlipoproteinemic that binds with bile acids in the intestine, forming an insoluble complex. Binding results in partial removal of bile acid from enterohepatic circulation.
Therapeutic Effect: Blocks absorption of cholesterol from GI tract.

USES
Treatment of primary hypercholesterolemia, pruritus associated with biliary obstruction, diarrhea caused by excess bile acid, digitalis toxicity, xanthomas

PHARMACOKINETICS
Not absorbed from the GI tract. Decreases in serum LDL apparent in 5–7 days and in serum cholesterol in 1 mo. Serum cholesterol returns to baseline levels about 1 mo after drug is discontinued.

INDICATIONS AND DOSAGES

▸ **Primary Hypercholesterolemia**

PO

Adults, Elderly. 3–4 g 3–4 times a day. Maximum: 16–32 g/day in 2–4 divided doses.

Children older than 10 yr. 2 g/day. Maximum: 8 g/day in 2 or more divided doses.

Children 10 yr and younger. Initially, 2 g/day. Range: 1–4 g/day.

▸ **Pruritus**

PO

Adults, Elderly. 4 g 1–2 times a day. Maintenance: Up to 24 g/day in divided doses.

SIDE EFFECTS/ADVERSE REACTIONS

Frequent

Constipation (may lead to fecal impaction), nausea, vomiting, abdominal pain, indigestion

Occasional

Diarrhea, belching, bloating, headache, dizziness

Rare

Gallstones, peptic ulcer disease, malabsorption syndrome

PRECAUTIONS AND CONTRAINDICATIONS

Complete biliary obstruction, hypersensitivity to cholestyramine or tartrazine (frequently seen in aspirin hypersensitivity)

Caution:

Lactation, children

DRUG INTERACTIONS OF CONCERN TO DENTISTRY

• Decreased absorption of tetracyclines, cephalexin, phenobarbital, corticosteroids, clindamycin, penicillins; administer doses several hours apart

SERIOUS REACTIONS

! GI tract obstruction, hyperchloremic acidosis, and osteoporosis secondary to calcium excretion may occur.

! High dosage may interfere with fat absorption, resulting in steatorrhea.

DENTAL CONSIDERATIONS

General:

• Consider semisupine chair position for patient comfort because of GI side effects of disease.

ciclesonide

sye-**kles**′-oh-nide

(Alvesco, Omnaris)

CATEGORY AND SCHEDULE

Pregnancy Risk Category: C

Drug Class: Glucocorticoid

MECHANISM OF ACTION

The exact mechanism of action of corticosteroids in asthma is unknown. Ciclesonide is a non-halogenated glucocorticoid prodrug, hydrolyzed to a pharmacologically-active metabolite, C21-desisobutyryl-ciclesonide (des-ciclesonide or RM1) following oral inhalation. Has antiinflammatory and inhibitory activities against various mediators (e.g., histamine) and cell types (e.g., mast cells).

PHARMACOKINETICS

Absorption: minimal systemic absorption (intranasal); about 52% following oral inhalation. Protein binding: 99% or higher. Metabolized in the liver by CYP 3A4 and 2D6. It is hydrolyzed into active metabolites, des-ciclesonide by esterases enzymes in nasal mucosa and lungs. Excreted primarily in feces (66% [intranasal]); partially in urine (20% [intranasal]); Oral inhalation: feces (78%). ***Half-life***: Oral inhalation: 5–7 hr (metabolites); less than 1 hr (parent compound).

INDICATIONS AND DOSAGES

▸ **Asthma**

Oral Inhalation (Alvesco)

Adults, Children 12 yr and older. Prior therapy with bronchodilators alone: 80 mcg twice daily (max: 160 mcg twice day). Prior therapy with inhaled corticosteroids: 80 mcg twice daily (max: 320 mcg twice daily). Prior therapy with oral corticosteroids: 320 mcg twice daily (max: 320 mcg twice daily).

▸ **Allergic Rhinitis**

Nasal (Omnaris)

Adults, Children 6 yr and older. 200 mcg daily (2 sprays [50 mcg/spray]) in each nostril once daily. Do not exceed a total daily dose of 2 sprays in each nostril.

SIDE EFFECTS/ADVERSE REACTIONS

Frequent

Nasal: Mild nasopharyngeal irritation, burning, stinging, or dryness; headache, cough

Oral inhalation: Flu-like symptoms, headache, pharyngitis

Occasional

Nasal: Dry mouth, dyspepsia, rebound congestion, rhinorrhea, loss of taste

Inhalation: Back pain, vomiting, altered taste, voice changes, abdominal pain, nausea, dyspepsia

Rare

Facial edema, oral candidiasis, arthralgia, back pain, weight gain, cough, rash, rhinorrhea

PRECAUTIONS AND CONTRAINDICATIONS

Hypersensitivity to ciclesonide, corticosteroids, or any component of the formulations

Acute asthma and status asthmaticus (oral inhalation)

Untreated fungal, bacterial, or tuberculosis infections of the respiratory tract

Hypertension, diabetes mellitus, osteoporosis, peptic ulcer, glaucoma, cataracts, suppression of the hypothalamic-pituitary-adrenal (HPA) axis

DRUG INTERACTIONS OF CONCERN TO DENTISTRY

- Antifungals (azole): May increase levels of ciclesonide.
- CYP3A4 inhibitors (e.g., azole antifungals): May increase the levels and effects of ciclesonide.
- Quinolone antibiotics: May enhance the adverse effects of corticosteroids.

SERIOUS REACTIONS

! May cause adrenocortical suppression, which can lead to adrenal crisis, especially in younger children or in patients receiving high doses for prolonged periods.

DENTAL CONSIDERATIONS

General:

- Determine frequency and severity of asthmatic attacks.
- Assess salivary flow as a factor in caries, periodontal disease, and candidiasis.
- Mid-day appointments are suggested with stress-reduction protocol for anxious patients.
- Place on frequent recall because of oral side effects, including oropharyngeal candidiasis.

- Acute asthmatic episodes may be precipitated in dental office. Rapid-acting sympathomimetic inhalants should be available for emergency use.

Consultations:

- Medical consultation may be required to assess disease control and ability of patient to tolerate dental treatment.

Teach Patient/Family to:

- Encourage effective oral hygiene to prevent soft tissue inflammation.
- When chronic dry mouth occurs, advise patient to:
  - Avoid mouth rinses with high alcohol content because of drying effects.
  - Use daily home fluoride products for anticaries effect.
  - Use sugarless gum, frequent sips of water or artificial saliva substitutes.

ciclopirox

sye-kloe-**peer′**-ox
(Loprox, Penlac)
Do not confuse with ciprofloxacin.

CATEGORY AND SCHEDULE

Pregnancy Risk Category: B

Drug Class: Topical antifungal

MECHANISM OF ACTION

An antifungal that inhibits the transport of essential elements in the fungal cell, thereby interfering with biosynthesis in fungi.
Therapeutic Effect: Results in fungal cell death.

USES

Treatment of tinea cruris, tinea corporis, tinea pedis, tinea versicolor, cutaneous candidiasis, nail solution for immunocompetent patients with mild to moderate onychomycosis of nails without lunula involvement; caused by *T. rubrum*

PHARMACOKINETICS

Absorbed through intact skin. Distributed to epidermis, dermis, including hair, hair follicles, and sebaceous glands. Protein binding: 98%. Primarily excreted in urine and to a lesser extent in feces. ***Half-life:*** 1.7 hr.

INDICATIONS AND DOSAGES

▸ Tinea Pedis

Topical
Adults, Elderly, Children 10 yr and older. Apply 2 times a day until signs and symptoms significantly improve.

▸ Tinea Cruris, Tinea Corporis

Topical
Adults, Elderly, Children 10 yr and older. Apply 2 times a day until signs and symptoms significantly improve.

▸ Onychomycosis

Topical (Solution)
Adults, Elderly, Children 10 yr and older. Apply to the affected area (nails) daily. Remove with alcohol every 7 days.

▸ Seborrheic Dermatitis

Shampoo
Adults, Elderly, Children 10 yr and older. Apply to affected scalp areas 2 times a day, in the morning and evening for 4 wk.

SIDE EFFECTS/ADVERSE REACTIONS

Rare
Topical: Irritation, burning, redness, pain at the site of application

C

PRECAUTIONS AND CONTRAINDICATIONS

Hypersensitivity to ciclopirox or any one of its components

Caution:

Lactation, children younger than 10 yr

DRUG INTERACTIONS OF CONCERN TO DENTISTRY

- None reported

SERIOUS REACTIONS

! None known

DENTAL CONSIDERATIONS

General:

- There are neither dental drug interactions nor relevant considerations to dentistry for this drug.

cimetidine

sye-**met′**-ih-deen

(Apo-Cimetidine[CAN], Cimehexal[AUS], Magicul[AUS], Novocimetine[CAN], Peptol[CAN], Sigmetadine[AUS], Tagamet, Tagamet HB)

Do not confuse cimetidine with simethicone.

CATEGORY AND SCHEDULE

Pregnancy Risk Category: B

Drug Class: H_2 histamine receptor antagonist

OTC (100 mg tablets)

MECHANISM OF ACTION

An antiulcer agent and gastric acid secretion inhibitor that inhibits histamine action at H_2 receptor sites of parietal cells.

Therapeutic Effect: Inhibits gastric acid secretion during fasting, at night, or when stimulated by food, caffeine, or insulin.

USES

Short-term treatment of duodenal and benign gastric ulcers and maintenance; gastroesophageal reflux disease (GERD), upper GI bleeding, pathologic hypersecretory diseases and heartburn with acid indigestion

PHARMACOKINETICS

Well absorbed from the GI tract. Protein binding: 15%–20%. Widely distributed. Metabolized in the liver. Primarily excreted in urine. Not removed by hemodialysis. ***Half-life:*** 2 hr; increased with impaired renal function.

INDICATIONS AND DOSAGES

▸ Active Ulcer

PO

Adults, Elderly. 300 mg 4 times a day or 400 mg twice a day or 800 mg at bedtime.

IV, IM

Adults, Elderly. 300 mg q6h or 150 mg as single dose followed by 37.5 mg/hr continuous infusion.

▸ Prevention of Duodenal Ulcer

PO

Adults, Elderly. 400–800 mg at bedtime.

▸ Gastric Hypersecretory Secretions

PO, IV, IM

Adults, Elderly. 300–600 mg q6h. Maximum: 2400 mg/day.

Children. 20–40 mg/kg/day in divided doses q6h.

Infants. 10–20 mg/kg/day in divided doses q6–12h.

Neonates. 5–10 mg/kg/day in divided doses q8–12h.

▸ **GERD**
PO
Adults, Elderly. 800 mg twice a day or 400 mg 4 times a day for 12 wk.
▸ **OTC Use**
PO
Adults, Elderly. 100 mg up to 30 min before meals. Maximum: 2 doses a day.
▸ **Prevention of Upper GI Bleeding**
IV Infusion
Adults, Elderly. 50 mg/hr.
▸ **Dosage in Renal Impairment**
Dosage is based on a 300-mg dose in adults. Dosage interval is modified on the basis of creatinine clearance.

Creatinine Clearance	Dosage Interval
Greater than 40 ml/min	q6h
20–40 ml/min	q8h or decrease dose by 25%
Less than 20 ml/min	q12h or decrease dose by 50%

Give after hemodialysis and q12h between dialysis sessions.

SIDE EFFECTS/ADVERSE REACTIONS

Occasional
Headache
Elderly and severely ill patients, patients with impaired renal function: Confusion, agitation, psychosis, depression, anxiety, disorientation, hallucinations. Effects reverse 3–4 days after discontinuance
Rare
Diarrhea, dizziness, somnolence, nausea, vomiting, gynecomastia, rash, impotence

PRECAUTIONS AND CONTRAINDICATIONS

Hypersensitivity to other H_2-antagonists
Caution:
Lactation, children younger than 12 yr, organic brain syndrome, hepatic disease, renal disease, smoking

DRUG INTERACTIONS OF CONCERN TO DENTISTRY

- GI ulceration, bleeding: aspirin, NSAIDs
- Decreased absorption: sodium bicarbonate, anticholinergics
- Decreased absorption of fluconazole, ketoconazole, tetracycline (take doses 2 hr apart), ferrous salts
- Increased blood levels of metronidazole, alcohol, lidocaine, narcotic analgesics, benzodiazepines, carbamazepine

SERIOUS REACTIONS

! Rapid IV administration may produce cardiac arrhythmias and hypotension.

DENTAL CONSIDERATIONS

General:
- Monitor vital signs at every appointment because of cardiovascular side effects.
- Consider semisupine chair position for patient comfort because of GI side effects of disease.
- Avoid prescribing aspirin- or NSAID-containing products in patients with active upper GI disease; risk of irritation and ulceration exists.
- Sodium bicarbonate products can be used 1 hr before or 1 hr after cimetidine dose.

Teach Patient/Family to:
- Encourage effective oral hygiene to prevent soft tissue inflammation.
- Use caution to prevent injury when using oral hygiene aids.

ciprofloxacin hydrochloride

sip-ro-**floks**′-ah-sin
hi-droe-**klor**′-ide
(C-Flox[AUS], Ciloquin[AUS], Ciloxan, Cipro, Ciproxin[AUS])
Do not confuse ciprofloxacin or Ciproxin with Ciloxan, cinoxacin, or Cytoxan.

CATEGORY AND SCHEDULE

Pregnancy Risk Category: C

Drug Class: Topical fluoroquinolone antiinfective

MECHANISM OF ACTION

A fluoroquinolone that inhibits the enzyme DNA gyrase in susceptible bacteria, interfering with bacterial cell replication.
Therapeutic Effect: Bactericidal.

USES

Infections caused by susceptible strains of microorganisms in conjunctivitis or corneal ulcers

PHARMACOKINETICS

Well absorbed from the GI tract (food delays absorption). Protein binding: 20%–40%. Widely distributed (including to CSF). Metabolized in the liver to active metabolite. Primarily excreted in urine. Minimal removal by hemodialysis. ***Half-life:*** 4–6 hr (increased in impaired renal function and the elderly).

INDICATIONS AND DOSAGES

▸ Mild to Moderate UTIs

PO
Adults, Elderly. 250 mg q12h.
IV
Adults, Elderly. 200 mg q12h.

▸ Complicated UTIs; Mild to Moderate Respiratory Tract, Bone, Joint, Skin, and Skin-Structure Infections; Infectious Diarrhea

PO
Adults, Elderly. 500 mg q12h.
IV
Adults, Elderly. 400 mg q12h.

▸ Severe, Complicated Infections

PO
Adults, Elderly. 750 mg q12h.
IV
Adults, Elderly. 400 mg q12h.

▸ Prostatitis

PO
Adults, Elderly. 500 mg q12h for 28 days.

▸ Uncomplicated Bladder Infection

PO
Adults. 100 mg twice a day for 3 days.

▸ Acute Sinusitis

PO
Adults. 500 mg q12h.

▸ Uncomplicated Gonorrhea

PO
Adults. 250 mg as a single dose.

▸ Cystic Fibrosis

IV
Children. 30 mg/kg/day in 2–3 divided doses. Maximum: 1.2 g/day.
PO
Children. 40 mg/kg/day. Maximum: 2 g/day.

▸ Corneal Ulcer

Ophthalmic
Adults, Elderly. 2 drops q15min for 6 hr, then 2 drops q30min for the remainder of first day, 2 drops q1h on second day, and 2 drops q4h on days 3–14.

▸ Conjunctivitis

Ophthalmic
Adults, Elderly. 1–2 drops q2h for 2 days, then 2 drops q4h for next 5 days.

▸ **Dosage in Renal Impairment**
Dosage and frequency are modified on the basis of creatinine clearance and the severity of the infection.

Creatinine Clearance	Dosage Interval
Less than 30 ml/min	Usual dose q18–24h

▸ **Hemodialysis**
Adults, Elderly. 250–500 mg q24h (after dialysis).
▸ **Peritoneal Dialysis**
Adults, Elderly. 250–500 mg q24h (after dialysis).

SIDE EFFECTS/ADVERSE REACTIONS

Frequent
Nausea, diarrhea, dyspepsia, vomiting, constipation, flatulence, confusion, crystalluria
Ophthalmic: Burning, crusting in corner of eye
Occasional
Abdominal pain or discomfort, headache, rash
Ophthalmic: Bad taste, sensation of something in eye, eyelid redness or itching
Rare
Dizziness, confusion, tremors, hallucinations, hypersensitivity reaction, insomnia, dry mouth, paresthesia

PRECAUTIONS AND CONTRAINDICATIONS

Hypersensitivity to ciprofloxacin or other quinolones; for ophthalmic administration: vaccinia, varicella, epithelial herpes simplex, keratitis, mycobacterial infection, fungal disease of ocular structure, use after uncomplicated removal of a foreign body

Caution:
Lactation, children, renal disease, tendon ruptures of shoulder, hand, and Achilles tendons, epilepsy, severe cerebral arteriosclerosis; monitor blood glucose levels, extended release tablets can be taken with meals, defects in glucose-6-phosphate dehydrogenase activity, myasthenia gravis

DRUG INTERACTIONS OF CONCERN TO DENTISTRY

- Decreased absorption: divalent, trivalent antacids, iron and zinc salts, calcium fortified juices.
- Increased serum levels: probenecid.
- Increased risk of bleeding with warfarin (monitor).
- Serious adverse effects with theophylline, caffeine.
- Specific studies have not been conducted with topical ciprofloxacin.

SERIOUS REACTIONS

! Superinfection (especially enterococcal or fungal), nephropathy, cardiopulmonary arrest, chest pain, and cerebral thrombosis may occur.
! Hypersensitivity reactions, including photosensitivity (as evidenced by rash, pruritus, blisters, edema, and burning skin), have occurred in patients receiving fluoroquinolones.
! Arthropathy may occur if the drug is given to children younger than 18 yr.
! Sensitization to the ophthalmic form of the drug may contraindicate later systemic use of ciprofloxacin.

C

DENTAL CONSIDERATIONS

General:

- Determine why the patient is taking the drug.
- Avoid dental light in patient's eyes; offer dark glasses for patient comfort.
- Minimize exposure to sunlight and wear sunscreen if sun exposure is planned.
- Ruptures of the shoulder, hand, and Achilles tendon requiring surgical repair or resulting in prolonged disability have been reported with this drug.
- Protect patient's eyes from accidental spatter during dental treatment.
- Avoid dental light in patient's eyes; offer dark glasses for patient comfort.

Consultations:

- Consult with patient's physician if an acute dental infection occurs and another antiinfective is required.

Teach Patient/Family to:

- Discontinue treatment and inform dentist immediately if patient experiences pain or inflammation of a tendon, and to rest and refrain from exercise.

cisplatin

sis-**plah'**-tin
(Platinol-AQ)
Do not confuse cisplatin with carboplatin, or Platinol with Paraplatin or Patanol.

CATEGORY AND SCHEDULE

Pregnancy Risk Category: D

Drug Class: Platinum coordination complex; antineoplastic

MECHANISM OF ACTION

A platinum coordination complex that inhibits DNA and to a lesser extent, RNA, protein synthesis by cross-linking with DNA strands, preventing cell division. Cell cycle-phase nonspecific.
Therapeutic Effect: Interferes with DNA function.

USES

Treatment of metastatic testicular tumors, metastatic ovarian tumors, advanced bladder carcinoma

PHARMACOKINETICS

Widely distributed. Protein binding: greater than 90%. Undergoes rapid nonenzymatic conversion to inactive metabolite. Excreted in urine. Removed by hemodialysis. ***Half-life:*** 58–73 hr (increased with impaired renal function).

INDICATIONS AND DOSAGES

▸ **Advanced Bladder Carcinoma, Metastatic Ovarian Tumors, Metastatic Testicular Tumors**

IV

Adults, Elderly, Children. For intermittent dosage schedule, 37–75 mg/m^2 once every 2–3 wk or 50–100 mg/m^2 over 4–8 hr once every 21–28 days. For daily dosage schedule, 15–20 mg/m^2/day for 5 days every 3–4 wk.

▸ **Dosage in Renal Impairment**

Dosage is modified on the basis of creatinine clearance.

Creatinine Clearance	Dosage Interval
10–50 ml/min	75%
Less than 10 ml/min	50%

SIDE EFFECTS/ADVERSE REACTIONS

Frequent

Nausea, vomiting (generally beginning 1–4 hr after administration and lasting up to 24 hr); myelosuppression (affecting 25%–30% of patients with recovery generally occurring in 18–23 days)

Occasional

Peripheral neuropathy (with prolonged therapy [4–7 mo]). Pain or redness at injection site, loss of taste or appetite

Rare

Hemolytic anemia, blurred vision, stomatitis

PRECAUTIONS AND CONTRAINDICATIONS

Hearing impairment, myelosuppression, pregnancy

DRUG INTERACTIONS OF CONCERN TO DENTISTRY

- Risk of masking ototoxicity: antihistamines

SERIOUS REACTIONS

! An anaphylactic reaction manifested as angioedema, wheezing, tachycardia, and hypotension, may occur in the first few minutes of IV administration in patients previously exposed to cisplatin.

! Nephrotoxicity occurs in 28%–36% of patients treated with a single dose of cisplatin, usually during the second week of therapy.

! Ototoxicity, including tinnitus and hearing loss, occurs in 31% of patients treated with a single dose of cisplatin. It may be more severe in children and may become more frequent or severe with repeated doses.

DENTAL CONSIDERATIONS

General:

- Determine why patient is taking the drug.
- If additional analgesia is required for dental pain, consider alternative analgesics (NSAIDs) in patients taking narcotics for acute or chronic pain.
- Examine for oral manifestation of opportunistic infection.
- Avoid prescribing aspirin-containing products.
- This drug may be used in the hospital or on an outpatient basis. Confirm the patient's disease and treatment status.
- Chlorhexidine mouth rinse prior to and during chemotherapy may reduce severity of mucositis.
- Patient on chronic drug therapy may rarely present with symptoms of blood dyscrasias, which can include infection, bleeding, and poor healing. If dyscrasia is present, caution patient to prevent oral tissue trauma when using oral hygiene aids.
- Palliative medication may be required for management of oral side effects.
- Short appointments and a stress-reduction protocol may be required for anxious patients.
- Patients may have received other chemotherapy or radiation; confirm medical and drug history.
- Patients may be at risk of bleeding; check for oral signs.
- Oral infections should be eliminated and/or treated aggressively.
- Patients may be at risk of infection.

Consultations:

- Medical consultation should include routine blood counts

including platelet counts and bleeding time.
• Consult physician; prophylactic or therapeutic antiinfectives may be indicated if surgery or periodontal treatment is required.
• Medical consultation may be required to assess immunologic status during cancer chemotherapy and determine safety risk, if any, posed by the required dental treatment.
• Medical consultation may be required to assess disease control and patient's ability to tolerate stress.

Teach Patient/Family to:
• See dentist immediately if secondary oral infection occurs.
• Be aware of oral side effects.
• Encourage effective oral hygiene to prevent soft tissue inflammation.
• Report oral lesions, soreness, or bleeding to dentist.
• Prevent trauma when using oral hygiene aids.
• Update health and medication history if physician makes any changes in evaluation or drug regimens; include OTC, herbal, and nonherbal remedies in the update.

clarithromycin

clare-ih-thro-**mye′**-sin
(Biaxin, Biaxin XL, Klacid[AUS])

CATEGORY AND SCHEDULE

Pregnancy Risk Category: C

Drug Class: Macrolide antibiotic

MECHANISM OF ACTION

A macrolide that binds to ribosomal receptor sites of susceptible organisms, inhibiting protein synthesis of the bacterial cell wall.
Therapeutic Effect: Bacteriostatic; may be bactericidal with high dosages or very susceptible microorganisms.

USES

Treatment of mild-to-moderate infections of the upper and lower respiratory tract; community-acquired pneumonia caused by *H. influenzae*; uncomplicated skin and skin structure infections caused by *S. pneumoniae, M. pneumoniae, C. diphtheriae, B. pertussis, L. monocytogenes, H. influenzae, S. pyogenes*, and *S. aureus*; otitis media; maxillary sinusitis, bronchitis (XL dose form); middle ear infection; disseminated *Mycobacterium avium* complex (MAC); in combination with other drugs for *H. pylori* duodenal ulcer

PHARMACOKINETICS

Well absorbed from the GI tract. Protein binding: 65%–75%. Widely distributed. Metabolized in the liver to active metabolite. Primarily excreted in urine. Not removed by hemodialysis.
Half-life: 3–7 hr; metabolite 5–7 hr (increased in impaired renal function).

INDICATIONS AND DOSAGES

▸ **Bronchitis**

PO

Adults, Elderly. 500 mg q12h for 7–14 days.

▸ **Skin, Soft Tissue Infections**

PO

Adults, Elderly. 250 mg q12h for 7–14 days.

Children. 7.5 mg/kg q12h for 10 days.

▸ **MAC Prophylaxis**
PO
Adults, Elderly. 500 mg 2 times a day.
Children. 7.5 mg/kg q12h. Maximum: 500 mg 2 times a day.

▸ **MAC Treatment**
PO
Adults, Elderly. 500 mg 2 times a day in combination.
Children. 7.5 mg/kg q12h in combination. Maximum: 500 mg 2 times a day.

▸ **Pharyngitis, Tonsillitis**
PO
Adults, Elderly. 250 mg q12h for10 days.
Children. 7.5 mg/kg q12h for 10 days.

▸ **Pneumonia**
PO
Adults, Elderly. 250 mg q12h for 7–14 days.
Children. 7.5 mg/kg q12h.

▸ **Maxillary Sinusitis**
PO
Adults, Elderly. 500 mg q12h for 14 days.
Children. 7.5 mg/kg q12h. Maximum: 500 mg 2 times a day.

▸ ***H. pylori***
PO
Adults, Elderly. 500 mg q12h for 10–14 days in combination.

▸ **Acute Otitis Media**
PO
Children. 7.5 mg/kg q12h for 10 days.

▸ **Dosage in Renal Impairment**
For patients with creatinine clearance less than 30 ml/min, reduce dose by 50% and administer once or twice a day.

SIDE EFFECTS/ADVERSE REACTIONS

Occasional
Diarrhea, nausea, altered taste, abdominal pain

Rare
Headache, dyspepsia

PRECAUTIONS AND CONTRAINDICATIONS

Hypersensitivity to clarithromycin or other macrolide antibiotics
Caution:
Lactation, hepatic and renal disease

DRUG INTERACTIONS OF CONCERN TO DENTISTRY

- Decreased effect: anticholinergic drugs
- Use with caution, possible reduced metabolism: drugs metabolized by CYP3A4 isoenzymes
- Increased effects of cyclosporine, warfarin, cilostazol, tacrolimus, pimozide, methylprednisolone, fluconazole, buspirone
- Decreased action of clindamycin, penicillins, lincomycin, rifabutin, rifampin, zidovudine
- Increased serum levels of carbamazepine, theophylline, digoxin
- Contraindicated with indinavir
- Increased CNS depression with alprazolam, diazepam, midazolam, triazolam
- Suspected increase in plasma levels of repaglinide
- Risk of severe myopathy or rhabdomyolysis: atorvastatin, fluvastatin, lovastatin, pravastatin

SERIOUS REACTIONS

! Antibiotic-associated colitis and other superinfections may result from altered bacterial balance.
! Hepatotoxicity and thrombocytopenia occur rarely.

C

DENTAL CONSIDERATIONS

General:

- Determine why the patient is taking the drug.
- May prove to be an alternative drug of choice for mild infections caused by a susceptible organism in patients who are allergic to penicillin.

Teach Patient/Family to:

- Encourage effective oral hygiene to prevent soft tissue inflammation.
- When used for dental infection, advise patient to:
  - Report sore throat, oral burning sensation, fever, and fatigue, any of which could indicate superinfection.
  - Take at prescribed intervals and complete dosage regimen.
  - Immediately notify the dentist if signs or symptoms of infection increase.

clemastine fumarate

klem′-as-teen **fyoo′**-mer-ate
(Dayhistol Allergy, Tavist Allergy)

CATEGORY AND SCHEDULE

Pregnancy Risk Category: B

Drug Class: Antihistamine, H_1-receptor antagonist

MECHANISM OF ACTION

An ethanolamine that competes with histamine on effector cells in the GI tract, blood vessels, and respiratory tract.

Therapeutic Effect: Relieves allergy symptoms, including urticaria, rhinitis, and pruritus.

USES

Treatment of allergy symptoms, rhinitis, angioedema, urticaria, common cold

PHARMACOKINETICS

Route	Onset	Peak	Duration
PO	15–60 min	5–7 hr	10–12 hr

Well absorbed from the GI tract. Metabolized in the liver. Excreted primarily in urine.

INDICATIONS AND DOSAGES

▸ **Allergic Rhinitis, Urticaria**

PO

Adults, Children older than 11 yr. 1.34 mg twice a day up to 2.68 mg 3 times a day. Maximum: 8.04 mg/day.

Children 6–11 yr. 0.67–1.34 mg twice a day. Maximum: 4.02 mg/day.

Children younger than 6 yr. 0.05 mg/kg/day divided into 2–3 doses per day. Maximum: 1.34 mg/day.

Elderly. 1.34 mg 1–2 times a day.

SIDE EFFECTS/ADVERSE REACTIONS

Frequent

Somnolence, dizziness, urine retention, thickening of bronchial secretions, dry mouth, nose, or throat; in elderly, sedation, dizziness, hypotension

Occasional

Epigastric distress, flushing, blurred vision, tinnitus, paresthesia, diaphoresis, chills

PRECAUTIONS AND CONTRAINDICATIONS

Angle-closure glaucoma, hypersensitivity to clemastine, use within 14 days of MAOIs

Caution:
Increased intraocular pressure, renal disease, cardiac disease, hypertension, bronchial asthma, seizure disorder, stenosed peptic ulcers, hyperthyroidism, prostatic hypertrophy, bladder neck obstruction, elderly

DRUG INTERACTIONS OF CONCERN TO DENTISTRY

- Increased CNS depression: all CNS depressants, alcohol
- Increased anticholinergic effect of anticholinergics, phenothiazines, tricyclic antidepressants

SERIOUS REACTIONS

! A hypersensitivity reaction, marked by eczema, pruritus, rash, cardiac disturbances, angioedema, and photosensitivity, may occur.
! Overdose symptoms may vary from CNS depression, including sedation, apnea, cardiovascular collapse, and death to severe paradoxical reaction, such as hallucinations, tremors, and seizures.
! Children may experience paradoxical reactions, such as restlessness, insomnia, euphoria, nervousness, and tremors.
! Overdose in children may result in hallucinations, seizures, and death.

DENTAL CONSIDERATIONS

General:

- Assess salivary flow as a factor in caries, periodontal disease, and candidiasis.
- Determine why the patient is taking the drug.

Teach Patient/Family to:

- Encourage effective oral hygiene to prevent soft tissue inflammation.
- Use caution to prevent injury when using oral hygiene aids.
- When chronic dry mouth occurs, advise patient to:
  - Avoid mouth rinses with high alcohol content because of drying effects.
  - Use daily home fluoride products for anticaries effect.
  - Use sugarless gum, frequent sips of water, or saliva substitutes.

clevidipine

klev-**id**-i-peen
(Cleviprex)

CATEGORY AND SCHEDULE

Pregnancy Risk Category: C

Drug Class: Antihypertensive; Calcium Channel Blocker, third-generation dihydropyridine

MECHANISM OF ACTION

A short-acting dihydropyridine calcium channel antagonist that selectively relaxes smooth muscle cells that line the small arteries. Decreases systemic vascular resistance; does not reduce preload. It is associated with greater inotropic versus chronotropic selectivity; increase in stroke volume.
Therapeutic Effect: Reduces blood pressure.

USES

Hypertension when oral therapy is not feasible or desired, perioperative hypertension, hypertensive urgency, and hypertensive emergency

PHARMACOKINETICS

IV administration results in complete bioavailability. Protein

C

binding: 99.5%. Rapidly metabolized by hydrolysis, primarily esterases in plasma and tissue to inactive metabolites; metabolites are excreted in urine (63%–74%) and feces (7%–22%). ***Half-life:*** 1 min (initial phase); 15 min (terminal phase).

INDICATIONS AND DOSAGES

▸ Hypertension when Oral Therapy Is Not Feasible or Desired, Perioperative Hypertension, Hypertensive Urgency, and Hypertensive Emergency

IV

Adults. Initial dose: 1–2 mg/hr; Dose titration: Double dose every 90 sec initially; as blood pressure approaches goal, increase dose by less than double and lengthen the time between dose adjustments to every 5–10 min. Usual dose required is 4–6 mg/hr. Severe hypertensive patients may require higher doses with a maximum of 16 mg/hr or less. Doses up to 32 mg/hr have been used, but generally should not exceed 21 mg/hr in a 24-hr period due to lipid load.

SIDE EFFECTS/ADVERSE REACTIONS

Frequent

Atrial fibrillation, nausea, fever, insomnia

Occasional

Headache, CHF, hypotension, rebound hypertension, reflex tachycardia, vomiting, arthralgia, acute renal failure

PRECAUTIONS AND CONTRAINDICATIONS

Hypersensitivity to clevidipine or any component of the formulation

Allergy to soybeans or eggs/egg products

Defective lipid metabolism including pathologic hyperlipidemia, lipoid nephrosis or acute pancreatitis

Severe aortic stenosis

Caution:

Elderly

Heart failure

Concurrent β-blocker use; gradually reduce dose

DRUG INTERACTIONS OF CONCERN TO DENTISTRY

• Other antihypertensives: May increase risk of hypotension.

• Anesthetics: General anesthetics may be potentiated by calcium-channel blockers' additive hypotension, depression of cardiac contractility, conductivity, and automaticity. Local anesthetics may cause additive hypotension as well.

• Reduced response to antihypertensive agents.

SERIOUS REACTIONS

! Hypotension and reflex tachycardia may occur with rapid upward titration.

DENTAL CONSIDERATIONS

General:

• Monitor vital signs at every appointment because of cardiovascular side effects.

• After supine positioning, have patient sit upright for at least 2 min before standing to avoid orthostatic hypotension.

• Assess salivary flow as a factor in caries, periodontal disease, and candidiasis.

• Stress from dental procedures may compromise cardiovascular function; determine patient risk.

Consultations:
• Medical consultation may be required to assess disease control.
Teach Patient/Family to:
• Report oral lesions, soreness, or bleeding to dentist.
• When chronic dry mouth occurs, advise patient to:
  • Avoid mouth rinses with high alcohol content because of drying effects.
  • Use daily home fluoride products for anticaries effect.
  • Use sugarless gum, frequent sips of water, or saliva substitutes.

clindamycin

klin-da-**mye′**-sin
(Cleocin, Cleocin HCl[AUS], Clindesse, Dalacin[CAN], Dalacin C[AUS])

CATEGORY AND SCHEDULE

Pregnancy Risk Category: B

Drug Class: Lincomycin derivative antiinfective

MECHANISM OF ACTION

A lincosamide antibiotic that inhibits protein synthesis of the bacterial cell wall by binding to bacterial ribosomal receptor sites. Topically, it decreases fatty acid concentration on the skin.
Therapeutic Effect: Bacteriostatic, anti-acne.

USES

Indications for use include serious infections caused by susceptible anaerobic bacteria and the treatment of serious infections caused by susceptible strains of pneumococci and streptococci; includes infections of the respiratory tract, serious skin and soft tissue infections, intraabdominal abscess, and infections of the female GU tract.

PHARMACOKINETICS

Rapidly absorbed from the GI tract. Protein binding: 92%–94%. Widely distributed. Metabolized in the liver to some active metabolites. Primarily excreted in urine. Not removed by hemodialysis. ***Half-life:*** 2.4–3 hr (increased in impaired renal function and premature infants).

INDICATIONS AND DOSAGES

▸ **Chronic Bone and Joint, Respiratory Tract, Skin and Soft Tissue, Intraabdominal, and Female GU Infections; Endocarditis; Septicemia**
PO
Adults, Elderly. 150–450 mg/dose q6–8h.
Children. 10–30 mg/kg/day in 3–4 divided doses. Maximum: 1.8 g/day.
IV, IM
Adults, Elderly. 1.2–1.8 g/day in 2–4 divided doses.
Children. 25–40 mg/kg/day in 3–4 divided doses. Maximum: 4.8 g/day.
▸ **Bacterial Vaginosis**
PO
Adults, Elderly. 300 mg twice a day for 7 days.
▸ **Intravaginal**
Adults. One full applicator at bedtime for 3–7 days or 1 suppository at bedtime for 3 days.
▸ **Acne Vulgaris**
Topical
Adults. Apply thin layer to affected area twice a day.

SIDE EFFECTS/ADVERSE REACTIONS

Frequent

Systemic: Abdominal pain, nausea, vomiting, diarrhea

Topical: Dry scaly skin

Vaginal: Vaginitis, pruritus

Occasional

Systemic: Phlebitis or thrombophlebitis with IV administration, pain and induration at IM injection site, allergic reaction, urticaria, pruritus

Topical: Contact dermatitis, abdominal pain, mild diarrhea, burning, or stinging

Vaginal: Headache, dizziness, nausea, vomiting, abdominal pain

Rare

Vaginal: Hypersensitivity reaction

PRECAUTIONS AND CONTRAINDICATIONS

History of antibiotic-associated colitis, regional enteritis, or ulcerative colitis; hypersensitivity to clindamycin or lincomycin

Caution:

Renal disease, liver disease, GI disease, elderly, lactation, tartrazine sensitivity

DRUG INTERACTIONS OF CONCERN TO DENTISTRY

- Decreased action: erythromycin, absorbent antidiarrheals (e.g., aluminum salts)
- Increased effects of nondepolarizing muscle relaxants, hydrocarbon inhalation anesthetics
- Avoid antiperistaltic drugs if diarrhea occurs
- Possible reduced blood levels of cyclosporine

SERIOUS REACTIONS

! Antibiotic-associated colitis and other superinfections may occur during and several weeks after clindamycin therapy (including the topical form).

! Blood dyscrasias (leukopenia, thrombocytopenia) and nephrotoxicity (proteinuria, azotemia, oliguria) occur rarely.

DENTAL CONSIDERATIONS

General:

- Determine why the patient is taking the drug.

Consultations:

- Medical consultation may be required to assess disease control.

Teach Patient/Family to:

- Encourage effective oral hygiene to prevent soft tissue inflammation.
- Use caution to prevent injury when using oral hygiene aids.
- When used for dental infection, advise patient to:
  - Report sore throat, oral burning sensation, fever, diarrhea, and fatigue, any of which could indicate superinfection.
  - Take at prescribed intervals and complete dosage regimen.
  - Immediately notify the dentist if signs or symptoms of infection increase.

C

clindamycin + tretinoin

klin-da-**mye′**-sin & tret-i-noyn
(Veltin; Ziana)

CATEGORY AND SCHEDULE

Pregnancy Risk Category: C

Drug Class: Acne products; antiinfective, retinoic acid derivative

MECHANISM OF ACTION

Clindamycin reversibly binds to 50S ribosomal subunits, inhibiting bacterial protein synthesis. Topical tretinoin decreases follicular epithelial cells' cohesiveness, resulting in decreased formation and increased expulsion of comedones. ***Therapeutic Effect:*** Prevents outbreaks of acne vulgaris, causes expulsion of comedomes.

USES

Treatment of acne vulgaris

PHARMACOKINETICS

Clindamycin: low but variable systemic absorption. Tretinoin: minimal systemic absorption. ***Half-life:*** None reported.

INDICATIONS AND DOSAGES

▸ **Acne Vulgaris**

Topical

Adults, Children 12 yr and older: Apply once daily.

SIDE EFFECTS/ADVERSE REACTIONS

Frequent

Burning, dryness, erythema, scaling

Occasional

Exfoliation, irritation, pruritus, stinging, sunburn, nasopharyngitis

PRECAUTIONS AND CONTRAINDICATIONS

Patients with regional enteritis, ulcerative colitis, or history of antibiotic-associated colitis. Additive diarrhea and photosensitivity may occur with other agents.

DRUG INTERACTIONS OF CONCERN TO DENTISTRY

- Macrolide (e.g., erythromycin) antibiotics: reduced efficacy of Veltin
- Neuromuscular blocking drugs: enhanced neuromuscular blockade with Veltin

SERIOUS REACTIONS

! None known

DENTAL CONSIDERATIONS

General:

- Veltin is a topical gel used to treat skin problems. Dental personnel should be cognizant of areas of adverse skin reactions at the application site(s) and position patient accordingly.

Teach Patient/Family to:

- Report changes in medical condition and drug therapy to dental personnel.

clobazam

kloe-ba-zam
(Onfi)
Do not confuse with clonazepam.

CATEGORY AND SCHEDULE

Pregnancy Risk Category: D

Drug Class: Anticonvulsant, benzodiazepine

C

MECHANISM OF ACTION

A benzodiazepine that binds to receptors on the postsynaptic GABA neuron within the central nervous system, including the limbic system, reticular formation, enhancing the inhibitory effect of GABA on neuronal excitability and increased neuronal membrane stabilization. ***Therapeutic Effect:*** Decreases seizure activity in patients with Lennox-Gastaut syndrome.

USES

Adjunctive treatment of seizures associated with Lennox-Gastaut syndrome

PHARMACOKINETICS

Well absorbed from the GI tract. Peak plasma concentrations reached in 0.5–4 hr. 80% to 90% plasma protein bound. Hepatic metabolism via CYP3A4 and to a lesser extent via CYP2C19 and 2B6 to N-desmethyl metabolite. Excreted 94% via urine (as metabolites). ***Half-life:*** 36–42 hr.

INDICATIONS AND DOSAGES

▸ **Lennox-Gastaut (adjunctive)**

PO

Adults, Children 2 yr or older weighing less than 30 kg. Initially, 5 mg once daily for ≥1 wk, then increase to 5 mg twice daily for ≥1 wk, then increase to 10 mg twice daily thereafter.

Children weighing more than 30 kg. Initially, 5 mg twice daily for ≥1 wk, then increase to 10 mg twice daily for ≥1 wk, then increase to 20 mg twice daily thereafter.

Elderly weighing less than 30 kg. Initially, 5 mg once daily for ≥2 wk, then increase to 5 mg twice daily; after ≥1 wk may increase to 10 mg twice daily based on patient tolerability and response.

Elderly weighing more than 30 kg. Initially, 5 mg once daily for ≥1 wk, then increase to 5 mg twice daily for ≥1 wk, then increase to 10 mg twice daily; after ≥1 wk may increase to 20 mg twice daily based on patient tolerability and response.

SIDE EFFECTS/ADVERSE REACTIONS

Frequent

Somnolence, fever, lethargy, upper respiratory tract infection

Occasional

Ataxia, fatigue, insomnia, sedation, increased salivation, vomiting, constipation, dysphagia, urinary tract infection, dysarthria, cough, bronchitis

PRECAUTIONS AND CONTRAINDICATIONS

May cause anterograde amnesia, hyperactive or aggressive behavior, suicidal ideation. Use with caution in patients with history of drug abuse, impaired gag reflex, muscle weakness and poor coordination, psychiatric disease, respiratory disease.

DRUG INTERACTIONS OF CONCERN TO DENTISTRY

- Increased risk of CNS depression: all CNS depressants, alcohol. May potentiate mental impairment and somnolence, postural hypotension, avoid alcohol.
- Bioavailability increased if administered with CYP 2C19 inhibitors (e.g., barbiturates).
- Reduced doses of drugs metabolized by CYP2D6 may be necessary (e.g., opioid analgesics).

SERIOUS REACTIONS

! Abrupt withdrawal may result in pronounced restlessness, irritability, insomnia, hand tremors, abdominal or muscle cramps, diaphoresis, vomiting, and status epilepticus. Overdose results in somnolence, confusion, diminished reflexes, and coma.

DENTAL CONSIDERATIONS

General:

- Monitor patient for signs/ symptoms of seizure activity.
- Assess salivary flow as a factor in caries, periodontal disease, and candidiasis.
- Beware of possible impaired coordination when seating and discharging patient.
- Constipation may be worsened by coadministration of opioid analgesics.

Consultations:

- Consult physician to determine degree of seizure control and ability of patient to tolerate dental procedures.
- Consult physician if evidence of drug dependence or suicidal tendencies are exhibited.

Teach Patient/Family to:

- Report changes in seizure control.
- Avoid mouth rinses with high alcohol content because of drying effect.
- Use home fluoride products for anticaries effect.
- Use sugarless/xylitol gum, frequent sips of water, or saliva substitutes if dry mouth occurs.

C

clobetasol

klo-**bet′**-ah-sol
(Alti-Clobetasol[CAN], Cormax, Dermovate[CAN], Gen-Clobetasol[CAN], Olux, Novo-Clobetasol[CAN], Temovate)

CATEGORY AND SCHEDULE

Pregnancy Risk Category: C

Drug Class: Topical corticosteroid, very high potency

MECHANISM OF ACTION

A corticosteroid that inhibits accumulation of inflammatory cells at inflammation sites, phagocytosis, lysosomal enzyme release, and synthesis or release of mediators of inflammation.
Therapeutic Effect: Decreases or prevents tissue response to inflammatory process.

USES

Treatment of inflammatory and pruritic manifestations of moderate to severe corticosteroid-responsive dermatitis of the scalp; other uses include psoriasis.

PHARMACOKINETICS

May be absorbed from intact skin. Metabolized in liver. Excreted in the urine.

INDICATIONS AND DOSAGES

▸ **Antiinflammatory, Corticosteroid Replacement Therapy**

Topical
Adults, Elderly, Children 12 yr and older: Apply 2 times a day for 2 wk.
Foam
Adults, Elderly, Children 12 yr and older: Apply 2 times a day for 2 wk.

C

SIDE EFFECTS/ADVERSE REACTIONS

Frequent
Local irritation, dry skin, itching, redness
Occasional
Allergic contact dermatitis
Rare
Cushing's syndrome, numbness of fingers, skin atrophy

PRECAUTIONS AND CONTRAINDICATIONS

Hypersensitivity to clobetasol or other corticosteroids
Caution:
Lactation, bacterial infections

DRUG INTERACTIONS OF CONCERN TO DENTISTRY

- None reported

SERIOUS REACTIONS

! Overdosage can occur from topically applied clobetasol propionate absorbed in sufficient amounts to produce systemic effects producing reversible adrenal suppression, manifestations of Cushing's syndrome, hyperglycemia, and glucosuria in some patients.

DENTAL CONSIDERATIONS

Clobetasol Propionate (Topical Foam)

General:
- Determine why patient is taking the drug.
- Avoid use of systemic corticosteroids unless a consultation is made.

Clobetasol Propionate

General:
- Place on frequent recall to evaluate healing response.
- Topical adrenocorticosteroids are not indicated for treating plaque-related gingivitis, which should be treated by removal of local irritants and improved oral hygiene.

Teach Patient/Family to:
- Encourage effective oral hygiene to prevent soft tissue inflammation.
- Use on oral herpetic ulcerations is contraindicated.
- Apply at bedtime or after meals for maximum effect.
- Apply with cotton-tipped applicator by pressing, not rubbing, paste on lesion.
- Return for oral evaluation if response of oral tissues has not occurred in 7–14 days.

clocortolone

klo-**kort′**-oh-lone
(Cloderm, Cloderm[CAN])

CATEGORY AND SCHEDULE

Pregnancy Risk Category: C

Drug Class: Topical corticosteroid, group III medium potency

MECHANISM OF ACTION

A topical corticosteroid that inhibits accumulation of inflammatory cells at inflammation sites, suppresses mitotic activity, and causes vasoconstriction.
Therapeutic Effect: Decreases or prevents tissue response to inflammatory process.

USES

Psoriasis, eczema, contact dermatitis, pruritus

PHARMACOKINETICS

Absorption is variable and dependent upon many factors including integrity of skin, dose, vehicle used, and use of occlusive dressings. Small amounts may be absorbed from the skin. Metabolized in liver. Excreted in the urine and feces.

INDICATIONS AND DOSAGES

▸ **Dermatoses**

Topical

Adults, Elderly, Children 12 yr and older: Apply 1–4 times a day.

SIDE EFFECTS/ADVERSE REACTIONS

Occasional

Local irritation, burning, itching, redness

Allergic contact dermatitis

Rare

Hypertrichosis, hypopigmentation, maceration of skin, miliaria, perioral dermatitis, skin atrophy, striae

PRECAUTIONS AND CONTRAINDICATIONS

Hypersensitivity to clocortolone pivalate or other corticosteroids; viral, fungal, or tubercular skin lesions

Caution:

Lactation, viral infections, bacterial infections

DRUG INTERACTIONS OF CONCERN TO DENTISTRY

- None reported

SERIOUS REACTIONS

! Overdosage can occur from topically applied clocortolone pivalate absorbed in sufficient amounts to produce systemic effects in some patients.

DENTAL CONSIDERATIONS

General:

- Determine why the patient is taking the drug.
- Place on frequent recall to evaluate healing response if used on a chronic basis.
- Apply lubricant to dry lips for patient comfort before dental procedures.

clofarabine

kloe-**far′**-ah-been

(Clolar)

CATEGORY AND SCHEDULE

Pregnancy Risk Category: D

Drug Class: Antineoplastic

MECHANISM OF ACTION

An antineoplastic agent that inhibits DNA synthesis by decreasing deoxynucleotide triphosphate pools. It inhibits ribonucleoside reductase, terminates elongation of the DNA chain, and inhibits repair through incorporation into the DNA chain by competitive inhibition of DNA polymerases.

Therapeutic Effect: Inhibits synthesis of DNA.

USES

Treatment of acute lymphoid leukemia (ALL) in patients who have failed prior regimens

PHARMACOKENETICS

Protein binding: 47%. Negligible liver metabolism. Primarily excreted in urine. ***Half-life:*** 5.2 hr.

INDICATIONS AND DOSAGES

▸ **ALL**

IV

Adults. 52 mg/m^2 over 2 hr daily for 5 consecutive days. Repeat every 2–6 wk following recovery or return to baseline organ function.

Children. 52 mg/m^2 over 2 hr daily for 5 consecutive days. Repeat every 2–6 wk following recovery or return to baseline organ function.

SIDE EFFECTS/ADVERSE REACTIONS:

Frequent

Infection, vomiting, nausea, febrile neutropenia, diarrhea, pruritus, headache, ALT increased, dermatitis, pyrexia, AST increased, rigors, abdominal pain, fatigue, pericardial effusion, tachycardia, epistaxis, anorexia, petechiae, hypotension, pain in limb, left ventricular systolic dysfunction, anxiety, constipation, edema, pain, cough, erythema, flushing, mucosal inflammation, hematuria, dizziness, bilirubin increased, jaundice, gingival bleeding, hepatomegaly, injection site pain, myalgia, respiratory distress, palmar-plantar sore throat, back pain, dyspnea, erythrodysesthesia syndrome, staphylococcal infection, oral candidiasis, appetite decreased, cellulitis, depression, irritability, arthralgia, herpes simplex, hypertension, lethargy

Occasional

Somnolence, weight gain, tremor, pleural effusion, pneumonia, systemic inflammatory response syndrome (SIRS)/capillary leak syndrome, transfusion reaction, bacteremia, creatinine increased

PRECAUTIONS AND CONTRAINDICATIONS

Hypersensitivity to clofarabine or its components

Caution:

Do not breast-feed, renal or hepatic impairment

DRUG INTERACTIONS OF CONCERN TO DENTISTRY

- CNS depressants, alcohol: may increase CNS depression and dizziness.

SERIOUS REACTIONS

! Tumor lysis syndrome may occur.

! Severe bone marrow suppression, including neutropenia, anemia, and thrombocytopenia, have been observed.

DENTAL CONSIDERATIONS

General:

- Monitor vital signs at every appointment because of cardiovascular side effects.
- Avoid NSAIDs for pain control.
- Examine for oral manifestation of opportunistic infection.
- This drug may be used in the hospital or on an outpatient basis. Confirm the patient's disease and treatment status.
- Chlorhexidine mouth rinse prior to and during chemotherapy may reduce severity of mucositis.
- Determine presence, type, and severity of blood dyscrasias prior to undertaking any dental treatment and modify therapy accordingly.
- Consider effects of drug on healing and susceptibility to infection.
- Palliative measures may be required for management of oral side effects.

Consultations:

- Consult physician to determine disease control and ability of patient to tolerate dental procedures.
- Consult physician to determine need for prophylactic antiinfectives if invasive dental procedures are needed.

• Consult physician about patient's immunologic status during cancer chemotherapy and determine safety risk, if any, posed by required dental treatment.

Teach Family/Patient to:

• Be aware of oral side effects of medication.

• Practice effective oral hygiene to prevent soft-tissue inflammation and prevent trauma when using oral hygiene aids.

• Report oral lesions, soreness, or bleeding to dentist.

• Update health and medication history if physician makes any changes in evaluation or drug regimens, including the use of OTC drugs, herbal products, and dietary supplements.

clofazimine

kloe-**faz′**-ih-meen
(Lamprene)

CATEGORY AND SCHEDULE

Pregnancy Risk Category: C

Drug Class: Leprostatic

MECHANISM OF ACTION

An antibiotic that binds to mycobacterial DNA.

Therapeutic Effect: Inhibits mycobacterial growth and produces antiinflammatory action.

USES

Treatment of lepromatous leprosy, dapsone-resistant leprosy, lepromatous leprosy complicated by erythema nodosum leprosum

PHARMACOKINETICS

Deposited in fatty tissue, reticuloendothelial system; small amount excreted in feces, sputum, sweat. ***Half-life:*** 70 days.

INDICATIONS AND DOSAGES

▸ **Leprosy**

PO

Adults, Elderly. 100 mg/day in combination with dapsone and rifampin for 3 yr, then 100 mg/day as monotherapy.

Children. 1 mg/kg/day in combination with dapsone and rifampin.

▸ **Erythema Nodosum**

PO

Adults, Elderly. 100–200 mg/day for up to 3 mo, then 100 mg/day.

SIDE EFFECTS/ADVERSE REACTIONS

Frequent

Dry skin, abdominal pain, nausea, vomiting, diarrhea, skin discoloration (pink to brownish-black)

Occasional

Rash; pruritus; eye irritation; discoloration of sputum; sweat and urine

PRECAUTIONS AND CONTRAINDICATIONS

Caution:

Lactation, children, abdominal pain, diarrhea, depression

DRUG INTERACTIONS OF CONCERN TO DENTISTRY

• None reported

SERIOUS REACTIONS

! None significant

DENTAL CONSIDERATIONS

General:

• Develop awareness of the patient's disease.

C

Teach Patient/Family to:
• Encourage effective oral hygiene to prevent soft tissue inflammation.
• Avoid mouth rinses with high alcohol content because of drying effects.

clofibrate

kloe-**fye**′-brate
(Abitrate, Atromid-S, Claripex[CAN], Novofibrate[CAN])

CATEGORY AND SCHEDULE

Pregnancy Risk Category: C

Drug Class: Antihyperlipidemic

MECHANISM OF ACTION

An antihyperlipidemic that enhances synthesis of lipoprotein lipase and reduces triglyceride-rich lipoproteins and VLDLs.
Therapeutic Effect: Increases VLDL catabolism and reduces total plasma triglyceride levels.

USES

Treatment of hyperlipidemia (types III, IV, V)

PHARMACOKINETICS

Well absorbed from the GI tract. Protein binding: 95%–97%. Metabolized in liver. Excreted primarily in urine, lesser amount in feces. ***Half-life:*** 14–35 hr.

INDICATIONS AND DOSAGES

▸ **Hypercholesterolemia**
PO
Adults, Elderly. 2 g/day in divided doses. Some patients may respond to a lower dosage.

SIDE EFFECTS/ADVERSE REACTIONS

Frequent
Nausea, vomiting, loose stools, dyspepsia, flatulence, abdominal distress
Occasional
Headache, dizziness, fatigue
Rare
Muscle cramping, aching, weakness; skin rash, urticaria, pruritus; dry brittle hair, alopecia

PRECAUTIONS AND CONTRAINDICATIONS

Hypersensitivity to clofibrate, severe renal or hepatic dysfunction, pregnancy, nursing women, rhabdomyolysis, severe hyperkalemia, primary biliary cirrhosis
Caution:
Peptic ulcer

DRUG INTERACTIONS OF CONCERN TO DENTISTRY

• None reported

SERIOUS REACTIONS

! May increase excretion of cholesterol into bile, leading to cholelithiasis.
! Various cardiac arrhythmias have been reported.
! Anemia and, more frequently, leukopenia have been reported.

DENTAL CONSIDERATIONS

General:
• Consider semisupine chair position for patient comfort if GI side effects occur.
• Patients on chronic drug therapy may rarely have symptoms of blood dyscrasias, which can include infection, bleeding, and poor healing.

Consultations:

• In a patient with symptoms of blood dyscrasias, request a medical consultation for blood studies and postpone treatment until normal values are reestablished.

Teach Patient/Family to:

• Encourage effective oral hygiene to prevent soft tissue inflammation.

clomiphene

kloe′-mi-feen

(Clomhexal[AUS], Clomid, Clomid[CAN], Milophene, Milophene[CAN], Serophene, Serophene[CAN])

Do not confuse with clomipramine.

CATEGORY AND SCHEDULE

Pregnancy Risk Category: X

Drug Class: Nonsteroidal ovulatory stimulant, antiestrogen

MECHANISM OF ACTION

An ovulation stimulator that promotes release of pituitary gonadotropins.

Therapeutic Effect: Stimulates ovulation.

USES

Treatment of female infertility

PHARMACOKINETICS

Readily absorbed. Time to peak occurs within 6.5 hr. Undergoes enterohepatic recirculation. Primarily excreted in feces. ***Half-life:*** 5–7 days.

INDICATIONS AND DOSAGES

▸ **Ovulatory Failure, Females**

PO

Adults. 50 mg/day for 5 days (first course); start the regimen on the fifth day of cycle. Increase dose only if unresponsive to cyclic 50 mg. Maximum: 100 mg/day for 5 days.

SIDE EFFECTS/ADVERSE REACTIONS

Frequent

Hot flashes, ovarian enlargement

Occasional

Abdominal/pelvic discomfort, bloating, nausea, vomiting, breast discomfort (females)

Rare

Vision disturbances, abnormal menstrual flow, breast enlargement (males), headache, mental depression, ovarian cyst formation, thromboembolism, uterine fibroid enlargement

PRECAUTIONS AND CONTRAINDICATIONS

Liver dysfunction, abnormal uterine bleeding, enlargement or development of ovarian cyst, uncontrolled thyroid or adrenal dysfunction in the presence of an organic intracranial lesion such as pituitary tumor, pregnancy, hypersensitivity to clomiphene

Caution:

Hypertension, depression, convulsions, diabetes mellitus

DRUG INTERACTIONS OF CONCERN TO DENTISTRY

• None reported

SERIOUS REACTIONS

! Thrombophlebitis, alopecia, and polyuria occurs rarely.

C

DENTAL CONSIDERATIONS

General:

- Consider semisupine chair position for patient comfort if GI side effects occur.
- Avoid dental light in patient's eyes; offer dark glasses for patient comfort.
- Be aware that patient may be in early stage of pregnancy.

clomipramine hydrochloride

klom-**ip′**-ra-meen hi-droh-**klor′**-ide

(Anafranil, Apo-Clomipramine[CAN], Clopram[AUS], Novo-Clopamine[CAN], Placil[AUS])

Do not confuse clomipramine with chlorpromazine, clomiphene, or imipramine, or Anafranil with alfentanil, enalapril, or nafarelin.

CATEGORY AND SCHEDULE

Pregnancy Risk Category: C

Drug Class: Tricyclic antidepressant

MECHANISM OF ACTION

A tricyclic antidepressant that blocks the reuptake of neurotransmitters, such as norepinephrine and serotonin, at CNS presynaptic membranes, increasing their availability at postsynaptic receptor sites.

Therapeutic Effect: Reduces obsessive-compulsive behavior.

USES

Treatment of obsessive-compulsive disorder; unapproved: depression, panic disorder, narcolepsy, and neurogenic pain

PHARMACOKINETICS

Well absorbed from GI tract. Protein binding: 97%. Principally bound to albumin. Distributed into cerebrospinal fluid. Metabolized in the liver. Undergoes extensive first-pass effect. Excreted in urine and feces. ***Half-life:*** 19–37 hr.

INDICATIONS AND DOSAGES

▸ **Obsessive-Compulsive Disorder**

PO

Adults, Elderly. Initially, 25 mg/day. May gradually increase to 100 mg/day in the first 2 wk. Maximum: 250 mg/day.

Children 10 yr and older. Initially, 25 mg/day. May gradually increase up to maximum of 200 mg/day.

SIDE EFFECTS/ADVERSE REACTIONS

Frequent

Somnolence, fatigue, dry mouth, blurred vision, constipation, sexual dysfunction, ejaculatory failure, impotence, weight gain, delayed micturition, orthostatic hypotension, diaphoresis, impaired concentration, increased appetite, urine retention

Occasional

GI disturbances (such as nausea, GI distress, and metallic taste), asthenia, aggressiveness, muscle weakness

Rare

Paradoxical reactions (agitation, restlessness, nightmares, insomnia), extrapyramidal symptoms, (particularly fine hand tremor), laryngitis, seizures

PRECAUTIONS AND CONTRAINDICATIONS

Acute recovery period after MI, use within 14 days of MAOIs

Caution:

Seizures, suicidal patients, elderly, MAOIs, not for use in children younger than 10 yr, renal or hepatic dysfunction

DRUG INTERACTIONS OF CONCERN TO DENTISTRY

• Increased anticholinergic effects: muscarinic blockers, antihistamines, phenothiazines
• Increased effects of direct-acting sympathomimetics (epinephrine, levonordefrin)
• Potential risk of CNS depression: alcohol, barbiturates, benzodiazepines, and other CNS depressants
• Decreased antihypertensive effects: clonidine, guanadrel, guanethidine
• Use with caution, possible reduced metabolism: drugs metabolized by CYP2D6 isoenzymes
• Avoid concurrent use with St. John's wort (herb)

SERIOUS REACTIONS

! Overdose may produce seizures; cardiovascular effects, such as severe orthostatic hypotension, dizziness, tachycardia, palpitations, and arrhythmias; and altered temperature regulation, including hyperpyrexia or hypothermia.
! Abrupt discontinuation after prolonged therapy may produce headache, malaise, nausea, vomiting, and vivid dreams.
! Anemia and agranulocytosis have been noted.

DENTAL CONSIDERATIONS

General:
• Take vital signs at every appointment because of cardiovascular side effects.
• Assess salivary flow as a factor in caries, periodontal disease, and candidiasis.
• Patients on chronic drug therapy may rarely have symptoms of blood dyscrasias, which can include infection, bleeding, and poor healing.
• After supine positioning, have patient sit upright for at least 2 min before standing to avoid orthostatic hypotension.
• Use vasoconstrictor with caution, in low doses, and with careful aspiration. Avoid use of gingival retraction cord with epinephrine.
• Place on frequent recall because of oral side effects.
• A stress-reduction protocol may be required.

Consultations:
• In a patient with symptoms of blood dyscrasias, request a medical consultation for blood studies and postpone dental treatment until normal values are reestablished.
• Physician should be informed if significant xerostomic side effects occur (e.g., increased caries, sore tongue, problems eating or swallowing, difficulty wearing prosthesis) so that a medication change can be considered.
• Medical consultation may be required to assess disease control.

Teach Patient/Family to:
• Encourage effective oral hygiene to prevent soft tissue inflammation.
• Prevent injury when using oral hygiene aids.
• When chronic dry mouth occurs, advise patient to:
  • Avoid mouth rinses with high alcohol content because of drying effects.
  • Use daily home fluoride products for anticaries effect.
  • Use sugarless gum, frequent sips of water, or saliva substitutes.

C

clonazepam

kloe-**na**′-zi-pam
(Apo-Clonazepam[CAN], Clonapam[CAN], Klonopin, Paxam[AUS], Rivotril[CAN])
Do not confuse clonazepam with clonidine or lorazepam.

CATEGORY AND SCHEDULE

Pregnancy Risk Category: D
Controlled Substance Schedule IV

Drug Class: Anticonvulsant, benzodiazepine

MECHANISM OF ACTION

A benzodiazepine that depresses all levels of the CNS; inhibits nerve impulse transmission in the motor cortex and suppresses abnormal discharge in petit mal seizures. ***Therapeutic Effect:*** Produces anxiolytic and anticonvulsant effects.

USES

Absence, atypical absence, akinetic, myoclonic seizures; unlabeled uses: Parkinson's dysarthria, adjunct in schizophrenia, neuralgias

PHARMACOKINETICS

Well absorbed from the GI tract. Protein binding: 85%. Metabolized in the liver. Excreted in urine. Not removed by hemodialysis. ***Half-life:*** 18–50 hr.

INDICATIONS AND DOSAGES

▸ **Adjunctive Treatment of Lennox-Gastaut Syndrome (Petit Mal Variant) and Akinetic, Myoclonic, and Absence (Petit Mal) Seizures**

PO

Adults, Elderly, Children 10 yr and older. 1.5 mg/day; may be increased in 0.5- to 1-mg increments every 3 days until seizures are controlled. Do not exceed maintenance dosage of 20 mg/day.

Infants, Children younger than 10 yr or weighing less than 30 kg. 0.01–0.03 mg/kg/day in 2–3 divided doses; may be increased by up to 0.5 mg every 3 days until seizures are controlled. Don't exceed maintenance dosage of 0.2 mg/kg/day.

▸ **Panic Disorder**

PO

Adults, Elderly. Initially, 0.25 mg twice a day; increased in increments of 0.125–0.25 mg twice a day every 3 days. Maximum: 4 mg/day.

SIDE EFFECTS/ADVERSE REACTIONS

Frequent

Mild, transient drowsiness; ataxia; behavioral disturbances (aggression, irritability, agitation), especially in children

Occasional

Rash, ankle or facial edema, nocturia, dysuria, change in appetite or weight, dry mouth, sore gums, nausea, blurred vision

Rare

Paradoxical CNS reactions, including hyperactivity or nervousness in children and excitement or restlessness in the elderly (particularly in the presence of uncontrolled pain)

PRECAUTIONS AND CONTRAINDICATIONS

Narrow-angle glaucoma, significant hepatic disease

Caution:

Open-angle glaucoma, chronic respiratory disease, renal, hepatic disease, elderly, interferes with cognitive and motor performance, withdrawal symptoms

DRUG INTERACTIONS OF CONCERN TO DENTISTRY

• Increased sedation: alcohol, all CNS depressants, indinavir, kava (herb)
• Risk of increased serum levels: drugs that inhibit CYP3A4 isoenzymes, ketoconazole, itraconazole, fluconazole, protease inhibitor, nefazodone
• Risk of decreased effect: St. John's wort (herb)

SERIOUS REACTIONS

! Abrupt withdrawal may result in pronounced restlessness, irritability, insomnia, hand tremors, abdominal or muscle cramps, diaphoresis, vomiting, and status epilepticus.
! Overdose results in somnolence, confusion, diminished reflexes, and coma.

DENTAL CONSIDERATIONS

General:
• Patients on chronic drug therapy may rarely have symptoms of blood dyscrasias, which can include infection, bleeding, and poor healing.
• Assess salivary flow as a factor in caries, periodontal disease, and candidiasis.
• Psychologic and physical dependence may occur with chronic administration.
• Geriatric patients are more susceptible to drug effects; use lower dose.
• Ask about type of epilepsy, seizure frequency, and quality of seizure control.

Consultations:
• Medical consultation may be required to assess disease control.
• In a patient with symptoms of blood dyscrasias, request a medical consultation for blood studies and postpone dental treatment until normal values are reestablished.

Teach Patient/Family to:
• Encourage effective oral hygiene to prevent soft tissue inflammation.
• Use caution to prevent injury when using oral hygiene aids.
• When chronic dry mouth occurs, advise patient to:
  • Avoid mouth rinses with high alcohol content because of drying effects.
  • Use daily home fluoride products for anticaries effect.
  • Use sugarless gum, frequent sips of water, or saliva substitutes.

clonidine

klon′-ih-deen
(Catapres, Catapres TTS, Dixarit[CAN], Duraclon)
Do not confuse clonidine with clomiphene, Klonopin, or quinidine, or Catapres with Cetapred.

CATEGORY AND SCHEDULE

Pregnancy Risk Category: C

Drug Class: Antihypertensive, central α-adrenergic agonist

MECHANISM OF ACTION

An antiadrenergic, sympatholytic agent that prevents pain signal transmission to the brain and produces analgesia at pre- and post-α-adrenergic receptors in the spinal cord.
Therapeutic Effect: Reduces peripheral resistance; decreases B/P and heart rate.

C

USES

Hypertension, severe pain in combination with opioids for cancer patients; unapproved: opioid abstinence syndrome, nicotine withdrawal, vascular headache, alcohol withdrawal, ADHD, postherpetic neuralgia

PHARMACOKINETICS

Route	Onset	Peak	Duration
PO	0.5–1 hr	2–4 hr	Up to 8 hr

Well absorbed from the GI tract. Transdermal best absorbed from the chest and upper arm; least absorbed from the thigh. Protein binding: 20%–40%. Metabolized in the liver. Primarily excreted in urine. Minimally removed by hemodialysis. ***Half-life:*** 12–16 hr (increased with impaired renal function).

INDICATIONS AND DOSAGES

▸ **Hypertension**

PO

Adults. Initially, 0.1 mg twice a day. Increase by 0.1–0.2 mg q2–4 days. Maintenance: 0.2–1.2 mg/day in 2–4 divided doses up to maximum of 2.4 mg/day.

Elderly. Initially, 0.1 mg at bedtime. May increase gradually.

Children. 5–25 mcg/kg/day in divided doses q6h. Increase at 5- to 7-day intervals. Maximum: 0.9 mg/day.

Transdermal

Adults, Elderly. System delivering 0.1 mg/24 hr up to 0.6 mg/24 hr q7 days.

▸ **Attention Deficit Hyperactivity Disorder (ADHD)**

PO

Children. Initially 0.05 mg/day. May increase by 0.05 mg/day q3–7 days. Maximum: 0.3–0.4 mg/day.

▸ **Severe Pain**

Epidural

Adults, Elderly. 30–40 mcg/hr.

Children. Initially, 0.5 mcg/kg/hr, not to exceed adult dose.

SIDE EFFECTS/ADVERSE REACTIONS

Frequent

Dry mouth, somnolence, dizziness, sedation, constipation

Occasional

Tablets, injection: Depression, swelling of feet, loss of appetite, decreased sexual ability, itching eyes, dizziness, nausea, vomiting, nervousness

Transdermal: Itching, reddening, or darkening of skin

Rare

Nightmares, vivid dreams, cold feeling in fingers and toes

PRECAUTIONS AND CONTRAINDICATIONS

Epidural contraindicated in those patients with bleeding diathesis or infection at the injection site, and in those receiving anticoagulation therapy

Caution:

MI (recent), cerebrovascular disease, chronic renal failure, Raynaud's disease, thyroid disease, depression, COPD, children younger than 12 yr (patches), asthma, lactation, elderly

DRUG INTERACTIONS OF CONCERN TO DENTISTRY

• Increased CNS depression: alcohol, all CNS depressants

• Decreased hypotensive effects: NSAIDs, sympathomimetics, tricyclic antidepressants

SERIOUS REACTIONS

! Overdose produces profound hypotension, irritability, bradycardia, respiratory depression, hypothermia, miosis (pupillary constriction), arrhythmias, and apnea.

! Abrupt withdrawal may result in rebound hypertension associated with nervousness, agitation, anxiety, insomnia, hand tingling, tremor, flushing, and diaphoresis.

DENTAL CONSIDERATIONS

General:

- Monitor vital signs at every appointment because of cardiovascular side effects.
- After supine positioning, have patient sit upright for at least 2 min before standing to avoid orthostatic hypotension.
- Limit use of sodium-containing products, such as saline IV fluids, for patients with a dietary salt restriction.
- Observe appropriate limitations of vasoconstrictor doses.
- Assess salivary flow as a factor in caries, periodontal disease, and candidiasis.
- Stress from dental procedures may compromise cardiovascular function; determine patient risk.
- Short appointments and a stress-reduction protocol may be required for anxious patients.
- Consider drug in diagnosis of taste alterations.

Consultations:

- Medical consultation may be required to assess disease control.

Teach Patient/Family:

- When chronic dry mouth occurs, advise patient to:
  - Avoid mouth rinses with high alcohol content because of drying effects.
  - Use daily home fluoride products for anticaries effect.
  - Use sugarless gum, frequent sips of water, or saliva substitutes.

C

clopidogrel

clo-**pid′**-oh-grill

(Iscover[AUS], Plavix)

Do not confuse Plavix with Paxil.

CATEGORY AND SCHEDULE

Pregnancy Risk Category: B

Drug Class: Platelet aggregation inhibitor

MECHANISM OF ACTION

A thienopyridine derivative that inhibits binding of the enzyme adenosine phosphate (ADP) to its platelet receptor and subsequent ADP-mediated activation of a glycoprotein complex.

Therapeutic Effect: Inhibits platelet aggregation.

USES

Adjunctive treatment in recent MI, ischemic stroke, and peripheral vascular disease in patients with atherosclerosis; treatment of acute coronary syndrome (unstable angina with non-Q wave MI)

PHARMACOKINETICS

Route	Onset	Peak	Duration
PO	1 hr	2 hr	N/A

Rapidly absorbed. Protein binding: 98%. Extensively metabolized by the liver. Eliminated equally in the urine and feces. ***Half-life:*** 8 hr.

INDICATIONS AND DOSAGES

▸ **MI, Stroke Reduction**

PO

Adults, Elderly. 75 mg once a day.

▸ **Acute Coronary Syndrome**

PO

Adults, Elderly. Initially, 300 mg loading dose, then 75 mg once a day (in combination with aspirin).

SIDE EFFECTS/ADVERSE REACTIONS

Frequent

Skin disorders

Occasional

Upper respiratory tract infection, chest pain, flu-like symptoms, headache, dizziness, arthralgia

Rare

Fatigue, edema, hypertension, abdominal pain, dyspepsia, diarrhea, nausea, epistaxis, dyspnea, rhinitis

PRECAUTIONS AND CONTRAINDICATIONS

Active bleeding, coagulation disorders, severe hepatic disease

Caution:

Hepatic impairment, renal impairment, hypertension, history of bleeding disorders, major surgery, safety and efficacy during lactation or use in children not established

DRUG INTERACTIONS OF CONCERN TO DENTISTRY

• Caution in use with NSAIDs

SERIOUS REACTIONS

! None known

DENTAL CONSIDERATIONS

General:

• Avoid discontinuation for dental procedures because of increased risk of thromboembolism.

• Effects on platelet aggregation return to normal in 5–7 days.

• Patients on chronic drug therapy may rarely have symptoms of blood dyscrasias, which can include infection, bleeding, and poor healing.

• Consider local hemostasis measures to prevent excessive bleeding.

• Question patient about concurrent aspirin use.

• Monitor vital signs at every appointment because of cardiovascular disease.

• Consider semisupine chair position for patient comfort if GI side effects occur.

Consultations:

• Medical consultation may be required to assess disease control and patient's ability to tolerate stress.

• Consultation should include data on bleeding time.

• In a patient with symptoms of blood dyscrasias, request a medical consultation for blood studies and postpone treatment until normal values are reestablished.

Teach Patient/Family to:

• Update health and drug history if physician makes any changes in evaluation or drug regimens.

• Use caution to prevent trauma when using oral hygiene aids.

• Report any unusual or prolonged bleeding episodes after dental treatment.

clorazepate dipotassium

klor-**az**′-e-pate di-poe-**tass**′-ee-um (Novoclopate[CAN], Tranxene, Tranxene SD, Tranxene SD Half-Strength, T-Tab)
Do not confuse clorazepate with clofibrate.

CATEGORY AND SCHEDULE

Pregnancy Risk Category: D
Controlled Substance Schedule IV

Drug Class: Benzodiazepine

MECHANISM OF ACTION

A benzodiazepine that depresses all levels of the CNS, including limbic and reticular formation, by binding to benzodiazepine receptor sites on the gamma-aminobutyric acid (GABA) receptor complex. Modulates GABA, a major inhibitory neurotransmitter in the brain.
Therapeutic Effect: Produces anxiolytic effect, suppresses seizure activity.

USES

Anxiety, acute alcohol withdrawal, adjunctive treatment of partial seizures

PHARMACOKINETICS

Well absorbed after oral administration rapidly metabolized by liver to nordazepam, which is slowly eliminated. ***Half-life:*** 40–50 hr. Protein binding of nordazepam: 97%–98%. Metabolites (nordazepam, oxazepam, and glucuronide conjugates) excreted in urine.

INDICATIONS AND DOSAGES

▸ **Anxiety**

PO (Regular-Release)
Adults, Elderly. 7.5–15 mg 2–4 times a day.
PO (Sustained-Release)
Adults, Elderly. 11.25 mg or 22.5 mg once a day at bedtime.

▸ **Anticonvulsant**

PO
Adults, Elderly, Children older than 12 yr. Initially, 7.5 mg 2–3 times a day. May increase by 7.5 mg at weekly intervals. Maximum: 90 mg/day.
Children 9–12 yr. Initially, 3.75–7.5 mg twice a day. May increase by 2.75 mg at weekly intervals. Maximum: 60 mg/day.

▸ **Alcohol Withdrawal**

PO
Adults, Elderly. Initially, 30 mg, then 15 mg 2–4 times a day on first day. Gradually decrease dosage over subsequent days. Maximum: 90 mg/day.

SIDE EFFECTS/ADVERSE REACTIONS

Frequent
Somnolence
Occasional
Dizziness, GI disturbances, nervousness, blurred vision, dry mouth, headache, confusion, ataxia, rash, irritability, slurred speech
Rare
Paradoxical CNS reactions, such as hyperactivity or nervousness in children and excitement or restlessness in the elderly or debilitated (generally noted during first 2 wk of therapy, particularly in presence of uncontrolled pain)

PRECAUTIONS AND CONTRAINDICATIONS

Acute narrow-angle glaucoma

C

Caution:
Elderly, debilitated, hepatic disease, renal disease

DRUG INTERACTIONS OF CONCERN TO DENTISTRY

• Increased effects: CNS depressants, alcohol, opioid analgesics, general anesthetics, indinavir
• Increased serum levels and prolonged effect of benzodiazepines: fluconazole, ketoconazole, itraconazole, miconazole (systemic)
• Possible increase in CNS side effects: kava kava (herb)
• Contraindicated with saquinavir

SERIOUS REACTIONS

! Abrupt or too-rapid withdrawal may result in pronounced restlessness, irritability, insomnia, hand tremors, abdominal or muscle cramps, diaphoresis, vomiting, and seizures.
! Overdose results in somnolence, confusion, diminished reflexes, and coma.

DENTAL CONSIDERATIONS

General:
• Monitor vital signs at every appointment because of cardiovascular side effects.
• Assess salivary flow as a factor in caries, periodontal disease, and candidiasis.
• After supine positioning, have patient sit upright for at least 2 min to avoid orthostatic hypotension.
• Psychologic and physical dependence may occur with chronic administration.
• Geriatric patients are more susceptible to drug effects; use a lower dose.
• Short appointments and a stress-reduction protocol may be required for anxious patients.
• Seizure: Ask about type of epilepsy, seizure frequency, and degree of seizure control.
Consultations:
• Medical consultation may be required to assess disease control and the patient's ability to tolerate stress.
Teach Patient/Family:
• When chronic dry mouth occurs, advise patient to:
  • Avoid mouth rinses with high alcohol content because of drying effects.
  • Use daily home fluoride products for anticaries effect.
  • Use sugarless gum, frequent sips of water, or saliva substitutes.

clotrimazole

kloe-try′-mah-zole
(Canesten[CAN], Clotrimaderm[CAN], Mycelex, Mycelex OTC, Lotrimin, Gyne-Lotrimin, Trivagizole 3)

CATEGORY AND SCHEDULE

Pregnancy Risk Category: B (topical), C (troches)

Drug Class: Imidazole antifungal

MECHANISM OF ACTION

An antifungal that binds with phospholipids in fungal cell membrane. Damages the fungal cell membrane, altering its function.
Therapeutic Effect: Inhibits yeast growth.

USES

Treatment of tinea pedis; tinea cruris; tinea corporis; tinea versicolor; *C. albicans* infection of the vagina, vulva, throat, mouth

PHARMACOKINETICS

Poorly, erratically absorbed from GI tract. Bound to oral mucosa. Absorbed portion metabolized in liver. Eliminated in feces. Topical: Minimal systemic absorption (highest concentration in stratum corneum). Intravaginal: Small amount systemically absorbed. ***Half-life:*** 3.5–5 hr.

INDICATIONS AND DOSAGES

▸ **Oropharyngeal Candidiasis Treatment**

PO

Adults, Elderly. 10 mg 5 times a day for 14 days.

▸ **Oropharyngeal Candidiasis Prophylaxis**

PO

Adults, Elderly. 10 mg 3 times a day.

▸ **Dermatophytosis, Cutaneous Candidiasis**

Topical

Adults, Elderly. 2 times a day. Therapeutic effect may take up to 8 wk.

▸ **Vulvovaginal Candidiasis**

Vaginal (Tablets)

Adults, Elderly. 1 tablet (100 mg) at bedtime for 7 days; 2 tablets (200 mg) at bedtime for 3 days; or 500 mg tablet one time.

Vaginal (Cream)

Adults, Elderly. 1 full applicator at bedtime for 7–14 days.

SIDE EFFECTS/ADVERSE REACTIONS

Frequent

Oral: Nausea, vomiting, diarrhea, abdominal pain

Occasional

Topical: Itching, burning, stinging, erythema, urticaria

Vaginal: Mild burning (tablets/cream); irritation, cystitis (cream)

Rare

Vaginal: Itching, rash, lower abdominal cramping, headache

PRECAUTIONS AND CONTRAINDICATIONS

Hypersensitivity to clotrimazole or any component of the formulation, children younger than 3 yr

DRUG INTERACTIONS OF CONCERN TO DENTISTRY

• None reported

SERIOUS REACTIONS

! None reported

DENTAL CONSIDERATIONS

General:

• Determine why the patient is taking the drug.

• Examine oral mucous membranes for signs of fungal infection.

Teach Patient/Family to:

• Soak full or partial dentures in an antifungal solution overnight until lesions are absent; prolonged infections may require fabrication of new prosthesis.

• Dispose of tooth brush used during oral infection after oral lesions are absent to prevent reinoculation.

• Complete entire course of medication; long-term therapy may be necessary to completely eradicate infection.

C

clozapine

klo′-za-peen
(Clopine[AUS], Clozaril, FazaClo)
Do not confuse clozapine with Cloxapen or clofazimine, or Clozaril with Clinoril or Colazal.

CATEGORY AND SCHEDULE

Pregnancy Risk Category: B

Drug Class: Antipsychotic, atypical

MECHANISM OF ACTION

A dibenzodiazepine derivative that interferes with the binding of dopamine at dopamine receptor sites; binds primarily at nondopamine receptor sites. ***Therapeutic Effect:*** Diminishes schizophrenic behavior.

USES

Management of psychotic symptoms in schizophrenic patients for whom other antipsychotics have failed (available only through the Clozaril Patient Management System)

PHARMACOKINETICS

Absorbed rapidly and almost completely. Distributed rapidly and extensively. Crosses the blood-brain barrier. Protein binding: 95%. Metabolized in the liver. Excreted in urine and feces. ***Half-life:*** 8 hr.

INDICATIONS AND DOSAGES

▸ Schizophrenic Disorders, Reduce Suicidal Behavior

PO

Adults. Initially, 25 mg once or twice a day. May increase by 25–50 mg/day over 2 wk until dosage of 300–450 mg/day is achieved. May further increase by 50–100 mg/day no more than once or twice a wk. Range: 200–600 mg/day. Maximum: 900 mg/day.

Elderly. Initially, 25 mg/day. May increase by 25 mg/day. Maximum: 450 mg/day.

SIDE EFFECTS/ADVERSE REACTIONS

Frequent

Somnolence, salivation, tachycardia, dizziness, constipation

Occasional

Hypotension, headache, tremors, syncope, diaphoresis, dry mouth, nausea, visual disturbances, nightmares, restlessness, akinesia, agitation, hypertension, abdominal discomfort or heartburn, weight gain

Rare

Rigidity, confusion, fatigue, insomnia, diarrhea, rash

PRECAUTIONS AND CONTRAINDICATIONS

Coma, concurrent use of other drugs that may suppress bone marrow function, history of clozapine-induced agranulocytosis or severe granulocytopenia, myeloproliferative disorders, severe CNS depression

Caution:

Lactation; children younger than 16 yr; hepatic, renal, cardiac disease; seizures; prostatic enlargement; elderly; increased incidence of cardiomyopathy

DRUG INTERACTIONS OF CONCERN TO DENTISTRY

- Increased anticholinergic effects: anticholinergics
- Increased CNS depression: alcohol, all CNS depressant drugs
- Increased serum concentration, leukocytosis: erythromycin base
- Possible decreased effects: carbamazepine
- Increased plasma levels: ciprofloxacin

SERIOUS REACTIONS

! Blood dyscrasias, particularly agranulocytosis and mild leukopenia, may occur.

! Seizures occur in about 3% of patients.

! Overdose produces CNS depression (including sedation, coma, and delirium), respiratory depression, and hypersalivation.

DENTAL CONSIDERATIONS

General:

- Monitor vital signs at every appointment because of cardiovascular and respiratory side effects.
- Patients on chronic drug therapy may rarely have symptoms of blood dyscrasias, which can include infection, bleeding, and poor healing.
- After supine positioning, have patient sit upright for at least 2 min before standing to avoid orthostatic hypotension.
- Assess salivary flow as a factor in caries, periodontal disease, and candidiasis.
- Determine why the patient is taking the drug.
- Place on frequent recall because of oral side effects.

Consultations:

- In a patient with symptoms of blood dyscrasias, request a medical consultation for blood studies and postpone dental treatment until normal values are reestablished.
- Medical consultation may be required to assess disease control and stress tolerance of patient.
- Physician should be informed if significant xerostomic side effects occur (e.g., increased caries, sore tongue, problems eating or swallowing, difficulty wearing prosthesis) so that a medication change can be considered.

Teach Patient/Family to:

- Encourage effective oral hygiene to prevent soft tissue inflammation.
- Use caution to prevent injury when using oral hygiene aids.
- Use powered tooth brush if patient has difficulty holding conventional devices.
- When chronic dry mouth occurs, advise patient to:
  - Avoid mouth rinses with high alcohol content because of drying effects.
  - Use daily home fluoride products for anticaries effect.
  - Use sugarless gum, frequent sips of water, or saliva substitutes.

cocaine hydrochloride

koe-**kane′** hi-droh-**klor′**-ide

(Cocaine[CAN], Cocaine HCl)

CATEGORY AND SCHEDULE

Pregnancy Risk Category: C

Controlled Substance: Schedule II

Drug Class: Ester; topical anesthetic

MECHANISM OF ACTION

A topical anesthetic that decreases membrane permeability, increases norepinephrine at postsynaptic receptor sites, producing intense vasoconstriction.

Therapeutic Effect: Blocks conduction of nerve impulses.

USES

Topical anesthesia for mucous membranes of orolaryngeal, nasal areas; minor, uncomplicated facial lacerations

PHARMACOKINETICS

Readily absorbed from all mucous membranes. Cocaine penetrates the CNS but is rapidly metabolized. Rapidly hydrolyzed in blood by serum cholinesterases. Metabolized in liver. Excreted in urine. ***Half-life:*** 1–1.5 hr.

INDICATIONS AND DOSAGES

▸ **Anesthesia**

Topical

Adults, Elderly, Children. 1%–4% to mucous membranes. Maximum: 1–3 mg/kg. Dosage varies depending upon the area to be anesthetized, vascularity of the tissues, individual tolerance, and anesthetic technique. Administer lowest effective dose.

SIDE EFFECTS/ADVERSE REACTIONS

Frequent

Loss of sense of smell and taste

Occasional

Anxiety, CNS stimulation or depression

PRECAUTIONS AND CONTRAINDICATIONS

Hypersensitivity to cocaine or any component of the formulation

DRUG INTERACTIONS OF CONCERN TO DENTISTRY

- Sensitization to catecholamines, such as epinephrine; risk of serious adverse cardiovascular events
- Avoid ester-type local anesthetics in patients with allergic reactions to cocaine

SERIOUS REACTIONS

! Repeated nasal application may produce stuffy nose and chronic rhinitis.

! Early signs of overdosage are increased B/P, increased pulse, irregular heartbeat, chills or fever, agitation, nervousness, confusion, inability to remain still, nausea, vomiting, abdominal pain, increased sweating, rapid breathing, and large pupils.

! Advanced signs of overdosage are arrhythmias, CNS hemorrhage, CHF, convulsions, delirium, hyperreflexia, loss of bladder or bowel control, and respiratory weakness.

! Late signs of overdosage are loss of reflexes, muscle paralysis, dilated pupils, LOC, cyanosis, pulmonary edema, cardiac and respiratory failure.

DENTAL CONSIDERATIONS

General:

- Acute-use drug for medical topical anesthesia (not for injection).
- Abusers of cocaine may present with oral or nasal mucosal lesions and dry mucous membranes, nervousness, and anxiety.
- Caution: drug interactions in chronic abusers of cocaine.
- Determine why patient is taking the drug.
- Monitor vital signs at every appointment because of cardiovascular side effects.
- Assess salivary flow as a factor in caries, periodontal disease, and candidiasis.
- If additional analgesia is required for dental pain, consider alternative analgesics (NSAIDs) in patients taking narcotics for acute or chronic pain.
- Use vasoconstrictor with caution, in low doses, and with careful aspiration. Avoid using gingival retraction cord containing epinephrine.
- Examine for oral manifestation of opportunistic infection.

- Psychologic and physical dependence may occur with chronic administration.
- Dental local anesthetics will not interfere with urine test for cocaine abuse.

Consultations:

- Notify recovery program director if controlled substances may be required for a patient in recovery from cocaine use.

Teach Patient/Family:

- When chronic dry mouth occurs, advise patient to:
  - Avoid mouth rinses with high alcohol content because of drying effects.
  - Use daily home fluoride products for anticaries effect.
  - Use sugarless gum, frequent sips of water, or saliva substitutes.
  - Report oral lesions, soreness, or bleeding to dentist.

codeine phosphate/ codeine sulfate

koe′-deen **foss′**-fate/**koe′**-deen **sull′**-fate

(codeine phosphate) Actacode[AUS], Codeine Phosphate Injection, Codeine Linctus[AUS](codeine sulfate) Contin[CAN]

Do not confuse codeine with Cardene or Lodine.

CATEGORY AND SCHEDULE

Pregnancy Risk Category: C (D if used for prolonged periods or at high dosages at term)

Controlled Substance: Schedule II (single drug), III (combination form)

Drug Class: Opioid analgesic

MECHANISM OF ACTION

An opioid agonist that binds to opioid receptors at many sites in the CNS, particularly in the medulla. This action inhibits the ascending pain pathways.

Therapeutic Effect: Alters the perception of and emotional response to pain, suppresses cough reflex.

USES

Treatment of mild-to-moderate pain, non-productive cough

PHARMACOKINETICS

Well absorbed after oral administration; rapidly metabolized by liver; 10% methylated to the active analgesic morphine. ***Half-life:*** 2.5–3 hr. Metabolites excreted in urine.

INDICATIONS AND DOSAGES

▸ Analgesia

PO, IM, subcutaneous

Adults, Elderly. 30 mg q4–6h. Range: 15–60 mg.

Children. 0.5–1 mg/kg q4–6h. Maximum: 60 mg/dose.

▸ Cough

PO

Adults, Elderly, Children 12 yr and older. 10–20 mg q4–6h.

Children 6–11 yr. 5–10 mg q4–6h.

Children 2–5 yr. 2.5–5 mg q4–6h.

▸ Dosage in Renal Impairment

Dosage is modified on the basis of creatinine clearance.

Creatinine Clearance	Dosage
10–50 ml/min	75% of usual dose
Less than 10 ml/min	50% of usual dose

C

SIDE EFFECTS/ADVERSE REACTIONS

Frequent
Constipation, somnolence, nausea, vomiting
Occasional
Paradoxical excitement, confusion, palpitations, facial flushing, decreased urination, blurred vision, dizziness, dry mouth, headache, hypotension (including orthostatic hypotension), decreased appetite, injection site redness, burning, or pain
Rare
Hallucinations, depression, abdominal pain, insomnia

PRECAUTIONS AND CONTRAINDICATIONS

Caution:
Elderly, cardiac dysrhythmias

DRUG INTERACTIONS OF CONCERN TO DENTISTRY

- Increased sedation with other CNS depressants and alcohol
- Increased effects of anticholinergics

SERIOUS REACTIONS

! Too-frequent use may result in paralytic ileus.
! Overdose may produce cold and clammy skin, confusion, seizures, decreased B/P, restlessness, pinpoint pupils, bradycardia, respiratory depression, decreased LOC, and severe weakness.
! The patient who uses codeine repeatedly may develop a tolerance to the drug's analgesic effect, as well as physical dependence.

DENTAL CONSIDERATIONS

General:
- Monitor vital signs at every appointment because of cardiovascular and respiratory side effects.
- After supine positioning, have patient sit upright for at least 2 min to avoid orthostatic hypotension.
- Assess salivary flow as a factor in caries, periodontal disease, and candidiasis.
- Psychologic and physical dependence may occur with chronic administration.

Teach Patient/Family:
- When chronic dry mouth occurs, advise patient to:
  - Avoid mouth rinses with high alcohol content because of drying effects.
  - Use daily home fluoride products for anticaries effect.
  - Use sugarless gum, frequent sips of water, or saliva substitutes.

colchicine

kol′-chi-seen
(Colchicine, Colgout[AUS])

CATEGORY AND SCHEDULE

Pregnancy Risk Category: D

Drug Class: Antigout agent

MECHANISM OF ACTION

An alkaloid that decreases leukocyte motility, phagocytosis, and lactic acid production.
Therapeutic Effect: Decreases urate crystal deposits and reduces inflammatory process.

USES

Gout, gouty arthritis (prevention, treatment); unlabeled uses: hepatic cirrhosis, Behçet's disease, scleroderma, Sweet's syndrome

C

PHARMACOKINETICS

Rapidly absorbed from the GI tract. Highest concentration is in the liver, spleen, and kidney. Protein binding: 30%–50%. Reenters the intestinal tract by biliary secretion and is reabsorbed from the intestines. Partially metabolized in the liver. Eliminated primarily in feces.

INDICATIONS AND DOSAGES

▸ Acute Gouty Arthritis

PO

Adults, Elderly. 0.6–1.2 mg; then 0.6 mg q1–2h or 1–1.2 mg q2h, until pain is relieved or nausea, vomiting, or diarrhea occurs. Total dose: 4–8 mg.

IV

Adults, Elderly. Initially, 2 mg; then 0.5 mg q6h until satisfactory response. Maximum: 4 mg/wk or 4 mg/one course of treatment. If pain recurs, may give 1–2 mg/day for several days but no sooner than 7 days after a full course of IV therapy (total of 4 mg).

▸ Chronic Gouty Arthritis

PO

Adults, Elderly. 0.5–.6 mg once a wk up to once a day, depending on number of attacks per year.

SIDE EFFECTS/ADVERSE REACTIONS

Frequent

PO: Nausea, vomiting, abdominal discomfort

Occasional

PO: Anorexia

Rare

Hypersensitivity reaction, including angioedema

Parenteral: Nausea, vomiting, diarrhea, abdominal discomfort, pain or redness at injection site, neuritis in injected arm

PRECAUTIONS AND CONTRAINDICATIONS

Blood dyscrasias; severe cardiac, GI, hepatic, or renal disorders

Caution:

Severe renal disease, blood dyscrasias, hepatic disease, elderly, lactation, children, retards B_{12} absorption

DRUG INTERACTIONS OF CONCERN TO DENTISTRY

- Increased risk of GI side effects: NSAIDs, alcohol
- Possible increased serum levels: erythromycin

SERIOUS REACTIONS

! Bone marrow depression, including aplastic anemia, agranulocytosis, and thrombocytopenia, may occur with long-term therapy.

! Overdose initially causes a burning feeling in the skin or throat, severe diarrhea, and abdominal pain. The patient then experiences fever, seizures, delirium, and renal impairment, marked by hematuria and oliguria. The third stage of overdose causes hair loss, leukocytosis, and stomatitis.

DENTAL CONSIDERATIONS

General:

- Consider drug in diagnosis of taste alteration.
- Patients on chronic drug therapy may rarely have symptoms of blood dyscrasias, which can include infection, bleeding, and poor healing.
- Avoid prescribing aspirin-containing products.

Consultations:

- Medical consultation may be required to assess disease control.

C

• In a patient with symptoms of blood dyscrasias, request a medical consultation for blood studies and postpone dental treatment until normal values are reestablished.

Teach Patient/Family to:

• Encourage effective oral hygiene to prevent soft tissue inflammation.

• Use caution to prevent injury when using oral hygiene aids.

• Avoid mouth rinses with high alcohol content because of drying effects.

coleseveIam

ko-lee-**sev′**-a-lam
(WelChol [U.S.], Cholestagel [intl.])

CATEGORY AND SCHEDULE

Pregnancy Risk Category: B

Drug Class: Antihyperlipidemic, bile acid sequestrant, lipid-lowering agent

MECHANISM OF ACTION

Non-absorbed polymer that binds to bile acids in the intestine to prevent their absorption. As bile acid is reduced, the hepatic enzyme cholesterol 7-alpha hydroxylase is upregulated, increasing the demand for cholesterol in the liver and increasing the clearance of LDL-cholesterol from the blood. The mechanism by which blood glucose control is achieved is unknown.

Therapeutic Effect: Partially removes bile acid from enterohepatic circulation, increases clearance of LDL-cholesterol from the blood and improves glycemic control in patients with Type 2 diabetes mellitus.

USES

Adjunct to diet and exercise to reduce low-density lipoprotein cholesterol (LDL-C) in patients with primary hyperlipidemia (as monotherapy or in combination with an HMG-CoA reductase inhibitor/statin); also used to improve glycemic control in Type 2 diabetes mellitus.

PHARMACOKINETICS

Not absorbed from GI tract; not metabolized; excreted primarily in feces.

INDICATIONS AND DOSAGES

▸ Primary Hyperlipidemia (Used as Monotherapy or in Combinations with an HMG COA Reductase Inhibitor, or "Statin")

Adult. PO 6 tablets once daily or 3 tablets twice daily, taken with a meal and liquid.

▸ Type 2 Diabetes Mellitus

Adult. PO 6 tablets once daily or 3 tablets twice daily, taken with a meal and liquid.

SIDE EFFECTS/ADVERSE REACTIONS

Frequent

Constipation, nausea, vomiting, abdominal pain, dyspepsia

Occasional

Nasopharyngitis, hypoglycemia, nausea, hypertension

Rare

Myocardial infarction, aortic stenosis, bradycardia

PRECAUTIONS AND CONTRAINDICATIONS

Elevated serum triglycerides
Vitamin K or fat-soluble vitamin deficiencies (A, D, E, K)
Gastroparesis, GI tract surgery, patients at risk for bowel obstruction
Dysphagia, swallowing disorders

DRUG INTERACTIONS OF CONCERN TO DENTISTRY
• None reported

SERIOUS REACTIONS
! GI tract obstruction, hyperchloremic acidosis, osteoporosis secondary to excessive calcium excretion
! High doses may interfere with fat absorption and result in steatorrhea

DENTAL CONSIDERATIONS
General:
• Monitor vital signs at every appointment because of underlying disease and cardiovascular side effects of drug.
• Position patient for comfort if GI adverse effects occur.
• Assess glycemic control to avoid possible hypoglycemic emergency.
Consultations:
• Consult with physician to determine disease control and ability to tolerate dental procedures.
Teach Patient/Family to:
• Update medical history as changes in medication or disease status occur.

colestipol
koe-**les′**-ti-pole
(Colestid, Colestid[CAN])

CATEGORY AND SCHEDULE
Pregnancy Risk Category: C

Drug Class: Antihyperlipidemic

MECHANISM OF ACTION
An antihyperlipoproteinemic that binds with bile acids in the intestine, forming an insoluble complex. Binding results in partial removal of bile acid from enterohepatic circulation.
Therapeutic Effect: Removes LDL and cholesterol from plasma.

USES
Adjunctive therapy to diet and exercise for the reduction of elevated serum total and LDL cholesterol in patients with primary hypercholesterolemia

PHARMACOKINETICS
Not absorbed from the GI tract. Excreted in the feces.

INDICATIONS AND DOSAGES
▸ **Primary Hypercholesterolemia**
PO, Granules
Adults, Elderly. Initially, 5 g 1–2 times a day. Range: 5–30 g/day once or in divided doses.
PO, Tablets
Adults, Elderly. Initially, 2 g 1–2 times a day. Range: 2–16 g/day.

SIDE EFFECTS/ADVERSE REACTIONS
Frequent
Constipation (may lead to fecal impaction), nausea, vomiting, stomach pain, indigestion
Occasional
Diarrhea, belching, bloating, headache, dizziness
Rare
Gallstones, peptic ulcer, malabsorption syndrome

PRECAUTIONS AND CONTRAINDICATIONS
Complete biliary obstruction, hypersensitivity to bile acid sequestering resins
Caution:
Lactation, children, bleeding disorders

DRUG INTERACTIONS OF CONCERN TO DENTISTRY

• Decreased absorption of tetracyclines, cephalexin, phenobarbital, corticosteroids, clindamycin, penicillins; administer doses several hours apart.

SERIOUS REACTIONS

! GI tract obstruction, hyperchloremic acidosis, and osteoporosis secondary to calcium excretion may occur.
! High dosage may interfere with fat absorption, resulting in steatorrhea.

DENTAL CONSIDERATIONS

General:
• Consider semisupine chair position for patient comfort because of GI side effects of disease.

conivaptan

con-ih-**vap′**-tan
(Vaprisol)

CATEGORY AND SCHEDULE

Pregnancy Risk Category: C

Drug Class: Vasopressin antagonist

MECHANISM OF ACTION

An arginine vasopressin (AVP) V1A and V2 selective antagonist that inhibits vasopressin binding V1A in the liver and V1 and V2 sites in renal collecting ducts. Results in excretion of free water.
Therapeutic Effect: Restores normal fluid and electrolyte status.

USES

Treatment of euvolemic hyponatremia in hospitalized patients

PHARMACOKINETICS

Protein binding: 99%. Metabolized in liver; CYP3A4 is responsible for primary metabolism. Primarily eliminated in feces (approximately 83%); minimal excretion in urine (about 12%). ***Half-life:*** 3.6–8.6 hr.

INDICATIONS AND DOSAGES

▸ **Hyponatremia**

IV

Adults. Initially, a loading dose of 20 mg given over 30 min. Maintenance: 20 mg/day as continuous infusion over 24 hr for an additional 1–3 days. May titrate to maximum dose of 40 mg/day; total duration should not exceed 4 days after loading dose. Safety and efficacy have not been established in children.

SIDE EFFECTS/ADVERSE REACTIONS

Frequent
Injection site reaction, headache
Occasional
Hypokalemia, thirst, vomiting, diarrhea, hypertension, orthostatic hypotension, polyuria, phlebitis, constipation, dry mouth, anemia, fever, nausea, confusion, erythema, insomnia, atrial fibrillation, hyper- or hypoglycemia, hyponatremia, pneumonia, UTI, hypomagnesemia, pain, dehydration, oral candidiasis, hematuria

PRECAUTIONS AND CONTRAINDICATIONS

Hypersensitivity to conivaptan or its components
Use with ketoconazole, itraconazole, clarithromycin, ritonavir, and indinavir is contraindicated
Caution:
Hyponatremia with underlying CHF, renal, or hepatic impairment

DRUG INTERACTIONS OF CONCERN TO DENTISTRY

• CYP3A4 inducers: may decrease the levels and effects of conivaptan.
• CYP3A4 inhibitors (e.g., erythromycin): may increase the levels and effects of conivaptan.
• CYP3A4 substrates: conivaptan may increase the levels and effects of CYP3A4 substrates.
• Digoxin: may increase the levels of digoxin.

SERIOUS REACTIONS

! Atrial fibrillation has been reported.

DENTAL CONSIDERATIONS

• Monitor vital signs at every appointment because of cardiovascular side effects.
• Avoid NSAIDs because of renal side effects.
• After supine positioning, have patient sit upright for at least 2 min before standing to avoid orthostatic hypotension.
• Patients taking this medication are treated on an inpatient basis.

Consultations:

• Consult physician to determine disease control and ability of patient to tolerate dental procedures, if needed while receiving drug.

Teach Patient/Family to:

• Report signs and symptoms of dry mouth and candidiasis.

C

cortisone acetate

kor′-ti-sone **ass′**-eh-tayte (Cortate[AUS], Cortone[CAN])
Do not confuse cortisone with Cort-Dome.

CATEGORY AND SCHEDULE

Pregnancy Risk Category: C (D if used in the first trimester)

Drug Class: Glucocorticoid, short-acting

MECHANISM OF ACTION

An adrenocortical steroid that inhibits the accumulation of inflammatory cells at inflammation sites, phagocytosis, lysosomal enzyme release and synthesis, and release of mediators of inflammation.
Therapeutic Effect: Prevents or suppresses cell-mediated immune reactions. Decreases or prevents tissue response to inflammatory process.

USES

Treatment of inflammation, severe allergy, adrenal insufficiency, collagen disorders, respiratory, dermatologic disorders

PHARMACOKINETICS

Well absorbed after oral administration. ***Half-life:*** 60–90 min. Metabolized in liver and kidneys, approximately one-third excreted in urine as metabolites.

INDICATIONS AND DOSAGES

Dosage is dependent on the condition being treated and patient response.

C

▸ **Antiinflammation, Immunosuppression**
PO
Adults, Elderly. 25–300 mg/day in divided doses q12–24h.
Children. 2.5–10 mg/kg/day in divided doses q6–8h.
▸ **Physiologic Replacement**
PO
Adults, Elderly. 25–35 mg/day.
Children. 0.5–0.75 mg/kg/day in divided doses q8h.

SIDE EFFECTS/ADVERSE REACTIONS

Frequent
Insomnia, heartburn, anxiety, abdominal distention, increased diaphoresis, acne, mood swings, increased appetite, facial flushing, delayed wound healing, increased susceptibility to infection, diarrhea or constipation
Occasional
Headache, edema, change in skin color, frequent urination
Rare
Tachycardia, allergic reaction (such as rash and hives), psychological changes, hallucinations, depression

PRECAUTIONS AND CONTRAINDICATIONS

Hypersensitivity to corticosteroids, administration of live virus vaccine, peptic ulcers (except in life-threatening situations), systemic fungal infection
Caution:
Diabetes mellitus, glaucoma, osteoporosis, seizure disorders, ulcerative colitis, CHF, myasthenia gravis, renal disease, esophagitis, peptic ulcer, rifampin

DRUG INTERACTIONS OF CONCERN TO DENTISTRY

- Decreased action: barbiturates, rifabutin, rifampin
- Increased GI side effects: alcohol, salicylates, NSAIDs
- Increased action: ketoconazole, macrolide antibiotics
- Hepatotoxicity: acetaminophen (chronic, high doses)

SERIOUS REACTIONS

! Long-term therapy may cause hypocalcemia, hypokalemia, muscle wasting in arms and legs, osteoporosis, spontaneous fractures, amenorrhea, cataracts, glaucoma, peptic ulcer disease, and CHF.
! Abrupt withdrawal following long-term therapy may cause anorexia, nausea, fever, headache, joint pain, rebound inflammation, fatigue, weakness, lethargy, dizziness, and orthostatic hypotension.

DENTAL CONSIDERATIONS

General:
- Monitor vital signs at every appointment because of cardiovascular side effects.
- Patients on chronic drug therapy may rarely have symptoms of blood dyscrasias, which can include infection, bleeding, and poor healing.
- Assess salivary flow as a factor in caries, periodontal disease, and candidiasis.
- Avoid prescribing aspirin-containing products.
- Symptoms of oral infections may be masked.
- Place on frequent recall to evaluate healing response.
- Prophylactic antibiotics may be indicated to prevent infection if surgery or deep scaling is planned.
- Determine dose and duration of steroid therapy for each patient to assess risk for stress tolerance and immunosuppression.

• Patients who have been or are currently on chronic steroid therapy (>2 wk) may require supplemental steroids for dental treatment.
• Determine why the patient is taking the drug.

Consultations:

• In a patient with symptoms of blood dyscrasias, request a medical consultation for blood studies and postpone dental treatment until normal values are reestablished.
• Medical consultation may be required to assess disease control and stress tolerance of patient.
• Consultation may be required to confirm steroid dose and duration of use.

Teach Patient/Family to:

• Encourage effective oral hygiene to prevent soft tissue inflammation.
• Prevent injury when using oral hygiene aids.
• When chronic dry mouth occurs, advise patient to:
  • Avoid mouth rinses with high alcohol content because of drying effects.
  • Use daily home fluoride products for anticaries effect.
  • Use sugarless gum, frequent sips of water, or saliva substitutes.

cottonseed oil

OTHER NAMES

Numoisyn

Drug Class: Prescription nonherbal remedy

MAJOR INGREDIENTS

Hydrogenated cottonseed oil, sorbitol, polyethylene glycol, malic acid, sodium citrate, calcium phosphate, citric acid, magnesium stearate, silicon dioxide in lozenge dose form

CLAIMED ACTIONS

Exerts an oral demulcent (coating) effect in the oral cavity.

USES

For oral lubrication for the relief of dry mouth (xerostomia) associated with medication use, chemotherapy, head-and-neck irradiation involving the salivary glands, or Sjögren's syndrome. It is also recommended for radiation- or chemotherapy-induced mucositis (this indication is not supported by randomized clinical trials).

ADMINISTRATION

The lozenge is dissolved slowly in the mouth as needed (not to exceed 16/day).

SIDE EFFECTS

Excessive consumption can cause minor digestive problems.

DRUG INTERACTIONS

None reported

DENTAL CONSIDERATIONS

Patients with xerostomia must be monitored carefully for periodontal inflammation and caries and treated accordingly with saliva substitutes, xylitol chewing gum, non-alcoholic mouth rinses and topical fluorides. Patients with a history of head-and-neck irradiation may develop osteoradionecrosis from invasive dental procedures, and patients with a history of the use of antineoplastic drugs should be monitored for oral signs and symptoms of recurrences of certain tumors, mucositis, and blood dyscrasias.

C

cromolyn sodium

kroe′-moe-lin **so′**-dee-um
(Apo-Cromolyn[CAN], Crolom, Gastrocom, Intal, Nasalcrom, Opticrom, Rynacrom[AUS])

CATEGORY AND SCHEDULE

Pregnancy Risk Category: B

Drug Class: Antiasthmatic, mast cell stabilizer

MECHANISM OF ACTION

An antiasthmatic and antiallergic agent that prevents mast cell release of histamine and formation of other mediators (leukotrienes) of anaphylaxis by inhibiting degranulation after contact with antigens.

Therapeutic Effect: Helps prevent symptoms of asthma, allergic rhinitis, mastocytosis, and exercise-induced bronchospasm.

USES

Treatment of allergic rhinitis, severe perennial bronchial asthma, exercise-induced bronchospasm (prevention), prevention of acute bronchospasm induced by environmental pollutants, mastocytosis

PHARMACOKINETICS

Minimal absorption after PO, inhalation, or nasal administration. Absorbed portion excreted in urine or by biliary system. ***Half-life:*** 80–90 min.

INDICATIONS AND DOSAGES

▸ **Asthma**

Inhalation (Nebulization)

Adults, Elderly, Children older than 2 yr. 20 mg 3–4 times a day.

Aerosol spray

Adults, Elderly, Children 12 yr and older. Initially, 2 sprays 4 times a day. Maintenance: 2–4 sprays 3–4 times a day.

Children 5–11 yr. Initially, 2 sprays 4 times a day, then 1–2 sprays 3–4 times a day.

▸ **Prevention of Bronchospasm**

Inhalation (Nebulization)

Adults, Elderly, Children older than 2 yr. 20 mg 1 hr before exercise or exposure to allergens.

Aerosol spray

Adults, Elderly, Children older than 5 yr. 2 sprays 1 hr before exercise or exposure to allergens.

▸ **Food Allergy, Inflammatory Bowel Disease**

PO

Adults, Elderly, Children older than 12 yr. 200–400 mg 4 times a day.

Children 2–12 yr. 100–200 mg 4 times a day. Maximum: 40 mg/kg/day.

▸ **Allergic Rhinitis**

Intranasal

Adults, Elderly, Children older than 6 yr. 1 spray each nostril 3–4 times a day. May increase up to 6 times a day.

▸ **Systemic Mastocytosis**

PO

Adults, Elderly, Children older than 12 yr. 200 mg 4 times a day.

Children 2–12 yr. 100 mg 4 times a day. Maximum: 40 mg/kg/day.

Children younger than 2 yr. 20 mg/kg/day in 4 divided doses. Maximum: 30 mg/kg/day (children 6 mo–2 yr).

▸ **Conjunctivitis**

Ophthalmic

Adults, Elderly, Children older than 4 yr. 1–2 drops in both eyes 4–6 times a day.

SIDE EFFECTS/ADVERSE REACTIONS

Frequent

PO: Headache, diarrhea
Inhalation: Cough, dry mouth and throat, stuffy nose, throat irritation, unpleasant taste
Nasal: Nasal burning, stinging, or irritation; increased sneezing
Ophthalmic: Eye burning or stinging

Occasional

PO: Rash, abdominal pain, arthralgia, nausea, insomnia
Inhalation: Bronchospasm, hoarseness, lacrimation
Nasal: Cough, headache, unpleasant taste, postnasal drip
Ophthalmic: Lacrimation and itching of eye

Rare

Inhalation: Dizziness, painful urination, arthralgia, myalgia, rash
Nasal: Epistaxis, rash
Ophthalmic: Chemosis or edema of conjunctiva, eye irritation

PRECAUTIONS AND CONTRAINDICATIONS

Status asthmaticus

Caution:

Lactation, renal disease, hepatic disease, children younger than 5 yr

DRUG INTERACTIONS OF CONCERN TO DENTISTRY

• None reported

SERIOUS REACTIONS

! Anaphylaxis occurs rarely when cromolyn is given by the inhalation, nasal, or oral route.

DENTAL CONSIDERATIONS

General:

• Determine why patient is taking the drug.
• Protect patient's eyes from accidental spatter during dental treatment.
• Avoid dental light in patient's eyes; offer dark glasses for patient comfort.
• Assess salivary flow as a factor in caries, periodontal disease, and candidiasis.
• Consider semisupine chair position for patients with respiratory disease.
• A stress-reduction protocol may be required.
• Midday appointments and a stress-reduction protocol may be required for anxious patients.
• Be aware that aspirin or sulfite preservatives in vasoconstrictor-containing products can exacerbate asthma.

Consultations:

• Consider drug in diagnosis of taste alteration and burning mouth syndrome.
• Medical consultation may be required to assess disease control and stress tolerance of patient.

Teach Patient/Family to:

• Rinse mouth with water after each inhaled dose to prevent dryness.
• When chronic dry mouth occurs, advise patient to:
  • Avoid mouth rinses with high alcohol content because of drying effects.
  • Use daily home fluoride products for anticaries effect.
  • Use sugarless gum, frequent sips of water, or saliva substitutes.

C

cyanocobalamin (vitamin B_{12})

sye-an-oh-koe-**bal′**-ah-min
(Bedoz[CAN], Cytamen[AUS], Nascobal)

CATEGORY AND SCHEDULE

Pregnancy Risk Category: A (C if used in doses above recommended daily allowance)

Drug Class: Vitamin B_{12}, water-soluble vitamin

MECHANISM OF ACTION

Acts as a coenzyme for various metabolic functions, including fat and carbohydrate metabolism and protein synthesis.
Therapeutic Effect: Necessary for cell growth and replication, hematopoiesis, and myelin synthesis.

USES

Vitamin B_{12} deficiency, pernicious anemia, vitamin B_{12} malabsorption syndrome, Schilling test, increased requirements with pregnancy thyrotoxicosis, hemolytic anemia, hemorrhage, renal and hepatic disease; intranasal gel: maintaining vitamin B_{12} levels in patients with HIV, multiple sclerosis, or Crohn's disease

PHARMACOKINETICS

In the presence of calcium, absorbed systemically in lower half of ileum. Initially, bound to intrinsic factor; this complex passes down intestine, binding to receptor sites on ileal mucosa. Protein binding: High. Metabolized in the liver. Primarily eliminated unchanged in urine.
Half-life: 6 days.

INDICATIONS AND DOSAGES

▸ **Pernicious Anemia**

IM, Subcutaneous
Adults, Elderly. 100 mcg/day for 7 days, then every other day for 7 days, then every 3–4 days for 2–3 wk. Maintenance: 100 mcg/mo (oral 1000–2000 mcg/day).
Children. 30–50 mcg/day for 2 or more wk. Maintenance: 100 mcg/mo.
Neonates. 1000 mcg/day for 2 or more wk. Maintenance: 50 mcg/mo.
Intranasal
Adults, Elderly. 500 mcg once a wk.

▸ **Uncomplicated Vitamin B_{12} Deficiency**

PO
Adults, Elderly. 1000–2000 mcg/day.
IM, Subcutaneous
Adults, Elderly. 100 mcg/day for 5–10 days, followed by 100–200 mcg/mo.

▸ **Complicated Vitamin B_{12} Deficiency**

IM, Subcutaneous
Adults, Elderly. 1000 mcg (with IM or IV folic acid 15 mg) as a single dose, then 1000 mcg/day plus oral folic acid 5 mg/day for 7 days.

SIDE EFFECTS/ADVERSE REACTIONS

Occasional
Diarrhea, pruritus

PRECAUTIONS AND CONTRAINDICATIONS

Folic acid deficiency anemia, hereditary optic nerve atrophy, history of allergy to cobalamins
Caution:
Lactation, children

DRUG INTERACTIONS OF CONCERN TO DENTISTRY

- Increased absorption: prednisone

SERIOUS REACTIONS

! Impurities in preparation may cause a rare allergic reaction.
! Peripheral vascular thrombosis, pulmonary edema, hypokalemia, and CHF may occur.

DENTAL CONSIDERATIONS

General:

- Deficiency in vitamin B_{12} and other B-complex vitamins may cause oral symptomatology.

cyclobenzaprine hydrochloride

sye-kloe-**ben**′-za-preen hi-droh-**klor**′-ide
(Flexeril, Flexitec[CAN], Novo-Cycloprine[CAN])
Do not confuse cyclobenzaprine with cycloserine or cyproheptadine, or Flexeril with Floxin.

CATEGORY AND SCHEDULE

Pregnancy Risk Category: B

Drug Class: Skeletal muscle relaxant, centrally-acting tricyclic

MECHANISM OF ACTION

A centrally-acting skeletal muscle relaxant that reduces tonic somatic muscle activity at the level of the brainstem.
Therapeutic Effect: Relieves local skeletal muscle spasm.

USES

Adjunct for relief of muscle spasm and pain in musculoskeletal conditions

PHARMACOKINETICS

Route	Onset	Peak	Duration
PO	1 hr	3–4 hr	12–24 hr

Well but slowly absorbed from the GI tract. Protein binding: 93%. Metabolized in the GI tract and the liver. Primarily excreted in urine.
Half-life: 1–3 days.

INDICATIONS AND DOSAGES

▸ **Acute, Painful Musculoskeletal Conditions**

PO

Adults. Initially, 5 mg 3 times a day. May increase to 10 mg 3 times a day.
Elderly. 5 mg 3 times a day.

▸ **Dosage in Hepatic Impairment**

Mild. 5 mg 3 times a day.
Moderate and severe. Not recommended.

PRECAUTIONS AND CONTRAINDICATIONS

Acute recovery phase of MI, arrhythmias, CHF, heart block, conduction disturbances, hyperthyroidism, use within 14 days of MAOIs

Caution:

Renal disease, hepatic disease, addictive personality, elderly

SIDE EFFECTS/ADVERSE REACTIONS

Frequent

Somnolence, dry mouth, dizziness

Rare

Fatigue, asthenia, blurred vision, headache, nervousness, confusion, nausea, constipation, dyspepsia, unpleasant taste

PRECAUTIONS AND CONTRAINDICATIONS

Acute recovery phase of MI, dysrhythmias, heart block, CHF,

C

hypersensitivity, children younger than 12 yr, intermittent porphyria, thyroid disease, concomitant use with or within 14 days of discontinuing MAOIs, renal disease, hepatic disease, addictive personality, elderly

DRUG INTERACTIONS OF CONCERN TO DENTISTRY

- Increased CNS depression: alcohol, narcotics, barbiturates, sedatives, hypnotics
- Increased effects of anticholinergic drugs
- Increased effects of direct-acting sympathomimetics (epinephrine, levonordefrin)

SERIOUS REACTIONS

! Overdose may result in visual hallucinations, hyperactive reflexes, muscle rigidity, vomiting, and hyperpyrexia.

DENTAL CONSIDERATIONS

General:

- Monitor vital signs at every appointment because of cardiovascular side effects.
- Assess salivary flow as a factor in caries, periodontal disease, and candidiasis.
- After supine positioning, have patient sit upright for at least 2 min to avoid orthostatic hypotension.
- Use vasoconstrictors with caution, in low doses, and with careful aspiration. Avoid use of gingival retraction cord with epinephrine.
- Place on frequent recall because of oral side effects.
- Consider drug in diagnosis of taste alterations.

Consultations:

- Medical consultation may be required to assess disease control.

Teach Patient/Family:

- When chronic dry mouth occurs, advise patient to:
  - Avoid mouth rinses with high alcohol content because of drying effects.
  - Use daily home fluoride products for anticaries effect.
  - Use sugarless gum, frequent sips of water, or saliva substitutes.

cyclopentolate hydrochloride

sye-kloe-**pen**′-toe-late
hi-droh-**klor**′-ide
(AK-Pentolate, Cyclogyl, Cylate, Diopentolate[CAN], Ocu-Pentolate, Pentolair)

CATEGORY AND SCHEDULE

Pregnancy Risk Category: C

Drug Class: Cycloplegic; mydriatic

MECHANISM OF ACTION

An antimuscarinic similar to atropine that competes with acetylcholine. Blocks the responses of the sphincter muscle of the iris and the accommodative muscle of the ciliary body to cholinergic stimulation.

Therapeutic Effect: Results in mydriasis and cycloplegia.

USES

Used to dilate (enlarge) the pupil for eye examination.

PHARMACOKINETICS

Rapid systemic absorption following ophthalmic administration. Shorter duration of action than atropine. Complete recovery takes 6–24 hr.

INDICATIONS AND DOSAGES

▸ **Cycloplegia Induction, Mydriasis Induction**

Ophthalmic

Adults, Elderly, Children. Instill 1–2 drops of 0.5%–2% solution in eye(s). May repeat with 0.5% or 1% solution in 5–10 min as needed.

Neonates, infants. Instill 1 drop of 0.5%–2% solution in eye(s) followed by 1 drop of 0.5% or 1% in 5 min as needed.

SIDE EFFECTS/ADVERSE REACTIONS

Occasional

Blurred vision, burning of eye, photophobia

Rare

Conjunctivitis, increased intraocular pressure

PRECAUTIONS AND CONTRAINDICATIONS

Narrow-angle glaucoma, anatomical narrow angles, hypersensitivity to cyclopentolate or any component of the formulation

DRUG INTERACTIONS OF CONCERN TO DENTISTRY

• None reported

SERIOUS REACTIONS

! Systemic absorption, which includes signs and symptoms of confusion, psychosis, and ataxia; tachycardia and vasodilation occur rarely.

DENTAL CONSIDERATIONS

General:

• Not likely to be encountered in the dental office; used for diagnostic procedures.

• Question patient about eye health, including the presence of glaucoma.

cyclophosphamide

sye-kloe-**foss′**-fa-mide

(Cycloblastin[AUS], Cytoxan, Endoxan Asta[AUS], Endoxon Asta[AUS], Neosar, Procytox[CAN])

Do not confuse Cytoxan with cefoxitin, Ciloxan, cyclosporine, or Cytotec.

CATEGORY AND SCHEDULE

Pregnancy Risk Category: D

Drug Class: Antineoplastic alkylating agent

MECHANISM OF ACTION

An alkylating agent that inhibits DNA and RNA protein synthesis by cross-linking with DNA and RNA strands, preventing cell growth. Cell cycle-phase nonspecific.

Therapeutic Effect: Potent immunosuppressant.

USES

Treatment of Hodgkin's disease; lymphomas; leukemia; cancer of female reproductive tract, lung, prostate; multiple myeloma; neuroblastoma, retinoblastoma; Ewing's sarcoma; Burkitt's lymphoma; advanced mycosis fungoides; nephrotic syndrome (children)

PHARMACOKINETICS

Well absorbed from the GI tract. Protein binding: Low. Crosses the blood-brain barrier. Metabolized in the liver to active metabolites. Primarily excreted in urine. Removed by hemodialysis. ***Half-life:*** 3–12 hr.

C

C

INDICATIONS AND DOSAGES

▸ **Ovarian Adenocarcinoma, Breast Carcinoma, Hodgkin's Disease, Non-Hodgkin's Lymphoma, Multiple Myeloma, Leukemia (Acute Lymphoblastic, Acute Myelogenous, Acute Monocytic, Chronic Granulocytic, Chronic Lymphocytic), Mycosis Fungoides, Disseminated Neuroblastoma, Retinoblastoma**

PO

Adults. 1–5 mg/kg/day.

Children. Initially, 2–8 mg/kg/day. Maintenance: 2–5 mg/kg twice a wk.

IV

Adults. 40–50 mg/kg in divided doses over 2–5 days; or 10–15 mg/kg every 7–10 days or 3–5 mg/kg twice a wk.

Children. 2–8 mg/kg/day for 6 days or total dose for 7 days once a wk.

▸ **Biopsy-Proven Minimal-Change Nephrotic Syndrome**

PO

Adults, Children. 2.5–3 mg/kg/day for 60–90 days.

SIDE EFFECTS/ADVERSE REACTIONS

Expected

Marked leukopenia 8–15 days after initial therapy

Frequent

Nausea, vomiting (beginning about 6 hr after administration and lasting about 4 hr), alopecia

Occasional

Diarrhea, darkening of skin and fingernails, stomatitis, headache, diaphoresis

Rare

Pain or redness at injection site

PRECAUTIONS AND CONTRAINDICATIONS

Lactation

Caution:

Radiation therapy

DRUG INTERACTIONS OF CONCERN TO DENTISTRY

• Increased blood dyscrasia: NSAIDs, dapsone, phenothiazines, corticosteroids

• Increased metabolism: phenobarbital

SERIOUS REACTIONS

! Major toxic effect is myelosuppression resulting in blood dyscrasias, such as leukopenia, anemia, thrombocytopenia, and hypoprothrombinemia.

! Expect leukopenia to resolve in 17–28 days. Anemia generally occurs after large doses or prolonged therapy. Thrombocytopenia may occur 10–15 days after drug initiation.

! Hemorrhagic cystitis occurs commonly in long-term therapy, especially in pediatric patients.

! Pulmonary fibrosis and cardiotoxicity have been noted with high doses.

! Amenorrhea, azoospermia, and hyperkalemia may also occur.

DENTAL CONSIDERATIONS

General:

• Monitor vital signs at every appointment because of cardiovascular and respiratory side effects.

• Patients on chronic drug therapy may rarely have symptoms of blood dyscrasias, which can include infection, bleeding, and poor healing.

• Avoid prescribing aspirin-containing products.

• Prophylactic antibiotics may be indicated to prevent infection if surgery or deep scaling is planned because of leukopenic drug side effects.

• Patients receiving chemotherapy may require palliative treatment for stomatitis.

Consultations:

• In a patient with symptoms of blood dyscrasias, request a medical consultation for blood studies and postpone dental treatment until normal values are reestablished.

• Take precautions if dental surgery is anticipated and anesthesia is required.

Teach Patient/Family to:

• Encourage effective oral hygiene to prevent soft tissue inflammation.

• Prevent injury when using oral hygiene aids.

cycloserine

sye-kloe-**ser**′-een

(Closina[AUS], Seromycin)

CATEGORY AND SCHEDULE

Pregnancy Risk Category: C

Drug Class: Antitubercular

MECHANISM OF ACTION

An antitubercular that inhibits cell wall synthesis by competing with the amino acid, D-alanine, for incorporation into the bacterial cell wall.

Therapeutic Effect: Causes disruption of bacterial cell wall. Bactericidal or bacteriostatic.

USES

Treatment of pulmonary TB, extrapulmonary as adjunctive

PHARMACOKINETICS

Readily absorbed from the GI tract. No protein binding. Widely distributed (including CSF). Metabolized in liver. Primarily excreted in urine. Removed by hemodialysis. ***Half-life:*** 10 hr.

INDICATIONS AND DOSAGES

▸ **TB**

Adults, Elderly. 250 mg q12h for 14 days, then 500 mg to 1g/day in 2 divided doses for 18–24 mo. Maximum: 1 g as a single daily dose.

Children. 10–20 mg/kg/day in 2 divided doses. Maximum: 1000 mg/day for 18–24 mo.

▸ **Dosage in Renal Impairment**

Creatinine Clearance	Dosage Interval
10–50 ml/min	q24h
Less than 10 ml/min	q36–48h

SIDE EFFECTS/ADVERSE REACTIONS

Occasional

Drowsiness, headache, dizziness, vertigo, seizures, confusion, psychosis, paresis, tremor, vitamin B_{12} deficiency, folate deficiency, cardiac arrhythmias, increased liver enzymes

PRECAUTIONS AND CONTRAINDICATIONS

Epilepsy, depression, severe anxiety, psychosis, severe renal insufficiency, excessive concurrent use of alcohol, history of hypersensitivity reactions with previous cycloserine therapy

DRUG INTERACTIONS OF CONCERN TO DENTISTRY

• Seizures: alcohol

• Drowsiness is a common side effect; although no drug interactions with sedatives are reported, increased drowsiness is possible

C

SERIOUS REACTIONS/ADVERSE REACTIONS

! Neurotoxicity, as evidenced by confusion, agitation, CNS depression, psychosis, coma, and seizures, occur rarely.
! Neurotoxic effects of cycloserine may be treated and prevented with the administration of 200–300 mg of pyridoxine daily.

DENTAL CONSIDERATIONS

General:
• Patients on chronic drug therapy may rarely have symptoms of blood dyscrasias, which can include infection, bleeding, and poor healing.
• Examine for evidence of oral signs of disease.
• Determine why the patient is taking the drug (i.e., for preventive or therapeutic therapy).
Consultation:
• Medical consultation may be required to assess patient's ability to tolerate stress.
• In a patient with symptoms of blood dyscrasias, request a medical consultation for blood studies and postpone dental treatment until normal values are reestablished.
• Determine that noninfectious status exists by ensuring that:
  • Anti-TB drugs have been taken for more than 3 wk.
  • Culture confirms antibiotic susceptibility to TB microorganism.
  • Patient has had three consecutive negative sputum smears.
  • Patient is not in the coughing stage.
Teach Patient/Family to:
• Avoid mouth rinses with high alcohol content.
• Use caution to prevent injury when using oral hygiene aids.
• Encourage effective oral hygiene to prevent soft tissue inflammation.
• Take medication for full length of prescribed therapy to ensure effectiveness of treatment and prevent the emergence of resistant forms of microbe.

cyclosporine

sye-kloe-**spor′**-in
(Cysporin[AUS], Gengraf, Neoral, Restasis, Sandimmune, Sandimmune Neoral[AUS])
Do not confuse cyclosporine with cycloserine, cyclophosphamide, or Cyklokapron.

CATEGORY AND SCHEDULE

Pregnancy Risk Category: C

Drug Class: Immunosuppressant

MECHANISM OF ACTION

A cyclic polypeptide that inhibits both cellular and humoral immune responses by inhibiting interleukin-2, a proliferative factor needed for T-cell activity.
Therapeutic Effect: Prevents organ rejection and relieves symptoms of psoriasis and arthritis.

USES

Prevent rejection of tissues/allogeneic organ transplants; severe recalcitrant psoriasis; rheumatoid arthritis (Neoral only). Note: Sandimmune and Neoral are not bioequivalent.

PHARMACOKINETICS

Variably absorbed from the GI tract. Protein binding: 90%. Widely distributed. Metabolized in the liver.

Eliminated primarily by biliary or fecal excretion. Not removed by hemodialysis. ***Half-life:*** Adults, 10–27 hr; children, 7–19 hr.

INDICATIONS AND DOSAGES

▸ **Transplantation, Prevention of Organ Rejection**

PO

Adults, Elderly, Children. 10–18 mg/kg/dose given 4–12 hr prior to organ transplantation. Maintenance: 5–15 mg/kg/day in divided doses then tapered to 3–10 mg/kg/day.

IV

Adults, Elderly, Children. Initially, 5–6 mg/kg/dose given 4–12 hr prior to organ transplantation. Maintenance: 2–10 mg/kg/day in divided doses.

▸ **Rheumatoid Arthritis**

PO

Adults, Elderly. Initially, 2.5 mg/kg a day in 2 divided doses. May increase by 0.5–0.75 mg/kg/day. Maximum: 4 mg/kg/day.

▸ **Psoriasis**

PO

Adults, Elderly. Initially, 2.5 mg/kg/day in 2 divided doses. May increase by 0.5 mg/kg/day. Maximum: 4 mg/kg/day.

▸ **Dry Eye**

Ophthalmic

Adults, Elderly. Instill 1 drip in each affected eye q12h.

SIDE EFFECTS/ADVERSE REACTIONS

Frequent

Mild-to-moderate hypertension, hirsutism, tremors

Occasional

Acne, leg cramps, gingival hyperplasia (marked by red, bleeding, and tender gums), paresthesia, diarrhea, nausea, vomiting, headache

Rare

Hypersensitivity reaction, abdominal discomfort, gynecomastia, sinusitis

PRECAUTIONS AND CONTRAINDICATIONS

History of hypersensitivity to cyclosporine or polyoxyethylated castor oil

Caution:

Severe renal disease, severe hepatic disease

DRUG INTERACTIONS OF CONCERN TO DENTISTRY

Systemic Form

• Hepatotoxicity/nephrotoxicity: erythromycin, azithromycin, clarithromycin

• Decreased action: barbiturates, carbamazepine

• Possibly reduced blood levels: clindamycin

• Increased infection and immunosuppression: corticosteroids

• Increased blood levels and risk of toxicity: fluconazole, ketoconazole, and itraconazole

Ophthalmic-Dose Form

• None reported

SERIOUS REACTIONS

! Mild nephrotoxicity occurs in 25% of renal transplant patients, 38% of cardiac transplant patients, and 37% of liver transplant patients, generally 2 to 3 months after transplantation (more severe toxicity generally occurs soon after transplantation). Hepatotoxicity occurs in 4% of renal transplant patients, 7% of cardiac transplant patients, and 4% of liver transplant patients, generally within the first month after transplantation. Both toxicities usually respond to dosage reduction.

! Severe hyperkalemia and hyperuricemia occur occasionally.

C

DENTAL CONSIDERATIONS

Systemic Form

General:

- Monitor vital signs at every appointment because of cardiovascular side effects.
- Patients on chronic drug therapy may rarely have symptoms of blood dyscrasias, which can include infection, bleeding, and poor healing.
- Examine for gingival enlargement (place on frequent recall to evaluate gingival condition and healing response).
- Monitor time since organ/tissue transplant.

Consultations:

- Antibiotic prophylaxis usually is recommended in patients with organ transplants and immunosuppression.
- In a patient with symptoms of blood dyscrasias, request a medical consultation for blood studies and postpone dental treatment until normal values are reestablished.
- Request baseline B/P in renal transplant patients for patient evaluation before dental treatment.

Teach Patient/Family to:

- Encourage effective oral hygiene to prevent soft tissue inflammation.
- Use caution to prevent injury when using oral hygiene aids.

Ophthalmic-Dose Form

General:

- Determine why the patient is taking the drug.
- Protect the patient's eyes from accidental spatter during dental treatment.
- Avoid dental light in the patient's eyes; offer dark glasses for patient comfort.

Teach Patient/Family:

- When chronic dry mouth occurs, advise patient to:
- Avoid mouth rinses with high alcohol content because of drying effects.
- Use daily home fluoride products for anticaries effect.
- Use sugarless gum, frequent sips of water, or saliva substitutes.

cyproheptadine

si-proe-**hep**′-ta-deen
(Periactin)

CATEGORY AND SCHEDULE

Pregnancy Risk Category: B

Drug Class: Antihistamine, H_1-receptor antagonist

MECHANISM OF ACTION

An antihistamine that competes with histamine at histaminic receptor sites. Anticholinergic effects cause drying of nasal mucosa.
Therapeutic Effect: Relieves allergic conditions (urticaria, pruritus).

USES

Allergy symptoms, rhinitis, pruritus, cold urticaria

PHARMACOKINETICS

Well absorbed from GI tract. Metabolized in liver. Primarily eliminated in feces. ***Half-life:*** 16 hr.

INDICATIONS AND DOSAGES

▸ **Allergic Condition**

PO

Adults, Children older than 15 yr. 4 mg 3 times a day. May increase dose but do not exceed 0.5 mg/kg/day.

Children 7–14 yr. 4 mg 2–3 times a day, or 0.25 mg/kg daily in divided doses.
Children 2–6 yr. 2 mg 2–3 times a day, or 0.25 mg/kg daily in divided doses.

▸ **Usual Elderly Dosage**
PO
Initially, 4 mg 2 times a day.

SIDE EFFECTS/ADVERSE REACTIONS

Frequent
Drowsiness, dizziness, muscular weakness, dry mouth/nose/throat/lips, urinary retention, thickening of bronchial secretions
Frequent
Sedation, dizziness, hypotension
Occasional
Epigastric distress, flushing, visual disturbances, hearing disturbances, paresthesia, sweating, chills

PRECAUTIONS AND CONTRAINDICATIONS

Acute asthmatic attack, patients receiving MAOIs, history of hypersensitivity to antihistamines
Caution:
Increased intraocular pressure, renal disease, cardiac disease, hypertension, bronchial asthma, seizure disorder, stenosed peptic ulcers, hyperthyroidism, prostatic hypertrophy, bladder neck obstruction, elderly

DRUG INTERACTIONS OF CONCERN TO DENTISTRY

• Increased CNS depression: alcohol, CNS depressants
• Increased effect of anticholinergic drugs

SERIOUS REACTIONS

! Children may experience dominant paradoxical reaction (restlessness, insomnia, euphoria, nervousness, tremors).
! Overdose in children may result in hallucinations, convulsions, death.
! Hypersensitivity reaction (eczema, pruritus, rash, cardiac disturbances, angioedema, photosensitivity) may occur.
! Overdose may vary from CNS depression (sedation, apnea, cardiovascular collapse, death) to severe paradoxical reaction (hallucinations, tremor, seizures).

DENTAL CONSIDERATIONS

General:
• Assess salivary flow as a factor in caries, periodontal disease, and candidiasis.
• Determine why the patient is taking the drug.

cysteamine bitartrate

sis-**tee**′-ah-meen bye-**tar**′-trate
(Cystagon)

CATEGORY AND SCHEDULE

Pregnancy Risk Category: C

Drug Class: Nephropathic cystinosis therapy

MECHANISM OF ACTION

An aminothiol that participates within lysosomes in a thiol-disulfide interchange reaction converting cystine into cysteine and cysteine-cysteamine mixed disulfide, both of which can exit cystinotic lysosomes.
Therapeutic Effect: Lowers the cystine content in cells.

C

USES

Used to prevent damage that may be caused by the buildup of cystine crystals in organs such as the kidneys.

PHARMACOKINETICS

Poorly bound to plasma proteins. ***Half-life:*** Unknown.

INDICATIONS AND DOSAGES

▸ **Cystinosis**

PO

Adults. Initially, ¼–⅙ of maintenance dose. Gradually, increase dose over 4–6 wk. Maintenance. 2 g/day in 4 divided doses.

Children older than 12 yr and weighing more than 110 lb. 2 g/day in 4 divided doses.

Children 6–12 yr. 1.30 g/m^2/day of the free base, given in 4 divided doses.

SIDE EFFECTS/ADVERSE REACTIONS

Frequent

Rash, loss of appetite, fever, vomiting, diarrhea, lethargy

Occasional

Dehydration, hypertension, nausea, abdominal pain, somnolence, nervousness, nightmares, urticaria

PRECAUTIONS AND CONTRAINDICATIONS

Hypersensitivity to cysteamine or penicillamine

DRUG INTERACTIONS OF CONCERN TO DENTISTRY

• Dental drug interactions have not been studied.

SERIOUS REACTIONS

! Leukopenia, abnormal liver function, and anemia occur rarely.

! Sudden deaths have been reported.

DENTAL CONSIDERATIONS

General:

• Patients taking this medication may have significant renal disease; thoroughly review medical and drug history.

Consultations:

• Specific consultation depends on type of renal disease.

Teach Patient/Family to:

• Encourage effective oral hygiene to prevent soft tissue inflammation.

• Prevent trauma when using oral hygiene aids.

• Update health and medication history if physician makes any changes in evaluation or drug regimens; include OTC, herbal, and nonherbal remedies in the update.

cytarabine

sigh-**tar′**-ah-bean

(Ara-C, Cytosar[CAN], Cytosar-U)

Do not confuse cytarabine with Cytadren, Cytovene, or vidarabine.

CATEGORY AND SCHEDULE

Pregnancy Risk Category: D

Drug Class: Antimetabolite; antineoplastic

MECHANISM OF ACTION

An antimetabolite that is converted intracellularly to a nucleotide. Cell cycle-specific for S phase of cell division.

Therapeutic Effect: May inhibit DNA synthesis. Potent immunosuppressive activity.

USES

Treatment of acute and chronic myelocytic leukemia, acute lymphocytic leukemia, meningeal leukemia, non-Hodgkin's lymphoma in children. Off label: Treatment of Hodgkin's lymphoma, myelodysplastic syndrome

PHARMACOKINETICS

Widely distributed; moderate amount crosses the blood-brain barrier. Protein binding: 15%. Primarily excreted in urine. ***Half-life:*** 1–3 hr.

INDICATIONS AND DOSAGES

▸ To Induce Remission in Acute Lymphocytic Leukemia, Acute and Chronic Myelocytic Leukemia, Meningeal Leukemia, or Non-Hodgkin's Lymphoma in Children

IV

Adults, Elderly, Children. 200 mg/m^2/day for 5 days q2wk as monotherapy or 100–200 mg/m^2/day for 5- to 10-day course of therapy every q2–4wk in combination therapy.

Intrathecal

Adults, Elderly, Children. 5–7.5 mg/m^2 every 2–7 days.

▸ To Maintain Remission in Acute Lymphocytic Leukemia, Acute and Chronic Myelocytic Leukemia, Meningeal Leukemia, or Non-Hodgkin's Lymphoma in Children

IV

Adults, Elderly, Children. 70–200 mg/m^2/day for 2–5 days every month.

IM, Subcutaneous

Adults, Elderly, Children. 1–1.5 mg/m^2 as single dose q1–4wk.

Intrathecal

Adults, Elderly, Children. 5–7.5 mg/m^2 every 2–7 days.

SIDE EFFECTS/ADVERSE REACTIONS

Frequent

IV, Subcutaneous: Asthenia, fever, pain, altered taste and smell, nausea, vomiting (risk greater with IV push than with continuous IV infusion)
Intrathecal: Headache, asthenia, altered taste and smell, confusion, somnolence, nausea, vomiting

Occasional

IV, Subcutaneous: Abnormal gait, somnolence, constipation, back pain, urinary incontinence, peripheral edema, headache, confusion
Intrathecal: Peripheral edema, back pain, constipation, abnormal gait, urinary incontinence

PRECAUTIONS AND CONTRAINDICATIONS

None known

DRUG INTERACTIONS OF CONCERN TO DENTISTRY

- Increased risk of bleeding: drugs that interfere with coagulation or platelet function, such as NSAIDs and aspirin
- Increased risk of infection; glucocorticoids

SERIOUS REACTIONS

! Myelosuppression may result in blood dyscrasias, such as leukopenia, anemia, thrombocytopenia, megaloblastosis, and reticulocytopenia, after a single IV dose.

! Leukopenia, anemia, and thrombocytopenia should be expected with daily or continuous IV therapy.

! Cytarabine syndrome, (as evidenced by fever, myalgia, rash, conjunctivitis, malaise, and chest pain) and hyperuricemia may occur.

! High-dose cytarabine therapy may produce severe CNS, GI, and pulmonary toxicity.

DENTAL CONSIDERATIONS

General:

• Determine why patient is taking the drug.
• If additional analgesia is required for dental pain, consider alternative analgesics (acetaminophen) in patients taking narcotics for acute or chronic pain.
• Avoid prescribing aspirin-containing products.
• This drug may be used in the hospital or on an outpatient basis. Confirm the patient's disease and treatment status.
• Patient on chronic drug therapy may rarely present with symptoms of blood dyscrasias, which can include infection, bleeding, and poor healing. If dyscrasia is present, caution patient to prevent oral tissue trauma when using oral hygiene aids.
• Short appointments and a stress-reduction protocol may be required for anxious patients.
• Patients may have received other chemotherapy or radiation; confirm medical and drug history.
• Patients may be at risk of infection.
• Patients may be taking a prophylactic antiinfective.
• Patients are at risk of bleeding; check for oral signs of blood loss.
• Oral infections should be eliminated and/or treated aggressively.

Consultations:

• Medical consultation should include routine blood counts including platelet counts and bleeding time.
• Consult physician; prophylactic or therapeutic antiinfectives may be indicated if surgery or periodontal treatment is required.
• Medical consultation may be required to assess immunologic status during cancer chemotherapy and determine safety risk, if any, posed by the required dental treatment.
• Medical consultation may be required to assess disease control and patient's ability to tolerate stress.

Teach Patient/Family to:

• Encourage effective oral hygiene to prevent soft tissue inflammation.
• Report oral lesions, soreness, or bleeding to dentist.
• Prevent trauma when using oral hygiene aids.
• Update health and medication history if physician makes any changes in evaluation or drug regimens; include OTC, herbal, and nonherbal remedies in the update.

dabigatran

da-**big**′-a tran
(Pradaxa)
Do not confuse Pradaxa with Plavix.

CATEGORY AND SCHEDULE

Pregnancy Risk Category: C

Drug Class: Anticoagulant, thrombin inhibitor

MECHANISM OF ACTION

A direct thrombin inhibitor that inhibits coagulation by preventing thrombin-mediated effects and by inhibition of thrombin-induced platelet aggregation.
Therapeutic Effect: Produces anticoagulation.

USES

Prevention of stroke and systemic embolism in patients with nonvalvular atrial fibrillation

PHARMACOKINETICS

Rapidly absorbed following oral administration. Peak plasma concentrations reached in 1 hr (2 hr if given with food). 35% plasma protein bound. Dabigatran etexilate is a prodrug, converted to active form by plasma and hepatic esterases. Hepatic glucuronidation to active metabolites. Excreted 80% via urine. ***Half-life:*** 12–17 hr; elderly: 14–17 hr; mild-to-moderate renal impairment: 15–18 hr; severe renal impairment: 28 hr.

INDICATIONS AND DOSAGES

▸ Nonvalvular Atrial Fibrillation

PO

Adults. 150 mg twice daily. Conversion from a parenteral anticoagulant: Initiate dabigatran ≤2 hr prior to the time of the next scheduled dose of the parenteral anticoagulant or at the time of discontinuation for a continuously administered parenteral drug; discontinue parenteral anticoagulant at the time of dabigatran initiation.
Elderly older than 65 yr. No dosage adjustment required unless renal impairment exists; however, increased risk of bleeding has been observed, particularly in elderly patients with low body weight and/or concomitant renal impairment.

▸ Secondary Prevention of Cardioembolic Stroke or TIA

PO

Adults. 150 mg twice daily initiated within 1–2 wk after stroke onset or earlier in patients at low bleeding risk.

Do not break, chew, or open capsules, as this will lead to 75% increase in absorption and potentially serious adverse reactions. May be taken without regard to meals.

SIDE EFFECTS/ADVERSE REACTIONS

Frequent

Dyspepsia, abdominal discomfort and pain, bleeding

Occasional

GERD, esophagitis, anemia, hematuria, hematoma, epistaxis, wound secretion, anaphylaxis

PRECAUTIONS AND CONTRAINDICATIONS

Hypersensitivity to dabigatran or any component of the formulation. May cause fatal bleeding. No specific antidote exists for dabigatran reversal; protamine and vitamin K do not reverse or impact anticoagulant effects of dabigatran. Use in patients with severe renal and hepatic impairment and valvular heart disease is not recommended. Use with extreme caution in elderly patients. Avoid use in patients taking other anticoagulants and P-glycoprotein inducers/inhibitors.

DRUG INTERACTIONS OF CONCERN TO DENTISTRY

- Increased risk of bleeding: NSAIDs, aspirin
- P-gp inducers (e.g., carbamazepine, barbiturates, St. John's wort): reduced blood levels and effectiveness of dabigatran
- P-gp inhibitors and CYP3A4 inhibitors (e.g., macrolide antibiotics, azole antifungals): increased blood levels and adverse effects of dabigatran

SERIOUS REACTIONS

! Discontinuing dabigatran, for elective and/or invasive procedures, increases the risk of stroke, which is sometimes fatal.

DENTAL CONSIDERATIONS

General:

- Increased intra- and postoperative bleeding, additional hemostatic measures are indicated.
- Monitor vital signs at every visit due to existing cardiovascular disease.
- Avoid discontinuation of drug therapy for routine dental procedures without consulting patient's prescribing physician.

Consultations:

- Consult physician to determine patient's coagulation status and risk for complications.

Teach Patient/Family to:

- Report changes in drug regimen.
- Report signs and symptoms of excessive postoperative bleeding.

daclizumab

day-**cly**′-zu-mab
(Zenapax)

CATEGORY AND SCHEDULE

Pregnancy Risk Category: C

Drug Class: Immunosuppressive, IgG1 monoclonal antibody

MECHANISM OF ACTION

A monoclonal antibody that binds to the interleukin-2 (IL-2) receptor complex, inhibiting the IL-2-mediated activation of T lymphocytes, a critical pathway in the cellular immune response involved in allograft rejection.
Therapeutic Effect: Prevents organ rejection.

USES

Prophylaxis of acute organ rejection in patients with renal transplants; used in combination with cyclosporine and glucocorticoids.

PHARMACOKINETICS

Half-life: Adults, 20 days.

INDICATIONS AND DOSAGES

▸ Prevention of Acute Renal Transplant Rejection (in combination with an immunosuppressive)

IV

Adults, Children. 1 mg/kg over 15 min q14 days for 5 doses, beginning no more than 24 hr before transplantation. Maximum: 100 mg.

SIDE EFFECTS/ADVERSE REACTIONS

Occasional

Constipation, nausea, diarrhea, vomiting, abdominal pain, edema, headache, dizziness, fever, pain, fatigue, insomnia, weakness, arthralgia, myalgia, diaphoresis

PRECAUTIONS AND CONTRAINDICATIONS

Caution:
Risk of lymphoproliferative disease and opportunistic infections, anaphylaxis risk unknown, long-term effects unknown, lactation, children, geriatric patients

DRUG INTERACTIONS OF CONCERN TO DENTISTRY

- None reported

SERIOUS REACTIONS

! Hypersensitivity reaction, which occurs rarely, is characterized by dyspnea, tachycardia, dysphagia, peripheral edema, rash, and pruritus.

DENTAL CONSIDERATIONS

General:
- This is a hospital-type drug, but because some dosing is continued, patients may appear in the dental office while receiving this drug.
- Transplant patients may also be taking cyclosporine and glucocorticoids; review each transplant patient's medications.
- Short appointments and a reduction protocol may be required for anxious patients.

Consultations:
- Antibiotic prophylaxis usually is recommended in patients with organ transplants and immunosuppression.
- Medical consultation may be required to assess disease control and patient's ability to tolerate stress.

Teach Patient/Family to:
- Encourage effective oral hygiene to prevent soft tissue inflammation.
- Prevent trauma when using oral hygiene aids.
- Update health and drug history if physician makes any changes in evaluation or drug regimens.

dalfampridine

dal-**fam**-pri-deen
(Ampyra)

CATEGORY AND SCHEDULE

Pregnancy Risk Category: C

Drug Class: Potassium channel blocker

MECHANISM OF ACTION

A potassium channel blocker that increases conduction of action potentials in demyelinated axons.
Therapeutic Effect: Improved walking speed.

USES

Multiple sclerosis

PHARMACOKINETICS

Rapidly and completely absorbed after PO administration. Unbound to plasma proteins. Well distributed in saliva. Minimally metabolized in liver. Primarily excreted unchanged (90%) in urine. CYP2E1 is the major isoenzyme responsible for the 3-hydroxylation of dalfampridine. ***Half-life:*** 5.2–6.5 hr.

INDICATIONS AND DOSAGES

▸ **Multiple Sclerosis**

PO

Adults. 10 mg twice a day, 12 hr apart. Max: 20 mg/day.

SIDE EFFECTS/ADVERSE REACTIONS

Frequent
Nausea, vomiting, urinary tract infection

Occasional
Abdominal pain, abnormal gait, backache, asthenia, dizziness, headache, insomnia, anxiety

Rare
Constipation, indigestion, multiple sclerosis relapse, paresthesia, seizure, nasopharyngitis, pain in throat

PRECAUTIONS AND CONTRAINDICATIONS

Hypersensitivity to dalfampridine or its components
Renal impairment, moderate or severe (CrCl ≤ 50 mL/min)
History of seizures
Caution:
Concomitant use with 4-aminopyridine derivatives
Mild renal impairment

DRUG INTERACTIONS OF CONCERN TO DENTISTRY

• None reported

SERIOUS REACTIONS

! Seizures have been observed and appear to be dose related.

DENTAL CONSIDERATIONS

General:
• Consider semisupine chair position for patient comfort if GI side effects occur.
Consultations:
• Medical consultation may be required to assess disease control.
Teach Patient/Family to:
• Encourage effective oral hygiene to prevent soft tissue inflammation.
• Prevent trauma when using oral hygiene aids.
• Be alert for the possibility of secondary oral infection and the need to see dentist immediately if signs of infection occur.

dalteparin sodium

doll′-teh-pare-in **so′**-dee-um
(Fragmin)

CATEGORY AND SCHEDULE

Pregnancy Risk Category: B

Drug Class: Heparin-type anticoagulant

MECHANISM OF ACTION

An antithrombin that inhibits factor Xa and thrombin in the presence of low-molecular-weight heparin. Only slightly influences platelet aggregation, PT, and aPTT.
Therapeutic Effect: Produces anticoagulation.

USES

Prevention of deep vein thrombosis (DVT) following abdominal surgery, treatment of life-threatening conditions such as unstable angina, non–Q-wave MI; prevention of ischemia complications caused by blood clot formation in patients on aspirin therapy; in combination with warfarin in deep vein thrombosis with or without pulmonary embolism (PE)

PHARMACOKINETICS

Route	Onset	Peak	Duration
Subcutaneous	N/A	4 hr	N/A

Protein binding: less than 10%.
Half-life: 3–5 hr.

INDICATIONS AND DOSAGES

▸ **Low- to Moderate-Risk Abdominal Surgery**
Subcutaneous
Adults, Elderly. 2500 international units 1–2 hr before surgery, then daily for 5–10 days.

▸ High-Risk Abdominal Surgery
Subcutaneous
Adults, Elderly. 5000 international units 1–2 hr before surgery, then daily for 5–10 days.
▸ Total Hip Surgery
Subcutaneous
Adults, Elderly. 2500 international units 1–2 hr before surgery, then 2500 units 6 hr after surgery, then 5000 units/day for 7–10 days.
▸ Unstable Angina, Non–Q-Wave MI
Subcutaneous
Adults, Elderly. 120 international units/kg q12h (maximum: 10,000 international units/dose) given with aspirin until clinically stable.
▸ Prevention of DVT or PE in the Acutely Ill Patient
Subcutaneous
Adults, Elderly. 5000 international units once a day.

SIDE EFFECTS/ADVERSE REACTIONS

Occasional
Hematoma at injection site
Rare
Hypersensitivity reaction (chills, fever, pruritus, urticaria, asthma, rhinitis, lacrimation, headache); mild, local skin irritation

PRECAUTIONS AND CONTRAINDICATIONS

Active major bleeding; concurrent heparin therapy; hypersensitivity to dalteparin, heparin, or pork products; thrombocytopenia associated with positive in vitro test for antiplatelet antibody
Caution:
Hemorrhage, cannot be used interchangeably with other forms of heparin, lactation, children, requires monitoring, GI bleeding

DRUG INTERACTIONS OF CONCERN TO DENTISTRY

- Avoid concurrent use of aspirin (except as noted), NSAIDs, dipyridamole, and sulfinpyrazone.

SERIOUS REACTIONS

! Overdose may lead to bleeding complications ranging from local ecchymoses to major hemorrhage.
! Thrombocytopenia occurs rarely.

DENTAL CONSIDERATIONS

General:
- Product may be used in outpatient therapy. Delay elective dental treatment until patient completes anticoagulant therapy; do not discontinue dalteparin.
- Determine why patient is taking the drug.
- Consider local hemostasis measures to prevent excessive bleeding.
- Avoid prescribing aspirin-containing products.

Consultations:
- Medical consultation should include routine blood counts, including platelet counts and aggegration tests.

Teach Patient/Family to:
- Encourage effective oral hygiene to prevent soft tissue inflammation.
- Prevent trauma when using oral hygiene aids.
- Report oral lesions, soreness, or bleeding to dentist.

danaparoid

da-**nah′**-pah-roid
(Orgaran k)

CATEGORY AND SCHEDULE

Pregnancy Risk Category: B

Drug Class: Heparinoid-type anticoagulant

D

D

MECHANISM OF ACTION
An antithrombotic agent that inhibits thrombin formation through factor antiXa and antiIIa effects. Does not significantly influence bleeding time, PT, aPTT, or platelet function. Possesses greater antithrombotic activity than anticoagulant activity.

USES
Prevention of deep vein thrombosis (DVT) following hip or knee replacement surgery; unapproved: thromboembolism, hemodialysis, and cardiovascular surgery

PHARMACOKINETICS
Well absorbed following subcutaneous administration. Eliminated primarily in the urine. ***Half-life:*** 24 hr (half-life prolonged with severe renal impairment).

INDICATIONS AND DOSAGES
Note: Give initial dose as soon as possible after surgery but not more than 24 hr after surgery.

▸ **Prevention of DVT**

Subcutaneous

Adults, Elderly. 750 anti-Xa units twice daily beginning 1–4 hr preoperatively and then not sooner than 2 hr after surgery. Continue treatment throughout postoperative care until risk of DVT has diminished (average duration 7–14 days).

SIDE EFFECTS/ADVERSE REACTIONS
Frequent

Injection site pain

Occasional

Fever, pain, nausea, UTI, constipation

Rare

Rash, pruritus, infection

PRECAUTIONS AND CONTRAINDICATIONS
Severe hemorrhagic diathesis (hemophilia, idiopathic thrombocytopenic purpura), active major bleeding state, including hemorrhagic stroke in the acute phase, type II phase thrombocytopenia associated with positive in vitro test for antiplatelet antibody in presence of danaparoid, hypersensitivity to pork products, danaparoid, or any component of the formulation

Caution:

Cannot interchange with heparin, hemorrhage, thrombocytopenia, renal or hepatic impairment, lactation, children, antidotes not available, GI bleeding

DRUG INTERACTIONS OF CONCERN TO DENTISTRY
- Avoid concurrent use of platelet aggregation antagonist, such as aspirin; NSAIDs; dipyridamole.

SERIOUS REACTIONS
! Accidental overdosage may lead to bleeding complications ranging from minor ecchymosis to major hemorrhage. An unexplained fall in HCT or fall in B/P should lead to consideration of a hemorrhagic event. The antidote protamine sulfate only partially neutralizes danaparoid activity and is incapable of reducing severe nonsurgical bleeding during treatment. If serious bleeding occurs, discontinue danaparoid; give blood or blood product transfusions.

DENTAL CONSIDERATIONS
General:

- Determine why patient is taking the drug.

• Do not discontinue danaparoid.
• Consider local hemostasis measures to prevent excessive bleeding if dental treatment must be performed.
• Delay elective dental treatment until patient completes danaparoid therapy.

Consultations:

• Medical consultation should include routine blood counts, including platelet counts and bleeding time.

Teach Patient/Family to:

• Encourage effective oral hygiene to prevent soft tissue inflammation.
• Use caution to prevent trauma when using oral hygiene aids.
• Report oral lesions, soreness, or bleeding to dentist.

danazol

da′-na-zole
(Cyclomen[CAN], Danocrine)

CATEGORY AND SCHEDULE

Pregnancy Risk Category: X

Drug Class: Androgen, α-ethinyl testosterone derivative

MECHANISM OF ACTION

A testosterone derivative that suppresses the pituitary-ovarian axis by inhibiting the output of pituitary gonadotropins. Causes atrophy of both normal and ectopic endometrial tissue in endometriosis. Follicle-stimulating hormone (FSH) and luteinizing hormone (LH) are depressed in fibrocystic breast disease. Inhibits steroid synthesis and binding of steroids to their receptors in breast tissues. Increases serum levels of esterase inhibitor.
Therapeutic Effect: Produces anovulation and amenorrhea, reduces the production of estrogen, corrects biochemical deficiency as seen in hereditary angioedema.

USES

Treatment of endometriosis, prevention of hereditary angioedema, fibrocystic breast disease

PHARMACOKINETICS

Well absorbed from GI tract. Metabolized in liver, primarily to 2-hydroxymethylethisterone. Excreted in urine. ***Half-life:*** 4.5 hr.

INDICATIONS AND DOSAGES

▸ **Endometriosis**

PO

Adults. 200–800 mg/day in 2 divided doses for 3–9 mo.

▸ **Fibrocystic Breast Disease**

PO

Adults. 100–400 mg/day in 2 divided doses.

▸ **Hereditary Angioedema**

PO

Adults. Initially, 200 mg 2–3 times a day. Decrease dose by 50% or less at 1–3 mo intervals. If attack occurs, increase dose by up to 200 mg/day.

SIDE EFFECTS/ADVERSE REACTIONS

Frequent

Females: Amenorrhea, breakthrough bleeding/spotting, decreased breast size, increased weight, irregular menstrual period.

Occasional

Males/females: Edema, rhabdomyolysis (muscle cramps, unusual fatigue), virilism (acne, oily skin), flushed skin, altered moods

D

Rare
Males/females: Hematuria, gingivitis, carpal tunnel syndrome, cataracts, severe headache, vomiting, rash, photosensitivity
Females: Enlarged clitoris, hoarseness, deepening voice, hair growth, monilial vaginitis
Males: Decreased testicle size

PRECAUTIONS AND CONTRAINDICATIONS
Cardiac impairment, hypercalcemia, pregnancy, prostatic or breast cancer in males, severe liver or renal disease
Caution:
Migraine headaches, seizure disorders

DRUG INTERACTIONS OF CONCERN TO DENTISTRY
• Increased serum concentration of carbamazepine; consider avoiding concurrent administration.

SERIOUS REACTIONS
! Jaundice may occur in those receiving 400 mg/day or more. Liver dysfunction, eosinophilia, thrombocytopenia, pancreatitis occur rarely.

DENTAL CONSIDERATIONS
General:
• Patients on chronic drug therapy may rarely have symptoms of blood dyscrasias, which can include infection, bleeding, and poor healing.
Consultations:
• In a patient with symptoms of blood dyscrasias, request a medical consultation for blood studies and postpone dental treatment until normal values are reestablished.
Teach Patient/Family to:
• Encourage effective oral hygiene to prevent soft tissue inflammation.
• Avoid mouth rinses with high alcohol content because of drying and irritating effects.

dantrolene sodium
dan′-troe-leen **so′**-dee-um
(Dantrium)
Do not confuse Dantrium with Daraprim.

CATEGORY AND SCHEDULE
Pregnancy Risk Category: C

Drug Class: Skeletal muscle relaxant, direct-acting

MECHANISM OF ACTION
A skeletal muscle relaxant that reduces muscle contraction by interfering with release of calcium ion. Reduces calcium ion concentration.
Therapeutic Effect: Dissociates excitation-contraction coupling. Interferes with catabolic process associated with malignant hyperthermic crisis.

USES
Treatment of spasticity in multiple sclerosis, stroke, spinal cord injury, cerebral palsy, malignant hyperthermia

PHARMACOKINETICS
Poorly absorbed from the GI tract. Protein binding: High. Metabolized in the liver. Primarily excreted in urine. ***Half-life:*** IV: 4–8 hr; PO: 8.7 hr.

INDICATIONS AND DOSAGES
▸ **Spasticity**
PO
Adults, Elderly. Initially, 25 mg/day. Increase to 25 mg 2–4 times a day,

then by 25-mg increments up to 100 mg 2–4 times a day.
Children. Initially, 0.5 mg/kg twice a day. Increase to 0.5 mg/kg 3–4 times a day, then in increments of 0.5 mg/kg/day up to 3 mg/kg 2–4 times a day. Maximum: 400 mg/day.

▸ **Prevention of Malignant Hyperthermic Crisis**
PO
Adults, Elderly, Children. 4–8 mg/kg/day in 3–4 divided doses 1–2 days before surgery; give last dose 3–4 hr before surgery.
IV
Adults, Elderly, Children. 2.5 mg/kg about 1.25 hr before surgery.

▸ **Management of Malignant Hyperthermic Crisis**
IV
Adults, Elderly, Children. Initially, a minimum of 1 mg/kg rapid IV; may repeat up to total cumulative dose of 10 mg/kg. May follow with 4–8 mg/kg/day PO in 4 divided doses up to 3 days after crisis.

SIDE EFFECTS/ADVERSE REACTIONS

Frequent
Drowsiness, dizziness, weakness, general malaise, diarrhea (mild)
Occasional
Confusion, diarrhea (may be severe), headache, insomnia, constipation, urinary frequency
Rare
Paradoxical CNS excitement or restlessness, paresthesia, tinnitus, slurred speech, tremors, blurred vision, dry mouth, nocturia, impotence, rash, pruritus

PRECAUTIONS AND CONTRAINDICATIONS

Active hepatic disease
Caution:
Peptic ulcer disease, renal disease, hepatic disease, stroke, seizure disorder, diabetes mellitus, elderly; monitor liver enzymes

DRUG INTERACTIONS OF CONCERN TO DENTISTRY

• None reported

SERIOUS REACTIONS

! There is a risk of liver toxicity, most notably in females, those 35 yr of age and older, and those taking other medications concurrently.
! Overt hepatitis noted most frequently between 3rd and 12th mo of therapy.
! Overdosage results in vomiting, muscular hypotonia, muscle twitching, respiratory depression, and seizures.

DENTAL CONSIDERATIONS

General:
• Monitor vital signs at every appointment because of cardiovascular and respiratory side effects.
• Patients on chronic drug therapy may rarely have symptoms of blood dyscrasias, which can include infection, bleeding, and poor healing.
• Requires proficiency in IV administration technique when used for emergency treatment of malignant hyperthermia.
Consultations:
• In a patient with symptoms of blood dyscrasias, request a medical consultation for blood studies and postpone dental treatment until normal values are reestablished.
Teach Patient/Family to:
• Encourage effective oral hygiene to prevent soft tissue inflammation.
• Avoid mouth rinses with high alcohol content because of drying effects.

D

dapiprazole hydrochloride

da-**pip**′-rah-zohl hi-droh-**klor**′-ide
(Rev-Eyes)

CATEGORY AND SCHEDULE

Pregnancy Risk Category: B

Drug Class: Antimydriatic

MECHANISM OF ACTION

An α-adrenergic blocker that primarily affects α-1 adrenoceptors. Does not significantly affect intraocular pressure.
Therapeutic Effect: Induces miosis via relaxation of the smooth dilator (radial) muscle of the iris, which causes papillary constriction.

USES

Reduction of pupil size after certain kinds of eye examinations

PHARMACOKINETICS

Well absorbed. Mydriasis reversal begins in 1 hr and occurs in about 6 hr.

INDICATIONS AND DOSAGES

▸ **Drug-Induced Mydriasis**

Ophthalmic
Adults, Elderly, Children. 2 drops applied topically to the conjunctiva of each eye. Repeat after 5 min. Do not use more than once a week.

SIDE EFFECTS/ADVERSE REACTIONS

Occasional
Burning, eyelid edema, photophobia

PRECAUTIONS AND CONTRAINDICATIONS

Acute iritis, hypersensitivity to dapiprazole or any component of the formulation

DRUG INTERACTIONS OF CONCERN TO DENTISTRY

- None reported

SERIOUS REACTIONS

! None reported

DENTAL CONSIDERATIONS

General:

- Used in ophthalmic examinations.
- Protect patient's eyes from accidental spatter during dental treatment.
- Avoid dental light in patient's eyes; offer dark glasses for patient comfort.

dapsone

dap′-sone
(Dapsone)

CATEGORY AND SCHEDULE

Pregnancy Risk Category: C

Drug Class: Leprostatic, antibacterial

MECHANISM OF ACTION

An antibiotic that is a competitive antagonist of para-aminobenzoic acid (PABA); it prevents normal bacterial utilization of PABA for synthesis of folic acid.
Therapeutic Effect: Inhibits bacterial growth.

USES

Treatment of leprosy (Hansen's disease); dermatitis herpetiformis; unapproved: cicatricial pemphigoid, LE, pemphigoid, malaria, *Pneumocystis carinii* pneumonia (PCP)

PHARMACOKINETICS
Rapid complete absorption; highly bound to plasma protein; metabolized in liver; excreted in urine. ***Half-life:*** 10–50 hr.

INDICATIONS AND DOSAGES
▸ **Leprosy**
PO
Adults, Elderly. 50–100 mg/day for 3–10 yr.
Children. 1–2 mg/kg/24 hr. Maximum: 100 mg/day.
▸ **Dermatitis Herpetiformis**
PO
Adults, Elderly. Initially, 50 mg/day. May increase up to 300 mg/day.
▸ **PCP**
PO
Adults, Elderly. 100 mg/day in combination with trimethoprim for 21 days.
▸ **Prevention of PCP**
PO
Adults, Elderly. 100 mg/day.
Children older than 1 mo. 2 mg/kg/day. Maximum: 100 mg/day.

SIDE EFFECTS/ADVERSE REACTIONS
Frequent
Hemolytic anemia, methemoglobinemia, rash
Occasional
Hemolysis, photosensitivity reaction

PRECAUTIONS AND CONTRAINDICATIONS
Hypersensitivity to sulfones, severe anemia
Caution:
Renal disease, hepatic disease, G6PD deficiency, lactation

DRUG INTERACTIONS OF CONCERN TO DENTISTRY
• None reported

SERIOUS REACTIONS
! Agranulocytosis and blood dyscrasias may occur.

DENTAL CONSIDERATIONS
General:
• Patients on chronic drug therapy may rarely have symptoms of blood dyscrasias, which can include infection, bleeding, and poor healing.
• Avoid dental light in patient's eyes; offer dark glasses for patient comfort.
• Advise patient if dental drugs prescribed have a potential for photosensitivity.
Consultations:
• In a patient with symptoms of blood dyscrasias, request a medical consultation for blood studies and postpone dental treatment until normal values are reestablished.
Teach Patient/Family to:
• Encourage effective oral hygiene to prevent soft tissue inflammation.
• Use caution to prevent injury when using oral hygiene aids.

daptomycin
dap′-toe-my-sin
(Cubicin)

CATEGORY AND SCHEDULE
Pregnancy Risk Category: B

Drug Class: Antiinfective (polypeptide)

MECHANISM OF ACTION
A lipopeptide antibacterial agent that binds to bacterial membranes and causes a rapid depolarization of the membrane potential. The loss of membrane potential leads to

inhibition of protein, DNA, and RNA synthesis.
Therapeutic Effect: Bactericidal.

USES

Treatment of complicated skin and skin-structure infections caused by susceptible strains of *S. aureus* (including methicillin-resistant *S. aureus*), *S. pyogenes, S. agalactiae, S. dysgalactiae, E. coli,* and *E. faecalis* (vancomycin-susceptible strains only)

PHARMACOKINETICS

Widely distributed. Protein binding: 90%. Primarily excreted unchanged in urine. Moderately removed by hemodialysis. ***Half-life:*** 7–8 hr (increased in impaired renal function).

INDICATIONS AND DOSAGES

▸ Complicated Skin and Skin-Structure Infections

IV

Adults, Elderly. 4 mg/kg every 24 hr for 7–14 days.

▸ Dosage in Renal Impairment

For patients with creatinine clearance of less than 30 ml/min, dosage is 4 mg/kg q48h for 7–14 days.

SIDE EFFECTS/ADVERSE REACTIONS

Frequent

Constipation, nausea, peripheral injection site reactions, headache, diarrhea

Occasional

Insomnia, rash, vomiting

Rare

Pruritus, dizziness, hypotension

PRECAUTIONS AND CONTRAINDICATIONS

Hypersensitivity

Caution:

Reduce dose in renal impairment, risk of superinfection, monitor for muscle weakness, pain, and CPK levels, lactation, elderly, safety and efficacy in children younger than 18 yr not established

DRUG INTERACTIONS OF CONCERN TO DENTISTRY

• None reported

SERIOUS REACTIONS

! Skeletal muscle myopathy, characterized by muscle pain and weakness, particularly of the distal extremities, occurs rarely.
! Antibiotic-associated colitis and other superinfections may result from altered bacterial balance.

DENTAL CONSIDERATIONS

General:

• Used in the hospital environment for serious infections.
• Determine why patient is taking the drug.
• Monitor vital signs, including temperature, B/P, and respiration characteristics and rate, at every appointment.

Consultations:

• Consult with patient's physician if an acute dental infection occurs and another antiinfective is required.

darbepoetin alfa

dar-beh-**poe**′-ee-tin **al**′-fah
(Aranesp)
Do not confuse Aranesp with Aricept.

CATEGORY AND SCHEDULE

Pregnancy Risk Category: C

Drug Class: Hematopoietic agent

MECHANISM OF ACTION
A glycoprotein that stimulates formation of RBCs in bone marrow; increases serum half-life of epoetin. ***Therapeutic Effect:*** Induces erythropoiesis and release of reticulocytes from bone marrow.

USES
An erythropoiesis-stimulating protein; stimulates the division and differentiation of erythroid progenitors in bone marrow

PHARMACOKINETICS
Well absorbed after subcutaneous administration. ***Half-life:*** 48.5 hr.

INDICATIONS AND DOSAGES
▸ Anemia in Chronic Renal Failure
IV Bolus, Subcutaneous
Adults, Elderly. Initially, 0.45 mcg/kg once a wk. Adjust dosage to achieve and maintain a target Hgb not to exceed 12 g/dl. Do not increase dosage more frequently than once a mo. Limit increases in Hgb by less than 1 g/dl over any 2-wk period.
▸ Anemia Associated with Chemotherapy
IV, Subcutaneous
Adults, Elderly. 2.25 mcg/kg/dose once a wk.

SIDE EFFECTS/ADVERSE REACTIONS
Frequent
Myalgia, hypertension or hypotension, headache, diarrhea
Occasional
Fatigue, edema, vomiting, reaction at administration site, asthenia, dizziness

PRECAUTIONS AND CONTRAINDICATIONS
History of sensitivity to mammalian cell-derived products or human albumin, uncontrolled hypertension
Caution:
Increased risk of serious cardiovascular events, seizures in CRF, albumin formula has risk of viral diseases, safety in lactation or pediatric patients has not been established

DRUG INTERACTIONS OF CONCERN TO DENTISTRY
- No studies reported

SERIOUS REACTIONS
! Vascular access thrombosis, CHF, sepsis, arrhythmias, and anaphylactic reaction occur rarely.

DENTAL CONSIDERATIONS
General:
- Monitor vital signs at every appointment because of cardiovascular side effects.
- Consider semisupine chair position for patient comfort if GI side effects occur.
- Monitor disease control and date of last dialysis.
- Prophylactic antibiotics may be indicated to prevent infection if invasive procedure is planned.

Consultations:
- Medical consultation may be required to assess disease control and patient's ability to tolerate stress.

Teach Patient/Family to:
- Encourage effective oral hygiene to prevent soft tissue inflammation, infection.
- Update health and drug history if physician makes any changes in evaluation or drug regimens.

D

D

darifenacin

dar-i-fen′-a-sin
(Enablex)
Do not confuse Enablex with Celebrex.

CATEGORY AND SCHEDULE

Pregnancy Risk Category: C

Drug Class: Anticholinergic agent

MECHANISM OF ACTION

A selective muscarinic antagonist that limits bladder contractions, reducing the symptoms of bladder irritability and overactivity.
Therapeutic Effect: Reduces bladder overactivity, improves bladder capacity.

USES

Management of symptoms of bladder overactivity

PHARMACOKINETICS

Well absorbed following PO administration. Protein binding: 98%. Hepatic metabolism via CYP3A4 (major) and CYP2D6 (minor) enzyme systems. Excreted in urine (60%) and feces (40%) as inactive metabolites. ***Half-life:*** 13–19 hr.

INDICATIONS AND DOSAGES

▸ **Symptoms of Bladder Overactivity**

PO

Adults. Initially, 7.5 mg once daily. May increase to 15 mg a day, based upon individual response and tolerability.

Patients with moderate hepatic insufficiency (Child-Pugh class B) or those taking concomitant potent CYP3A4 inhibitors (azole antifungals, erythromycin, isoniazid, protease inhibitors) should not use doses greater than 7.5 mg a day.

SIDE EFFECTS/ADVERSE REACTIONS

Frequent

Dry mouth, dry eye, constipation, dysuria

Occasional

Dizziness, headache, dry throat, dry eye, abdominal pain, diarrhea, dyspepsia, nausea, insomnia

PRECAUTIONS AND CONTRAINDICATIONS

Hypersensitivity to darifenacin or any component of the formulation. Avoid use in patients with urinary retention, gastric retention, and uncontrolled narrow-angle glaucoma. Use with caution in patients with bladder outlet obstruction, decreased gastrointestinal motility, controlled narrow-angle glaucoma, and myasthenia gravis.

DRUG INTERACTIONS OF CONCERN TO DENTISTRY

- CYP2D6 and CYP3A4 substrates (e.g., opioid analgesics, macrolide antibiotics): increased frequency of adverse effects of darifenacin
- CNS depressants, alcohol: may potentiate mental impairment and somnolence; avoid products with alcohol
- Anticholinergic drugs (e.g., atropine, glycopyrrolate): increased likelihood of dry mouth, constipation, blurred vision, and other anticholinergic adverse effects

SERIOUS REACTIONS

! None reported

DENTAL CONSIDERATIONS

General:

• Plan for breaks in treatment associated with urinary frequency.
• Assess salivary flow as a factor in caries, periodontal disease, and candidiasis.

Teach Patient/Family to:

• Avoid mouth rinses with high alcohol content because of drying effect.
• Use home fluoride products for anticaries effect.
• Use sugarless/xylitol gum, frequent sips of water, or saliva substitutes if dry mouth occurs.

darunavir

dar-**oo**′-na-veer
(Prezista)

CATEGORY AND SCHEDULE

Pregnancy Risk Category: B

Drug Class: Antiretroviral agent, protease inhibitor

MECHANISM OF ACTION

An antiretroviral agent that inhibits HIV-1 protease. Prevents the cleavage of HIV encoded Gag-Pol polyproteins in infected cells.
Therapeutic Effect: Impedes HIV replication, slowing the progression of HIV infection.

USES

Treatment of HIV infection

PHARMACOKENETICS

Absorption increased 30% with food. Protein binding: 95%. Extensively metabolized in liver, primarily by CYP450 3A4. Primarily eliminated in feces (about 80%, 41% unchanged); partial excretion in urine (approximately 14%, 8% unchanged). ***Half-life:*** 15 hr.

INDICATIONS AND DOSAGES

▸ HIV Infection (in combination with ritonavir)

PO

Adults. 600 mg twice a day taken with ritonavir 100 mg twice a day with food. Safety and efficacy have not been established in children.

SIDE EFFECTS/ADVERSE REACTIONS

Frequent

Hypertriglyceridemia, diarrhea, nausea, increased amylase level, headache, nasopharyngitis

Occasional

Hypercholesterolemia, rash, hypoglycemia, hypocalcemia, thrombocytopenia, hyponatremia, vomiting, abdominal pain

Rare

Constipation, anxiety, acute renal failure, fat redistribution, confusional state, disorientation, irritability, altered mood, nightmares, dyspnea, cough, hiccups, night sweats, diabetes mellitus, Stevens-Johnson syndrome

PRECAUTIONS AND CONTRAINDICATIONS

• Hypersensitivity to darunavir or its components
• Sulfa allergy, diabetes mellitus
• Multiple drug interactions

DRUG INTERACTIONS OF CONCERN TO DENTISTRY

• Anticonvulsants: may decrease concentrations of darunavir
• Antihistamines: increased risk of arrhythmias
• Benzodiazepines: may cause increased sedation or respiratory depression

- Clarithromycin: may increase concentrations of clarithromycin
- Corticosteroids: may increase levels and effects of these drugs
- CYP3A4 inducers: may decrease levels and effects of darunavir
- CYP3A4 substrates: may increase levels and effects of CYP3A4 substrates
- Estrogens, oral contraceptives: may decrease concentrations of these drugs; may reduce contraceptive effectiveness
- Immunosuppressants: may increase concentrations of these drugs
- Ketoconazole: may increase levels and effects of darunavir and ketoconazole
- Methadone: may decrease concentrations of methadone
- Neuroleptic agents: increased risk of arrhythmias
- Rifampin: may decrease concentrations of darunavir
- Sedatives/hypnotics: increased sedation and risk of respiratory depression
- SSRIs: may decrease the levels and effects of SSRIs
- St. John's wort: may decrease the levels of darunavir
- Trazodone: may increase concentrations of trazodone

SERIOUS REACTIONS

! Protease inhibitors have been associated with severe dermatologic reactions, including Stevens-Johnson syndrome.

DENTAL CONSIDERATIONS

General:

- Monitor vital signs at every appointment because of cardiovascular side effects.
- Examine for oral manifestation of opportunistic infection.
- Place on frequent recall to evaluate healing response.
- Assess salivary flow as a factor in caries, periodontal disease, and candidiasis.
- Consider semisupine chair position for patient comfort because of GI effects of drug.

Consultations:

- Medical consultation may be required to assess disease control.

Teach Patient/Family to:

- Encourage effective oral hygiene to prevent soft tissue inflammation.
- See dentist immediately if secondary oral infection occurs.
- When chronic dry mouth occurs, advise patient to:
  - Avoid mouth rinses with high alcohol content because of drying effects.
  - Use daily home fluoride products for anticaries effect.
  - Use sugarless gum, frequent sips of water, or saliva substitutes.

dasatinib

da-**sa**′-ti-nib
(Sprycel)

CATEGORY AND SCHEDULE

Pregnancy Risk Category: D

Drug Class: Antineoplastic

MECHANISM OF ACTION

Inhibits BCR-ABL tyrosine kinase, an enzyme created by the Philadelphia chromosome abnormality found in patients with chronic myeloid leukemia (CML). Also inhibits SRC family kinases. ***Therapeutic Effect:*** Suppresses tumor growth during the three stages of CML: blast crisis, accelerated phase, and chronic phase.

USES

Treatment in CML-blast crisis, accelerated phase, and chronic phase-resistant or intolerant to prior therapy. Also used in treatment of Philadelphia chromosome-positive acute lymphoblastic leukemia (ALL) with resistance or intolerance to prior therapy.

PHARMACOKENETICS

Protein binding: 96%. Metabolized in liver, primarily by CYP450 3A4. Primarily eliminated in feces (85%, 19% as unchanged); minimal excretion in urine (4%, 0.1% unchanged). ***Half-life:*** 3–5 hr.

INDICATIONS AND DOSAGES

▸ ALL, Philadelphia Chromosome-Positive, Resistant or Intolerant to Prior Therapy

PO

Adults. 70 mg twice a day (morning and evening), with or without food.

▸ CML, Blast Crisis

Adults. 70 mg twice a day (morning and evening), with or without food.

▸ CML, Accelerated Phase

Adults. 70 mg twice a day (morning and evening), with or without food.

▸ CML, Chronic Phase

Adults. 70 mg twice a day (morning and evening), with or without food.

Safety and efficacy have not been established in children.

SIDE EFFECTS/ADVERSE REACTIONS (ADULT)

Frequent

Neutropenia, thrombocytopenia, diarrhea, headache, musculoskeletal pain, fatigue, fever, superficial edema, rash, nausea, dyspnea, upper respiratory infection, abdominal pain, pleural effusion, vomiting, arthralgia, asthenia, loss of appetite, inflammatory disease of mucous membrane, GI hemorrhage, constipation, weight loss, dizziness, chest pain, neuropathy, myalgia, weight increased, cardiac dysrhythmia, pruritus, pneumonia, swollen abdomen, pneumonia, shivering

Occasional

Febrile neutropenia, CHF, pericardial effusion, pulmonary edema, prolonged QT interval, anemia

Rare

Pulmonary hypertension, CNS hemorrhage, ascites

PRECAUTIONS AND CONTRAINDICATIONS

Hypersensitivity to dasatinib or its components, hypokalemia, hypomagnesemia, use with antiarrhythmic medication, patients at risk for fluid retention

DRUG INTERACTIONS OF CONCERN TO DENTISTRY

- NSAIDs: increased risk of bleeding
- CYP3A4 inhibitors (e.g., clarithromycin, erythromycin, azole antifungals): may increase the levels and adverse effects of dasatinib
- CYP3A4 substrates (midazolam, triazolam): increased plasma concentrations of these drugs with increased CNS depression
- Vasoconstrictors: may increase the risk of potentially fatal arrhythmias

SERIOUS REACTIONS

! Severe CNS hemorrhage, including fatalities, have been reported.

! Dasatinib may cause severe bone marrow suppression (thrombocytopenia, neutropenia, anemia).

! Fluid retention, including pleural and pericardial effusion, severe ascites, and generalized edema, has been reported.

DENTAL CONSIDERATIONS

General:

• Monitor vital signs at every appointment because of cardiovascular adverse effects.
• Determine why patient is taking drug.
• Avoid aspirin and NSAIDs.
• Consider semisupine chair position for patients with GI or respiratory adverse effects.
• Consider blood dyscrasias as factors in infection, bleeding, and poor healing.
• If blood dyscrasia present, caution patient to prevent oral tissue trauma when using oral hygiene aids.
• Examine for oral manifestations of opportunistic infection.
• Consider local hemostatic measures to prevent excessive bleeding.
• Use caution with potentially hepatotoxic drugs (e.g., telithromycin).

Consultations:

• Consult physician to determine disease control and ability of patient to tolerate dental procedures.
• Medical consultation should include routine blood counts, including platelets and bleeding time, and postpone dental therapy until values are in acceptable range.
• Consult physician to determine possible need for prophylactic antibiotics.

Teach Patient/Family to:

• Use effective, atraumatic oral hygiene to prevent soft-tissue inflammation.
• Update health and medication history if physician makes any changes in evaluation or drug regimen; include over-the-counter, herbal products, and dietary supplements.
• Report oral lesions, soreness, or bleeding to dentist.

daunorubicin citrate liposome

dawn-oh-**rue**′-bih-sin
(DaunoXome)
Do not confuse with dactinomycin or doxorubicin.

CATEGORY AND SCHEDULE

Pregnancy Risk Category: D

Drug Class: Anthracycline antibiotic; antineoplastic

MECHANISM OF ACTION

An anthracycline antibiotic that is cell cycle-phase nonspecific. Most active in S phase of cell division. Appears to bind to DNA.
Therapeutic Effect: Inhibits DNA, DNA-dependent RNA synthesis.

USES

Treatment of advanced AIDS-associated Kaposi's sarcoma (KS), a skin cancer

PHARMACOKINETICS

Widely distributed. Does not cross blood-brain barrier. Protein binding: High. Metabolized in liver to active metabolite. Excreted in urine, eliminated by biliary excretion.
Half-life: 18.5 hr; metabolite: 26.7 hr.

INDICATIONS AND DOSAGES

▸ KS

IV

Adults. 20–40 mg/m^2 over 1 hr. Repeat q2wk or 100 mg/m^2 q3wk.

SIDE EFFECTS/ADVERSE REACTIONS

Frequent
Mild to moderate nausea, fatigue, fever
Occasional
Diarrhea, abdominal pain, esophagitis, stomatitis (redness or burning of oral mucous membranes, inflammation of gums or tongue), transverse pigmentation of fingernails and toenails
Rare
Transient fever, chills

PRECAUTIONS AND CONTRAINDICATIONS

Arrhythmias, CHF, left ventricular ejection fraction less than 40%, preexisting bone marrow suppression

DRUG INTERACTIONS OF CONCERN TO DENTISTRY

• Dental drug interactions have not been studied.

SERIOUS REACTIONS

! Bone marrow depression manifested as hematologic toxicity (severe leukopenia, anemia, and thrombocytopenia) may occur.
! Decreases in platelet and white blood cell (WBC) counts occur in 10–14 days and return to normal levels by the third wk of daunorubicin treatment.
! Cardiotoxicity noted as either acute with transient abnormal ECG findings or as chronic with cardiomyopathy manifested as CHF. The risk of cardiotoxicity increases when the cumulative dose exceeds 550 mg/m^2 in adults and 300 mg/m^2 in children older than 2 yr or when the total dosage is greater than 10 mg/kg in children younger than 2 yr.

DENTAL CONSIDERATIONS

General:
• Determine why patient is taking the drug.
• Assess salivary flow as a factor in caries, periodontal disease, and candidiasis.
• Administered in the hospital; AIDS patients will be taking many other medications; confirm medical and drug history.
Consultations:
• In a patient with symptoms of blood dyscrasias, request a medical consultation for blood studies and postpone treatment until normal values are reestablished.
• Medical consultation may be required to assess disease control and patient's ability to tolerate stress.
Teach Patient/Family to:
• Encourage effective oral hygiene to prevent soft tissue inflammation.
• Prevent trauma when using oral hygiene aids.
• Report oral lesions, soreness, or bleeding to dentist.
• When chronic dry mouth occurs, advise patient to:
  • Avoid mouth rinses with high alcohol content because of drying effects.
  • Use daily home fluoride products for anticaries effect.
  • Use sugarless gum, frequent sips of water, or saliva substitutes.
  • Update health and medication history if physician makes any changes in evaluation or drug regimens; include OTC, herbal, and nonherbal remedies in the update.

decitabine

de-**sye**′-ta-been
(Dacogen)

CATEGORY AND SCHEDULE

Pregnancy Risk Category: D

Drug Class: Antineoplastic

MECHANISM OF ACTION

A pyrimidine antimetabolite that is incorporated into DNA and inhibits DNA methyltransferase causing hypomethylation and subsequent cell death.
Therapeutic Effect: Restores normal function to tumor-suppressor genes regulating cellular differentiation and proliferation.

USES

Treatment of myelodysplastic syndrome (MDS)

PHARMACOKINETICS

No information is available regarding the pharmacokinetics of decitabine.

INDICATIONS AND DOSAGES

▸ MDS

IV
Adults. 15 mg/m^2 over 3 hr, repeat every 8 hr for 3 days; repeat cycle every 6 wk for a minimum of 4 cycles.

SIDE EFFECTS/ADVERSE REACTIONS

Frequent
Neutropenia, thrombocytopenia, anemia, fever, nausea, cough, petechiae, constipation, diarrhea, hyperglycemia, headache, febrile neutropenia, leukopenia, insomnia, peripheral edema, hypomagnesemia, hypoalbuminemia, vomiting, pallor, bruising, hypokalemia, rigors, pneumonia, arthralgia, rash, limb pain, edema, dizziness, back pain, cardiac murmur, anorexia, pharyngitis, appetite decreased, abdominal pain, lung crackles, hyperbilirubinemia, erythema, pain, hyperkalemia, hyponatremia, oral mucosal lymphadenopathy, confusion, lethargy, cellulitis, stomatitis, dyspepsia, anxiety, hypoesthesia, lesions, pruritus, alkaline phosphatase increased, tenderness
Occasional
Candidal infection, ascites, AST increased, breath sounds diminished, hyperuricemia, hypoxia, rales, LDH increased, hemorrhoids, alopecia, catheter infection, gingival bleeding, chest discomfort, UTI, chest wall pain, loose stools, staphylococcal infection, transfusion reaction, tongue ulceration, dysphagia, oral candidiasis, dysuria, facial swelling, hypotension, musculoskeletal discomfort, blurred vision, bicarbonate increased, dehydration, hypochloremia, pulmonary edema, urticaria, malaise, hematoma, thrombocythemia, bacteremia, polyuria, hypobilirubinemia, site erythema, catheter site pain, injection site swelling, lip ulceration, abdominal, bicarbonate decreased, hypoproteinemia, crepitation, myalgia, gastroesophageal reflux, glossodynia, postnasal drip, sinusitis
Rare
Anaphylactic reaction, atrial fibrillation, cardiomyopathy, CHF, cholecystitis, dyspnea, fungal infection, hemorrhage, gingival pain, mental status change, mucosal inflammation, mycobacterium avium complex infection, peridiverticular abscess, pseudomonal lung infection, pulmonary embolism, renal failure, respiratory arrest,

respiratory tract infection, sepsis, splenomegaly, supraventricular tachycardia, weakness

PRECAUTIONS AND CONTRAINDICATIONS

Hypersensitivity to decitabine or its components; do not breast-feed, bone marrow depression, renal or hepatic impairment

DRUG INTERACTIONS OF CONCERN TO DENTISTRY

• None reported

SERIOUS REACTIONS

! Neutropenia and thrombocytopenia are expected to occur.

DENTAL CONSIDERATIONS

General:

• Monitor vital signs at every appointment because of cardiovascular side effects.
• Avoid aspirin and NSAIDs.
• Consider immunosuppression as a factor in oral opportunistic infections.
• Consider semisupine chair position if GI or respiratory adverse effects occur.
• Chlorhexidine mouth rinse before and during chemotherapy may reduce severity of mucositis.
• Consider blood dyscrasias as a factor in infection, bleeding, and delayed healing.
• Palliative medication may be required of oral adverse effects.
• Assess salivary flow as a factor in caries, periodontal disease, and candidiasis.
• Obtain CBCs, including platelets and bleeding time, prior to initiating invasive dental procedures and postpone dental treatment as needed.

Consultations:

• Consult physician to determine why patient is taking drug.
• Consult physician to determine disease control and ability of patient to tolerate dental procedures.
• Consult physician(s) to determine if prophylactic antibiotics are required prior to dental procedures.

Teach Patient/Family to:

• Use effective atraumatic oral hygiene measures to prevent soft tissue inflammation.
• Report oral lesions, soreness, or bleeding to dentist.
• Update health history when physician changes drug regimen and/or report use of over-the-counter medications, herbal products, and dietary supplements.
• When chronic dry mouth occurs, advise patient to:
  • Avoid mouth rinses with high alcohol content because of drying effect.
  • Use daily home fluoride products for anticaries effects.
  • Use sugarless gum, frequent sips of water, or artificial saliva substitutes.

deferiprone

de-**fer**-i-prone

(Ferriprox)

Do not confuse deferiprone with deferoxamine or deferasirox.

CATEGORY AND SCHEDULE

Pregnancy Risk Category: D

Drug Class: Chelating agent

MECHANISM OF ACTION

Iron-chelating agent with affinity for ferric ion; binds to ferric ion and forms a complex that is excreted in the urine. Has a lower affinity for other metals such as copper, aluminum, and zinc.

Therapeutic Effect: Promotes urinary excretion of iron.

D

USES

Treatment of transfusional iron overload due to thalassemia syndromes with inadequate response to other chelation therapy

PHARMACOKINETICS

Rapid absorption following oral administration. Less than 10% protein binding. Metabolized primarily by glucuronidation. Excreted primarily in urine (75%–90%). ***Half-life:*** 1.9 hr.

INDICATIONS AND DOSAGES

▸ Transfusional Iron Overload

PO

Adults. Initially, 25 mg/kg 3 times/day (75 mg/kg/day). Dose should be individualized based on response and therapeutic goal. Maximum dose is 33 mg/kg 3 times/day (99 mg/kg/day).

Dose adjustment for toxicity:

ANC <1500/mm^3: Interrupt treatment

ANC <500/mm^3: In addition to treatment interruption, consider hospitalization

SIDE EFFECTS/ADVERSE REACTIONS

Frequent

Nausea, chromaturia

Occasional

Headache, agranulocytosis, abdominal pain, vomiting, diarrhea, dyspepsia, neutropenia, arthralgia, back pain

PRECAUTIONS AND CONTRAINDICATIONS

Hypersensitivity to deferiprone or any component of the formulation. Use with caution in patients at risk for QT prolongation and those taking concomitant neutropenic agents. Deferiprone may bind with polyvalent cations (aluminum, zinc). Allow at least 4 hr between other medications or supplements containing polyvalent cations.

DRUG INTERACTIONS OF CONCERN TO DENTISTRY

• No studies of dental drug interactions reported

SERIOUS REACTIONS

! May cause agranulocytosis, which could lead to serious infections (some fatal)

DENTAL CONSIDERATIONS

General:

• Avoid interruption of patient's drug regimen.

• Monitor for signs and symptoms of possible agranulocytosis and neutropenia (e.g., infection).

delavirdine mesylate

deh-**la′**-ver-deen **mess′**-ah-late

(Rescriptor)

Do not confuse Rescriptor with Retrovir or Ritonavir.

CATEGORY AND SCHEDULE

Pregnancy Risk Category: C

Drug Class: Antiviral, nonnucleoside

MECHANISM OF ACTION

A nonnucleoside reverse transcriptase inhibitor that binds directly to HIV-1 reverse transcriptase and blocks RNA- and DNA-dependent DNA polymerase activities.

Therapeutic Effect: Interrupts HIV replication, slowing the progression of HIV infection.

USES
Treatment of HIV infection in combination with appropriate antiretroviral agents when therapy is warranted

PHARMACOKINETICS
Rapidly absorbed after PO administration. Protein binding: 98%. Primarily distributed in plasma. Metabolized in the liver. Eliminated in feces and urine. ***Half-life:*** 2–11 hr.

INDICATIONS AND DOSAGES
▸ **HIV Infection (in combination with other antiretrovirals)**
PO
Adults. 400 mg 3 times a day.

SIDE EFFECTS/ADVERSE REACTIONS
Frequent
Rash, pruritus
Occasional
Headache, nausea, diarrhea, fatigue, anorexia

PRECAUTIONS AND CONTRAINDICATIONS
Hypersensitivity
Caution:
Modify dose in liver disease; children younger than 16 yr, lactation; rapid development of viral resistance if used as a single drug

DRUG INTERACTIONS OF CONCERN TO DENTISTRY
- Reduced absorption: antacids, cimetidine, other H_2-receptor antagonists
- Increased plasma levels of both delavirdine and clarithromycin
- Increased plasma levels of alprazolam, triazolam, midazolam
- Avoid coadministration with carbamazepine, phenobarbital, ketoconazole, fluoxetine

SERIOUS REACTIONS
! None known

DENTAL CONSIDERATIONS
General:
- Examine for oral manifestation of opportunistic infection.
- Patients on chronic drug therapy may rarely have symptoms of blood dyscrasias, which can include infection, bleeding, and poor healing.
- Assess salivary flow as a factor in caries, periodontal disease, and candidiasis.
- After supine positioning, have patient sit upright for at least 2 min before standing to avoid orthostatic hypotension.
- Do not use ingestible sodium bicarbonate products, such as the Prophy-Jet air polishing system, within 2 hr of drug use.

Consultations:
- In a patient with symptoms of blood dyscrasias, request a medical consultation for blood studies and postpone treatment until normal values are reestablished.
- Medical consultation may be required to assess disease control and patient's ability to tolerate stress.

Teach Patient/Family to:
- Encourage effective oral hygiene to prevent soft tissue inflammation.
- Use caution to prevent trauma when using oral hygiene aids.
- See dentist immediately if secondary oral infection occurs.
- When chronic dry mouth occurs, advise patient to:
  - Avoid mouth rinses with high alcohol content because of drying effects.
  - Use daily home fluoride products for anticaries effect.

- Use sugarless gum, frequent sips of water, or saliva substitutes.

D

demecarium bromide

de-mi-**kare**′-ee-um **bro**′-mide
(Humorsol Ocumeter)

CATEGORY AND SCHEDULE

Pregnancy Risk Category: X

Drug Class: Antiglaucoma agent, ophthalmic; cyclostimulant, accommodative esotropia

MECHANISM OF ACTION

A cholinesterase inhibitor that increases the concentration of acetylcholine at cholinergic receptor sites and produces effects equivalent to excessive stimulation of cholinergic receptors.
Therapeutic Effect: Reduces intraocular pressure (IOP) because of facilitation of outflow of aqueous humor.

USES

Treatment of certain types of glaucoma and other eye conditions, such as accommodative esotropia. Also used in the diagnosis of certain eye conditions, such as accommodative esotropia.

PHARMACOKINETICS

Decreases intraocular pressure within a few hours. The duration is variable among individuals.

INDICATIONS AND DOSAGES

▸ **Glaucoma**

Ophthalmic, Topical
Adults, Elderly. 1–2 drops of the 0.125% or 0.25% solution in affected eye(s) twice a day to twice a wk.

▸ **Cyclostimulant**

Ophthalmic, Topical
Adults, Elderly. 1 drop of 0.125% or 0.25% solution in each eye daily for 2–3 wk, followed by 1 drop every 2 days for 4 wk.

▸ **Diagnostic Aid (accommodative esotropia)**

Ophthalmic, Topical
Adults, Elderly. 1 drop of 0.125% or 0.25% solution once a day for 2 wk, then 1 drop every 2 days for 2–3 wk.

SIDE EFFECTS/ADVERSE REACTIONS

Occasional

Brow ache, nausea, vomiting, abdominal cramps, diarrhea, hypersalivation, urinary incontinence, lid muscle twitching, redness, myopia blurred vision, increase in IOP, iris cysts, breathing difficulties, increased sweating

PRECAUTIONS AND CONTRAINDICATIONS

Pregnancy, active uveal inflammation and/or glaucoma associated with iridocyclitis, hypersensitivity to demecarium or any component of the formulation.

DRUG INTERACTIONS OF CONCERN TO DENTISTRY

- Avoid use of succinylcholine in general anesthesia
- Possible inhibition of the metabolism of ester-type local and topical anesthetics
- Avoid use of anticholinergics, such as systemic atropine or related drugs

SERIOUS REACTIONS

! Systemic absorption has been associated with demecarium resulting in anticholinesterase toxicity.
! Overdosage can produce cholinergic crisis characterized by

cardiac arrhythmias, diarrhea, muscle weakness, profuse sweating, respiratory difficulties, urinary incontinence, and shock.

DENTAL CONSIDERATIONS

General:

- Determine why patient is taking the drug.
- Avoid drugs with anticholinergic activity, such as antihistamines, opioids, benzodiazepines, propantheline, atropine, and scopolamine.
- Avoid dental light in patient's eyes; offer dark glasses for patient comfort.
- Question glaucoma patient about compliance with prescribed drug regimen.

Consultations:

- Medical consultation may be required to assess disease control.

Teach Patient/Family to:

- Update health and medication history if physician makes any changes in evaluation or drug regimens; include OTC, herbal, and nonherbal remedies in the update.

demeclocycline hydrochloride

dem-eh-kloe-**sye**′-kleen
hi-droh-**klor**′-ide
(Declomycin, Ledermycin[AUS])

CATEGORY AND SCHEDULE

Pregnancy Risk Category: D

Drug Class: Tetracycline

MECHANISM OF ACTION

A tetracycline antibiotic that inhibits bacterial protein synthesis by binding to ribosomal receptor sites; also inhibits ADH-induced water reabsorption.

Therapeutic Effect: Bacteriostatic; also produces diuresis.

USES

Treatment of a wide variety of gram-positive and gram-negative bacteria, protozoa, *Rickettsia, Mycoplasma,* agents of psittacosis and ornithosis, *Actinomyces* species

PHARMACOKINETICS

PO: Peak 3–6 hr, duration 48–72 hr, ***Half-life:*** 10–17 hr; 36%–91% bound to serum protein; crosses placenta; excreted in urine, breast milk

INDICATIONS AND DOSAGES

▸ Mild-to-Moderate Infections, Including Acne, Pertussis, Chronic Bronchitis, and UTIs

PO

Adults, Elderly. 150 mg 4 times a day or 300 mg 2 times a day.

Children older than 8 yr. 8–12 mg/kg/day in 2–4 divided doses.

▸ Uncomplicated Gonorrhea

PO

Adults. Initially, 600 mg, then 300 mg q12h for 4 days for total of 3 g.

▸ Syndrome of Inappropriate ADH Secretion (SIADH)

PO

Adults, Elderly. Initially, 900–1200 mg/day in 3–4 divided doses, then decrease dose to 600–900 mg/day in divided doses.

SIDE EFFECTS/ADVERSE REACTIONS

Frequent

Anorexia, nausea, vomiting, diarrhea, dysphagia, possibly severe photosensitivity (with moderate to high demeclocycline dosage)

Occasional
Urticaria, rash; diabetes insipidus syndrome, marked by polydipsia, polyuria, and weakness (with long-term therapy)

D

PRECAUTIONS AND CONTRAINDICATIONS

Children 8 yr and younger, last half of pregnancy.
The use of tetracycline drugs during tooth development (last half of pregnancy, infancy, and childhood up to the age of 8 may cause permanent discoloration of the teeth (yellow-gray-brown). Enamel hypoplasia has also been reported. May also cause retardation of skeletal development and deformations.

Caution:
Renal disease, hepatic disease, lactation, nephrogenic diabetes insipidus

DRUG INTERACTIONS OF CONCERN TO DENTISTRY

- Decreased effect of penicillins, cephalosporins, oral contraceptives
- Contraindicated with isotretinoin (Accutane)

SERIOUS REACTIONS

! Superinfection (especially fungal), anaphylaxis, and benign intracranial hypertension occur rarely.
! Bulging fontanelles occur rarely in infants.

DENTAL CONSIDERATIONS

General:

- Examine oral cavity for side effects if on long-term drug therapy.
- Determine why the patient is taking the drug.
- Do not prescribe during pregnancy or before age 8 yr because of tooth discoloration.
- Absorption is reduced by dairy products, metals, and antacids.
- Dental staining or enamel hypoplasia may be associated with exposure to this drug before birth or up to the age of 8. Tetracycline stains may be extremely resistant to ordinary tooth-whitening procedures.

Consultations:

- Medical consultation may be required to assess disease control.

Teach Patient/Family to:

- Encourage effective oral hygiene to prevent soft tissue inflammation.
- Use caution to prevent injury when using oral hygiene aids.
- When used for dental infection, advise patient to:
  - Report sore throat, oral burning sensation, fever, and fatigue, any of which could indicate superinfection.
  - Take at prescribed intervals and complete dosage regimen.
  - Immediately notify the dentist if signs or symptoms of infection increase.

desipramine hydrochloride

dess-**ip′**-ra-meen hi-droh-**klor′**-ide
(Apo-Desipramine [CAN], Norpramin, Novo-Desipramine [CAN], Pertofran[AUS])
Do not confuse desipramine with clomipramine, disopyramide, imipramine, or nortriptyline.

CATEGORY AND SCHEDULE

Pregnancy Risk Category: C

Drug Class: Antidepressant, tricyclic

MECHANISM OF ACTION
A tricyclic antidepressant that blocks the reuptake of neurotransmitters, such as norepinephrine and serotonin, at presynaptic membranes, increasing their availability at postsynaptic receptor sites. Also has strong anticholinergic activity.
Therapeutic Effect: Relieves depression.

USES
Treatment of depression; unapproved: neurogenic pain

PHARMACOKINETICS
Rapidly and well absorbed from the GI tract. Protein binding: 90%. Metabolized in the liver. Primarily excreted in urine. Minimally removed by hemodialysis. ***Half-life:*** 12–27 hr.

INDICATIONS AND DOSAGES
▸ Depression
PO
Adults. 75 mg/day. May gradually increase to 150–200 mg/day. Maximum: 300 mg/day.
Elderly. Initially, 10–25 mg/day. May gradually increase to 75–100 mg/day. Maximum: 300 mg/day.
Children older than 12 yr. Initially, 25–50 mg/day. May gradually increase to 100 mg/day. Maximum: 150 mg/day.
Children 6–12 yr. 1–3 mg/kg/day. Maximum: 5 mg/kg/day.

SIDE EFFECTS/ADVERSE REACTIONS
Frequent
Somnolence, fatigue, dry mouth, blurred vision, constipation, delayed micturition, orthostatic hypotension, diaphoresis, impaired concentration, increased appetite, urine retention
Occasional
GI disturbances (such as nausea, GI distress, metallic taste)
Rare
Paradoxical reactions (agitation, restlessness, nightmares, insomnia), extrapyramidal symptoms (particularly fine hand tremor)

PRECAUTIONS AND CONTRAINDICATIONS
Angle-closure glaucoma, use within 14 days of MAOIs.
Caution:
Suicidal patients, severe depression, increased intraocular pressure, narrow-angle glaucoma, elderly, MAOIs

DRUG INTERACTIONS OF CONCERN TO DENTISTRY
- Increased anticholinergic effects: muscarinic blockers, antihistamines, phenothiazines
- Increased effects of direct-acting sympathomimetics: epinephrine, levonordefrin
- Potential risk for increased CNS depression: alcohol, barbiturates, benzodiazepines, and other CNS depressants
- Decreased antihypertensive effects: clonidine, guanadrel, guanethidine
- At higher tricyclic doses, serum levels of fluconazole and ketoconazole may be elevated
- Avoid concurrent use with St. John's wort (herb)

SERIOUS REACTIONS
! Overdose may produce confusion, seizures, somnolence, arrhythmias, fever, hallucinations, dyspnea, vomiting, and unusual fatigue or weakness.
! Abrupt discontinuation after prolonged therapy may produce severe headache, malaise, nausea, vomiting, and vivid dreams.

D

DENTAL CONSIDERATIONS

General:

• Take vital signs at every appointment because of cardiovascular side effects.
• Assess salivary flow as a factor in caries, periodontal disease, and candidiasis.
• Patients on chronic drug therapy may rarely have symptoms of blood dyscrasias, which can include infection, bleeding, and poor healing.
• After supine positioning, have patient sit upright for at least 2 min to avoid orthostatic hypotension.
• Use vasoconstrictors with caution, in low doses, and with careful aspiration. Avoid use of gingival retraction cord with epinephrine.
• Place on frequent recall because of oral side effects.

Consultations:

• In a patient with symptoms of blood dyscrasias, request a medical consultation for blood studies and postpone dental treatment until normal values are reestablished.
• Medical consultation may be required to assess disease control.
• Physician should be informed if significant xerostomic side effects occur (e.g., increased caries, sore tongue, problems eating or swallowing, difficulty wearing prosthesis) so that a medication change can be considered.

Teach Patient/Family to:

• Encourage effective oral hygiene to prevent soft tissue inflammation.
• Use caution to prevent injury when using oral hygiene aids.
• When chronic dry mouth occurs, advise patient to:
  • Avoid mouth rinses with high alcohol content because of drying effects.
  • Use daily home fluoride products for anticaries effect.
  • Use sugarless gum, frequent sips of water, or saliva substitutes.

desirudin

deh-**sear′**-ew-din
(Iprivask)

CATEGORY AND SCHEDULE

Pregnancy Risk Category: C

Drug Class: Anticoagulant; thrombin inhibitor

MECHANISM OF ACTION

An anticoagulant that binds specifically and directly to thrombin, inhibiting free-circulating and clot-bound thrombin.
Therapeutic Effect: Prolongs the clotting time of human plasma.

USES

Prophylaxis for deep vein thrombosis (DVT) in those undergoing hip replacement

PHARMACOKINETICS

Completely absorbed. Distributed in extracellular space. Metabolized and eliminated by the kidney. ***Half-life:*** 2–3 hr.

INDICATIONS AND DOSAGES

▸ **Prevention of DVT in Patients Undergoing Hip Replacement Surgery**

Subcutaneous

Adults, Elderly. Initially, 15 mg q12h given 5–15 min before surgery but following induction of regional block anesthesia, if used. May administer up to 12 days after surgery.

▸ **Moderate Renal Impairment (creatinine clearance 31–60 ml/min or higher)**
Subcutaneous
Adults, Elderly. 5 mg q12h.

▸ **Severe Renal Impairment (creatinine clearance less than 31 ml/min)**
Subcutaneous
Adults, Elderly. 1.7 mg q12h.

SIDE EFFECTS/ADVERSE REACTIONS

Frequent
Hematoma
Occasional
Injection site mass, wound secretion, nausea, hypersensitivity reaction

PRECAUTIONS AND CONTRAINDICATIONS

Hypersensitivity to natural or recombinant hirudins (anticoagulation factors), active bleeding, irreversible coagulation disorders

DRUG INTERACTIONS OF CONCERN TO DENTISTRY

- Increased risk of bleeding: salicylates, NSAIDs, or any drug that affects coagulation

SERIOUS REACTIONS

! Serious or major hemorrhage and anaphylactic reaction occur rarely.

DENTAL CONSIDERATIONS

General:
- Patients are at risk of bleeding, so check for oral signs.
- Product may be used in outpatient therapy. Delay elective dental treatment until patient completes anticoagulant therapy.
- Determine why patient is taking the drug.
- Do not discontinue desirudin.
- Avoid products that affect platelet function, such as aspirin and NSAIDs.
- Consider local hemostasis measures to prevent excessive bleeding.

Consultations:
- Medical consultation should include PPT or INR.
- Medical consultation may be required to assess disease control and patient's ability to tolerate stress.

Teach Patient/Family to:
- Use soft tooth brush to reduce risk of bleeding.
- Encourage effective oral hygiene to prevent soft tissue inflammation.
- Report oral lesions, soreness, or bleeding to dentist.
- Prevent trauma when using oral hygiene aids.
- Update health and medication history if physician makes any changes in evaluation or drug regimens; include OTC, herbal, and nonherbal remedies in the update.

desloratadine

des-loer-**at**′-ah-deen
(Aerius [CAN], Clarinex, Clarinex Redi-Tabs)

CATEGORY AND SCHEDULE

Pregnancy Risk Category: C
Do not confuse Clarinex with Claritin.

Drug Class: Antihistamine, histamine H_1-receptor antagonist

MECHANISM OF ACTION

A nonsedating antihistamine that exhibits selective peripheral histamine H_1 receptor blocking action. Competes with histamine at receptor sites.

D

Therapeutic Effect: Prevents allergic responses mediated by histamine, such as rhinitis and urticaria.

USES

Treatment of seasonal allergic rhinitis; chronic idiopathic urticaria

PHARMACOKINETICS

Rapidly and almost completely absorbed from the GI tract. Distributed mainly in liver, lungs, GI tract, and bile. Metabolized in the liver to active metabolite and undergoes extensive first-pass metabolism. Eliminated in urine and feces. ***Half-life:*** 27 hr (increased in the elderly and in renal or hepatic impairment).

INDICATIONS AND DOSAGES

▸ Allergic Rhinitis, Urticaria

PO

Adults, Elderly, Children older than 12 yr. 5 mg once a day.

▸ Dosage in Hepatic or Renal Impairment

Dosage is decreased to 5 mg every other day.

SIDE EFFECTS/ADVERSE REACTIONS

Frequent

Headache

Occasional

Dry mouth, somnolence

Rare

Fatigue, dizziness, diarrhea, nausea

PRECAUTIONS AND CONTRAINDICATIONS

Hypersensitivity to this drug or loratadine

Caution:

Distributed to breast milk (caution in nursing), incomplete dosing studies in the elderly, safety has not been established in children younger than 12 yr, dosage adjustment required in hepatic impairment

DRUG INTERACTIONS OF CONCERN TO DENTISTRY

- Limited studies with concurrent doses of erythromycin; ketoconazole and azithromycin show slight elevations of plasma levels but no clinically relevant changes in electrocardiographic parameters.
- One report indicated a potential for increased anticholinergic effects with other anticholinergic drugs and increased somnolence with CNS depressants; however, data are lacking.

SERIOUS REACTIONS

! None known

DENTAL CONSIDERATIONS

General:

- Assess salivary flow as a factor in caries, periodontal disease, and candidiasis.

Teach Patient/Family to:

- Encourage effective oral hygiene to prevent soft tissue inflammation.
- When chronic dry mouth occurs, advise patient to:
  - Avoid mouth rinses with high alcohol content because of drying effects.
  - Use sugarless gum, frequent sips of water, or saliva substitutes.
  - Use daily home fluoride products for anticaries effect.

D

desmopressin

des-moe-**press′**-in
(DDAVP, Minirin[AUS], Octostim[CAN], Stimate)

CATEGORY AND SCHEDULE

Pregnancy Risk Category: B

Drug Class: Antidiuretic, central diabetes insipidus; antidiuretic, primary nocturnal enuresis; antihemorrhagic

MECHANISM OF ACTION

A synthetic pituitary hormone that increases reabsorption of water by increasing permeability of collecting ducts of the kidneys. Also serves as a plasminogen activator.
Therapeutic Effect: Increases plasma factor VIII (antihemophilic factor). Decreases urinary output.

USES

Prevents or controls the frequent urination, increased thirst, and loss of water associated with diabetes insipidus (water diabetes). It is used also to control bed-wetting and frequent urination and increased thirst associated with certain types of brain injuries or brain surgery.

PHARMACOKINETICS

Route	Onset	Peak	Duration
PO	1 hr	2–7 hr	6–8 hr
IV	15–30 min	1.5–3 hr	N/A
Intranasal	15 min–1 hr	1–5 hr	5–21 hr

Poorly absorbed after oral or nasal administration. Metabolism: Unknown. ***Half-life:*** Oral: 1.5–2.5 hr. Intranasal: 3.3–3.5 hr. IV: 0.4–4 hr.

INDICATIONS AND DOSAGES

▸ **Primary Nocturnal Enuresis**

PO

Children 12 yr and older. 0.2–0.6 mg once before bedtime.
Intranasal. Initially, 20 mcg (0.2 ml) at bedtime; use one-half dose in each nostril. Adjust to maximum of 40 mcg/day.

▸ **Central Cranial Diabetes Insipidus**

PO

Adults, Elderly, Children 12 yr and older. Initially, 0.05 mg twice a day. Range: 0.1–1.2 mg/day in 2–3 divided doses.
Children younger than 12 yr. Initially, 0.05 mg; then twice a day. Range: 0.1–0.8 mg daily.

IV, Subcutaneous

Adults, Elderly, Children 12 yr and older. 2–4 mcg/day in 2 divided doses or 1/10 of maintenance intranasal dose.

Intranasal

Adults, Elderly, Children older than 12 yr. 5–40 mcg (0.05–0.4 ml) in 1–3 doses/day.
Children 3 mo–12 yr. Initially, 5 mcg (0.05 ml)/day. Range: 5–30 mcg (0.05–0.3 ml)/day.

▸ **Hemophilia A, von Willebrand's Disease (Type I)**

IV Infusion

Adults, Elderly, Children weighing more than 10 kg. 0.3 mcg/kg diluted in 50 ml 0.9% NaCl.
Children weighing 10 kg and less. 0.3 mcg/kg diluted in 10 ml 0.9% NaCl.

Intranasal

Adults, Elderly, Children 12 yr and older weighing more than 50 kg. 300 mcg; use 1 spray in each nostril.
Adults, Elderly, Children 12 yr and older weighing 50 kg or less. 150 mcg as a single spray.

D

SIDE EFFECTS/ADVERSE REACTIONS

Occasional

IV: Pain, redness, or swelling at injection site; headache; abdominal cramps; vulval pain; flushed skin; mild B/P elevation; nausea with high dosages

Nasal: Rhinorrhea, nasal congestion, slight B/P elevation

PRECAUTIONS AND CONTRAINDICATIONS

Hemophilia A with factor VIII levels less than 5%; hemophilia B; severe type I, type IIB, or platelet-type von Willebrand's disease

Caution:

Lactation, hypertension

DRUG INTERACTIONS OF CONCERN TO DENTISTRY

- Decreased antidiuretic effects: demeclocycline
- Increased antidiuretic effects: carbamazepine

SERIOUS REACTIONS

! Water intoxication or hyponatremia, marked by headache, somnolence, confusion, decreased urination, rapid weight gain, seizures, and coma, may occur in overhydration. Children, elderly patients, and infants are especially at risk.

DENTAL CONSIDERATIONS

General:

- Monitor vital signs at every appointment because of cardiovascular side effects.
- Avoid prescribing aspirin-containing products if treatment is for bleeding disorder.
- Consider local hemostatic measures to prevent excessive bleeding.
- Determine why the patient is taking the drug.
- Consider semisupine chair position for patient comfort because of GI effects of disease.

Consultations:

- Medical consultation may be required to assess disease control; definite consultation for patients with chronic bleeding disorders.
- Medical consultation should include PTT or INR.

Teach Patient/Family to:

- Advise dentist if excessive bleeding occurs or continues after dental treatment.

desonide

dess'-oh-nide

(Delonide, Desocrot[CAN], DesOwen, Scheinpharm Desonide[CAN], Tridesilon)

CATEGORY AND SCHEDULE

Pregnancy Risk Category: C

Drug Class: Topical corticosteroid, group IV low potency

MECHANISM OF ACTION

A topical corticosteroid that has antiinflammatory, antipruritic, and vasoconstrictive properties. The exact mechanism of the antiinflammatory process is unclear.

Therapeutic Effect: Reduces or prevents tissue response to the inflammatory process.

USES

Treatment of psoriasis, eczema, contact dermatitis, pruritus

PHARMACOKINETICS
Large variation in absorption determined by many factors. Metabolized in the liver. Primarily excreted by the kidneys and small amounts in the bile.

INDICATIONS AND DOSAGES
▸ **Dermatoses**
Topical
Adults, Elderly. Apply sparingly 2–3 times a day.
▸ **Otitis Externa**
Aural
Adults, Elderly, Children. Instill 3–4 drops into the ear 3–4 times a day.

SIDE EFFECTS/ADVERSE REACTIONS
Occasional
Burning and stinging at site of application, dryness, skin peeling, contact dermatitis

PRECAUTIONS AND CONTRAINDICATIONS
Perforated eardrum, history of hypersensitivity to desonide or other corticosteroids
Caution:
Lactation, viral infections, bacterial infections

DRUG INTERACTIONS OF CONCERN TO DENTISTRY
• None listed

SERIOUS REACTIONS
! The serious reactions of long-term therapy and the addition of occlusive dressings are reversible hypothalamic-pituitary-adrenal (HPA) axis suppression, manifestations of Cushing's syndrome, hyperglycemia, and glucosuria.

DENTAL CONSIDERATIONS
General:
• Determine why the patient is taking the drug.
• Place on frequent recall to evaluate healing response if used on chronic basis.
• Apply lubricant to dry lips for patient comfort before dental procedures.

desoximetasone
des-ox-ih-**met′**-ah-sone
(Taro-Desoximetason[CAN], Topicort, Topicort-LP)
Do not confuse with dexamethasone.

CATEGORY AND SCHEDULE
Pregnancy Risk Category: C

Drug Class: Topical corticosteroid, group II potency (0.25%), group III potency (0.05%)

MECHANISM OF ACTION
A high-potency, fluorinated topical corticosteroid that has antiinflammatory, antipruritic, and vasoconstrictive properties. The exact mechanism of the antiinflammatory process is unclear.
Therapeutic Effect: Reduces tissue response to the inflammatory process.

USES
Treatment of psoriasis, eczema, contact dermatitis, pruritus

PHARMACOKINETICS
Large variation in absorption among sites. Protein binding in varying degrees. Metabolized in liver. Primarily excreted in urine.

D

INDICATIONS AND DOSAGES

▸ **Dermatoses**

Topical

Adults, Elderly. Apply sparingly 2 times a day.

Children. Apply sparingly 1–2 times a day.

SIDE EFFECTS/ADVERSE REACTIONS

Frequent

Itching, redness, irritation, burning at site of application

Occasional

Dryness, folliculitis, hypertrichosis, acneiform eruptions, hypopigmentation, perioral dermatitis

Rare

Allergic contact dermatitis, adrenal suppression, atrophy, striae, miliaria, photosensitivity

PRECAUTIONS AND CONTRAINDICATIONS

History of hypersensitivity to desoximetasone or other corticosteroids

Caution:

Lactation, viral infections, bacterial infections

SERIOUS REACTIONS

! Serious reactions of long-term therapy and addition of occlusive dressings are reversible hypothalamic-pituitary-adrenal (HPA) axis suppression, manifestations of Cushing's syndrome, hyperglycemia, and glucosuria.

! Abruptly withdrawing the drug after long-term therapy may require supplemental systemic corticosteroids.

DENTAL CONSIDERATIONS

General:

- Gel formulations are used in the treatment of oral lichen planus lesions when the diagnosis has been confirmed by immunofluorescent biopsy testing.
- Patient may require supplemented steroid prior to dental procedures.
- Place on frequent recall to evaluate healing response.

Teach Patient/Family to:

- Return for oral evaluation if response of oral tissues has not occurred in 7–14 days.
- Encourage effective oral hygiene to prevent soft tissue inflammation.
- Not for use on oral herpetic ulcerations.
- Apply at bedtime or after meals for maximum effect.
- Apply with cotton-tipped applicator, dabbing gently, not rubbing medication on lesion.

desvenlafaxine

des-ven-la-**fax**'een

(Pristiq)

CATEGORY AND SCHEDULE

Pregnancy Risk Category: C

Drug Class: Antidepressants

MECHANISM OF ACTION

The major active metabolite of the antidepressant venlafaxine that potentiates CNS neurotransmitter activity by inhibiting the reuptake of serotonin and norepinephrine.

Therapeutic Effect: Relieves depression.

USES

Major depressive disorder

PHARMACOKINETICS

Well absorbed from the GI tract. Bioavailability: approximately 80%. Protein binding: 30%. Metabolized by conjugation (mediated by UGT isoforms); minor extent through oxidative metabolism by CYP3A4.

Approximately 45% desvenlafaxine excreted unchanged in urine; approximately 19% excreted as the glucuronide metabolite, <5% as the oxidative metabolite (N,O-didesmethylvenlafaxine) in urine. ***Half-life:*** 11 hr.

INDICATIONS AND DOSAGES

▸ Major Depressive Disorder

PO

Adults. 50 mg once daily with or without food. Range: 50–400 mg/day.

▸ Dosage in Renal Impairment

Adults, moderate impairment.
50 mg once daily with or without food.

Adults, severe impairment and end-stage renal disease (ESRD).
50 mg every other day with or without food. Do not escalate dose.

▸ Dosage in Hepatic Impairment

Adults. 50 mg once daily with or without food. Do not exceed 100 mg/day.

SIDE EFFECTS/ADVERSE REACTIONS

Frequent

Hypertension, nausea, dry mouth, diarrhea, fatigue, decreased appetite, dizziness, somnolence, headache, constipation, hyperhidrosis

Occasional

Palpitations, vomiting, chills, jittery, anxiety, abnormal dreams, yawning, mydriasis, irritability, tinnitus, dysgeusia, hot flush, sexual dysfunction (men), proteinuria

Rare

Tachycardia, asthenia, weight decrease, disturbed attention, nervousness, sexual dysfunction (women), mania, seizure, hyponatremia/SIADH, interstitial lung disease, eosinophilic pneumonia, abnormal bleeding, cholesterol and triglyceride elevations

PRECAUTIONS AND CONTRAINDICATIONS

Hypersensitivity to desvenlafaxine, venlafaxine or any component of the formulation

Use within 14 days of MAOIs

Caution:

Suicide risk, hypertension, abnormal bleeding

Narrow-angle glaucoma

Renal impairment

Seizure disorder

Hyperlipidemia, hypertriglyceridemia

Hepatic dysfunction

DRUG INTERACTIONS OF CONCERN TO DENTISTRY

- MAOIs: May cause neuroleptic malignant syndrome, autonomic instability (including rapid fluctuations of vital signs), extreme agitation, hyperthermia, mental status changes, myoclonus, rigidity, and coma.
- Serotonergic drugs: May increase the risk of serotonin syndrome.
- Anticoagulants/antiplatelets, NSAIDs: May increase the risk of bleeding.
- CYP3A4 inhibitors: May increase drug concentration levels of desvenlafaxine.

SERIOUS REACTIONS

! Increased risk of suicidal thinking and behavior in children, adolescents, and young adults have been reported.

! Seizures have been reported.

! Serotonin syndrome or neuroleptic malignant syndrome (NMS)-like reactions have been reported.

! When discontinuing desvenlafaxine, plan to taper the dosage slowly over 2 wk.

! Allow at least 14 days to elapse before switching the patient from a MAOI to desvenlafaxine and at least 7 days to elapse before switching the patient from desvenlafaxine to a MAOI.

DENTAL CONSIDERATIONS

D

General:

• Monitor vital signs at every appointment because of cardiovascular side effects.

Consultations:

• Medical consultation may be required to assess disease control.

Teach Patient/Family to:

• Report oral lesions, soreness, or bleeding to dentist.

• When chronic dry mouth occurs, advise patient to:

  • Avoid mouth rinses with high alcohol content because of drying effects.

  • Use daily home fluoride products for anticaries effect.

  • Use sugarless gum, frequent sips of water, or saliva substitutes.

dexamethasone

dex-ah-**meth**′-ah-sone
(Decadron, Desamethasone Intensol, Dexasone, Dexasone LA, Dexmethsone[AUS], Diodex[CAN], Hexadrol[CAN], Maxidex, Solurex, Solurex LA)
Do not confuse dexamethasone with desoximetasone or dextromethorphan, or Maxidex with Maxzide.

CATEGORY AND SCHEDULE

Pregnancy Risk Category: C (D if used in the first trimester)

Drug Class: Synthetic topical corticosteroid

MECHANISM OF ACTION

A long-acting glucocorticoid that inhibits accumulation of inflammatory cells at inflammation sites, phagocytosis, lysosomal enzyme release and synthesis, and release of mediators of inflammation.
Therapeutic Effect: Prevents and suppresses cell and tissue immune reactions and inflammatory process.

USES

Treatment of corticosteroid-responsive dermatoses, oral ulcerative inflammatory lesions

PHARMACOKINETICS

Rapidly, completely absorbed from the GI tract after oral administration. Widely distributed. Protein binding: High. Metabolized in the liver. Primarily excreted in urine. Minimally removed by hemodialysis.
Half-life: 3–4.5 hr.

INDICATIONS AND DOSAGES

▸ **Antiinflammatory**

PO, IV, IM

Adults, Elderly. 0.75–9 mg/day in divided doses q6–12h.
Children. 0.08–0.3 mg/kg/day in divided doses q6–12h.

▸ **Cerebral Edema**

IV

Adults, Elderly. Initially, 10 mg, then 4 mg (IV or IM) q6h.

PO, IV, IM

Children. Loading dose of 1–2 mg/kg, then 1–1.5 mg/kg/day in divided doses q4–6h.

▸ **Nausea and Vomiting in Chemotherapy Patients**

IV

Adults, Elderly. 8–20 mg once, then 4 mg (PO) q4–6h or 8 mg q8h.
Children. 10 mg/m^2/dose (Maximum: 20 mg), then 5 mg/m^2/dose q6h.

▸ **Physiologic Replacement**

PO, IV, IM

Children. 0.03–0.15 mg/kg/day in divided doses q6–12h.

▸ **Usual Ophthalmic Dosage, Ocular Inflammatory Conditions**

Ointment

Adults, Elderly, Children. Thin coating 3–4 times a day.

Suspension

Adults, Elderly, Children. Initially, 2 drops q1h while awake and q2h at night for 1 day, then reduce to 3–4 times a day.

SIDE EFFECTS/ADVERSE REACTIONS

Frequent

Inhalation: Cough, dry mouth, hoarseness, throat irritation

Intranasal: Burning, mucosal dryness

Ophthalmic: Blurred vision

Systemic: Insomnia, facial swelling or cushingoid appearance, moderate abdominal distention, indigestion, increased appetite, nervousness, facial flushing, diaphoresis

Occasional

Inhalation: Localized fungal infection, such as thrush

Intranasal: Crusting inside nose, nosebleed, sore throat, ulceration of nasal mucosa

Ophthalmic: Decreased vision, watering of eyes, eye pain, burning, stinging, redness of eyes, nausea, vomiting

Systemic: Dizziness, decreased or blurred vision

Topical: Allergic contact dermatitis, purpura or blood-containing blisters, thinning of skin with easy bruising, telangiectasis or raised dark red spots on skin

Rare

Inhalation: Increased bronchospasm, esophageal candidiasis

Intranasal: Nasal and pharyngeal candidiasis, eye pain

Systemic: General allergic reaction (such as rash and hives); pain, redness, or swelling at injection site; psychological changes; false sense of well-being; hallucinations; depression

PRECAUTIONS AND CONTRAINDICATIONS

Active untreated infections, fungal, tuberculosis, or viral diseases of the eye

Caution:

Lactation, viral infections, bacterial infections

SERIOUS REACTIONS

! Long-term therapy may cause muscle wasting (especially in the arms and legs), osteoporosis, spontaneous fractures, amenorrhea, cataracts, glaucoma, peptic ulcer disease, and CHF.

! The ophthalmic form may cause glaucoma, ocular hypertension, and cataracts.

! Abrupt withdrawal following long-term therapy may cause severe joint pain, severe headache, anorexia, nausea, fever, rebound inflammation, fatigue, weakness, lethargy, dizziness, and orthostatic hypotension.

DENTAL CONSIDERATIONS

General:

- Monitor vital signs at every appointment because of cardiovascular side effects.
- Patients on chronic drug therapy may rarely have symptoms of blood dyscrasias, which can include infection, bleeding, and poor healing.
- Symptoms of oral infections may be masked.
- Patients who have been or are currently on chronic steroid therapy (longer than 2 wk) may require supplemental steroids for dental treatment.

• Avoid prescribing aspirin-containing products.
• Place on frequent recall to evaluate healing response.
• Prophylactic antibiotics may be indicated to prevent infection if surgery or deep scaling is planned.

Consultations:

• In a patient with symptoms of blood dyscrasias, request a medical consultation for blood studies and postpone dental treatment until normal values are reestablished.
• Medical consultation may be required to assess disease control.
• Consultation may be required to confirm steroid dose and duration of use.

Teach Patient/Family to:

• Encourage effective oral hygiene to prevent soft tissue inflammation.
• Use caution to prevent injury when using oral hygiene aids.
• Avoid mouth rinses with high alcohol content because of drug interaction.

dexamethasone sodium phosphate

dex-ah-**meth′**-ah-sone **soe′**-dee-um **foss′**-fate
(AK-Dex, Decadron Phosphate Ophthalmic, Dexamethasone Ophthalmic, Maxidex, Ocu-Dex, Diodex[CAN])
Do not confuse dexamethasone with desoximetasone, dextromethorphan, or Maxzide.

CATEGORY AND SCHEDULE

Pregnancy Risk Category: C (D if used in the first trimester)

Drug Class: Synthetic topical corticosteroid

MECHANISM OF ACTION

A corticosteroid that inhibits accumulation of inflammatory cells at inflammation sites, phagocytosis, lysosomal enzyme release, and synthesis and release of mediators of inflammation.

Therapeutic Effect: Prevents and suppresses cell and tissue immune reactions, inflammatory process.

USES

Treatment of corticosteroid-responsive dermatoses, oral ulcerative inflammatory lesions

PHARMACOKINETICS

Absorbed into aqueous humor, cornea, iris, choroids, ciliary body, and retina. Systemic absorption may occur and is more likely at higher doses or in pediatric therapy.

INDICATIONS AND DOSAGES

▸ **Ocular Inflammatory Conditions**

Ophthalmic, Ointment

Adults, Elderly. Apply thin strip 3–4 times a day.

Ophthalmic, Solution and Suspension

Adults, Elderly. Instill 1 or 2 drops up to 6 times a day.

SIDE EFFECTS/ADVERSE REACTIONS

Frequent

Blurred vision, increased intraocular pressure

Occasional

Decreased vision, watering of eyes, eye pain, burning, stinging, redness of eyes, nausea, vomiting

Rare

Optic nerve damage, posterior subcapsular cataract formation, delayed wound healing

PRECAUTIONS AND CONTRAINDICATIONS

Epithelial herpes simplex keratitis (dendritic keratitis), vaccinia, varicella or other viral diseases of the cornea and conjunctiva, mycobacterial infection of the eye, fungal diseases of ocular structures, hypersensitivity to any component of the medication

Caution:

Diabetes mellitus, glaucoma, osteoporosis, seizure disorders, ulcerative colitis, CHF, myasthenia gravis, renal disease, peptic ulcer, esophagitis

DRUG INTERACTIONS OF CONCERN TO DENTISTRY

- Decreased action: barbiturates
- Increased side effects: alcohol, salicylates, other NSAIDs
- Increased action: ketoconazole, macrolide antibiotics

SERIOUS REACTIONS

! The serious reactions of the ophthalmic form of dexamethasone sodium phosphate are glaucoma, ocular hypertension, and cataracts.

! May promote development and spread of secondary infection (usually fungal).

DENTAL CONSIDERATIONS

General:

- Place on frequent recall to evaluate healing response.

Teach Patient/Family to:

- Return for oral evaluation if response of oral tissues has not occurred in 7–14 days.
- Encourage effective oral hygiene to prevent soft tissue inflammation.
- Apply approximately 0.25 inch; measure and apply with cotton-tipped applicator by gently dabbing, not rubbing, medication on lesion.
- Apply at bedtime or after meals for maximum effect.
- Avoid use on oral herpetic lesions.

D

dexchlorpheniramine

dex-klor-fen-**eer**′-ah-meen (Polaramine, Polaramine Repetabs)

CATEGORY AND SCHEDULE

Pregnancy Risk Category: B

Drug Class: Antihistamine

MECHANISM OF ACTION

A propylamine derivative that competes with histamine for H_1-receptor sites on effector cells in the GI tract, blood vessels, and respiratory tract.

Dexchlorpheniramine is the dextro-isomer of chlorpheniramine and is approximately 2 times more active.

Therapeutic Effect: Prevents allergic response, produces mild bronchodilation, blocks histamine-induced bronchitis.

USES

Treatment of allergy symptoms, rhinitis, pruritus, contact dermatitis

PHARMACOKINETICS

Route	Onset	Peak	Duration
PO	0.5 hr	1–2 hr	3–6 hr

Well absorbed from the GI tract. Protein binding: 70%. Widely distributed. Metabolized in liver to active metabolite, undergoes extensive first-pass metabolism.

Excreted primarily in urine. Not removed by hemodialysis. ***Half-life:*** 20 hr.

INDICATIONS AND DOSAGES

▸ Allergic Rhinitis, Common Cold

PO

Adults, Elderly, Children 12 yr or older. 2 mg q4–6h or 4–6 mg timed release at bedtime or q8–10h.
Children 6–11 yr. 4 mg timed release at bedtime or 1 mg q4–6h.
Children 2–5 yr. 0.5 mg q4–6h. Do not use timed release.

SIDE EFFECTS/ADVERSE REACTIONS

Frequent

Drowsiness, dizziness, headache, dry mouth, nose, or throat, urinary retention, thickening of bronchial secretions, sedation, hypotension

Occasional

Epigastric distress, flushing, blurred vision, tinnitus, paresthesia, sweating, chills

PRECAUTIONS AND CONTRAINDICATIONS

History of hypersensitivity to antihistamines, newborn or premature infants, nursing mothers, third trimester of pregnancy

Caution:

Increased intraocular pressure, renal disease, cardiac disease, hypertension, bronchial asthma, seizure disorder, stenosed peptic ulcers, hyperthyroidism, prostatic hypertrophy, bladder neck obstruction, elderly

DRUG INTERACTIONS OF CONCERN TO DENTISTRY

- Increased CNS depression: barbiturates, opioids, hypnotics, tricyclic antidepressants, alcohol
- Increased anticholinergic effect: anticholinergic drugs

SERIOUS REACTIONS

! Children may experience dominant paradoxical reactions, including restlessness, insomnia, euphoria, nervousness, and tremors.

! Hypersensitivity reaction, such as eczema, pruritus, rash, cardiac disturbances, and photosensitivity, may occur.

! Overdosage may vary from CNS depression, including sedation, apnea, hypotension, cardiovascular collapse, or death to severe paradoxical reaction, such as hallucinations, tremors, and seizures.

DENTAL CONSIDERATIONS

General:

- Assess salivary flow as a factor in caries, periodontal disease, and candidiasis.
- Consider semisupine chair position for patient comfort because of respiratory effects of disease.

Teach Patient/Family:

- When chronic dry mouth occurs, advise patient to:
  - Avoid mouth rinses with high alcohol content because of drying effects.
  - Use sugarless gum, frequent sips of water, or saliva substitutes.
  - Use daily home fluoride products for anticaries effect.

dexlansoprazole

dex-lan-**soe**-prah-zole

(Kapidex)

Do not confuse with dexamethasone or lansoprazole.

CATEGORY AND SCHEDULE

Pregnancy Risk Category: B

Drug Class: Antisecretory, proton pump inhibitor

MECHANISN OF ACTION

A proton pump inhibitor that selectively inhibits the parietal cell membrane enzyme system in the GI tract (hydrogen-potassium adenosine triphosphatase), or proton pump.

Therapeutic effect: Suppresses gastric acid secretion.

USES

Healing all grades of erosive esophagitis, maintenance of healing of erosive esophagitis, and treatment of heartburn due to gastroesophageal reflux disease (GERD)

PHARMACOKINETICS

Well absorbed orally, peak concentrations reached in 1–2 hr and 4–5 hr. Widely distributed. Protein binding: 96%. Extensively metabolized in the liver by oxidation (CYP 2C19 and CYP3A4).

Half-life: 1–2 hr. Metabolites excreted by the kidneys.

INDICATIONS AND DOSAGES

▸ **Erosive Esophagitis**

PO

Adult, Elderly. 60 mg once daily for up to 8 wk.

▸ **Maintenance of Healing of Erosive Esophagitis**

PO

Adult, Elderly. 30 mg once daily.

▸ **Symptomatic, Non-Erosive GERD**

PO

Adult, Elderly. 30 mg once daily for 4 wk.

SIDE EFFECTS/ADVERSE REACTIONS

Frequent

Diarrhea, abdominal pain, nausea, upper respiratory tract infections, vomiting, flatulence

PRECAUTIONS AND CONTRAINDICATIONS

Hypersensitivity to dexlansoprazole or its ingredients, children under the age of 18, pregnancy, lactation

Caution:

Symptomatic improvement with dexlansoprazole does not preclude the possibility of gastric malignancy

DRUG INTERACTIONS OF CONCERN TO DENTISTRY

- Drug interactions in dentistry not established but dexlansoprazole may interfere with the absorption of ampicillin esters and ketoconazole.

SERIOUS REACTIONS

! None established in dental patients

DENTAL CONSIDERATIONS

General:

- Consider semisupine chair position for patient comfort because of GI effects of disease.
- Question the patient about tolerance of NSAIDs or aspirin related to GI adverse effects.
- Patients with GERD may have oral symptoms of acid reflux, including dental erosion, or TMJ dysfunction that may require appropriate dental treatment.

Teach patient/family to:

- Seek medical care for worsening or unrelieved GI symptoms.
- Use fluoridated toothpaste and effective oral hygiene measures to minimize sensitivity and caries associated with dental erosion.

D

dexmethylphenidate hydrochloride

dex-meth-ill-**fen**′-ih-date hi-droh-**klor**′-ide
(Focalin)

CATEGORY AND SCHEDULE

Pregnancy Risk Category: C
Controlled Substance: Schedule II

Drug Class: CNS stimulant; related to the amphetamines

MECHANISM OF ACTION

A CNS stimulant that blocks the reuptake of norepinephrine and dopamine into presynaptic neurons, increasing the release of these neurotransmitters into the synaptic cleft.
Therapeutic Effect: Decreases motor restlessness and fatigue; increases motor activity, mental alertness, and attention span; elevates mood.

USES

Treatment of attention-deficit/hyperactivity disorder (ADHD)

PHARMACOKINETICS

Route	Onset	Peak	Duration
PO	N/A	N/A	4–5 hr

Readily absorbed from the GI tract. Plasma concentrations increase rapidly. Metabolized in the liver. Excreted unchanged in urine. ***Half-life:*** 2.2 hr.

INDICATIONS AND DOSAGES

▸ **ADHD**

PO

Patients new to dexmethylphenidate or methylphenidate. 2.5 mg twice a day (5 mg/day). May adjust dosage in 2.5- to 5-mg increments. Maximum: 20 mg/day.
Patients currently taking methylphenidate. Half the methylphenidate dosage. Maximum: 20 mg/day.

SIDE EFFECTS/ADVERSE REACTIONS

Frequent
Abdominal pain, nausea, anorexia, fever
Occasional
Tachycardia, arrhythmias, palpitations, insomnia, twitching
Rare
Blurred vision, rash, arthralgia

PRECAUTIONS AND CONTRAINDICATIONS

Diagnosis or family history of Tourette syndrome; glaucoma; history of marked agitation, anxiety, or tension; motor tics; use within 14 days of MAOIs
Caution:
Long-term effect on growth in children unknown, exacerbation of psychotic behavior, history of seizures, hypertension, heart failure, recent MI, hyperthyroidism, use in children younger than 6 yr not established, drug dependence, lactation

DRUG INTERACTIONS OF CONCERN TO DENTISTRY

• May inhibit metabolism of phenobarbital, tricyclic antidepressants, and SSRIs
• Increased effects of anticholinergics, CNS stimulants, tricyclic antidepressants, and sympathomimetics

SERIOUS REACTIONS

! Withdrawal after prolonged therapy may unmask symptoms of the underlying disorder.

! Dexmethylphenidate may lower the seizure threshold in those with a history of seizures.
! Overdose produces excessive sympathomimetic effects, including vomiting, tremor, hyperreflexia, seizures, confusion, hallucinations, and diaphoresis.
! Prolonged administration to children may delay growth.

DENTAL CONSIDERATIONS

General:
- Monitor vital signs at every appointment because of cardiovascular side effects.
- Assess salivary flow as a factor in caries, periodontal disease, and candidiasis.
- Patients on chronic drug therapy may rarely have symptoms of blood dyscrasias, which can include infection, bleeding, and poor healing.
- Use vasoconstrictor with caution, in low doses, and with careful aspiration.
- Determine why the patient is taking the drug.

Consultations:
- In a patient with symptoms of blood dyscrasias, request a medical consultation for blood studies and postpone treatment until normal values are reestablished.
- Medical consultation may be required to assess disease control.

Teach Patient/Family to:
- Encourage effective oral hygiene to prevent soft tissue inflammation, infection.
- Use caution to prevent injury when using oral hygiene aids.
- Update health and drug history if physician makes any changes in evaluation or drug regimens.
- When chronic dry mouth occurs, advise patient to:
  - Avoid mouth rinses with high alcohol content because of drying effects.
  - Use daily home fluoride products for anticaries effect.
  - Use sugarless gum, frequent sips of water, or saliva substitutes.

D

dextroamphetamine sulfate

dex-troe-am-**fet′**-ah-meen sull′-fate
(Dexamphetamine[AUS], Dexedrine, Dexedrine Spansule, DextroStat)
Do not confuse dextroamphetamine with dextromethorphan, or Dexedrine with Dextran or Excedrin.

CATEGORY AND SCHEDULE

Pregnancy Risk Category: C
Controlled Substance: Schedule II

Drug Class: Amphetamine

MECHANISM OF ACTION

An amphetamine that enhances the action of dopamine and norepinephrine by blocking their reuptake from synapses; also inhibits monoamine oxidase and facilitates the release of catecholamines.
Therapeutic Effect: Increases motor activity and mental alertness; decreases motor restlessness, drowsiness, and fatigue; suppresses appetite.

USES

Treatment of narcolepsy, attention-deficit/hyperactivity disorder (ADHD)

PHARMACOKINETICS

PO: Onset 30 min, peak 1–3 hr, duration 4–20 hr. ***Half-life:*** 10–30 hr; metabolized by liver; urine excretion pH dependent; crosses placenta, excreted in breast milk.

INDICATIONS AND DOSAGES

▸ **Narcolepsy**

PO

Adults, Children older than 12 yr. Initially, 10 mg/day. Increase by 10 mg/day at weekly intervals until therapeutic response is achieved.

Children 6–12 yr. Initially, 5 mg/day. Increase by 5 mg/day at weekly intervals until therapeutic response is achieved. Maximum: 60 mg/day.

▸ **ADHD**

PO

Children 6 yr and older. Initially, 5 mg once or twice a day. Increase by 5 mg/day at weekly intervals until therapeutic response is achieved.

Children 3–5 yr. Initially, 2.5 mg/ day. Increase by 2.5 mg/day at weekly intervals until therapeutic response is achieved. Maximum: 40 mg/day.

▸ **Appetite Suppressant**

PO

Adults. 5–30 mg daily in divided doses of 5–10 mg each, given 30–60 min before meals; or 1 extended-release capsule in the morning.

SIDE EFFECTS/ADVERSE REACTIONS

Frequent

Irregular pulse, increased motor activity, talkativeness, nervousness, mild euphoria, insomnia

Occasional

Headache, chills, dry mouth, GI distress, worsening depression in patients who are clinically depressed, tachycardia, palpitations, chest pain, dizziness, decreased appetite

PRECAUTIONS AND CONTRAINDICATIONS

Advanced arteriosclerosis, agitated states, glaucoma, history of drug abuse, hypersensitivity to sympathomimetic amines, hyperthyroidism, moderate to severe hypertension, symptomatic cardiovascular disease, use within 14 days of MAOIs

Caution:

Gilles de la Tourette's syndrome, lactation, children younger than 3 yr

DRUG INTERACTIONS OF CONCERN TO DENTISTRY

- Increased risk of serious side effects: meperidine, propoxyphene, tricyclic antidepressants

SERIOUS REACTIONS

! Overdose may produce skin pallor or flushing, arrhythmias, and psychosis.

! Abrupt withdrawal after prolonged use of high doses may produce lethargy lasting for weeks.

! Prolonged administration to children with ADHD may inhibit growth.

DENTAL CONSIDERATIONS

General:

- Monitor vital signs at every appointment because of cardiovascular side effects.
- Assess salivary flow as a factor in caries, periodontal disease, and candidiasis.
- Psychologic and physical dependence may occur with chronic administration.

Consultations:

- Medical consultation may be required to assess disease control.

Teach Patient/Family:

- When chronic dry mouth occurs, advise patient to:
  - Avoid mouth rinses with high alcohol content because of drying effects.
  - Use daily home fluoride products for anticaries effect.
  - Use sugarless gum, frequent sips of water, or saliva substitutes.

dextromethorphan

dex-troe-meth-**or**′-fan

(Babee Cof Syrup, Benylin Adult, Benylin Pediatric, Creomulsion Cough, Creomulsion for Children, Creo-Terpin, Delsym, DexAlone, ElixSure Cough, Hold DM, PediaCare Infants' Long-Acting Cough, [AUS], Robitussin CoughGels, Robitussin Honey Cough, Robitussin Maximum Strength Cough, Robitussin Pediatric Cough, Scot-Tussin DM Cough Chasers, Silphen DM, Simply Cough, Vicks 44 Cough Relief)

CATEGORY AND SCHEDULE

Pregnancy Risk Category: C
OTC

Drug Class: Antitussive, nonnarcotic

MECHANISM OF ACTION

A chemical relative of morphine without the opioid properties that acts on the cough center in the medulla oblongata by elevating the threshold for coughing.
Therapeutic Effect: Suppresses cough.

USES

Treatment of nonproductive cough

PHARMACOKINETICS

Rapidly absorbed from the GI tract. Distributed into CSF. Extensively and poorly metabolized in liver to dextrorphan (active metabolite). Excreted unchanged in urine.
Half-life: 1.4–3.9 hr (parent compound), 3.4–5.6 hr (dextrorphan).

INDICATIONS AND DOSAGES

▸ **Cough**

PO

Adults, Elderly, Children 12 yr and older. 10–20 mg q4h. Maximum: 120 mg/day.
Children 6–12 yr. 5–10 mg q4h. Maximum: 60 mg/day.
Children 2–5 yr. 2.5–5 mg q4h. Maximum: 30 mg/day.

SIDE EFFECTS/ADVERSE REACTIONS

Rare

Abdominal discomfort, constipation, dizziness, drowsiness, GI upset, nausea

PRECAUTIONS AND CONTRAINDICATIONS

Coadministration with MAOIs, hypersensitivity to dextromethorphan or its components

Caution:

Nausea, vomiting, increased temperature, persistent headache, drug abuse

DRUG INTERACTIONS OF CONCERN TO DENTISTRY

- Inhibition of metabolism: terbinafine

D

SERIOUS REACTIONS

! Overdosage may result in muscle spasticity, increase or decrease in B/P.

! Blurred vision, blue fingernails and lips, nausea, vomiting, hallucinations, and respiratory depression.

DENTAL CONSIDERATIONS

General:

• Consider semisupine chair position for patients with respiratory disease.

dextromethorphan + quinidine

deks-troe-meth-**or′**-fan & **kwin**-i-deen

(Nuedexta)

CATEGORY AND SCHEDULE

Pregnancy Risk Category: C

Drug Class: N-methyl-d-aspartate receptor antagonist

MECHANISM OF ACTION

Dextromethorphan may relieve the symptoms of pseudobulbar affect by binding to receptors in the brain that may be involved in behavior; however, the exact mechanism of action is not known. Quinidine is used to block the rapid metabolism of dextromethorphan, thereby increasing serum concentrations. ***Therapeutic Effect:*** Diminishes manifestations of psuedobulbar affect.

USES

Treatment of pseudobulbar affect (PBA)

PHARMACOKINETICS

Bioavailability of dextromethorphan is increased approximately 20-fold when administered with quinidine. Plasma protein binding: dextromethorphan: 60%–70%; quinidine: 80%–89%.

Hepatic metabolism: dextromethorphan via CYP2D6 to active metabolite (dextrorphan) and quinidine via CYP3A4 to active metabolite (3-hydroxyquinidine) and other metabolites. Excreted primarily in urine. ***Half-life:*** Dextromethorphan: 13 hr in extensive metabolizers. Quinidine: 7 hr in extensive metabolizers.

INDICATIONS AND DOSAGES

▸ **Pseudobulbar Affect (PBA)**

PO

Adults. 1 capsule once daily for 7 days, then increase to 1 capsule twice daily. May be administered with or without food. Administer twice-daily doses every 12 hr. Avoid grapefruit juice.

SIDE EFFECTS/ADVERSE REACTIONS

Frequent

Dizziness, diarrhea

Occasional

Peripheral edema, vomiting, flatulence, urinary tract infection, weakness, cough

PRECAUTIONS AND CONTRAINDICATIONS

Hypersensitivity to dextromethorphan, quinidine, quinine, mefloquine, or any component of the formulation. Avoid concomitant use with quinidine or other medications containing quinidine, quinine, or mefloquine. Avoid use in patients with history of quinine-, mefloquine-, or quinidine-induced thrombocytopenia; hepatitis;

bone marrow depression; or lupus-like syndrome. Avoid concurrent administration with, or use within 2 wk of discontinuing, an MAO inhibitor. Avoid use in patients with prolonged QT interval, congenital QT syndrome, or history of torsades de pointes. Avoid concurrent use with drugs that prolong the QT interval and are metabolized by CYP2D6 (pimozide, thioridazine). Avoid use in patients with complete AV block without an implanted pacemaker or patients at high risk of complete AV block. Avoid use in patients with severe hepatic and renal impairment.

DRUG INTERACTIONS OF CONCERN TO DENTISTRY

• Increased effect of CYP2D6 substrates (e.g., opioid analgesics)
• Increased effect of anticholinergic drugs (e.g., atropine)
• Contraindicated with azole antifungals

SERIOUS REACTIONS

! Possible cardiotoxic events, including complete AV block

DENTAL CONSIDERATIONS

General:

• Monitor for possible dizziness and take precautions when seating and dismissing patient from the operatory.
• Monitor vital signs at every appointment because of possible adverse cardiovascular effects.
• Avoid in patients taking MAOIs or selective serotonin reuptake inhibitors (SSRIs).
• Possible increased tendency for vomiting (e.g., during sedation).

Teach Patient/Family to:

• Report changes in disease status and drug regimen.

diazepam

dye-**az**′-eh-pam
(Antenex[AUS], Apo-Diazepam[CAN], Diastat, Diazemuls[CAN], Dizac, Ducene[AUS], Valium, Valpam[AUS], Vivol[CAN])
Do not confuse diazepam with diazoxide or Ditropan, or Valium with Valcyte.

CATEGORY AND SCHEDULE

Pregnancy Risk Category: D
Controlled Substance: Schedule IV

Drug Class: Benzodiazepine, anxiolytic

MECHANISM OF ACTION

A benzodiazepine that depresses all levels of the CNS by enhancing the action of gamma-aminobutyric acid, a major inhibitory neurotransmitter in the brain.

Therapeutic Effect: Produces anxiolytic effect, elevates the seizure threshold, produces skeletal muscle relaxation.

USES

Anxiety, acute alcohol withdrawal, adjunct in seizure disorders, skeletal muscle spasm; conscious sedation in dentistry

PHARMACOKINETICS

Route	Onset	Peak	Duration
PO	30 min	1–2 hr	2–3 hr
IV	1–5 min	15 min	15–60 min
IM	15 min	30–90 min	30–90 min

Well absorbed from the GI tract. Widely distributed. Protein binding: 98%. Metabolized in the liver to active metabolite. Excreted in urine.

Minimally removed by hemodialysis. ***Half-life:*** 20–70 hr (increased in hepatic dysfunction and the elderly).

D

INDICATIONS AND DOSAGES

▸ Anxiety, Skeletal Muscle Relaxation

PO

Adults. 2–10 mg 2–4 times a day.
Elderly. 2.5 mg twice a day.
Children. 0.12–0.8 mg/kg/day in divided doses q6–8h.

IV, IM

Adults. 2–10 mg repeated in 3–4 hr.
Children. 0.04–0.3 mg/kg/dose q2–4h. Maximum: 0.5 mg/kg in an 8-hr period.

▸ Preanesthesia

IV

Adults, Elderly. 5–15 mg 5–10 min before procedure.
Children. 0.2–0.3 mg/kg. Maximum: 10 mg.

▸ Alcohol Withdrawal

PO

Adults, Elderly. 10 mg 3–4 times during first 24 hr, then reduced to 5–10 mg 3–4 times a day as needed.

IV, IM

Adults, Elderly. Initially, 10 mg, followed by 5–10 mg q3–4h.

▸ Status Epilepticus

IV

Adults, Elderly. 5–10 mg q10–15min up to 30 mg/8 hr.
Children 5 yr and older. 0.05–0.3 mg/kg/dose q15–30min. Maximum: 10 mg/dose.
Children 1 mo to younger than 5 yr. 0.05–0.3 mg/kg/dose q15–30min. Maximum: 5 mg/dose.

▸ Control of Increased Seizure Activity in Patients with Refractory Epilepsy Who Are on Stable Regimens of Anticonvulsants

Rectal Gel

Adults, Children 12 yr and older. 0.2 mg/kg; may be repeated in 4–12 hr.
Children 6–11 yr. 0.3 mg/kg; may be repeated in 4–12 hr.
Children 2–5 yr. 0.5 mg/kg; may be repeated in 4–12 hr.

SIDE EFFECTS/ADVERSE REACTIONS

Frequent

Pain with IM injection, somnolence, fatigue, ataxia

Occasional

Slurred speech, orthostatic hypotension, headache, hypoactivity, constipation, nausea, blurred vision

Rare

Paradoxical CNS reactions, such as hyperactivity or nervousness in children and excitement or restlessness in the elderly or debilitated (generally noted during first 2 wk of therapy, particularly in presence of uncontrolled pain)

PRECAUTIONS AND CONTRAINDICATIONS

Angle-closure glaucoma, coma, preexisting CNS depression, respiratory depression, severe, uncontrolled pain

Caution:

Elderly, debilitated, hepatic disease, renal disease

DRUG INTERACTIONS OF CONCERN TO DENTISTRY

- Increased CNS depression of diazepam: alcohol, all CNS depressants, kava kava (herb), opioids
- Increased serum levels and prolonged effect of benzodiazepines: erythromycin, clarithromycin, ketoconazole, itraconazole, fluconazole, miconazole (systemic), cimetidine, rifamycin
- Contraindicated with saquinavir
- Possible increase in CNS side effects: kava kava (herb)

SERIOUS REACTIONS

! IV administration may produce pain, swelling, thrombophlebitis, and carpal tunnel syndrome.
! Abrupt or too-rapid withdrawal may result in pronounced restlessness, irritability, insomnia, hand tremor, abdominal or muscle cramps, diaphoresis, vomiting, and seizures.
! Abrupt withdrawal in patients with epilepsy may produce an increase in the frequency or severity of seizures.
! Overdose results in somnolence, confusion, diminished reflexes, and coma.

DENTAL CONSIDERATIONS

General:

- Assess salivary flow as a factor in caries, periodontal disease, and candidiasis.
- After supine positioning, have patient sit upright for at least 2 min before standing to avoid orthostatic hypotension.
- Psychologic and physical dependence may occur with chronic administration.
- Geriatric patients are more susceptible to drug effects; use lower dose.
- Have someone drive patient to and from dental appointment when drug used for conscious sedation.
- Provide assistance when escorting patient to and from dental chair when dizziness occurs.
- Avoid use of this drug in a patient with a history of drug abuse or alcoholism.

Teach Patient/Family to:

- Encourage effective oral hygiene to prevent soft tissue inflammation.
- When chronic dry mouth occurs, advise patient to:
  - Avoid mouth rinses with high alcohol content because of drying effects.
  - Use daily home fluoride products for anticaries effect.
  - Use sugarless gum, frequent sips of water, or saliva substitutes.

D

diclofenac

dye-**kloe′**-fen-ak
(Cataflam, Diclohexal[AUS], Diclotek[CAN], Fenac[AUS], Novo-Difenac[CAN], Solaraze, Voltaren, Voltaren Emulgel[AUS], Voltaren Ophthalmic, Voltaren Rapid[AUS], Voltaren XR)
Do not confuse diclofenac with Diflucan or Duphalac, or Voltaren with Verelan.

CATEGORY AND SCHEDULE

Pregnancy Risk Category: X

Drug Class: Nonsteroidal antiinflammatory

MECHANISM OF ACTION

An NSAID that inhibits prostaglandin synthesis, reducing the intensity of pain. Also constricts the iris sphincter. May inhibit angiogenesis (the formation of blood vessels) by inhibiting substance P or blocking the angiogenic effects of prostaglandin E.
Therapeutic Effect: Produces analgesic and antiinflammatory effects. Prevents miosis during cataract surgery. May reduce angiogenesis in inflamed tissue.

USES

Treatment of acute, chronic rheumatoid arthritis, osteoarthritis, ankylosing spondylitis, analgesia

PHARMACOKINETICS

Route	Onset	Peak	Duration
PO	30 min	2–3 hr	Up to 8 hr

Completely absorbed from the GI tract; penetrates cornea after ophthalmic administration (may be systemically absorbed). Protein binding: greater than 99%. Widely distributed. Metabolized in the liver. Primarily excreted in urine. Minimally removed by hemodialysis. ***Half-life:*** 1.2–2 hr.

INDICATIONS AND DOSAGES

▸ **Osteoarthritis**

PO (Cataflam, Voltaren)

Adults, Elderly. 50 mg 2–3 times a day.

PO (Voltaren XR)

Adults, Elderly. 100 mg/day as a single dose.

▸ **Rheumatoid Arthritis**

PO (Cataflam, Voltaren)

Adults, Elderly. 50 mg 2–4 times a day. Maximum: 225 mg/day.

PO (Voltaren XR)

Adults, Elderly. 100 mg once a day. Maximum: 100 mg twice a day.

▸ **Ankylosing Spondylitis**

PO (Voltaren)

Adults, Elderly. 100–125 mg/day in 4–5 divided doses.

▸ **Analgesia, Primary Dysmenorrhea**

PO (Cataflam)

Adults, Elderly. 30 mg 3 times a day.

▸ **Usual Pediatric Dosage**

Children. 2–3 mg/kg/day in 2–4 divided doses.

▸ **Actinic Keratoses**

Topical

Adults, Adolescents. Apply twice a day to lesion for 60–90 days.

▸ **Cataract Surgery**

Ophthalmic

Adults, Elderly. Apply 1 drop to eye 4 times a day commencing 24 hr after cataract surgery. Continue for 2 wk afterward.

▸ **Pain, Relief of Photophobia in Patients Undergoing Corneal Refractive Surgery**

Ophthalmic

Adults, Elderly. Apply 1 drop to affected eye 1 hr before surgery, within 15 min after surgery, then 4 times a day for 3 days.

SIDE EFFECTS/ADVERSE REACTIONS

Frequent

PO: Headache, abdominal cramps, constipation, diarrhea, nausea, dyspepsia

Ophthalmic: Burning or stinging on instillation, ocular discomfort

Occasional

PO: Flatulence, dizziness, epigastric pain

Ophthalmic: Ocular itching or tearing

Rare

PO: Rash, peripheral edema or fluid retention, visual disturbances, vomiting, drowsiness

PRECAUTIONS AND CONTRAINDICATIONS

Hypersensitivity to aspirin, diclofenac, and other NSAIDs; porphyria

Caution:

Lactation, children, bleeding disorders, GI disorders, cardiac disorders, hypersensitivity to other antiinflammatory agents

DRUG INTERACTIONS OF CONCERN TO DENTISTRY

- Use with caution in patients with cardiovascular disease at risk of thromboembolism
- GI ulceration, bleeding: aspirin, alcohol, corticosteroids, potassium supplements
- Nephrotoxicity: acetaminophen (prolonged use)
- Possible risk of decreased renal function: cyclosporine

- When prescribed for dental pain:
- Risk of increased effects: oral anticoagulants, oral antidiabetics, lithium, methotrexate
- Decreased antihypertensive effects of diuretics, β-adrenergic blockers, and ACE inhibitors
- First-time users of SSRIs also taking NSAIDs may have a higher risk of GI side effects; until more data are available, it may be advisable to avoid use of NSAIDs in these patients (*Br J Clin Pharmacol* 55:591–595, 2003)

Diclofenac Sodium (Voltaren)

- None reported

SERIOUS REACTIONS

! Overdose may result in acute renal failure.

! Rare reactions with long-term use include peptic ulcer disease, GI bleeding, gastritis, a severe hepatic reaction (jaundice), nephrotoxicity (hematuria, dysuria, proteinuria), and a severe hypersensitivity reaction (bronchospasm or angioedema).

DENTAL CONSIDERATIONS

General:

- Patients on chronic drug therapy may rarely have symptoms of blood dyscrasias, which can include infection, bleeding, and poor healing.
- Assess salivary flow as a factor in caries, periodontal disease, and candidiasis.
- Avoid prescribing for dental use in pregnancy.
- Avoid prescribing aspirin-containing products.
- Consider semisupine chair position for patients with rheumatic disease.
- Increased risk of thromboembolism in patients with history of stroke or MI.
- Advise patient if dental drugs prescribed have a potential for photosensitivity.
- Severe stomach bleeding may occur in patients who regularly use NSAIDs in recommended doses, when the patient is also taking another NSAID, a blood thinning, or steroid drug, if the patient has GI or peptic ulcer disease, if they are 60 years or older, or when NSAIDs are taken longer than directed. Warn patients of the potential for severe stomach bleeding.
- Warn patient of potential risks of NSAIDs.

Consultations:

- In a patient with symptoms of blood dyscrasias, request a medical consultation for blood studies and postpone dental treatment until normal values are reestablished.
- Medical consultation may be required to assess disease control.

Teach Patient/Family to:

- Encourage effective oral hygiene to prevent soft tissue inflammation.
- Use caution to prevent injury when using oral hygiene aids.
- When chronic dry mouth occurs, advise patient to:
  - Avoid mouth rinses with high alcohol content because of drying effects.
  - Use daily home fluoride products for anticaries effect.
  - Use sugarless gum, frequent sips of water, or saliva substitutes.

Diclofenac Sodium (Voltaren)

General:

- Determine why patient is taking the drug.
- Protect patient's eyes from accidental spatter during dental treatment.
- Avoid dental light in patient's eyes; offer dark glasses for patient comfort.

D

dicloxacillin sodium

dye-**klox**′-ah-sill-in **soe**′-dee-um
(Dycil, Pathocil)

CATEGORY AND SCHEDULE

Pregnancy Risk Category: B

Drug Class: Penicillinase-resistant penicillin

MECHANISM OF ACTION

A penicillin that acts as a bactericidal in susceptible microorganisms.
Therapeutic Effect: Inhibits bacterial cell wall synthesis.

USES

Treatment of infections caused by penicillinase-producing *Staphylococcus*

PHARMACOKINETICS

Well absorbed from GI tract. Rate and extent reduced by food. Distributed throughout body including CSF. Protein binding: 96%. Partially metabolized in liver. Primarily excreted in feces and urine. Not removed by hemodialysis. ***Half-life:*** 0.7 hr.

INDICATIONS AND DOSAGE

▸ **Respiratory Tract Infection, Staphylococcal and Streptococcal Infections**

PO

Adults, Elderly, Children weighing more than 40 kg. 125–250 mg q6h.
Children weighing less than 40 kg. 12.5–25 mg/kg/day q6h.

SIDE EFFECTS/ADVERSE REACTIONS

Frequent

GI disturbances (mild diarrhea, nausea, or vomiting), headache

Occasional

Generalized rash, urticaria

PRECAUTIONS AND CONTRAINDICATIONS

Hypersensitivity to any penicillin
Caution:
Hypersensitivity to cephalosporins

DRUG INTERACTIONS OF CONCERN TO DENTISTRY

• Tetracyclines: reduced effectiveness of dicloxacillin

SERIOUS REACTIONS

! Altered bacterial balance may result in potentially fatal superinfections and antibiotic-associated colitis as evidenced by abdominal cramps, watery or severe diarrhea, and fever.
! Severe hypersensitivity reactions, including anaphylaxis and acute interstitial nephritis, occur rarely.

DENTAL CONSIDERATIONS

General:
• Take precautions regarding allergy to medication.
• Determine why the patient is taking the drug.
Consultations:
• Concern for drug of choice if dental infection is also present.
Teach Patient/Family to:
• Encourage effective oral hygiene to prevent soft tissue inflammation.
• Use caution to prevent trauma when using oral hygiene aids.
• When used for dental infection, advise patient to:
  • Report sore throat, oral burning sensation, fever, and fatigue, any of which could indicate superinfection.
  • Take at prescribed intervals and complete dosage regimen.

• Immediately notify the dentist if signs or symptoms of infection increase.

dicyclomine hydrochloride

dye-**sye′**-kloe-meen
hye-droe-**klor′**-ide
(Bentyl, Bentylol[CAN], Formulex[CAN], Lomine[CAN], Merbentyl[AUS])
Do not confuse dicyclomine with doxycycline or dyclonime, or Bentyl with Aventyl or Benadryl.

CATEGORY AND SCHEDULE

Pregnancy Risk Category: B

Drug Class: GI anticholinergic

MECHANISM OF ACTION

A GI antispasmodic and anticholinergic agent that directly acts as a relaxant on smooth muscle. ***Therapeutic Effect:*** Reduces tone and motility of GI tract.

USES

Treatment of irritable bowel syndrome

PHARMACOKINETICS

Route	Onset	Peak	Duration
PO	1–2 hr	N/A	4 hr

Readily absorbed from the GI tract. Widely distributed. Metabolized in the liver. ***Half-life:*** 9–10 hr.

INDICATIONS AND DOSAGES

▸ Functional Disturbances of GI Motility

PO

Adults. 10–20 mg 3–4 times a day up to 40 mg 4 times a day.
Children older than 2 yr. 10 mg 3–4 times a day.
Children 6 mo–2 yr. 5 mg 3–4 times a day.
Elderly. 10–20 mg 4 times a day. May increase up to 160 mg/day.

IM

20 mg q4–6h.

SIDE EFFECTS/ADVERSE REACTIONS

Frequent

Dry mouth (sometimes severe), constipation, diminished sweating ability

Occasional

Blurred vision; photophobia; urinary hesitancy; somnolence (with high dosage); agitation, excitement, confusion, or somnolence noted in elderly (even with low dosages); transient light-headedness (with IM route), irritation at injection site (with IM route)

Rare

Confusion, hypersensitivity reaction, increased intraocular pressure, nausea, vomiting, unusual fatigue

PRECAUTIONS AND CONTRAINDICATIONS

Bladder neck obstruction because of prostatic hyperplasia, coronary vasospasm, intestinal atony, myasthenia gravis in patients not treated with neostigmine, narrow-angle glaucoma, obstructive disease of the GI tract, paralytic ileus, severe ulcerative colitis, tachycardia secondary to cardiac insufficiency or thyrotoxicosis, toxic megacolon, unstable cardiovascular status in acute hemorrhage

Caution:

Hyperthyroidism, CAD, dysrhythmias, CHF, ulcerative colitis, hypertension, hiatal hernia, hepatic disease, renal disease, urinary retention, prostatic hypertrophy

D

DRUG INTERACTIONS OF CONCERN TO DENTISTRY

- Increased anticholinergic effect: atropine, scopolamine, other anticholinergics, meperidine
- Decreased effect of ketoconazole

SERIOUS REACTIONS

! Overdose may produce temporary paralysis of ciliary muscle; pupillary dilation; tachycardia; palpitations; hot, dry, or flushed skin; absence of bowel sounds; hyperthermia; increased respiratory rate; ECG abnormalities; nausea; vomiting; rash over face or upper trunk; CNS stimulation; and psychosis (marked by agitation, restlessness, rambling speech, visual hallucinations, paranoid behavior, and delusions, followed by depression).

DENTAL CONSIDERATIONS

General:

- Assess salivary flow as a factor in caries, periodontal disease, and candidiasis.
- Avoid dental light in patient's eyes; offer dark glasses for patient comfort.

Consultation:

- Physician should be informed if significant xerostomic side effects occur (e.g., increased caries, sore tongue, problems eating or swallowing, difficulty wearing prosthesis) so that a medication change can be considered.

Teach Patient/Family to:

- Encourage effective oral hygiene to prevent soft tissue inflammation.
- When chronic dry mouth occurs, advise patient to:
  - Avoid mouth rinses with high alcohol content because of drying effects.
  - Use daily home fluoride products for anticaries effect.
  - Use sugarless gum, frequent sips of water, or saliva substitutes.

didanosine

dye-**dan**′-oh-seen
(Videx, Videx-EC)

CATEGORY AND SCHEDULE

Pregnancy Risk Category: B

Drug Class: Synthetic antiviral, nucleoside analogue

MECHANISM OF ACTION

A purine nucleoside analogue that is intracellularly converted into a triphosphate, which interferes with RNA-directed DNA polymerase (reverse transcriptase).
Therapeutic Effect: Inhibits replication of retroviruses, including HIV.

USES

Treatment of advanced HIV infections in adults and children who have been unable to use zidovudine or who have not responded to treatment; used in combination with other antiretroviral drugs.

PHARMACOKINETICS

Variably absorbed from the GI tract. Protein binding: less than 5%. Rapidly metabolized intracellularly to active form. Primarily excreted in urine. Partially (20%) removed by hemodialysis. ***Half-life:*** 1.5 hr; metabolite: 8–24 hr.

INDICATIONS AND DOSAGES

▸ **HIV Infection (in combination with other antiretrovirals)**

PO (Chewable Tablets)

Adults, Children 13 yr and older weighing 60 kg or more. 200 mg q12h or 400 mg once a day.
Adults, Children 13 yr and older weighing 60 kg or less. 125 mg q12h or 250 mg once a day.
Children 3 mo to less than 13 yr. 180–300 mg/m^2/day in divided doses q12h.
Children younger than 3 mo. 50 mg/m^2/day in divided doses q12h.
PO (Delayed-Release Capsules)
Adults, Children 13 yr and older, weighing 60 kg or more. 400 mg once a day.
Adults, Children 13 yr and older, weighing 60 kg or less. 250 mg once a day.
PO (Oral Solution)
Adults, Children 13 yr and older weighing 60 kg or more. 250 mg q12h.
Adults, Children 13 yr and older weighing 60 kg or less. 167 mg q12h.
PO (Pediatric Powder for Oral Solution)
Children 3 mo to younger than 13 yr. 180–300 mg/m^2/day in divided doses q12h.
Children younger than 3 mo. 50 mg/m^2/day in divided doses q12h.

▸ **Dosage in Renal Impairment**

CrCl	Tablets	Oral Solution	Delayed Release Capsules
30–59 ml/min	75 mg twice a day	100 mg twice a day	125 mg once a day
10–29 ml/min	100 mg once a day	100 mg once a day	125 mg once a day
Less than 10 ml/min	75 mg once a day	100 mg once a day	N/A

*CrCl = creatinine clearance

Patients weighing 60 kg or more:

CrCl	Tablets	Oral Solution	Delayed Release Capsules
30–59 ml/min	100 mg twice a day	10 mg twice a day	200 mg once a day
10–29 ml/min	150 mg once a day	167 mg once a day	125 mg once a day
Less than 10 ml/min	100 mg once a day	100 mg once a day	125 mg once a day

*CrCl = creatinine clearance

SIDE EFFECTS/ADVERSE REACTIONS

Frequent

Adults: Diarrhea, neuropathy, chills and fever
Children: Chills, fever, decreased appetite, pain, malaise, nausea, vomiting, diarrhea, abdominal pain, headache, nervousness, cough, rhinitis, dyspnea, asthenia, rash, pruritus

Occasional

Adults: Rash, pruritus, headache, abdominal pain, nausea, vomiting, pneumonia, myopathy, decreased appetite, dry mouth, dyspnea
Children: Failure to thrive, weight loss, stomatitis, oral thrush, ecchymosis, arthritis, myalgia, insomnia, epistaxis, pharyngitis

PRECAUTIONS AND CONTRAINDICATIONS

Hypersensitivity to didanosine or any of its components

Caution:

Renal disease, hepatic disease, lactation, children, sodium-restricted diets; pancreatitis (in combination with stavudine); lactic acidosis, severe hepatomegaly

D

DRUG INTERACTIONS OF CONCERN TO DENTISTRY

- Decreased absorption of the following drugs: ketoconazole, dapsone, itraconazole, tetracyclines, fluoroquinolone antibiotics
- Increased risk of pancreatitis: metronidazole, sulfonamides, sulindac, tetracyclines
- Increased risk of peripheral neuropathy: metronidazole, nitrous oxide

SERIOUS REACTIONS

! Pneumonia and opportunistic infections occur occasionally.
! Peripheral neuropathy, potentially fatal pancreatitis, retinal changes, and optic neuritis are the major toxic effects.

DENTAL CONSIDERATIONS

General:

- Monitor vital signs at every appointment because of cardiovascular side effects.
- Avoid dental light in patient's eyes; offer dark glasses for patient comfort.
- Patients on chronic drug therapy may rarely have symptoms of blood dyscrasias, which can include infection, bleeding, and poor healing.

Consultations:

- Medical consultation may be required to assess patient's ability to tolerate stress.
- In a patient with symptoms of blood dyscrasias, request a medical consultation for blood studies and postpone dental treatment until normal values are reestablished.

Teach Patient/Family to:

- Encourage effective oral hygiene to prevent soft tissue inflammation.
- Use caution to prevent injury when using oral hygiene aids.
- When chronic dry mouth occurs, advise patient to:
  - Avoid mouth rinses with high alcohol content because of drying effects.
  - Use daily home fluoride products for anticaries effect.
  - Use sugarless gum, frequent sips of water, or saliva substitutes.

diethylpropion

die-ethyl-**prop′**-ion
(Tenuate, Tenuate Dospan)

CATEGORY AND SCHEDULE

Pregnancy Risk Category: B
Controlled Substance: Schedule IV

Drug Class: Anorexiant, amphetamine-like

MECHANISM OF ACTION

A sympathomimetic amine that stimulates the release of norepinephrine and dopamine.
Therapeutic Effect: Decreases appetite.

USES

Treatment of exogenous obesity

PHARMACOKINETICS

Rapidly absorbed from the GI tract. Widely distributed. Metabolized in liver to active metabolite and undergoes extensive first-pass metabolism. Excreted in urine. Unknown if removed by hemodialysis. ***Half-life:*** 4–6 hr.

INDICATIONS AND DOSAGES

▸ **Obesity**

PO

Adults. 25 mg 3 times a day before meals. Extended-release: 75 mg at midmorning.

SIDE EFFECTS/ADVERSE REACTIONS

Frequent
Elevated B/P, nervousness, insomnia
Occasional
Dizziness, drowsiness, tremors, headache, nausea, stomach pain, fever, rash
Rare
Agranulocytosis, leukopenia, blurred vision, psychosis, CVA, seizure

PRECAUTIONS AND CONTRAINDICATIONS

Agitated states, use of MAOIs within 14 days, glaucoma, history of drug abuse, hyperthyroidism, advanced arteriosclerosis or severe cardiovascular disease, severe hypertension, and hypersensitivity to sympathomimetic amines
Caution:
Convulsive disorders, lactation

DRUG INTERACTIONS OF CONCERN TO DENTISTRY

- Dysrhythmia: hydrocarbon inhalation anesthetics
- Decreased effects: barbiturates, tricyclic antidepressants, phenothiazines

SERIOUS REACTIONS

! Overdose may produce agitation, tachycardia, palpitations, cardiac irregularities, chest pain, psychotic episode, seizures, and coma.
! Hypersensitivity reactions and blood dyscrasias occur rarely.

DENTAL CONSIDERATIONS

General:
- Monitor vital signs at every appointment because of cardiovascular and respiratory side effects.
- Examine for evidence of oral manifestations of blood dyscrasias (infection, bleeding, poor healing).
- Assess salivary flow as a factor in caries, periodontal disease, and candidiasis.
- Psychologic and physical dependence may occur with chronic administration.
- Consider semisupine chair position for patient comfort because of GI effects of disease.

Consultations:
- Medical consultation for blood studies (e.g., CBC); leukopenic or thrombocytopenic side effects may result in infection, delayed healing, and excessive bleeding. Postpone dental treatment until normal values are maintained.

Teach Patient/Family to:
- Encourage effective oral hygiene to prevent soft tissue inflammation.
- Use caution in use of oral hygiene aids to prevent injury.
- When chronic dry mouth occurs, advise patient to:
  - Avoid mouth rinses with high alcohol content because of drying effects.
  - Use daily home fluoride products for anticaries effect.
  - Use sugarless gum, frequent sips of water, or saliva substitutes.

diflorasone

die-**floor′**-ah-sone
(Florone[CAN], Maxiflor, Psorcon, Psorcon-e)

CATEGORY AND SCHEDULE

Pregnancy Risk Category: C

Drug Class: Topical corticosteroid, group II high potency

D

MECHANISM OF ACTION

A high-potency, fluorinated corticosteroid that decreases inflammation by suppression of migration of polymorphonuclear leukocytes and reversal of increased capillary permeability. The exact mechanism of the antiinflammatory process is unclear.
Therapeutic Effect: Decreases or prevents tissue response to the inflammatory process.

USES

Treatment of psoriasis, eczema, contact dermatitis, pruritus

PHARMACOKINETICS

Poor absorption; occlusive dressings increase absorption. Metabolized in liver. Primarily excreted in urine.

INDICATIONS AND DOSAGES

▸ **Dermatoses**

Topical
Adults, Elderly. (Cream) Apply sparingly 2–4 times a day. (Ointment) Apply sparingly 1–3 times a day.

SIDE EFFECTS/ADVERSE REACTIONS

Rare
Itching, redness, dryness, irritation, burning at site of application, arthralgia, folliculitis, maceration, muscle atrophy, secondary infection

PRECAUTIONS AND CONTRAINDICATIONS

History of hypersensitivity to diflorasone or other corticosteroids
Caution:
Lactation, viral infections, bacterial infections

SERIOUS REACTIONS

! Overdosage symptoms include moon face, central obesity, hypertension, diabetes, hyperlipidemia, peptic ulcer, increased susceptibility to infection, electrolyte and fluid imbalance, psychosis, and hallucinations.
! The serious reactions of long-term therapy and the addition of occlusive dressings are reversible hypothalamic-pituitary-adrenal (HPA) axis suppression, manifestations of Cushing's syndrome, hyperglycemia, and glucosuria.

DENTAL CONSIDERATIONS

General:
• Determine why the patient is taking the drug.
• Apply lubricant to dry lips for patient comfort before dental procedures.
• Place on frequent recall to evaluate healing response if used on chronic basis.

diflunisal

die-**floo**′-ni-sal
(Apo-Diflunisal[CAN], Dolobid, Novo-Diflunisal[CAN])
Do not confuse diflunisal with Dicarbosil or Dolobid with Slo-bid.

CATEGORY AND SCHEDULE

Pregnancy Risk Category: C

Drug Class: Salicylate derivative, nonsteroidal antiinflammatory

MECHANISM OF ACTION

A nonsteroidal antiinflammatory drug that inhibits prostaglandin synthesis, reducing inflammatory response and intensity of pain stimulus reaching sensory nerve endings.

Therapeutic Effect: Produces analgesic and antiinflammatory effect.

USES

Treatment of mild-to-moderate pain, symptoms of rheumatoid arthritis and osteoarthritis

PHARMACOKINETICS

Route	Onset	Peak	Duration
PO	1 hr	2–3 hr	8–12 hr

Completely absorbed from the GI tract. Widely distributed. Protein binding: greater than 99%. Metabolized in liver. Primarily excreted in urine. Not removed by hemodialysis. ***Half-life:*** 8–12 hr.

INDICATIONS AND DOSAGES

▸ Mild-to-Moderate Pain

PO

Adults, Elderly. Initially, 0.5–1 g, then 250–500 mg q8–12h. Maximum: 1.5 g/day.

▸ Rheumatoid Arthritis, Osteoarthritis

PO

Adults, Elderly. 0.5–1 g/day in 2 divided doses. Maximum: 1.5 g/day.

SIDE EFFECTS/ADVERSE REACTIONS

Side effects are less common with short-term treatment.

Occasional

Nausea, dyspepsia (heartburn, indigestion, epigastric pain), diarrhea, headache, rash

Rare

Vomiting, constipation, flatulence, dizziness, somnolence, insomnia, fatigue, tinnitus

PRECAUTIONS AND CONTRAINDICATIONS

Active GI bleeding, factor VII or factor IX deficiencies, hypersensitivity to aspirin or NSAIDs

Caution:

Anemia, hepatic disease, renal disease, Hodgkin's disease, lactation

DRUG INTERACTIONS OF CONCERN TO DENTISTRY

- Increased risk of GI ulceration and bleeding: aspirin, steroids, alcohol, indomethacin, other NSAIDs
- Hepatotoxicity, nephrotoxicity: acetaminophen (prolonged use)
- Suspected increase in potential toxic effects: probenecid

SERIOUS REACTIONS

! Overdosage may produce drowsiness, vomiting, nausea, diarrhea, hyperventilation, tachycardia, diaphoresis, stupor, and coma.

! Peptic ulcer, GI bleeding, gastritis, and severe hepatic reaction, including cholestasis, jaundice occur rarely.

! Nephrotoxicity, including dysuria, hematuria, proteinuria, and nephrotic syndrome, and severe hypersensitivity reaction, marked by bronchospasm and angioedema, occur rarely.

DENTAL CONSIDERATIONS

General:

- Patients on chronic drug therapy may rarely have symptoms of blood dyscrasias, which can include infection, bleeding, and poor healing.

• Assess salivary flow as a factor in caries, periodontal disease, and candidiasis.
• Avoid prescribing for dental use in first and last trimester of pregnancy.
• Use with caution in patients with cardiovascular disease at risk for thromboembolism.
• Severe stomach bleeding may occur in patients who regularly use NSAIDs in recommended doses, when the patient is also taking another NSAID, anticoagulant/antiplatelet, or steroid drug, if the patient has GI or peptic ulcer disease, if they are 60 years or older, or when NSAIDs are taken longer than directed. Warn patients of the potential for severe stomach bleeding.

Consultations:
• Medical consultation may be required to assess disease control.
• In a patient with symptoms of blood dyscrasias, request a medical consultation for blood studies and postpone dental treatment until normal values are reestablished.

Teach Patient/Family to:
• Encourage effective oral hygiene to prevent soft tissue inflammation.
• Prevent injury when using oral hygiene aids.
• Warn patient of potential risks of NSAIDs.
• When chronic dry mouth occurs, advise patient to:
  • Avoid mouth rinses with high alcohol content because of drying effects.
  • Use daily home fluoride products for anticaries effect.
  • Use sugarless gum, frequent sips of water, or saliva substitutes.

digoxin

di-**jox′**-in
(Digitek, Lanoxicaps, Lanoxin, Sigmaxin[AUS])
Do not confuse digoxin with Desoxyn or doxepin, or Lanoxin with Levsinex or Lonox.

CATEGORY AND SCHEDULE

Pregnancy Risk Category: C

Drug Class: Cardiac glycoside

MECHANISM OF ACTION

A cardiac glycoside that increases the influx of calcium from extracellular to intracellular cytoplasm.
Therapeutic Effect: Potentiates the activity of the contractile cardiac muscle fibers and increases the force of myocardial contraction. Slows the heart rate by decreasing conduction through the SA and AV nodes.

USES

Treatment of CHF, atrial fibrillation, atrial flutter, paroxysmal atrial tachycardia, rapid digitalization in these disorders

PHARMACOKINETICS

Route	Onset	Peak	Duration
PO	0.5–2 hr	28 hr	3–4 days
IV	5–30 hr	1–4 hr	3–4 days

Readily absorbed from the GI tract. Widely distributed. Protein binding: 30%. Partially metabolized in the liver. Primarily excreted in urine. Minimally removed by hemodialysis. ***Half-life:*** 36–48 hr (increased with impaired renal function and in the elderly).

INDICATIONS AND DOSAGES

▸ Rapid Loading Dose for the Management and Treatment of CHF; Control of Ventricular Rate in Patients with Atrial Fibrillation; Treatment and Prevention of Recurrent Paroxysmal Atrial Tachycardia

PO

Adults, Elderly. Initially, 0.5–0.75 mg, additional doses of 0.125–0.375 mg at 6- to 8-hr intervals. Range: 0.75–1.25 mg.
Children 10 yr and older. 10–15 mcg/kg.
Children 5–9 yr. 20–35 mcg/kg.
Children 2–4 yr. 30–40 mcg/kg.
Children 1–23 mo. 35–60 mcg/kg.
Neonate, full-term. 25–35 mcg/kg.
Neonate, premature. 20–30 mcg/kg.

IV

Adults, Elderly. 0.6–1 mg.
Children 10 yr and older. 8–12 mcg/kg.
Children 5–9 yr. 15–30 mcg/kg.
Children 2–4 yr. 25–35 mcg/kg.
Children 1–23 mo. 30–50 mcg/kg.
Neonates, full-term. 20–30 mcg/kg.
Neonates, premature. 15–25 mcg/kg.

▸ Maintenance Dosage for CHF; Control of Ventricular Rate in Patients with Atrial Fibrillation; Treatment and Prevention of Recurrent Paroxysmal Atrial Tachycardia

PO, IV

Adults, Elderly. 0.125–0.375 mg/day.
Children. 25%–35% loading dose (20%–30% for premature neonates).

▸ Dosage in Renal Impairment

Dosage adjustment is based on creatinine clearance. Total digitalizing dose: decrease by 50% in end-stage renal disease.

Creatinine Clearance	Dosage
10–50 ml/min	25%–75% usual
Less than 10 ml/min	10%–25% usual

SIDE EFFECTS/ADVERSE REACTIONS

There is a very narrow margin of safety between a therapeutic and toxic result, cardiac dysrhythmias, nausea, vomiting, visual scotomas.

PRECAUTIONS AND CONTRAINDICATIONS

! Ventricular fibrillation, ventricular tachycardia unrelated to CHF

Caution:

Renal disease, acute MI, AV block, severe respiratory disease, hypothyroidism, elderly, sinus nodal disease, lactation, hypokalemia

DRUG INTERACTIONS OF CONCERN TO DENTISTRY

- Hypokalemia: corticosteroids
- Increased digoxin blood levels: erythromycin, clarithromycin, tetracyclines, itraconazole, propantheline
- Cardiac dysrhythmias: adrenergic agonists, succinylcholine

SERIOUS REACTIONS

! The most common early manifestations of digoxin toxicity are GI disturbances (anorexia, nausea, vomiting) and neurologic abnormalities (fatigue, headache, depression, weakness, drowsiness, confusion, nightmares).

! Facial pain, personality change, and ocular disturbances (photophobia, light flashes, halos around bright objects, yellow or green color perception) may be noted.

DENTAL CONSIDERATIONS

General:

- Monitor vital signs at every appointment because of cardiovascular side effects.

• After supine positioning, have patient sit upright for at least 2 min to avoid orthostatic hypotension.
• Avoid dental light in patient's eyes; offer dark glasses for patient comfort.
• An increased gag reflex may make dental procedures, such as taking radiographs or impressions, difficult.
• Use vasoconstrictors with caution, in low doses, and with careful aspiration. Avoid use of gingival retraction cord with epinephrine.

Consultations:

• Stress from dental procedures may compromise cardiovascular function; determine patient risk.
• Use stress-reduction protocol.
• Medical consultation may be required to assess disease control and patient's ability to tolerate stress.

dihydrotachysterol

dye-hye-droe-tak-ee-**ster′**-ole
(DHT, DHT Intensol, Hytakerol)

CATEGORY AND SCHEDULE

Pregnancy Risk Category: A (D if used in doses above RDA)

Drug Class: Vitamin D analogue

MECHANISM OF ACTION

A fat-soluble vitamin that is essential for absorption, utilization of calcium phosphate, and normal calcification of bone.
Therapeutic Effect: Stimulates calcium and phosphate absorption from small intestine, promotes secretion of calcium from bone to blood, promotes renal tubule phosphate resorption, acts on bone cells to stimulate skeletal growth and on parathyroid gland to suppress hormone synthesis and secretion.

USES

Nutritional supplement, treatment of rickets, hypoparathyroidism, pseudo-hypoparathyroidism, postoperative tetany

PHARMACOKINETICS

Well absorbed from small intestine. Metabolized in liver. Eliminated via biliary system; excreted in urine. ***Half-life:*** Unknown.

INDICATIONS AND DOSAGES

▸ Hypoparathyroidism

PO

Adults, Elderly, Older Children. Initially, 0.8–2.4 mg/day for several days. Maintenance: 0.2–1 mg/day.
Infants, Young Children. Initially, 1–5 mg/day for 4 days, then 0.1–0.5 mg/day.

▸ Nutritional Rickets

PO

Adults, Elderly, Children. 0.5 mg as a single dose or 13–50 mcg/day until healing occurs.

▸ Renal Osteodystrophy

PO

Adults, Elderly. 0.25–0.6 mg/24 hr adjusted as needed to achieve normal serum calcium levels and promote bone healing.

SIDE EFFECTS/ADVERSE REACTIONS

Occasional

Nausea, vomiting

PRECAUTIONS AND CONTRAINDICATIONS

Hypercalcemia, malabsorption syndrome, vitamin D toxicity, hypersensitivity to vitamin D products or analogues

Caution:
Renal calculi, lactation, cardiovascular disease

DRUG INTERACTIONS OF CONCERN TO DENTISTRY

• Decreased effect of dihydrotachysterol: prolonged use of corticosteroids, barbiturates

SERIOUS REACTIONS

! Early signs of overdosage are manifested as weakness, headache, somnolence, nausea, vomiting, dry mouth, constipation, muscle and bone pain, and metallic taste sensation.
! Later signs of overdosage are evidenced by polyuria, polydipsia, anorexia, weight loss, nocturia, photophobia, rhinorrhea, pruritus, disorientation, hallucinations, hyperthermia, hypertension, and cardiac arrhythmias.

DENTAL CONSIDERATIONS

General:
• Consider semisupine chair position for patient comfort because of GI effects of drug.
• Assess salivary flow as a factor in caries, periodontal disease, and candidiasis.
Teach Patient/Family:
• When chronic dry mouth occurs, advise patient to:
  • Avoid mouth rinses with high alcohol content because of drying effects.
  • Use daily home fluoride products for anticaries effect.
  • Use sugarless gum, frequent sips of water, or saliva substitutes.

diltiazem hydrochloride

dil-**tye′**-ah-zem hi-droh-**klor′**-ide
(Apo-Diltiaz[CAN], Auscard[AUS], Cardcal[AUS], Cardizem, Cardizem CD, Cardizem LA, Cardizem SR, Cartia, Coras[AUS], Dilacor XR, Diltahexal[AUS], Diltia XT, Diltiamax[AUS], Dilzem[AUS], Novo-Diltiazem[CAN], Taztia XT, Tiazac, Vasocardal CD[AUS])
Do not confuse Cardizem with Cardene or Cardene SR, or Tiazac with Ziac.

CATEGORY AND SCHEDULE

Pregnancy Risk Category: C

Drug Class: Calcium channel blocker

MECHANISM OF ACTION

An antianginal, antihypertensive, and antiarrhythmic agent that inhibits calcium movement across cardiac and vascular smooth-muscle cell membranes. This action causes the dilation of coronary arteries, peripheral arteries, and arterioles.
Therapeutic Effect: Decreases heart rate and myocardial contractility, slows SA and AV conduction, and decreases total peripheral vascular resistance by vasodilation.

USES

Treatment of chronic stable angina pectoris, vasospastic angina, coronary artery spasm, hypertension, supraventricular tachydysrhythmias

PHARMACOKINETICS

Route	Onset	Peak	Duration
PO	0.5–1 hr	N/A	
PO (extended release)	2–3 hr	N/A	
IV	3 min	N/A	

Well absorbed from the GI tract. Protein binding: 70%–80%. Undergoes first-pass metabolism in the liver to active metabolite. Primarily excreted in urine. Not removed by hemodialysis. ***Half-life:*** 3–8 hr.

INDICATIONS AND DOSAGES

▸ Angina Related to Coronary Artery Spasm (Prinzmetal's Variant), Chronic Stable Angina (Effort-Associated)

PO

Adults, Elderly. Initially, 30 mg 4 times a day. Increase up to 180–360 mg/day in 3–4 divided doses at 1- to 2-day intervals.

PO (Cardizem LA)

Adults, Elderly. Initially, 180 mg/day. May increase at intervals of 7–14 days up to 360 mg/day.

PO (Cardizem CD)

Adults, Elderly. Initially, 120–180 mg/day; titrate over 7–14 days. Range: Up to 480 mg/day.

▸ Essential Hypertension

PO (Cardizem CD, Cartia XT)

Adults, Elderly. Initially, 180–240 mg once a day. May increase at 2-wk intervals. Maintenance 240–360 mg/day. Maximum: 480 mg once a day.

PO (Cardizem SR)

Adults, Elderly. Initially, 60–120 mg twice a day. May increase at 2-wk intervals. Maintenance: 240–360 mg/day.

PO (Cardizem LA)

Adults, Elderly. Initially, 180–240 mg once a day. May increase at 2-wk intervals. Maintenance: 120–540 mg/day.

PO (Dilacor XR)

Adults, Elderly. 180–240 mg once a day.

PO (Dilacor XT)

Adults, Elderly. Initially, 180–240 mg a day. May increase at 2-wk intervals. Maximum: 540 mg once a day.

PO (Taztia XT)

Adults, Elderly. Initially, 120–240 mg once a day. May increase at 2-wk intervals. Maximum: 540 mg once a day.

▸ Temporary Control of Rapid Ventricular Rate in Atrial Fibrillation or Flutter, Rapid Conversion of Paroxysmal Supraventricular Tachycardia to Normal Sinus Rhythm.

IV Push

Adults, Elderly. Initially, 0.25 mg/kg actual body weight over 2 min. May repeat in 15 min at dose of 0.35 mg/kg actual body weight. Subsequent doses individualized.

IV Infusion

Adults, Elderly. After initial bolus injection, may begin infusion at 5–10 mg/hr; may increase by 5 mg/hr up to a maximum of 15 mg/hr. Infusion duration should not exceed 24 hr.

SIDE EFFECTS/ADVERSE REACTIONS

Frequent

Peripheral edema, dizziness, light-headedness, headache, bradycardia, asthenia (loss of strength, weakness)

Occasional
Nausea, constipation, flushing, ECG changes
Rare
Rash, micturition disorder (polyuria, nocturia, dysuria, frequency of urination), abdominal discomfort, somnolence

PRECAUTIONS AND CONTRAINDICATIONS

Acute MI, pulmonary congestion, severe hypotension (less than 90 mm Hg, systolic), sick sinus syndrome, second- or third-degree AV block (except in the presence of a pacemaker)
Caution:
CHF, hypotension, hepatic injury, lactation, children, renal disease

DRUG INTERACTIONS OF CONCERN TO DENTISTRY

- Decreased effect: indomethacin, possibly other NSAIDs, phenobarbital
- Increased effect: parenteral and inhalational general anesthetics, other drugs with hypotensive actions
- Increased effects of carbamazepine, midazolam, triazolam, buspirone

SERIOUS REACTIONS

! Abrupt withdrawal may increase frequency or duration of angina.
! CHF and second- and third-degree AV block occur rarely.
! Overdose produces nausea, somnolence, confusion, slurred speech, and profound bradycardia.

DENTAL CONSIDERATIONS

General:
- Monitor cardiac status; take vital signs at each appointment because of cardiovascular side effects. Consider a stress-reduction protocol to prevent angina during the dental appointment.
- After supine positioning, have patient sit upright for at least 2 min to avoid orthostatic hypotension.
- Place on frequent recall to monitor possible gingival enlargement.
- Limit use of sodium-containing products, such as saline IV fluids, for patients with a dietary salt restriction.
- Assess salivary flow as a factor in caries, periodontal disease, and candidiasis.
- Consider drug in diagnosis of taste alterations.

Consultations:
- Medical consultation may be required to assess disease control.

Teach Patient/Family to:
- Encourage effective oral hygiene to prevent soft tissue inflammation and minimize gingival overgrowth.
- Schedule frequent oral prophylaxis if gingival overgrowth occurs.
- When chronic dry mouth occurs, advise patient to:
  - Avoid mouth rinses with high alcohol content because of drying effects.
  - Use daily home fluoride products for anticaries effect.
  - Use sugarless gum, frequent sips of water, or saliva substitutes.

D

dimenhydrinate

dye-men-**hye**′-dri-nate
(Dramamine)

CATEGORY AND SCHEDULE

Pregnancy Risk Category: B

Drug Class: H_1-receptor antagonist (equal parts diphenhydramine and chlorotheophylline)

MECHANISM OF ACTION

An antihistamine and anticholinergic that competes for H_1 receptor sites on effector cells of the GI tract, blood vessels, and respiratory tract. The anticholinergic action diminishes vestibular stimulation and depresses labyrinthine function.
Therapeutic Effect: Prevents symptoms of motion sickness.

USES

Treatment of motion sickness, nausea, vomiting, vertigo

PHARMACOKINETICS

IM/PO: Duration 4–6 hr.

INDICATIONS AND DOSAGES

▸ **Motion Sickness**

PO

Adults, Elderly, Children older than 12 yr. 50–100 mg q4–6h. Maximum: 400 mg/day.
Children 6–12 yr. 25–50 mg q6–8h. Maximum: 150 mg/day.
Children 2–5 yr. 12.5–25 mg q6–8h. Maximum: 75 mg/day.

SIDE EFFECTS/ADVERSE REACTIONS

Frequent

Dry mouth

Occasional

Hypotension, palpitations, tachycardia, headache, somnolence, dizziness, paradoxical stimulation (especially in children), anorexia, constipation, dysuria, blurred vision, tinnitus, wheezing, chest tightness

Rare

Photosensitivity, rash, urticaria

PRECAUTIONS AND CONTRAINDICATIONS

Hypersensitivity to narcotics, shock

Caution:

Children, cardiac dysrhythmias, elderly, asthma, prostatic hypertrophy, bladder neck obstruction, narrow-angle glaucoma, stenosing peptic ulcer, pyloroduodenal obstruction, may mask ototoxicity of ototoxic antibiotics

DRUG INTERACTIONS OF CONCERN TO DENTISTRY

- Increased photosensitization: tetracycline
- Increased effects of alcohol, other CNS depressants, anticholinergics

SERIOUS REACTIONS

! None significant

DENTAL CONSIDERATIONS

General:

- Assess salivary flow as a factor in caries, periodontal disease, and candidiasis.

Teach Patient/Family to:

- When chronic dry mouth occurs, advise patient to:
  - Avoid mouth rinses with high alcohol content because of drying effects.
  - Use daily home fluoride products for anticaries effect.
  - Use sugarless gum, frequent sips of water, or saliva substitutes.

diphenhydramine

dye-fen-**hye**′-dra-meen
(Allerdryl[CAN], Banophen, Benadryl, Diphen, Diphenhist, Genahist, Nytol[CAN], Unisom Sleepgels[AUS])
Do not confuse diphenhydramine with dimenhydrinate or Benadryl with benazepril, Bentyl, or Benylin, or Banophen with baclofen.

CATEGORY AND SCHEDULE

Pregnancy Risk Category: B
OTC (capsules, tablets, chewable tablets, syrup, elixir, cream, spray)

Drug Class: Antihistamine, H_1-receptor antagonist

MECHANISM OF ACTION

An ethanolamine that competitively blocks the effects of histamine at peripheral H_1 receptor sites.
Therapeutic Effect: Produces anticholinergic, antipruritic, antitussive, antiemetic, antidyskinetic, and sedative effects.

USES

Allergy symptoms, rhinitis, motion sickness, antiparkinsonism, nighttime sedation, infant colic, nonproductive cough; unlabeled use for dental local anesthesia

PHARMACOKINETICS

Route	Onset	Peak	Duration
PO	15–30 min	1–4 hr	4–6 hr
IV, IM	Less than 15 min	1–4 hr	4–6 hr

Well absorbed after PO or parenteral administration. Protein binding: 98%–99%. Widely distributed. Metabolized in the liver. Primarily excreted in urine. ***Half-life:*** 1–4 hr.

INDICATIONS AND DOSAGES

▸ **Moderate to Severe Allergic Reaction, Dystonic Reaction**
PO, IV, IM
Adults, Elderly. 25–50 mg q4h. Maximum: 400 mg/day.
Children. 5 mg/kg/day in divided doses q6–8h. Maximum: 300 mg/day.

▸ **Motion Sickness, Minor Allergic Rhinitis**
PO, IV, IM
Adults, Elderly, Children 12 yr and older. 25–50 mg q4–6h. Maximum: 300 mg/day.
Children 6–11 yr. 12.5–25 mg q4–6h. Maximum: 150 mg/day.
Children 2–5 yr. 6.25 mg q4–6h. Maximum: 37.5 mg/day.

▸ **Antitussive**
PO
Adults, Elderly, Children 12 yr and older. 25 mg q4h. Maximum: 150 mg/day.
Children 6–11 yr. 12.5 mg q4h. Maximum: 75 mg/day.
Children 2–5 yr. 6.25 mg q4h. Maximum: 37.5 mg/day.

▸ **Nighttime Sleep Aid**
PO
Adults, Elderly, Children 12 yr and older. 50 mg at bedtime.
Children 2–11 yr. 1 mg/kg/dose. Maximum: 50 mg.

▸ **Pruritus**
Topical
Adults, Elderly, Children 12 yr and older. Apply 1% or 2% cream or spray 3–4 times a day.
Children 2–11 yr. Apply 1% cream or spray 3–4 times a day.

SIDE EFFECTS/ADVERSE REACTIONS

Frequent
Somnolence, dizziness, muscle weakness, hypotension, urine

retention, thickening of bronchial secretions, dry mouth, nose, throat, or lips; in elderly, sedation, dizziness, hypotension
Occasional
Epigastric distress, flushing, visual or hearing disturbances, paresthesia, diaphoresis, chills

D

PRECAUTIONS AND CONTRAINDICATIONS

Acute exacerbation of asthma, use within 14 days of MAOIs
Caution:
Increased intraocular pressure, renal disease, cardiac disease, hypertension, bronchial asthma, seizure disorder, stenosed peptic ulcers, hyperthyroidism, prostatic hypertrophy, bladder neck obstruction

DRUG INTERACTIONS OF CONCERN TO DENTISTRY

- Increased CNS depression: all CNS depressants, alcohol
- Increased anticholinergic effect: anticholinergics
- Increased plasma levels of labetalol

SERIOUS REACTIONS

! Hypersensitivity reactions, such as eczema, pruritus, rash, cardiac disturbances, and photosensitivity, may occur.
! Overdose symptoms may vary from CNS depression, including sedation, apnea, hypotension, cardiovascular collapse, and death, to severe paradoxical reactions, such as hallucinations, tremors, and seizures.
! Children and neonates may experience paradoxical reactions, including restlessness, insomnia, euphoria, nervousness, and tremors.
! Overdosage in children may result in hallucinations, seizures, and death.

DENTAL CONSIDERATIONS

General:
- Patients on chronic drug therapy may rarely have symptoms of blood dyscrasias, which can include infection, bleeding, and poor healing.
- Assess salivary flow as a factor in caries, periodontal disease, and candidiasis.
- Consider semisupine chair position for patients with respiratory disease.

Consultations:
- In a patient with symptoms of blood dyscrasias, request a medical consultation for blood studies and postpone dental treatment until normal values are reestablished.

Teach Patient/Family to:
- Encourage effective oral hygiene to prevent soft tissue inflammation.
- Use caution to prevent injury when using oral hygiene aids.
- When chronic dry mouth occurs, advise patient to:
  - Avoid mouth rinses with high alcohol content because of drying effects.
  - Use daily home fluoride products for anticaries effect.
  - Use sugarless gum, frequent sips of water, or saliva substitutes.

dipivefrin hydrochloride

die-pih-vef′-rin hi-droh-**klor**′-ide
(Propine)

CATEGORY AND SCHEDULE

Pregnancy Risk Category: B

Drug Class: Adrenergic agonist

MECHANISM OF ACTION

A prodrug of epinephrine that penetrates into anterior chamber of

the eye through its lipophilic character.
Therapeutic Effect: Reduces intraocular pressure.

USES
Treatment of open-angle glaucoma

PHARMACOKINETICS
Onset of action occurs within 30 min and peak effect in 1 hr. Dipivefrin is more lipophilic than epinephrine. Distributed to cornea. Dipivefrin is converted to epinephrine inside the eye by enzyme hydrolysis.

INDICATIONS AND DOSAGES
▸ **Glaucoma, Open-Angle**
Ophthalmic, Topical
Adults, Elderly. Instill 1 drop of 0.1% solution in affected eye(s) q12h.

SIDE EFFECTS/ADVERSE REACTIONS
Occasional
Blurred vision, burning or stinging of eye, mydriasis, headache
Rare
Follicular conjunctivitis

PRECAUTIONS AND CONTRAINDICATIONS
Narrow-angle glaucoma, hypersensitivity to dipivefrin or any component of the formulation
Caution:
Lactation, children, aphakia

DRUG INTERACTIONS OF CONCERN TO DENTISTRY
• Avoid use of anticholinergics such as atropine, scopolamine, and propantheline; use benzodiazepines with caution.

SERIOUS REACTIONS
! Signs of systemic absorption include hypertension, arrhythmias, and tachycardia.
! Follicular conjunctivitis has been reported.

DENTAL CONSIDERATIONS
General:
• Avoid dental light in patient's eyes; offer dark glasses for patient comfort.

dipyridamole
die-peer-**id**′-ah-mole
(Apo-Dipyridamole[CAN], Novodipiradol[CAN], Persantin[AUS], Persantin 100[AUS], Persantin SR[AUS], Persantine)
Do not confuse Aggrenox with Aggrastat, or dipyridamole with disopyramide, or Persantin with Periactin.

CATEGORY AND SCHEDULE
Pregnancy Risk Category: C

Drug Class: Platelet aggregation inhibitor

MECHANISM OF ACTION
A blood modifier and platelet aggregation inhibitor that inhibits the activity of adenosine deaminase and phosphodiesterase, enzymes causing accumulation of adenosine and cyclic adenosine monophosphate.
Therapeutic Effect: Inhibits platelet aggregation; may cause coronary vasodilation.

USES
Adjunctive therapy with warfarin in prosthetic heart valve replacement

D

PHARMACOKINETICS

Slowly, variably absorbed from the GI tract. Widely distributed. Protein binding: 91%–99%. Metabolized in the liver. Primarily eliminated via biliary excretion. ***Half-life:*** 10–15 hr.

INDICATIONS AND DOSAGES

▸ Prevention of Thromboembolic Disorders

PO

Adults, Elderly. 75–400 mg/day in combination with other medications.
Children. 3–6 mg/kg/day in 3 divided doses.

▸ Diagnostic Aid

IV

Adults, Elderly (based on weight). 0.142 mg/kg/min infused over 4 min; although a maximum hasn't been determined, doses greater than 60 mg have been determined to be unnecessary for any patient.

SIDE EFFECTS/ADVERSE REACTIONS

Frequent

Dizziness

Occasional

Abdominal distress, headache, rash

Rare

Diarrhea, vomiting, flushing, pruritus

PRECAUTIONS AND CONTRAINDICATIONS

Hypersensitivity, hypotension

Caution:

Children younger than 12 yr

DRUG INTERACTIONS OF CONCERN TO DENTISTRY

• Additive antiplatelet effects: aspirin, other NSAIDs

SERIOUS REACTIONS

! Overdose produces peripheral vasodilation, resulting in hypotension.

DENTAL CONSIDERATIONS

General:

• Monitor vital signs at every appointment because of cardiovascular side effects.
• After supine positioning, have patient sit upright for at least 2 min to avoid orthostatic hypotension.
• Avoid prescribing NSAIDs and aspirin-containing products, even though ASA/dipyridamole combination drugs are used in some patients.
• Patients with prosthetic valves require antibiotic prophylaxis.
• Evaluate for clotting ability during gingival instrumentation because inhibition of platelet aggregation may occur.
• Do not discontinue dipyridamole.
• Consider local hemostatic measures to prevent excessive bleeding during instrumentation.

Consultations:

• Medical consultation should include PTT or INR.
• Medical consultation may be required to assess disease control.

Teach Patient/Family to:

• Encourage effective oral hygiene to prevent gingival inflammation.

dirithromycin

die-rith-ro-**my'**-sin
(Dynabac)
Do not confuse Dynabac with Dynacin or DynaCirc.

CATEGORY AND SCHEDULE

Pregnancy Risk Category: C

Drug Class: Macrolide antibiotic

MECHANISM OF ACTION

A macrolide that binds to ribosomal receptor sites of susceptible

organisms, inhibiting bacterial protein synthesis.
Therapeutic Effect: Bactericidal or bacteriostatic, depending on drug dosage.

USES

Treatment of acute and secondary bacterial infection of acute bronchitis, community-acquired pneumonia, streptococcal pharyngitis, and uncomplicated skin and skin-structure infections

PHARMACOKINETICS

Rapidly absorbed from the GI tract. Protein binding: 15%–30%. Widely distributed into tissues and within cells. Eliminated primarily unchanged by biliary excretion. Not removed by hemodialysis. ***Half-life:*** 30–44 hr.

INDICATIONS AND DOSAGES

▸ Pharyngitis, Tonsillitis
PO
Adults, Elderly, Children 12 yr and older. 500 mg once a day for 10 days.

▸ Acute or Chronic Bronchitis, Skin and Skin-Structure Infections
PO
Adults, Elderly, Children 12 yr and older. 500 mg once a day for 7 days.

▸ Community-Acquired Pneumonia
PO
Adults, Elderly, Children 12 yr and older. 500 mg once a day for 14 days.

SIDE EFFECTS/ADVERSE REACTIONS

Frequent
Abdominal pain, headache, nausea, diarrhea

Occasional
Vomiting, dyspepsia, dizziness, nonspecific pain, asthenia

Rare
Increased cough, flatulence, rash, dyspnea, pruritus and urticaria, insomnia

PRECAUTIONS AND CONTRAINDICATIONS

Hypersensitivity to dirithromycin or other macrolide antibiotics

Caution:
Not for *H. influenzae* or *S. pyogenes* infections, lactation, children younger than 12 yr

DRUG INTERACTIONS OF CONCERN TO DENTISTRY

• Other drug interactions: data are limited; antacids and histamine H_2 antagonists tend to enhance absorption; refer to erythromycin for potential interacting drugs.
• Other antibiotics: reduced effectiveness of dirithromycin.

SERIOUS REACTIONS

! Antibiotic-associated colitis and other superinfections may result from altered bacterial balance.

DENTAL CONSIDERATIONS

General:
• Do not use in patients at risk for bacteremias caused by inadequate serum levels.
• Potential value in dental infections is unknown.
• Determine why the patient is taking the drug.
• Examine for oral manifestations of opportunistic infections.

Consultations:
• Medical consultation may be required to assess disease control.

Teach Patient/Family to:
• Be aware of the possibility of secondary oral infection and the need to see dentist immediately if infection occurs.

D

disopyramide phosphate

die-soe-**peer**′-ah-mide
(Norpace, Norpace CR, Rythmodan[CAN])
Do not confuse disopyramide with desipramine, dipyridamole, or Rythmol.

CATEGORY AND SCHEDULE

Pregnancy Risk Category: C

Drug Class: Antidysrhythmic (class Ia)

MECHANISM OF ACTION

An antiarrhythmic that prolongs the refractory period of the cardiac cell by direct effect, decreasing myocardial excitability and conduction velocity.
Therapeutic Effect: Depresses myocardial contractility. Has anticholinergic and negative inotropic effects.

USES

Treatment of premature ventricular contractions (PVCs), ventricular tachycardia

PHARMACOKINETICS

PO: Peak 30 min–3 hr, duration 6–12 hr. ***Half-life:*** 4–10 hr; metabolized in liver; excreted in feces, urine, breast milk; crosses placenta.

INDICATIONS AND DOSAGES

▸ **Suppression and Prevention of Ventricular Ectopy, Unifocal or Multifocal Premature Ventricular Contractions, Paired Ventricular Contractions (Couplets), and Episodes of Ventricular Tachycardia**
PO
Adults, Elderly weighing 50 kg and more. 150 mg q6h (300 mg ql2h with extended-release).
Adults, Elderly weighing less than 50 kg. 100 mg q6h (200 mg q12h with extended-release).

▸ **Rapid Control of Arrhythmias**
PO
Adults, Elderly weighing 50 kg and more. Initially, 300 mg, then 150 mg q6h or 300 mg (controlled release) q12h.
Adults, Elderly weighing less than 50 kg. Initially, 200 mg, then 100 mg q6h or 200 mg (controlled release) q12h.

▸ **Severe Refractory Arrhythmias**
PO
Adults, Elderly. Up to 400 mg q6h.
Children 12–18 yr. 6–15 mg/kg/day in divided doses q6h.
Children 5–11 yr. 10–15 mg/kg/day in divided doses q6h.
Children 1–4 yr. 10–20 mg/kg/day in divided doses q6h.
Children younger than 1 yr. 10–30 mg/kg/day in divided doses q6h.

▸ **Dosage in Renal Impairment**
With or without loading dose of 150 mg:

Creatinine Clearance	Dosage
40 ml/min and higher	100 mg q6h (extended-release 200 mg q12h)
30–39 ml/min	100 mg q8h
15–29 ml/min	100 mg q12h
Less than 15 ml/min	100 mg q24h

▸ **Dosage in Liver Impairment**
Adults, Elderly weighing 50 kg and more. 100 mg q6h (200 mg q12h with extended-release).

▸ **Dosage in Cardiomyopathy, Cardiac Decompensation**
Adults, Elderly weighing 50 kg and more. No loading dose; 100 mg q6–8h with gradual dosage adjustments.

SIDE EFFECTS/ADVERSE REACTIONS

Frequent

Dry mouth (32%), urinary hesitancy, constipation

Occasional

Blurred vision, dry eyes, nose, or throat, urinary retention, headache, dizziness, fatigue, nausea

Rare

Impotence, hypotension, edema, weight gain, shortness of breath, syncope, chest pain, nervousness, diarrhea, vomiting, decreased appetite, rash, itching

PRECAUTIONS AND CONTRAINDICATIONS

Cardiogenic shock, narrow-angle glaucoma (unless patient is undergoing cholinergic therapy), preexisting second- or third-degree AV block, preexisting urinary retention

Caution:

Lactation, diabetes mellitus, renal disease, children, hepatic disease, myasthenia gravis, narrow-angle glaucoma, cardiomyopathy, conduction abnormalities

DRUG INTERACTIONS OF CONCERN TO DENTISTRY

- Possible increased risk of prolonged QT interval: clarithromycin, erythromycin
- Increased side effects: anticholinergics, alcohol
- Decreased effects: barbiturates, corticosteroids

SERIOUS REACTIONS

! May produce or aggravate CHF.

! May produce severe hypotension, shortness of breath, chest pain, syncope (especially in patients with primary cardiomyopathy or CHF).

! Hepatotoxicity occurs rarely.

DENTAL CONSIDERATIONS

General:

- Monitor vital signs at every appointment because of cardiovascular side effects.
- Consider a stress-reduction protocol.
- After supine positioning, have patient sit upright for at least 2 min before standing to avoid orthostatic hypotension.
- Patients on chronic drug therapy may rarely have symptoms of blood dyscrasias, which can include infection, bleeding, and poor healing.
- Assess salivary flow as a factor in caries, periodontal disease, and candidiasis.

Consultations:

- In a patient with symptoms of blood dyscrasias, request a medical consultation for blood studies and postpone dental treatment until normal values are reestablished.
- Medical consultation may be required to assess disease control and patient's ability to tolerate stress.

Teach Patient/Family to:

- Encourage effective oral hygiene to prevent soft tissue inflammation.
- When chronic dry mouth occurs, advise patient to:
    - Avoid mouth rinses with high alcohol content because of drying effects.
    - Use daily home fluoride products for anticaries effect.
    - Use sugarless gum, frequent sips of water, or saliva substitutes.

disulfiram

die-**sul′**-fi-ram
(Antabuse)

D

CATEGORY AND SCHEDULE

Pregnancy Risk Category: C

Drug Class: Aldehyde dehydrogenase inhibitor

MECHANISM OF ACTION

A thiuram derivative and an irreversible aldehyde dehydrogenase inhibitor. When taken with alcohol, there is an increase in serum acetaldehyde levels.
Therapeutic Effect: Produces an acute sensitivity to alcohol.

USES

Treatment of chronic alcoholism (as adjunct)

PHARMACOKINETICS

Slowly absorbed from GI tract. Metabolized in liver. Primarily excreted in urine. Up to 20% of dose remains in body for at least 1 wk. ***Half-life:*** Unknown.

INDICATIONS AND DOSAGES

▸ **Adjunct in Management of Selected Chronic Alcoholic Patients Who Want to Remain in State of Enforced Sobriety**

PO

Adults, Elderly. Initially, administer maximum of 500 mg daily given as a single dose for 1–2 wk. Maintenance: 250 mg daily (normal range: 125–500 mg). Do not exceed maximum daily dose of 500 mg.

SIDE EFFECTS/ADVERSE REACTIONS

Frequent
Drowsiness

Occasional
Headache, restlessness, optic neuritis (impaired color perception, altered vision), peripheral neuropathy, metallic or garlic taste, rash

PRECAUTIONS AND CONTRAINDICATIONS

Severe heart disease, psychosis, hypersensitivity to disulfiram or any component of the formulation
Caution:
Hypothyroidism, hepatic disease, diabetes mellitus, seizure disorders, nephritis, cerebral damage

DRUG INTERACTIONS OF CONCERN TO DENTISTRY

- Increased CNS depression: long-acting benzodiazepines
- Increased disulfiram reaction: alcohol
- Risk of psychosis: metronidazole (do not use), tricyclic antidepressants

SERIOUS REACTIONS

! Disulfiram-alcohol reactions to ingestion of alcohol in any form include flushing/throbbing in head and neck, throbbing headache, nausea, copious vomiting, diaphoresis, dyspnea, hyperventilation, tachycardia, hypotension, marked uneasiness, vertigo, blurred vision, confusion, and death

DENTAL CONSIDERATIONS

General:
- Be aware of the needs of patients who are in recovery from substance abuse.
- Avoid other addictive drugs, including opioids and benzodiazepines.

Consultations:
- Medical consultation may be required to assess disease control.

Teach Patient/Family to:
• Avoid mouth rinses with alcohol because of drying effects and drug-drug interaction.

dobutamine hydrochloride

doe-**bute**′-a-meen hi-droh-**klor**′-ide
(Dobutrex)
Do not confuse dobutamine with dopamine.

CATEGORY AND SCHEDULE

Pregnancy Risk Category: B

Drug Class: Adrenergic direct-acting β_1-agonist, cardiac stimulant; Catecholamine

MECHANISM OF ACTION

A direct-acting inotropic agent acting primarily on β_1-adrenergic receptors.
Therapeutic Effect: Decreases preload and afterload, and enhances myocardial contractility, stroke volume, and cardiac output. Improves renal blood flow and urine output.

USES

Treatment of cardiac decompensation caused by organic heart disease or cardiac surgery

PHARMACOKINETICS

Metabolized in the liver. Primarily excreted in urine. Not removed by hemodialysis. ***Half-life:*** 2 min.

INDICATIONS AND DOSAGES

▸ **Short-Term Management of Cardiac Decompensation**
IV Infusion
Adults, Elderly, Children. 2.5–15 mcg/kg/min. Rarely, drug can be infused at a rate of up to 40 mcg/kg/min to increase cardiac output.
Neonates. 2–15 mcg/kg/min.

SIDE EFFECTS/ADVERSE REACTIONS

Frequent
Increased heart rate, increased B/P
Occasional
Pain at injection site
Rare
Nausea, headache, anginal pain, shortness of breath, fever

PRECAUTIONS AND CONTRAINDICATIONS

Hypovolemia patients, idiopathic hypertrophic subaortic stenosis, sulfite sensitivity

DRUG INTERACTIONS OF CONCERN TO DENTISTRY

• None reported

SERIOUS REACTIONS

! Overdose may produce a marked increase in heart rate (by 30 beats/min or higher), marked increase in B/P (by 50 mm Hg or higher), anginal pain, and premature ventricular contractions (PVCs).

DENTAL CONSIDERATIONS

General:
• Acute-use drug for use in hospitals, cardiac labs, or emergency rooms.

D

D

docetaxel

doe-ceh-**tax**′-el
(Taxotere)
Do not confuse docetaxel with Taxol.

CATEGORY AND SCHEDULE

Pregnancy Risk Category: D

Drug Class: Miscellaneous antineoplastic

MECHANISM OF ACTION

An antimitotic agent belonging to the toxoid family that disrupts the microtubular cell network, which is essential for cellular function.
Therapeutic Effect: Inhibits cellular mitosis.

USES

Locally advanced or metastatic breast cancer, non-small-cell lung cancer, androgen independent metastatic prostate cancer, post-surgery operable node-positive breast cancer

PHARMACOKINETICS

Distributed into peripheral compartments. Protein binding: 94%. Extensively metabolized. Excreted primarily in feces, with lesser amount in urine. ***Half-life:*** 11.1 hr.

INDICATIONS AND DOSAGES

▸ **Breast Carcinoma**

IV

Adults. 60–100 mg/m^2 given over 1 hr q3wk. If patient develops febrile neutropenia, a neutrophil count less than 500 cells/mm^3 for longer than 1 wk, severe or cumulative cutaneous reactions, or severe peripheral neuropathy with initial dose of 100 mg/m^2, dosage should be decreased to 75 mg/m^2. If reaction continues, dosage should be further reduced to 55 mg/m^2 or therapy should be discontinued. Patients who don't experience the above symptoms at a dose of 60 mg/m^2 may tolerate an increased docetaxel dose.

▸ **Non-Small-Cell Lung Carcinoma**

IV

Adults. 75 mg/m^2 q3wk. Adjust dosage if toxicity occurs.

SIDE EFFECTS/ADVERSE REACTIONS

Frequent

Alopecia, asthenia, hypersensitivity reaction such as dermatitis (59%, decreases to 16% in those pretreated with oral corticosteroids), fluid retention, stomatitis, nausea and diarrhea, fever, nail changes, vomiting, myalgia

Occasional

Hypotension, edema, anorexia, headache, weight gain, infection (urinary tract, injection site, indwelling catheter tip), dizziness

Rare

Dry skin, sensory disorders (vision, speech, taste), arthralgia, weight loss, conjunctivitis, hematuria, proteinuria

PRECAUTIONS AND CONTRAINDICATIONS

History of severe hypersensitivity to docetaxel or other drugs formulated with polysorbate 80, neutrophil count less than 1500 cells/mm^3

DRUG INTERACTIONS OF CONCERN TO DENTISTRY

• Significant risk of increased effects: drugs that inhibit CYP3A4 isoenzymes (including ketoconazole, itraconazole, erythromycin)
• Caution in use of any drugs that induce CYP3A4 isoenzymes

SERIOUS REACTIONS

! In patients with normal liver function tests, neutropenia (neutrophil count 2000 cells/mm^3) and leukopenia (WBC count less than 4000 cells/mm^3) occur in 96% of patients; anemia (hemoglobin level less than 11 g/dl) occurs in 90% of patients; thrombocytopenia (platelet count less than 100,000 cells/mm^3) occurs in 8% of patients; and infection occurs in 28% of patients.

! Neurosensory and neuromotor effects, such as distal paresthesias and weakness, occur in 54% and 13% of patients, respectively.

DENTAL CONSIDERATIONS

General:

- If additional analgesia is required for dental pain, consider alternative analgesics in patients taking opioids for acute or chronic pain.
- Examine for oral manifestation of opportunistic infection.
- Avoid products that affect platelet function, such as aspirin and NSAIDs.
- This drug may be used in the hospital or on an outpatient basis. Confirm the patient's disease and treatment status.
- Chlorhexidine mouth rinse prior to and during chemotherapy may reduce severity of mucositis.
- Patient on chronic drug therapy may rarely present with symptoms of blood dyscrasias, which can include infection, bleeding, and poor healing. If dyscrasia is present, caution patient to prevent oral tissue trauma when using oral hygiene aids.
- Palliative medication may be required for management of oral side effects.
- Short appointments and a stress-reduction protocol may be required for anxious patients.
- Patients may be at risk of bleeding; check for oral signs.
- Oral infections should be eliminated and/or treated aggressively.

Consultations:

- Medical consultation should include routine blood counts including platelet counts and bleeding time.
- Consult physician; prophylactic or therapeutic antiinfectives may be indicated if surgery or periodontal treatment is required.
- Medical consultation may be required to assess immunologic status during cancer chemotherapy and determine safety risk, if any, posed by the required dental treatment.
- Medical consultation may be required to assess disease control and patient's ability to tolerate stress.

Teach Patient/Family to:

- Be aware of oral side effects.
- Encourage effective oral hygiene to prevent soft tissue inflammation.
- Report oral lesions, soreness, or bleeding to dentist.
- Use caution to prevent trauma when using oral hygiene aids.
- Update health and medication history if physician makes any changes in evaluation or drug regimens; include OTC, herbal, and nonherbal remedies in the update.

D

docosanol
do-**cos**′-ah-nole
(Abreva)

CATEGORY AND SCHEDULE
Pregnancy Risk Category: B

Drug Class: Synthetic lipophilic alcohol

MECHANISM OF ACTION
A highly lipophilic, fatty alcohol that prevents fusion of lipid-enveloped viruses with cell membranes, thereby blocking viral replication

USES
Treatment of recurrent herpes labialis (cold sores, fever blisters) on the face or lips; appears to shorten healing time by at least 1 day.

PHARMACOKINETICS
Topical: Negligible absorption.

INDICATIONS AND DOSAGES
▸ **Recurrent Herpes Labialis**
Topical
Adult, Children older than 12 yr. Apply small amount to affected area on face or lips or at the first sign of lesion 5 times a day until healed.

SIDE EFFECTS/ADVERSE REACTIONS
CNS: Headache
INTEG: Site reaction, rash, pruritus, dry skin, acne

PRECAUTIONS AND CONTRAINDICATIONS
Hypersensitivity
Caution:
Avoid application to eyes, external use only (not for intraoral use), children younger than 12 yr

DRUG INTERACTIONS OF CONCERN TO DENTISTRY
• None reported

DENTAL CONSIDERATIONS
Teach Patient/Family to:
• Apply with finger cot; wash hands before and after use.
• Not share this medication to prevent potential cross contamination of virus.
• Replace tooth brush after resolution of lesion to prevent reinfection of virus.

docusate
dok′-yoo-sate
(Apo-Docusate[CAN], Colace, Colax-C[CAN], Coloxyl[AUS], Diocto, Docusoft-S, Novo-Ducosate[CAN], PMS-Docusate[CAN], Pro-Cal-Sof, Regulex[CAN], Selax[CAN], Soflax[CAN], Surfak)

CATEGORY AND SCHEDULE
Pregnancy Risk Category: C
OTC

Drug Class: Bulk-producing laxative; stool softener

MECHANISM OF ACTION
A bulk-producing laxative that decreases surface film tension by mixing liquid and bowel contents. ***Therapeutic Effect:*** Increases infiltration of liquid to form a softer stool.

USES
Stool softener for those who need to avoid straining during defecation; treatment of constipation associated with hard, dry stools

PHARMACOKINETICS

Minimal absorption from the GI tract. Acts in small and large intestines. Results usually occur 1–2 days after first dose, but may take 3–5 days.

INDICATIONS AND DOSAGES

▸ **Stool Softener**

PO

Adults, Elderly, Children 12 yr and older. 50–500 mg/day in 1–4 divided doses.
Children 6–11 yr. 40–150 mg/day in 1–4 divided doses.
Children 3–5 yr. 20–60 mg/day in 1–4 divided doses.
Children younger than 3 yr. 10–40 mg in 1–4 divided doses.

SIDE EFFECTS/ADVERSE REACTIONS

Occasional

Mild GI cramping, throat irritation (with liquid preparation)

Rare

Rash

PRECAUTIONS AND CONTRAINDICATIONS

Acute abdominal pain, concomitant use of mineral oil, intestinal obstruction, nausea, vomiting

DRUG INTERACTIONS OF CONCERN TO DENTISTRY

- None reported

SERIOUS REACTIONS

! None known

DENTAL CONSIDERATIONS

General:

- Determine why patient is taking the drug.
- Use caution when prescribing medications that may aggravate constipation.

dofetilide

doe-**fet′**-ill-ide
(Tikosyn)

CATEGORY AND SCHEDULE

Pregnancy Risk Category: C

Drug Class: Antidysrhythmic (class III)

MECHANISM OF ACTION

A selective potassium channel blocker that prolongs repolarization without affecting conduction velocity by blocking one or more time-dependent potassium currents. Dofetilide has no effect on sodium channels or adrenergic alpha or beta receptors.
Therapeutic Effect: Terminates reentrant tachyarrhythmias, preventing reinduction.

USES

Maintenance of normal sinus rhythm in patients with atrial fibrillation or atrial flutter longer than 1 wk duration, who have been converted to normal sinus rhythm; conversion of atrial fibrillation or atrial flutter to normal sinus rhythm

PHARMACOKINETICS

PO: Bioavailability greater than 90%, peak plasma levels 2–3 hr, steady-state levels 2–3 days, plasma protein binding 60%–70%, excreted (80%) in urine unchanged, excretion involves both glomerular filtration and active tubular secretion, limited metabolism by CYP450 3A4 isoenzymes

D

INDICATIONS AND DOSAGES

▸ Maintain Normal Sinus Rhythm after Conversion from Atrial Fibrillation or Flutter

PO

Adults, Elderly. Individualized using a 7-step dosing algorithm dependent upon calculated creatinine clearance and QT interval measurements.

SIDE EFFECTS/ADVERSE REACTIONS

Occasional

Headache, chest pain, dizziness, dyspnea, nausea, insomnia, back and abdominal pain, diarrhea, rash

PRECAUTIONS AND CONTRAINDICATIONS

Concurrent use of drugs that prolong the QT interval; concurrent use of amiodarone, megestrol, prochlorperazine, or verapamil; congenital or acquired prolonged QT syndrome; paroxysmal atrial fibrillation; severe renal impairment

Caution:

Requires dose adjustment in renal impairment, can cause life-threatening ventricular arrhythmias, caution in use with CYP450 3A4 isoenzyme inhibitors, hepatic impairment, abnormal serum potassium or magnesium levels, lactation, children younger than 18 yr

DRUG INTERACTIONS OF CONCERN TO DENTISTRY

- Use NSAIDs with caution in patients at risk for thromboembolism
- Decreased renal excretion: ketoconazole (contraindicated use)
- Not recommended with concurrent use of phenothiazines, tricyclic antidepressants, SSRIs, macrolide antiinfectives (erythromycin, clarithromycin), azole antifungals, or other drugs that inhibit CYP3A4 isoenzymes
- Contraindicated with cimetidine, trimethoprim, ketoconazole, prochlorperazine, megestrol, or verapamil

SERIOUS REACTIONS

! Angioedema, bradycardia, cerebral ischemia, facial paralysis, and serious ventricular arrhythmias or various forms of heart block may be noted.

DENTAL CONSIDERATIONS

General:

- Monitor vital signs at every appointment because of cardiovascular side effects.
- Consider a stress-reduction protocol.
- Delay or avoid dental treatment if patient shows signs of cardiac symptoms or respiratory distress.
- Ensure that the patient is compliant with drug therapy.

Consultations:

- Patient's physician should be informed about use of any dental drugs.
- Medical consultation may be required to assess disease control and patient's ability to tolerate stress.

Teach Patient/Family to:

- Update health and drug history if physician makes any changes in evaluation or drug regimens.

dolasetron

doe-**lass′**-eh-tron
(Anzemet)
Do not confuse Anzemet with Aldomdet.

CATEGORY AND SCHEDULE

Pregnancy Risk Category: B

Drug Class: Antinauseant and antiemetic

MECHANISM OF ACTION

A 5-HT_3 receptor antagonist that acts centrally in the chemoreceptor trigger zone and peripherally at the vagal nerve terminals.
Therapeutic Effect: Prevents nausea and vomiting.

USES

Control of nausea and vomiting associated with cancer chemotherapy and prevention of postoperative nausea and vomiting

PHARMACOKINETICS

Readily absorbed from the GI tract after PO administration. Protein binding: 69%–77%. Metabolized in the liver. Primarily excreted in urine. Unknown if removed by hemodialysis. ***Half-life:*** 5–10 hr.

INDICATIONS AND DOSAGES

▸ Prevention of Chemotherapy-Induced Nausea and Vomiting

PO

Adults. 100 mg within 1 hr of chemotherapy.
Children 2–16 yr. 1.8 mg/kg within 1 hr of chemotherapy. Maximum: 100 mg.

IV

Adults, Children 1–16 yr. 1.8 mg/kg as a single dose 30 min before chemotherapy. Maximum: 100 mg.

▸ Treatment or Prevention of Postoperative Nausea or Vomiting

PO

Adults. 100 mg within 2 hr of surgery.
Children 2–16 yr. 1.2 mg/kg within 2 hr of surgery. Maximum: 100 mg.

IV

Adults. 12.5 mg 15 min before cessation of anesthesia or as soon as nausea occurs.
Children 2–16 yr. 0.35 mg/kg 15 min before cessation of anesthesia or as soon as nausea occurs. Maximum: 12.5 mg.

SIDE EFFECTS/ADVERSE REACTIONS

Frequent
Headache, diarrhea, fatigue
Occasional
Fever, dizziness, tachycardia, dyspepsia

PRECAUTIONS AND CONTRAINDICATIONS

Hypersensitivity
Caution:
Previous hypersensitivity to other 5-HT_3 antagonists, cardiovascular disease, seizure disorders, ECG changes, hypokalemia, hypomagnesemia, diuretics, antiarrhythmics, lactation

DRUG INTERACTIONS OF CONCERN TO DENTISTRY

- None reported.

SERIOUS REACTIONS

! Overdose may produce a combination of CNS stimulant and depressant effects.

D

DENTAL CONSIDERATIONS

General:

- Monitor patients in recovery to avoid untoward events.
- Patients taking opioids for acute or chronic pain should be given alternative analgesics for dental pain.
- Chlorhexidine mouth rinse before and during chemotherapy may reduce severity of mucositis.
- Palliative medication may be required for management of oral side effects from chemotherapy.

Teach Patient/Family to:

- Be aware of possible oral side effects from concurrent cancer chemotherapy.
- Report to dentist excessive nausea and vomiting in patients recovering from anesthesia after dental treatment.

donepezil hydrochloride

dah-**nep′**-eh-zil hi-droh-**klor′**-ide
(Aricept)
Do not confuse Aricept with AcipHex or Ascriptin.

CATEGORY AND SCHEDULE

Pregnancy Risk Category: C

Drug Class: Cholinesterase inhibitor

MECHANISM OF ACTION

A cholinesterase inhibitor that inhibits the enzyme acetylcholinesterase, thus increasing the concentration of acetylcholine at cholinergic synapses and enhancing cholinergic function in the CNS.

Therapeutic Effect: Slows the progression of Alzheimer's disease.

USES

Treatment of mild-to-moderate dementia associated with Alzheimer's disease

PHARMACOKINETICS

Well absorbed after PO administration. Protein binding: 96%. Extensively metabolized. Eliminated in urine and feces. ***Half-life:*** 70 hr. Tablets (Orally Disintegrating): 5 mg, 10 mg.

INDICATIONS AND DOSAGES

▸ **Alzheimer's Disease**

PO

Adults, Elderly. 5–10 mg/day as a single dose. If initial dose is 5 mg, do not increase to 10 mg for 4–6 wk.

SIDE EFFECTS/ADVERSE REACTIONS

Frequent

Nausea, diarrhea, headache, insomnia, nonspecific pain, dizziness

Occasional

Mild muscle cramps, fatigue, vomiting, anorexia, ecchymosis

Rare

Depression, abnormal dreams, weight loss, arthritis, somnolence, syncope, frequent urination

PRECAUTIONS AND CONTRAINDICATIONS

History of hypersensitivity to donepezil or piperidine derivatives

Caution:

Bradycardia, sick sinus syndrome, GI ulcer disease, bladder obstruction, seizures, asthma, obstructive pulmonary disease, lactation, children, hepatic impairment

DRUG INTERACTIONS OF CONCERN TO DENTISTRY

• Enhanced succinylcholine muscle relaxation during anesthesia
• Increased risk of GI side effects: NSAIDs
• Action may be inhibited by anticholinergic drugs or enhanced by cholinergic agonists
• Increased blood levels: ketoconazole, paroxetine
• Use with caution drugs that inhibit CYP3A4 or CYP2D6 isoenzymes

SERIOUS REACTIONS

! Overdose may result in cholinergic crisis, characterized by severe nausea, increased salivation, diaphoresis, bradycardia, hypotension, flushed skin, abdominal pain, respiratory depression, seizures, and cardiorespiratory collapse. Increasing muscle weakness may result in death if respiratory muscles are involved.
! The antidote is 1–2 mg IV atropine sulfate with subsequent doses based on therapeutic response.

DENTAL CONSIDERATIONS

General:
• Determine why patient is taking the drug.
• Monitor vital signs at every appointment because of cardiovascular side effects.
• After supine positioning, have patient sit upright for at least 2 min before standing to avoid orthostatic hypotension.
• Use caution if sedation or general anesthesia is required.
• Patients on chronic drug therapy may rarely have symptoms of blood dyscrasias, which can include infection, bleeding, and poor healing.
• Drug is used early in the disease; ensure that patient or caregiver understands informed consent.
• Place on frequent recall because early attention to dental health is important for Alzheimer's patients.
• Assess salivary flow as factor in caries, periodontal disease, and candidiasis.
• Consider semisupine chair position for patient comfort if GI side effects occur.

Consultations:
• Consultation with physician may be necessary if sedation or general anesthesia is required.
• Medical consultation may be required to assess disease control and patient's ability to tolerate stress.
• In a patient with symptoms of blood dyscrasias, request a medical consultation for blood studies and postpone treatment until normal values are reestablished.

Teach Patient/Family to:
• Encourage effective oral hygiene to prevent soft tissue inflammation.
• Prevent trauma when using oral hygiene aids.
• Use powered tooth brush if patient has difficulty holding conventional devices.
• When chronic dry mouth occurs, advise patient to:
  • Avoid mouth rinses with high alcohol content because of drying effects.
  • Use daily home fluoride products for anticaries effect.
  • Use sugarless gum, frequent sips of water, or saliva substitutes.

D

doripenem

(door-eh-**pee′**-nam)
(Doribax [U.S.], Finibax [JAPAN])

CATEGORY AND SCHEDULE

Pregnancy Risk Category: B

Drug Class: Broad-spectrum, carbapenem antibiotic

MECHANISM OF ACTION

Beta-lactam that binds to and inhibits bacterial cell wall synthesis. Doripenem inactivates multiple penicillin-binding proteins (PBPs), resulting in defective cell walls and bacterial death.

Therapeutic Effect: Broad-spectrum, bactericidal action treats complicated intraabdominal and urinary infections (including pyelonephritis).

USES

Serious systemic infections, particularly those caused by susceptible strains of *Pseudomonas aeruginosa* and *E. coli*

PHARMACOKINETICS

Completely absorbed after parenteral administration. Protein binding: 8%. Metabolized by non-hepatic pathways (dehydropeptidase-I). Excreted primarily in unchanged form by the kidneys.

INDICATIONS AND DOSAGES

▸ Complicated Intraabdominal Infection

Adult. 500 mg IV q8h over 1 hr, for 5–14 days.

▸ Complicated Urinary Tract Infection, Including Pyelonephritis

Adult. 500 mg IV q8h over 1 hr, for 10 days.

SIDE EFFECTS/ADVERSE REACTIONS

Frequent

Headache, nausea, diarrhea, rash, phlebitis

Occasional

Anemia, renal impairment, pruritus, rash, hepatic enzyme elevations, oral and vaginal fungal infections

Rare

Anaphylaxis

PRECAUTIONS

- Hypersensitivity
- Reductions of blood levels of sodium valproate (with possible loss of seizure control)
- *Clostridium difficile*–associated diarrhea and colitis
- Development of drug-resistant bacteria

DRUG INTERACTIONS OF CONCERN TO DENTISTRY

- Bacteriostatic antibiotics can theoretically reduce the effectiveness of doripenem.

SERIOUS REACTIONS

! Hypersensitivity, anaphylaxis

DENTAL CONSIDERATIONS

General:

- Determine why patient is receiving drug.
- Avoid administration of antibiotics that could reduce effectiveness of doripenem.

Consultations:

- Consult with physician to determine disease control and ability to tolerate dental procedures.

Teach Patient/Family to:

- Update medical history as changes in disease or drug regimen occur.

dornase alfa

door′-nace al′-fa
(Pulmozyme)

CATEGORY AND SCHEDULE

Pregnancy Risk Category: B

Drug Class: Recombinant human deoxyribonuclease (rh DNase)

MECHANISM OF ACTION

An enzyme that selectively splits and hydrolyzes DNA in sputum.
Therapeutic Effect: Reduces sputum viscosity and elasticity.

USES

Treatment of cystic fibrosis; reduces incidence of pulmonary infections; improves pulmonary function.

PHARMACOKINETICS

Inhalation: Peak sputum levels 15 min

INDICATIONS AND DOSAGES

▸ To Improve Management of Pulmonary Function in Patients with Cystic Fibrosis

Nebulization

Adults, Children older than 5 yr. 2.5 mg (1 ampule) once daily by recommended nebulizer. May increase to 2.5 mg twice daily.

SIDE EFFECTS/ADVERSE REACTIONS

Frequent

Pharyngitis, chest pain or discomfort, voice changes

Occasional

Conjunctivitis, hoarseness, rash

PRECAUTIONS AND CONTRAINDICATIONS

Sensitivity to dornase alfa or epoetin alfa

Caution:

Lactation, children younger than 5 yr

DRUG INTERACTIONS OF CONCERN TO DENTISTRY

• None documented

SERIOUS REACTIONS

! None significant

DENTAL CONSIDERATIONS

General:

• Consider semisupine chair position for patients with respiratory disease.
• Monitor vital signs at every appointment because of respiratory and cardiovascular side effects.
• Stress-reduction protocol may be required.

Consultations:

• Medical consultation may be required to assess disease control.

Teach Patient/Family to:

• Encourage effective oral hygiene to prevent soft tissue inflammation.

dorzolamide hydrochloride

door-**zol**′-ah-mide
hi-droh-**klor**′-ide
(Trusopt)

CATEGORY AND SCHEDULE

Pregnancy Risk Category: C

Drug Class: Carbonic anhydrase inhibitor

D

MECHANISM OF ACTION

An ophthalmic agent that inhibits carbonic anhydrase.
Therapeutic Effect: Reduces intraocular pressure (IOP).

USES

Treatment of ocular hypertension, open-angle glaucoma

PHARMACOKINETICS

Peak response occurs in 2 hr and the duration of action is 8–12 hr. Systemically absorbed to some degree. Protein binding: 33%. Distributed in red blood cells. Sites of metabolism have not been established. Metabolized to active metabolite, N-desethyldorzolamide. Excreted in urine. ***Half-life:*** Unknown; 147 days (terminal red blood cell).

INDICATIONS AND DOSAGES

▸ Glaucoma, Ocular Hypertension

Ophthalmic
Adults, Elderly. 1 drop in affected eye(s) 3 times a day.

SIDE EFFECTS/ADVERSE REACTIONS

Frequent
Ocular burning, bitter taste
Occasional
Superficial punctuate keratitis, ocular allergic reaction

PRECAUTIONS AND CONTRAINDICATIONS

Hypersensitivity to dorzolamide or any other component of the formulation
Caution:
Allergy to sulfonamides, renal or hepatic impairment, lactation, children, oral carbonic anhydrase inhibitors, contact lenses

DRUG INTERACTIONS OF CONCERN TO DENTISTRY

- Avoid drugs that may exacerbate glaucoma (anticholinergic drugs)
- High-dose salicylates to avoid systemic toxicity

SERIOUS REACTIONS

! Iridocyclitis, skin rash, and urolithiasis occur rarely.
! Electrolyte imbalance, development of an acidotic state, and possible CNS effects may occur.

DENTAL CONSIDERATIONS

General:
- Avoid dental light in patient's eyes; offer dark glasses for patient comfort.
- Protect patient's eyes from accidental spatter during dental treatment.
- Check patient's compliance with prescribed drug regimen for glaucoma.

Consultations:
- Medical consultation may be required to assess disease control.

doxazosin mesylate

dox-**ay′**-zoe-sin **mess′**-ah-late
(Apo-Doxazosin[CAN], Cardura)
Do not confuse doxazosin with doxapram, doxepin, or doxorubicin, or Cardura with Cardene, Cordarone, Coumadin, K-Dur, or Ridaura.

CATEGORY AND SCHEDULE

Pregnancy Risk Category: C

Drug Class: α-adrenergic blocker

MECHANISM OF ACTION

An antihypertensive that selectively blocks α_1-adrenergic receptors, decreasing peripheral vascular resistance.

Therapeutic Effect: Causes peripheral vasodilation and lowers of B/P. Also relaxes smooth muscle of bladder and prostate.

USES

Treatment of benign prostatic hyperplasia (BPH)

PHARMACOKINETICS

54%–59% absorbed; peak blood levels 8–9 hr. 99% protein binding. Primarily metabolized in the liver by the CYP 3A4 isoenzyme. 63% excreted in feces, 9% in urine.

Route	Onset	Peak	Duration
PO	N/A	2–6 hr	24 hr

Well absorbed from the GI tract. Protein binding: 98%–99%. Metabolized in the liver. Primarily eliminated in feces. Not removed by hemodialysis. ***Half-life:*** 19–22 hr.

INDICATIONS AND DOSAGES

▸ Mild-to-Moderate Hypertension

PO

Adults. Initially, 1 mg once a day. May increase to a maximum of 16 mg/day.

Elderly. Initially, 0.5 mg once a day.

▸ Benign Prostatic Hyperplasia, Alone or in Combination with Finasteride (Proscar)

PO

Adults, Elderly. Initially, 1 mg/day. May increase q1–2 wk. Maximum: 8 mg/day.

SIDE EFFECTS/ADVERSE REACTIONS

Frequent

Dizziness, asthenia, headache, edema

Occasional

Nausea, pharyngitis, rhinitis, pain in extremities, somnolence

Rare

Palpitations, diarrhea, constipation, dyspnea, myalgia, altered vision, dizziness, nervousness

PRECAUTIONS AND CONTRAINDICATIONS

Hypersensitivity to other quinazolines

Caution:

Children, lactation, hepatic disease

DRUG INTERACTIONS OF CONCERN TO DENTISTRY

- Increased hypotensive effects: all CNS depressants
- Reduced effects with indomethacin, NSAIDs, sympathomimetics
- Caution in use of drugs that may cause urinary retention: anticholinergics, opioids

SERIOUS REACTIONS

! First-dose syncope (hypotension with sudden loss of consciousness) may occur 30–90 min following initial dose of 2 mg or greater, a too-rapid increase in dosage, or addition of another antihypertensive agent to therapy. First-dose syncope may be preceded by tachycardia (pulse rate of 120–160 beats/min).

D

D

DENTAL CONSIDERATIONS

General:

- Monitor vital signs at every appointment because of cardiovascular side effects.
- After supine positioning, have patient sit upright for at least 2 min before standing to avoid orthostatic hypotension.
- Consider a stress-reduction protocol.
- Assess salivary flow as a factor in caries, periodontal disease, and candidiasis.

Consultations:

- Medical consultation may be required to assess disease control and patient's ability to tolerate stress.

Teach Patient/Family to:

- When chronic dry mouth occurs, advise patient to:
  - Avoid mouth rinses with high alcohol content because of drying effects.
  - Use daily home fluoride products for anticaries effect.
  - Use sugarless gum, frequent sips of water, or saliva substitutes.

doxepin hydrochloride

dox′-eh-pin hye-droe-**klor**′-ide (Apo-Doxepin[CAN], Deptran[AUS], Novo-Doxepin[CAN], Prudoxin, Sinequan, Zonalon)

Do not confuse doxepin with doxapram, doxazosin, or Doxidan, or Sinequan with saquinavir.

CATEGORY AND SCHEDULE

Pregnancy Risk Category: C (B for topical form)

Drug Class: Antidepressant, tricyclic

MECHANISM OF ACTION

A tricyclic antidepressant, antianxiety agent, antineuralgic agent, antipruritic, and antiulcer agent that increases synaptic concentrations of norepinephrine and serotonin.

Therapeutic Effect: Produces antidepressant and anxiolytic effects.

USES

Treatment of major depression, anxiety; unapproved: panic disorders

PHARMACOKINETICS

Rapidly and well absorbed from the GI tract. Protein binding: 80%–85%. Metabolized in the liver to active metabolite. Primarily excreted in urine. Not removed by hemodialysis. ***Half-life:*** 6–8 hr. Topical: Absorbed through the skin. Distributed to body tissues. Metabolized to active metabolite. Excreted in urine.

INDICATIONS AND DOSAGES

▸ Depression, Anxiety

PO

Adults. 30–150 mg/day at bedtime or in 2–3 divided doses. May increase to 300 mg/day.

Elderly. Initially, 10–25 mg at bedtime. May increase by 10–25 mg/day every 3–7 days. Maximum: 75 mg/day.

Adolescents. Initially, 25–50 mg/day as a single dose or in divided doses. May increase to 100 mg/day.

Children 12 yr and younger. 1–3 mg/kg/day.

▸ Pruritus Associated with Eczema

Topical

Adults, Elderly. Apply thin film 4 times a day.

SIDE EFFECTS/ADVERSE REACTIONS

Frequent

Oral: Orthostatic hypotension, somnolence, dry mouth, headache, increased appetite, weight gain, nausea, unusual fatigue, unpleasant taste

Topical: Edema; increased pruritus and eczema; burning, tingling, or stinging at application site; altered taste; dizziness; drowsiness; dry skin; dry mouth; fatigue; headache; thirst

Occasional

Oral: Blurred vision, confusion, constipation, hallucinations, difficult urination, eye pain, irregular heartbeat, fine muscle tremors, nervousness, impaired sexual function, diarrhea, diaphoresis, heartburn, insomnia

Topical: Anxiety, skin irritation or cracking, nausea

Rare

Oral: Allergic reaction, alopecia, tinnitus, breast enlargement

Topical: Fever, photosensitivity

PRECAUTIONS AND CONTRAINDICATIONS

Angle-closure glaucoma, hypersensitivity to other tricyclic antidepressants, urine retention

Caution:

Suicidal patients, elderly, MAOIs

DRUG INTERACTIONS OF CONCERN TO DENTISTRY FOR TOPICAL FORM

- Potential for interactions depends on how much drug is absorbed and duration of use (longer than 8 days)
- Increased anticholinergic effects: anticholinergics, antihistamines, phenothiazines, other tricyclic antidepressants
- Potential risk for increased CNS depression: all CNS depressants
- Increased effects of direct-acting sympathomimetics: epinephrine, levonordefrin
- Avoid concurrent use with St. John's wort (herb)

DRUG INTERACTIONS OF CONCERN TO DENTISTRY FOR SYSTEMIC-DOSE FORM

- Increased anticholinergic effects: anticholinergic blockers, antihistamines, phenothiazines
- Increased effects of direct-acting sympathomimetics (epinephrine, levonordefrin)
- Potential risk of increased CNS depression: alcohol, barbiturates, benzodiazepines, other CNS depressants, opioids
- Decreased antihypertensive effects: clonidine, guanadrel, guanethidine

SERIOUS REACTIONS

! Abrupt or too-rapid withdrawal may result in headache, malaise, nausea, vomiting, and vivid dreams.

! Overdose may produce seizures, dizziness, and cardiovascular effects, such as severe orthostatic hypotension, tachycardia, palpitations, and arrhythmias.

DENTAL CONSIDERATIONS

▸ Topical Form

General:

- Doxepin may be absorbed and produce typical systemic side effects of tricyclic drugs.
- Monitor vital signs at every appointment because of cardiovascular side effects.
- Use vasoconstrictors with caution, in low doses, and with careful aspiration.
- Place on frequent recall because of oral side effects.
- Apply lubricant to dry lips for patient comfort before dental procedures.
- Assess salivary flow as a factor in caries, periodontal disease, and candidiasis.

Consultations:

- Medical consultation may be required to assess disease control.

Teach Patient/Family to:

- Avoid mouth rinses with high alcohol content because of interaction with alcohol (see precautions) and drying effects.
- When chronic dry mouth occurs, advise patient to:
  - Use daily home fluoride products for anticaries effect.
  - Use sugarless gum, frequent sips of water, or saliva substitutes.

▸ Systemic-Dose Form

General:

- Monitor vital signs at every appointment because of cardiovascular side effects.
- Assess salivary flow as a factor in caries, periodontal disease, and candidiasis.
- Patients on chronic drug therapy may rarely have symptoms of blood dyscrasias, which can include infection, bleeding, and poor healing.
- After supine positioning, have patient sit upright for at least 2 min before standing to avoid orthostatic hypotension.
- Use vasoconstrictors with caution, in low doses, and with careful aspiration. Avoid use of gingival retraction cord with epinephrine.
- Place on frequent recall because of oral side effects.

Consultations:

- In a patient with symptoms of blood dyscrasias, request a medical consultation for blood studies and postpone dental treatment until normal values are reestablished.
- Medical consultation may be required to assess disease control.
- Physician should be informed if significant xerostomic side effects occur (e.g., increased caries, sore tongue, problems eating or swallowing, difficulty wearing prosthesis) so that a medication change can be considered.

Teach Patient/Family to:

- Encourage effective oral hygiene to prevent soft tissue inflammation.
- When chronic dry mouth occurs, advise patient to:
  - Avoid mouth rinses with high alcohol content because of drying effects.
  - Use daily home fluoride products for anticaries effect.
  - Use sugarless gum, frequent sips of water, or saliva substitutes.

doxorubicin

dox-oh-**roo′**-bi-sin
(Doxil)
Do not confuse doxorubicin with Daunorubicin, Idamycin, or Idarubicin.

CATEGORY AND SCHEDULE

Pregnancy Risk Category: D

Drug Class: Anthracycline antibiotic; antineoplastic

MECHANISM OF ACTION

An anthracycline antibiotic that inhibits DNA and DNA-dependent RNA synthesis by binding with DNA strands. Liposomal encapsulation increases uptake by tumors, prolongs action, and may decrease toxicity.
Therapeutic Effect: Prevents cellular division.

USES

Treatment of some kinds of cancer

PHARMACOKINETICS

Widely distributed. Protein binding: Unknown. Metabolized in liver. Minimal excretion in urine.
Half-life: 45–55 hr.

INDICATIONS AND DOSAGES

▸ **AIDS-Related Kaposi's Sarcoma**
IV Infusion
Adults. 20 mg/m^2 over 30 min q3wk.
▸ **Ovarian Cancer**
IV Infusion
Adults. 50 mg/m^2 q4wk.
▸ **Dosage in Liver Impairment**

Serum Bilirubin Concentration	Dosage
1.2–3 mg/dl	50% usual dose
More than 3 mg/dl	25% usual dose

SIDE EFFECTS/ADVERSE REACTIONS

Frequent
Nausea
Occasional
Anorexia, diarrhea, hyperpigmentation of nailbeds, phalangeal and dermal creases
Rare
Fever, chills, conjunctivitis, lacrimation

PRECAUTIONS AND CONTRAINDICATIONS

Nursing mothers, hypersensitivity to doxorubicin compounds or daunorubicin

DRUG INTERACTIONS OF CONCERN TO DENTISTRY

• None reported

SERIOUS REACTIONS

! Bone marrow depression manifested as hematologic toxicity (principally leukopenia and, to lesser extent, anemia, thrombocytopenia) may occur.
! Cardiotoxicity noted as either acute, transient abnormal ECG findings or cardiomyopathy manifested as CHF may occur.

DENTAL CONSIDERATIONS

General:
• If additional analgesia is required for dental pain, consider alternative analgesics (NSAIDs) in patients taking narcotics for acute or chronic pain.
• Avoid prescribing aspirin-containing products.
• Examine for oral manifestation of opportunistic infection.
• This drug usually is administered in a hospital, a cancer treatment center, or possibly a home IV service. Dentists are involved in the

management of oral mucositis associated with the chemotherapy.
• Chlorhexidine mouth rinse prior to and during chemotherapy may reduce severity of mucositis.
• Patient on chronic drug therapy may rarely present with symptoms of blood dyscrasias, which can include infection, bleeding, and poor healing. If dyscrasia is present, caution patient to prevent oral tissue trauma when using oral hygiene aids.
• Palliative medication may be required for management of oral side effects.
• Consider local hemostasis measures to prevent excessive bleeding.
• Patient may be at risk of bleeding; check oral signs.

Consultations:
• Medical consultation should include routine blood counts including platelet counts and bleeding time.
• Consult physician; prophylactic or therapeutic antiinfectives may be indicated if surgery or periodontal treatment is required.
• Medical consultation may be required to assess immunologic status during cancer chemotherapy and determine safety risk, if any, posed by the required dental treatment.
• Medical consultation may be required to assess disease control and patient's ability to tolerate stress.
• In a patient with symptoms of blood dyscrasias, request a medical consultation for blood studies and postpone treatment until normal values are reestablished.

Teach Patient/Family to:
• Be aware of oral side effects.
• Encourage effective oral hygiene to prevent soft tissue inflammation.
• See dentist immediately if signs of secondary oral infection occur.
• Prevent trauma when using oral hygiene aids.
• Update health and medication history if physician makes any changes in evaluation or drug regimens; include OTC, herbal, and nonherbal remedies in the update.

doxycycline

dox-ih-**sye′**-kleen
(Adoxa, Apo-Doxy[CAN], Doryx, Doxsig[AUS], Doxy-100, Doxycin[CAN], Doxyhexal[AUS], Doxylin[AUS], Monodox, Vibramycin, Vibra-Tabs)
Do not confuse doxycycline with Dicyclomine or doxylamine, or Monodox with Monopril.

CATEGORY AND SCHEDULE

Pregnancy Risk Category: D

Drug Class: Tetracycline, broad-spectrum antiinfective

MECHANISM OF ACTION

A tetracycline antibiotic that inhibits bacterial protein synthesis by binding to ribosomes.
Therapeutic Effect: Bacteriostatic.

USES

Treatment of syphilis, *C. trachomatis,* gonorrhea, lymphogranuloma venereum, uncommon gram-negative and gram-positive organisms, necrotizing ulcerative gingivostomatitis; cutaneous or inhalational anthrax exposure

PHARMACOKINETICS

PO: Peak 1.5–4 hr, ***Half-life:*** 15–22 hr; 25%–93% protein bound; excreted in bile.

INDICATIONS AND DOSAGES

▸ **Respiratory, Skin, and Soft-Tissue Infections; UTIs; Pelvic Inflammatory Disease (PID); Brucellosis; Trachoma; Rocky Mountain Spotted Fever; Typhus; Q Fever; Rickettsia; Severe Acne (Adoxa); Smallpox; Psittacosis; Ornithosis; Granuloma Inguinale; Lymphogranuloma Venereum; Intestinal Amebiasis (Adjunctive Treatment); Prevention of Rheumatic Fever**

PO

Adults, Elderly. Initially, 100 mg q12h, then 100 mg/day as single dose or 50 mg q12h for severe infections.

Children 8 yr and older and weighing more than 45 kg. 2–4 mg/kg/day divided q12–24h. Maximum: 200 mg/day.

IV

Adults, Elderly. Initially, 200 mg as 1–2 infusions; then 100–200 mg/day in 1–2 divided doses.

Children 8 yr and older. 2–4 mg/kg/day divided q12–24h. Maximum: 200 mg/day.

▸ **Acute Gonococcal Infections**

PO

Adults. Initially, 200 mg, then 100 mg at bedtime on first day; then 100 mg twice a day for 14 days.

▸ **Syphilis**

PO, IV

Adults. 200 mg/day in divided doses for 14–28 days.

▸ **Traveler's Diarrhea**

PO

Adults, Elderly. 100 mg/day during a period of risk (up to 14 days) and for 2 days after returning home.

▸ **Periodontitis**

PO

Adults. 20 mg twice a day as an adjunct to scaling and root planning; may be administered for up to 9 mo; exceeding the recommended dosage may increase risk of side effects, including the development of resistant organisms.

SIDE EFFECTS/ADVERSE REACTIONS

Frequent

Anorexia, nausea, vomiting, diarrhea, dysphagia, possibly severe photosensitivity

Occasional

Rash, urticaria

PRECAUTIONS AND CONTRAINDICATIONS

Children 8 yr and younger, hypersensitivity to tetracyclines or sulfites, last half of pregnancy, severe hepatic dysfunction.

The use of tetracycline drugs during tooth development (last half of pregnancy, infancy and childhood up to the age of 8 may cause permanent discoloration of the teeth (yellow-gray-brown). Enamel hypoplasia has also been reported. May also cause retardation of skeletal development and deformations.

Caution:

Hepatic disease, lactation

DRUG INTERACTIONS OF CONCERN TO DENTISTRY

• No data reported for this dose form; see doxycycline hyclate monograph for drug interactions reported with tetracyclines.

DRUG INTERACTIONS OF CONCERN TO DENTISTRY FOR SYSTEMIC FORM

• Decreased absorption: $NaHCO_3$, other antacids

• Increased rate of metabolism: barbiturates, carbamazepine, hydantoins

• Decreased effect of penicillins, cephalosporins

- May increase the effectiveness of anticoagulants, methotrexate, digoxin
- Contraindicated with isotretinoin (Accutane)

SERIOUS REACTIONS

! Superinfection (especially fungal) and benign intracranial hypertension (headache, visual changes) may occur.

! Hepatotoxicity, fatty degeneration of the liver, and pancreatitis occur rarely.

DENTAL CONSIDERATIONS

▸ Doxycycline Hyclate (Dental-Systemic)

General:

- Examine for oral manifestation of opportunistic infection.
- Should be administered at least 1 hr before or 2 hr after morning or evening meals.

Teach Patient/Family to:

- Avoid using ingestible sodium bicarbonate products, such as the Prophy-Jet air polishing system, within 2 hr of drug use.

▸ Doxycycline Hyclate/Doxycycline Calcium (Systemic Form)

General:

- Determine why the patient is taking tetracycline.
- Broad-spectrum antibiotics may promote oral or vaginal fungal infection.
- Dental staining or enamel hypoplasia may be associated with exposure to this drug before birth or up to the age of 8. Tetracycline stains may be extremely resistant to ordinary tooth-whitening procedures.

Consultations:

- Medical consultation may be required to assess disease control.

Teach Patient/Family:

- That tetracycline can be taken with milk, food; take with a full glass of water.
- To take tetracycline doses 1 hr before or 2 hr after air polishing device (Prophy-Jet), if used.
- When used for dental infection, advise patient:
  - To report sore throat, oral burning sensation, fever, and fatigue, any of which could indicate superinfection.
  - To take at prescribed intervals and complete dosage regimen.
  - To immediately notify the dentist if signs or symptoms of infection increase.

doxycycline hyclate (dental-systemic)

dox-ih-**sye**′-kleen

(Periostat)

CATEGORY AND SCHEDULE

Pregnancy Risk Category: D

Drug Class: Tetracycline derivative for nonantibacterial use

MECHANISM OF ACTION

Reduces collagenase activity in gingival tissues of patients with adult periodontitis; no antibacterial effect reported at this dose.

USES

Adjunct to scaling and root planing to promote attachment level gain and reduce pocket depth in adult periodontitis

PHARMACOKINETICS

No data available.

INDICATIONS AND DOSAGES

PO

Adult. 20 mg twice daily as an adjunct to scaling and root planing; may be administered for up to 9 mo; exceeding the recommended dosage may increase risk of side effects, including the development of resistant organisms.

SIDE EFFECTS/ADVERSE REACTIONS

Note: In a clinical study of 428 patients, there was little to no difference in the incidence of side effects reported between this drug and a placebo. See doxycycline hyclate monograph for typical side effects associated with oral administration. Whether these side effects would occur at doses used in this product is unknown.

PRECAUTIONS AND CONTRAINDICATIONS

Hypersensitivity to tetracyclines

Caution:

Children younger than 8 yr, pregnant and nursing mothers, predisposition to oral or vaginal candidiasis; not to be used for antimicrobial effect in periodontitis

DRUG INTERACTIONS OF CONCERN TO DENTISTRY

- No data reported for this dose form; see doxycycline hyclate monograph for drug interactions reported with tetracyclines.

SERIOUS REACTIONS

! Pregnancy (permanent tooth discoloration), fetal toxicity

DENTAL CONSIDERATIONS

General:

- Examine for oral manifestation of opportunistic infection.
- Should be administered at least 1 hr before or 2 hr after morning or evening meals.

Teach Patient/Family to:

- Avoid using ingestible sodium bicarbonate products, such as the air polishing system Prophy Jet, within 2 hr of drug use.

doxycycline hyclate gel

dox-ih-**sye**′-kleen

(Atridox)

CATEGORY AND SCHEDULE

Pregnancy Risk Category: D

Drug Class: Tetracycline, antiinfective

MECHANISM OF ACTION

Inhibits bacterial protein synthesis by disruption of transfer RNA and messenger RNA.

USES

Adjunctive treatment of chronic adult periodontitis to increase clinical attachment, reduce probing depth, and reduce bleeding on probing

PHARMACOKINETICS

Gingival crevicular fluid levels peak at 2 hr, sustained levels up to 18 hr and decline over 7 days; low serum levels not exceeding 0.1 g/ml.

INDICATIONS AND DOSAGES

Topical

Adult. Mix contents of syringes according to detailed instructions, completing 100 cycles; attach blunt cannula to syringe A and fill the pocket; after it becomes firm, the mixture may be packed further into the pocket with a dental instrument.

D

SIDE EFFECTS/ADVERSE REACTIONS

Oral: Gingival discomfort, pain, loss of attachment, toothache, periodontal abscess, exudate, infection, drainage, swelling, thermal tooth sensitivity, extreme mobility, localized allergic reaction
CNS: Headache
CV: High B/P
GI: Diarrhea
GU: PMS
EENT: Skin infection, photosensitivity
MS: Muscle aches, backache

PRECAUTIONS AND CONTRAINDICATIONS

Hypersensitivity
Caution:
Children (tooth staining), lactation, photosensitivity, predisposition to candidiasis

DRUG INTERACTIONS OF CONCERN TO DENTISTRY

- None specifically identified for this product; unknown whether typical tetracycline interactions occur.

SERIOUS REACTIONS

! Pregnancy (permanent tooth discoloration), fetal toxicity

DENTAL CONSIDERATONS

General:
- Examine for oral manifestation of opportunistic infection.

Teach Patient/Family to:
- Be alert to the possibility of secondary oral infection and the need to see dentist immediately if signs of infection occur.
- Avoid oral hygiene procedures in treated areas of mouth for 7 days to avoid dislodging product.

dronabinol

droe-**nab′**-ih-nol
(Marinol)
Do not confuse dronabinol with droperidol.

CATEGORY AND SCHEDULE

Pregnancy Risk Category: C
Controlled Substance Schedule: III

Drug Class: Antiemetic, appetite stimulant

MECHANISM OF ACTION

An antiemetic and appetite stimulant that may act by inhibiting vomiting control mechanisms in the medulla oblongata.
Therapeutic Effect: Inhibits vomiting and stimulates appetite.

USES

Control of nausea, vomiting in selected patients receiving emetogenic cancer chemotherapy; stimulate appetite in AIDS-associated anorexia

PHARMACOKINETICS

Well absorbed after PO administration. Protein binding: 97%. Undergoes first-pass metabolism. Is highly lipid soluble. Primarily excreted in feces.
Half-life: 4 hr.

INDICATIONS AND DOSAGES

▸ Prevention of Chemotherapy-Induced Nausea and Vomiting
PO
Adults, Children. Initially, 5 mg/m^2 1–3 hr before chemotherapy, then q2–4h after chemotherapy for total of 4–6 doses a day. May increase by 2.5 mg/m^2 up to 15 mg/m^2 per dose.

▸ **Appetite Stimulant**

PO

Adults. Initially, 2.5 mg twice a day (before lunch and dinner). Range: 2.5–20 mg/day.

SIDE EFFECTS/ADVERSE REACTIONS

Frequent

Euphoria, dizziness, paranoid reaction, somnolence

Occasional

Asthenia, ataxia, confusion, abnormal thinking, depersonalization

Rare

Diarrhea, depression, nightmares, speech difficulties, headache, anxiety, tinnitus, flushed skin

PRECAUTIONS AND CONTRAINDICATIONS

Treatment of nausea and vomiting not caused by chemotherapy, hypersensitivity to sesame oil or tetrahydrocannabinol products

Caution:

Lactation, children, elderly, cardiac disorders, drug abuse, alcoholism, hypertension, manic or depressive state, schizophrenia

DRUG INTERACTIONS OF CONCERN TO DENTISTRY

- Increased CNS depression: alcohol, CNS depressants, tricyclic antidepressants
- Additive hypertension, tachycardia, possible cardiotoxicity: tricyclic antidepressants, amphetamines, other sympathomimetics
- Additive tachycardia, drowsiness: atropine, scopolamine, antihistamines, anticholinergic drugs

SERIOUS REACTIONS

! Mild intoxication may produce increased sensory awareness (including taste, smell, and sound), altered time perception, reddened conjunctiva, dry mouth, and tachycardia.

! Moderate intoxication may produce memory impairment and urine retention.

! Severe intoxication may produce lethargy, decreased motor coordination, slurred speech, and orthostatic hypotension.

DENTAL CONSIDERATIONS

General:

- Monitor vital signs at every appointment because of cardiovascular side effects.
- After supine positioning, have patient sit upright for at least 2 min to avoid orthostatic hypotension.
- Patients taking opioids for acute or chronic pain should be given alternative analgesics for dental pain.
- Assess salivary flow as a factor in caries, periodontal disease, and candidiasis.
- Consider semisupine chair position for patient comfort if GI side effects occur.

Teach Patient/Family to:

- When chronic dry mouth occurs, advise patient to:
  - Avoid mouth rinses with high alcohol content because of drying effects.
  - Use daily home fluoride products for anticaries effect.
  - Use sugarless gum, frequent sips of water, or saliva substitutes.

D

dronedarone

droe-**ne**-da-rone
(Multaq)

CATEGORY AND SCHEDULE

Pregnancy Risk Category: X

Drug Class: Antiarrhythmic agents

MECHANISM OF ACTION

A non-iodinated amiodarone analogue with unknown mechanism of action. Properties of all four Vaughan-Williams classes; inhibits calcium, sodium, and potassium channels; α- and β-adrenergic receptor antagonist.
Therapeutic Effect: Suppresses atrial fibrillation or atrial flutter.

USES

Atrial fibrillation
Atrial flutter

PHARMACOKINETICS

Route	Onset	Peak	Duration
PO	Unknown	3–6 hr	12 hr

Poor bioavailability. Protein binding: >98%. Extensive first pass hepatic metabolism, mostly by CYP3A. Primarily excreted in feces; minimal excretion in urine. Food increases bioavailability. ***Half-life:*** 13–19 hr.

INDICATIONS AND DOSAGES

▸ **Atrial Fibrillation**

PO

Adults. 400 mg twice a day, with morning and evening meals.

▸ **Atrial Flutter**

PO

Adults. 400 mg twice a day, with morning and evening meals.

SIDE EFFECTS/ADVERSE REACTIONS

Frequent

Prolonged QT interval, elevated serum creatinine

Occasional

Dermatitis, eczema, pruritus, rash, diarrhea, nausea, asthenia

Rare

Bradyarrhythmia, photosensitivity, hypokalemia, hypomagnesemia, abdominal pain, indigestion, altered taste, vomiting

PRECAUTIONS AND CONTRAINDICATIONS

Hypersensitivity to dronedarone or its components
Bradycardia (<50 bpm)
Concomitant use of strong CYP3A inhibitors
Heart failure, Class II or III, with recent decompensation requiring hospitalization
Heart failure, Class IV
Severe hepatic impairment
Pregnancy
Nursing mothers
Concomitant use of QT prolonging agents
QTc Bazett interval ≥ 500 ms
Second- or third-degree atrioventricular block or sick sinus syndrome

Caution:

- Concurrent use with CYP450 3A inducers, antiarrhythmic agents, or β-blockers
- Women of childbearing potential
- New or worsening heart failure
- Hypokalemia or hypomagnesemia
- QT prolongation (discontinue dronedarone if QTc Bazett ≥ 500 ms)
- Moderate hepatic impairment
- Patients of Asian decent

DRUG INTERACTIONS OF CONCERN TO DENTISTRY

- QT prolonging agents: May increase the risk of QT prolongation.
- CYP450 3A4 inhibitors: May increase dronedarone levels and risk of adverse effects.
- CYP450 3A4 substrates: May increase drug concentrations of CYP3A4 substrates and risk of adverse effects.
- CYP450 3A4 inducers: May decrease dronedarone levels and effectiveness.
- Antiarrhythmics: May increase the risk of adverse cardiovascular effects.
- β-blocker: May increase risk of bradycardia.
- Digoxin: May increase digoxin levels and risk of toxicity; discontinue or reduce dose by 50%.
- Grapefruit juice: May increase dronedarone levels and risk of toxicity.
- HMG-CoA reductase inhibitors: May increase the drug levels of HMG-CoA reductase inhibitors and risk of toxicity.
- Calcium channel blockers: May increase the drug levels of dronedarone and/or calcium channel blockers and risk of toxicity.
- Photosensitizers: May increase the risk of photosensitivity.
- Potassium-depleting agents: May increase the risk of hypokalemia.
- SSRIs, TCA antidepressants: May increase drug levels of SSRIs and TCA antidepressants and effects.

SERIOUS REACTIONS

! Black box warning: patients with NYHA Class IV heart failure or NYHA Class II-III heart failure with recent decompensation require hospitalization or referral to specialized clinic.
! QT prolongation may occur.
! Heart failure may develop; existing heart failure may worsen during treatment.
! Raised serum creatinine may occur.

D

DENTAL CONSIDERATIONS

General:
- Avoid or limit use of vasoconstrictors.
- Monitor vital signs at every appointment because of cardiovascular side effects.
- Consider semisupine chair position for patient if GI side effects occur.

Consultations:
- Medical consultation may be required to assess disease control.

Teach Patient/Family to:
- Encourage effective oral hygiene to prevent soft tissue inflammation.
- Prevent trauma when using oral hygiene aids.
- Be alert for the possibility of secondary oral infection and the need to see dentist immediately if signs of infection occur.
- Women of childbearing potential should avoid pregnancy.

droperidol

droe-**pear′**-ih-dall
(Inapsine)

CATEGORY AND SCHEDULE

Pregnancy Risk Category: C

Drug Class: General anesthetic; anesthesia adjunct, antiemetic

MECHANISM OF ACTION

A general anesthetic and antiemetic agent that antagonizes dopamine neurotransmission at synapses by blocking postsynaptic dopamine receptor sites; partially blocks adrenergic receptor binding sites.

Therapeutic Effect: Produces tranquilization, antiemetic effect.

D

USES

Treatment of nausea and vomiting associated with surgical and diagnostic procedures.

PHARMACOKINETICS

Onset of action occurs within 30 min. Well absorbed. Metabolized in liver. Excreted in urine and feces. ***Half-life:*** 2.3 hr.

INDICATIONS AND DOSAGES

▸ **Preoperative**

IM/IV

Adults, Elderly, Children 12 yr and older. 2.5–10 mg 30–60 min before induction of general anesthesia.

Children 2–12 yr. 0.088–0.165 mg/kg.

▸ **Adjunct for Induction of General Anesthesia**

IV

Adults, Elderly, Children 12 yr and older. 0.22–0.275 mg/kg.

Children 2–12 yr. 0.088–0.165 mg/kg.

▸ **Adjunct for Maintenance of General Anesthesia**

IV

Adults, Elderly. 1.25–2.5 mg.

▸ **Diagnostic Procedures without General Anesthesia**

IM

Adults, Elderly. 2.5–10 mg 30–60 min before procedure. If needed, may give additional doses of 1.25–2.5 mg (usually by IV injection).

SIDE EFFECTS/ADVERSE REACTIONS

Frequent

Mild-to-moderate hypotension

Occasional

Tachycardia, postoperative drowsiness, dizziness, chills, shivering

Rare

Postoperative nightmares, facial sweating, bronchospasm

PRECAUTIONS AND CONTRAINDICATIONS

Known or suspected QT prolongation, hypersensitivity to droperidol or any component of the formulation

DRUG INTERACTIONS OF CONCERN TO DENTISTRY

- Increased frequency of nausea/vomiting: propofol
- Increased CNS depression: all CNS depressants
- Prolonged QT interval: intravenous narcotics
- Increased hypotension: anesthetics, systemic or local
- Risk of hypotension: epinephrine
- Orthostatic hypotension: antihypertensive medications

SERIOUS REACTIONS

! Extrapyramidal symptoms may appear as akathisia (motor restlessness) and dystonias: torticollis (neck muscle spasm), opisthotonos (rigidity of back muscles), and oculogyric crisis (rolling back of eyes).

! Overdosage includes symptoms of hypotension, tachycardia, hallucinations, and extrapyramidal symptoms.

! Prolonged QT interval, seizures, and arrhythmias have been reported.

DENTAL CONSIDERATIONS

General:
- Used in a hospital, emergency room, or cancer treatment center for acute need.
- Caution in the use of drugs that prolong the QT interval.
- Use caution if sedation or general anesthesia is required; risk of hypotensive episode.
- After supine positioning, have patient sit upright for at least 2 min before standing to avoid orthostatic hypotension.
- Monitor vital signs at every appointment because of cardiovascular side effects.

Consultations:
- Consultation with physician may be necessary if sedation or general anesthesia is required.
- Medical consultation may be required to assess disease control.

duloxetine

doo-**lox**′-eh-teen
(Cymbalta)

CATEGORY AND SCHEDULE

Pregnancy Risk Category: C

Drug Class: Antidepressant

MECHANISM OF ACTION

Selectively inhibits the reuptake of serotonin (5-HT) and norepinephrine in the brain.

USES

Treatment of major depressive disorder; diabetic peripheral neuropathic pain

PHARMACOKINETICS

Peak 6 hr, plasma protein binding greater than 90%; metabolized in liver by CYP2D6 and CYP1A2 isoenzymes; excreted in urine (70%) and feces (30%) ***Half-life:*** 8–17 hr.

INDICATIONS AND DOSAGES

▸ **Depression**

PO

Adult. 40 mg per day (20 mg twice daily) to 60 mg/day (once daily or 30 mg twice daily).

▸ **Diabetic Peripheral Neuropathic Pain**

PO

Adult. Up to a total dose of 60 mg per day (once a day).

Available forms include Caplets 20, 30, and 60 mg.

SIDE EFFECTS/ADVERSE REACTIONS

Dry mouth, insomnia, anxiety, decreased appetite, dizziness, somnolence, tremors, fatigue, decreased libido, hot flushes, elevated B/P, nausea, constipation, diarrhea, vomiting, dyspepsia, cough, nasopharyngitis, erectile and ejaculation dysfunction, polyuria, blurred vision, pharyngolaryngeal pain, sweating, muscle cramps, myalgia, fatigue, asthenia, pyrexia

PRECAUTIONS AND CONTRAINDICATIONS

Hypersensitivity, MAOIs, uncontrolled narrow-angle glaucoma, hepatotoxicity, elevated B/P, psychiatric changes, seizures, glaucoma, physical and psychological symptoms of withdrawal, renal impairment

D

DRUG INTERACTIONS OF CONCERN TO DENTISTRY

• Potentiation of anticholinergic effects by antisialagogues used in dentistry (e.g., atropine, glycopyrrolate)
• Increased fluoxetine blood levels and toxicity with some fluoroquinolone antibacterials
• Centrally acting drugs (e.g., sedatives) may enhance CNS adverse effects
• Caution: can inhibit CYP2D6 isoenzymes, use phenothiazines with caution (see Appendix I)
• Avoid administration with alcohol or alcohol-containing agents (e.g., elixirs)

SERIOUS REACTIONS

! Hepatotoxicity
! Worsening of suicide risk
! Activation of mania seizures
! Increased intraocular pressure
! Withdrawal symptoms if abruptly discontinued

DENTAL CONSIDERATIONS

General:
• Monitor vital signs at every appointment because of cardiovascular side effects.
• Assess salivary flow as a factor in caries, periodontal disease, candidiasis, denture sore mouth.
• Assess salivary flow as a factor in reduced retention and/or increased irritation of removable prostheses.
Consultations:
• Medical consultation may be required to assess disease control and patient's ability to tolerate stress.
• Inform physician of potential adverse effects of dry mouth and possible need to change medications if severe.
Teach Patient/Family to:
• Encourage effective oral hygiene measures to minimize effects of reduced salivary flow.
• Avoid mouth rinses with high alcohol content because of drying effects.
• Use daily home fluoride products for anticaries effect.
• Use sugarless or xylitol chewing gums, frequent sips of water, and/or saliva substitutes if dry mouth occurs.

dutasteride

do-tah-**stir′**-eyed
(Avodart)

CATEGORY AND SCHEDULE

Pregnancy Risk Category: X

Drug Class: Synthetic steroid

MECHANISM OF ACTION

An androgen hormone inhibitor that inhibits 5-alpha reductase, an intracellular enzyme that converts testosterone into dihydrotestosterone (DHT) in the prostate gland, reducing the serum DHT level.
Therapeutic Effect: Reduces size of the prostate gland.

USES

Treatment of benign prostate hyperplasia (BPH) in men to improve symptoms, reduce the risk of urinary retention, and reduce the need for BPH-related surgery

PHARMACOKINETICS

Route	Onset	Peak	Duration
PO	24 hr	N/A	3–8 wk

Moderately absorbed after PO administration. Widely distributed. Protein binding: 99%. Metabolized in the liver. Primarily excreted in feces. ***Half-life:*** Up to 5 wk.

INDICATIONS AND DOSAGES

▸ BPH

PO

Adults, Elderly. 0.5 mg once a day.

SIDE EFFECTS/ADVERSE REACTIONS

Occasional

Gynecomastia, sexual dysfunction (decreased libido, impotence, and decreased volume of ejaculate)

PRECAUTIONS AND CONTRAINDICATIONS

Females, physical handling of tablets by those who are or may be pregnant

Caution:

Hepatic impairment, men cannot donate blood until at least 6 mo after last dose, drug also found in semen, no data on use in patients younger than 18 yr or in renal impairment, nursing mothers (not used in women)

DRUG INTERACTIONS OF CONCERN TO DENTISTRY

- No drug interaction studies have been conducted; however, caution should be observed when used in combination with potent and chronically used CYP3A4 inhibitors.
- Opioids and anticholinergic drugs may enhance urinary retention; use alternative analgesics (NSAIDs).

SERIOUS REACTIONS

! Toxicity may be manifested as rash, diarrhea, and abdominal pain.

DENTAL CONSIDERATIONS

General:

- Determine why patient is taking the drug.

Consultations:

- Medical consultation may be required to assess disease control.

Teach Patient/Family to:

- Update health and drug history if physician makes any changes in evaluation or drug regimens.

D

dutasteride + tamsulosin

doo-**tas′**-teer-ide &
tam-**soo**-loe-sin
(Jalyn)

CATEGORY AND SCHEDULE

Pregnancy Risk Category: X

Drug Class: 5-Alpha-reductase inhibitor; alpha-1 blocker

MECHANISM OF ACTION

Dutasteride is an androgen hormone inhibitor that inhibits 5-alpha reductase, an intracellular enzyme that converts testosterone into dihydrotestosterone (DHT) in the prostate gland, reducing the serum DHT level. Tamsulosin is an α_1 antagonist that targets receptors around the bladder neck and prostate capsule, which relaxes smooth muscle and improves urinary flow and symptoms of prostatic hypertrophy.

Therapeutic Effect: Reduces size of prostate gland and symptoms of BPH.

USES

Treatment of symptomatic benign prostatic hyperplasia (BPH)

PHARMACOKINETICS

Dutasteride: Moderately absorbed and widely distributed after oral administration. Protein binding is 99%. Metabolized in the liver. Primarily excreted in feces. Tamsulosin: Well absorbed and widely distributed after oral administration. Protein binding is 94%–99%. Metabolized in the liver. Primarily excreted in urine.
Half-life: Dutasteride: up to 5 wk. Tamsulosin: 9–13 hr.

INDICATIONS AND DOSAGES

▸ Benign Prostatic Hyperplasia (BPH)

PO
Adults. 1 capsule (0.5 mg dutasteride/0.4 mg tamsulosin) once daily. Take 30 min after the same meal each day. Capsules should be swallowed whole; do not crush, chew, or open. Oropharyngeal contact with capsule contents may result in irritation of the mucosa.

SIDE EFFECTS/ADVERSE REACTIONS

Frequent
Dizziness, somnolence, gynecomastia, sexual dysfunction (decreased libido, impotence, and decreased volume of ejaculate)
Occasional
Headache, anxiety, insomnia, orthostatic hypotension, nasal congestion, pharyngitis, rhinitis, nausea, vertigo, impotence

PRECAUTIONS AND CONTRAINDICATIONS

Hypersensitivity to dutasteride, tamsulosin, other 5α-reductase inhibitors (finasteride), or any component of the formulation. Potential syncope risk caused by hypotension, vertigo, dizziness, carcinoma of prostate. Avoid use with other adrenoreceptor antagonists. Not for use in women, children or during lactation. Avoid in patients with previous severe allergic reaction to sulfonamides.

DRUG INTERACTIONS OF CONCERN TO DENTISTRY

- CYP3A4 inhibitors (e.g., macrolide antibiotics): increased risk of adverse effects of Jalyn.
- Opioids and anticholinergics may increase urinary retention.

SERIOUS REACTIONS

! First-dose syncope (hypotension with sudden loss of consciousness) may occur within 30–90 min after administration of initial dose and may be preceded by tachycardia (pulse rate of 120–160 beats/min).

DENTAL CONSIDERATIONS

General:
- Expect interruptions in treatment due to urinary frequency.
- Monitor vital signs at every appointment due to cardiovascular and respiratory adverse effects.
- After supine positioning, have patient sit upright for at least 2 min before standing to avoid orthostatic hypotension.
- Consider semisupine chair position for patient comfort when GI side effects occur.

dyphylline

die′-fih-lin
(Dilor, Lufyllin)
Do not confuse with Dilacor.

CATEGORY AND SCHEDULE

Pregnancy Risk Category: C

Drug Class: Xanthine derivative

MECHANISM OF ACTION

A xanthine derivative that acts as a bronchodilator by directly relaxing smooth muscle of the bronchial airway and pulmonary blood vessels similar to theophylline.
Therapeutic Effect: Relieves bronchospasm, increases vital capacity, produces cardiac arrhythmias, and skeletal muscle stimulation.

USES

Treatment of bronchial asthma, bronchospasm in chronic bronchitis, COPD, emphysema

PHARMACOKINETICS

Rapid absorption after PO administration. Excreted in urine.
Half-life: 2 hr.

INDICATIONS AND DOSAGES

▸ **Chronic Bronchospasm, Asthma**

PO

Adults, Elderly. 15 mg/kg 4 times a day.

IM

Adults, Elderly. 250–500 mg. Maximum: 15 mg/kg q6h.
Children. 4.4–6.6 mg/kg/day in divided doses.

▸ **Dosage in Renal Impairment**

Creatinine Clearance	Dosage Percent
50–80 ml/min	Administer 75% of dose
10–50 ml/min	Administer 50% of dose
Less than 10 ml/min	Administer 25% of dose

SIDE EFFECTS/ADVERSE REACTIONS

Frequent
Tachycardia, nervousness, restlessness
Occasional
Heartburn, vomiting, headache, mild diuresis, insomnia, nausea

PRECAUTIONS AND CONTRAINDICATIONS

Uncontrolled arrhythmias, hyperthyroidism, history of hypersensitivity to dyphylline, related xanthine derivatives, or any component of the formulation
Caution:
Elderly, CHF, cor pulmonale, hepatic disease, active peptic ulcer disease, diabetes mellitus, hyperthyroidism, hypertension, children, renal disease, glaucoma

DRUG INTERACTIONS OF CONCERN TO DENTISTRY

- Increased action: erythromycin, ciprofloxacin, tetracyclines
- Increased risk of cardiac dysrhythmia: halothane-inhalation anesthesia, CNS stimulants
- Decreased effect: barbiturates, carbamazepine, ketoconazole
- May decrease sedative effects of benzodiazepines

SERIOUS REACTIONS

! Ventricular arrhythmias, hypotension, circulatory failure, seizures, hyperglycemia, and syndrome of inappropriate antidiuretic hormone (SIADH) have been reported.

DENTAL CONSIDERATIONS

General:
- Monitor vital signs at every appointment because of cardiovascular and respiratory side effects.
- Consider semisupine chair position for patients with respiratory disease.

echothiophate iodide

ek-oh-**thye**′-oh-fate **eye**′-oh-dide
(Phospholine iodide)

E

CATEGORY AND SCHEDULE

Pregnancy Risk Category: C

Drug Class: Antiglaucoma agent, ophthalmic; cyclostimulant, accommodative esotropia; diagnostic aid, accommodative esotropia

MECHANISM OF ACTION

A cholinesterase inhibitor that causes acetylcholine to accumulate at cholinergic receptor sites and produce effects like excessive stimulation of cholinergic receptors.
Therapeutic Effect: Causes conjunctival hyperemia and constriction of the sphincter pupillae and ciliary muscles, which results in miosis and paralysis of accommodation.

USES

Treatment of certain types of glaucoma and other eye conditions, such as accommodative esotropia. They may also be used in the diagnosis of certain eye conditions, such as accommodative esotropia.

PHARMACOKINETICS

None reported

INDICATIONS AND DOSAGES

▸ Glaucoma

Ophthalmic

Adults, Elderly. Instill 1 drop twice daily into eyes with 1 dose prior to bedtime.

▸ Accommodative Esotropia, Diagnosis

Ophthalmic

Children. Instill 1 drop once daily into both eyes at bedtime for 2–3 wk.

▸ Accommodative Esotropia, Treatment

Ophthalmic

Children. Instill 1 drop once daily.

SIDE EFFECTS/ADVERSE REACTIONS

Occasional

Headache, brow ache, blurred vision, burning and stinging of eyes, decreased night vision, intraocular pressure changes, iritis, uveitis

PRECAUTIONS AND CONTRAINDICATIONS

Active uveal inflammation, angle-closure glaucoma, hypersensitivity to echothiophate products

DRUG INTERACTIONS OF CONCERN TO DENTISTRY

- Avoid use of succinylcholine in general anesthesia
- Possible inhibition of the metabolism of ester-type local and topical anesthetics
- Avoid use of anticholinergics, such as systemic atropine or related drugs, benzodiazepine sedatives

SERIOUS REACTIONS

! Cardiac irregularities have been reported.

DENTAL CONSIDERATIONS

General:

- Determine why patient is taking the drug.
- Avoid drugs with anticholinergic activity, such as antihistamines,

opioids, benzodiazepines, propantheline, atropine, and scopolamine.
• Avoid dental light in patient's eyes; offer dark glasses for patient comfort.
• Question glaucoma patient about compliance with prescribed drug regimen.

Consultations:
• Medical consultation may be required to assess disease control.

Teach Patient/Family to:
• Update health and medication history if physician makes any changes in evaluation or drug regimens; include OTC, herbal, and nonherbal remedies in the update.

efalizumab

ef-ah-**liz′**-yoo-mab
(Raptiva)

CATEGORY AND SCHEDULE

Pregnancy Risk Category: C

Drug Class: Monoclonal antibody

MECHANISM OF ACTION

A monoclonal antibody that interferes with lymphocyte activation by binding to the lymphocyte antigen, inhibiting the adhesion of leukocytes to other cell types.
Therapeutic Effect: Prevents the release of cytokines and the growth and migration of circulating total lymphocytes, predominant in psoriatic lesions.

USES

Treatment of chronic moderate to severe plaque psoriasis in patients (older than 18 yr) who are candidates for systemic therapy or phototherapy

PHARMACOKINETICS

Clearance is affected by body weight, not by gender or race, after subcutaneous injection. Serum concentration reaches steady state at 4 wk. Mean time to elimination: 25 days.

INDICATIONS AND DOSAGES

▸ **Psoriasis**

Subcutaneous

Adults, Elderly. Initially, 0.7 mg/kg followed by weekly doses of 1 mg/kg. Maximum: 200 mg (single dose).

SIDE EFFECTS/ADVERSE REACTIONS

Frequent

Headache, chills, nausea, injection site pain

Occasional

Myalgia, flu-like symptoms, fever

Rare

Back pain, acne

PRECAUTIONS AND CONTRAINDICATIONS

Concurrent use of immunosuppressive agents

Caution:

Increased risk of infections, malignancies, worsening of psoriasis, use in elderly, safety and efficacy have not been established in lactation or children

DRUG INTERACTIONS OF CONCERN TO DENTISTRY

• None reported

SERIOUS REACTIONS

! Hypersensitivity reaction, malignancies, serious infections (abscess, cellulitis, postoperative wound infection, pneumonia), thrombocytopenia and worsening of psoriasis occur rarely.

DENTAL CONSIDERATIONS

General:

- Understand the disease and the patient's need to use this drug.
- Rarely, oral lesions and geographic tongue may occur in patients with psoriasis.

efavirenz

e-**fav**′-er-inz

(Stocrin[AUS], Sustiva)

Do not confuse Sustiva with Survanta.

CATEGORY AND SCHEDULE

Pregnancy Risk Category: C.

Drug Class: Antiviral (nonnucleoside)

MECHANISM OF ACTION

A nonnucleoside reverse transcriptase inhibitor that inhibits the activity of HIV reverse transcriptase of HIV-1 and the transcription of HIV-1 RNA to DNA.

Therapeutic Effect: Interrupts HIV replication, slowing the progression of HIV infection.

USES

Treatment in HIV-1 infection, only in combination with other HIV-1 antiretroviral agents

PHARMACOKINETICS

Rapidly absorbed after PO administration. Protein binding: 99%. Metabolized to major isoenzymes in the liver. Eliminated in urine and feces. ***Half-life:*** 40–55 hr.

INDICATIONS AND DOSAGES

▸ HIV Infection (in Combination with Other Antiretrovirals)

PO

Adults, Elderly, Children 3 yr and older weighing 40 kg or more. 600 mg once a day at bedtime.

Children 3 yr and older weighing 32.5 kg to less than 40 kg. 400 mg once a day.

Children 3 yr and older weighing 25 kg to less than 32.5 kg. 350 mg once a day.

Children 3 yr and older weighing 20 kg to less than 25 kg. 300 mg once a day.

Children 3 yr and older weighing 15 kg to less than 20 kg. 250 mg once a day.

Children 3 yr and older weighing 10 kg to less than 15 kg. 200 mg once a day.

SIDE EFFECTS/ADVERSE REACTIONS

Frequent

Mild to severe: Dizziness, vivid dreams, insomnia, confusion, impaired concentration, amnesia, agitation, depersonalization, hallucinations, euphoria, somnolence (mild symptoms don't interfere with daily activities; severe symptoms interrupt daily activities)

Occasional

Mild to moderate: Maculopapular rash; nausea, fatigue, headache, diarrhea, fever, cough (moderate symptoms may interfere with daily activities)

PRECAUTIONS AND CONTRAINDICATIONS

Concurrent use with ergot derivatives, midazolam, or triazolam;

efavirenz as monotherapy; hypersensitivity to efavirenz
Caution:
Must not be used as a single agent for HIV, avoid pregnancy with use, lactation, mental illness, substance abuse, caution with alcohol or psychotropic drugs, driving or other hazardous tasks, monitor cholesterol, hepatic impairment

DRUG INTERACTIONS OF CONCERN TO DENTISTRY

- Contraindicated drugs: midazolam, triazolam
- Decreased plasma levels of clarithromycin, carbamazepine, St. John's wort (herb)
- Potential for increased levels with ketoconazole, itraconazole
- Increased risk of CNS side effects with CNS depressants

SERIOUS REACTIONS

! None known

DENTAL CONSIDERATIONS

General:
- Examine for oral manifestations of opportunistic infection.
- Monitor vital signs at every appointment because of cardiovascular and respiratory side effects.
- Consider semisupine chair position for patient comfort because of GI side effects of drug.
- Assess salivary flow as a factor in caries, periodontal disease, and candidiasis.
- Short appointments and a stress-reduction protocol may be required for anxious patients.

Consultations:
- Medical consultation may be required to assess disease control.

Teach Patient/Family to:
- Prevent trauma when using oral hygiene aids.
- Encourage effective oral hygiene to prevent soft tissue inflammation.
- Be alert for the possibility of secondary oral infection and to see dentist immediately if signs of infection occur.
- When chronic dry mouth occurs, advise patient to:
  - Avoid mouth rinses with high alcohol content because of drying effects.
  - Use daily home fluoride products for anticaries effect.
  - Use sugarless gum, frequent sips of water, or saliva substitutes.

eletriptan

el-eh-**trip′**-tan
(Relpax)

CATEGORY AND SCHEDULE

Pregnancy Risk Category: C

Drug Class: Serotonin receptor agonist

MECHANISM OF ACTION

A serotonin receptor agonist that binds selectively to vascular receptors, producing a vasoconstrictive effect on cranial blood vessels.
Therapeutic Effect: Relieves migraine headache.

USES

Treatment of acute migraine with or without aura in adults

PHARMACOKINETICS

Well absorbed after PO administration. Metabolized by the

liver to inactive metabolite. Eliminated in urine. ***Half-life:*** 4.4 hr (increased in hepatic impairment and the elderly [older than 65 yr]).

E

INDICATIONS AND DOSAGES

▸ Acute Migraine Headache

PO

Adults, Elderly. 20–40 mg. If headache improves but then returns, dose may be repeated after 2 hr. Maximum: 80 mg/day.

SIDE EFFECTS/ADVERSE REACTIONS

Occasional

Dizziness, somnolence, asthenia, nausea

Rare

Paresthesia, headache, dry mouth, warm or hot sensation, dyspepsia, dysphagia

PRECAUTIONS AND CONTRAINDICATIONS

Arrhythmias associated with conduction disorders, coronary artery disease, ischemic heart disease, severe hepatic impairment, uncontrolled hypertension

Caution:

Do not use within 72 hr of treatment with CYP3A4 enzyme inhibitors, caution in lactation, safety and use in children younger than 18 yr has not been established

DRUG INTERACTIONS OF CONCERN TO DENTISTRY

• Avoid use of CYP3A4 inhibitors concurrently or within 72 hr of use of eletriptan: ketoconazole, itraconazole, erythromycin, clarithromycin, others

SERIOUS REACTIONS

! Cardiac reactions (including ischemia, coronary artery vasospasm and MI) and noncardiac vasospasm-related reactions (such as hemorrhage and CVA) occur rarely, particularly in patients with hypertension, diabetes, or a strong family history of coronary artery disease; obese patients; smokers; males older than 40 yr; and postmenopausal women.

DENTAL CONSIDERATIONS

General:

• This is an acute-use drug; it is doubtful that patients will seek dental treatment during acute migraine attacks.

• Be aware of the patient's disease, its severity and its frequency, when known.

• Monitor vital signs at every appointment because of cardiovascular side effects.

• Assess salivary flow as a factor in caries, periodontal disease, and candidiasis.

• Consider semisupine chair position for patient comfort if GI side effects occur.

Consultations:

• If treating chronic orofacial pain, consult with patient's physician.

Teach Patient/Family to:

• Be aware that oral symptoms will disappear when drug is discontinued.

emedastine

eh-med-**ah′**-steen

(Emadine)

CATEGORY AND SCHEDULE

Pregnancy Risk Category: B

Drug Class: Ophthalmic antihistamine

MECHANISM OF ACTION

An ophthalmic H_1-receptor antagonist that inhibits histamine-stimulated vascular permeability in the conjunctiva.
Therapeutic Effect: Relieves ocular itching associated with allergic conjunctivitis.

USES

Temporary relief of signs and symptoms of allergic conjunctivitis

PHARMACOKINETICS

Negligible absorption after ophthalmic administration. Metabolized into inactive metabolites. Excreted in urine.
Half-life: 6.6 hr.

INDICATIONS AND DOSAGES

▸ **Allergic Conjunctivitis**

Ophthalmic

Adults, Elderly, Children 3 yr and older. 1–2 drops in affected eye(s) twice daily.

SIDE EFFECTS/ADVERSE REACTIONS

Frequent

Headache

Occasional

Abnormal dreams, asthenia (loss of strength, energy), bad taste, blurred vision, burning or stinging, dry eyes, foreign body sensation, tearing

PRECAUTIONS AND CONTRAINDICATIONS

Hypersensitivity to emedastine or any other component of the formulation

Caution:

Avoid wearing contact lens if eye is red, wait at least 10 min after application to insert contact lens, lactation, no data for use in children younger than 3 yr

DRUG INTERACTIONS OF CONCERN TO DENTISTRY

- None reported

SERIOUS REACTIONS

! Somnolence and malaise occurs rarely.

E

emtricitabine

em-trih-**sit′**-ah-bean

(Emtriva)

CATEGORY AND SCHEDULE

Pregnancy Risk Category: B

Drug Class: Antiviral, nucleoside reverse transcriptase inhibitor

MECHANISM OF ACTION

An antiretroviral that inhibits HIV-1 reverse transcriptase by incorporating itself into viral DNA, resulting in chain termination.
Therapeutic Effect: Interrupts HIV replication, slowing the progression of HIV infection.

USES

Treatment of HIV-1 infection in adults; used in combination with other antiretroviral medications

PHARMACOKINETICS

Rapidly and extensively absorbed from the GI tract. Excreted primarily in urine (86%) and, to a lesser extent, in feces (14%); 30% removed by hemodialysis. Unknown if removed by peritoneal dialysis.
Half-life: 10 hr.

E

INDICATIONS AND DOSAGES

▸ **HIV Infection (in Combination with Other Antiretrovirals)**

PO

Adults, Elderly. 200 mg once a day.

▸ **Dosage in Renal Impairment**

Dosage and frequency are modified on the basis of creatinine clearance.

Creatinine Clearance	Dosage
30–49 ml/min	200 mg q48h
15–29 ml/min	200 mg q72h
Less than 15 ml/min, hemodialysis patients	200 mg q96h

SIDE EFFECTS/ADVERSE REACTIONS

Frequent

Headache, rhinitis, rash, diarrhea, nausea

Occasional

Cough, vomiting, abdominal pain, insomnia, depression, paresthesia, dizziness, peripheral neuropathy, dyspepsia, myalgia

Rare

Arthralgia, abnormal dreams

PRECAUTIONS AND CONTRAINDICATIONS

Hypersensitivity

Caution:

Possible risk of lactic acidosis, severe hepatomegaly with steatosis, use not established in HIV/HBV infections, renal impairment (dose reduction required), avoid nursing when taking this drug, safety and efficacy in pediatric patients have not been established

DRUG INTERACTIONS OF CONCERN TO DENTISTRY

- None reported

SERIOUS REACTIONS

! Lactic acidosis and hepatomegaly with steatosis occur rarely and may be severe.

DENTAL CONSIDERATIONS

General:

- Examine for oral manifestations of opportunistic infection.
- Consider semisupine chair position for patient comfort if GI side effects occur.
- Patient history should include all medications and herbal or nonherbal remedies taken by the patient.

Consultations:

- Medical consultation may be required to assess disease control and patient's ability to tolerate stress.

Teach Patient/Family to:

- Encourage effective oral hygiene to prevent soft tissue inflammation, infection.
- Prevent trauma when using oral hygiene aids.
- Update health and drug history, reporting changes in health status, drug regimen changes or disease/treatment status.

emtricitabine + rilpivirine + tenofovir disoproxil

em-tri-**site′**-uh-been, ril-pi-**vir′**-een, & te noe fo veer

(Complera)

CATEGORY AND SCHEDULE

Pregnancy Risk Category: B

Drug Class: Antiretroviral agent, reverse transcriptase inhibitor (nonnucleoside); antiretroviral agent, reverse transcriptase inhibitor (nucleoside); antiretroviral agent, reverse transcriptase inhibitor (nucleotide)

MECHANISM OF ACTION

Nonnucleoside, nucleoside, and nucleotide reverse transcriptase inhibitor combination; rilpivirine binds to reverse transcriptase, emtricitabine is a cytosine analogue, and tenofovir is an analogue of adenosine 5'-monophosphate. Each drug interferes with HIV viral RNA dependent DNA polymerase activities, resulting in inhibition of viral replication.
Therapeutic Effect: Slows HIV replication and reduces viral load.

USES

Treatment of human immunodeficiency virus type 1 (HIV-1) infection in antiretroviral treatment-naive adult patients

PHARMACOKINETICS

Emtricitabine: Rapidly and extensively absorbed after oral administration. Less than 4% plasma protein bound. Eliminated by a combination of glomerular filtration and active tubular secretion. Excreted primarily in urine (86%) and, to a lesser extent, in feces (14%). Rilpivirine: Rapid absorption after oral administration. 99% plasma protein bound. Hepatic metabolism via CYP3A enzymes. Eliminated in feces (85%) and urine (6%). Tenofovir: Moderate absorption following oral administration. Plasma protein binding less than 7%; minimal systemic metabolism; excreted by glomerular filtration and active tubular secretion. ***Half-life:*** Emtricitabine: 10 hr. Rilpivirine: 50 hr. Tenofovir: 17 hr.

INDICATIONS AND DOSAGES

▸ **HIV**

PO

Adults. 1 tablet once daily. Administer with a meal (preferably high fat).

SIDE EFFECTS/ADVERSE REACTIONS

Frequent

Increased serum cholesterol and LDL, increased ALT and AST

Occasional

Anxiety, depression, diarrhea, dizziness, fatigue, nausea, rash, somnolence, sleep disorders

PRECAUTIONS AND CONTRAINDICATIONS

Not recommended for use in patients with severe hepatic and renal impairment. May cause immune reconstitution syndrome, depressive disorder, renal toxicity, and decreased bone mineral density.

DRUG INTERACTIONS OF CONCERN TO DENTISTRY

• CYP3A4 inhibitors (e.g., macrolide antibiotics): increased risk of adverse effects of Complera
• CYP3A4 inducers (e.g., barbiturates): reduced blood levels and effectiveness of Complera

SERIOUS REACTIONS

! Lactic acidosis and severe hepatomegaly have been reported with nucleoside analogues (e.g., tenofovir), including fatal cases. Safety and efficacy during coinfection of HIV and HBV have not been established; acute, severe exacerbations of HBV have been reported following discontinuation of antiretroviral therapy.

E

E

DENTAL CONSIDERATIONS

General:

• Monitor for possible dizziness and take precautions when seating and dismissing patient.

• Consider adverse effects of Complera when prescribing drugs with CNS actions.

• Monitor for oral manifestations of opportunistic infections.

Teach Patient/Family to:

• Report changes in disease status and drug regimen.

enalapril maleate

en-**al**′-ah-pril **ma**′-lee-ate

(Alphapril[AUS], Amprace[AUS], Apo-Enalapril[CAN], Auspril[AUS], Renitec[AUS], Vasotec)

Do not confuse enalapril with Anafranil, Eldepryl, or ramipril.

CATEGORY AND SCHEDULE

Pregnancy Risk Category: D (C if used in first trimester)

Drug Class: Angiotensin-converting enzyme (ACE) inhibitor

MECHANISM OF ACTION

This ACE inhibitor suppresses the renin-angiotensin-aldosterone system and prevents conversion of angiotensin I to angiotensin II, a potent vasoconstrictor; may inhibit angiotensin II at local vascular, renal sites. Decreases plasma angiotensin II, increases plasma renin activity, decreases aldosterone secretion.

Therapeutic Effect: In hypertension, reduces peripheral arterial resistance. In CHF, increases cardiac output; decreases peripheral vascular resistance, B/P, pulmonary capillary wedge pressure, heart size.

USES

Treatment of hypertension, heart failure adjunct, asymptomatic left ventricular dysfunction

PHARMACOKINETICS

Route	Onset	Peak	Duration
PO	1 hr	4–6 hr	24 hr
IV	15 min	1–4 hr	6 hr

Readily absorbed from the GI tract (not affected by food). Protein binding: 50%–60%. Converted to active metabolite. Primarily excreted in urine. Removed by hemodialysis. ***Half-life:*** 11 hr (half-life is increased with impaired renal function).

INDICATIONS AND DOSAGES

▸ **Hypertension Alone or in Combination with Other Antihypertensives**

PO

Adults, Elderly. Initially, 2.5–5 mg/day. Range: 10–40 mg/day in 1–2 divided doses.

Children. 0.1 mg/kg/day in 1–2 divided doses. Maximum: 0.5 mg/kg/day.

Neonates. 0.1 mg/kg/day q24h.

IV

Adults, Elderly. 0.625–1.25 mg q6h up to 5 mg q6h.

Children, Neonates. 5–10 mcg/kg/dose q8–24h.

▸ **Adjunctive Therapy for CHF**

PO

Adults, Elderly. Initially, 2.5–5 mg/day. Range: 5–20 mg/day in 2 divided doses.

▸ **Dosage in Renal Impairment**

Dosage is modified on the basis of creatinine clearance.

Creatinine Clearance	% of Usual Dose
10–50 ml/min	75–100
Less than 10 ml/min	50

SIDE EFFECTS/ADVERSE REACTIONS

Frequent
Headache, dizziness
Occasional
Orthostatic hypotension, fatigue, diarrhea, cough, syncope
Rare
Angina, abdominal pain, vomiting, nausea, rash, asthenia (loss of strength, energy), syncope

PRECAUTIONS AND CONTRAINDICATIONS

History of angioedema from previous treatment with ACE inhibitors
Caution:
Renal disease, hyperkalemia

DRUG INTERACTIONS OF CONCERN TO DENTISTRY

• Increased hypotension: alcohol, phenothiazines
• Decreased hypotensive effects: indomethacin, possibly other NSAIDs, sympathomimetics
• Suspected reduction in the antihypertensive and vasodilator effects by salicylates; monitor B/P if used concurrently

SERIOUS REACTIONS

! Excessive hypotension (“first-dose syncope”) may occur in patients with CHF and in those who are severely salt or volume depleted.
! Angioedema (swelling of face, lips) and hyperkalemia occur rarely.
! Agranulocytosis and neutropenia may be noted in patients with collagen vascular diseases, including scleroderma and systemic lupus erythematosus and impaired renal function.
! Nephrotic syndrome may be noted in those with history of renal disease.

DENTAL CONSIDERATIONS

General:
• Monitor vital signs at every appointment because of cardiovascular side effects.
• After supine positioning, have patient sit upright for at least 2 min before standing to avoid orthostatic hypotension.
• Patients on chronic drug therapy may rarely have symptoms of blood dyscrasias, which can include infection, bleeding, and poor healing.
• Assess salivary flow as a factor in caries, periodontal disease, and candidiasis.
• Limit use of sodium-containing products, such as saline IV fluids, for those patients with a dietary salt restriction.
• Use vasoconstrictors with caution, in low doses and with careful aspiration.
• Stress from dental procedures may compromise cardiovascular function; determine patient risk.
• Short appointments and a stress-reduction protocol may be required for anxious patients.
Consultations:
• Medical consultation may be required to assess patient’s ability to tolerate stress.
• In a patient with symptoms of blood dyscrasias, request a medical consultation for blood studies and postpone dental treatment until normal values are reestablished.
• Take precautions if dental surgery is anticipated and sedation or general anesthesia is required; risk of hypotensive episode.
Teach Patient/Family to:
• Encourage effective oral hygiene to prevent soft tissue inflammation.

- When chronic dry mouth occurs, advise patient to:
  - Avoid mouth rinses with high alcohol content because of drying effects.
  - Use daily home fluoride products for anticaries effect.
  - Use sugarless gum, frequent sips of water, or saliva substitutes.

enfuvirtide

en-**few**′-vir-tide

(Fuzeon)

Do not confuse Fuzeon with Furoxone.

CATEGORY AND SCHEDULE

Pregnancy Risk Category: B

Drug Class: Antiviral

MECHANISM OF ACTION

A fusion inhibitor that interferes with the entry of HIV-1 into CD4+ cells by inhibiting the fusion of viral and cellular membranes.

Therapeutic Effect: Impairs HIV replication, slowing the progression of HIV infection.

USES

Treatment, in combination with other antiretroviral agents, of HIV-1 infection in treatment-experienced patients with HIV-1 replication despite ongoing antiretroviral therapy

PHARMACOKINETICS

Comparable absorption when injected into subcutaneous tissue of abdomen, arm, or thigh. Protein binding: 92%. Undergoes catabolism to amino acids. ***Half-life:*** 3.8 hr.

INDICATIONS AND DOSAGES

▸ **HIV Infection (in combination with other antiretrovirals)**

Subcutaneous

Adults, Elderly. 90 mg (1 ml) twice a day.

Children 6–16 yr. 2 mg/kg twice a day. Maximum 90 mg twice a day.

Pediatric dosing guidelines

Weight: lb (kg)	Dose: mg (ml)
11–15.5 (24–34)	27 (0.3)
15.6–20 (35–44)	36 (0.4)
20.1–24.5 (45–54)	45 (0.5)
24.6–29 (55–64)	54 (0.6)
29.1–33.5 (65–74)	63 (0.7)
33.6–38 (75–84)	72 (0.8)
38.1–42.5 (85–94)	81 (0.9)
Greater than 42.5 (greater than 94)	90 (1)

SIDE EFFECTS/ADVERSE REACTIONS

Expected

Local injection site reactions (pain, discomfort, induration, erythema, nodules, cysts, pruritus, ecchymosis)

Frequent

Diarrhea, nausea, fatigue

Occasional

Insomnia, peripheral neuropathy, depression, cough, decreased appetite or weight loss, sinusitis, anxiety, asthenia, myalgia, cold sores

Rare

Constipation, influenza, upper abdominal pain, anorexia, conjunctivitis

PRECAUTIONS AND CONTRAINDICATIONS

Hypersensitivity; patients should be instructed in recognizing local injection site reactions and trained in aseptic technique, HIV-infected mothers must not nurse, use in children younger than 6 yr has not been established

DRUG INTERACTIONS OF CONCERN TO DENTISTRY

- None reported

SERIOUS REACTIONS

! Enfuvirtide use may potentiate bacterial pneumonia.
! Hypersensitivity (rash, fever, chills, rigors, hypotension), thrombocytopenia, neutropenia, and renal insufficiency or failure may occur rarely.

DENTAL CONSIDERATIONS

General:

- Patients taking this drug will be taking other antiviral drugs that may interact with some dental drugs. Be sure to take a complete drug history.
- Patients on chronic drug therapy may rarely have symptoms of blood dyscrasias, which can include infection, bleeding, and poor healing.
- Examine for oral manifestation of opportunistic infection.

Consultations:

- Medical consultation may be required to assess disease control in the patient.
- In a patient with symptoms of blood dyscrasias, request a medical consultation for blood studies and postpone treatment until normal values are reestablished.

Teach Patient/Family to:

- Encourage effective oral hygiene to prevent soft tissue inflammation.
- Prevent trauma when using oral hygiene aids.
- Update health and drug history if physician makes any changes in evaluation or drug regimens.

enoxaparin sodium

ee-nox-**ap′**-air-in **soe′**-dee-um
(Clexane[AUS], Klexane[CAN], Lovenox)
Do not confuse Lovenox with Lotronex.

CATEGORY AND SCHEDULE

Pregnancy Risk Category: B

Drug Class: Heparin-type anticoagulant

MECHANISM OF ACTION

A low-molecular-weight heparin that potentiates the action of antithrombin III and inactivates coagulation factor Xa.
Therapeutic Effect: Produces anticoagulation. Does not significantly influence bleeding time, PT, or aPTT.

USES

Prevention and treatment of deep vein thrombosis (DVT) following hip or knee replacement surgery; also used in abdominal and gynecologic surgery; with aspirin in the prevention of ischemic complications of unstable angina and non–Q-wave MI; in combination with warfarin for DVT, with or without pulmonary embolism

PHARMACOKINETICS

Route	Onset	Peak	Duration
Subcutaneous	N/A	3–5 hr	12 hr

Well absorbed after subcutaneous administration. Eliminated primarily in urine. Not removed by hemodialysis. ***Half-life:*** 4.5 hr.

INDICATIONS AND DOSAGES

▸ **Prevention of DVT after Hip and Knee Surgery**

Subcutaneous

Adults, Elderly. 30 mg twice a day, generally for 7–10 days.

▸ **Prevention of DVT after Abdominal Surgery**

Subcutaneous

Adults, Elderly. 40 mg a day for 7–10 days.

▸ **Prevention of Long-Term DVT in Nonsurgical Acute Illness**

Subcutaneous

Adults, Elderly. 40 mg once a day for 3 wk.

▸ **Prevention of Ischemic Complications of Unstable Angina and Non–Q-Wave MI (with Oral Aspirin Therapy)**

Subcutaneous

Adults, Elderly. 1 mg/kg q12h.

▸ **Acute DVT**

Subcutaneous

Adults, Elderly. 1 mg/kg q12h or 1.5 mg/kg once daily.

▸ **Usual Pediatric Dosage**

Subcutaneous

Children. 0.5 mg/kg q12h (prophylaxis); 1 mg/kg q12h (treatment).

▸ **Dosage in Renal Impairment**

Clearance of enoxaparin is decreased when creatinine clearance is less than 30 ml/min. Monitor patient and adjust dosage as necessary. When enoxaparin is used in abdominal, hip, or knee surgery or acute illness, the dosage in renal impairment is 30 mg once a day. When enoxaparin is used to treat DVT, angina, or MI the dosage in renal impairment is 1 mg/kg once a day.

SIDE EFFECTS/ADVERSE REACTIONS

Occasional

Injection site hematoma, nausea, peripheral edema

PRECAUTIONS AND CONTRAINDICATIONS

Active major bleeding, concurrent heparin therapy, hypersensitivity to heparin or pork products, thrombocytopenia associated with positive in vitro test for antiplatelet antibodies

Caution:

Hemorrhage, thrombocytopenia, renal impairment, elderly, lactation, children, requires monitoring, GI bleeding

DRUG INTERACTIONS OF CONCERN TO DENTISTRY

- Avoid concurrent use of aspirin, NSAIDs, dipyridamole, sulfinpyrazone
- Use with caution in patients taking olanzapine

SERIOUS REACTIONS

! Overdose may lead to bleeding complications ranging from local ecchymoses to major hemorrhage. Antidote: Protamine sulfate (1% solution) equal to the dose of enoxaparin injected. 1 mg protamine sulfate neutralizes 1 mg enoxaparin. A second dose of 0.5 mg protamine sulfate per 1 mg enoxaparin may be given if aPTT tested 2–4 hr after first injection remains prolonged.

DENTAL CONSIDERATIONS

General:

- Determine why patient is taking the drug.
- Product may be used in outpatient therapy. Delay elective dental

treatment until patient completes enoxaparin therapy.
• Do not discontinue enoxaparin.
• Consider local hemostasis measures to prevent excessive bleeding if dental treatment must be performed.
• Avoid products that affect platelet function, such as aspirin and NSAIDs.
Consultations:
• Medical consultation should include routine blood counts, including platelet counts and bleeding time.
Teach Patient/Family to:
• Encourage effective oral hygiene to prevent soft tissue inflammation.
• Use caution to prevent trauma when using oral hygiene aids.
• Report oral lesions, soreness, or bleeding to dentist.

entacapone

en-**tak**′-ah-pone
(Comtan)

CATEGORY AND SCHEDULE

Pregnancy Risk Category: C

Drug Class: Antiparkinsonian

MECHANISM OF ACTION

An antiparkinson agent that inhibits the enzyme catechol-O-methyltransferase (COMT), potentiating dopamine activity and increasing the duration of action of levodopa.
Therapeutic Effect: Decreases signs and symptoms of Parkinson's disease.

USES

Adjunct to levodopa/carbidopa in the treatment of Parkinson's disease, not used alone

PHARMACOKINETICS

Rapidly absorbed after PO administration. Protein binding: 98%. Metabolized in the liver. Primarily eliminated by biliary excretion. Not removed by hemodialysis. ***Half-life:*** 2.4 hr.

INDICATIONS AND DOSAGES

▸ Adjunctive Treatment of Parkinson's Disease

PO

Adults, Elderly. 200 mg concomitantly with each dose of carbidopa and levodopa up to a maximum of 8 times a day (1600 mg).

SIDE EFFECTS/ADVERSE REACTIONS

Frequent

Dyskinesia, nausea, dark yellow or orange urine and sweat, diarrhea

Occasional

Abdominal pain, vomiting, constipation, dry mouth, fatigue, back pain

Rare

Anxiety, somnolence, agitation, dyspepsia, flatulence, diaphoresis, asthenia, dyspnea

PRECAUTIONS AND CONTRAINDICATIONS

Hypersensitivity, use within 14 days of MAOIs

Caution:

Enhanced orthostatic hypotension with levodopa and carbidopa, hepatic impairment, caution in driving, lactation, children

DRUG INTERACTIONS OF CONCERN TO DENTISTRY

• Increased heart rate, arrhythmias, hypertension: epinephrine, norepinephrine, levonordefrin, other sympathomimetics metabolized by COMT
• Possible decrease in urinary excretion: erythromycin

SERIOUS REACTIONS

! None known

DENTAL CONSIDERATIONS

General:
• Monitor vital signs at every appointment because of cardiovascular side effects.
• Short appointments and a stress-reduction protocol may be required for anxious patients.
• Consider semisupine chair position for patient comfort if GI side effects occur.
• Use vasoconstrictor with caution, in low doses and with careful aspiration. Avoid using gingival retraction cord containing epinephrine.
• Assess for presence of extrapyramidal motor symptoms, such as tardive dyskinesia and akathisia. Extrapyramidal motor activity may complicate dental treatment.
• After supine positioning, have patient sit upright for at least 2 min to avoid orthostatic hypotension.
• Assess salivary flow as a factor in caries, periodontal disease and candidiasis.

Consultations:
• Medical consultation may be required to assess disease control and patient's ability to tolerate stress.

Teach Patient/Family to:
• Use powered tooth brush if patient has difficulty holding conventional devices.
• Update health and drug history if physician makes any changes in evaluation or drug regimens.
• When chronic dry mouth occurs, advise patient to:
  • Avoid mouth rinses with high alcohol content because of drying effects.
  • Use daily home fluoride products for anticaries effect.
  • Use sugarless gum, frequent sips of water, or saliva substitutes.

ephedrine

eh-**fed**′-rin
(Pretz-D)
Do not confuse ephedrine with epinephrine.

CATEGORY AND SCHEDULE

Pregnancy Risk Category: C

Drug Class: Adrenergic, mixed direct and indirect effects

MECHANISM OF ACTION

An adrenergic agonist that stimulates alpha-adrenergic receptors causing vasoconstriction and pressor effects, β_1-adrenergic receptors, resulting in cardiac stimulation, and β_2-adrenergic receptors, resulting in bronchial dilation and vasodilation.
Therapeutic Effect: Increases B/P and pulse rate, reduces nasal congestion.

USES

Treatment of shock, increased perfusion, hypotension, bronchodilation, nasal decongestant

PHARMACOKINETICS

Well absorbed after nasal and parenteral absorption. Metabolized in liver. Excreted in urine. ***Half-life:*** 3–6 hr.

INDICATIONS AND DOSAGES

▸ **Asthma**

PO

Adults. 25–50 mg q3–4h as needed.
Children. 3 mg/kg/day in 4 divided doses.

▸ **Hypotension**

IM

Adults. 25–50 mg as a single dose. Maximum 150 mg/day.
Children. 0.2–0.3 mg/kg/dose q4–6h.

IV

Adults. 5 mg/dose slow IVP as prevention. 10–25 mg/dose slow IVP repeated q5–10 min as treatment. Maximum: 150 mg/day.
Children. 0.2–0.3 mg/kg/dose slow IVP q4–6h.

Subcutaneous

Adults. 25–50 q4–6h. Maximum 150 mg/day.
Children. 3 mg/kg/day q4–6h.

▸ **Nasal Congestion**

PO

Adults. 25–50 mg q6h as needed.
Children. 3 mg/kg/day in 4 divided doses.

Nasal

Adults, Children 12 yr and older. 2–3 sprays into each nostril q4h.
Children 6–12 yr. 1–2 sprays into each nostril q4h.

SIDE EFFECTS/ADVERSE REACTIONS

Frequent

Hypertension, anxiety

Occasional

Nausea, vomiting, palpitations, tremor
Nasal: Burning, stinging, runny nose

Rare

Psychosis, decreased urination, necrosis at injection site from repeated injections

PRECAUTIONS AND CONTRAINDICATIONS

Anesthesia with cyclopropane or halothane, diabetes (ephedrine injection), hypersensitivity to ephedrine or other sympathomimetic amines, hypertension or other cardiovascular disorders, pregnancy with maternal B/P above 130/80, thyrotoxicosis

Caution:

Cardiac disorders, hyperthyroidism, diabetes mellitus, prostatic hypertrophy

DRUG INTERACTIONS OF CONCERN TO DENTISTRY

• Decreased pressor effect: haloperidol, phenothiazines, thioxanthenes
• Dysrhythmia: halogenated general anesthetics

SERIOUS REACTIONS

! Excessive doses may cause hypertension, intracranial hemorrhage, anginal pain, and fatal arrhythmias.
! Prolonged or excessive use may result in metabolic acidosis due to increased serum lactic acid concentrations.
! Observe for disorientation, weakness, hyperventilation, headache, nausea, vomiting, and diarrhea.

DENTAL CONSIDERATIONS

General:

• Monitor vital signs at every appointment because of cardiovascular side effects.

E

- Avoid or limit dose of vasoconstrictor.
- Assess salivary flow as a factor in caries, periodontal disease, and candidiasis.
- Consider semisupine chair position for patients with respiratory disease.
- Consider short appointments and a stress-reduction protocol for anxious patients.

Consultations:

- Medical consultation may be required to assess disease control and patient's tolerance for stress.

Teach Patient/Family:

- When chronic dry mouth occurs, advise patient to:
  - Avoid mouth rinses with high alcohol content because of drying effects.
  - Use daily home fluoride products for anticaries effect.
  - Use sugarless gum, frequent sips of water, or saliva substitutes.

epinastine

eh-pin-**ass**′-teen
(Elestat)

CATEGORY AND SCHEDULE

Pregnancy Risk Category: C

Drug Class: Ophthalmic antihistamine

MECHANISM OF ACTION

An ophthalmic H_1 receptor antagonist that inhibits the release of histamine from the mast cell.
Therapeutic Effect: Prevents pruritus associated with allergic conjunctivitis.

USES

Prevention of itching associated with allergic conjunctivitis

PHARMACOKINETICS

Low systemic exposure. Protein binding: 64%. Less than 10% is metabolized. Excreted primarily in urine and, to a lesser extent, in feces. ***Half-life:*** 12 hr.

INDICATIONS AND DOSAGES

▸ **Allergic Conjunctivitis**

Ophthalmic

Adults, Elderly, Children 3 yr and older. 1 drop in each eye twice a day. Continue treatment until period of exposure (pollen season, exposure to offending allergen) is over.

SIDE EFFECTS/ADVERSE REACTIONS

Occasional

Ocular (10%–1%): Burning sensation in the eye, hyperemia, pruritus
Nonocular (10%): Cold symptoms, upper respiratory tract infection

Rare

Headache, rhinitis, sinusitis, increased cough, pharyngitis

PRECAUTIONS AND CONTRAINDICATIONS

Hypersensitivity

Caution:

Do not wear contact lens if the eye is red, otherwise contact may be placed in eye 10 min after dosing; use in nursing and in children younger than 3 yr has not been established

DRUG INTERACTIONS OF CONCERN TO DENTISTRY

- None reported

SERIOUS REACTIONS

! None known

DENTAL CONSIDERATIONS

General:

• Avoid dental light in patient's eyes; offer dark glasses for patient comfort.

epinephrine

ep-ih-**nef'**-rin

(Adrenalin, Adrenaline Injection[AUS], EpiPen, EpiPen Jr. 0.15 Adrenaline Autoinjector[AUS], Primatene)

Do not confuse epinephrine with ephedrine.

CATEGORY AND SCHEDULE

Pregnancy Risk Category: C

Drug Class: Adrenergic agonist, catecholamine

MECHANISM OF ACTION

A sympathomimetic, adrenergic agonist that stimulates alpha-adrenergic receptors causing vasoconstriction and pressor effects, β_1-adrenergic receptors, resulting in cardiac stimulation, and β_2-adrenergic receptors, resulting in bronchial dilation and vasodilation. With ophthalmic form, increases outflow of aqueous humor from anterior eye chamber.

Therapeutic Effect: Relaxes smooth muscle of the bronchial tree, produces cardiac stimulation and dilates skeletal muscle vasculature. The ophthalmic form dilates pupils and constricts conjunctival blood vessels.

USES

Treatment of acute asthmatic attacks, hemostasis, bronchospasm, anaphylaxis, allergic reactions, cardiac arrest, vasopressor, open-angle glaucoma, nasal congestion

PHARMACOKINETICS

Route	Onset	Peak	Duration
IM	5–10 min	20 min	1–4 hr
Subcutaneous	5–10 min	20 min	1–4 hr
Inhalation	3–5 min	20 min	1–3 hr
Ophthalmic	1 hr	4–8 hr	12–24 hr

Well absorbed after parenteral administration; minimally absorbed after inhalation. Metabolized in the liver, other tissues and sympathetic nerve endings. Excreted in urine. The ophthalmic form may be systemically absorbed as a result of drainage into nasal pharyngeal passages. Mydriasis occurs within several min and persists several hr; vasoconstriction occurs within 5 min and lasts less than 1 hr.

INDICATIONS AND DOSAGES

▸ **Asystole**

IV

Adults, Elderly. 1 mg q3–5 min up to 0.1 mg/kg q3–5 min.

Children. 0.01 mg/kg (0.1 ml/kg of 1:10,000 solution). May repeat q3–5 min. Subsequent doses of 0.1 mg/kg (0.1 ml/kg) of a 1:1000 solution q3–5 min.

▸ **Bradycardia**

IV Infusion

Adults, Elderly. 1–10 mcg/min titrated to desired effect.

IV

Children. 0.01 mg/kg (0.1 mg/kg of 1:10,000 solution) q3–5 min. Maximum: 1 mg/10 ml.

▸ **Bronchodilation**

IM, Subcutaneous

Adults, Elderly. 0.3 mg (1:1000) q10–15 min to 4 hr.

Subcutaneous

Children. 10 mcg/kg (0.01 ml/kg of 1:1,000) Maximum: 0.5 mg or suspension (1:200) 0.005 ml/kg/dose (0.025 mg/kg/dose) to a maximum of 0.15 ml (0.75 mg for single dose) q8–12h.

▸ **Hypersensitivity Reaction**

IM, Subcutaneous

Adults, Elderly. 0.3 mg q15–20 min.

Subcutaneous

Children. 0.01 mg/kg q15 min for 2 doses, then q4h. Maximum single dose: 0.5 mg.

Inhalation

Adults, Elderly, Children 4 yr and older. 1 inhalation, may repeat in at least 1 min. Give subsequent doses no sooner than 3 hr.

Nebulizer

Adults, Elderly, Children 4 yr and older. 1–3 deep inhalations. Give subsequent doses no sooner than 3 hr.

▸ **Glaucoma**

Ophthalmic

Adults, Elderly. 1–2 drops 1–2 times a day.

SIDE EFFECTS/ADVERSE REACTIONS

Frequent

Systemic: Tachycardia, palpitations, nervousness

Ophthalmic: Headache, eye irritation, watering of eyes

Occasional

Systemic: Dizziness, lightheadedness, facial flushing, headache, diaphoresis, increased B/P, nausea, trembling, insomnia, vomiting, fatigue

Ophthalmic: Blurred or decreased vision, eye pain

Rare

Systemic: Chest discomfort or pain, arrhythmias, bronchospasm, dry mouth or throat

PRECAUTIONS AND CONTRAINDICATIONS

Cardiac arrhythmias, cerebrovascular insufficiency, hypertension, hyperthyroidism, ischemic heart disease, narrow-angle glaucoma, shock

Caution:

Cardiac disorders, hyperthyroidism, diabetes mellitus, prostatic hypertrophy

DRUG INTERACTIONS OF CONCERN TO DENTISTRY

- Hypotension, tachycardia: haloperidol, loxapine, phenothiazines, thioxanthenes
- Ventricular dysrhythmia: hydrocarbon-inhalation anesthetics, CNS stimulants, tricyclic antidepressants
- With larger doses of epinephrine, risk of hypertension followed by bradycardia with non-cardioselective β-adrenergic antagonists

SERIOUS REACTIONS

! Excessive doses may cause acute hypertension or arrhythmias.

! Prolonged or excessive use may result in metabolic acidosis because of increased serum lactic acid concentrations. Metabolic acidosis may cause disorientation, fatigue, hyperventilation, headache, nausea, vomiting, and diarrhea.

DENTAL CONSIDERATIONS

General:

- Monitor vital signs at every appointment because of cardiovascular side effects.
- Assess salivary flow as a factor in caries, periodontal disease, and candidiasis.
- Consider semisupine chair position for patients with respiratory disease.

• Acute asthmatic episodes may be precipitated in the dental office. Sympathomimetic inhalants should be available for emergency use; a stress-reduction protocol may be required.

epinephryl borate

ep-ih-**nef**′-rill **bor**′-ate

(Epifrin, Epinal, Eppy/N)

CATEGORY AND SCHEDULE

Pregnancy Risk Category: C

Drug Class: Antiglaucoma agent, ophthalmic; surgical aid, ophthalmic

MECHANISM OF ACTION

A direct-acting sympathomimetic amine whose mechanism of action is unknown.

Therapeutic Effect: Increases outflow of aqueous humor from anterior eye chamber.

USES

Treatment of certain types of glaucoma. It may also be used in eye surgery.

PHARMACOKINETICS

May have systemic absorption from drainage into nasal pharyngeal passages. Mydriasis occurs within several min, persists several hr; vasoconstriction occurs within 5 min, lasts less than 1 hr.

INDICATIONS AND DOSAGES

▸ **Glaucoma**

Ophthalmic

Adults, Elderly. Instill 1 drop 1–2 times a day.

SIDE EFFECTS/ADVERSE REACTIONS

Frequent

Headache, stinging, burning or other eye irritation, watering of eyes

Occasional

Blurred or decreased vision, eye pain

PRECAUTIONS AND CONTRAINDICATIONS

Cardiac arrhythmias, cerebrovascular insufficiency, hypertension, hyperthyroidism, ischemic heart disease, narrow-angle glaucoma, shock, hypersensitivity to epinephryl borate or any component of the formulation

DRUG INTERACTIONS OF CONCERN TO DENTISTRY

• Risk of arrhythmias: halogenated hydrocarbon anesthetics, tricyclic antidepressants, amphetamine-like drugs

SERIOUS REACTIONS

! Systemic absorption occurs rarely. These effects include fast, irregular, or pounding heartbeat, feeling faint, increased sweating, paleness, trembling and increased B/P.

DENTAL CONSIDERATIONS

General:

• Determine why patient is taking the drug.

• Avoid drugs with anticholinergic activity, such as antihistamines, opioids, benzodiazepines, propantheline, atropine, and scopolamine.

• Avoid dental light in patient's eyes; offer dark glasses for patient comfort.

• Question glaucoma patient about compliance with prescribed drug regimen.

Consultations:

• Medical consultation may be required to assess disease control.

Teach Patient/Family to:

• Update health and medication history if physician makes any changes in evaluation or drug regimens; include OTC, herbal, and nonherbal remedies in the update.

E

epirubicin

eh-pea-**rew′**-bih-sin
(Ellence, Pharm Rubicin)

CATEGORY AND SCHEDULE

Pregnancy Risk Category: D

Drug Class: Anthracycline antibiotic; antineoplastic

MECHANISM OF ACTION

An anthracycline antibiotic whose exact mechanism is unknown but may include formation of a complex with DNA and subsequent inhibition of DNA, RNA, and protein synthesis. Also inhibits DNA helicase activity, preventing enzymatic separation of double-stranded DNA and interfering with replication and transcription.
Therapeutic Effect: Produces antiproliferative and cytotoxic activity.

USES

Treatment of some kinds of cancers of the breast, lung, lymph system, stomach, and ovaries

PHARMACOKINETICS

Widely distributed into tissues. Protein binding: 77%. Metabolized in the liver and RBCs. Primarily eliminated through biliary excretion. Not removed by hemodialysis.
Half-life: 33 hr.

INDICATIONS AND DOSAGES

▸ **Breast Cancer**

IV

Adults. Initially, 100–120 mg/m^2 in repeated cycles of 3–4 wk, in combination with fluorouracil (5-FU) and Cytoxan. Total dose may be given on day 1 of each cycle or in equally divided doses on days 1 and 8 of each cycle.

SIDE EFFECTS/ADVERSE REACTIONS

Frequent

Nausea, vomiting, alopecia, amenorrhea

Occasional

Stomatitis, diarrhea, hot flashes

Rare

Rash, pruritus, fever, lethargy, conjunctivitis

PRECAUTIONS AND CONTRAINDICATIONS

Baseline neutrophil count less than 1500/mm^3, hypersensitivity to epirubicin, previous treatment with anthracyclines up to maximum cumulative dose, recent MI, severe hepatic impairment, severe myocardial insufficiency

DRUG INTERACTIONS OF CONCERN TO DENTISTRY

• None reported

SERIOUS REACTIONS

! The risk of cardiotoxicity (either acute, manifested as transient ECG abnormalities, or chronic, manifested as CHF) increases when the total cumulative dose exceeds 900 mg/m^2.

! Extravasation during administration may result in severe local tissue necrosis.

! Myelosuppression may cause hematologic toxicity, manifested principally as leukopenia and, to a lesser extent, anemia and thrombocytopenia.

DENTAL CONSIDERATIONS

General:

• If additional analgesia is required for dental pain, consider alternative analgesics (NSAIDs) in patients taking opioids for acute or chronic pain.
• Examine for oral manifestations of opportunistic infection.
• This drug may be used in the hospital or on an outpatient basis. Confirm the patient's disease and treatment status.
• Chlorhexidine mouth rinse prior to and during chemotherapy may reduce severity of mucositis.
• Patient on chronic drug therapy may rarely present with symptoms of blood dyscrasias, which can include infection, bleeding, and poor healing. If dyscrasia is present, caution patient to prevent oral tissue trauma when using oral hygiene aids.
• Palliative medication may be required for management of oral side effects.
• Patient may be at risk of bleeding; check oral signs.
• Patient may be at risk of infection.

Consultations:

• Medical consultation should include routine blood counts including platelet counts and aggregation tests.
• In a patient with symptoms of blood dyscrasias, request a medical consultation for blood studies and postpone treatment until normal values are reestablished.
• Consult physician; prophylactic or therapeutic antiinfectives may be indicated if surgery or periodontal treatment is required.
• Medical consultation may be required to assess immunologic status during cancer chemotherapy and determine safety risk, if any, posed by the required dental treatment.
• Medical consultation may be required to assess disease control and patient's ability to tolerate stress.

Teach Patient/Family to:

• Be aware of oral side effects.
• Encourage effective oral hygiene to prevent soft tissue inflammation.
• Report oral lesions, soreness, or bleeding to dentist.
• Prevent trauma when using oral hygiene aids.
• Update health and medication history if physician makes any changes in evaluation or drug regimens; include OTC, herbal, and nonherbal remedies in the update.

eplerenone

eh-**plear′**-ah-nown
(Inspra)

CATEGORY AND SCHEDULE

Pregnancy Risk Category: B

Drug Class: Antihypertensive, aldosterone antagonist

MECHANISM OF ACTION

An aldosterone receptor antagonist that binds to the mineralocorticoid receptors in the kidney, heart, blood vessels and brain, blocking the binding of aldosterone.

Therapeutic Effect: Reduces B/P.

USES

Treatment of hypertension as a single drug or in combination with other antihypertensive drugs; improved survival of CHF patients following an acute heart attack

PHARMACOKINETICS

Absorption unaffected by food. Protein binding: 50%. No active metabolites. Excreted in the urine with a lesser amount eliminated in the feces. Not removed by hemodialysis. ***Half-life:*** 4–6 hr.

INDICATIONS AND DOSAGES

▸ Hypertension

PO

Adults, Elderly. 50 mg once a day. If 50 mg once a day produces an inadequate B/P response, may increase dosage to 50 mg twice a day. If patient is concurrently receiving erythromycin, saquinavir, verapamil, or fluconazole, reduce initial dose to 25 mg once a day.

▸ CHF Following MI

PO

Adults, Elderly. Initially, 25 mg once a day. If tolerated, titrate up to 50 mg once a day within 4 wk.

SIDE EFFECTS/ADVERSE REACTIONS

Rare

Dizziness, diarrhea, cough, fatigue, flu-like symptoms, abdominal pain

PRECAUTIONS AND CONTRAINDICATIONS

Concurrent use of potassium supplements or potassium-sparing diuretics (such as amiloride, spironolactone and triamterene), or inhibitors of the cytochrome P450 3A4 enzyme system (including erythromycin, ketoconazole and itraconazole), creatinine clearance less than 50 ml/min, serum creatinine level greater than 2 mg/dl in males or 1.8 mg/dl in females, serum potassium level greater than 5.5 mEq/L, type 2 diabetes mellitus with microalbuminuria

Caution:

Hyperkalemia, monitor serum potassium periodically, impaired hepatic or renal function, angiotensin-converting enzyme (ACE) inhibitors, angiotensin II antagonists, lactation, use in children has not been established

DRUG INTERACTIONS OF CONCERN TO DENTISTRY

- See contraindications; use with caution in patients taking strong inhibitors of CYP3A4 isoenzymes (erythromycin)
- Monitor blood pressure if NSAIDs are required

SERIOUS REACTIONS

! Hyperkalemia may occur, particularly in patients with Type 2 diabetes mellitus and microalbuminuria.

DENTAL CONSIDERATIONS

General:

- Monitor vital signs at every appointment because of cardiovascular side effects.
- Avoid or limit dose of vasoconstrictor.
- Short appointments and a stress-reduction protocol may be required for anxious patients.
- Take precautions if dental surgery is anticipated and general anesthesia is required.

Consultations:

- Medical consultation may be required to assess disease control and patient's ability to tolerate stress.

• Consultation with physician may be necessary if sedation or general anesthesia is required.

Teach Patient/Family to:

• Update health and drug history if physician makes any changes in evaluation or drug regimens.

epoetin alfa

eh-**poh′**-ee-tin **al′**-fa

(Epogen, Eprex[CAN], Procrit)

Do not confuse Epogen with Neupogen.

CATEGORY AND SCHEDULE

Pregnancy Risk Category: C

Drug Class: Hematinic, antianemic

MECHANISM OF ACTION

A glycoprotein that stimulates division and differentiation of erythroid progenitor cells in bone marrow.

Therapeutic Effect: Induces erythropoiesis and releases reticulocytes from bone marrow.

USES

Anemia of chronic renal failure, end-stage renal disease, anemia in zidovudine-treated HIV patients, anemia in cancer patients on chemotherapy, reduction of allogenic blood transfusion in surgery patients

PHARMACOKINETICS

Well absorbed after subcutaneous administration. Following administration, an increase in reticulocyte count occurs within 10 days and increases in Hgb, Hct, and RBC count are seen within 2–6 wk. ***Half-life:*** 4–13 hr.

INDICATIONS AND DOSAGES

▸ Treatment of Anemia in Chemotherapy Patients

IV, Subcutaneous

Adults, Elderly, Children. 150 units/kg/dose 3 times a wk. Maximum: 1200 units/kg/wk.

▸ Reduction of Allogenic Blood Transfusions in Elective Surgery

Subcutaneous

Adults, Elderly. 300 units/kg/day 10 days before day of and 4 days after surgery.

▸ Chronic Renal Failure

IV Bolus, Subcutaneous

Adults, Elderly. Initially, 50–100 units/kg 3 times a wk. Target Hct range: 30%–36%. Adjust dosage no earlier than 1-mo intervals unless prescribed. Decrease dosage if Hct is increasing and approaching 36%. Plan to temporarily withhold doses if Hct continues to rise and to reinstate lower dosage when Hct begins to decrease. If Hct increases by more than 4 points in 2 wk, monitor Hct twice a wk for 2–6 wk. Increase dose if Hct does not increase 5–6 points after 8 wk (with adequate iron stores) and if Hct is below target range. Maintenance: For patients on dialysis: 75 units/kg 3 times a wk. Range: 12.5–525 units/kg. For patients not on dialysis: 75–150 units/kg/wk.

▸ HIV Infection in Patients Treated with AZT

IV, Subcutaneous

Adults. Initially, 100 units/kg 3 times a wk for 8 wk; may increase by 50–100 units/kg 3 times a wk. Evaluate response q4–8wk thereafter. Adjust dosage by 50–100 units/kg 3 times a wk. If dosages larger than 300 units/kg 3 times a wk are not eliciting response, it is unlikely patient will respond. Maintenance: Titrate to maintain desired Hct.

SIDE EFFECTS/ADVERSE REACTIONS

▸ Patients Receiving Chemotherapy

Frequent
Fever, diarrhea, nausea, vomiting, edema
Occasional
Asthenia, shortness of breath, paresthesia
Rare
Dizziness, trunk pain

▸ Patients with Chronic Renal Failure

Frequent
Hypertension, headache, nausea, arthralgia
Occasional
Fatigue, edema, diarrhea, vomiting, chest pain, skin reactions at administration site, asthenia, dizziness

▸ Patients with HIV Infection Treated with AZT

Frequent
Fever, fatigue, headache, cough, diarrhea, rash, nausea
Occasional
Shortness of breath, asthenia, skin reaction at injection site, dizziness

PRECAUTIONS AND CONTRAINDICATIONS

History of sensitivity to mammalian cell-derived products or human albumin, uncontrolled hypertension
Caution:
Contains benzyl alcohol (risk of complications in premature infants), increased thrombosis risk in CHF, ischemic heart disease, coronary artery bypass, pure red cell aplasia, monitor and control B/P, seizures in CRF, thrombosis during hemodialysis, porphyria, lactation, safety and efficacy in children younger than 1 mo have not been established, monitor renal function, monitor hematocrit

DRUG INTERACTIONS OF CONCERN TO DENTISTRY

- None reported

SERIOUS REACTIONS

! Hypertensive encephalopathy, thrombosis, cerebrovascular accident, MI, and seizures have occurred rarely.
! Hyperkalemia occurs occasionally in patients with chronic renal failure, usually in those who do not conform to medication regimen, dietary guidelines, and frequency of dialysis regimen.

DENTAL CONSIDERATIONS

General:
- Patient's disease, treatment history, and use of other drugs will affect patient evaluation and management.
- Determine why patient is taking the drug.
- Monitor vital signs at every appointment because of cardiovascular and respiratory side effects.
- Take precautions if dental surgery is anticipated and general anesthesia is required.
- Patient history should include all medications and herbal or nonherbal remedies taken by the patient.
- Consider semisupine chair position for patient comfort if GI side effects occur.
- Place on frequent recall because of oral side effects, depending on chemotherapy regimen or HIV immunologic status.

Consultations:
- Medical consultation should include hematocrit and routine blood counts, including platelet counts and bleeding time.
- Consultation with physician may be necessary if sedation or general anesthesia is required.

• Medical consultation may be required to assess disease control and patient's ability to tolerate stress.

Teach Patient/Family to:

• Encourage effective oral hygiene to prevent soft tissue inflammation, infection.

epoprostenol sodium, prostacyclin

eh-poe-pros′-ten-ol soe′-dee-um, pros-ta-sih′-klin

(Flolan)

CATEGORY AND SCHEDULE

Pregnancy Risk Category: B

Drug Class: Vasodilator; antihypertensive

MECHANISM OF ACTION

An antihypertensive that directly dilates pulmonary and systemic arterial vascular beds and inhibits platelet aggregation.

Therapeutic Effect: Reduces right and left ventricular afterload; increases cardiac output and stroke volume.

USES

Treatment of the symptoms of primary pulmonary hypertension, or the high B/P that occurs in the main artery that carries blood from the right side of the heart (the ventricle) to the lungs

INDICATIONS AND DOSAGES

▸ **Long-Term Treatment of New York Heart Association Class III and IV Primary Pulmonary Hypertension**

IV Infusion

Adults, Elderly. Procedure to determine dose range: Initially, 2 ng/kg/min, increased in increments of 2 ng/kg/min q15 min until dose-limiting adverse effects occur. Chronic infusion: Start at 4 ng/kg/min less than the maximum dose rate tolerated during acute dose ranging (or one-half of the maximum rate if rate was less than 5 ng/kg/min).

SIDE EFFECTS/ADVERSE REACTIONS

Frequent

Acute phase: Flushing, headache, nausea, vomiting, hypotension, anxiety, chest pain, dizziness

Chronic phase: Dyspnea, asthenia, dizziness, headache, chest pain, nausea, vomiting, palpitations, edema, jaw pain, tachycardia, flushing, myalgia, nonspecific muscle pain, paresthesia, diarrhea, anxiety, chills, fever, or flu-like symptoms

Occasional

Acute phase: Bradycardia, abdominal pain, muscle pain, dyspnea, back pain

Chronic phase: Rash, depression, hypotension, pallor, syncope, bradycardia, ascites

Rare

Acute phase: Paresthesia

Chronic phase: Diaphoresis, dyspepsia, tachycardia

PRECAUTIONS AND CONTRAINDICATIONS

Long-term use in patients with CHF (severe ventricular systolic dysfunction)

DRUG INTERACTIONS OF CONCERN TO DENTISTRY

• Increased risk of bleeding: drugs which interfere with coagulation or platelet function; such as NSAIDs and aspirin

SERIOUS REACTIONS

! Overdose may cause hyperglycemia or ketoacidosis manifested as increased urination, thirst, and fruit-like breath odor.
! Angina, MI, and thrombocytopenia occur rarely.
! Abrupt withdrawal, including a large reduction in dosage or interruption in drug delivery, may produce rebound pulmonary hypertension as evidenced by dyspnea, dizziness, and asthenia.

DENTAL CONSIDERATIONS

General:

- Continuous-use drug for patients with severe cardiovascular disease. Provide palliative emergency dental care as required.
- Determine why patient is taking the drug.
- Monitor vital signs at every appointment because of cardiovascular side effects.
- Avoid products that affect platelet function, such as aspirin and NSAIDs.
- Stress from dental procedures may compromise cardiovascular function, determine patient risk.
- Postpone elective dental treatment if patient shows signs of cardiac symptoms or respiratory distress.
- Use vasoconstrictor with caution, in low doses and with careful aspiration. Avoid using gingival retraction cord containing epinephrine.

Consultations:

- Medical consultation may be required to assess disease control and patient's ability to tolerate stress.
- Medical consultation should include routine blood counts including platelet counts and bleeding time.

Teach Patient/Family to:

- Encourage effective oral hygiene to prevent soft tissue inflammation.
- Prevent trauma when using oral hygiene aids.
- Update health and medication history if physician makes any changes in evaluation or drug regimens; include OTC, herbal, and nonherbal remedies in the update.

eprosartan

eh-pro-**sar′**-tan
(Teveten)

CATEGORY AND SCHEDULE

Pregnancy Risk Category: C (D if used in second or third trimester)

Drug Class: Antihypertensive, angiotensin II receptor (AT_1) antagonist

MECHANISM OF ACTION

An angiotensin II receptor antagonist that blocks the vasoconstrictor and aldosterone-secreting effects of angiotensin II, inhibiting the binding of angiotensin II to the AT_1 receptors.
Therapeutic Effect: Causes vasodilation, decreases peripheral resistance, and decreases B/P.

USES

Treatment of hypertension as a single drug or in combination with other antihypertensive drugs

PHARMACOKINETICS

Rapidly absorbed after PO administration. Protein binding: 98%. Undergoes first-pass metabolism in the liver to active metabolites. Excreted in urine and biliary system. Minimally removed by hemodialysis. ***Half-life:*** 5–9 hr.

INDICATIONS AND DOSAGES

▸ **Hypertension**

PO

Adults, Elderly. Initially, 600 mg/day. Range: 400–800 mg/day.

SIDE EFFECTS/ADVERSE REACTIONS

Occasional

Headache, cough, dizziness

Rare

Muscle pain, fatigue, diarrhea, upper respiratory tract infection, dyspepsia

PRECAUTIONS AND CONTRAINDICATIONS

Bilateral renal artery stenosis, hyperaldosteronism

Caution:

Renal impairment maximum daily dose is 600 mg, risk of renal impairment, pregnancy category C (first trimester) and pregnancy category D (second and third trimesters); safety and efficacy in lactation and patients younger than 18 yr have not been established

DRUG INTERACTIONS OF CONCERN TO DENTISTRY

- None reported

SERIOUS REACTIONS

! Overdosage may manifest as hypotension and tachycardia. Bradycardia occurs less often.

DENTAL CONSIDERATIONS

General:

- Monitor vital signs at every appointment because of cardiovascular side effects.
- Avoid or limit dose of vasoconstrictor.
- Stress from dental procedures may compromise cardiovascular function; determine patient risk.
- Limit use of sodium-containing products, such as saline IV fluids, for those patients with a dietary salt restriction.
- Short appointments and a stress-reduction protocol may be required for anxious patients.
- Use precaution if sedation or general anesthesia is required; risk of hypotensive episode.
- Assess salivary flow as a factor in caries, periodontal disease, and candidiasis.
- After supine positioning, have patient sit upright for at least 2 min before standing to avoid orthostatic hypotension.

Consultations:

- Medical consultation may be required to assess disease control and patient's ability to tolerate stress.

Teach Patient/Family to:

- Update health and drug history if physician makes any changes in evaluation or drug regimens.
- When chronic dry mouth occurs, advise patient to:
  - Avoid mouth rinses with high alcohol content because of drying effects.
  - Use daily home fluoride products for anticaries effect.
  - Use sugarless gum, frequent sips of water, or saliva substitutes.

eptifibatide

ep-tih-**fib**′-ah-tide

(Integrilin)

CATEGORY AND SCHEDULE

Pregnancy Risk Category: B

Drug Class: Glycoprotein IIb/IIIa inhibitor; antiplatelet, antithrombotic

E

E

MECHANISM OF ACTION
A glycoprotein IIb/IIIa inhibitor that rapidly inhibits platelet aggregation by preventing binding of fibrinogen to receptor sites on platelets.
Therapeutic Effect: Prevents closure of treated coronary arteries. Also prevents acute cardiac ischemic complications.

USES
Treatment of patients with acute coronary syndrome (ACS), including those managed medically and those undergoing percutaneous coronary intervention (PCI)

PHARMACOKINETICS
Half-life 2.5 hr, steady state 4–6 hr, metabolism limited, excretion via kidneys.

INDICATIONS AND DOSAGES
▸Adjunct to Percutaneous Coronary Intervention
IV Bolus, IV Infusion
Adults, Elderly. 180 mcg/kg before PCI initiation; then continuous drip of 2 mcg/kg/min and a second 180 mcg/kg bolus 10 min after the first. Maximum: 15 mg/h. Continue until hospital discharge or for up to 18–24 hr. Minimum 12 hr is recommended. Concurrent aspirin and heparin therapy is recommended.
▸ Acute Coronary Syndrome
IV Bolus, IV Infusion
Adults, Elderly. 180 mcg/kg bolus then 2 mcg/kg/min until discharge or coronary artery bypass graft, up to 72 hr. Maximum: 15 mg/hr. Concurrent aspirin and heparin therapy is recommended.
▸ Dosage in Renal Impairment
Creatinine clearance less than 50 ml/min. Use 180 mcg/kg bolus (maximum 22.6 mg) and 1 mcg/kg/min infusion (maximum: 7.5 mg/hr).

SIDE EFFECTS/ADVERSE REACTIONS
Occasional
Hypotension

PRECAUTIONS AND CONTRAINDICATIONS
Active internal bleeding, AV malformation or aneurysm, history of cerebrovascular accident (CVA) within 2 yr or CVA with residual neurologic defect, history of vasculitis, intracranial neoplasm, oral anticoagulant use within last 7 days unless PT is less than 1.22 times the control, recent (6 wk) GI or GU bleeding, recent (6 wk) surgery or trauma, prior IV dextran use before or during PTCA, severe uncontrolled hypertension, thrombocytopenia (fewer than 100,000 cells/mcl)

DRUG INTERACTIONS OF CONCERN TO DENTISTRY
• Increased risk of bleeding: drugs that interfere with coagulation or platelet function, such as NSAIDs and aspirin

SERIOUS REACTIONS
! Minor to major bleeding complications may occur, most commonly at arterial access site for cardiac catheterization.

DENTAL CONSIDERATIONS
General:
• Monitor vital signs at every appointment because of cardiovascular side effects.
• Avoid products that affect platelet function, such as aspirin and NSAIDs.
• Consider local hemostasis measures to prevent excessive bleeding.
• Do not discontinue eptifibatide.

• For acute use in emergency rooms or hospitals.
• Provide palliative emergency dental care only during drug use.
• Patients may be at risk of bleeding; check for oral signs.
• Confirm patient's medical and drug history.

Consultations:

• Medical consultation may be required to assess disease control and patient's ability to tolerate stress.
• Medical consultation should include routine blood counts including platelet counts and aggregation tests.
• Medical consultation should include INR.

Teach Patient/Family to:

• Encourage effective oral hygiene to prevent soft tissue inflammation.
• Prevent trauma when using oral hygiene aids.
• Report oral lesions, soreness, or bleeding to dentist.
• Update health and medication history if physician makes any changes in evaluation or drug regimens; include OTC, herbal, and nonherbal remedies in the update.
• Use soft tooth brush to reduce risk of bleeding.

ergoloid mesylates

ur′-go-loyd **mess**′-ah-lates
(Gerimal, Hydergine, Hydergine[CAN])

CATEGORY AND SCHEDULE

Pregnancy Risk Category: C

Drug Class: Ergot alkaloids

MECHANISM OF ACTION

An ergot alkaloid that centrally acts on and decreases vascular tone, slows heart rate. Peripheral action blocks alpha adrenergic receptors. ***Therapeutic Effect:*** Improved O_2 uptake and improves cerebral metabolism.

USES

Senile dementia, Alzheimer's dementia, multiinfarct dementia, primary progressive dementia

PHARMACOKINETICS

Rapidly, incompletely absorbed from GI tract. Metabolized in liver. Eliminated primarily in feces. ***Half-life:*** 2–5 hr.

INDICATIONS AND DOSAGES

▸ Age-Related Decline in Mental Capacity

PO

Adults, Elderly. Initially, 1 mg 3 times a day. Range: 1.5–12 mg/day.

SIDE EFFECTS/ADVERSE REACTIONS

Occasional

GI distress, transient nausea, sublingual irritation

PRECAUTIONS AND CONTRAINDICATIONS

Acute or chronic psychosis (regardless or etiology), hypersensitivity to ergoloid mesylates or any component of the formulation.

Caution:

Acute intermittent porphyria

SERIOUS REACTIONS

! Overdose may produce blurred vision, dizziness, syncope, headache, flushed face, nausea, vomiting, decreased appetite, stomach cramps, and stuffy nose.

DENTAL CONSIDERATIONS

General:

- Monitor vital signs at every appointment because of cardiovascular side effects.
- After supine positioning, have patient sit upright for at least 2 min before standing to avoid orthostatic hypotension.
- Consider semisupine chair position for patient comfort because of GI effects of drug.
- Emphasize preventive oral home care.

Teach Patient/Family to:

- Use powered tooth brush if patient is unable to carry out oral hygiene procedures.

ergotamine tartrate/ dihydroergotamine

er-**got**′-ah-meen **tahr**′-treyt/ dahy-hahy-droh-ur-**got**′-uh-meen

ergotamine tartrate (Cafergot[CAN], Ergodryl Mono[AUS], Ergomar, Ergostat, Gynergen)

dihydroergotamine: (D.H.E. 45, Dihydergot[AUS], Dihydroergotamine Sandoz[CAN], Migranal)

CATEGORY AND SCHEDULE

Pregnancy Risk Category: X

Drug Class: α-Adrenergic blocker

MECHANISM OF ACTION

An ergotamine derivative that directly stimulates vascular smooth muscle, resulting in peripheral and cerebral vasoconstriction. May also have antagonist effects on serotonin. ***Therapeutic Effect:*** Suppresses vascular headaches.

USES

Treatment of vascular headache (migraine or histamine), cluster headache

PHARMACOKINETICS

Slowly and incompletely absorbed from the GI tract; rapidly and extensively absorbed after rectal administration. Protein binding: greater than 90%. Undergoes extensive first-pass metabolism in the liver to active metabolite. Eliminated in feces by the biliary system. ***Half-life:*** 21 hr.

INDICATIONS AND DOSAGES

▸ Vascular Headaches

PO (Cafergot [Fixed-Combination of Ergotamine and Caffeine])

Adults, Elderly. 2 mg at onset of headache, then 1–2 mg q30 min. Maximum: 6 mg/episode; 10 mg/wk.

PO, Sublingual

Children. 1 mg at onset of headache, then 1 mg q30 min. Maximum: 3 mg/episode.

IV

Adults, Elderly. 1 mg at onset of headache; may repeat hourly. Maximum: 2 mg/day; 6 mg/wk.

Sublingual

Adults, Elderly. 1 tablet at onset of headache, then 1 tablet q30 min. Maximum: 3 tablets/24 hr; 5 tablets/wk.

IM, Subcutaneous (Dihydroergotamine)

Adults, Elderly. 1 mg at onset of headache; may repeat hourly. Maximum: 3 mg/day; 6 mg/wk.

Intranasal

Adults, Elderly. 1 spray (0.5 mg) into each nostril; may repeat in 15 min. Maximum: 4 sprays/day; 8 sprays/wk.

Rectal
Adults, Elderly. 1 suppository at onset of headache; may repeat dose in 1 hr. Maximum: 2 suppositories/episode; 5 suppositories/wk.

SIDE EFFECTS/ADVERSE REACTIONS

Occasional
Cough, dizziness
Rare
Myalgia, fatigue, diarrhea, upper respiratory tract infection, dyspepsia

PRECAUTIONS AND CONTRAINDICATIONS

Coronary artery disease, hypertension, impaired hepatic or renal function, malnutrition, peripheral vascular diseases (such as thromboangiitis obliterans, syphilitic arteritis, severe arteriosclerosis, thrombophlebitis, and Raynaud's disease), sepsis, severe pruritus
Caution:
Lactation, children, anemia

DRUG INTERACTIONS OF CONCERN TO DENTISTRY

- Vasoconstrictor in local anesthetics
- Suspected increased risk of ergotism: erythromycin, clarithromycin, troleandomycin
- Use anticholinergics with caution in the elderly

SERIOUS REACTIONS

! Prolonged administration or excessive dosage may produce ergotamine poisoning, manifested as nausea and vomiting; paresthesia, muscle pain or weakness; precordial pain; tachycardia or bradycardia; and hypertension or hypotension. Vasoconstriction of peripheral arteries and arterioles may result in localized edema and pruritus. Muscle pain will occur when walking and later, even at rest. Other rare effects include confusion, depression, drowsiness, seizures, and gangrene.

DENTAL CONSIDERATIONS

General:
- This is an acute-use drug; patients are unlikely to seek dental treatment while using this drug.
- Monitor vital signs at every appointment because of cardiovascular side effects.

Teach Patient/Family to:
- Use powered tooth brush if patient has difficulty holding conventional devices.

erlotinib

er-**low**′-tih-nib
(Tarceva)

CATEGORY AND SCHEDULE

Pregnancy Risk Category: D

Drug Class: Antineoplastic

MECHANISM OF ACTION

A human epidermal growth factor that inhibits tyrosine kinases (TK) associated with transmembrane cell surface receptors found on both normal and cancer cells. One such receptor is epidermal growth factor receptor (EGFR).
Therapeutic Effect: TK activity appears to be vitally important to cell proliferation and survival.

USES

Treatment of non–small-cell lung cancer after the failure of other chemotherapy treatment. It is also used together with another medicine called gemcitabine (e.g., Gemzar) to treat cancer of the pancreas

E

PHARMACOKINETICS

Slowly absorbed, peak 3–7 hr, excreted in feces (86%), urine (less than 4%), metabolized by CYP3A4. ***Terminal Half-Life:*** 36 hr.

INDICATIONS AND DOSAGES

▸ **Non–Small-Cell Lung Pancreatic Cancer**

PO

Adults, Elderly. Initially, 7.5 mg once a day. If response is not adequate after a minimum of 2 wk, dosage may be increased to 15 mg once a day. Do not exceed 7.5 mg once a day in patients with moderate hepatic impairment.

SIDE EFFECTS/ADVERSE REACTIONS

Frequent

Dry mouth, constipation

Occasional

Dyspepsia, headache, nausea, abdominal pain

Rare

Asthenia, diarrhea, dizziness, ocular dryness

PRECAUTIONS AND CONTRAINDICATIONS

Pregnancy

DRUG INTERACTIONS OF CONCERN TO DENTISTRY

• Increased blood levels and effects: potent inhibitors of CYP3A4 isoenzymes (ketoconazole, itraconazole, erythromycin, clarithromycin, diclofenac, doxycycline, protease inhibitors)
• Decreased effects: potent inducers of CYP3A4 isoenzymes (carbamazepine, phenobarbital, St. John's wort [herb])

SERIOUS REACTIONS

! UTI occurs occasionally.

DENTAL CONSIDERATIONS

General:

• For longer dental appointments, offer patient frequent breaks.
• Consider semisupine chair position for patient comfort if GI side effects occur.
• Avoid dental light in patient's eyes; offer dark glasses for patient comfort.
• Examine for oral manifestation of opportunistic infection.
• Assess salivary flow as a factor in caries, periodontal disease, and candidiasis.
• Place on frequent recall because of oral side effects.

Consultations:

• Physician should be informed if significant xerostomic side effects occur (increased caries, sore tongue, problems eating or swallowing, difficulty wearing prosthesis) so that a medication change can be considered.

Teach Patient/Family to:

• Encourage effective oral hygiene to prevent soft tissue inflammation.
• Update health and medication history if physician makes any changes in evaluation or drug regimens; include OTC, herbal, and nonherbal remedies in the update.
• When chronic dry mouth occurs advise patient to:
  • Avoid mouth rinses with high alcohol content because of drying effects.
  • Use daily home fluoride products for anticaries effect.
  • Use sugarless gum, frequent sips of water, or saliva substitutes.

ertapenem

er-ta-**pen′**-em
(Invanz)

CATEGORY AND SCHEDULE

Pregnancy Risk Category: B

Drug Class: Antiinfective-miscellaneous; carbapenem

MECHANISM OF ACTION

A carbapenem that penetrates the bacterial cell wall of microorganisms and binds to penicillin-binding proteins, inhibiting cell wall synthesis.
Therapeutic Effect: Produces bacterial cell death.

USES

Treatment of infections caused by bacteria

PHARMACOKINETICS

Almost completely absorbed after IM administration. Protein binding: 85%–95%. Widely distributed. Primarily excreted in urine with smaller amount eliminated in feces. Removed by hemodialysis. ***Half-life:*** 4 hr.

INDICATIONS AND DOSAGES

▸ **Intraabdominal Infection**
IV, IM
Adults, Elderly. 1 g/day for 5–14 days.
▸ **Skin and Skin Structure Infection**
IV, IM
Adults, Elderly. 1 g/day for 7–14 days.
▸ **Pneumonia, UTI**
IV, IM
Adults, Elderly. 1 g/day for 10–14 days.
▸ **Pelvic Infection**
IV, IM
Adults, Elderly. 1 g/day for 3–10 days.
▸ **Dosage in Renal Impairment**
For adults and elderly patients with creatinine clearance less than 30 ml/min, dosage is 500 mg once a day.

SIDE EFFECTS/ADVERSE REACTIONS

Frequent
Diarrhea, nausea, headache
Occasional
Altered mental status, insomnia, rash, abdominal pain, constipation, vomiting, edema, fever
Rare
Dizziness, cough, oral candidiasis, anxiety, tachycardia, phlebitis at IV site

PRECAUTIONS AND CONTRAINDICATIONS

History of hypersensitivity to beta-lactams (imipenem and cilastin, meropenem), hypersensitivity to amide-type local anesthetics (IM)

DRUG INTERACTIONS OF CONCERN TO DENTISTRY

- Increased or prolonged plasma levels: probenecid
- Dental drug interactions have not been studied

SERIOUS REACTIONS

! Antibiotic-associated colitis and other superinfections may occur.
! Anaphylactic reactions have been reported.
! Seizures may occur in those with CNS disorders (including patients with brain lesions or a history of seizures), bacterial meningitis, or severe renal impairment.

E

DENTAL CONSIDERATIONS

General:

• For selected infections in the hospital setting; provide palliative emergency dental treatment only.
• Examine for oral manifestation of opportunistic infection.
• Determine why patient is taking the drug.
• Caution regarding allergy to medication.

Consultations:

• Medical consultation may be required to assess disease control and patient's ability to tolerate stress.

Teach Patient/Family to:

• Encourage effective oral hygiene to prevent soft tissue inflammation.
• Report sore throat, oral burning sensation, fever, or fatigue, any of which could indicate presence of a superinfection.

erythromycin

er-ith-roe-**mye**′-sin

(A/T/S, Akne-Mycin, Apo-Erythro Base[CAN], EES, Emgel, Eryacne[AUS], Erybid[CAN], Eryc, Eryc LD[AUS], EryDerm, Erygel, EryPed, Ery-Tab, Erythra-Derm, Erythrocin, Erythromid[CAN], PCE)

Do not confuse erythromycin with azithromycin or Ethmozine, or Eryc with Emct.

CATEGORY AND SCHEDULE

Pregnancy Risk Category: B

Drug Class: Antiinfective

MECHANISM OF ACTION

A macrolide that reversibly binds to bacterial ribosomes, inhibiting bacterial protein synthesis.

Therapeutic Effect: Bacteriostatic.

USES

Treatment of infection of external eye, prophylaxis of neonatal conjunctivitis and ophthalmia neonatorum; acne vulgaris; infections caused by *N. gonorrhoeae;* mild-to-moderate respiratory tract, skin, soft tissue infections caused by *S. pneumoniae, M. pneumoniae, C. diphtheriae, B. pertussis, L. monocytogenes, S. pyogenes;* syphilis; legionnaires' disease; *C. trachomatis; H. influenzae;* endocarditis prophylaxis

PHARMACOKINETICS

Variably absorbed from the GI tract (depending on dosage form used). Protein binding: 70%–90%. Widely distributed. Metabolized in the liver. Primarily eliminated in feces by bile. Not removed by hemodialysis.

Half-life: 1.4–2 hr (increased in impaired renal function).

INDICATIONS AND DOSAGES

▸ **Mild-to-Moderate Infections of the Upper and Lower Respiratory Tract, Pharyngitis, Skin Infections**

PO

Adults, Elderly. 500 mg q6h, or 333 mg q8h. Maximum: 2 g/day.

Children. 30–50 mg/kg/day in divided doses up to 60–100 mg/kg/day for severe infections.

Neonates. 20–40 mg/kg/day in divided doses q6–12h.

IV

Adults, Elderly, Children. 15–20 mg/kg/day in divided doses. Maximum: 4 g/day.

▸ **Preoperative Intestinal Antisepsis**
PO
Adults, Elderly. 1 g at 1 PM, 2 PM, and 11 PM on day before surgery (with neomycin).
Children. 20 mg/kg at 1 PM, 2 PM, and 11 PM on day before surgery (with neomycin).
▸ **Acne Vulgaris**
Topical
Adults. Apply thin layer to affected area twice a day.
▸ **Gonococcal Ophthalmia Neonatorum**
Ophthalmic
Neonates. 0.5–2 cm no later than 1 hr after delivery.

SIDE EFFECTS/ADVERSE REACTIONS

Frequent
IV: Abdominal cramping or discomfort, phlebitis or thrombophlebitis
Topical: Dry skin
Occasional
Nausea, vomiting, diarrhea, rash, urticaria
Rare
Ophthalmic: Sensitivity reaction with increased irritation, burning, itching, and inflammation
Topical: Urticaria

PRECAUTIONS AND CONTRAINDICATIONS

Administration of fixed-combination product, Pediazole, to infants younger than 2 mo; history of hepatitis because of macrolides; hypersensitivity to macrolides; preexisting hepatic disease.
Caution:
Hepatic disease, lactation

DRUG INTERACTIONS OF CONCERN TO DENTISTRY

- Increased duration of alfentanil, cyclosporine
- Increased serum levels: indinavir, digoxin
- Decreased action of clindamycin, penicillins, lincomycin
- Increased serum levels of alfentanil, carbamazepine, theophylline (and other methylxanthines) and felodipine (possibly with other calcium blockers in the dihydropyridine class), ergot alkaloids, oral anticoagulants, buspirone, tacrolimus
- Risk of rhabdomyolysis: HMG-CoA reductase inhibitors
- May increase the effects of certain benzodiazepines (e.g., midazolam, triazolam)
- Risk of prolonged QT interval; use with caution in patients taking gatifloxacin, moxifloxacin, pimozide, disopyramide
- Possible serotonin syndrome with SSRIs
- Suspected increase in plasma levels of repaglinide

SERIOUS REACTIONS

! Antibiotic-associated colitis and other superinfections may occur.
! High dosages in patients with renal impairment may lead to reversible hearing loss.
! Anaphylaxis and hepatotoxicity occur rarely.
! Ventricular arrhythmias and prolonged QT interval occur rarely with the IV drug form.

DENTAL CONSIDERATIONS

▸ **Erythromycin (Ophthalmic)**
General:
- Avoid dental light in patient's eyes; offer dark glasses for patient comfort.

▸ **Erythromycin (Topical)**
- None indicated

E

▸ **Erythromycin Base/Erythromycin Estolate/Erythromycin Ethylsuccinate/Erythromycin Gluceptate/Erythromycin Lactobionate/Erythromycin Stearate**

General:

• Alternative drug of choice for mild infection caused by a susceptible organism in patients who are allergic to penicillin.
• Determine why the patient is taking the drug.
• Estolate salt form is not indicated because of risk of cholestatic jaundice.

Teach Patient/Family to:

• Take oral drug with full glass of water.
• When used for dental infection, advise patient to:
  • Report sore throat, oral burning sensation, fever and fatigue, any of which could indicate superinfection.
  • Take at prescribed intervals and complete dosage regimen.
  • Immediately notify the dentist if signs or symptoms of infection increase.

escitalopram

es-sy-**tal′**-oh-pram
(Lexapro)

CATEGORY AND SCHEDULE

Pregnancy Risk Category: C

Drug Class: Antidepressant, selective serotonin reuptake inhibitor

MECHANISM OF ACTION

A selective serotonin reuptake inhibitor that blocks the uptake of the neurotransmitter serotonin at neuronal presynaptic membranes, increasing its availability at postsynaptic receptor sites.
Therapeutic Effect: Relieves depression.

USES

Treatment of major depressive disorder; maintenance treatment of major depressive disorder

PHARMACOKINETICS

Well absorbed after PO administration. Primarily metabolized in the liver. Primarily excreted in feces with a lesser amount eliminated in urine.
Half-life: 35 hr.

INDICATIONS AND DOSAGES

▸ **Depression, General Anxiety Disorder (GAD)**

PO

Adults. Initially, 10 mg once a day in the morning or evening. May increase to 20 mg after a minimum of 1 wk.

Elderly. Patients with hepatic impairment. 10 mg/day.

SIDE EFFECTS/ADVERSE REACTIONS

Frequent

Nausea, dry mouth, somnolence, insomnia, diaphoresis

Occasional

Tremor, diarrhea, abnormal ejaculation, dyspepsia, fatigue, anxiety, vomiting, anorexia

Rare

Sinusitis, sexual dysfunction, menstrual disorder, abdominal pain, agitation, decreased libido

PRECAUTIONS AND CONTRAINDICATIONS

Breast-feeding, use within 14 days of MAOIs

Caution:

Hyponatremia, activation of mania/hypomania, seizures, suicide, hepatic impairment, renal impairment, concurrent use of citalopram, lactation; use in children has not been established

DRUG INTERACTIONS OF CONCERN TO DENTISTRY

- Increased sedation: alcohol, other CNS depressants
- Drugs that inhibit CYP3A4 or other CYP isoenzymes may or may not affect plasma levels; should be used with observation and caution
- Modest inhibitor of CYP2D6
- NSAIDs may have a higher risk of GI side effects

SERIOUS REACTIONS

! Overdose is manifested as dizziness, drowsiness, tachycardia, somnolence, confusion, and seizures.

DENTAL CONSIDERATIONS

General:

- Assess salivary flow as a factor in caries, periodontal disease, and candidiasis.
- Consider semisupine chair position for patient comfort if GI side effects occur.
- Question patient about tolerance of NSAIDs or aspirin related to GI disease.
- Evaluate respiration characteristics and rate.

Consultations:

- Medical consultation may be required to assess disease control and patient's ability to tolerate stress.
- Physician should be informed if significant xerostomia occurs (e.g., increased caries, sore tongue, problems eating or swallowing, difficulty wearing prosthesis) so that a medication change can be considered.

Teach Patient/Family to:

- Encourage effective oral hygiene to prevent soft tissue inflammation, infection.
- When chronic dry mouth occurs, advise patient to:
  - Avoid mouth rinses with high alcohol content because of drying effects.
  - Use daily home fluoride products for anticaries effect.
  - Use sugarless gum, frequent sips of water, or saliva substitutes.
  - Comply with recommended regimens for oral care.

esomeprazole

es-oh-**mep′**-rah-zole
(Nexium, Nexium IV)

CATEGORY AND SCHEDULE

Pregnancy Risk Category: B

Drug Class: Antisecretory, proton pump inhibitor

MECHANISM OF ACTION

A proton pump inhibitor that is converted to active metabolites that irreversibly bind to and inhibit hydrogen-potassium adenosine triphosphates, an enzyme on the surface of gastric parietal cells. Inhibits hydrogen ion transport into gastric lumen.

Therapeutic Effect: Increases gastric pH, reduces gastric acid production.

E

USES

Treatment of gastroesophageal reflux disease (GERD), healing and maintenance of erosive esophagitis and *H. pylori* eradication in combination with antibiotics

PHARMACOKINETICS

Well absorbed after oral administration. Protein binding: 97%. Extensively metabolized by the liver. Primarily excreted in urine. ***Half-life:*** 1–1.5 hr.

INDICATIONS AND DOSAGES

▸ **Erosive Esophagitis**

PO

Adults, Elderly. 20–40 mg once daily for 4–8 wk.

IV

Adults, Elderly. 20 or 40 mg once daily by IV injection over at least 3 min or IV infusion over 10–30 min.

▸ **To Maintain Healing of Erosive Esophagitis**

PO

Adults, Elderly. 20 mg/day.

▸ **GERD, to Reduce the Risk of NSAID-Induced Gastric Ulcer**

PO

Adults, Elderly. 20 mg once a day for 4 wk.

▸ **Duodenal Ulcer Caused by *H. pylori***

PO

Adults, Elderly. 40 mg (esomeprazole) once a day, with amoxicillin 1000 mg and clarithromycin 500 mg twice a day for 10 days.

SIDE EFFECTS/ADVERSE REACTIONS

Frequent

Headache

Occasional

Diarrhea, abdominal pain, nausea

Rare

Dizziness, asthenia or loss of strength, vomiting, constipation, rash, cough

PRECAUTIONS AND CONTRAINDICATIONS

Hypersensitivity to benzimidazoles

Caution:

Presence of gastric malignancy, atrophic gastritis, lactation, use in pediatric patients has not been studied, severe hepatic impairment, allergic reactions to related proton pump inhibitors

DRUG INTERACTIONS OF CONCERN TO DENTISTRY

• May interfere with absorption of drugs where gastric pH is an important factor in bioavailability (e.g., iron products, ketoconazole, trovafloxacin, ampicillin)

SERIOUS REACTIONS

! None known

DENTAL CONSIDERATIONS

General:

• Assess salivary flow as a factor in caries, periodontal disease, and candidiasis.

• Question patient about tolerance of NSAIDs or aspirin related to GI disease.

• Consider semisupine chair position for patient comfort because of GI side effects of disease.

• Patients on chronic drug therapy may rarely have symptoms of blood dyscrasias, which can include infection, bleeding, and poor healing.

• Place on frequent recall because of oral side effects and oral effects of reflux disease.

Consultations:

- In a patient with symptoms of blood dyscrasias, request a medical consult for blood studies and postpone treatment until normal values are reestablished.

Teach Patient/Family to:

- Be aware of oral side effects and potential sequelae.
- Prevent trauma when using oral hygiene aids.
- Encourage effective oral hygiene to prevent soft tissue inflammation, infection.
- When chronic dry mouth occurs, advise patient to:
  - Avoid mouth rinses with high alcohol content because of drying effects.
  - Use daily home fluoride products for anticaries effect.
  - Use sugarless gum, frequent sips of water, or saliva substitutes.

estazolam

es-**tay**′-zoe-lam
(ProSom)

CATEGORY AND SCHEDULE

Pregnancy Risk Category: X
Controlled Substance: Schedule IV

Drug Class: Benzodiazepine, sedative hypnotic

MECHANISM OF ACTION

A benzodiazepine that enhances action of gamma-aminobutyric acid (GABA) neurotransmission in the CNS.
Therapeutic Effect: Produces depressant effect at all levels of CNS, relieves insomnia.

USES

Treatment of insomnia

PHARMACOKINETICS

Rapidly absorbed from GI tract. Protein binding: 93%. Metabolized in liver. Primarily excreted in urine, minimal in feces. ***Half-life:*** 10–24 hr.

INDICATIONS AND DOSAGES

▸ Insomnia

PO

Adults (older than 18 yr). 1–2 mg at bedtime.
Elderly, debilitated, liver disease, low serum albumin. 0.5–1 mg at bedtime.

SIDE EFFECTS/ADVERSE REACTIONS

Frequent

Drowsiness, sedation, rebound insomnia (may occur for 1–2 nights after drug is discontinued), dizziness, confusion, euphoria

Occasional

Weakness, anorexia, diarrhea

Rare

Paradoxical CNS excitement, restlessness (particularly noted in elderly/debilitated)

PRECAUTIONS AND CONTRAINDICATIONS

Pregnancy, hypersensitivity to other benzodiazepines

Caution:

Hepatic disease, renal disease, suicidal individuals, drug abuse, elderly, psychosis, children younger than 18 yr, lactation, depression, pulmonary insufficiency, narrow-angle glaucoma

DRUG INTERACTIONS OF CONCERN TO DENTISTRY

- Increased CNS depression: alcohol, all CNS depressants

• Increased serum levels and prolonged effect of benzodiazepines: ketoconazole, itraconazole, fluconazole, miconazole (systemic), indinavir
• Contraindicated with saquinavir
• Possible increase in CNS side effects: kava kava (herb)
• Decreased plasma levels: St. John's wort (herb)

SERIOUS REACTIONS

! Overdosage results in somnolence, confusion, diminished reflexes, and coma.

DENTAL CONSIDERATIONS

General:

• Psychologic and physical dependence may occur with chronic administration.
• Geriatric patients are more susceptible to drug effects; use lower dose.
• Avoid the use of this drug in a patient with a history of drug abuse or alcoholism.

Teach Patient/Family to:

• Avoid mouth rinses with high alcohol content because of drying effects.

estradiol

ess-tra-**dye**′-ole
(Aerodil[AUS], Alora, Climara, Delestrogen, Depo-Estradiol, Esclim, Estrace, Estraderm, Estraderm MX[AUS], Estradot[CAN], Estrasorb, EstroGel, Estring, Evamist, Femring, Kliovance[AUS], Menostar, Oesclim[CAN], Primogyn Depot[AUS], Progynova[AUS], Sandrena Gel[AUS], Vagifem, Vivelle, Vivelle Dot, Zumenon[AUS])
Do not confuse Estraderm with Testoderm.

CATEGORY AND SCHEDULE

Pregnancy Risk Category: X

Drug Class: Estrogen

MECHANISM OF ACTION

An estrogen that increases synthesis of DNA, RNA, and proteins in target tissues; reduces release of gonadotropin-releasing hormone from the hypothalamus; and reduces follicle-stimulating hormone and luteinizing hormone (LH) release from the pituitary.
Therapeutic Effect: Promotes normal growth, promotes development of female sex organs and maintains GU function and vasomotor stability. Prevents accelerated bone loss by inhibiting bone resorption, restoring balance of bone resorption and formation. Inhibits LH and decreases serum testosterone concentration.

USES

Treatment of menopause, breast cancer, prostatic cancer, atrophic vaginitis, kraurosis vulvae, hypogonadism, ovariectomy, primary ovarian failure, prevention of osteoporosis, and menopause-related vasomotor symptoms

PHARMACOKINETICS

Well absorbed from the GI tract. Widely distributed. Protein binding: 50%–80%. Metabolized in the liver. Primarily excreted in urine. ***Half-life:*** Unknown.

INDICATIONS AND DOSAGES

▸ Prostate Cancer

IM (Estradiol Valerate)
Adults, Elderly. 30 mg or more q1–2wk.
PO
Adults, Elderly. 10 mg 3 times a day for at least 3 mo.

▸ Breast Cancer

PO
Adults, Elderly. 10 mg 3 times a day for at least 3 mo.

▸ Osteoporosis Prophylaxis in Postmenopausal Females

PO
Adults, Elderly. 0.5 mg/day cyclically (3 wk on, 1 wk off).
Transdermal (Climara)
Adults, Elderly. Initially, 0.025 mg/wk, adjust dose as needed.
Transdermal (Alora, Vivelle, Vivelle-Dot)
Adults, Elderly. Initially, 0.025 mg patch twice a wk, adjust dose as needed.
Transdermal (Estraderm)
Adults, Elderly. 0.05 mg twice a wk.
Transdermal (Menostar)
Adults, Elderly. 1 mg a wk.

▸ Female Hypoestrogenism

PO
Adults, Elderly. 1–2 mg/day, adjust dose as needed.
IM (Cypionate)
Adults, Elderly. 1.5–2 mg/mo.
IM (Estradiol Valerate)
Adults, Elderly. 10–20 mg q4wk.

▸ Vasomotor Symptoms Associated with Menopause

PO
Adults, Elderly. 1–2 mg/day cyclically (3 wk on, 1 wk off), adjust dose as needed.
IM (Estradiol Cypionate)
Adults, Elderly. 1–5 mg q3–4wk.
IM (Estradiol Valerate)
Adults, Elderly. 10–20 mg q4wk.
Topical Emulsion (Estrasorb)
Adults, Elderly. 3.84 g once a day in the morning.
Topical Gel (EstroGel)
Adults, Elderly. 1.25 g/day.
Transdermal (Climara)
Adults, Elderly. 0.025 mg/wk. Adjust dose as needed.
Transdermal (Alora, Esclim, Estraderm, Vivelle-Dot)
Adults, Elderly. 0.05 mg twice a wk.
Transdermal (Vivelle)
Adults, Elderly. 0.0375 mg twice a wk.
Vaginal Ring (Femring)
Adults, Elderly. 0.05 mg. May increase to 0.1 mg if needed.

▸ Vaginal Atrophy

Vaginal Ring (Estring)
Adults, Elderly. 2 mg.

▸ Atrophic Vaginitis

Vaginal Tablet (Vagifem)
Adults, Elderly. Initially, 1 tablet/day for 2 wk. Maintenance: 1 tablet twice a wk.

SIDE EFFECTS/ADVERSE REACTIONS

Frequent

Anorexia, nausea, swelling of breasts, peripheral edema marked by swollen ankles and feet
Transdermal: Skin irritation, redness

Occasional

Vomiting, especially with high doses; headache that may be severe; intolerance to contact lenses; hypertension; glucose intolerance; brown spots on exposed skin

Vaginal: Local irritation, vaginal discharge, changes in vaginal bleeding, including spotting and breakthrough or prolonged bleeding

Rare

Chorea or involuntary movements, hirsutism or abnormal hairiness, loss of scalp hair, depression

PRECAUTIONS AND CONTRAINDICATIONS

Abnormal vaginal bleeding, active arterial thrombosis, blood dyscrasias, estrogen-dependent cancer, known or suspected breast cancer, pregnancy, thrombophlebitis or thromboembolic disorders, thyroid dysfunction

Caution:

Hypertension, asthma, blood dyscrasias, gallbladder disease, CHF, diabetes mellitus, bone disease, depression, migraine headache, convulsive disorders, hepatic disease, renal disease, family history of cancer of breast or reproductive tract

DRUG INTERACTIONS OF CONCERN TO DENTISTRY

• Increased action of corticosteroids

SERIOUS REACTIONS

! Estrogen therapy may increase the risk of developing coronary artery disease, hypercalcemia, gallbladder disease, cerebrovascular disease, and breast cancer.

! Prolonged administration increases the risk of gallbladder disease, thromboembolic disease and breast, cervical, vaginal, endometrial, and hepatic carcinoma.

! Cholestatic jaundice occurs rarely.

DENTAL CONSIDERATIONS

General:

• Place on frequent recall to evaluate gingival condition.

• Monitor vital signs because of cardiovascular side effects.

Teach Patient/Family to:

• Encourage effective oral hygiene to prevent gingival inflammation.

estradiol valerate + dienogest

es-tra-dye′-ole & dye-en′-oh-jest

(Natazia)

CATEGORY AND SCHEDULE

Pregnancy Risk Category: X

Drug Class: Contraceptive; estrogen and progestin combination

MECHANISM OF ACTION

Combination hormonal contraceptives inhibit ovulation and may also cause changes in the cervical mucus, rendering it unfavorable for sperm penetration even if ovulation occurs. The four-phasic formulation provides the estrogen in decreasing concentrations and the progestin in increasing concentrations over the 28-day cycle.

Therapeutic Effect: Prevents pregnancy, diminishes heavy menstrual bleeding.

USES

Prevention of pregnancy; treatment of heavy menstrual bleeding

PHARMACOKINETICS

Moderately absorbed following oral administration. Plasma protein binding: estradiol: 98%, dienogest: 90%. Hepatic metabolism via CYP3A4 enzymes to active and inactive metabolites. Excreted in the urine and feces. ***Half-life:*** Estradiol: 14 hr. Dienogest: 11 hr.

INDICATIONS AND DOSAGES

▸ **Contraception or Treatment of Heavy Menstrual Bleeding**

PO

Adults (Females). Take 1 tablet daily in the order presented in the blister pack.

SIDE EFFECTS/ADVERSE REACTIONS

Frequent

Headache

Occasional

Mood changes, acne, irregular menstruation, nausea, and weight gain

PRECAUTIONS AND CONTRAINDICATIONS

Avoid use in women with breast cancer or other estrogen- or progestin-dependent neoplasms (current or a history of), hepatic tumors or disease, pregnancy, undiagnosed abnormal uterine bleeding. Use is also contraindicated in women at high risk of arterial or venous thrombotic diseases including cerebrovascular disease, coronary artery disease, diabetes mellitus with vascular disease, DVT or PE, hypercoagulopathies, headaches with focal neurological symptoms, hypertension (uncontrolled), migraine headaches if over 35 yr of age, thrombogenic valvular or rhythm diseases of the heart, and women over 35 yr who smoke.

Avoid use in hepatic and renal impairment.

DRUG INTERACTIONS OF CONCERN TO DENTISTRY

• Inducers of CYP3A4 (e.g., carbamazepine, St. John's wort): decreased effectiveness of Natazia.

SERIOUS REACTIONS

! The risk of cardiovascular side effects is increased in women who smoke cigarettes.

DENTAL CONSIDERATIONS

General:

• Monitor vital signs because of possible cardiovascular adverse effects.

• Counsel patients who smoke about smoking cessation therapy to improve oral health and reduce risks of adverse effects of Natazia.

• Monitor for possible increased potential for vomiting (e.g., during sedation).

estramustine phosphate sodium

es-trah-**mew′**-steen **foss′**-fate **soe′**-dee-um

(Emcyt)

Do not confuse Emcyt with Eryc.

CATEGORY AND SCHEDULE

Pregnancy Risk Category: C

Drug Class: Antineoplastic

MECHANISM OF ACTION

An alkylating agent, estrogen and nitrogen mustard that binds to microtubule-associated proteins, causing their disassembly.

Therapeutic Effect: Reduces serum testosterone concentration.

USES

Treatment of metastatic prostate cancer

PHARMACOKINETICS

Well absorbed from the GI tract. Highly localized in prostatic tissue. Rapidly dephosphorylated during absorption into peripheral circulation. Metabolized in the liver. Primarily eliminated in feces by biliary system. ***Half-life:*** 20 hr.

INDICATIONS AND DOSAGES

▸ Prostatic Carcinoma

PO

Adults, Elderly. 10–16 mg/kg/day or 140 mg 4 times a day.

SIDE EFFECTS/ADVERSE REACTIONS

Frequent

Peripheral edema of lower extremities, breast tenderness or enlargement, diarrhea, flatulence, nausea

Occasional

Increase in B/P, thirst, dry skin, ecchymosis, flushing, alopecia, night sweats

Rare

Headache, rash, fatigue, insomnia, vomiting

PRECAUTIONS AND CONTRAINDICATIONS

Active thrombophlebitis or thromboembolic disorders (unless the tumor is the cause of the thromboembolic disorder and the benefits outweigh the risk), hypersensitivity to estradiol or nitrogen mustard

DRUG INTERACTIONS OF CONCERN TO DENTISTRY

- Increased risk of hepatotoxicity: hepatotoxic drugs
- Impaired absorption: calcium-containing products

SERIOUS REACTIONS

! Estramustine use may exacerbate CHF and increase the risk of pulmonary emboli, thrombophlebitis and cerebrovascular accident.

DENTAL CONSIDERATIONS

General:

- Patients with prostate disease may experience urinary retention; caution with use of anticholinergic drugs that could aggravate urinary retention.
- Patients may have received other chemotherapy or radiation; confirm medical and drug history.
- Determine why patient is taking the drug.
- Monitor vital signs at every appointment because of cardiovascular side effects.
- Consider semisupine chair position for patient comfort if GI side effects occur.
- Patient may need assistance in getting into and out of dental chair. Adjust chair position for patient comfort.
- Short appointments and a stress-reduction protocol may be required for anxious patients.

Consultations:

- Consultation with physician may be needed if sedation or general anesthesia is required.
- Medical consultation may be required to assess disease control.

Teach Patient/Family to:

- Encourage effective oral hygiene to prevent soft tissue inflammation.
- Update health and medication history if physician makes any changes in evaluation or drug regimens; include OTC, herbal, and nonherbal remedies in the update.

estrogens, conjugated; medroxyprogesterone acetate

ess′-troe-jens, **kon′**-joo-gay-ted; me-**drox′**-ee-proe-**jes′**-ter-rone **ass′**-eh-tayte
(Premphase, Prempro, Prempro Low Dose)

CATEGORY AND SCHEDULE

Pregnancy Risk Category: X

Drug Class: Estrogens

MECHANISM OF ACTION

Conjugated estrogens are estrogens that increase synthesis of DNA, RNA and various proteins in responsive tissues; reduces release of gonadotropin-releasing hormone, reducing follicle-stimulating hormone (FSH) and leuteinizing hormone (LH).
Medroxyprogesterone acetate is a hormone that transforms endometrium from proliferative to secretory in an estrogen-primed endometrium; inhibits secretion of pituitary gonadotropins.
Therapeutic Effect: Conjugated estrogens promote vasomotor stability, maintain GU function, normal growth, development of female sex organs; prevents accelerated bone loss by inhibiting bone resorption, restoring balance of bone resorption and formation; inhibits LH, decreases serum concentration of testosterone.
Medroxyprogesterone acetate prevents follicular maturation and ovulation; stimulates growth of mammary alveolar tissue; relaxes uterine smooth muscle; restores hormonal imbalance.

USES

Treatment of symptoms associated with menopause, inoperable breast cancer, prostatic cancer, abnormal uterine bleeding, hypogonadism, primary ovarian failure, prevention of osteoporosis

PHARMACOKINETICS

Conjugated estrogens are well absorbed from the GI tract. Widely distributed. Protein binding: 50%–80%. Metabolized in liver. Primarily excreted in urine. ***Half-life:*** 4–10 hr.
Medroxyprogesterone's absorption varies depending on the patient but is generally low. Binds mainly to albumin or other plasma proteins. Metabolized in liver. Primarily excreted in urine. ***Half-life:*** 2–4 hr.

INDICATIONS AND DOSAGES

▸ Menopausal Symptoms, Osteoporosis, Vulvar/Vaginal Atrophy

PO

(Prempro) Adults, Elderly. 1 tablet once daily.

▸ Menopausal Symptoms, Osteoporosis, Vulvar/Vaginal Atrophy

PO

(Premphase) Adults, Elderly. 1 maroon conjugated estrogen tablet on days 1–14 and 1 light blue conjugated estrogens/medroxyprogesterone tablet on days 15–28.

SIDE EFFECTS/ADVERSE REACTIONS

Frequent

Change in vaginal bleeding, such as spotting or breakthrough bleeding, breast pain or tenderness, gynecomastia

Occasional
Headache, increased B/P, intolerance to contact lenses, nausea, edema, weight change, breast tenderness, nervousness, insomnia, fatigue, dizziness
Rare
Loss of scalp hair, mental depression, dermatologic changes, headache, fever

PRECAUTIONS AND CONTRAINDICATIONS

Breast cancer with some exceptions, liver disease, thrombophlebitis, undiagnosed vaginal bleeding, estrogen-dependent neoplasia (known or suspected), pregnancy (known or suspected), hypersensitivity to conjugated estrogens, medroxyprogesterone acetate, or any component of the formulation
Caution:
Hypertension, asthma, blood dyscrasias, gallbladder disease, CHF, diabetes mellitus, bone disease, depression, migraine headache, convulsive disorders, hepatic disease, renal disease, family history of cancer of breast or reproductive tract

DRUG INTERACTIONS OF CONCERN TO DENTISTRY

• Increased action of corticosteroids

SERIOUS REACTIONS

Estrogens A, Conjugated Synthetic
! Prolonged administration may increase risk of gallbladder, thromboembolic disease, or breast, cervical, vaginal, endometrial, and liver carcinoma.

DENTAL CONSIDERATIONS

▸ Estrogens A, Conjugated Synthetic
General:
• Place on frequent recall to evaluate gingival condition.
• Monitor vital signs because of cardiovascular side effects.
• Consider semisupine chair position for patient comfort if GI side effects occur.
Teach Patient/Family to:
• Encourage effective oral hygiene to prevent gingival soft tissue inflammation.

estropipate

es-tro-**pip**′-ate
(Genoral[AUS], Ogen, Ortho-Est)

CATEGORY AND SCHEDULE

Pregnancy Risk Category: X

Drug Class: Estrogen (piperazine estrone sulfate)

MECHANISM OF ACTION

An estrogen that increases synthesis of DNA, RNA, and proteins in target tissues; reduces release of gonadotropin-releasing hormone from the hypothalamus; and reduces follicle-stimulating hormone (FSH) and luteinizing hormone (LH) from the pituitary.
Therapeutic Effect: Promotes normal growth, promotes development of female sex organs and maintains GU function and vasomotor stability. Prevents accelerated bone loss by inhibiting bone resorption, restoring balance of bone resorption and formation. Inhibits LH and decreases serum testosterone concentration.

USES

Treatment of vasomotor symptoms of menopause, atrophic vaginitis, primary female hypogonadism, primary ovarian failure, estrogen imbalance, ovariectomy

PHARMACOKINETICS

PO: Well absorbed; moderate-to-high protein binding; hepatic metabolism with primary renal excretion

INDICATIONS AND DOSAGES

▸ **Vasomotor Symptoms, Atrophic Vaginitis, Kraurosis Vulvae**

PO

Adults, Elderly. 0.625–5 mg/day cyclically.

▸ **Atrophic Vaginitis, Kraurosis Vulvae**

Intravaginal

Adults, Elderly. 2–4 g/day cyclically.

▸ **Female Hypogonadism, Castration, Primary Ovarian Failure**

PO

Adults, Elderly. 1.25–7.5 mg/day for 21 days; then off for 8–10 days. Repeat if bleeding does not occur by end of off cycle.

▸ **Prevention of Osteoporosis**

PO

Adults, Elderly. 0.625 mg/day (25 days of 31-day cycle/mo).

SIDE EFFECTS/ADVERSE REACTIONS

Frequent

Anorexia, nausea, swelling of breasts, peripheral edema marked by swollen ankles and feet

Occasional

Vomiting, especially with high doses; headache that may be severe; intolerance to contact lenses; hypertension; glucose intolerance; brown spots on exposed skin

Vaginal: Local irritation, vaginal discharge, changes in vaginal bleeding, including spotting and breakthrough or prolonged bleeding

Rare

Chorea or involuntary movements, hirsutism or abnormal hairiness, loss of scalp hair, depression

PRECAUTIONS AND CONTRAINDICATIONS

Abnormal vaginal bleeding, active arterial thrombosis, blood dyscrasias, estrogen-dependent cancer, known or suspected breast cancer, pregnancy, thrombophlebitis or thromboembolic disorders, thyroid dysfunction

Caution:

Hypertension, asthma, blood dyscrasias, gallbladder disease, CHF, diabetes mellitus, bone disease, depression, migraine headache, convulsive disorders, hepatic disease, renal disease, family history of cancer of breast or reproductive tract

DRUG INTERACTIONS OF CONCERN TO DENTISTRY

• Increased action of corticosteroids

SERIOUS REACTIONS

! Prolonged administration increases the risk of gallbladder disease, thromboembolic disease and breast, cervical, vaginal, endometrial, and hepatic carcinoma.

! Cholestatic jaundice occurs rarely.

DENTAL CONSIDERATIONS

General:

• Place on frequent recall to evaluate gingival condition.

• Monitor vital signs because of cardiovascular side effects.

Teach Patient/Family to:

• Encourage effective oral hygiene to prevent gingival inflammation.

E

eszopiclone

es-**zoe**′-pih-clone
(Lunesta)

CATEGORY AND SCHEDULE

Pregnancy Risk Category: C
Controlled Substance: Schedule IV

Drug Class: Sedative-hypnotic

MECHANISM OF ACTION

A nonbenzodiazepine that enhances the action of the inhibitory neurotransmitter gamma-aminobutyric acid (GABA).

USES

Treatment of insomnia

PHARMACOKINETICS

Rapidly absorbed, peak 1 hr. ***Half-life:*** 6 hr, metabolized in liver by CYP3A4 and CYP 2E1, weak protein binding (52%–59%), unchanged drug (10%) and metabolites (75%) excreted in urine.

INDICATIONS AND DOSAGES

▸ **Insomnia**

PO

Adult. 2 mg per day at bedtime.

SIDE EFFECTS/ADVERSE REACTIONS

ORAL: Dry mouth, taste alterations
CNS: Somnolence, nervousness, anxiety, confusion, depression, dizziness, hallucinations, decreased libido
GI: Dyspepsia, nausea, vomiting
RESP: Infection
GU: Dysmenorrhea (females), gynecomastia (males)
INTEG: Rash
SYST: Headache, chest pain, viral infection

PRECAUTIONS AND CONTRAINDICATIONS

Mental impairment, behavior and mood changes (depression), use lower doses in elderly and patients with renal/hepatic impairment

DRUG INTERACTIONS OF CONCERN TO DENTISTRY

• Increased CNS depression: all CNS depressants, alcohol
• Inhibitors of CYP3A4 (azole antifungals, macrolide antibiotics, e.g., erythromycin/clarithromycin): increased blood levels and CNS depression
• Food: Effects delayed by taking with or immediately after heavy/fatty meal

DENTAL CONSIDERATIONS

General:

• Assess salivary flow as a factor in caries, periodontal disease, and candidiasis.
• Differentiate taste changes because of drug from those associated with restorative materials.
• Use all appropriate precautions if prescribing for preoperative sedation.
• After supine positioning, allow patient to sit upright for 2 min before standing to avoid dizziness.

Consultations:

• Medical consultation may be required to assess disease control.

Teach Patient/Family to:

• Avoid mouth rinses with high alcohol content because of drying effect.
• Use home fluoride products to prevent caries.
• Use sugarless chewing gum, frequent sips of water, or saliva substitutes if dry mouth occurs.

etanercept

eh-**tan**′-er-cept
(Enbrel)

CATEGORY AND SCHEDULE

Pregnancy Risk Category: B

Drug Class: Antiinflammatory and immunomodulator; biologic response modifier

MECHANISM OF ACTION

A protein that binds to tumor necrosis factor (TNF), blocking its interaction with cell surface receptors. Elevated levels of TNF, which is involved in inflammatory and immune responses, are found in the synovial fluid of rheumatoid arthritis patients.
Therapeutic Effect: Relieves symptoms of rheumatoid arthritis.

USES

Reduction in signs and symptoms of moderately to severely active rheumatoid arthritis in patients with an inadequate response to one or more disease-modifying antirheumatic drugs; polyarticular-course juvenile rheumatoid arthritis; psoriatic arthritis; also approved for initial therapy

PHARMACOKINETICS

Well absorbed after subcutaneous administration. ***Half-life:*** 115 hr.

INDICATIONS AND DOSAGES

▸ **Rheumatoid Arthritis, Psoriatic Arthritis, Ankylosing Spondylitis**
Subcutaneous
Adults, Elderly. 25 mg twice weekly, given 72–96 hr apart. Alternative weekly dosing: 0.8 mg/kg/dose once a wk. Maximum: 50 mg/wk. Maximum: 25 mg/dose.

▸ **Juvenile Rheumatoid Arthritis**
Subcutaneous
Children 4–17 yr. 0.4 mg/kg (Maximum: 25 mg dose) twice a wk given 72–96 hr apart. Alternative weekly dosing: 50 mg once a wk. Maximum: 25 mg/dose.

▸ **Plaque Psoriasis**
Subcutaneous
Adults, Elderly. 50 mg twice a wk (give 3–4 days apart) for 3 mo. Maintenance: 50 mg once a wk.

SIDE EFFECTS/ADVERSE REACTIONS

Frequent
Injection site erythema, pruritus, pain, and swelling; abdominal pain, vomiting (more common in children than adults)
Occasional
Headache, rhinitis, dizziness, pharyngitis, cough, asthenia, abdominal pain, dyspepsia
Rare
Sinusitis, allergic reaction

PRECAUTIONS AND CONTRAINDICATIONS

Serious active infection or sepsis
Caution:
Risk of new malignancies and infrequent severe cardiovascular events, discontinue if serious infection occurs, immunosuppression risk, caution with preexisting demyelinating disorders, lactation, viral infections, children younger than 4 yr

DRUG INTERACTIONS OF CONCERN TO DENTISTRY

No studies have been conducted.

SERIOUS REACTIONS

! Infections (such as pyelonephritis, cellulitis, osteomyelitis, wound infection, leg ulcer, septic arthritis, diarrhea, bronchitis, and

pneumonia), occur in 29%–38% of patients.
! Rare adverse effects include heart failure, hypertension, hypotension, pancreatitis, GI hemorrhage, and dyspnea.
! The patient also may develop autoimmune antibodies.

E

DENTAL CONSIDERATIONS

General:
- Monitor vital signs at every appointment because of potential cardiovascular side effects.
- Consider semisupine chair position for patient comfort because of GI side effects of drug.
- If acute oral infection occurs, inform physician.
- Note elevated antinuclear antibody (ANA) levels if diagnosing Sjögren's syndrome.

Consultations:
- Medical consultation if needed.

Teach Patient/Family to:
- Encourage effective oral hygiene to prevent soft tissue inflammation.
- Use powered tooth brush if patient has difficulty holding conventional devices.

ethambutol

eh-**tham′**-byoo-tole
(Etibi[CAN], Myambutol)
Do not confuse ethambutol or Myambutol with Nembutal.

CATEGORY AND SCHEDULE

Pregnancy Risk Category: B

Drug Class: Antitubercular

MECHANISM OF ACTION

An isonicotinic acid derivative that interferes with RNA synthesis.

Therapeutic Effect: Suppresses the multiplication of mycobacteria.

USES

Treatment of pulmonary tuberculosis (TB), as an adjunct

PHARMACOKINETICS

Rapidly and well absorbed from the GI tract. Protein binding: 20%–30%. Widely distributed. Metabolized in the liver. Primarily excreted in urine. Removed by hemodialysis. ***Half-life:*** 3–4 hr (increased in impaired renal function).

INDICATIONS AND DOSAGES

▸ **TB**

PO

Adults, Elderly, Children. 15–25 mg/kg/day as a single dose or 50 mg/kg 2 times a wk. Maximum: 2.5 g/dose.

▸ **Atypical Mycobacterial Infections**

PO

Adults, Elderly, Children. 15 mg/kg/day. Maximum: 1 g/day.

▸ **Dosage in Renal Impairment**

Dosage interval is modified on the basis of creatinine clearance.

Creatinine Clearance	Dosage Interval
10–50 ml/ min	q24–36h
Less than 10 ml/min	q48h

SIDE EFFECTS/ADVERSE REACTIONS

Occasional

Acute gouty arthritis (chills, pain, swelling of joints with hot skin), confusion, abdominal pain, nausea, vomiting, anorexia, headache

Rare

Rash, fever, blurred vision, eye pain, red-green color blindness

PRECAUTIONS AND CONTRAINDICATIONS

Optic neuritis

Caution:

Renal disease, diabetic retinopathy, cataracts, ocular defects, hepatic disorders, hematopoietic disorders

DRUG INTERACTIONS OF CONCERN TO DENTISTRY

- None reported

SERIOUS REACTIONS

! Optic neuritis (more common with high-dosage or long-term ethambutol therapy), peripheral neuritis, thrombocytopenia, and an anaphylactoid reaction occur rarely.

DENTAL CONSIDERATIONS

General:

- Examine for evidence of oral signs of disease.
- Avoid dental light in patient's eyes; offer dark glasses for patient comfort.
- Determine why the patient is taking the drug.
- Do not treat patients with active tuberculosis.

Consultations:

- Medical consultation is required to assess patient's current status; avoid elective dental procedures in active infections.
- Determine that noninfectious status exists by ensuring the following:
  - Anti-TB drugs have been taken for longer than 3 wk.
  - Culture confirms antibiotic susceptibility to TB microorganisms.
  - Patient has had three consecutive negative sputum smears.
  - Patient is not in the coughing stage.

Teach Patient/Family to:

- Take medication for full length of prescribed therapy to ensure effectiveness of treatment and to prevent the emergence of resistant forms of microbes.

E

ethionamide

eh-thye-**on**′-am-ide

(Trecator)

Do not confuse with TriCor.

CATEGORY AND SCHEDULE

Pregnancy Risk Category: C

Drug Class: Antitubercular

MECHANISM OF ACTION

An antitubercular agent that inhibits peptide synthesis.

Therapeutic Effect: Suppresses mycobacterial multiplication. Bactericidal.

USES

Treatment of pulmonary, extrapulmonary tuberculosis (TB) when other antitubercular drugs have failed

PHARMACOKINETICS

Rapidly absorbed from the GI tract. Widely distributed. Protein binding: 10%. Metabolized in liver. Primarily excreted in urine. Removed by hemodialysis. ***Half-life:*** 2–3 hr (half-life is increased with impaired renal function).

INDICATIONS AND DOSAGES

▸ **TB**

PO

Adults, Elderly. 500–1000 mg/day as a single to 3 divided doses.

Children. 15–20 mg/kg/day. Maximum 1 g/day.

Dosage in Renal Impairment
Creatinine clearance less than 50 ml/min. Reduce dose by 50%.

SIDE EFFECTS/ADVERSE REACTIONS

Occasional
Abdominal pain, nausea, vomiting, weakness, postural hypotension, psychiatric disturbances, drowsiness, dizziness, headache, confusion, metallic taste, anorexia, diarrhea, stomatitis, peripheral neuritis
Rare
Rash, fever, blurred vision, optic neuritis, seizures, hypothyroidism, hypoglycemia, gynecomastia, thrombocytopenia, jaundice

PRECAUTIONS AND CONTRAINDICATIONS

Severe hepatic impairment, hypersensitivity to ethionamide
Caution:
Lactation, renal disease, diabetic retinopathy, cataracts, ocular defects, children younger than 12 yr; pyridoxine concurrent use is recommended, resistance may develop

DRUG INTERACTIONS OF CONCERN TO DENTISTRY

• None reported

SERIOUS REACTIONS

! Peripheral neuropathy, anorexia, and joint pain rarely occur.

DENTAL CONSIDERATIONS

General:
• Monitor vital signs at every appointment because of cardiovascular side effects.
• After supine positioning, have patient sit upright for at least 2 min before standing to avoid orthostatic hypotension.
• Consider semisupine chair position for patient comfort because of GI effects of disease.
• Evaluate for clotting ability during gingival instrumentation.
• Examine for evidence of oral manifestations of blood dyscrasias (infection, bleeding, poor healing).
• Palliative treatment may be required for oral side effects.
• Examine for evidence of oral signs of disease.
Consultations:
• Medical consultation for blood studies (CBC); leukopenic or thrombocytopenic side effects may result in infection, delayed healing, and excessive bleeding. Postpone elective dental treatment until normal values are maintained. Instruct patient to take with meals to decrease GI symptoms.
• Medical consultation may be required to assess disease control and determine infectious nature of disease.
• Confirm that patient is non-infectious prior to dental treatment.
Teach Patient/Family to:
• Encourage effective oral hygiene to prevent soft tissue inflammation.
• Use caution in use of oral hygiene aids to prevent injury.

ethosuximide

eth-oh-**sux**′-ih-mide
(Zarontin)
Do not confuse with Zaroxolyn or Neurontin.

CATEGORY AND SCHEDULE

Pregnancy Risk Category: C

Drug Class: Anticonvulsant

MECHANISM OF ACTION

An anticonvulsant that increases the seizure threshold and suppresses paroxysmal spike-and-wave pattern in absence seizures; depresses nerve transmission in the motor cortex. ***Therapeutic Effect:*** Produces anticonvulsant activity.

USES

Treatment of absence seizures (petit mal); unapproved: complex partial seizures

PHARMACOKINETICS

Well absorbed from the GI tract. Metabolized in liver. Excreted in urine. Removed by hemodialysis. ***Half-life:*** 50–60 hr (in adults); 30 hr (in children).

INDICATIONS AND DOSAGES

▸ Absence Seizures

PO

Adults, Elderly, Children older than 6 yr. Initially, 250 mg/day or 15 mg/kg/day in 2 divided doses. Maintenance: 15–40 mg/kg/day in 2 divided doses.

Children 3–6 yr. Initially, 250 mg in 2 divided doses, increased by 250 mg as needed every 4–7 days. Maintenance: 20–40 mg/kg/day in 2 divided doses. Use with caution in patients with renal impairment.

SIDE EFFECTS/ADVERSE REACTIONS

Occasional

Dizziness, drowsiness, double vision, headache, ataxia, nausea, diarrhea, vomiting, somnolence, urticaria

Rare

Agranulocytosis, gum hypertrophy, leucopenia, myopia, swelling of the tongue, systemic lupus erythematosus, vaginal bleeding

PRECAUTIONS AND CONTRAINDICATIONS

Hypersensitivity to succinimides

Caution:

Lactation, hepatic disease, renal disease

DRUG INTERACTIONS OF CONCERN TO DENTISTRY

- Enhanced CNS depression
- CNS depressants, alcohol

SERIOUS REACTIONS

! Abrupt withdrawal may increase seizure frequency.

! Overdosage results in nausea, vomiting, and CNS depression including coma with respiratory depression.

DENTAL CONSIDERATIONS

General:

- Patients on chronic drug therapy may rarely have symptoms of blood dyscrasias, which can include infection, bleeding, and poor healing.
- Talk with patient to ascertain seizure frequency and how well seizures are controlled. A stress reduction protocol may be required.

Consultations:

- In a patient with symptoms of blood dyscrasias, request a medical consultation for blood studies, and postpone dental treatment until normal values are reestablished.
- Medical consultation may be required to assess disease control and patient's ability to tolerate stress.

Teach Patient/Family to:

- Encourage effective oral hygiene to prevent gingival inflammation.
- Avoid mouth rinses with high alcohol content because of drying effects.

E

etidronate disodium

ee-**tid**′-roe-nate die-**soe**′-dee-um
(Didronel)
Do not confuse etidronate with etidocaine or etomidate.

CATEGORY AND SCHEDULE

Pregnancy Risk Category: C (parenteral), B (oral)

Drug Class: Antihypercalcemic

MECHANISM OF ACTION

A bisphosphonate that decreases mineral release and matrix in bone and inhibits osteocytic osteolysis. ***Therapeutic Effect:*** Decreases bone resorption.

USES

Treatment of Paget's disease, heterotopic ossification, hypercalcemia of malignancy

PHARMACOKINETICS

Therapeutic response: 1–3 mo; not metabolized; excreted in urine.

INDICATIONS AND DOSAGES

▸ Paget's Disease

PO

Adults, Elderly. Initially, 5–10 mg/kg/day not to exceed 6 mo, or 11–20 mg/kg/day not to exceed 3 mo. Repeat only after drug-free period of at least 90 days.

▸ Heterotopic Ossification Caused by Spinal Cord Injury

PO

Adult, Elderly. 20 mg/kg/day for 2 wk; then 10 mg/kg/day for 10 wk.

▸ Heterotopic Ossification Complicating Total Hip Replacement

PO

Adults, Elderly. 20 mg/kg/day for 1 mo before surgery; then 20 mg/kg/day for 3 mo after surgery.

▸ Hypercalcemia Associated with Malignancy

IV

Adults, Elderly. 7.5 mg/kg/day for 3 days. For retreatment, allow 7 days between treatment courses. Follow with oral therapy on day after last infusion. Begin with 20 mg/kg/day for 30 days; may extend up to 90 days.

SIDE EFFECTS/ADVERSE REACTIONS

Frequent

Nausea; diarrhea; continuing or more frequent bone pain in patients with Paget's disease

Occasional

Bone fractures, especially of the femur

Parenteral: Metallic, altered taste

Rare

Hypersensitivity reaction

PRECAUTIONS AND CONTRAINDICATIONS

Clinically overt osteomalacia

Caution:

Renal disease, lactation, adequate intake of vitamin D and calcium, safety and efficacy in children have not been established

DRUG INTERACTIONS OF CONCERN TO DENTISTRY

• Possible increased risk of gastric ulceration: NSAIDs

SERIOUS REACTIONS

! Nephrotoxicity, including hematuria, dysuria, and proteinuria, has occurred with parenteral route.

! Osteonecrosis of the jaw

DENTAL CONSIDERATIONS

General:

• Evaluate for signs and symptoms of osteonecrosis.

• Be aware of oral manifestations of Paget's disease (macrognathia, alveolar pain).
• Emphasize atraumatic and effective oral hygiene.
Consultations:
• Medical consultation may be required to assess disease control.

etodolac

eh-toe-**doe**′-lak
(Apo-Etodolac[CAN], Lodine, Lodine XL, Ultradol[CAN])
Do not confuse Lodine with codeine or iodine.

CATEGORY AND SCHEDULE

Pregnancy Risk Category: C (D if used in third trimester or near delivery)

Drug Class: Nonsteroidal antiinflammatory

MECHANISM OF ACTION

An NSAID that produces analgesic and antiinflammatory effects by inhibiting prostaglandin synthesis. ***Therapeutic Effect:*** Reduces the inflammatory response and intensity of pain.

USES

Mild-to-moderate pain, osteoarthritis, rheumatoid arthritis

PHARMACOKINETICS

Route	Onset	Peak	Duration
PO (analgesic)	30 min	N/A	4–12 hr

Completely absorbed from the GI tract. Protein binding: greater than 99%. Widely distributed. Metabolized in the liver. Primarily excreted in urine. Not removed by hemodialysis. ***Half-life:*** 6–7 hr.

INDICATIONS AND DOSAGES

▸ Osteoarthritis, Rheumatoid Arthritis

PO (Immediate-Release)
Adults, Elderly. Initially, 300 mg 2–3 times a day or 400–500 mg twice a day. Maintenance: 600–1000 mg/day in 2–4 divided doses.
PO (Extended-Release)
Adults, Elderly. 400–1000 mg once daily. Maximum: 1200 mg/day.

▸ Juvenile Rheumatoid Arthritis

PO (Extended-Release)
Children 6–16 yr. 1000 mg in children weighing more than 60 kg, 800 mg once daily in children weighing 46–60 kg, 600 mg once daily in children weighing 31–45 kg, 400 mg once daily in children weighing 20–30 kg.

▸ Analgesia

PO
Adults, Elderly. 200–400 mg q6–8h as needed. Maximum: 1200 mg/day.

SIDE EFFECTS/ADVERSE REACTIONS

Occasional
Dizziness, headache, abdominal pain or cramps, bloated feeling, diarrhea, nausea, indigestion
Rare
Constipation, rash, pruritus, visual disturbances, tinnitus

PRECAUTIONS AND CONTRAINDICATIONS

Active peptic ulcer disease, chronic inflammation of GI tract, GI bleeding or ulceration, history of hypersensitivity to aspirin or NSAIDs
Caution:
Lactation, children, bleeding disorders, GI disorders, cardiac

disorders, elderly, renal, hepatic disorders

DRUG INTERACTIONS OF CONCERN TO DENTISTRY

- GI ulceration, bleeding: aspirin, alcohol, corticosteroids, bisphosphonates
- Decreased action: salicylates
- Nephrotoxicity: acetaminophen (prolonged use)
- Possible risk of decreased renal function: cyclosporine
- NSAIDs may have a higher risk of GI side effects
- When prescribed for dental pain:
  - Risk of increased effects: oral anticoagulants, oral antidiabetics, lithium, methotrexate
  - Decreased effects of diuretics
  - Increased risk of methotrexate toxicity

SERIOUS REACTIONS

! Overdose may result in acute renal failure.

! There is an increased risk of cardiovascular events (including MI and CVA) and serious and potentially life-threatening GI bleeding.

! Rare reactions with long-term use include peptic ulcer disease, GI bleeding, gastritis, severe hepatic reactions (jaundice), nephrotoxicity (hematuria, dysuria, proteinuria), and a severe hypersensitivity reaction (bronchospasm, angioedema).

DENTAL CONSIDERATIONS

General:

- Possible increase in adverse cardiovascular events in patients at risk for thromboembolism.
- Patients on chronic drug therapy may rarely have symptoms of blood dyscrasias, which can include infection, bleeding, and poor healing.
- Assess salivary flow as a factor in caries, periodontal disease, and candidiasis.
- Avoid prescribing in pregnancy.
- Avoid prescribing with aspirin-containing products.
- Consider semisupine chair position for patients with arthritic disease.
- Severe stomach bleeding may occur in patients who regularly use NSAIDs in recommended doses, when the patient is also taking another NSAID, a blood thinning, or steroid drug, if the patient has GI or peptic ulcer disease, if they are 60 yr or older, or when NSAIDs are taken longer than directed. Warn patients of the potential for severe stomach bleeding.

Consultations:

- In a patient with symptoms of blood dyscrasias, request a medical consultation for blood studies and postpone dental treatment until normal values are reestablished.
- Medical consultation may be required to assess disease control.

Teach Patient/Family to:

- Avoid mouth rinses with high alcohol content because of drying effects.
- Warn patient of potential risks of NSAIDs.

etoposide, VP-16

eh-**toe**′-poe-side

(Etopophos, Toposar, VePesid)

Do not confuse VePesid with Pepcid or Versed.

CATEGORY AND SCHEDULE

Pregnancy Risk Category: D

Drug Class: Antineoplastic-miscellaneous; semisynthetic podophyllotoxin

MECHANISM OF ACTION
An epipodophyllotoxin that induces single-and double-stranded breaks in DNA. Cell cycle–dependent and phase-specific; most effective in the S and G2 phases of cell division. ***Therapeutic Effect:*** Inhibits or alters DNA synthesis.

USES
Leukemias, testicular cancer, lymphomas, small cell carcinoma of the lung

PHARMACOKINETICS
Variably absorbed from the GI tract. Rapidly distributed, low concentrations in CSF. Protein binding: 97%. Metabolized in the liver. Primarily excreted in urine. Not removed by hemodialysis. ***Half-life:*** 3–12 hr.

INDICATIONS AND DOSAGES
▸ Refractory Testicular Tumors
IV
Adults. 50–100 mg/m^2/day on days 1–5, or 100 mg/m^2/day on days 1, 3, and 5 (as combination therapy).
▸ Acute Myelocytic Leukemia
IV
Children. 150 mg/m^2/day for 2–3 days and 2–3 cycles.
▸ Brain Tumor
IV
Children. 150 mg/m^2/day on days 2 and 3 of treatment course.
▸ Neuroblastoma
IV
Children. 100 mg/m^2/day on days 1–5 of treatment course; repeated q4wk.
▸ Small-Cell Lung Carcinoma
PO
Adults. Twice the IV dose rounded to nearest 50 mg. Give once a day for doses 400 mg or less, in divided doses for dosages greater than 400 mg.
IV
Adults. 35 mg/m^2/day for 4 consecutive days up to 50 mg/m^2/day for 5 consecutive days (as combination therapy).
Children. 60–150 mg/m^2/day for 2–5 days q3–6wk.
▸ Dosage in Renal Impairment
Creatinine clearance 10–50 ml/min. 75% of normal dose. Creatinine clearance less than 10 ml/min. 50% of normal dose.

SIDE EFFECTS/ADVERSE REACTIONS
Frequent
Mild to moderate nausea and vomiting, alopecia
Occasional
Diarrhea, anorexia, stomatitis
Rare
Hypotension, peripheral neuropathy

PRECAUTIONS AND CONTRAINDICATIONS
Pregnancy

DRUG INTERACTIONS OF CONCERN TO DENTISTRY
• None reported

SERIOUS REACTIONS
! Myelosuppression may result in hematologic toxicity, manifested as anemia, leukopenia (occurring 7–14 days after drug administration), thrombocytopenia (occurring 9–16 days after administration) and, to a lesser extent, pancytopenia. Bone marrow recovery occurs by day 20.
! Hepatotoxicity occurs occasionally.

DENTAL CONSIDERATIONS
General:
• Determine why patient is taking the drug.
• If additional analgesia is required for dental pain, consider alternative

analgesics (NSAIDs) in patients taking narcotics for acute or chronic pain.

• Examine for oral manifestations of opportunistic infection.

• Avoid products that affect platelet function, such as aspirin and NSAIDs.

• This drug may be used in the hospital or on an outpatient basis. Confirm the patient's disease and treatment status.

• Chlorhexidine mouth rinse prior to and during chemotherapy may reduce severity of mucositis.

• Patient on chronic drug therapy may rarely present with symptoms of blood dyscrasias, which can include infection, bleeding, and poor healing. If dyscrasia is present, caution patient to prevent oral tissue trauma when using oral hygiene aids.

• Palliative medication may be required for management of oral side effects.

• Short appointments and a stress-reduction protocol may be required for anxious patients.

• Consider semisupine chair position for patient comfort if GI side effects occur.

• Patients may be at risk of bleeding; check for oral signs.

• Oral infections should be eliminated and/or treated aggressively.

Consultations:

• Medical consultation should include routine blood counts including platelet counts and bleeding time.

• Consult physician; prophylactic or therapeutic antiinfectives may be indicated if surgery or periodontal treatment is required.

• Medical consultation may be required to assess immunologic status during cancer chemotherapy and determine safety risk, if any, posed by the required dental treatment.

• Medical consultation may be required to assess disease control and patient's ability to tolerate stress.

Teach Patient/Family to:

• Encourage effective oral hygiene to prevent soft tissue inflammation.

• Report oral lesions, soreness, or bleeding to dentist.

• Prevent trauma when using oral hygiene aids.

• Update health and medication history if physician makes any changes in evaluation or drug regimens; include OTC, herbal, and nonherbal remedies in the update.

etravirine

et-ra-**vir**′-een
(Intelence)

CATEGORY AND SCHEDULE

Pregnancy Risk Category: B

Drug Class: Antiretroviral agent, reverse transcriptase inhibitor

MECHANISM OF ACTION

Non-nucleoside reverse transcriptase inhibitor (NNRTI) of human immunodeficiency virus type 1 (HIV-1). Binds directly to reverse transcriptase and blocks the RNA-dependent and DNA-dependent DNA polymerase activities. Does not inhibit the human DNA polymerases alpha, beta, and gamma.

USES

HIV-1 infection in combination with at least two additional antiretroviral agents in treatment-experienced patients exhibiting viral replication.

PHARMACOKINETICS

Food increases systemic exposure by 50%. Protein binding 99.9%. Metabolized by the liver via CYP 3A4, 2C9, and 2C19. Primarily excreted in feces (94%, up to 86% as unchanged drug), urine (1%). ***Half-life***: 41 hr.

INDICATIONS AND DOSAGES

PO

Adult. HIV-1 infection: 200 mg twice daily after meals.

Renal Impairment: No dose adjustment necessary.

Hepatic Impairment: No dose adjustment necessary for mild-to-moderate impairment.

SIDE EFFECTS/ADVERSE REACTIONS

Frequent

Rash, nausea, hyperglycemia

Occasional

Peripheral neuropathy, hypertension, abdominal pain

PRECAUTIONS AND CONTRAINDICATIONS

Contraindications have not been determined.

Skin reactions (severe and life threatening, including Stevens-Johnson syndrome), opportunistic infections, inflammatory response (immune reconstitution syndrome) and redistribution of fat may occur. Coadministration with other non-nucleoside reverse transcriptase inhibitors is not recommended. Coadministration of protease inhibitors administered without ritonavir is not recommended.

DRUG INTERACTIONS OF CONCERN TO DENTISTRY

- CYP3A4, 2C9, and 2C19 substrates (e.g., triazolam): Etravirine may increase the levels and effects of these drugs.
- CYP3A4, 2C9, and 2C19 inducers: May decrease the levels and effects of etravirine.
- Macrolides: Etravirine may decrease the levels and effects of clarithromycin.
- Methadone: Etravirine may decrease the levels and effects of methadone. Monitor for opioid withdrawal symptoms.

SERIOUS REACTIONS

! Rash including Stevens-Johnson syndrome (blisters, peeling of the skin, loosening of skin and mucous membranes, and fever may occur) and hypersensitivity reaction may occur.

! Immune reconstitution syndrome may occur.

! Fat redistribution has been reported.

DENTAL CONSIDERATIONS

General:

- Examine for oral manifestations of opportunistic infection.
- Patient on chronic drug therapy may rarely have symptoms of blood dyscrasias, which include infection and poor healing.
- Place on frequent recall because of oral side effects.
- Consider semisupine chair position for patient comfort if GI side effects occur.
- Palliative medication may be required for management of oral side effects.
- Stomatitis as an adverse effect with relation to dental treatment.

Consultations:

- In a patient with symptoms of blood dyscrasias, request a medical consultation for blood studies and

postpone treatment until normal values are reestablished.
• Medical consultation may be required to assess disease control and patient's ability to tolerate stress.

Teach Patient/Family to:
• Encourage effective oral hygiene to prevent soft tissue inflammation.
• Prevent trauma when using oral hygiene aids.
• Update health and drug history if physician makes any changes in evaluation or drug regimens.
• See dentist immediately if secondary oral infection occurs.
• Stomatitis and the need to see dentist as soon as symptoms occur.

everolimus

e-ver-oh′-li-mus
(Afinitor)
Do not confuse everolimus with sirolimus, tacrolimus, or temsirolimus.

CATEGORY AND SCHEDULE

Pregnancy Risk Category: D

Drug Class: Antineoplastic agent, mTOR kinase inhibitor; immunosuppressant agent

MECHANISM OF ACTION

Everolimus is a macrolide immunosuppressant and an m-TOR inhibitor that has antiproliferative and antiangiogenic properties, and also reduces lipoma volume in patients with angiomyolipoma.
Therapeutic Effect: Anti-cancer effect by reducing cell proliferation, angiogenesis.

USES

Treatment of advanced hormone receptor-positive, HER2-negative breast cancer in postmenopausal women (in combination with exemestane and after letrozole or anastrozole failure); treatment of advanced renal cell cancer (RCC), after sunitinib or sorafenib failure; treatment of renal angiomyolipoma with tuberous sclerosis complex (TSC) not requiring immediate surgery; treatment of subependymal giant cell astrocytoma (SEGA) associated with TSC that requires intervention but cannot be curatively resected; treatment of advanced, metastatic, or unresectable pancreatic neuroendocrine tumors (PNETs)

PHARMACOKINETICS

Rapid but moderate absorption after oral administration. 74% plasma protein bound. Extensively metabolized in the liver via CYP3A4; forms 6 weak metabolites. Excreted primarily via feces.
Half-life: 30 hr.

INDICATIONS AND DOSAGES

▸ **Breast Cancer, Advanced, Hormone Receptor-Positive, HER2-Negative**

PO

Adults. 10 mg once daily (in combination with exemestane); continue treatment until no longer clinically beneficial or until unacceptable toxicity. Avoid grapefruit juice. May be taken with or without food, although should be administered consistently with regard to food.

▸ **Pancreatic Neuroendocrine Tumors (PNETs), Advanced**
PO
Adults. 10 mg once daily; continue treatment until no longer clinically beneficial or until unacceptable toxicity.

▸ **Renal Angiomyolipoma**
PO
Adults. 10 mg once daily; continue treatment until no longer clinically beneficial or until unacceptable toxicity.

▸ **Renal Cell Cancer, Advanced (RCC)**
PO
Adults. 10 mg once daily; continue treatment until no longer clinically beneficial or until unacceptable toxicity.

▸ **Renal Transplantation, Rejection Prophylaxis**
PO
Adults. 0.75 mg twice daily; adjust maintenance dose if needed at a 4- to 5-day interval (from prior dose adjustment) based on serum concentrations, tolerability, and response; administer in combination with basiliximab induction and concurrently with cyclosporine (dose adjustment required) and corticosteroids.

▸ **Subependymal Giant Cell Astrocytoma (SEGA)**
PO
Adults. Initially, 4.5 mg/m^2 once daily; round to nearest tablet (tablet or tablet for oral suspension) size. Assess trough concentrations 2 wk after initiation or dosage modification; adjust maintenance dose if needed at 2-wk intervals to achieve and maintain serum trough concentrations between 5 and 15 ng/ml; monitor trough concentrations routinely; once stable dose is attained and BSA is stable throughout treatment, monitor trough concentrations every 6–12 mo; monitor every 3–6 mo if BSA is changing. Continue until disease progression or unacceptable toxicity.
If trough <5 ng/ml: Increase dose by 2.5 mg/day (tablets) or 2 mg/day (tablets for oral suspension)
If trough >15 ng/ml: Reduce dose by 2.5 mg/day (tablets) or 2 mg/day (tablets for oral suspension)
If dose reduction necessary in patients receiving the lowest strength available, administer every other day.

SIDE EFFECTS/ADVERSE REACTIONS

Frequent
Peripheral edema , hypertension, fatigue, fever, headache, anxiety/aggression/behavioral disturbance, insomnia, dizziness, rash, acneiform dermatitis, cellulitis, pruritus, contact dermatitis, hypercholesterolemia, hyperglycemia, hypophosphatemia, hypocalcemia, hypoglycemia, hypokalemia, amenorrhea, taste alteration, stomatitis, diarrhea, nausea, xerostomia, urinary tract infection, anemia, leukopenia, thrombocytopenia, neutropenia, weakness, arthralgia, back pain, otitis, hematuria, upper respiratory infection, sinusitis, cough, dyspnea, epistaxis, nasal congestion, rhinitis, pharyngitis
Occasional
Chest pain, tachycardia, angina, depression, migraine, eczema, alopecia, hirsutism, incision complications, hyperhydrosis, hypertrichosis, menstrual irregularities, diabetes mellitus,

gastritis, dysphagia, hemorrhage, muscle spasm, tremor, jaw pain, eyelid edema, renal failure, pleural effusion, bronchitis, nasopharyngitis

E

PRECAUTIONS AND CONTRAINDICATIONS

Hypersensitivity to everolimus, sirolimus, other rapamycin derivatives, or any component of the formulation. May cause angioedema, bone marrow suppression, edema, nephrotoxicity, pneumonitis, wound healing complication. Use with caution in patients with carcinoid tumors, diabetes, heart transplantation, hepatic impairment, hyperlipidemia, renal impairment, renal transplantation.

DRUG INTERACTIONS OF CONCERN TO DENTISTRY

• CYP3A4 inhibitors and/or P-gp inhibitors (e.g., macrolide antibiotics, azole antifungals): potential increased risk of adverse effects of everolimus
• CYP3A4 inducers: possible need to increase dose of everolimus

SERIOUS REACTIONS

! An increased risk of renal arterial and venous thrombosis has been reported with use of everolimus in renal transplantation, generally within the first 30 days after transplant; may result in graft loss. Everolimus has immunosuppressant properties that may result in infection; the risk of developing bacterial (including mycobacterial), viral, fungal, and protozoal infections and local, opportunistic (including polyomavirus), systemic infections, and/or sepsis is increased. Immunosuppressant use may result in the development of malignancy, including lymphoma and skin cancer.

DENTAL CONSIDERATIONS

General:
• Monitor patient for stomatitis, mucositis, and oral ulcerations.
• Monitor for gastrointestinal adverse effects, including possible increased likelihood of vomiting (e.g., during sedation).
• Avoid irritation of oral mucosa during dental treatment.

Teach Patient/Family to:
• Avoid mouth rinses with high alcohol content because of irritating effect. Use palliative therapies for stomatitis and oral ulcerations (see section on "Therapeutic Management of Common Oral Lesions").

exemestane

ex-eh-**mess′**-tane
(Aromasin)

CATEGORY AND SCHEDULE

Pregnancy Risk Category: D

Drug Class: Antineoplastic; aromatase inhibitor

MECHANISM OF ACTION

Inactivates aromatase, the principal enzyme that converts androgens to estrogens in both premenopausal and postmenopausal women, thereby lowering the circulating estrogen level.
Therapeutic Effect: Inhibits the growth of breast cancers that are stimulated by estrogens.

USES

Treatment of advanced breast carcinoma not responsive to other therapy (postmenopausal)

PHARMACOKINETICS

Rapidly absorbed after PO administration. Protein binding: 90%. Distributed extensively into tissues. Metabolized in the liver; eliminated in urine and feces. ***Half-life:*** 24 hr.

INDICATIONS AND DOSAGES

▸ **Breast Cancer**

PO

Adults, Elderly. 25 mg once a day after a meal.

SIDE EFFECTS/ADVERSE REACTIONS

Frequent

Fatigue, nausea, depression, hot flashes, pain, insomnia, anxiety, dyspnea

Occasional

Headache, dizziness, vomiting, peripheral edema, abdominal pain, anorexia, flu-like symptoms, diaphoresis, constipation, hypertension

Rare

Diarrhea

PRECAUTIONS AND CONTRAINDICATIONS

Hypersensitivity to exemestane

DRUG INTERACTIONS OF CONCERN TO DENTISTRY

- Data not available; however, possible reduction in plasma levels by inducers of CYP3A4 isoenzymes

SERIOUS REACTIONS

! None known

DENTAL CONSIDERATIONS

General:

- Monitor vital signs at every appointment because of cardiovascular side effects.
- If additional analgesia is required for dental pain, consider alternative analgesics (NSAIDs) in patients taking narcotics for acute or chronic pain.
- Product may be used in outpatient therapy.
- If used in prostate cancer, consider urinary retention concern and avoid anticholinergic drugs that may aggravate retention.

Consultations:

- Medical consultation may be required to assess disease control and patient's ability to tolerate stress.

Teach Patient/Family to:

- Encourage effective oral hygiene to prevent soft tissue inflammation.
- Prevent trauma when using oral hygiene aids.
- Update health and medication history if physician makes any changes in evaluation or drug regimens; include OTC, herbal, and nonherbal remedies in the update.

exenatide

ex-**en**′-a-tide

(Byetta)

CATEGORY AND SCHEDULE

Pregnancy Risk Category: C

Drug Class: Antidiabetic agent, incretin mimetic

MECHANISM OF ACTION

An analog of the hormone incretin (glucagon-like peptide 1 or GLP-1) which enhances insulin secretion; suppresses elevated glucagon secretion; slows gastric emptying; decreases food intake.

Therapeutic Effect: Improves glycemic control; decreases hemoglobin $A1_c$.

E

USES
Treatment of Type 2 diabetes mellitus (noninsulin dependent, NIDDM), adjunct or monotherapy

PHARMACOKINETICS
Bioavailability: 65%–76%. Minimal systemic metabolism. Primarily excreted in urine. ***Half-life:*** 2.4 hr.

INDICATIONS AND DOSAGES
▸ Treatment of Type 2 Diabetes Mellitus (NIDDM), Adjunct or Monotherapy

SC

Adults. Initially, 5 mcg twice a day for 1 month. Maintenance: 10 mcg twice a day after one month of therapy. Administer within 60 min prior to a meal in upper arm, thigh, or abdomen.

SIDE EFFECTS/ADVERSE REACTIONS
Frequent

Hypoglycemia, nausea, vomiting, diarrhea, anti-exenatide antibodies

Occasional

Dizziness, headache, hyperhidrosis, reduced appetite, dyspepsia, GERD, weakness, feeling jittery

PRECAUTIONS AND CONTRAINDICATIONS
Hypersensitivity to exenatide or its components

Renal insufficiency (Cl_{cr} <30 ml/min), end-stage renal disease

Type 1 diabetes

Caution:

Renal transplantation, moderate renal impairment (Cl_{cr} 30–50 ml/min)

Gastrointestinal disease

Pancreatitis

Diabetic patients with gastroparesis

DRUG INTERACTIONS OF CONCERN TO DENTISTRY
- Insulin secretagogues (e.g., sulfonylurea, meglitinide): May increase the risk of hypoglycemia.
- Oral medications: May reduce the rate and extent of absorption of orally administered drugs.
- Ethanol: May increase the risk of hypoglycemia.

SERIOUS REACTIONS
! Altered renal function, including renal insufficiency, acute renal failure, and worsening chronic renal failure may occur.

! Acute pancreatitis has been reported.

! Severe hypersensitivity (e.g., anaphylaxis, angioedema) has been reported.

DENTAL CONSIDERATIONS
General:
- Short appointments and a stress-reduction protocol may be required for anxious patients.
- Patients with diabetes may be more susceptible to infection and have delayed wound healing.
- Question the patient about self-monitoring of drug's antidiabetic effect including blood glucose values or finger-stick records.
- Avoid prescribing aspirin-containing products.
- Consider semisupine chair position for patient comfort if GI side effects occur.

Consultations:
- Medical consultation may include data from patient's blood glucose monitoring, including glycosylated hemoglobin or HbA_{1c} testing.

• Medical consultation may be required to assess disease control.

Teach Patient/Family to:

• Encourage effective oral hygiene to prevent soft tissue inflammation.

• Prevent trauma when using oral hygiene aids.

• Avoid mouth rinses with high alcohol content because of drying effects.

• Instruct patients to take antibiotics at least 1 hr prior to administering exenatide.

ezetimibe

eh-**zet**-eh-mibe

(Zetia)

Do not confuse Zetia with Zestril.

CATEGORY AND SCHEDULE

Pregnancy Risk Category: C

Drug Class: Antihyperlipidemics

MECHANISM OF ACTION

An antihyperlipidemic that inhibits cholesterol absorption in the small intestine, leading to a decrease in the delivery of intestinal cholesterol to the liver.

Therapeutic Effect: Reduces total serum cholesterol, LDL cholesterol, and triglyceride levels; and increases HDL cholesterol concentration.

USES

Hypercholesterolemia

PHARMACOKINETICS

Well absorbed following oral administration. Protein binding: greater than 90%. Metabolized in the small intestine and liver. Excreted by the kidneys and bile. ***Half-life:*** 22 hr.

INDICATIONS AND DOSAGES

▸ Hypercholesterolemia

PO

Adults, Elderly. 10 mg once a day, given with or without food. If the patient is also receiving a bile acid sequestrant, give ezetimibe at least 2 hr before or at least 4 hr after the bile acid sequestrant.

SIDE EFFECTS/ADVERSE REACTIONS

Occasional

Back pain, diarrhea, arthralgia, sinusitis, abdominal pain, nasopharyngitis, myalgia, upper respiratory tract infection, pain in extremities, cough, fatigue

PRECAUTIONS AND CONTRAINDICATIONS

Hypersensitivity to ezetimibe or any component of the formulation

Concurrent use of an HMG-CoA reductase inhibitor (atorvastatin, fluvastatin, lovastatin, pravastatin, or simvastatin) in patients with active liver disease, pregnancy, or nursing mothers

Active hepatic disease or unexplained persistent elevations in serum transaminase levels

Caution:

Moderate or severe hepatic insufficiency

Chronic renal failure; CrCl ≤ 30ml/min

Diabetes

Hypothyroidism

Concurrent use with cyclosporine

DRUG INTERACTIONS OF CONCERN TO DENTISTRY

• Aluminum and magnesium-containing antacids:

Increase ezetimibe plasma concentration.

SERIOUS REACTIONS

! Elevations in liver transaminases and hepatitis were reported.
! Hypersensitivity reactions, including angioedema and rash, have been reported.
! Myopathy and rhabdomyolysis occur rarely.

E

DENTAL CONSIDERATIONS

General:
- Consider semisupine chair position for patient comfort if GI side effects occur.
- Monitor vital signs at every appointment due to cardiovascular side effects.

Consultations:
- Update health and drug history if physician makes any changes in evaluation or drug regimens.

Teach Patient/Family to:
- Encourage effective oral hygiene to prevent soft tissue inflammation.
- Use soft tooth brush to reduce risk of bleeding.
- Immediately report any sign of infection to the dentist.

ezogabine

e-**zog**′-a-been
(Potiga)
Do not confuse Potiga with Portia.

CATEGORY AND SCHEDULE

Pregnancy Risk Category: C

Drug Class: Anticonvulsant, neuronal potassium channel opener

MECHANISM OF ACTION

Ezogabine binds voltage-gated potassium channels. As a result, neuronal excitability is regulated and epileptiform activity is suppressed.

Therapeutic Effect: Prevents seizure activity.

USES

Adjuvant treatment of partial-onset seizures

PHARMACOKINETICS

Rapid absorption after oral administration. 80% plasma protein bound. Metabolized via glucuronidation and acetylation. Excreted in urine (85%) as unchanged drug (36%) and active metabolite (18%) and in feces (14%) as unchanged drug (3%). ***Half-life:*** 7–11 hr.

INDICATIONS AND DOSAGES

▸ **Partial-Onset Seizures, Adjunct**

PO

Adults. Initially, 100 mg 3 times/day; may increase at weekly intervals in increments of ≤150 mg/day to a maintenance dose of 200–400 mg 3 times/day (maximum: 1200 mg/day).

Elderly. Initially, 50 mg 3 times/day; may increase at weekly intervals in increments of ≤150 mg/day to a maximum daily dose of 750 mg.

▸ **Renal Impairment**

Cl_{cr} <50 ml/min: Initially, 50 mg 3 times/day; may increase at weekly intervals in increments of ≤150 mg/day to a maximum daily dose of 600 mg.

▸ **Hepatic Impairment**

Moderate impairment (Child-Pugh 7–9): Initially, 50 mg 3 times/day; may increase at weekly intervals in increments of ≤150 mg/day to a maximum daily dose of 750 mg. Severe impairment (Child-Pugh >9): Initially, 50 mg 3 times/day; may increase at weekly intervals in increments of ≤150 mg/day to a maximum daily dose of 600 mg.

SIDE EFFECTS/ADVERSE REACTIONS

Frequent
Dizziness, somnolence, fatigue
Occasional
Confusion, vertigo, memory impairment, nausea, dysphagia, blurred vision, tremor, dysuria

PRECAUTIONS AND CONTRAINDICATIONS

May cause significant urinary retention. May cause suicidal thinking and neuropsychiatric disorders. May cause withdrawal symptoms upon abrupt discontinuation.

DRUG INTERACTIONS OF CONCERN TO DENTISTRY

- P-gb inducers (e.g., carbamazepine): reduced effectiveness of ezogabine
- Sedatives, alcohol: may potentiate dizziness, mental impairment, abnormal coordination, and somnolence

SERIOUS REACTIONS

! None known

DENTAL CONSIDERATIONS

General:
- Monitor patient for possible dizziness, somnolence, abnormal coordination, and dysarthria and take precautions when seating and dismissing patient.
- Monitor patients for signs and symptoms of partial-onset seizures.
- Consider memory impairment and disturbances of attention when communicating with patient.

Consultations:
- Consult patient's physician to determine disease control and ability of patient to tolerate dental procedures.

Teach Patient/Family to:
- Report changes in seizure activity and medical regimen.

famciclovir

fam-**si**′-klo-veer
(Famvir)
Do not confuse Famvir with Femhrt.

CATEGORY AND SCHEDULE

Pregnancy Risk Category: B

Drug Class: Antiviral

F

MECHANISM OF ACTION

A synthetic nucleoside that inhibits viral DNA synthesis.
Therapeutic Effect: Suppresses replication of herpes simplex virus and varicella-zoster virus.

USES

Treatment of acute herpes zoster (shingles) infection; recurrent genital herpes; recurrent herpes simplex virus infections in HIV-infected patients

PHARMACOKINETICS

Rapidly and extensively absorbed after PO administration. Protein binding: 20%–25%. Rapidly metabolized to penciclovir by enzymes in the GI wall, liver, and plasma. Eliminated unchanged in urine. Removed by hemodialysis.
Half-life: 2 hr.

INDICATIONS AND DOSAGES

▸ Herpes Zoster
PO
Adults. 500 mg q8h for 7 days.

▸ Recurrent Genital Herpes
PO
Adults. 125 mg twice a day for 5 days.

▸ Suppression of Recurrent Genital Herpes
PO
Adults. 250 mg twice a day for up to 1 yr.

▸ Recurrent Herpes Simplex
PO
Adults. 500 mg twice a day for 7 days.

▸ Dosage in Renal Impairment
Dosage and frequency are modified on the basis of creatinine clearance.

Creatinine Clearance	Herpes Zoster	Genital Herpes
40–59 ml/min	500 mg q12h	125 mg q12h
20–39 ml/min	500 mg q24h	125 mg q24h
Less than 20 ml/min	250 mg q24h	125 mg q24h

▸ Dosage in Hemodialysis Patients
For adults with herpes zoster, give 250 mg after each dialysis treatment; for adults with genital herpes, give 125 mg after each dialysis treatment.

SIDE EFFECTS/ADVERSE REACTIONS

Frequent
Headache, nausea
Occasional
Dizziness, somnolence, numbness of feet, diarrhea, vomiting, constipation, decreased appetite, fatigue, fever, pharyngitis, sinusitis, pruritus
Rare
Insomnia, abdominal pain, dyspepsia, flatulence, back pain, arthralgia

PRECAUTIONS AND CONTRAINDICATIONS

Hypersensitivity
Caution:
Children younger than 18 yr, lactation, elderly, hepatic and renal function impairment

DRUG INTERACTIONS OF CONCERN TO DENTISTRY

- None reported in otherwise uncompromised patients

SERIOUS REACTIONS

! None known

DENTAL CONSIDERATIONS

General:

- Determine why the patient is taking the drug.
- Consider semisupine chair position for patient comfort because of GI effects of drug.
- Be aware of general discomfort associated with shingles; acute symptoms may preclude patient's routine dental visit or mandate short appointments.

Consultations:

- Medical consultation may be required to assess disease control and patient's ability to tolerate stress.

famotidine

fam-**oh**'-tah-deen

(Amfamox[AUS], Novo-Famotidine[CAN] Pepcid, Pepcid AC, Pepcidine[AUS], Ulcidine[CAN])

CATEGORY AND SCHEDULE

Pregnancy Risk Category: B

OTC (10 mg tablets)

Drug Class: Histamine H_2-receptor antagonist

MECHANISM OF ACTION

An antiulcer agent and gastric acid secretion inhibitor that inhibits histamine action at H_2 receptors of parietal cells.

Therapeutic Effect: Inhibits gastric acid secretion when fasting, at night, or when stimulated by food, caffeine, or insulin.

USES

Short-term treatment of active duodenal ulcer, maintenance therapy for duodenal ulcer, Zollinger-Ellison syndrome, multiple endocrine adenomas, benign gastric ulcers, gastroesophageal reflux disease (GERD); OTC: heartburn, acid indigestion

PHARMACOKINETICS

Route	Onset	Peak	Duration
PO	1 hr	1–4 hr	10–12 hr
IV	1 hr	0.5–3 hr	10–12 hr

Rapidly, incompletely absorbed from the GI tract. Protein binding: 15%–20%. Partially metabolized in the liver. Primarily excreted in urine. Not removed by hemodialysis.

Half-life: 2.5–3.5 hr (increased with impaired renal function).

INDICATIONS AND DOSAGES

▸ **Acute Treatment of Duodenal and Gastric Ulcers**

PO

Adults, Elderly, Children 12 yr and older. 40 mg/day at bedtime.

Children 1–11 yr. 0.5 mg/kg/day at bedtime. Maximum: 40 mg/day.

▸ **Duodenal Ulcer Maintenance**

PO

Adults, Elderly. 20 mg/day at bedtime.

▸ **GERD**

PO

Adults, Elderly, Children 12 yr and older. 20 mg twice a day.

Children 1–11 yr. 1 mg/kg/day in 2 divided doses.

Children 3–11 mo. 0.5 mg/kg/dose twice a day.

Children younger than 3 mo. 0.5 mg/kg/dose once a day.

F

F

▸ **Esophagitis**
PO
Adults, Elderly, Children 12 yr and older. 2–40 mg twice a day.

▸ **Hypersecretory Conditions**
PO
Adults, Elderly, Children 12 yr and older. Initially, 20 mg q6h. May increase up to 160 mg q6h.

▸ **Acid Indigestion, Heartburn (OTC)**
PO
Adults, Elderly, Children 12 yr and older. 10–20 mg 15–60 min before eating. Maximum: 2 doses per day.

▸ **Usual Parenteral Dosage**
IV
Adults, Elderly, Children 12 yr and older. 20 mg q12h.

▸ **Dosage in Renal Impairment**
Dosing frequency is modified on the basis of creatinine clearance.

Creatinine Clearance	Dosage Interval
10–50 ml/min	q24h
Less than 10 ml/min	q36–48h

SIDE EFFECTS/ADVERSE REACTIONS

Occasional
Headache

Rare
Constipation, diarrhea, dizziness

PRECAUTIONS AND CONTRAINDICATIONS

Hypersensitivity

Caution:
Lactation, children, severe renal disease, severe hepatic function, elderly, RPD tablets contain aspartame (caution: phenylketonuria)

DRUG INTERACTIONS OF CONCERN TO DENTISTRY

- Decreased absorption of ketoconazole or itraconazole (take doses 2 hr apart)

SERIOUS REACTIONS

! None known

DENTAL CONSIDERATIONS

General:
- Avoid prescribing aspirin-containing products in patients with active GI disease.
- Consider semisupine chair position for patient comfort because of GI effects of disease.
- Assess salivary flow as a factor in caries, periodontal disease, and candidiasis.

Teach Patient/Family to:
- Encourage effective oral hygiene to prevent gingival inflammation.
- When chronic dry mouth occurs, advise patient to:
  - Avoid mouth rinses with high alcohol content because of drying effects.
  - Use daily home fluoride products for anticaries effect.
  - Use sugarless gum, frequent sips of water, or saliva substitutes.

febuxostat

feb-**ux**′-oh-stat
(Uloric)

CATEGORY AND SCHEDULE

Pregnancy Risk Category: C

Drug Class: Xanthine oxidase inhibitor

MECHANISM OF ACTION
A non-purine, selective inhibitor of xanthine oxidase.
Therapeutic Effect: Decreases serum uric acid.

USES
Hyperuricemia in patients with gout

PHARMACOKINETICS
Partially absorbed. Protein binding: 99.2%. Extensively metabolized by both conjugation via uridine diphosphate glucuronosyltransferase enzymes and oxidation via CYP enzymes, including CYP1A2, 2C8, and 2C9. Partially excreted in urine; partially excreted in feces. ***Half-life***: 5–8 hr.

INDICATIONS AND DOSAGES
▸ Hyperuricemia in Patients with Gout
PO
Adults. 40 mg a day. May increase to 80 mg/day in patients who do not achieve serum uric acid < 6 mg/dl after 2 wk of 40-mg treatment.

SIDE EFFECTS/ADVERSE REACTIONS
Rare (≤1%)
Dizziness, rash, nausea, abnormal liver function tests (LFTs), arthralgia

PRECAUTIONS AND CONTRAINDICATIONS
Hypersensitivity to febuxostat or its components
Drugs metabolized by xanthine oxidase (e.g., azathioprine, mercaptopurine, theophylline)
Caution:
Hepatic impairment
Renal impairment
Pregnancy
Cardiovascular disease

DRUG INTERACTIONS OF CONCERN TO DENTISTRY
- Drugs metabolized by xanthine oxidase (e.g., azathioprine, mercaptopurine, theophylline): May increase plasma concentrations of these agents.

SERIOUS REACTIONS
! Elevated transaminases have been reported.
! Cardiovascular thromboembolic events (cardiovascular deaths, non-fatal myocardial infarctions, and non-fatal strokes) may occur.
! Gout flares may occur during the initiation of treatment.

DENTAL CONSIDERATIONS
General:
- Patient on chronic drug therapy may rarely have symptoms of blood dyscrasias, which include infection, bleeding, and poor healing.

Consultations:
- In a patient with symptoms of blood dyscrasias, request a medical consultation for blood studies and postpone treatment until normal values are reestablished.
- Medical consultation may be required to assess disease control.

Teach Patient/Family to:
- Encourage effective oral hygiene to prevent soft tissue inflammation.
- Avoid mouth rinses with high alcohol content because of drying effects.

F

felbamate

fel′-ba-mate
(Felbatol)

CATEGORY AND SCHEDULE

Pregnancy Risk Category: C

Drug Class: Anticonvulsant (carbamate derivative)

MECHANISM OF ACTION

An anticonvulsant, structurally similar to meprobamate, that weakly blocks repetitive, sustained firing of neurons by enhancing the ability of γ-aminobutyric acid (GABA) and antagonizes the strychnine-insensitive glycine recognition site of the *N*-methyl-D-aspartate receptor-ionophore complex. ***Therapeutic Effect:*** Decreases seizure activity.

USES

Used alone or as adjunct therapy in partial seizures; also for partial seizures associated with Lennox-Gastaut syndrome in children; because of severe side effects use only for severe seizures when other therapy is inadequate

PHARMACOKINETICS

Rapidly and almost completely absorbed after PO administration. Protein binding: 22%–25%, primarily to albumin. Partially excreted unchanged in the urine. ***Half-life:*** 20–23 hr.

INDICATIONS AND DOSAGES

▸ Monotherapy or Adjunctive Therapy in the Treatment of Partial Seizures, with and without Generalization

PO

Adults, Children older than 14 yr. Initially, 1200 mg/day in divided doses 3–4 times a day. At week 2, increase the felbamate dosage to 2400 mg/day while reducing the dosage of other antiepileptic drugs (AEDs) up to an additional one-third of their original dosage. At week 3, increase the felbamate dosage up to 3600 mg/day and continue to reduce the dosage of other AEDs as clinically indicated.

▸ Adjunctive Therapy in the Treatment of Partial Seizures, with and without Generalization

PO

Adults, Children older than 14 yr. Add 1200 mg/day in divided doses 3–4 times a day while reducing present AEDs by 20% in order; control plasma concentrations of concurrent phenytoin, valproic acid, and carbamazepine and its metabolites. Increase dosage by 1200 mg/day increments at weekly intervals to 3600 mg/day.

SIDE EFFECTS/ADVERSE REACTIONS

Frequent

Somnolence, dizziness, headache, fatigue, nausea, anorexia, vomiting, constipation

Occasional

Chest pain, palpitations, tachycardia, depression and behavioral changes, anxiety, nervousness, ataxia, malaise, agitation, rash, acne, pruritus, diarrhea, weight gain, tremors, abnormal vision, diplopia, sinusitis, difficulty with coordination, taste perversion

Rare

Delusion, bradycardia, hallucinations, urinary retention, acute renal failure

PRECAUTIONS AND CONTRAINDICATIONS

History of any blood dyscrasia or hepatic dysfunction, hypersensitivity

to felbamate, its ingredients, or known sensitivity to other carbamates
Caution:
Lactation, warning of increased risk of aplastic anemia, hepatic failure; safety and efficacy in children with other types of seizures has not been established

DRUG INTERACTIONS OF CONCERN TO DENTISTRY

• Decreased effects of carbamazepine
• Increased photosensitization: drugs causing photosensitivity (e.g., tetracyclines)

SERIOUS REACTIONS

Alert
! Aplastic anemia has been reported during felbamate therapy.
! Hepatic failure resulting in death has been reported.

DENTAL CONSIDERATIONS

General:
• Examine for evidence of oral manifestations of blood dyscrasia (infection, bleeding, poor healing).
• Short appointments and a stress-reduction protocol may be required for anxious patients.
• Determine type of epilepsy, seizure frequency, and quality of seizure control. A stress reduction protocol may be required.
• Assess salivary flow as a factor in caries, periodontal disease, and candidiasis.
• Monitor vital signs at every appointment because of cardiovascular side effects.
• Advise patient if dental drugs prescribed have a potential for photosensitivity.
Consultations:
• Medical consultation may be required to assess disease control and patient's ability to tolerate stress.
Teach Patient/Family to:
• Encourage effective oral hygiene to prevent soft tissue inflammation.
• Use caution to prevent injury when using oral hygiene aids.
• Use powered tooth brush if patient has difficulty holding conventional devices.
• When chronic dry mouth occurs, advise patient to:
  • Avoid mouth rinses with high alcohol content because of drying effects.
  • Use daily home fluoride products for anticaries effect.
  • Use sugarless gum, frequent sips of water, or saliva substitutes.

felodipine

fell-**oh′**-da-peen
(AGON SR[AUS], Felodur ER[AUS], Plendil, Plendil ER[AUS], Renedil[CAN])
Do not confuse Plendil with Pletal, or Renedil with Prinivil.

CATEGORY AND SCHEDULE

Pregnancy Risk Category: C

Drug Class: Calcium channel blocker

MECHANISM OF ACTION

An antihypertensive and antianginal agent that inhibits calcium movement across cardiac and vascular smooth-muscle cell membranes. Potent peripheral vasodilator (does not depress SA or AV nodes).
Therapeutic Effect: Increases myocardial contractility, heart rate, and cardiac output; decreases peripheral vascular resistance and B/P.

USES

Essential hypertension, alone or with other antihypertensives, chronic angina pectoris

PHARMACOKINETICS

Route	Onset	Peak	Duration
PO	2–5 hr	N/A	N/A

Rapidly, completely absorbed from the GI tract. Protein binding: greater than 99%. Undergoes first-pass metabolism in the liver. Primarily excreted in urine. Not removed by hemodialysis. ***Half-life:*** 11–16 hr.

INDICATIONS AND DOSAGES

▸ **Hypertension**

PO

Adults. Initially, 5 mg/day as single dose.

Elderly, Patients with impaired hepatic function. Initially, 2.5 mg/day. Adjust dosage at no less than 2-wk intervals. Maintenance: 2.5–10 mg/day.

SIDE EFFECTS/ADVERSE REACTIONS

Frequent

Headache, peripheral edema

Occasional

Flushing, respiratory infection, dizziness, light-headedness, asthenia (loss of strength, weakness), gingival enlargement

Rare

Paresthesia, abdominal discomfort, nervousness, muscle cramping, cough, diarrhea, constipation

PRECAUTIONS AND CONTRAINDICATIONS

Hypersensitivity, sick sinus syndrome, second- or third-degree heart block

Caution:

CHF, hypotension less than 90 mm Hg systolic, hepatic injury, lactation, children, renal disease, elderly

DRUG INTERACTIONS OF CONCERN TO DENTISTRY

- Decreased effect: NSAIDs, phenobarbital, carbamazepine
- Increased effect: parenteral and inhalational general anesthetics, other drugs with hypotensive actions
- Increased effects of nondepolarizing muscle relaxants, diazepam, midazolam
- Increased plasma levels: itraconazole, erythromycin, carbamazepine

SERIOUS REACTIONS

! Overdose produces nausea, somnolence, confusion, slurred speech, hypotension and bradycardia.

DENTAL CONSIDERATIONS

General:

- Monitor cardiac status; take vital signs at each appointment because of cardiovascular side effects. Consider a stress reduction protocol to prevent stress-induced angina during the dental appointment.
- After supine positioning, have patient sit upright for at least 2 min before standing to avoid orthostatic hypotension at dismissal.
- Place on frequent recall to monitor gingival condition.
- Limit use of sodium-containing products, such as saline IV fluids, for patients with a dietary salt restriction.
- Assess salivary flow as a factor in caries, periodontal disease, and candidiasis.
- Use vasoconstrictors with caution, in low doses and with careful

aspiration. Avoid use of gingival retraction cord with epinephrine.

• Use precaution if sedation or general anesthesia is required; risk of hypotensive episode.

Consultations:

• Medical consultation may be required to assess disease control.

• Consultation with physician may be necessary if sedation or general anesthesia is required.

Teach Patient/Family to:

• Encourage effective oral hygiene to prevent gingival inflammation and minimize enlargement.

• Schedule frequent oral prophylaxis if enlargement occurs.

• When chronic dry mouth occurs, advise patient to:

  • Avoid mouth rinses with high alcohol content because of drying effects.
  • Use daily home fluoride products for anticaries effect.
  • Use sugarless gum, frequent sips of water, or saliva substitutes.

fenofibrate

fee-no-**fye′**-brate

(Apo-Fenofibrate[CAN], Lofibra, TriCor)

Do not confuse TriCor with Tracleer.

CATEGORY AND SCHEDULE

Pregnancy Risk Category: C

Drug Class: Antihyperlipidemic

MECHANISM OF ACTION

An antihyperlipidemic that enhances synthesis of lipoprotein lipase and reduces triglyceride-rich lipoproteins and VLDLs.

Therapeutic Effect: Increases VLDL catabolism and reduces total plasma triglyceride levels.

USES

Treatment of hyperlipidemia, types IV and V, as an adjunct to diet therapy

PHARMACOKINETICS

Well absorbed from the GI tract. Absorption increased when given with food. Protein binding: 99%. Rapidly metabolized in the liver to active metabolite. Excreted primarily in urine; lesser amount in feces. Not removed by hemodialysis. ***Half-life:*** 20 hr.

INDICATIONS AND DOSAGES

▸ Reduction of Very High Serum Triglyceride Levels in Patients at Risk for Pancreatitis

PO

Adults, Elderly. Initially, 67 mg/day (capsule); may increase to 200 mg/day. Or initially, 48 mg/day (tablet); may increase to 145 mg/day.

▸ Hypercholesterolemia

PO

Adults, Elderly. 200 mg/day (capsule) with meals. Or 145 mg/day (tablet) with meals.

SIDE EFFECTS/ADVERSE REACTIONS

Frequent

Pain, rash, headache, asthenia or fatigue, flu symptoms, dyspepsia, nausea or vomiting, rhinitis

Occasional

Diarrhea, abdominal pain, constipation, flatulence, arthralgia, decreased libido, dizziness, pruritus

Rare

Increased appetite, insomnia, polyuria, cough, blurred vision, eye floaters, earache

PRECAUTIONS AND CONTRAINDICATIONS

Gallbladder disease, hypersensitivity to fenofibrate, severe renal or hepatic dysfunction (including primary biliary cirrhosis, unexplained persistent liver function abnormality)

Caution:

Monitor liver function; may lead to cholelithiasis; can be associated with myositis, myopathy, or rhabdomyolysis; avoid if lactating; safe use in children unknown; discontinue use if no response in 2 mo; increased anticoagulant effect with oral anticoagulants

DRUG INTERACTIONS OF CONCERN TO DENTISTRY

- None reported

SERIOUS REACTIONS

! Fenofibrate may increase excretion of cholesterol into bile, leading to cholelithiasis.

! Pancreatitis, hepatitis, thrombocytopenia, and agranulocytosis occur rarely.

DENTAL CONSIDERATIONS

General:

- Monitor vital signs at every appointment because of cardiovascular and respiratory side effects.
- Consider semisupine chair position for patient comfort because of GI side effects of drug.
- Patients on chronic drug therapy may rarely have symptoms of blood dyscrasias, which can include infection, bleeding, and poor healing.
- Avoid dental light in patient's eyes; offer dark glasses for patient comfort.

Consultations:

- In a patient with symptoms of blood dyscrasias, request a medical consultation for blood studies and postpone treatment until normal values are reestablished.

Teach Patient/Family to:

- Use powered tooth brush if patient has difficulty holding conventional devices.
- Prevent trauma when using oral hygiene aids.

fenoprofen calcium

fen-oh-**proe′**-fen

(Nalfon)

Do not confuse Nalfon with Naldecon.

CATEGORY AND SCHEDULE

Pregnancy Risk Category: B (D if used in third trimester or near delivery)

Drug Class: Nonsteroidal antiinflammatory, propionic acid derivative

MECHANISM OF ACTION

An NSAID that produces analgesic and antiinflammatory effects by inhibiting prostaglandin synthesis. ***Therapeutic Effect:*** Reduces the inflammatory response and intensity of pain.

USES

Treatment of mild-to-moderate pain, osteoarthritis, rheumatoid arthritis, acute gout, arthritis, ankylosing spondylitis, nonrheumatic inflammation, dysmenorrhea

PHARMACOKINETICS

PO: Peak 2 hr. ***Half-life:*** 3–3.5 hr; 99% plasma protein binding;

metabolized in liver; excreted in urine (metabolites), breast milk.

INDICATIONS AND DOSAGES

▸ Mild-to-Moderate Pain

PO

Adults, Elderly. 200 mg q4–6h as needed.

▸ Rheumatoid Arthritis, Osteoarthritis

PO

Adults, Elderly. 300–600 mg 3–4 times a day.

SIDE EFFECTS/ADVERSE REACTIONS

Frequent

Headache, somnolence, dyspepsia, nausea, vomiting, constipation

Occasional

Dizziness, pruritus, nervousness, asthenia, diarrhea, abdominal cramps, flatulence, tinnitus, blurred vision, peripheral edema and fluid retention

PRECAUTIONS AND CONTRAINDICATIONS

Active peptic ulcer disease, chronic inflammation of GI tract, GI bleeding or ulceration, history of hypersensitivity to aspirin or NSAIDs, significant renal impairment

Caution:

Lactation, children, bleeding disorders, GI disorders, cardiac disorders, hypersensitivity to other antiinflammatory agents

DRUG INTERACTIONS OF CONCERN TO DENTISTRY

• GI bleeding, ulceration: salicylates, alcohol, corticosteroids, other NSAIDs, bisphosphonates
• May decrease effects of fenoprofen: phenobarbital
• Nephrotoxicity: acetaminophen (prolonged use)
• Possible risk of decreased renal function: cyclosporine
• Probable increased bleeding risk: warfarin
• Suspected increased risk for methotrexate toxicity
• First-time users of SSRIs also taking NSAIDs may have a higher risk of GI side effects; avoid use of NSAIDs in these patients

F

SERIOUS REACTIONS

! Overdose may result in acute hypotension and tachycardia.

! Rare reactions with long-term use include peptic ulcer disease, GI bleeding, gastritis, severe hepatic reaction (jaundice), nephrotoxicity (hematuria, dysuria, proteinuria) and a severe hypersensitivity reaction (bronchospasm, angioedema).

DENTAL CONSIDERATIONS

General:

• Assess salivary flow as a factor in caries, periodontal disease, and candidiasis.
• Avoid prescribing in pregnancy.
• Possibility of cross-allergenicity when patient is allergic to aspirin.
• Severe stomach bleeding may occur in patients who regularly use NSAIDs in recommended doses, when the patient is also taking another NSAID, a blood thinning, or steroid drug, if the patient has GI or peptic ulcer disease, if they are 60 years or older, or when NSAIDs are taken longer than directed. Warn patients of the potential for severe stomach bleeding.

Consultations:

• Medical consultation may be required to assess disease control.

Teach Patient/Family to:

• Encourage effective oral hygiene to prevent gingival inflammation.

- Use caution to prevent injury when using oral hygiene aids.
  - Warn patient of potential risks of NSAIDs.
- When chronic dry mouth occurs, advise patient to:
  - Avoid mouth rinses with high alcohol content because of drying effects.
  - Use daily home fluoride products for anticaries effect.
  - Use sugarless gum, frequent sips of water, or saliva substitutes.

F

fentanyl, buccal

fen′ta nil **bu′ck**-al

(Onsolis)

Do not confuse fentanyl with alfentanil or sufentanil.

CATEGORY AND SCHEDULE

Pregnancy Risk Category: C

Drug Class: Opioid analgesic

MECHANISM OF ACTION

Interacts with opioid receptors in the CNS to alter pain perception. ***Therapeutic Effect:*** Alters pain perception and increases pain threshold.

USES

Management of breakthrough cancer pain in patients with malignancies who are using or tolerant to opioids

PHARMACOKINETICS

Rapid absorption of 50% from the buccal mucosa; remaining 50% swallowed with saliva and slowly absorbed from GI tract. 80%–85% plasma protein bound. Hepatic metabolism primarily via CYP3A4 enzymes. Excreted in urine (75%) and feces (9%). ***Half-life:*** 3–14 hr.

INDICATIONS AND DOSAGES

▸ Chronic Pain

Transmucosal form

Adults. Initial dose: 200 mcg for all patients. Note: Patients previously using another transmucosal product should be initiated at doses of 200 mcg; do not switch patients using any other fentanyl product on a mcg-per-mcg basis.

SIDE EFFECTS/ADVERSE REACTIONS

Frequent

Hypersensitivity to opiates

Occasional

Dry mouth, dizziness, delirium, euphoria, bradycardia, hypotension or hypertension, nausea, vomiting, respiratory depression, laryngospasm, blurred vision, miosis, muscle rigidity

PRECAUTIONS AND CONTRAINDICATIONS

Use with caution in elderly patients and patients with respiratory depression, increased intracranial pressure, seizure disorders, severe respiratory disorders, cardiac dysrhythmias.

DRUG INTERACTIONS OF CONCERN TO DENTISTRY

- Increased risk of CNS depression: CYP3A4 inhibitors, all CNS depressants, alcohol. Interaction may result in fatal respiratory depression. May potentiate mental impairment and somnolence, postural hypotension.

SERIOUS REACTIONS

! Fentanyl may cause life-threatening respiratory depression, cardiorespiratory arrest, generalized CNS depression, coma, death. Should be used only for the care of opioid-tolerant cancer patients with breakthrough pain and is intended for use by specialists who are knowledgeable in treating cancer pain.

DENTAL CONSIDERATIONS

General:

• Monitor patient for dizziness and somnolence and take precautions when seating and dismissing patient.
• Monitor for drug abuse and dependence. Drug is available only through a restricted program.
• Fentanyl buccal is not indicated for the management of acute or postoperative dental pain.
• Be prepared to manage respiratory depression, nausea, and vomiting.
• Mental impairment may limit patient's ability to understand instructions and to communicate with dental team.

Teach Patient/Family to:

• Report changes in disease status or medication regimen.

fentanyl transdermal system

fen′-ta-nil trans-**derr**′-mal **sis**′-tem

(Duragesic 25, 50, 75, 100 Transdermal Patches, Fentanyl Oralet oral: transmucosal fentanyl citrate: Actiq [lozenges])

CATEGORY AND SCHEDULE

Pregnancy Risk Category: C
Controlled Substance Schedule II

Drug Class: Opioid analgesics

MECHANISM OF ACTION

Interacts with opioid receptors in the CNS to alter pain perception.

USES

Management of chronic pain when opioids are necessary; transmucosal form: only for management of breakthrough cancer pain in patients with malignancies who are using or tolerant to opioids; not appropriate for acute postoperative pain

PHARMACOKINETICS

Transdermal: Dosage adjusted according to opioid tolerance if patient has been taking opioids (2.5 mg of transdermal fentanyl is equivalent to approximately 90 mg of oral morphine in 24 hr); peak serum levels take up to 24 hr after applied; liver metabolism; renal excretion of metabolites.

INDICATIONS AND DOSAGES

▸ Chronic Pain

Topical

Adult only. One patch every 72 hr; dose depends on need for pain control; titrate as required.

Transmucosal Form

Adult only. (Patch and lozenge on a stick only [Actiq].) Dose must be titrated starting with lowest dose size (must be kept secure from children).

Conscious Sedation or Anesthesia (Oralet Only) in Hospital Setting

Adult. Doses must match patient, usually no more than 5 mcg/kg (400 mcg); doses for children must be adjusted for weight; see package insert directions for use.

SIDE EFFECTS/ADVERSE REACTIONS

ORAL: Dry mouth
CNS: Dizziness, delirium, euphoria

CV: Bradycardia, arrest, hypotension, or hypertension
GI: Nausea, vomiting
RESP: Respiratory depression, arrest, laryngospasm
EENT: Blurred vision, miosis
MS: Muscle rigidity

F

PRECAUTIONS AND CONTRAINDICATIONS

Hypersensitivity to opiates, myasthenia gravis

Caution:

Elderly, respiratory depression, increased intracranial pressure, seizure disorders, severe respiratory disorders, cardiac dysrhythmias

DRUG INTERACTIONS OF CONCERN TO DENTISTRY

- Effects may be increased with other CNS depressants: alcohol, narcotics, sedative/hypnotics, skeletal muscle relaxants, chlorpromazine
- Additive hypotension: nitrous oxide, benzodiazepines, phenothiazines
- Increased anticholinergic effect: anticholinergics
- Contraindication: MAOIs

SERIOUS REACTIONS

! Life-threatening respiratory depression, cardiorespiratory arrest, generalized CNS depression, coma, death

DENTAL CONSIDERATIONS

General:

- Monitor vital signs at every appointment because of cardiovascular and respiratory side effects.
- After supine positioning, have patient sit upright for at least 2 min before standing to avoid orthostatic hypotension.
- Assess salivary flow as a factor in caries, periodontal disease, and candidiasis.
- Psychologic and physical dependence may occur with chronic administration.
- Determine why the patient is taking the drug.
- Consider alternative drugs to opioids and NSAIDs for management of dental pain.

Consultations:

- Medical consultation may be required to assess disease control.

Teach Patient/Family to:

- Encourage effective oral hygiene to prevent gingival inflammation.
- Avoid mouth rinses with high alcohol content because of drying effects.

ferrous fumarate/ ferrous gluconate/ ferrous sulfate

fer′-us **fume′**-ah-rate/**fer′**-us **glue′**-kuh-nate/**fer′**-us sul′-fate

ferrous fumarate
(Feostat, Femiron, Ferro-Sequels, Nephro-Fer, Palafer[CAN])

ferrous gluconate
(Apo-Ferrous Gluconate[CAN], Fergon)

ferrous sulfate
(Apo-Ferrous Sulfate[CAN], Fer-In-Sol, Fer-Iron, Ferro-Gradumet[AUS], Slow-Fe)

CATEGORY AND SCHEDULE

Pregnancy Risk Category: A
OTC

Drug Class: Hematinic, iron preparation

MECHANISM OF ACTION

An enzymatic mineral that is an essential component in the formation of Hgb, myoglobin and enzymes. Promotes effective erythropoiesis and transport and utilization of oxygen (O_2). ***Therapeutic Effect:*** Prevents iron deficiency.

USES

Treatment of iron deficiency anemia, prophylaxis for iron deficiency in pregnancy

PHARMACOKINETICS

Absorbed in the duodenum and upper jejunum. Ten percent absorbed in patients with normal iron stores; increased to 20%–30% in those with inadequate iron stores. Primarily bound to serum transferrin. Excreted in urine, sweat and sloughing of intestinal mucosa and by menses. ***Half-life:*** 6 hr.

INDICATIONS AND DOSAGES

▸ Iron Deficiency Anemia

Dosage is expressed in terms of milligrams of elemental iron, degree of anemia, patient weight and presence of any bleeding. Expect to use periodic hematologic determinations as guide to therapy.

PO (Ferrous Fumarate)
Adults, Elderly. 60–100 mg twice a day.
Children. 3–6 mg/kg/day in 2–3 divided doses.
PO (Ferrous Gluconate)
Adults, Elderly. 60 mg 2–4 times a day.
Children. 3–6 mg/kg/day in 2–3 divided doses.
PO (Ferrous Sulfate)
Adults, Elderly. 325 mg 2–4 times a day.
Children. 3–6 mg/kg/day in 2–3 divided doses.

▸ Prevention of Iron Deficiency

PO (Ferrous Fumarate)
Adults, Elderly. 60–100 mg/day.
Children. 1–2 mg/kg/day.
PO (Ferrous Gluconate)
Adults, Elderly. 60 mg/day.
Children. 1–2 mg/kg/day.
PO (Ferrous Sulfate)
Adults, Elderly. 325 mg/day.
Children. 1–2 mg/kg/day.

SIDE EFFECTS/ADVERSE REACTIONS

Occasional

Mild, transient nausea, extrinsic stain on teeth (liquid form)

Rare

Heartburn, anorexia, constipation, diarrhea

PRECAUTIONS AND CONTRAINDICATIONS

Hemochromatosis, hemosiderosis, hemolytic anemias, peptic ulcer disease, regional enteritis, ulcerative colitis

Caution:

Long-term anemia

DRUG INTERACTIONS OF CONCERN TO DENTISTRY

• Decreased absorption of tetracycline, zinc, ciprofloxacin

SERIOUS REACTIONS

! Large doses may aggravate existing GI tract disease, such as peptic ulcer disease, regional enteritis and ulcerative colitis.

! Severe iron poisoning occurs most often in children and is manifested as vomiting, severe abdominal pain, diarrhea, and dehydration, followed by hyperventilation, pallor or cyanosis, and cardiovascular collapse.

F

DENTAL CONSIDERATIONS

Teach Patient/Family to:

- Avoid frequent use if patient is using hydrogen peroxide as a dentifrice to remove extrinsic stain so that peroxide-related soft tissue injury does not occur.
- Take through straw followed by rinsing mouth to reduce staining.

F

fesoterodine

fes′-oh-**ter**′-oh-deen
(Toviaz)

CATEGORY AND SCHEDULE

Pregnancy Risk Category: C

Drug Class: Urinary antispasmodics

MECHANISM OF ACTION

An anticholinergic that antagonizes acetylcholine at muscarinic receptors and relaxes the detrusor smooth muscle of the bladder.
Therapeutic Effect: Reduces urinary frequency and urgency.

USES

Overactive bladder

PHARMACOKINETICS

Well absorbed following PO administration. Protein binding: 50%. Rapidly and extensively metabolized to its active metabolite, 5-hydroxymethyl derivative (5-HMT). 5-HMT is metabolized by CYP450 2D6 and 3A4. Primarily excreted in urine and smaller amounts in feces. ***Half-life:*** 7 hr (active metabolite).

INDICATIONS AND DOSAGES

▸ Overactive Bladder

PO

Adults. 4 mg a day. May increase to 8 mg a day, based upon individual response and tolerability.
Patients with severe renal insufficiency or those taking potent CYP3A4 inhibitors should not use doses greater than 4 mg a day.
Not recommended in patients with hepatic impairment.

SIDE EFFECTS/ADVERSE REACTIONS

Frequent

Dry mouth, dry eye, constipation, dysuria

Occasional

Dizziness, headache, dry throat, abdominal pain, diarrhea, dyspepsia, nausea, insomnia

PRECAUTIONS AND CONTRAINDICATIONS

Hypersensitivity to fesoterodine or its components
Urinary retention
Gastric retention
Uncontrolled narrow-angle glaucoma

Caution:

Bladder outlet obstruction
Decreased gastrointestinal motility
Controlled narrow-angle glaucoma
Myasthenia gravis
Severe hepatic impairment

DRUG INTERACTIONS OF CONCERN TO DENTISTRY

- Anticholinergic agents: Increased effects of anticholinergics.
- CYP3A4 inhibitors (e.g., ketoconazole, itraconazole, clarithromycin): May increase levels of fesoterodine; increased risk of adverse effects.

- CYP3A4 inducers (rifampin, carbamazepine): May decrease levels of fesoterodine.
- Orally administered drugs: May alter the GI absorption of concomitantly administered drug due to anticholinergic effects on GI motility.

SERIOUS REACTIONS

! None reported

DENTAL CONSIDERATIONS

General:

- Monitor vital signs at every appointment because of cardiovascular side effects.
- Assess salivary flow as a factor in caries, periodontal disease, and candidiasis.
- Avoid dental light in patient's eyes; offer dark glasses for patient comfort.
- Consider semisupine chair position for patient comfort if GI side effects occur.

Consultations:

- Physician should be informed if significant xerostomic side effects occur (e.g., increased caries, sore tongue, problems eating or swallowing, difficulty wearing prosthesis) so that medication change can be considered.
- Medical consultation may be required to assess disease control.

Teach Patient/Family to:

- Encourage effective oral hygiene to prevent soft tissue inflammation.
- When chronic dry mouth occurs, advise patient to:
  - Avoid mouth rinses with high alcohol content because of drying effects.
  - Use daily home fluoride products for anticaries effect.
  - Use sugarless gum, frequent sips of water, or saliva substitutes.

fexofenadine hydrochloride

fex-oh-**fen**′-eh-deen
hi-droh-klor′-ide
(Allegra, Telfast[AUS])

CATEGORY AND SCHEDULE

Pregnancy Risk Category: C

Drug Class: Antihistamine, nonsedating

F

MECHANISM OF ACTION

A piperidine that competes with histamine for H_1-receptor sites on effector cells.

Therapeutic Effect: Relieves allergic rhinitis symptoms.

USES

Treatment of seasonal allergic rhinitis, chronic idiopathic urticaria

PHARMACOKINETICS

Rapidly absorbed after PO administration. Protein binding: 60%–70%. Does not cross the blood-brain barrier. Minimally metabolized. Eliminated in feces and urine. Not removed by hemodialysis. ***Half-life:*** 14.4 hr (increased in renal impairment).

INDICATIONS AND DOSAGES

▸ Allergic Rhinitis, Urticaria

PO

Adults, Elderly, Children 12 yr and older. 60 mg twice a day or 180 mg once a day.

Children 6–11 yr. 30 mg twice a day.

▸ Dosage in Renal Impairment

Adults, Elderly and Children 12 yr and older. Dosage is reduced to 60 mg once a day.

Children 6–11 yr. Dosage is reduced to 30 mg once a day.

SIDE EFFECTS/ADVERSE REACTIONS

Rare

Somnolence, headache, fatigue, nausea, vomiting, abdominal distress, dysmenorrhea

PRECAUTIONS AND CONTRAINDICATIONS

Hypersensitivity; troglitazone

Caution:

Reduce dose in elderly, renally impaired, lactation, children younger than 12 yr

DRUG INTERACTIONS OF CONCERN TO DENTISTRY

• Elevated plasma levels with erythromycin, ketoconazole
• Decreased absorption: grapefruit juice
• Suspected decreased antihistaminic effects: rifampin

SERIOUS REACTIONS

! None known

DENTAL CONSIDERATIONS

General:

• Consider semisupine chair position for patient comfort because of GI effects of drug.

fidaxomicin

fye-dax-oh-**mye**′sin
(Dificid)
Do not confuse Dificid with Diflucan.

CATEGORY AND SCHEDULE

Pregnancy Risk Category: B

Drug Class: Macrolide antibiotic

MECHANISM OF ACTION

Inhibits protein synthesis and cell death in susceptible organisms including C. difficile.

Therapeutic Effect: Bactericidal

USES

Treatment of Clostridium difficile-associated diarrhea (CDAD)

PHARMACOKINETICS

Minimal systemic absorption. Metabolized via intestinal hydrolysis to less active metabolite. Excreted in feces (92%) as unchanged drug and metabolites. ***Half-life:*** 11.7 hr.

INDICATIONS AND DOSAGES

▸ Treatment of *Clostridium Difficile*-Associated Diarrhea (CDAD)

PO

Adults. 200 mg twice daily for 10 days.

SIDE EFFECTS/ADVERSE REACTIONS

Frequent

Nausea

Occasional

Abdominal pain, anemia

PRECAUTIONS AND CONTRAINDICATIONS

Because there is minimal systemic absorption, fidaxomicin is not effective for treatment of systemic infections.

DRUG INTERACTIONS OF CONCERN TO DENTISTRY

• Antibiotics: coadministration of other antibiotics with fidaxomicin could potentially reduce its effectiveness.

SERIOUS REACTIONS

! None known

DENTAL CONSIDERATIONS

General:

• Patients taking fidaxomicin are being treated for a serious infection (*C. difficile*-associated diarrhea).

• Fidaxomicin should not be used for systemic infections.

• Beware of serious gastrointestinal disturbances, including nausea, vomiting, gastrointestinal bleeding, anemia, and neutropenia, which may require medical intervention.

Teach Patient/Family to:

• Report changes in disease status and drug regimen.

filgrastim

fill-**grass'**-tim

(Neupogen)

Do not confuse Neupogen with Epogen or Nutramigen.

CATEGORY AND SCHEDULE

Pregnancy Risk Category: C

Drug Class: Biologic modifier; granulocyte colony-stimulating factor

MECHANISM OF ACTION

A biologic modifier that stimulates production, maturation, and activation of neutrophils to increase their migration and cytotoxicity.

Therapeutic Effect: Decreases incidence of infection.

USES

Stimulates the bone marrow to make new white blood cells

PHARMACOKINETICS

Readily absorbed after subcutaneous administration. Not removed by hemodialysis. ***Half-life:*** 3.5 hr.

INDICATIONS AND DOSAGES

▸ Myelosuppression

IV or Subcutaneous Infusion, Subcutaneous Injection

Adults, Elderly. Initially, 5 mcg/kg/day. May increase by 5 mcg/kg for each chemotherapy cycle on the basis of duration or severity of absolute neutrophil count nadir.

▸ Bone Marrow Transplant

IV or Subcutaneous Infusion

Adults, Elderly. 5–10 mcg/kg/day. Adjust dosage daily during period of neutrophil recovery on the basis of neutrophil response.

▸ Mobilization Progenitor Cells

IV or Subcutaneous Infusion

Adults. 10 mcg/kg/day beginning at least 4 days before first leukapheresis and continuing until last leukapheresis.

▸ Chronic Neutropenia, Congenital Neutropenia

Subcutaneous

Adults, Children. 6 mcg/kg/dose twice a day.

▸ Idiopathic or Cyclic Neutropenia

Subcutaneous

Adults, Children. 5 mcg/kg/dose once a day.

SIDE EFFECTS/ADVERSE REACTIONS

Frequent

Nausea or vomiting, mild to severe bone pain that occurs more frequently with high-dose IV form and less frequently with low-dose subcutaneous form; alopecia, diarrhea, fever, fatigue

Occasional

Anorexia, dyspnea, headache, cough, rash

Rare

Psoriasis, hematuria or proteinuria, osteoporosis

PRECAUTIONS AND CONTRAINDICATIONS

Hypersensitivity to *Escherichia coli*–derived proteins, 24 hr before or after cytotoxic chemotherapy, concurrent use of other drugs that may result in lowered platelet count

DRUG INTERACTIONS OF CONCERN TO DENTISTRY

- Dental drug interactions have not been studied.

SERIOUS REACTIONS

! Long-term administration occasionally produces chronic neutropenia and splenomegaly.
! Thrombocytopenia, MI, and arrhythmias occur rarely.
! Adult respiratory distress syndrome may occur in patients with sepsis.

DENTAL CONSIDERATIONS

General:

- Determine why patient is taking the drug.
- Examine for oral manifestations of opportunistic infection.
- Monitor vital signs at every appointment because of cardiovascular side effects.
- Patient may need assistance in getting into and out of dental chair. Adjust chair position for patient comfort.
- Patients are at risk for infection.
- Oral infections should be eliminated and/or treated aggressively.
- Patients may have been treated with radiation and/or chemotherapy; confirm medical and drug history.

Consultations:

- Medical consultation may be required to assess disease control and patient's ability to tolerate stress.
- In a patient with symptoms of blood dyscrasias, request a medical consultation for blood studies and postpone treatment until normal values are reestablished.
- Medical consultation should include routine blood counts including platelet counts and bleeding time.

Teach Patient/Family to:

- Encourage effective oral hygiene to prevent soft tissue inflammation.
- Prevent trauma when using oral hygiene aids.
- Update health and medication history if physician makes any changes in evaluation or drug regimens; include OTC, herbal, and nonherbal remedies in the update.

finasteride

fen-**as**′-ter-ide
(Propecia, Proscar)
Do not confuse Proscar with Posicor, ProSom, Prozac, or Psorcon.

CATEGORY AND SCHEDULE

Pregnancy Risk Category: X

Drug Class: Synthetic steroid

MECHANISM OF ACTION

An androgen hormone inhibitor that inhibits 5-alpha reductase, an intracellular enzyme that converts testosterone into dihydrotestosterone (DHT) in the prostate gland, resulting in a decreased serum DHT level.

Therapeutic Effect: Reduces size of the prostate gland.

USES

Proscar: Treatment of symptomatic benign prostatic hyperplasia (BPH),

reduce risk for acute urinary retention and surgery
Propecia: Treatment of male pattern baldness (androgenic alopecia) in men 18–41 yr

PHARMACOKINETICS

Route	Onset	Peak	Duration
PO	24 hr	1–2 days	5–7 days

Rapidly absorbed from the GI tract. Protein binding: 90%. Widely distributed. Metabolized in the liver. ***Half-life:*** 6–8 hr. Onset of clinical effect: 3–6 mo of continued therapy.

INDICATIONS AND DOSAGES

▸ BPH
PO
Adults, Elderly. 5 mg once a day (for a minimum of 6 mo).

▸ Hair Loss
PO
Adults. 1 mg/day.

SIDE EFFECTS/ADVERSE REACTIONS

Rare
Gynecomastia, sexual dysfunction (impotence, decreased libido, decreased volume of ejaculate)

PRECAUTIONS AND CONTRAINDICATIONS

Exposure to the patient's semen or handling of finasteride tablets by those who are or may be pregnant
Caution:
Lactation, lower PSA levels do not suggest absence of prostate cancer; women should avoid drug or semen contact, hepatic impairment

DRUG INTERACTIONS OF CONCERN TO DENTISTRY

• Opioids and anticholinergic drugs may enhance urinary retention; use alternative analgesics (NSAIDs)

SERIOUS REACTIONS

! None known

DENTAL CONSIDERATIONS

Consultations:
• Determine why patient is taking the drug (for prostatic hyperplasia or male pattern baldness).
• Medical consultation may be required to assess disease control.

F

fingolimod

fin-**gol**′i-mod
(Gilenya)

CATEGORY AND SCHEDULE

Pregnancy Risk Category: C

Drug Class: Sphingosine 1-phosphate (S1P) receptor modulator

MECHANISM OF ACTION

Fingolimod binds to sphingosine 1-phosphate receptors, which results in a decrease in the amount of lymphocytes available to the central nervous system and, thus, reduces central inflammation.
Therapeutic Effect: Reduces the frequency of relapses of multiple sclerosis.

USES

Treatment of relapsing forms of multiple sclerosis (MS) to reduce the frequency of clinical exacerbations and delay disability progression

PHARMACOKINETICS

Well distributed after oral administration. 99.7% plasma protein bound. Hepatic metabolism via CYP4F2, 2D6, 2E1, 3A4, and 4F12. Excreted primarily in urine as inactive metabolites. ***Half-life:*** 6–9 days.

INDICATIONS AND DOSAGES

▸ Multiple Sclerosis

PO

Adults. 0.5 mg once daily; doses >0.5 mg/day associated with increased adverse events and no additional benefit.

SIDE EFFECTS/ADVERSE REACTIONS

Frequent

Headache, diarrhea, back pain, flu-like syndrome

Occasional

Hypertension, bradycardia, depression, dizziness, alopecia, eczema, gastroenteritis, leukopenia, weakness, blurred vision, cough, dyspnea

PRECAUTIONS AND CONTRAINDICATIONS

May cause AV block, bradycardia, hypertension, reduced respiration, and macular edema. Use with caution in patients with cardiovascular disease and hepatic impairment. May cause immunosuppression; use with caution in patients receiving concomitant immunosuppressant, immune modulating, or antineoplastic medications.

DRUG INTERACTIONS OF CONCERN TO DENTISTRY

• CYP3A4 inhibitors (e.g., macrolide antibiotics, azole antifungals): increased risk of adverse effects caused by fingolimod.

SERIOUS REACTIONS

! May cause immunosuppression and increased risk of infection for up to 2 mo following discontinuation of therapy

DENTAL CONSIDERATIONS

General:

• Patients taking fingolimod may have impaired coordination. Caution should be used when seating and dismissing patient.

• Monitor vital signs for possible cardiovascular adverse effects (e.g., bradycardia).

• Monitor patient for development of infections associated with use of this drug.

• Drug may cause loss of vision, which should be considered when communicating with patient through documents, visual aids, models, etc.

Consultations:

• Consult physician to determine disease status, presence of cardiovascular adverse effects, and potential liver damage.

Teach Patient/Family to:

• Report changes in disease status and drug regimen.

flavocoxid

flay-voh-**cox**′-id

(Limbrel)

CATEGORY AND SCHEDULE

Pregnancy Risk Category: Not classified.

Drug Class: Oral nutritional supplement

MECHANISM OF ACTION

An oral nutritional supplement that inhibits prostaglandin synthesis and arachidonic acid metabolism, reducing the production of leukotrienes. Also acts through an antioxidant mechanism.

Therapeutic Effect: Produces antiinflammatory and analgesic effects and increases mobility.

USES

Dietary management of osteoarthritis

PHARMACOKINETICS

Undergoes hydrolysis at the gut mucosal border. Food decreases absorption. Little hepatic metabolism.

INDICATIONS AND DOSAGES

▸ Osteoarthritis

PO

Adults 18 yr and older, Elderly. One 250-mg capsule q12h.

SIDE EFFECTS/ADVERSE REACTIONS

Rare

Increase in varicose veins, psoriasis, mild hypertension

PRECAUTIONS AND CONTRAINDICATIONS

History of peptic ulcer

DRUG INTERACTIONS OF CONCERN TO DENTISTRY

- None reported

SERIOUS REACTIONS

! GI bleeding, perforation, and ulceration occur rarely in patients currently or previously treated with NSAIDs or COX-2 inhibitors.

DENTAL CONSIDERATIONS

General:

- Determine why patient is taking the drug.
- Patient may need assistance in getting into and out of dental chair. Adjust chair position for patient comfort.
- Patients presenting with a history of osteoarthritis will be taking other agents; confirm medical and drug/herbal and nonherbal history.

Consultations:

- Medical consultation may be required to assess disease control and patient's ability to tolerate stress.

Teach Patient/Family to:

- Use powered tooth brush if patient has difficulty holding conventional devices.
- Encourage effective oral hygiene to prevent soft tissue inflammation.
- Prevent trauma when using oral hygiene aids.
- Update health and medication history if physician makes any changes in evaluation or drug regimens; include OTC, herbal, and nonherbal remedies in the update.

flavoxate

fla-**vox**′-ate

(Urispas)

Do not confuse Urispas with Urised.

CATEGORY AND SCHEDULE

Pregnancy Risk Category: B

Drug Class: Antispasmodic

MECHANISM OF ACTION

An anticholinergic that relaxes detrusor and other smooth muscle by cholinergic blockade, counteracting muscle spasm in the urinary tract.

Therapeutic Effect: Produces anticholinergic, local anesthetic and analgesic effects, relieving urinary symptoms.

USES

Relief of nocturia, incontinence, suprapubic pain, dysuria, frequency associated with urologic conditions (symptomatic only)

PHARMACOKINETICS

Excreted in urine.

F

INDICATIONS AND DOSAGES

▸ To Relieve Symptoms of Cystitis, Prostatitis, Urethritis, Urethrocystitis, or Urethrotrigonitis

PO

Adults, Elderly, Adolescents. 100–200 mg 3–4 times a day.

SIDE EFFECTS/ADVERSE REACTIONS

Frequent

Somnolence, dry mouth and throat

Occasional

Constipation, difficult urination, blurred vision, dizziness, headache, increased light sensitivity, nausea, vomiting, abdominal pain

Rare

Confusion (primarily in elderly), hypersensitivity, increased intraocular pressure, leukopenia

PRECAUTIONS AND CONTRAINDICATIONS

Duodenal or pyloric obstruction, GI hemorrhage or obstruction, ileus, lower urinary tract obstruction

Caution:

Lactation, suspected glaucoma, children younger than 12 yr

DRUG INTERACTIONS OF CONCERN TO DENTISTRY

- Increased anticholinergic effect: anticholinergic drugs
- Drug may cause drowsiness or blurred vision: advise patients when other CNS depressants are used

SERIOUS REACTIONS

! Overdose may produce anticholinergic effects, including unsteadiness, severe dizziness, somnolence, fever, facial flushing, dyspnea, nervousness, and irritability.

DENTAL CONSIDERATIONS

General:

- Assess salivary flow as a factor in caries, periodontal disease, and candidiasis.

Teach Patient/Family to:

- Encourage effective oral hygiene to prevent gingival inflammation.
- Avoid mouth rinses with high alcohol content because of drying effects.

flecainide

fle′-kah-nide

(Flecatab[AUS], Tambocor)

CATEGORY AND SCHEDULE

Pregnancy Risk Category: C

Drug Class: Antidysrhythmic (Class IC)

MECHANISM OF ACTION

An antiarrhythmic that slows atrial, AV, His-Purkinje, and intraventricular conduction. Decreases excitability, conduction velocity, and automaticity.

Therapeutic Effect: Controls atrial, supraventricular, and ventricular arrhythmias.

USES

Prevention of life-threatening ventricular dysrhythmias, sustained supraventricular tachycardia; prevention of paroxysmal atrial flutter (PAF), fibrillation, or paroxysmal atrial tachycardia

PHARMACOKINETICS

PO: Peak 3 hr. ***Half-life:*** 12–27 hr; metabolized by liver; excreted unchanged by kidneys (10%); excreted in breast milk.

INDICATIONS AND DOSAGES

▸ Life-Threatening Ventricular Arrhythmias, Sustained Ventricular Tachycardia

PO

Adults, Elderly. Initially, 100 mg q12h, increased by 100 mg (50 mg twice a day) every 4 days until effective dose or maximum of 400 mg/day is attained.

▸ Paroxysmal Supraventricular Tachycardias (PSVT), PAF

PO

Adults, Elderly. Initially, 50 mg q12h, increased by 100 mg (50 mg twice a day) every 4 days until effective dose or maximum of 300 mg/day is attained.

SIDE EFFECTS/ADVERSE REACTIONS

Frequent

Dizziness, dyspnea, headache

Occasional

Nausea, fatigue, palpitations, chest pain, asthenia (loss of strength, energy), tremors, constipation

PRECAUTIONS AND CONTRAINDICATIONS

Cardiogenic shock, preexisting second- or third-degree AV block, right bundle-branch block (without presence of a pacemaker)

Caution:

Lactation, children, renal disease, liver disease, CHF, respiratory depression, myasthenia gravis

DRUG INTERACTIONS OF CONCERN TO DENTISTRY

- No specific interactions are reported with dental drugs; however, any drug that could affect the cardiac action of flecainide (e.g., other local anesthetics, vasoconstrictors, anticholinergics) should be used in the lowest effective dose.

SERIOUS REACTIONS

! Flecainide may worsen existing arrhythmias or produce new ones.

! CHF may occur or existing CHF may worsen.

! Overdose may increase QRS duration, prolong QT interval, cause conduction disturbances, reduce myocardial contractility and cause hypotension.

DENTAL CONSIDERATIONS

General:

- Monitor vital signs at every appointment because of cardiovascular and respiratory side effects.
- Assess salivary flow as a factor in caries, periodontal disease, and candidiasis.
- Stress from dental procedures may compromise cardiovascular function; determine patient risk, use a stress-reduction protocol.
- Use vasoconstrictors with caution, in low doses and with careful aspiration. Avoid use of gingival retraction cord with epinephrine.

Consultations:

- Medical consultation may be required to assess disease control and patient's ability to tolerate stress.

Teach Patient/Family to:

- Encourage effective oral hygiene to prevent gingival inflammation.
- Avoid mouth rinses with high alcohol content because of drying effects.

fluconazole

floo-**con'**-ah-zole

(Apo-Fluconazole[CAN], Diflucan)

Do not confuse Diflucan with diclofenac.

CATEGORY AND SCHEDULE

Pregnancy Risk Category: C

Drug Class: Antifungal

F

MECHANISM OF ACTION

A fungistatic antifungal that interferes with cytochrome P-450, an enzyme necessary for ergosterol formation.

Therapeutic Effect: Directly damages fungal membrane, altering its function.

USES

Treatment of oropharyngeal candidiasis, chronic mucocutaneous candidiasis, vaginal candidiasis, cryptococcal meningitis, esophageal candidiasis and prophylaxis in patients receiving bone marrow transplants with chemotherapy or radiation

PHARMACOKINETICS

Well absorbed from GI tract. Widely distributed, including to CSF. Protein binding: 11%. Partially metabolized in liver. Excreted unchanged primarily in urine. Partially removed by hemodialysis. ***Half-life:*** 20–30 hr (increased in impaired renal function).

INDICATIONS AND DOSAGES

▸ Oropharyngeal Candidiasis

PO, IV

Adults, Elderly. 200 mg once, then 100 mg/day for at least 14 days.

Children. 6 mg/kg/day once, then 3 mg/kg/day.

▸ Esophageal Candidiasis

PO, IV

Adults, Elderly. 200 mg once, then 100 mg/day (up to 400 mg/day) for 21 days and at least 14 days following resolution of symptoms.

Children. 6 mg/kg/day once, then 3 mg/kg/day (up to 12 mg/kg/day) for 21 days at least 14 days following resolution of symptoms.

▸ Vaginal Candidiasis

PO

Adults. 150 mg once.

▸ Prevention of Candidiasis in Patients Undergoing Bone Marrow Transplantation

PO

Adults. 400 mg/day.

▸ Systemic Candidiasis

PO, IV

Adults, Elderly. 400 mg once, then 200 mg/day (up to 400 mg/day) for at least 28 days and at least 14 days following resolution of symptoms.

Children. 6–12 mg/kg/day.

▸ Cryptococcal Meningitis

PO, IV

Adults, Elderly. 400 mg once, then 200 mg/day (up to 800 mg/day) for 10–12 wk after CSF becomes negative (200 mg/day for suppression of relapse in patients with AIDS).

Children. 12 mg/kg/day once, then 6–12 mg/kg/day (6 mg/kg/day for suppression of relapse in patients with AIDS).

▸ Onychomycosis

PO

Adults. 150 mg/wk.

▸ Dosage in Renal Impairment

After a loading dose of 400 mg, the daily dosage is based on creatinine clearance.

Creatinine Clearance	% of Recommended Dose
Greater than 50 ml/min	100
21–50 ml/min	50
11–20 ml/min	25
Dialysis	Dose after dialysis

SIDE EFFECTS/ADVERSE REACTIONS

Occasional

Hypersensitivity reaction (including chills, fever, pruritus, and rash), dizziness, drowsiness, headache, constipation, diarrhea, nausea, vomiting, abdominal pain

PRECAUTIONS AND CONTRAINDICATIONS

Hypersensitivity

Caution:

Renal disease

DRUG INTERACTIONS OF CONCERN TO DENTISTRY

- Caution: potent inhibitor of CYP3A4
- Increased plasma levels of oral hypoglycemics: theophylline, cyclosporine, tacrolimus, corticosteroids
- Inhibits metabolism of benzodiazepines: alprazolam, chlordiazepoxide, clonazepam, clorazepate, diazepam, estazolam, flurazepam, halazepam, midazolam, triazolam, quazepam, zolpidem
- Increased anticoagulant effect: may inhibit metabolism of warfarin
- Suspected risk of increased neurologic side effects: haloperidol, tricyclic antidepressants
- May increase levels and side effects of HMG-CoA reductase inhibitors
- Suspected increase in antihypertensive effects of losartan; monitor blood pressure if used concurrently
- Decreased renal clearance: hydrochlorothiazide
- Suspected decrease in oral contraceptive effectiveness; may want to suggest additional contraception

SERIOUS REACTIONS

! Exfoliative skin disorders, serious hepatic effects and blood dyscrasias (such as eosinophilia, thrombocytopenia, anemia, and leukopenia) have been reported rarely.

DENTAL CONSIDERATIONS

General:

- Culture may be required to confirm fungal organism.
- Patients on chronic drug therapy may rarely have symptoms of blood dyscrasias, which can include infection, bleeding, and poor healing.

Consultations:

- In a patient with symptoms of blood dyscrasias, request a medical consultation for blood studies and postpone treatment until normal values are reestablished.

Teach Patient/Family to:

- Be aware that long-term therapy may be necessary to clear infection.
- Prevent reinoculation of *Candida* infection by disposing of tooth brush or other contaminated oral hygiene devices used during period of infection.

flucytosine

floo-**sye**′-toe-seen
(Ancobon)

CATEGORY AND SCHEDULE

Pregnancy Risk Category: C

F

Drug Class: Antifungal

MECHANISM OF ACTION

An antifungal that penetrates fungal cells and is converted to fluorouracil which competes with uracil interfering with fungal RNA and protein synthesis.
Therapeutic Effect: Damages fungal membrane.

USES

Treatment of *Candida* infections (septicemia, endocarditis, pulmonary and UTIs), *Cryptococcus* (meningitis, pulmonary and urinary tract infections)

PHARMACOKINETICS

Well absorbed from GI tract. Widely distributed, including CSF. Protein binding: 2%–4%. Metabolized in liver. Partially removed by hemodialysis. ***Half-life:*** 3–8 hr (half-life is increased with impaired renal function).

INDICATIONS AND DOSAGES

▸ **Fungal Infections, Candidiasis, Cryptococcosis**

PO

Adults, Elderly, Children. 50–150 mg/kg/day in 4 equally divided doses.

▸ **Dosage in Renal Function Impairment**

Based on creatinine clearance:

Creatinine Clearance	Dosage Interval
20–40 ml/min	q12h
10–20 ml/min	q24h
0–10 ml/min	q24–48h

SIDE EFFECTS/ADVERSE REACTIONS

Occasional

Pruritus, rash, photosensitivity, dizziness, drowsiness, headache, diarrhea, nausea, vomiting, abdominal pain, increased liver enzymes, jaundice, increased BUN and creatinine, weakness, hearing loss

PRECAUTIONS AND CONTRAINDICATIONS

Hypersensitivity to flucytosine

Caution:

Renal disease, bone marrow depression, blood dyscrasias, radiation therapy, or chemotherapy

DRUG INTERACTIONS OF CONCERN TO DENTISTRY

- None reported

SERIOUS REACTIONS

! Hepatic dysfunction and severe bone marrow suppression occur rarely.

DENTAL CONSIDERATIONS

General:

- Patients on chronic drug therapy may rarely have symptoms of blood dyscrasias, which can include infection, bleeding, and poor healing.
- Examine for evidence of oral *Candida* infection.

Consultations:

- Medical consultation may be required to assess disease control.

• In a patient with symptoms of blood dyscrasias, request a medical consultation for blood studies and postpone dental treatment until normal values are reestablished.

Teach Patient/Family to:

• Encourage effective oral hygiene to prevent gingival inflammation.

fludarabine phosphate

flew-**dare′**-ah-bean **foss′**-fate

(Fludara)

Do not confuse Fludara with FUDR.

CATEGORY AND SCHEDULE

Pregnancy Risk Category: D

Drug Class: Antineoplastic, antimetabolite

MECHANISM OF ACTION

An antimetabolite that inhibits DNA synthesis by interfering with DNA polymerase alpha, ribonucleotide reductase and DNA primase.

Therapeutic Effect: Induces cell death.

USES

Treatment of chronic lymphocyte leukemia, non-Hodgkin's lymphoma

PHARMACOKINETICS

Rapidly dephosphorylated in serum, then phosphorylated intracellularly to active triphosphate. Primarily excreted in urine. ***Half-life:*** 7–20 hr.

INDICATIONS AND DOSAGES

▸ **Chronic Lymphocytic Leukemia**

IV

Adults. 25 mg/m^2 daily for 5 consecutive days. Continue for up to 3 additional cycles. Begin each course of treatment every 28 days.

▸ **Non-Hodgkin's Lymphoma**

IV

Adults, Elderly. Initially, 20 mg/m^2, then 30 mg/m^2/day for 48 hr.

▸ **Dosage in Renal Impairment**

Creatinine Clearance	Dosage
30–70 ml/min	Decrease dose by 20%
Less than 30 ml/min	Not recommended

SIDE EFFECTS/ADVERSE REACTIONS

Frequent

Fever, nausea and vomiting

Occasional

Chills, fatigue, generalized pain, rash, diarrhea, cough, asthenia, stomatitis, dyspnea, peripheral edema

Rare

Anorexia, sinusitis, dysuria, myalgia, paresthesia, headaches, visual disturbances

PRECAUTIONS AND CONTRAINDICATIONS

Concurrent use with pentostatin

DRUG INTERACTIONS OF CONCERN TO DENTISTRY

• None reported

SERIOUS REACTIONS

! Pneumonia occurs frequently.

! Severe hematologic toxicity (as evidenced by anemia, thrombocytopenia, and neutropenia) and GI bleeding may occur.

! Tumor lysis syndrome may start with flank pain and hematuria and may include hypercalcemia, hyperphosphatemia, hyperuricemia, and renal failure.

! High-dosage therapy may produce acute leukemia, blindness, and coma.

DENTAL CONSIDERATIONS

General:

- Monitor vital signs at every appointment because of cardiovascular side effects.
- If additional analgesia is required for dental pain, consider alternative analgesics in patients taking narcotics for acute or chronic pain.
- Examine for oral manifestation of opportunistic infection.
- Avoid products that affect platelet function, such as aspirin and NSAIDs.
- This drug may be used in the hospital or on an outpatient basis. Confirm the patient's disease and treatment status.
- Chlorhexidine mouth rinse prior to and during chemotherapy may reduce severity of mucositis.
- Patient on chronic drug therapy may rarely present with symptoms of blood dyscrasias, which can include infection, bleeding, and poor healing. If dyscrasia is present, caution patient to prevent oral tissue trauma when using oral hygiene aids.
- Palliative medication may be required for management of oral side effects.
- Patients may be at risk of infection.
- Patients may be at risk of bleeding; check for oral signs.
- Oral infections should be eliminated and/or treated aggressively.

Consultations:

- Medical consultation should include routine blood counts including platelet counts and bleeding time.
- Consult physician; prophylactic or therapeutic antiinfectives may be indicated if surgery or periodontal treatment is required.
- Medical consultation may be required to assess immunologic status during cancer chemotherapy and determine safety risk, if any, posed by the required dental treatment.
- Medical consultation may be required to assess disease control and patient's ability to tolerate stress.

Teach Patient/Family to:

- Be aware of oral side effects.
- Encourage effective oral hygiene to prevent soft tissue inflammation.
- Report oral lesions, soreness, or bleeding to dentist.
- Prevent trauma when using oral hygiene aids.
- Update health and medication history if physician makes any changes in evaluation or drug regimens; include OTC, herbal, and nonherbal remedies in the update.

fludrocortisone

floo-droe-**kor′**-ti-sone

(Florinef)

Do not confuse Florinef with Fioricet or Florinal.

CATEGORY AND SCHEDULE

Pregnancy Risk Category: C

Drug Class: Glucocorticoid and mineralocorticoid

MECHANISM OF ACTION

A mineralocorticoid that acts at distal renal tubules.

Therapeutic Effect: Increases potassium and hydrogen ion excretion. Replaces sodium loss and raises blood pressure (with low dosages). Inhibits endogenous adrenal cortical secretion, thymic activity, and secretion of corticotropin by pituitary gland (with higher dosages).

USES

Treatment of adrenal insufficiency (Addison's disease), salt-losing adrenogenital syndrome

PHARMACOKINETICS

Well absorbed from the GI tract. Protein binding: 42%. Widely distributed. Metabolized in the liver and kidney. Primarily excreted in urine. ***Half-life:*** 3.5 hr.

INDICATIONS AND DOSAGES

▸ Addison's Disease

PO

Adults, Elderly. 0.05–0.1 mg/day. Range: 0.1 mg 3 times a wk to 0.2 mg/day. Administration with cortisone or hydrocortisone preferred.

▸ Salt-Losing Adrenogenital Syndrome

PO

Adults, Elderly. 0.1–0.2 mg/day.

Usual Pediatric Dosage

Children. 0.05–0.1 mg/day.

SIDE EFFECTS/ADVERSE REACTIONS

Frequent

Increased appetite, exaggerated sense of well-being, abdominal distention, weight gain, insomnia, mood swings

High dosages, prolonged therapy, too rapid withdrawal: Increased susceptibility to infection with masked signs and symptoms, delayed wound healing, hypokalemia, hypocalcemia, GI distress, diarrhea or constipation, hypertension

Occasional

Headache, dizziness, menstrual difficulty or amenorrhea, gastric ulcer development

Rare

Hypersensitivity reaction

PRECAUTIONS AND CONTRAINDICATIONS

CHF, systemic fungal infection

Caution:

Lactation, osteoporosis, CHF, safety and use in children has not been established

DRUG INTERACTIONS OF CONCERN TO DENTISTRY

- Decreased action: barbiturates
- Increased side effects: sodium-containing food, sodium-containing polishing devices
- Decreased effects of salicylates

SERIOUS REACTIONS

! Long-term therapy may cause muscle wasting (especially in the arms and legs), osteoporosis, spontaneous fractures, amenorrhea, cataracts, glaucoma, peptic ulcer disease, and CHF.

! Abruptly withdrawing the drug after long-term therapy may cause anorexia, nausea, fever, headache, joint pain, rebound inflammation, fatigue, weakness, lethargy, dizziness, and orthostatic hypotension.

DENTAL CONSIDERATIONS

General:

- Patients with Addison's disease are more susceptible to stress and may require supplemental systemic glucocorticoids before dental treatment.
- Patients who have been or are currently on chronic steroid therapy (longer than 2 wk) may require supplemental steroids for dental treatment.
- Monitor vital signs at every appointment because of nature of disease.

• Short appointments and a stress-reduction protocol may be required for anxious patients.
• Patients with Addison's disease must be evaluated closely for presence of oral infection.
• Do not use ingestible sodium bicarbonate products, such as the Prophy-Jet air polishing system, or IV saline fluids for patients on a salt-restricted regimen.
• Use precautions if dental surgery is anticipated and conscious sedation or general anesthesia is required.
• Monitor patient for any signs of inadequate management of disease, such as potassium depletion, muscle weakness, paresthesia, fatigue, nausea, depression, polyuria, and edema.

Consultations:
• Medical consultation is required to assess disease control and patient's ability to tolerate stress.
• Consultation may be required to confirm steroid dose and duration of use.

Teach Patient/Family to:
• Carry identification as a steroid user.
• Report to the dental office any signs that might indicate an oral infection.

F

flumazenil

flew-**maz'**-ah-nil
(Anexate[CAN], Romazicon)

CATEGORY AND SCHEDULE

Pregnancy Risk Category: C

Drug Class: Benzodiazepine receptor antagonist

MECHANISM OF ACTION

An antidote that antagonizes the effect of benzodiazepines on the gamma-aminobutyric acid receptor complex in the CNS.
Therapeutic Effect: Reverses sedative effect of benzodiazepines.

USES

Reversal of the sedative effects of benzodiazepines

PHARMACOKINETICS

Route	Onset	Peak	Duration
IV	1–2 min	6–10 min	Less than 1 hr

Duration and degree of benzodiazepine reversal depend on dosage and plasma concentration. Protein binding: 50%. Metabolized by the liver; excreted in urine.

INDICATIONS AND DOSAGES

▸ Reversal of Conscious Sedation or General Anesthesia
IV
Adults, Elderly. Initially, 0.2 mg (2 ml) over 15 sec; may repeat dose in 45 sec; then at 60-sec intervals. Maximum: 1 mg (10-ml) total dose.
Children, Neonates. Initially, 0.01 mg/kg; may repeat in 45 sec, then at 60-sec intervals. Maximum: 0.2 mg single dose; 0.05 mg/kg or 1 mg cumulative dose.

▸ Benzodiazepine Overdose
IV
Adults, Elderly. Initially, 0.2 mg (2 ml) over 30 sec; if desired LOC is not achieved after 30 sec, 0.3 mg (3 ml) may be given over 30 sec. Further doses of 0.5 mg (5 ml) may be administered over 30 sec at 60-sec intervals. Maximum: 3 mg (30 ml) total dose.

Children, Neonates. Initially, 0.01 mg/kg; may repeat in 45 sec, then at 60-sec intervals. Maximum: 0.2 mg single dose; 1 mg cumulative dose.

SIDE EFFECTS/ADVERSE REACTIONS

Frequent
Agitation, anxiety, dry mouth, dyspnea, insomnia, palpitations, tremors, headache, blurred vision, dizziness, ataxia, nausea, vomiting, pain at injection site, diaphoresis
Occasional
Fatigue, flushing, auditory disturbances, thrombophlebitis, rash
Rare
Urticaria, pruritus, hallucinations

PRECAUTIONS AND CONTRAINDICATIONS

Anticholinergic signs (such as mydriasis, dry mucosa, and hypoperistalsis), arrhythmias, cardiovascular collapse, history of hypersensitivity to benzodiazepines, patients with signs of serious cyclic antidepressant overdose (such as motor abnormalities), patients who have been given a benzodiazepine for control of a potentially life-threatening condition (such as control of status epilepticus or increased intracranial pressure)
Caution:
Lactation, elderly, renal disease, seizure disorders, head injury, labor and delivery, hepatic disease, hypoventilation, panic disorder, drug and alcohol dependency, ambulatory patients; no risk-benefits have been established for children

DRUG INTERACTIONS OF CONCERN TO DENTISTRY

• May not be effective: mixed drug overdosage

SERIOUS REACTIONS

! Toxic effects, such as seizures and arrhythmias, of other drugs taken in overdose, especially tricyclic antidepressants, may emerge with reversal of sedative effect of benzodiazepines.
! Flumazenil may provoke a panic attack in those with a history of panic disorder.

DENTAL CONSIDERATIONS

General:
• Monitor vital signs at every appointment because of cardiovascular side effects.
• Monitor for resedation; duration of antagonism is short compared with benzodiazepines.
• IM administration delays onset of effect.
Teach Patient/Family to:
• Be alert for possible resedation when discharged from office.

flunisolide

floo-**niss**′-oh-lide
(AeroBid, Nasalide, Nasarel, Rhinalar[CAN])
Do not confuse flunisolide with fluocinonide, or Nasalide with NasalCrom.

CATEGORY AND SCHEDULE

Pregnancy Risk Category: C

Drug Class: Synthetic glucocorticoid

MECHANISM OF ACTION

An adrenocorticosteroid that controls the rate of protein synthesis, depresses migration of polymorphonuclear leukocytes, reverses capillary permeability, and stabilizes lysosomal membranes.

Therapeutic Effect: Prevents or controls inflammation.

USES

Oral inhalation for prophylaxis or maintenance treatment of chronic asthma; nasal solution for seasonal or perennial rhinitis

PHARMACOKINETICS

Aerosol: Effective response time 1–4 wk; metabolized in liver; excreted in urine and feces.

INDICATIONS AND DOSAGES

▸ Long-Term Control of Bronchial Asthma, Assists in Reducing or Discontinuing Oral Corticosteroid Therapy

Inhalation

Adults, Elderly. 2 inhalations twice a day, morning and evening. Maximum: 4 inhalations twice a day.

Children 6–15 yr. 2 inhalations twice a day.

▸ Relief of Symptoms of Perennial and Seasonal Rhinitis

Intranasal

Adults, Elderly. Initially, 2 sprays each nostril twice a day, may increase at 4–7 day intervals to 2 sprays 3 times a day. Maximum: 8 sprays in each nostril daily.

Children 6–14 yr. Initially, 1 spray 3 times a day or 2 sprays twice a day. Maximum: 4 sprays in each nostril daily. Maintenance: 1 spray into each nostril each day.

SIDE EFFECTS/ADVERSE REACTIONS

Frequent

Inhalation: Unpleasant taste, nausea, vomiting, sore throat, diarrhea, upset stomach, cold symptoms, nasal congestion

Occasional

Inhalation: Dizziness, irritability, nervousness, tremors, abdominal pain, heartburn, oropharynx candidiasis, edema

Nasal: Mild nasopharyngeal irritation or dryness, rebound congestion, bronchial asthma, rhinorrhea, altered taste

PRECAUTIONS AND CONTRAINDICATIONS

Hypersensitivity to any corticosteroid, persistently positive sputum cultures for *C. albicans,* primary treatment of status asthmaticus, systemic fungal infections

Caution:

Lactation; warning: switching patients from systemic steroids to inhalation must be done carefully to avoid severe adrenal insufficiency

SERIOUS REACTIONS

! An acute hypersensitivity reaction, marked by urticaria, angioedema and severe bronchospasm, occurs rarely.

! A transfer from systemic to local steroid therapy may unmask previously suppressed bronchial asthma condition.

DENTAL CONSIDERATIONS

General:

- Examine oral cavity for evidence of drug side effects.
- Assess salivary flow as a factor in caries, periodontal disease, and candidiasis.
- Evaluate respiration characteristics and rate.
- Consider semisupine chair position for patients with respiratory disease.
- Determine dose and duration of steroid therapy for each patient to assess risk for stress tolerance and immunosuppression.
- Acute asthmatic episodes may be precipitated in the dental office.

Sympathomimetic inhalants should be available for emergency use. A stress reduction protocol may be required.

• Consider the drug in the diagnosis of taste alterations.

Consultations:

• Medical consultation may be required to assess disease control.

Teach Patient/Family to:

• Encourage effective oral hygiene to prevent soft tissue inflammation.

• Use caution to prevent injury when using oral hygiene aids.

• Gargle, rinse mouth with water and expectorate after each aerosol dose.

• When chronic dry mouth occurs, advise patient to:

  • Use daily home fluoride products for anticaries effect.
  • Avoid mouth rinses with high alcohol content because of drying effects.
  • Use sugarless gum, frequent sips of water, or saliva substitutes.

fluocinolone acetonide

floo-oh-**sin′**-oh-lone ah-**seat′**-oh-nide

(Capex, Derma-Smooth/FS, Fluoderm[CAN], Synalar)

CATEGORY AND SCHEDULE

Pregnancy Risk Category: C

Drug Class: Antiinflammatory, steroidal, topical; corticosteroid, topical

MECHANISM OF ACTION

A fluorinated topical corticosteroid that controls the rate of protein synthesis; depresses migration of polymorphonuclear leukocytes and fibroblasts; reduces capillary permeability; prevents or controls inflammation.

Therapeutic Effect: Decreases tissue response to inflammatory process.

USES

Relief of redness, swelling, itching, and discomfort of inflammatory skin problems

PHARMACOKINETICS

Use of occlusive dressings may increase percutaneous absorption. Protein binding: more than 90%. Excreted in urine. ***Half-life:*** Unknown.

INDICATIONS AND DOSAGES

▸ **Atopic Dermatitis**

Topical

Adults, Elderly. Apply 3 times a day. *Children 2 yr and older.* Apply 2 times a day.

▸ **Scalp Psoriasis**

Topical

Adults, Elderly. Apply to damp or wet hair and leave on overnight or for at least 4 hr. Remove by washing hair with shampoo.

▸ **Seborrheic Dermatitis, Scalp**

Shampoo

Adults, Elderly. Apply once daily; allow to remain on scalp for at least 5 min.

SIDE EFFECTS/ADVERSE REACTIONS

Occasional

Burning, dryness, itching, stinging

Rare

Allergic contact dermatitis, purpura or blood-containing blisters, thinning of skin with easy bruising, telangiectasis or raised dark red spots on skin

PRECAUTIONS AND CONTRAINDICATIONS
Hypersensitivity to fluocinolone or other corticosteroids

DRUG INTERACTIONS OF CONCERN TO DENTISTRY
- None reported

SERIOUS REACTIONS
! When taken in excessive quantities, systemic hypercorticism and adrenal suppression may occur.

DENTAL CONSIDERATIONS
General:
- Determine why patient is taking the drug.

Teach Patient/Family to:
- Avoid use on oral herpetic ulcerations.

fluocinonide
floo-oh-**sin′**-oh-nide
(Lidex, Lidex-E)

CATEGORY AND SCHEDULE
Pregnancy Risk Category: C

Drug Class: Topical corticosteroid, synthetic fluorinated agent, group II potency

MECHANISM OF ACTION
A topical corticosteroid that has antiinflammatory, antipruritic, and vasoconstrictive properties. The exact mechanism of the antiinflammatory process is unclear.
Therapeutic Effect: Reduces or prevents tissue response to the inflammatory process.

USES
Treatment of psoriasis, eczema, contact dermatitis, pruritus, oral lichen planus lesions

PHARMACOKINETICS
Well absorbed systemically. Large variation in absorption among sites. Protein binding: varies. Metabolized in liver. Primarily excreted in urine.

INDICATIONS AND DOSAGES
▸ **Dermatoses**
Topical
Adults, Elderly. Apply sparingly 2–4 times a day.

SIDE EFFECTS/ADVERSE REACTIONS
Occasional
Itching, redness, irritation, burning at site of application, dryness, folliculitis, acneiform eruptions, hypopigmentation
Rare
Allergic contact dermatitis, maceration of the skin, secondary infection, skin atrophy

PRECAUTIONS AND CONTRAINDICATIONS
History of hypersensitivity to fluocinonide or other corticosteroids
Caution:
Lactation, viral infections, bacterial infections

DRUG INTERACTIONS OF CONCERN TO DENTISTRY
- None reported

SERIOUS REACTIONS
! The serious reactions of long-term therapy and the addition of occlusive dressings are reversible hypothalamic-pituitary-adrenal (HPA) axis suppression,

manifestations of Cushing's syndrome, hyperglycemia, and glucosuria.

DENTAL CONSIDERATIONS

General:
- Place on frequent recall to evaluate healing response.

Teach Patient/Family to:
- Return for oral evaluation if response of oral tissues has not occurred in 7–14 days.
- Avoid use on oral herpetic ulcerations.
- Encourage effective oral hygiene to prevent soft tissue inflammation.
- Apply at bedtime or after meals for maximum effect.
- Apply with cotton-tipped applicator by pressing, not rubbing, paste on lesion.

fluorometholone

flure-oh-**meth′**-oh-lone
(Eflone, Flarex, Fluor-Op, FML Forte Liquifilm, FML Liquifilm, FML S.O.P.)

CATEGORY AND SCHEDULE

Pregnancy Risk Category: C

Drug Class: Antiinflammatory, steroidal, ophthalmic; corticosteroid, ophthalmic

MECHANISM OF ACTION

An ophthalmic corticosteroid that decreases inflammation by suppression of migration of polymorphonuclear leukocytes and reversal of increased capillary permeability.
Therapeutic Effect: Decreased ocular inflammation.

USES

Prevention of permanent damage to the eye, which may occur with certain eye problems. They also provide relief from redness, irritation, and other discomfort.

PHARMACOKINETICS

Absorbed into aqueous humor with slight systemic absorption.

INDICATIONS AND DOSAGES

▸ **Treatment of Steroid-Responsive Inflammatory Conditions of the Eye**

Ophthalmic Ointment
Adults, Elderly. Apply thin strip to conjunctival sac every 4 hr in severe cases or 1–3 times a day in mild to moderate cases.

Ophthalmic Solution
Adults, Elderly, Children 2 yr and older. Instill 1–2 drops into conjunctival sac every hour during the day, every 2 hr at night until favorable response is obtained. Then use 1 drop every 4 hr. For mild to moderate inflammation, instill 1–2 drops into conjunctival sac 2–4 times a day.

SIDE EFFECTS/ADVERSE REACTIONS

Occasional
Burning, tearing, itching, blurred vision

Rare
Cataract formation, corneal ulcers, glaucoma with optic nerve damage

PRECAUTIONS AND CONTRAINDICATIONS

Viral diseases of the cornea and conjunctiva, mycobacterial or fungal infections of the eye, untreated eye infections that may be masked or enhanced by steroids, hypersensitivity to fluorometholone or any component of the formulation

F

DRUG INTERACTIONS OF CONCERN TO DENTISTRY

• None reported

SERIOUS REACTIONS

! Hypercorticoidism and taste perversion occurs rarely.
! Superinfections, particularly with fungi, may result from bacterial imbalance via any route of administration.

DENTAL CONSIDERATIONS

General:

• Determine why patient is taking the drug.
• Avoid dental light in patient's eyes; offer dark glasses for patient comfort.
• Protect patient's eyes from accidental spatter during dental treatment.

fluorouracil, 5FU

flure-oh-**yoor′**-ah-sill
(Adrucil, Carac, Efudex, Efudex[AUS], Fluoroplex)
Do not confuse Efudex with Efidac.

CATEGORY AND SCHEDULE

Pregnancy Risk Category: D

Drug Class: Topical antineoplastic

MECHANISM OF ACTION

An antimetabolite that blocks formation of thymidylic acid. Cell cycle–specific for S phase of cell division.
Therapeutic Effect: Inhibits DNA and RNA synthesis. Topical form destroys rapidly proliferating cells.

USES

Treatment of keratosis (multiple/actinic), basal cell carcinoma; unapproved: condyloma acuminatum

PHARMACOKINETICS

Widely distributed. Crosses the blood-brain barrier. Rapidly metabolized in tissues to active metabolite, which is localized intracellularly. Primarily excreted by lungs as carbon dioxide. Removed by hemodialysis. ***Half-life:*** 20 hr.

INDICATIONS AND DOSAGES

▸ **Carcinoma of Breast, Colon, Pancreas, Rectum, and Stomach; in Combination with Levamisole after Surgical Resection in Patients with Duke's Stage C Colon Cancer**
IV
Adults, Elderly, Children. Initially, 12 mg/kg/day for 4–5 days. Maximum: 800 mg/day.
Maintenance: 6 mg/kg every other day for 4 doses repeated in 4 wk; or 15 mg/kg as a single bolus dose; or 5–15 mg/kg/wk as a single dose, not to exceed 1 g.
▸ **Multiple Actinic or Solar Keratoses**
Topical (Carac)
Adults, Elderly. Apply once a day.
Topical (Efudex, Fluoroplex)
Adults, Elderly. Apply twice a day.
▸ **Basal Cell Carcinoma**
Topical (Efudex)
Adults, Elderly. Apply twice a day.

SIDE EFFECTS/ADVERSE REACTIONS

Occasional

Parenteral: Anorexia, diarrhea, minimal alopecia, fever, dry skin, skin fissures, scaling, erythema
Topical: Pain, pruritus, hyperpigmentation, irritation, inflammation, and burning at application site; photosensitivity

Rare
Nausea, vomiting, anemia, esophagitis, proctitis, GI ulcer, confusion, headache, lacrimation, visual disturbances, angina, allergic reactions

PRECAUTIONS AND CONTRAINDICATIONS

Major surgery within previous month, myelosuppression, poor nutritional status, potentially serious infections

Caution:
Occlusive dressings, lactation, children, excessive exposure to sunlight

DRUG INTERACTIONS OF CONCERN TO DENTISTRY

• None reported, but limit drugs that may also produce photosensitivity reaction.

SERIOUS REACTIONS

! The earliest sign of toxicity, which may occur 4–8 days after beginning therapy, is stomatitis (as evidenced by dry mouth, burning sensation, mucosal erythema, and ulceration at inner margin of lips).

! Hematologic toxicity may be manifested as leukopenia (generally within 9–14 days after drug administration but possibly as late as the 25th day), thrombocytopenia (within 7–17 days after administration), pancytopenia, or agranulocytosis.

! The most common dermatologic toxicity is a pruritic rash on the extremities or, less frequently, the trunk.

DENTAL CONSIDERATIONS

General:
• Be aware of patient's disease and avoid treated areas to prevent further irritation.

F

fluoxetine hydrochloride

floo-**ox′**-eh-teen hi-droh-**klor′**-ide
(Auscap[AUS], Fluohexal[AUS], Lovan[AUS], Novo-Fluoxetine [CAN], Prozac, Prozac Weekly, Sarafem, Zactin[AUS])
Do not confuse fluoxetine with fluvastatin, Prozac with Prilosec, Proscar, or ProSom; or Sarafem with Serophene.

CATEGORY AND SCHEDULE

Pregnancy Risk Category: C

Drug Class: Antidepressant

MECHANISM OF ACTION

A psychotherapeutic agent that selectively inhibits serotonin uptake in the CNS, enhancing serotonergic function. Selective serotonin reuptake inhibitor (SSRI).
Therapeutic Effect: Relieves depression; reduces obsessive-compulsive and bulimic behavior.

USES

Treatment of major depressive disorder, bulimia, obsessive-compulsive disorder, premenstrual tension, geriatric depression in patients older than 65 yr, panic disorder with or without agoraphobia; premenstrual dysphoric disorder (Sarafem)

PHARMACOKINETICS

Well absorbed from the GI tract. Crosses the blood-brain barrier. Protein binding: 94%. Metabolized in the liver to active metabolite. Primarily excreted in urine. Not removed by hemodialysis. ***Half-life:*** 2–3 days; metabolite 7–9 days.

F

INDICATIONS AND DOSAGES

▸ **Depression, Obsessive-Compulsive Disorder**

PO

Adults. Initially, 20 mg each morning. If therapeutic improvement does not occur after 2 wk, gradually increase to maximum of 80 mg/day in 2 equally divided doses in morning and at noon. Prozac Weekly: 90 mg/wk, begin 7 days after last dose of 20 mg.
Elderly. Initially, 10 mg/day. May increase by 10–20 mg q2wk.
Children 7–17 yr. Initially, 5–10 mg/day. Titrate upward as needed. Usual dosage is 20 mg/day.

▸ **Panic Disorder**

PO

Adults, Elderly. Initially, 10 mg/day. May increase to 20 mg/day after 1 wk. Maximum: 60 mg/day.

▸ **Bulimia Nervosa**

PO

Adults. 60 mg each morning.

▸ **Premenstrual Dysphoric Disorder**

PO

Adults. 20 mg/day.

SIDE EFFECTS/ADVERSE REACTIONS

Frequent

Headache, asthenia, insomnia, anxiety, nervousness, somnolence, nausea, diarrhea, decreased appetite

Occasional

Dizziness, tremors, fatigue, vomiting, constipation, dry mouth, abdominal pain, nasal congestion, diaphoresis, rash

Rare

Flushed skin, light-headedness, impaired concentration

PRECAUTIONS AND CONTRAINDICATIONS

Use within 14 days of MAOIs

Caution:

Lactation, children, elderly; treatment-emergent adverse effects, hepatic impairment, interference with cognitive or motor performance

DRUG INTERACTIONS OF CONCERN TO DENTISTRY

- Increased CNS depression: alcohol, all CNS depressants, tricyclic antidepressants, benzodiazepines, St. John's wort (herb)
- Increased side effects: highly protein-bound drugs (aspirin)
- Caution: can inhibit cytochrome CYP2D6 isoenzymes
- Increased serum levels of carbamazepine
- Possible "serotonin syndrome" with macrolide antibiotics
- NSAIDs: increased risk of GI side effects

SERIOUS REACTIONS

! Overdose may produce seizures, nausea, vomiting, agitation, and restlessness.

DENTAL CONSIDERATIONS

General:

- Monitor vital signs at every appointment because of cardiovascular side effects.
- Assess salivary flow as a factor in caries, periodontal disease, and candidiasis.

Consultations:

- Medical consultation may be required to assess disease control and patient's ability to tolerate stress.
- Physician should be informed if significant xerostomic side effects occur (e.g., increased caries, sore tongue, problems eating or swallowing, difficulty wearing

prosthesis) so that a medication change can be considered.

Teach Patient/Family to:

• Use powered tooth brush if patient has difficulty holding conventional devices.

• When chronic dry mouth occurs, advise patient to:

  • Avoid mouth rinses with high alcohol content because of drying effects.
  • Use daily home fluoride products for anticaries effect.
  • Use sugarless gum, frequent sips of water, or saliva substitutes.

fluoxymesterone

floo-ox-ih-**mes′**-teh-rone
(Android-F, Halotestin, Halotestin[CAN])

CATEGORY AND SCHEDULE

Pregnancy Risk Category: X
Controlled substance: Schedule III

Drug Class: Androgenic anabolic steroid

MECHANISM OF ACTION

An androgen that suppresses gonadotropin-releasing hormone, luteinizing hormone (LH) and follicle-stimulating hormone (FSH).
Therapeutic Effect: Stimulates spermatogenesis, development of male secondary sex characteristics, and sexual maturation at puberty. Stimulates production of red blood cells (RBCs).

USES

Treatment of impotence from testicular deficiency, hypogonadism, palliative treatment of female breast cancer

PHARMACOKINETICS

Rapidly absorbed from the GI tract. Protein binding: 98%. Metabolized in liver. Excreted in urine. ***Half-life:*** 9.2 hr.

INDICATIONS AND DOSAGES

▸ **Males (Hypogonadism)**

PO

Adults. 5–20 mg/day.

▸ **Males (Delayed Puberty)**

PO

Adults. 2.5–20 mg/day for 4–6 mo.

▸ **Females (Inoperable Breast Cancer)**

PO

Adults. 10–40 mg/day in divided doses for 1–3 mo.

▸ **Females (Prevent Postpartum Breast Pain/Engorgement)**

PO

Adults. Initially, 2.5 mg shortly after delivery, then 5–10 mg/day in divided doses for 4–5 days.

SIDE EFFECTS/ADVERSE REACTIONS

Frequent

Females: Amenorrhea, virilism (e.g., acne, decreased breast size, enlarged clitoris, male pattern baldness), deepening voice
Males: UTI, breast soreness, gynecomastia, priapism, virilism (e.g., acne, early pubic hair growth)

Occasional

Females: Edema, nausea, vomiting, mild acne, diarrhea, stomach pain
Males: Impotence, testicular atrophy

PRECAUTIONS AND CONTRAINDICATIONS

Serious cardiac, renal, or hepatic dysfunction, men with carcinomas of the breast or prostate, hypersensitivity to fluoxymesterone or any component of the formulation including tartrazine

F

Caution:
Diabetes mellitus, CV disease, MI

DRUG INTERACTIONS OF CONCERN TO DENTISTRY

- Edema: corticosteroids

SERIOUS REACTIONS

! Peliosis hepatitis (liver, spleen replaced with blood-filled cysts), hepatic neoplasms, and hepatocellular carcinoma have been associated with prolonged high dosage.

DENTAL CONSIDERATIONS

General:

- Monitor vital signs at every appointment because of cardiovascular side effects.
- Patients receiving chemotherapy may require palliative treatment for stomatitis.

Teach Patient/Family to:

- Encourage effective oral hygiene to prevent soft tissue inflammation.
- Prevent trauma when using oral hygiene aids.

fluphenazine decanoate

floo-**fen′**-ah-zeen
(Apo-Fluphenazine[CAN], Modecate[AUS], Prolixin); fluphenazine enanthate (Moditen[CAN], Prolixin); fluphenazine hydrochloride (Prolixin, Permitil)

CATEGORY AND SCHEDULE

Pregnancy Risk Category: C

Drug Class: Phenothiazine antipsychotic

MECHANISM OF ACTION

A phenothiazine that blocks dopamine at postsynaptic receptor sites. Possesses weak anticholinergic, sedative and antemetic effects, and strong extrapyramidal activity.
Therapeutic Effect: Decreases psychotic behavior.

USES

Treatment of psychotic disorders, schizophrenia

PHARMACOKINETICS

Erratic and variable absorption from the GI tract. Widely distributed. Metabolized in liver. Primarily excreted in urine. ***Half-life:*** 16.3–23.2 hr.

INDICATIONS AND DOSAGES

▸ **Psychotic Disorders**
PO
Adults. Initially, 0.5–10 mg/day fluphenazine HCl in divided doses q6–8h. Increase gradually until therapeutic response is achieved (usually under 20 mg daily); decrease gradually to maintenance level (1–5 mg/day).
Elderly. Initially, 1–2.5 mg/day.
IM
Adults. Initially, 1.25 mg, followed by 2.5–10 mg/day in divided doses q6–8h.
▸ **Chronic Schizophrenic Disorder**
IM
Adults. Initially, 12.5–25 mg of fluphenazine decanoate q1–6wk, or 25 mg fluphenazine enanthate q2wk.
▸ **Usual Elderly Dosage (Nonpsychotic)**
PO
Initially, 1–2.5 mg/day. May increase by 1–2.5 mg/day q4–7 days. Maximum: 20 mg/day.

SIDE EFFECTS/ADVERSE REACTIONS

Frequent

Hypotension, dizziness, and fainting occur frequently after first injection, occasionally after subsequent injections, and rarely with oral dosage

Occasional

Drowsiness during early therapy, dry mouth, blurred vision, lethargy, constipation or diarrhea, nasal congestion, peripheral edema, urinary retention

Rare

Ocular changes, skin pigmentation (those on high doses for prolonged periods)

PRECAUTIONS AND CONTRAINDICATIONS

Severe CNS depression, comatose states, severe cardiovascular disease, bone marrow depression, subcortical brain damage, hypersensitivity to fluphenazine or any component of the formulation including tartrazine

Caution:

Lactation, seizure disorders, hypertension, hepatic disease, cardiac disease

DRUG INTERACTIONS OF CONCERN TO DENTISTRY

- Increased sedation: other CNS depressants, alcohol, barbiturate anesthetics, opioid analgesics
- Hypotension, tachycardia: epinephrine
- Increased extrapyramidal effects: phenothiazines and related drugs (haloperidol, droperidol), metoclopramide
- Additive photosensitization: tetracyclines
- Increased anticholinergic effects: anticholinergics

SERIOUS REACTIONS

! Extrapyramidal symptoms appear dose related (particularly high dosage), divided into 3 categories: akathisia (inability to sit still, tapping of feet, urge to move around); parkinsonian symptoms (mask-like face, tremors, shuffling gait, hypersalivation); and acute dystonias: torticollis (neck muscle spasm), opisthotonos (rigidity of back muscles), and oculogyric crisis (rolling back of eyes).

! Dystonic reaction may also produce profuse sweating and pallor.

! Tardive dyskinesia (protrusion of tongue, puffing of cheeks, chewing/puckering of the mouth) occurs rarely (may be irreversible).

! Abrupt withdrawal after long-term therapy may precipitate nausea, vomiting, gastritis, dizziness, and tremors.

! Blood dyscrasias, particularly agranulocytosis, or mild leukopenia (sore mouth/gums/throat) may occur.

! May lower seizure threshold.

DENTAL CONSIDERATIONS

General:

- Monitor vital signs at every appointment because of cardiovascular side effects.
- Patients on chronic drug therapy may rarely have symptoms of blood dyscrasias, which can include infection, bleeding, and poor healing.
- After supine positioning, have patient sit upright for at least 2 min before standing to avoid orthostatic hypotension.
- Assess salivary flow as a factor in caries, periodontal disease, and candidiasis.
- Avoid dental light in patient's eyes; offer dark glasses for patient comfort.

• Assess for presence of extrapyramidal motor symptoms, such as tardive dyskinesia and akathisia. Extrapyramidal motor activity may complicate dental treatment.
• Geriatric patients are more susceptible to drug effects; use a lower dose.
• Use vasoconstrictors with caution, in low doses and with careful aspiration.

Consultations:

• In a patient with symptoms of blood dyscrasias, request a medical consultation for blood studies and postpone dental treatment until normal values are reestablished.
• Take precautions if dental surgery is anticipated and anesthesia is required.
• If signs of tardive dyskinesia or akathisia are present, refer to physician.
• Physician should be informed if significant xerostomic side effects occur (e.g., increased caries, sore tongue, problems eating or swallowing, difficulty wearing prosthesis) so that a medication change can be considered.

Teach Patient/Family to:

• Encourage effective oral hygiene to prevent soft tissue inflammation.
• Prevent injury when using oral hygiene aids.
• Use powered tooth brush if patient has difficulty holding conventional devices.
• When chronic dry mouth occurs, advise patient to:
  • Avoid mouth rinses with high alcohol content because of drying effects.
  • Use daily home fluoride products for anticaries effect.
  • Use sugarless gum, frequent sips of water, or saliva substitutes.

flurandrenolide

flure-an-**dren′**-oh-lide
(Cordran, Cordran SP)

CATEGORY AND SCHEDULE

Pregnancy Risk Category: C

Drug Class: Topical corticosteroid, group III medium potency

MECHANISM OF ACTION

A fluorinated corticosteroid that decreases inflammation by suppressing the migration of polymorphonuclear leukocytes and reversal of increased capillary permeability.
Therapeutic Effect: Decreases tissue response to inflammatory process.

USES

Treatment of corticosteroid-responsive dermatoses, pruritus

PHARMACOKINETICS

Repeated applications may lead to percutaneous absorption. Absorption is about 36% from scrotal area, 7% from the forehead, 4% from scalp, and 1% from forearm. Metabolized in liver. Excreted in urine. ***Half-life:*** Unknown.

INDICATIONS AND DOSAGES

▸ Antiinflammatory, Immunosuppressant, Corticosteroid Replacement Therapy

Topical
Adults, Elderly. Apply 2–3 times a day.
Children. Apply 1–2 times a day.

SIDE EFFECTS/ADVERSE REACTIONS

Occasional

Itching, dry skin, folliculitis

Rare

Intracranial hemorrhage, acne, striae, miliaria, allergic contact dermatitis, telangiectasis or raised dark red spots on skin

PRECAUTIONS AND CONTRAINDICATIONS

Hypersensitivity to flurandrenolide or any component of the formulation, viral, fungal, or tubercular skin lesions

Caution:

Lactation, viral infections, bacterial infections

DRUG INTERACTIONS OF CONCERN TO DENTISTRY

• None reported

SERIOUS REACTIONS

! When taken in excessive quantities, systemic hypercorticism and adrenal suppression may occur.

DENTAL CONSIDERATIONS

General:

• Determine why the patient is taking the drug.
• Apply lubricant to dry lips for patient comfort before dental procedures.
• Place on frequent recall to evaluate healing response when used on chronic basis.

flurazepam hydrochloride

flure-**az**′-eh-pam hi-droh-**klor**′-ide
(Apo-Flurazepam[Can], Dalmane)
Do not confuse Dalmane with Dialume.

CATEGORY AND SCHEDULE

Pregnancy Risk Category: X
Controlled Substance: Schedule IV

Drug Class: Benzodiazepine, sedative-hypnotic

MECHANISM OF ACTION

A benzodiazepine that enhances action of inhibitory neurotransmitter gamma-aminobutyric acid (GABA). ***Therapeutic Effect:*** Produces hypnotic effect because of CNS depression.

USES

Treatment of insomnia

PHARMACOKINETICS

Route	Onset	Peak	Duration
PO	15–20 min	3–6 hr	7–8 hr

Well absorbed from the GI tract. Protein binding: 97%. Crosses the blood-brain barrier. Widely distributed. Metabolized in liver to active metabolite. Primarily excreted in urine. Not removed by hemodialysis. ***Half-life:*** 2.3 hr; metabolite: 40–114 hr.

INDICATIONS AND DOSAGES

▸ **Insomnia**

PO

Adults. 15–30 mg at bedtime.
Elderly, debilitated, liver disease, low serum albumin, Children 15 yr and older. 15 mg at bedtime.

F

SIDE EFFECTS/ADVERSE REACTIONS

Frequent

Drowsiness, dizziness, ataxia, sedation

Morning drowsiness may occur initially

Occasional

GI disturbances, nervousness, blurred vision, dry mouth, headache, confusion, skin rash, irritability, slurred speech

Rare

Paradoxical CNS excitement or restlessness, particularly noted in elderly or debilitated

PRECAUTIONS AND CONTRAINDICATIONS

Acute alcohol intoxication, acute angle-closure glaucoma, pregnancy or breast-feeding

Caution:

Anemia, hepatic disease, renal disease, suicidal individuals, drug abuse, elderly, psychosis, children younger than 15 yr

DRUG INTERACTIONS OF CONCERN TO DENTISTRY

• Increased sedation: alcohol, CNS depressants

• Increased serum levels and prolonged effect of benzodiazepines: ketoconazole, itraconazole, fluconazole, miconazole (systemic), indinavir, macrolide antibiotics

• Contraindicated with saquinavir

• Possible increase in CNS side effects: kava kava (herb)

SERIOUS REACTIONS

! Abrupt or too-rapid withdrawal after long-term use may result in pronounced restlessness and irritability, insomnia, hand tremors, abdominal or muscle cramps, vomiting, diaphoresis, and seizures.

! Overdose results in somnolence, confusion, diminished reflexes, and coma.

DENTAL CONSIDERATIONS

General:

• Assess salivary flow as a factor in caries, periodontal disease, and candidiasis.

• Psychologic and physical dependence may occur with chronic administration.

• Geriatric patients are more susceptible to drug effects; use lower dose.

Consultations:

• Medical consultation may be required to assess disease control.

Teach Patient/Family to:

• Avoid mouth rinses with high alcohol content because of drying effects.

flurbiprofen

flure-**bi′**-proe-fen

(Ansaid, Froben[CAN], Ocufen, Strepfen[AUS])

Do not confuse Ocufen with Ocuflox.

CATEGORY AND SCHEDULE

Pregnancy Risk Category: B (D if used in third trimester or near delivery; C for ophthalmic solution)

Drug Class: Nonsteroidal antiinflammatory

MECHANISM OF ACTION

A phenylalkanoic acid that produces analgesic and antiinflammatory effect by inhibiting prostaglandin synthesis. Also relaxes the iris sphincter.

Therapeutic Effect: Reduces the inflammatory response and intensity of pain. Prevents or decreases miosis during cataract surgery.

USES

Acute, long-term treatment of rheumatoid arthritis, osteoarthritis

PHARMACOKINETICS

Well absorbed from the GI tract; ophthalmic solution penetrates cornea after administration, and may be systemically absorbed. Protein binding: 99%. Widely distributed. Metabolized in the liver. Primarily excreted in urine. ***Half-life:*** 3–4 hr.

INDICATIONS AND DOSAGES

▸ Rheumatoid Arthritis, Osteoarthritis

PO

Adults, Elderly. 200–300 mg/day in 2–4 divided doses. Maximum: 100 mg/dose or 300 mg/day.

▸ Dysmenorrhea, Pain

PO

Adults. 50 mg 4 times a day

▸ Usual Ophthalmic Dosage

Adults, Elderly, Children. Apply 1 drop q30min starting 2 hr before surgery for total of 4 doses.

SIDE EFFECTS/ADVERSE REACTIONS

Occasional

PO: Headache, abdominal pain, diarrhea, indigestion, nausea, fluid retention

Ophthalmic: Burning or stinging on instillation, keratitis, elevated intraocular pressure

Rare

PO: Blurred vision, flushed skin, dizziness, somnolence, nervousness, insomnia, unusual fatigue, constipation, decreased appetite, vomiting, confusion

PRECAUTIONS AND CONTRAINDICATIONS

Active peptic ulcer, chronic inflammation of GI tract, GI bleeding or ulceration, history of hypersensitivity to aspirin or NSAIDs

Caution:

Lactation, children, bleeding disorders, GI disorders, cardiac disorders, severe renal disease, severe hepatic disease

DRUG INTERACTIONS OF CONCERN TO DENTISTRY

- GI ulceration, bleeding: aspirin, alcohol, corticosteroids
- Decreased action: salicylates
- Nephrotoxicity: acetaminophen (prolonged use), excess dosage
- When prescribed for dental pain:
  - Risk of increased effects: oral anticoagulants, oral antidiabetics, lithium, methotrexate
  - Decreased effects of diuretics
  - SSRIs: increased risk of GI side effects

SERIOUS REACTIONS

! Overdose may result in acute renal failure.

! Rare reactions with long-term use include peptic ulcer disease, GI bleeding, gastritis, severe hepatic reaction (jaundice), nephrotoxicity (hematuria, dysuria, proteinuria), a severe hypersensitivity reaction (angioedema, bronchospasm), and cardiac arrhythmias.

DENTAL CONSIDERATIONS

General:

- Patients on chronic drug therapy may rarely have symptoms of blood dyscrasias, which can include infection, bleeding, and poor healing.

• Assess salivary flow as a factor in caries, periodontal disease, and candidiasis.
• Avoid prescribing for dental use in last trimester of pregnancy.
• Avoid prescribing aspirin-containing products.
• Consider semisupine chair position for patients with arthritic disease.
• Severe stomach bleeding may occur in patients who regularly use NSAIDs in recommended doses, when the patient is also taking another NSAID, anticoagulant/antiplatelet, or steroid drug, if the patient has GI or peptic ulcer disease, if they are 60 years or older, or when NSAIDs are taken longer than directed. Warn patients of the potential for severe stomach bleeding.

Consultations:
• Medical consultation may be required to assess disease control.
• In a patient with symptoms of blood dyscrasias, request a medical consultation for blood studies and postpone dental treatment until normal values are reestablished.

Teach Patient/Family to:
• Encourage effective oral hygiene to prevent soft tissue inflammation.
• Prevent injury when using oral hygiene aids.
• Warn patient of potential risks of NSAIDs.
• When chronic dry mouth occurs, advise patient to:
  • Avoid mouth rinses with high alcohol content because of drying effects.
  • Use daily home fluoride products for anticaries effect.
  • Use sugarless gum, frequent sips of water, or saliva substitutes.

flutamide

flew′-tah-myd
(Euflex[CAN], Eulexin, Flugerel[AUS], Flutamin[AUS], Fugerel[AUS], Novo-Flutamide[CAN])
Do not confuse flutamide with Flumadine.

CATEGORY AND SCHEDULE

Pregnancy Risk Category: D

Drug Class: Antineoplastic

MECHANISM OF ACTION

An antiandrogen hormone that inhibits androgen uptake and prevents androgen from binding to androgen receptors in target tissue. Used in conjunction with leuprolide to inhibit the stimulant effects of flutamide on serum testosterone levels.

Therapeutic Effect: Suppresses testicular androgen production and decreases growth of prostate carcinoma.

USES

Treatment of metastatic prostatic carcinoma, stage D2; early-stage prostate cancer, stages B2 and C, in combination with LHRH agonistic analogs (leuprolide) and radiation

PHARMACOKINETICS

Completely absorbed from the GI tract. Protein binding: 94%–96%. Metabolized in the liver to active metabolite. Primarily excreted in urine. Not removed by hemodialysis. ***Half-life:*** 6 hr (increased in elderly).

INDICATIONS AND DOSAGES

▸ **Prostatic Carcinoma (in Combination with Leuprolide)**
PO
Adults, Elderly. 250 mg q8h.

SIDE EFFECTS/ADVERSE REACTIONS

Frequent

Hot flashes; decreased libido, diarrhea; generalized pain; asthenia; constipation; nausea, nocturia

Occasional

Dizziness, paresthesia, insomnia, impotence, peripheral edema, gynecomastia

Rare

Rash, diaphoresis, hypertension, hematuria, vomiting, urinary incontinence, headache, flu-like syndromes, photosensitivity

PRECAUTIONS AND CONTRAINDICATIONS

Severe hepatic impairment

Caution:

Liver toxicity, monitoring requirements for hepatic injury, women

SERIOUS REACTIONS

! Hepatotoxicity, including hepatic encephalopathy and hemolytic anemia may be noted.

DENTAL CONSIDERATIONS

General:

- Possible increase in adverse cardiovascular events in patients at risk for thromboembolism.
- Talk with patient about any pain medication being taken.
- Avoid drugs (anticholinergics) that could exacerbate urinary retention (if present).

fluticasone propionate

flu-**tic**′-ah-zone **proh**′-pie-oh-neyt (Beconase Allergy 24 Hour[AUS], Beconase Hayfever[AUS], Cutivate, Flixotide Disks[AUS], Flixotide Inhaler[AUS], Flonase, Flovent, Flovent Diskus, Flovent HFA, Veramyst)

F

CATEGORY AND SCHEDULE

Pregnancy Risk Category: C

Drug Class: Synthetic corticosteroid, medium potency

MECHANISM OF ACTION

A corticosteroid that controls the rate of protein synthesis, depresses migration of polymorphonuclear leukocytes, reverses capillary permeability, and stabilizes lysosomal membranes.

Therapeutic Effect: Prevents or controls inflammation.

USES

Nasal spray: Management of nasal symptoms of seasonal and perennial allergic and nonallergic rhinitis in adults and pediatric patient 4 yr and older

Oral: inhalation: For maintenance treatment of asthma as prophylactic therapy; also indicated for patients requiring oral glucocorticoid therapy

PHARMACOKINETICS

Inhalation/intranasal: Protein binding: 91%. Undergoes extensive first-pass metabolism in liver. Excreted in urine. ***Half-life:*** 3–7.8 hr. ***Topical:*** Amount absorbed depends on affected area and skin condition (absorption increased with fever, hydration, inflamed or denuded skin).

F

INDICATIONS AND DOSAGES

▸ Allergic Rhinitis

Intranasal

Adults, Elderly. Initially, 200 mcg (2 sprays in each nostril once daily or 1 spray in each nostril q12h). Maintenance: 1 spray in each nostril once daily. Maximum: 200 mcg/day.

Children 4 yr and older. Initially, 100 mcg (1 spray in each nostril once daily). Maximum: 200 mcg/day.

▸ Relief of Inflammation and Pruritus associated with Steroid-Responsive Disorders, such as Contact Dermatitis and Eczema

Topical

Adults, Elderly, Children 3 mo and older. Apply sparingly to affected area once or twice a day.

▸ Maintenance Treatment for Asthma for Those Previously Treated with Bronchodilators

Inhalation Powder (Flovent Diskus)

Adults, Elderly, Children 12 yr and older. Initially, 100 mcg q12h. Maximum: 500 mcg/day.

Inhalation (Oral [Flovent])

Adults, Elderly, Children 12 yr and older. 88 mcg twice a day. Maximum: 440 mcg twice a day.

▸ Maintenance Treatment for Asthma for Those Previously Treated with Inhaled Steroids

Inhalation Powder (Flovent Diskus)

Adults, Elderly, Children 12 yr and older. Initially, 100–250 mcg q12h. Maximum: 500 mcg q12h.

Inhalation (Oral [Flovent])

Adults, Elderly, Children 12 yr and older. 88–220 mcg twice a day. Maximum: 440 mcg twice a day.

▸ Maintenance Treatment for Asthma for Those Previously Treated with Oral Steroids

Inhalation Powder (Flovent Diskus)

Adults, Elderly, Children 12 yr and older. 500–1000 mcg twice a day.

Inhalation (Oral [Flovent])

Adults, Elderly, Children 12 yr and older. 88 mcg twice a day.

SIDE EFFECTS/ADVERSE REACTIONS

Frequent

Inhalation: Throat irritation, hoarseness, dry mouth, cough, temporary wheezing, oropharyngeal candidiasis (particularly if mouth is not rinsed with water after each administration)

Intranasal: Mild nasopharyngeal irritation; nasal burning, stinging, or dryness; rebound congestion; rhinorrhea; loss of taste

Occasional

Inhalation: Oral candidiasis

Intranasal: Nasal and pharyngeal candidiasis, headache

Topical: Skin burning, pruritus

PRECAUTIONS AND CONTRAINDICATIONS

Primary treatment of status asthmaticus or other acute asthma episodes (inhalation); untreated localized infection of nasal mucosa

Caution:

Suppression of hypothalamic-pituitary-adrenal (HPA) axis, warning of manifestation of HPA suppression when switching drug from oral to inhaled steroids, suppression of growth in children younger than 4 yr; use is restricted for some dose forms to children older than 12 yr; lactation

DRUG INTERACTIONS OF CONCERN TO DENTISTRY

- No specific interactions reported

SERIOUS REACTIONS

! Deaths because of adrenal insufficiency have occurred in asthma patients during and after transfer from use of long-term systemic corticosteroids to less systemically available inhaled corticosteroids.

DENTAL CONSIDERATIONS

General:

• Examine oral cavity for evidence of opportunistic candidiasis in patients using the inhaler.

• Allergic rhinitis may be a factor in mouth breathing and drying of oral tissues.

• Be aware that aspirin or sulfite preservatives in vasoconstrictor-containing products can exacerbate asthma.

• Acute asthmatic episodes may be precipitated in the dental office. Rapid-acting sympathomimetic inhalants should be available for emergency use. A stress-reduction protocol may be required.

• Consider semisupine chair position for patients with respiratory disease.

Consultations:

• Consultation may be required to confirm steroid dose and duration of use, supplementation may be required.

Teach Patient/Family to:

• Update health and drug history if physician makes any changes in drug regimens.

• Gargle, rinse mouth with water, and expectorate after each aerosol use.

• Avoid use of topical preparations on fungal or herpetic lesions.

fluvastatin

floo′-va-sta-tin

(Lescol, Lescol XL, Vastin[Aus])

Do not confuse fluvastatin with fluoxetine.

CATEGORY AND SCHEDULE

Pregnancy Risk Category: X

Drug Class: Cholesterol-lowering agent, antihyperlipidemic

MECHANISM OF ACTION

An antihyperlipidemic that inhibits HMG-CoA reductase, the enzyme that catalyzes the early step in cholesterol synthesis.

Therapeutic Effect: Decreases low-density lipoprotein (LDL) cholesterol, very low-density lipoproteins (VLDLs), and plasma triglyceride levels. Slightly increases high-density lipoprotein (HDL) cholesterol concentration.

USES

As an adjunct in homozygous familial hypercholesterolemia, mixed hyperlipidemia, elevated serum triglyceride levels, and type IV hyperproteinemia, also reduces total cholesterol LDL-C, apo B, and triglyceride levels; patient should first be placed on cholesterol-lowering diet; to reduce risk in coronary artery revascularization procedures; prevention of secondary coronary events

PHARMACOKINETICS

Well absorbed from the GI tract and is unaffected by food. Does not cross the blood-brain barrier. Protein binding: greater than 98%. Primarily eliminated in feces. ***Half-life:*** 1.2 hr. Tablets (Extended-Release [Lescol XL]): 80 mg.

INDICATIONS AND DOSAGES

▸ **Hyperlipoproteinemia**

PO

Adults, Elderly. Initially, 20 mg/day (capsule) in the evening. May increase up to 40 mg/day. Maintenance: 20–40 mg/day in a single dose or divided doses.

Patients requiring more than a 25% decrease in LDL cholesterol. 40 mg (capsule) 1–2 times a day, or 80 mg tablet once a day.

SIDE EFFECTS/ADVERSE REACTIONS

Frequent

Headache, dyspepsia, back pain, myalgia, arthralgia, diarrhea, abdominal cramping, rhinitis

Occasional

Nausea, vomiting, insomnia, constipation, flatulence, rash, pruritus, fatigue, cough, dizziness

PRECAUTIONS AND CONTRAINDICATIONS

Active hepatic disease, unexplained increased serum transaminase levels

Caution:

Liver dysfunction; alcoholism; severe acute infection; metabolic, endocrine, or electrolyte disorders; uncontrolled seizures; alterations in liver function tests may be observed with use

DRUG INTERACTIONS OF CONCERN TO DENTISTRY

- Increased plasma levels: alcohol, fluconazole, itraconazole, ketoconazole, erythromycin

SERIOUS REACTIONS

! Myositis (inflammation of voluntary muscle) with or without increased CK and muscle weakness, occur rarely. These conditions may progress to frank rhabdomyolysis and renal impairment.

DENTAL CONSIDERATIONS

General:

- Consider semisupine chair position for patient comfort because of GI, musculoskeletal, and respiratory side effects.

fluvoxamine maleate

floo-**vox**′-ah-meen **mal**′-ee-ate

(Faverin[AUS], Luvox)

CATEGORY AND SCHEDULE

Pregnancy Risk Category: C

Drug Class: Selective serotonin reuptake inhibitor, antidepressant

MECHANISM OF ACTION

An antidepressant and antiobsessive agent that selectively inhibits neuronal reuptake of serotonin (SSRI).

Therapeutic Effect: Relieves depression and symptoms of obsessive-compulsive disorder.

USES

Obsessive-compulsive disorder and panic disorder

PHARMACOKINETICS

PO: Rapid absorption, peak plasma levels 5 hr; plasma protein binding 77%; hepatic metabolism; urinary excretion.

INDICATIONS AND DOSAGES

▸ **Obsessive-Compulsive Disorder**

PO

Adults. 50 mg at bedtime; may increase by 50 mg every 4–7 days. Dosages greater than 100 mg/day given in 2 divided doses. Maximum: 300 mg/day.

Children 8–17 yr. 25 mg at bedtime; may increase by 25 mg every 4–7 days. Dosages greater than 50 mg/day given in 2 divided doses. Maximum: 200 mg/day.

SIDE EFFECTS/ADVERSE REACTIONS

Frequent

Nausea, headache, somnolence, insomnia

Occasional
Dizziness, diarrhea, dry mouth, asthenia, weakness, dyspepsia, constipation, abnormal ejaculation
Rare
Anorexia, anxiety, tremors, vomiting, flatulence, urinary frequency, sexual dysfunction, altered taste

PRECAUTIONS AND CONTRAINDICATIONS

Use within 14 days of MAOIs
Caution:
Lactation, renal and hepatic impairment, epilepsy, elderly

DRUG INTERACTIONS OF CONCERN TO DENTISTRY

- Increased plasma levels of tricyclic antidepressants, carbamazepine, benzodiazepine; reduce doses of alprazolam, diazepam, midazolam, triazolam by half
- Risk of serotonin syndrome: SSRIs
- NSAIDs: increased risk of GI side effects

SERIOUS REACTIONS

! Overdose may produce seizures, nausea, vomiting, and extreme agitation and restlessness.

DENTAL CONSIDERATIONS

General:
- After supine positioning, have patient sit upright for at least 2 min to avoid orthostatic hypotension.
- Assess salivary flow as a factor in caries, periodontal disease, and candidiasis.
- Consider semisupine chair position for patient comfort because of GI effects of drug.

Consultations:
- Medical consultation may be required to assess patient's ability to tolerate stress.
- Physician should be informed if significant xerostomic side effects occur (e.g., increased caries, sore tongue, problems eating or swallowing, difficulty wearing prosthesis) so that a medication change can be considered.

Teach Patient/Family:
- When chronic dry mouth occurs, advise patient to:
  - Avoid mouth rinses with high alcohol content because of drying effects.
  - Use daily home fluoride products for anticaries effect.
  - Use sugarless gum, frequent sips of water, or saliva substitutes.

F

folic acid/sodium folate (vitamin B_9)

foe′-lik **ass**′-id/**soe**′-dee-um foe′-late
folic acid
(Apo-Folic[CAN], Folvite, Megafol[AUS])
sodium folate
(Folvite-parenteral)
Do not confuse Folvite with Florvite.

CATEGORY AND SCHEDULE

Pregnancy Risk Category: A (C if used in doses above the recommended daily allowance)
OTC (0.4- and 0.8-mg tablets only)

Drug Class: Water-soluble B vitamin

MECHANISM OF ACTION

A coenzyme that stimulates production of platelets, RBCs, and WBCs.

Therapeutic Effect: Essential for nucleoprotein synthesis and maintenance of normal erythropoiesis.

USES

Treatment of megaloblastic or macrocytic anemia caused by folic acid deficiency, liver disease, alcoholism, hemolysis, intestinal obstruction, pregnancy

PHARMACOKINETICS

PO form almost completely absorbed from the GI tract (upper duodenum). Protein binding: High. Metabolized in the liver and plasma to active form. Excreted in urine. Removed by hemodialysis.

INDICATIONS AND DOSAGES

▸ **Vitamin B_9 Deficiency**

PO, IV, IM, Subcutaneous

Adults, Elderly, Children 12 yr and older. Initially, 1 mg/day. Maintenance: 0.5 mg/day.

Children 1–11 yr. Initially 1 mg/day. Maintenance: 0.1–0.4 mg/day.

Infants. 50 mcg/day.

▸ **Dietary Supplement**

PO, IV, IM, Subcutaneous

Adults, Elderly, Children 4 yr and older. 0.4 mg/day.

Children at least 1 yr and younger than 4 yr. 0.3 mg/day.

Children younger than 1 yr. 0.1 mg/day.

Pregnant women. 0.8 mg/day.

SIDE EFFECTS/ADVERSE REACTIONS

None known

PRECAUTIONS AND CONTRAINDICATIONS

Anemias (aplastic, normocytic, pernicious, refractory)

DRUG INTERACTIONS OF CONCERN TO DENTISTRY

- Increased metabolism of phenobarbital

SERIOUS REACTIONS

! Allergic hypersensitivity occurs rarely with parenteral form. Oral folic acid is nontoxic.

DENTAL CONSIDERATIONS

General:

- Deficiency in folic acid; glossitis may be a symptom of folic acid deficiency.

formoterol fumarate

for-**moe**′-ter-ol **fyoo**′-muh-rate
(Foradil Aerolizer, Foradile[AUS], Oxis[AUS])

CATEGORY AND SCHEDULE

Pregnancy Risk Category: C

Drug Class: Selective β_2-adrenergic bronchodilator

MECHANISM OF ACTION

A long-acting bronchodilator that stimulates β_2-adrenergic receptors in the lungs, resulting in relaxation of bronchial smooth muscle. Also inhibits release of mediators from various cells in the lungs, including mast cells, with little effect on heart rate.

Therapeutic Effect: Relieves bronchospasm, reduces airway resistance. Improves bronchodilation, nighttime asthma control, and peak flow rates.

USES

Long-term treatment of asthma and prevention of bronchospasm in adults and children older than 5 yr;

prevention of exercise-induced bronchospasm in adults and children older than 12 yr; maintenance treatment of COPD

PHARMACOKINETICS

Route	Onset	Peak	Duration
Inhalation	1–3 min	0.5–1 hr	12 hr

Absorbed from bronchi after inhalation. Metabolized in the liver. Primarily excreted in urine. Unknown if removed by hemodialysis. ***Half-life:*** 10 hr.

INDICATIONS AND DOSAGES

▸ Asthma, COPD

Inhalation

Adults, Elderly, Children 5 yr and older. 12 mcg capsule q12h.

▸ Exercise-Induced Bronchospasm

Inhalation

Adults, Elderly, Children 5 yr and older. 12 mcg capsule at least 15 min before exercise. Do not repeat for another 12 hr.

SIDE EFFECTS/ADVERSE REACTIONS

Occasional

Tremors, muscle cramps, tachycardia, insomnia, headache, irritability, irritation of mouth or throat

PRECAUTIONS AND CONTRAINDICATIONS

Hypersensitivity

Caution:

Not for acute asthma symptoms, not for use in life-threatening situations; paradoxic bronchospasm may occur with use; not a substitute for corticosteroids; cardiovascular disease (coronary insufficiency, cardiac arrhythmias, hypertension), hyperthyroidism, seizures, hypokalemia, lactation

DRUG INTERACTIONS OF CONCERN TO DENTISTRY

- Avoid MAOIs, tricyclic antidepressants, and drugs that prolong the QT interval (phenothiazines, procainamide).
- Adrenergic agents/ sympathomimetics may potentiate effects.
- β-Adrenergic blockers may antagonize sympathomimetic effects.

SERIOUS REACTIONS

! Excessive sympathomimetic stimulation may produce palpitations, extrasystole, and chest pain.

DENTAL CONSIDERATIONS

General:

- Monitor vital signs at every appointment because of cardiovascular side effects.
- Assess salivary flow as a factor in caries, periodontal disease, and candidiasis.
- Consider semisupine chair position for patient comfort because of respiratory side effects of disease.
- Short midday appointments and a stress-reduction protocol may be required for anxious patients.
- Have patient bring personal short-acting bronchodilator to appointment for use in emergency.
- Acute asthmatic episodes may be precipitated in the dental office. Rapid-acting sympathomimetic inhalants should be available for emergency use.
- Avoid prescribing aspirin-containing products.

Consultations:

- Medical consultation may be required to assess disease control and patient's ability to tolerate stress.

Teach Patient/Family to:

- Gargle, rinse mouth with water, and expectorate after each aerosol dose.
- When chronic dry mouth occurs, advise patient to:
  - Avoid mouth rinses with high alcohol content because of drying effects.
  - Use daily home fluoride products for anticaries effect.
  - Use sugarless gum, frequent sips of water, or saliva substitutes.

fosamprenavir

foss-am-**pren**′-ah-vur
(Lexiva)

CATEGORY AND SCHEDULE

Pregnancy Risk Category: C

Drug Class: Antiretroviral; protease inhibitor

MECHANISM OF ACTION

An antiretroviral that is rapidly converted to amprenavir, which inhibits HIV-1 protease by binding to the enzyme's active site, thus preventing the processing of viral precursors and resulting in the formation of immature, noninfectious viral particles. ***Therapeutic Effect:*** Impairs HIV replication and proliferation.

USES

Treatment of HIV-1 infection in combination with antiretrovirals

PHARMACOKINETICS

Rapidly absorbed after PO administration. Protein binding: 90%. Metabolized in the liver. Excreted in urine and feces. ***Half-life:*** 7.7 hr.

INDICATIONS AND DOSAGES

▸ HIV Infection in Patients Who Have Not Had Previous Protease Inhibitor Therapy

PO

Adults, Elderly. 1400 mg twice daily without ritonavir; or 1400 mg twice daily plus ritonavir 200 mg once daily; or 700 mg twice daily plus ritonavir 100 mg twice daily.

▸ HIV Infection in Patients Who Have Had Previous Protease Inhibitor Therapy

PO

Adults, Elderly. 700 mg twice daily plus ritonavir 100 mg twice daily.

▸ Concurrent Therapy with Efavirenz

PO

Adults, Elderly. In patients receiving fosamprenavir plus once-daily ritonavir in combination with efavirenz, an additional 100 mg/day ritonavir (300 mg total/day) should be given.

SIDE EFFECTS/ADVERSE REACTIONS

Frequent

Nausea, rash, diarrhea

Occasional

Headache, vomiting, fatigue, depression

Rare

Pruritus, abdominal pain, perioral paresthesia

PRECAUTIONS AND CONTRAINDICATIONS

Concurrent use of amprenavir, dihydroergotamine, ergonovine, ergotamine, methylergonovine, pimozide, midazolam, or triazolam. If fosamprenavir is given concurrently with ritonavir, flecainide and propafenone are also contraindicated.

DRUG INTERACTIONS OF CONCERN TO DENTISTRY

- Contraindicated with midazolam, triazolam
- Increased plasma levels of: tricyclic antidepressants, lidocaine, alprazolam, clorazepate, diazepam, flurazepam, ketoconazole, itraconazole, sildenafil, vardenafil
- Reduced absorption: antacids, carbamazepine, phenobarbital, St. John's wort (herb)

SERIOUS REACTIONS

! Severe and possibly life-threatening dermatologic reactions occur rarely.

DENTAL CONSIDERATIONS

General:

- Caution significant drug interactions with drugs used in dentistry.
- Question patient about other drugs or herbals they may be taking.
- Patient on chronic drug therapy may rarely present with symptoms of blood dyscrasias, which can include infection, bleeding, and poor healing. If dyscrasia is present, caution patient to prevent oral tissue trauma when using oral hygiene aids.
- Consider semisupine chair position for patient comfort if GI side effects occur.

Consultations:

- In a patient with symptoms of blood dyscrasias, request a medical consultation for blood studies and postpone treatment until normal values are reestablished.
- Medical consultation may be required to assess disease control and patient's ability to tolerate stress.

Teach Patient/Family to:

- Encourage effective oral hygiene to prevent soft tissue inflammation.
- Prevent trauma when using oral hygiene aids.
- Update health and medication history if physician makes any changes in evaluation or drug regimens; include OTC, herbal, and nonherbal remedies in the update.

foscarnet sodium

foss-**car′**-net **soe′**-dee-um
(Foscavir)

CATEGORY AND SCHEDULE

Pregnancy Risk Category: C

Drug Class: Antiviral

MECHANISM OF ACTION

An antiviral that selectively inhibits binding sites on virus-specific DNA polymerase and reverse transcriptase.
Therapeutic Effect: Inhibits replication of herpes virus.

USES

Treatment of cytomegalovirus (CMV) retinitis in AIDS, acyclovir-resistant herpes simplex I mucocutaneous diseases, and acyclovir-resistant HSV in immunocompromised patients

PHARMACOKINETICS

Sequestered into bone and cartilage. Protein binding: 14%–17%. Primarily excreted unchanged in urine. Removed by hemodialysis. ***Half-life:*** 3.3–6.8 hr (increased in impaired renal function).

INDICATIONS AND DOSAGES

▸ CMV Retinitis

IV

Adults, Elderly. Initially, 60 mg/kg q8h or 100 mg/kg q12h for 2–3 wk.

Maintenance: 90–120 mg/kg/day as a single IV infusion.

▸ **Herpes Infection**

IV

Adults. 40 mg/kg q8–12h for 2–3 wk or until healed.

▸ **Dosage in Renal Impairment**

Dosages are individualized on the basis of creatinine clearance. Refer to the dosing guide provided by the manufacturer.

F

SIDE EFFECTS/ADVERSE REACTIONS

Frequent

Fever, nausea, vomiting, diarrhea

Occasional

Anorexia, pain and inflammation at injection site, fever, rigors, malaise, headache, paresthesia, dizziness, rash, diaphoresis, abdominal pain

Rare

Back or chest pain, edema, flushing, pruritus, constipation, dry mouth

PRECAUTIONS AND CONTRAINDICATIONS

Hypersensitivity

Caution:

Lactation, children, elderly, renal disease, seizure disorders, electrolyte/mineral imbalances, severe anemia; monitor for renal impairment

DRUG INTERACTIONS OF CONCERN TO DENTISTRY

- Avoid nephrotoxic drugs (amphotericin B)
- Possible increased risk of seizures: fluoroquinolones

SERIOUS REACTIONS

! Nephrotoxicity occurs to some extent in most patients.

! Seizures and serum mineral or electrolyte imbalances may be life-threatening.

DENTAL CONSIDERATIONS

General:

- Examine for oral manifestations of opportunistic infections.
- Examine for evidence of oral manifestations of blood dyscrasias (infection, bleeding, poor healing).
- Consider local hemostasis measures to prevent excessive bleeding.
- Assess salivary flow as a factor in caries, periodontal disease, and candidiasis.
- Monitor vital signs at every appointment because of cardiovascular and respiratory side effects.
- Place on frequent recall to evaluate healing response.

Consultations:

- Medical consultation for blood studies (CBC); leukopenic or thrombocytopenic side effects may result in infection, delayed healing, and excessive bleeding. Postpone elective dental treatment until normal values are maintained.
- Medical consultation may be required to assess disease control.

Teach Patient/Family to:

- Use oral hygiene aids carefully to prevent injury.
- See dentist immediately if secondary oral infection occurs.
- Encourage effective oral hygiene to prevent soft tissue inflammation.
- Use powered tooth brush if patient has difficulty holding conventional devices because of extrapyramidal side effects.
- When chronic dry mouth occurs, advise patient to:
    - Avoid mouth rinses with high alcohol content because of drying effects.
    - Use daily home fluoride products for anticaries effect.

• Use sugarless gum, frequent sips of water, or saliva substitutes.

fosfomycin tromethamine

foss-fo-**mye′**-sin troe-meth′-a-mine
(Monurol)
Do not confuse Monurol with Monopril.

CATEGORY AND SCHEDULE

Pregnancy Risk Category: B

Drug Class: Antiinfective (phosphonic acid derivative)

MECHANISM OF ACTION

An antibiotic that prevents bacterial cell wall formation by inhibiting the synthesis of peptidoglycan.
Therapeutic Effect: Bactericidal.

USES

Treatment of uncomplicated UTIs in women caused by susceptible strains of *E. coli* and *Enterococcus faecalis*

PHARMACOKINETICS

PO: Peak plasma levels after 2 hr; not plasma protein bound; widely distributed to GU tissues; excreted unchanged in urine and feces.

INDICATIONS AND DOSAGES

▸ **Uncomplicated UTIs**

PO

Females. 3 g mixed in 4 oz water as a single dose.
Males. 3 g/day for 2–3 days.

SIDE EFFECTS/ADVERSE REACTIONS

Occasional

Diarrhea, nausea, headache, back pain

Rare

Dysmenorrhea, pharyngitis, abdominal pain, rash

F

PRECAUTIONS AND CONTRAINDICATIONS

Hypersensitivity

Caution:

Renal impairment, one dose per single episode of cystitis, lactation, children younger than 12 yr

DRUG INTERACTIONS OF CONCERN TO DENTISTRY

• Lowered serum concentrations: metoclopramide

SERIOUS REACTIONS

! None known

DENTAL CONSIDERATIONS

General:

• Determine why patient is taking the drug.
• Consider semisupine chair position for patient comfort if GI side effects occur.

Teach Patient/Family:

• When chronic dry mouth occurs, advise patient to:
  • Avoid mouth rinses with high alcohol content because of drying effects.
  • Use daily home fluoride products for anticaries effect.
  • Use sugarless gum, frequent sips of water, or saliva substitutes.

fosinopril

fo-**sin**′-oh-pril
(Monopril)
Do not confuse Monopril with Monurol.

CATEGORY AND SCHEDULE

Pregnancy Risk Category: C (D if used in second or third trimester)

Drug Class: Angiotensin-converting enzyme (ACE) inhibitor

F

MECHANISM OF ACTION

An ACE inhibitor that suppresses the renin-angiotensin-aldosterone system and prevents conversion of angiotensin I to angiotensin II, a potent vasoconstrictor; may also inhibit angiotensin II at local vascular and renal sites. Decreases plasma angiotensin II, increases plasma renin activity and decreases aldosterone secretion.
Therapeutic Effect: Reduces peripheral arterial resistance, pulmonary capillary wedge pressure; improves cardiac output and exercise tolerance.

USES

Treatment of hypertension, alone or in combination with thiazide diuretics, management of heart failure

PHARMACOKINETICS

Route	Onset	Peak	Duration
PO	1 hr	2–6 hr	24 hr

Slowly absorbed from the GI tract. Protein binding: 97%–98%. Metabolized in the liver and GI mucosa to active metabolite. Primarily excreted in urine. Minimal removal by hemodialysis. ***Half-life:*** 11.5 hr.

INDICATIONS AND DOSAGES

▸ **Hypertension (Monotherapy)**
PO
Adults, Elderly. Initially, 10 mg/day. Maintenance: 20–40 mg/day. Maximum: 80 mg/day.
▸ **Hypertension (with Diuretic)**
PO
Adults, Elderly. Initially, 10 mg/day titrated to patient's needs.
▸ **Heart Failure**
PO
Adults, Elderly. Initially, 5–10 mg. Maintenance: 20–40 mg/day.

SIDE EFFECTS/ADVERSE REACTIONS

Frequent
Dizziness, cough
Occasional
Hypotension, nausea, vomiting, upper respiratory tract infection

PRECAUTIONS AND CONTRAINDICATIONS

History of angioedema from previous treatment with ACE inhibitors
Caution:
Impaired liver function, hypovolemia, blood dyscrasias, CHF, COPD, asthma, elderly

DRUG INTERACTIONS OF CONCERN TO DENTISTRY

- Increased hypotension: alcohol, phenothiazines
- Decreased hypotensive effects: indomethacin, possibly other NSAIDs, sympathomimetics
- Suspected reduction in the antihypertensive and vasodilator effects by salicylates; monitor B/P if used concurrently

SERIOUS REACTIONS

! Excessive hypotension ("first-dose syncope") may occur in patients with CHF and in those who are severely salt and volume depleted.
! Angioedema (swelling of face and lips) and hyperkalemia occur rarely.
! Agranulocytosis and neutropenia may be noted in those with collagen vascular disease, including scleroderma and systemic lupus erythematosus and impaired renal function.
! Nephrotic syndrome may be noted in those with history of renal disease.

DENTAL CONSIDERATIONS

General:

- Monitor vital signs at every appointment because of cardiovascular and respiratory side effects.
- After supine positioning, have patient sit upright for at least 2 min before standing to avoid orthostatic hypotension.
- Patients on chronic drug therapy may rarely have symptoms of blood dyscrasias, which can include infection, bleeding, and poor healing.
- Assess salivary flow as a factor in caries, periodontal disease, and candidiasis.
- Limit use of sodium-containing products, such as saline IV fluids, for patients with a dietary salt restriction.
- Stress from dental procedures may compromise cardiovascular function; determine patient risk.
- Short appointments and a stress-reduction protocol may be required for anxious patients.

Consultations:

- Medical consultation may be required to assess disease control and patient's ability to tolerate stress.
- In a patient with symptoms of blood dyscrasias, request a medical consultation for blood studies and postpone dental treatment until normal values are reestablished.
- Take precautions if dental surgery is anticipated and sedation or general anesthesia is required; risk of hypotensive episode.

Teach Patient/Family to:

- Encourage effective oral hygiene to prevent soft tissue inflammation.
- Use caution to prevent injury when using oral hygiene aids.
- When chronic dry mouth occurs, advise patient to:
  - Avoid mouth rinses with high alcohol content because of drying effects.
  - Use daily home fluoride products for anticaries effect.
  - Use sugarless gum, frequent sips of water, or saliva substitutes.

fosphenytoin

fos-**phen**′-ih- toyn
(Cerebyx)
Do not confuse Cerebyx with Celebrex or Celexa.

CATEGORY AND SCHEDULE

Pregnancy Risk Category: D

Drug Class:
Hydantoin-anticonvulsant

MECHANISM OF ACTION

A hydantoin-anticonvulsant that stabilizes neuronal membranes by decreasing sodium and calcium ion influx into the neurons. Also decreases post-tetanic potentiation and repetitive discharge.

Therapeutic Effect: Decreases seizure activity.

USES

Control of generalized convulsive status epilepticus; prevention and treatment of seizures during neurosurgery; short-term substitute for oral phenytoin

PHARMACOKINETICS

Completely absorbed after IM administration. Protein binding: 95%–99%. Rapidly and completely hydrolyzed to phenytoin after IM or IV administration. Time of complete conversion to phenytoin: 4 hr after IM injection; 2 hr after IV infusion. ***Half-life:*** 8–15 min (for conversion to phenytoin).

INDICATIONS AND DOSAGES

▸ Status Epilepticus

IV

Adults. Loading dose: 15–20 mg phenytoin equivalent (PE)/kg infused at rate of 100–150 mg PE/min.

▸ Nonemergent Seizures

IV, IM

Adults. Loading dose: 10–20 mg PE/kg. Maintenance: 4–6 mg PE/kg/day.

▸ Short-Term Substitution for Oral Phenytoin

IV, IM

Adults. May substitute for oral phenytoin at same total daily dose.

SIDE EFFECTS/ADVERSE REACTIONS

Frequent

Dizziness, paresthesia, tinnitus, pruritus, headache, somnolence

Occasional

Morbilliform rash

PRECAUTIONS AND CONTRAINDICATIONS

Adams-Stokes syndrome, hypersensitivity to fosphenytoin or phenytoin, second- or third-degree AV block, severe bradycardia, sinoatrial block

Caution:

IV: Do not exceed injection rate of 150 mg PE/min, risk of seizures with abrupt withdrawal; hypotension, severe myocardial insufficiency, phosphate restriction; thyroid, renal, or hepatic disease; elderly, lactation, pediatric use

DRUG INTERACTIONS OF CONCERN TO DENTISTRY

- Increased phenytoin levels: benzodiazepines (chlordiazepoxide, diazepam), halothane, salicylates
- Increased CNS depression: benzodiazepines, H_1-blocker antihistamines, opiate agonists
- Decreased phenytoin levels: carbamazepine, ciprofloxacin
- Decreased effectiveness of corticosteroids
- Suspected risk of hepatic toxicity: chronic use of acetaminophen and phosphenytoin

SERIOUS REACTIONS

! An elevated fosphenytoin blood concentration may produce ataxia, nystagmus, diplopia, lethargy, slurred speech, nausea, vomiting, and hypotension. As the drug level increases, extreme lethargy may progress to coma.

DENTAL CONSIDERATIONS

General:

- This drug is intended for short-term use in an emergency department or hospital setting. Patient probably will return to oral phenytoin or other anticonvulsant after hospital care.
- Use precaution if sedation or general anesthesia is required; risk of hypotensive episode.

Consultations:

- Determine type of epilepsy, seizure frequency and quality of seizure control. A stress reduction protocol may be required.
- Medical consultation may be required to assess disease control and patient's ability to tolerate stress.

Teach Patient/Family to:

- Update health and drug history if physician makes any changes in evaluation or drug regimens.

frovatriptan

fro-va-**trip′**-tan
(Frovan)

CATEGORY AND SCHEDULE

Pregnancy Risk Category: C

Drug Class: Antimigraine agent; $5HT_1$-receptor agonist

MECHANISM OF ACTION

A serotonin receptor agonist that binds selectively to vascular receptors, producing a vasoconstrictive effect on cranial blood vessels.

Therapeutic Effect: Relieves migraine headache.

USES

Acute treatment of migraine with or without aura

PHARMACOKINETICS

Well absorbed after PO administration. Metabolized by the liver to inactive metabolite. Eliminated in urine. ***Half-life:*** 26 hr (increased in hepatic impairment).

INDICATIONS AND DOSAGES

▸ **Acute Migraine Attack**

PO

Adults, Elderly. Initially 2.5 mg. If headache improves but then returns, dose may be repeated after 2 hr. Maximum: 7.5 mg/day.

SIDE EFFECTS/ADVERSE REACTIONS

Occasional

Dizziness, paresthesia, fatigue, flushing

Rare

Hot or cold sensation, dry mouth, dyspepsia

PRECAUTIONS AND CONTRAINDICATIONS

Basilar or hemiplegic migraine, cerebrovascular or peripheral vascular disease, coronary artery disease, ischemic heart disease (including angina pectoris, history of MI, silent ischemia, and Prinzmetal's angina), severe hepatic impairment (Child-Pugh grade C), uncontrolled hypertension, use within 24 hr of ergotamine-containing preparations or another serotonin receptor agonist, use within 14 days of MAOIs

DRUG INTERACTIONS OF CONCERN TO DENTISTRY

- Potential serotonin crisis: SSRIs, ergot-containing drugs (avoid use within 24 hr of taking this drug)
- Decreased plasma levels: cimetidine

SERIOUS REACTIONS

! Cardiac reactions (including ischemia, coronary artery vasospasm and MI) and noncardiac vasospasm-related reactions (such as hemorrhage and CVA) occur rarely, particularly in patients with hypertension, diabetes, or a strong family history of coronary artery disease; obese patients; smokers; males older than 40 yr; and postmenopausal women.

DENTAL CONSIDERATIONS

General:

- This is an acute-use drug; it is doubtful that patients will seek dental treatment during acute migraine attacks.
- Be aware of patient's disease, its severity and its frequency, when known.
- Advise patient if dental drugs prescribed have a potential for photosensitivity.

Consultations:

- If treating chronic orofacial pain, consult with physician of record.
- Medical consultation may be required to assess disease control and patient's ability to tolerate stress.

Teach Patient/Family to:

- Avoid mouth rinses with high alcohol content because of additional drying effects.
- Update health and drug history if physician makes any changes in evaluation or drug regimens.

furosemide

fur-**oh'**-se-mide

(Apo-Furosemide[CAN], Frusehexal[AUS], Frusid[AUS], Lasix, Uremide[AUS], Urex-M[AUS])

Do not confuse Lasix with Lidex, Luvox, or Luxiq, or furosemide with Torsemide.

CATEGORY AND SCHEDULE

Pregnancy Risk Category: C (D if used in pregnancy-induced hypertension)

Drug Class: Loop diuretic

MECHANISM OF ACTION

A loop diuretic that enhances excretion of sodium, chloride, and potassium by direct action at the ascending limb of the loop of Henle.

Therapeutic Effect: Produces diuresis and lowers B/P.

USES

Pulmonary edema, edema in CHF, liver disease, nephrotic syndrome, ascites, hypertension

PHARMACOKINETICS

Route	Onset	Peak	Duration
PO	30–60 min	1–2 hr	6–8 hr
IV	5 min	20–60 min	2 hr
IM	30 min	N/A	N/A

Well absorbed from the GI tract. Protein binding: 91%–97%. Partially metabolized in the liver. Primarily excreted in urine (nonrenal clearance increases in severe renal impairment). Not removed by hemodialysis. ***Half-life:*** 30–90 min (increased in renal or hepatic impairment and in neonates).

INDICATIONS AND DOSAGES

▸ **Edema, Hypertension**

PO

Adults, Elderly. Initially, 20–80 mg/dose; may increase by 20–40 mg/dose q6–8h. May titrate up to 600 mg/day in severe edematous states.

Children. 1–6 mg/kg/day in divided doses q6–12h.

IV, IM

Adults, Elderly. 20–40 mg/dose; may increase by 20 mg/dose q1–2h.

Children. 1–2 mg/kg/dose q6–12h.

Neonates. 1–2 mg/kg/dose q12–24h.

IV infusion
Adults, Elderly. Bolus of 0.1 mg/kg, followed by infusion of 0.1 mg/kg/hr; may double q2h. Maximum: 0.4 mg/kg/hr.
Children. 0.05 mg/kg/hr; titrate to desired effect.

SIDE EFFECTS/ADVERSE REACTIONS

Expected
Increased urinary frequency and urine volume
Frequent
Nausea, dyspepsia, abdominal cramps, diarrhea or constipation, electrolyte disturbances
Occasional
Dizziness, light-headedness, headache, blurred vision, paresthesia, photosensitivity, rash, fatigue, bladder spasm, restlessness, diaphoresis
Rare
Flank pain

PRECAUTIONS AND CONTRAINDICATIONS

Anuria, hepatic coma, severe electrolyte depletion
Caution:
Diabetes mellitus, dehydration, ascites, severe renal disease

DRUG INTERACTIONS OF CONCERN TO DENTISTRY

- Increased electrolyte imbalance: corticosteroids
- Masked ototoxicity: phenothiazines
- Decreased antihypertensive effect: NSAIDs, especially indomethacin

SERIOUS REACTIONS

! Vigorous diuresis may lead to profound water loss and electrolyte depletion, resulting in hypokalemia, hyponatremia, and dehydration.
! Sudden volume depletion may result in increased risk of thrombosis, circulatory collapse, and sudden death.
! Acute hypotensive episodes may occur, sometimes several days after beginning therapy.
! Ototoxicity—manifested as deafness, vertigo, or tinnitus—may occur, especially in patients with severe renal impairment.
! Furosemide use can exacerbate diabetes mellitus, systemic lupus erythematosus, gout, and pancreatitis.
! Blood dyscrasias have been reported.

DENTAL CONSIDERATIONS

General:
- Monitor vital signs at every appointment because of cardiovascular side effects.
- Patients on chronic drug therapy may rarely have symptoms of blood dyscrasias, which can include infection, bleeding, and poor healing.
- Assess salivary flow as a factor in caries, periodontal disease, and candidiasis.
- After supine positioning, have patient sit upright for at least 2 min before standing to avoid orthostatic hypotension.
- Patients on high-potency diuretics should be monitored for serum K levels.

Consultations:
- In a patient with symptoms of blood dyscrasias, request a medical consultation for blood studies and postpone dental treatment until normal values are reestablished.
- Medical consultation may be required to assess disease control.

Teach Patient/Family to:
- Encourage effective oral hygiene to prevent soft tissue inflammation.

- Use caution to prevent injury when using oral hygiene aids.
- When chronic dry mouth occurs, advise patient to:
  - Use daily home fluoride products for anticaries effect.
  - Avoid mouth rinses with high alcohol content because of drying effects.
  - Use sugarless gum, frequent sips of water, or saliva substitutes.

gabapentin

ga′-ba-**pen**-tin
(Neurontin, Pendine[AUS])
Do not confuse Neurontin with Noroxin.

CATEGORY AND SCHEDULE

Pregnancy Risk Category: C

Drug Class: Anticonvulsant, analgesic

MECHANISM OF ACTION

An anticonvulsant and antineuralgic agent whose exact mechanism unknown. May increase the synthesis or accumulation of gamma-aminobutyric acid (GABA) by binding to as-yet-undefined receptor sites in brain tissue. ***Therapeutic Effect:*** Reduces seizure activity and neuropathic pain.

USES

Adjunctive therapy in patients 12 yr or older with partial seizures with or without secondary generalization and as adjunctive therapy for partial seizures in children 3–12 yr; postherpetic neuralgia in adults

PHARMACOKINETICS

Well absorbed from the GI tract (not affected by food). Protein binding: less than 5%. Widely distributed. Crosses the blood-brain barrier. Primarily excreted unchanged in urine. Removed by hemodialysis. ***Half-life:*** 5–7 hr (increased in impaired renal function and the elderly).

INDICATIONS AND DOSAGES

▸ **Adjunctive Therapy for Seizure Control**

PO

Adults, Elderly, Children older than 12 yr. Initially, 300 mg 3 times a day. May titrate dosage. Range: 900–1800 mg/day in 3 divided doses. Maximum: 3600 mg/day.
Children 3–12 yr. Initially, 10–15 mg/kg/day in 3 divided doses. May titrate up to 25–35 mg/kg/day (for children 5–12 yr) and 40 mg/kg/day (for children 3–4 yr). Maximum: 50 mg/kg/day.

▸ **Adjunctive Therapy for Neuropathic Pain**

PO

Adults, Elderly. Initially, 100 mg 3 times a day; may increase by 300 mg/day at weekly intervals. Maximum: 3600 mg/day in 3 divided doses.
Children. Initially, 5 mg/kg/dose at bedtime, followed by 5 mg/kg/dose for 2 doses on day 2, then 5 mg/kg/dose for 3 doses on day 3. Range: 8–35 mg/kg/day in 3 divided doses.

▸ **Postherpetic Neuralgia**

PO

Adults, Elderly. 300 mg on day 1300 mg twice a day on day 2 and 300 mg 3 times a day on day 3. Titrate up to 1800 mg/day.

▸ **Dosage in Renal Impairment**

Dosage and frequency are modified on the basis of creatinine clearance:

Creatinine Clearance	Dosage
60 ml/min or higher	400 mg q8h
30–59 ml/min	300 mg q12h
16–29 ml/min	300 mg daily
Less than 16 ml/min	300 mg every other day
Hemodialysis	200–300 mg after each 4-hr hemodialysis session

G

SIDE EFFECTS/ADVERSE REACTIONS

Frequent
Fatigue, somnolence, dizziness, ataxia
Occasional
Nystagmus, tremors, diplopia, rhinitis, weight gain
Rare
Nervousness, dysarthria, memory loss, dyspepsia, pharyngitis, myalgia

PRECAUTIONS AND CONTRAINDICATIONS

Hypersensitivity
Caution:
Lactation, renal function impairment, children younger than 12 yr, elderly

DRUG INTERACTIONS OF CONCERN TO DENTISTRY

• None reported at this time, but, because CNS side effects are common, the use of anxiolytic sedative drugs may potentially increase the CNS side effects.

SERIOUS REACTIONS

! Abrupt withdrawal may increase seizure frequency.
! Overdosage may result in diplopia, slurred speech, drowsiness, lethargy, and diarrhea.

DENTAL CONSIDERATIONS

General:
• Early-morning appointments and a stress-reduction protocol may be required for anxious patients.
• Place on frequent recall because of oral side effects.
• Monitor vital signs at every appointment because of cardiovascular side effects.
• Assess salivary flow as a factor in caries, periodontal disease, and candidiasis.
• Determine type of epilepsy and quality of seizure control.
Consultations:
• Medical consultation may be required to assess disease control and patient's ability to tolerate stress.
Teach Patient/Family to:
• Encourage effective oral hygiene to prevent soft tissue inflammation.
• Use caution with oral hygiene aids to prevent injury.
• When chronic dry mouth occurs, advise patient to:
  • Avoid mouth rinses with high alcohol content because of drying effects.
  • Use daily home fluoride products for anticaries effect.
  • Use sugarless gum, frequent sips of water, or saliva substitutes.

galantamine

ga-**lan′**-ta-mene
(Reminyl)
Do not confuse Reminyl with Remeron, Remicade, or Robinul.

CATEGORY AND SCHEDULE

Pregnancy Risk Category: B

Drug Class: Cholinesterase inhibitor

MECHANISM OF ACTION

A cholinesterase inhibitor that inhibits the enzyme acetylcholinesterase, thus increasing the concentration of acetylcholine at cholinergic synapses and enhancing cholinergic function in the CNS.
Therapeutic Effect: Slows the progression of Alzheimer's disease.

USES

Treatment of mild-to-moderate dementia of Alzheimer's disease

PHARMACOKINETICS

Rapidly absorbed from the GI tract. Protein binding: 18%. Distributed to blood cells; binds to plasma proteins, mainly albumin. Metabolized in the liver. Excreted in urine. ***Half-life:*** 7 hr.

INDICATIONS AND DOSAGES

▸ Alzheimer's Disease

PO

Adults, Elderly. Initially, 4 mg twice a day (8 mg/day). After a minimum of 4 wk (if well tolerated), may increase to 8 mg twice a day (16 mg/day). After another 4 wk, may increase to 12 mg twice daily (24 mg/day). Range: 16–24 mg/day in 2 divided doses.

▸ Dosage in Renal Impairment

For moderate impairment, maximum dosage is 16 mg/day. Drug is not recommended for patients with severe impairment.

SIDE EFFECTS/ADVERSE REACTIONS

Frequent

Nausea, vomiting, diarrhea, anorexia, weight loss

Occasional

Abdominal pain, insomnia, depression, headache, dizziness, fatigue, rhinitis

Rare

Tremors, constipation, confusion, cough, anxiety, urinary incontinence

PRECAUTIONS AND CONTRAINDICATIONS

Severe hepatic or renal impairment

Caution:

Potentiation of succinylcholine-like neuromuscular blocking drugs, obstructive GI disease, Parkinson's disease, epilepsy, cardiac conduction disorders, AV block, bradycardia, history of GI ulcer, hypersecretory disorders (gastric), bladder outflow obstruction, COPD, asthma, moderate hepatic impairment, moderate renal impairment, lactation, pediatric use

DRUG INTERACTIONS OF CONCERN TO DENTISTRY

- Increased plasma levels: ketoconazole
- Increased bioavailability: cimetidine, paroxetine
- Enhanced succinylcholine muscle relaxation during anesthesia
- Action may be inhibited by anticholinergic drugs or enhanced by cholinergic agonists

SERIOUS REACTIONS

! Overdose may cause cholinergic crisis, characterized by increased salivation, lacrimation, severe nausea and vomiting, bradycardia, respiratory depression, hypotension, and increased muscle weakness. Treatment usually consists of supportive measures and an anticholinergic such as atropine.

DENTAL CONSIDERATIONS

General:

- Monitor vital signs at every appointment because of cardiovascular side effects.
- After supine positioning, have patient sit upright for at least 2 min to avoid orthostatic hypotension.
- Drug is used early in the disease; ensure that patient or caregiver understands informed consent.
- Place on frequent recall because early attention to dental health is important for Alzheimer's patients.
- Consider semisupine chair position for patient comfort if GI side effects occur.

Consultations:

• Consultation with physician may be necessary if sedation or general anesthesia is required.

• Medical consultation may be required to assess disease control and patient's ability to tolerate stress.

Teach Patient/Family to:

• Encourage effective oral hygiene to prevent soft tissue inflammation.

• Have caregiver assist patient with oral home-care regimen as cognitive ability declines.

• Use powered tooth brush if patient has difficulty holding conventional devices.

• Update health and drug history if physician makes any changes in evaluation or drug regimens.

galsulfase

gal-**sul**′-face

(Naglazyme)

CATEGORY AND SCHEDULE

Pregnancy Risk Category: B

Drug Class: Enzyme

MECHANISM OF ACTION

A recombinant normal variant form of a polymorphic enzyme (*N*-acetylgalactosamine 4-sulfatase), produced in Chinese hamster cells, that is taken up into lysosomes and increases the catabolism of glycosaminoglycans.

Therapeutic Effect: Replaces enzyme (*N*-acetylgalactosamine 4-sulfatase).

USES

Treatment of Maroteaux-Lamy syndrome

PHARMACOKINETICS

Half-life: wk 1: 6–21 hr; wk 24: 8–40 hr.

INDICATIONS AND DOSAGES

▸ **Maroteaux-Lamy Syndrome**

IV

Adults. 1 mg/kg once a wk.

Children (5 yr and older). 1 mg/kg once a wk.

SIDE EFFECTS/ADVERSE REACTIONS

Frequent

Antibody development, abdominal pain, ear pain, headache, fever, arthralgia, vomiting, upper respiratory infections, diarrhea, cough, otitis media, infusion-related reactions, pain, rigors, conjunctivitis, dyspnea, chest pain, pharyngitis, facial edema, hypertension, malaise, gastroenteritis, areflexia, corneal opacification, nasal congestion, umbilical hernia

Less frequent adverse effects were not described

PRECAUTIONS AND CONTRAINDICATIONS

Hypersensitivity to galsulfase or its components

Caution:

Respiratory illness

DRUG INTERACTIONS OF CONCERN TO DENTISTRY

• None reported

SERIOUS REACTIONS

! Respiratory distress has been reported.

DENTAL CONSIDERATIONS

General

• Monitor vital signs at every appointment because of cardiovascular side effects.

• Consider semisupine chair position for patient comfort because of respiratory complications.
• Avoid aspirin and NSAIDs.
• Consider visual disturbances when presenting instructions to patients.

Consultations:
• Consult physician to determine disease control and ability of patient to tolerate dental procedures.

Teach Patient/Family to:
• Update medication/health history whenever symptoms of disease or medication regimen is changed.
• Use effective, atraumatic oral hygiene measures to reduce soft tissue inflammation.
• Use home fluoride products for anticaries effect.

ganciclovir sodium

gan-**sy**′-clo-ver **soe**′-dee-um
(Cymevene[AUS], Cytovene, Vitrasert)
Do not confuse Cytovene with Cytosar.

CATEGORY AND SCHEDULE

Pregnancy Risk Category: C

Drug Class: Antiviral, nucleoside analogue

MECHANISM OF ACTION

This synthetic nucleoside competes with viral DNA polymerase and is incorporated into growing viral DNA chains.
Therapeutic Effect: Interferes with synthesis and replication of viral DNA.

USES

Prevention and treatment of cytomegalovirus (CMV) retinitis in patients with AIDS or organ transplants; life-threatening CMV disease

PHARMACOKINETICS

Widely distributed. Protein binding: 1%–2%. Undergoes minimal metabolism. Excreted unchanged primarily in urine. Removed by hemodialysis. ***Half-life:*** 2.5–3.6 hr (increased in impaired renal function).

G

INDICATIONS AND DOSAGES

▸ **CMV Retinitis**
IV
Adults, Children 3 mo and older. 10 mg/kg/day in divided doses q12h for 14–21 days, then 5 mg/kg/day as a single daily dose.

▸ **Prevention of CMV Disease in Transplant Patients**
IV
Adults, Children. 10 mg/kg/day in divided doses q12h for 7–14 days, then 5 mg/kg/day as a single daily dose.

▸ **Other CMV Infections**
IV
Adults. Initially, 10 mg/kg/day in divided doses q12h for 14–21 days, then 5 mg/kg/day as a single daily dose. Maintenance: 1000 mg 3 times a day or 500 mg q3h (6 times a day).
Children. Initially, 10 mg/kg/day in divided doses q12h for 14–21 days, then 5 mg/kg/day as a single daily dose. Maintenance: 30 mg/kg/dose q8h.

▸ **Intravitreal Implant**
Adults. 1 implant q6–9mo plus oral ganciclovir.
Children 9 yr and older. 1 implant q6–9mo plus oral ganciclovir (30 mg/dose q8h).

▸ **Adult Dosage in Renal Impairment**
Dosage and frequency are modified on the basis of CrCl.

CrCl	Induction Dosage	Maintenance Dosage	Oral
50–69 ml/min	2.5 mg/kg q12h	2.5 mg/kg q24h	1500 mg/day
25–49 ml/min	2.5 mg/kg q24h	1.25 mg/kg q24h	1000 mg/day
10–24 ml/min	1.25 mg/kg q24h	0.625 mg/kg q24h	500 mg/day
Less than 10 ml/min	1.25 mg/kg 3 times a wk	0.625 mg/kg 3 times a wk	500 mg 3 times a wk

CrCl = creatinine clearance

SIDE EFFECTS/ADVERSE REACTIONS

Frequent

Diarrhea, fever, nausea, abdominal pain, vomiting

Occasional

Diaphoresis, infection, paresthesia, flatulence, pruritus

Rare

Headache, stomatitis, dyspepsia, phlebitis

PRECAUTIONS AND CONTRAINDICATIONS

Hypersensitivity to acyclovir or ganciclovir

Caution:

Preexisting cytopenia, renal function impairment, lactation, children younger than 6 mo, elderly, platelet count less than 25,000/mm^3

DRUG INTERACTIONS OF CONCERN TO DENTISTRY

• Increased risk of blood dyscrasias: dapsone, carbamazepine, phenothiazines
• Increased risk of seizures: imipenem/cilastatin (Primaxin)
• Low platelet counts may prevent the use of aspirin, NSAIDs

SERIOUS REACTIONS

! Hematologic toxicity occurs commonly: leukopenia in 29%–41% of patients and anemia in 19%–25%.
! Intraocular insertion occasionally results in visual acuity loss, vitreous hemorrhage, and retinal detachment.
! GI hemorrhage occurs rarely.

DENTAL CONSIDERATIONS

General:

• Examine for oral manifestations of opportunistic infection.
• Examine for evidence of oral manifestations of blood dyscrasias (infection, bleeding, poor healing).
• Place on frequent recall to evaluate healing response.
• Consider local hemostasis measures to prevent excessive bleeding.
• Monitor vital signs at every appointment because of cardiovascular and respiratory side effects.

Consultations:

• Medical consultation for blood studies (CBC); leukopenic or thrombocytopenic side effects may result in infection, delayed healing, and excessive bleeding. Postpone elective dental treatment until normal values are maintained.
• Medical consultation may be required to assess disease control.

Teach Patient/Family to:

• Use caution in use of oral hygiene aids to prevent injury.
• See dentist immediately if secondary oral infection occurs.
• Encourage effective oral hygiene to prevent soft tissue inflammation.

gatifloxacin

gah-tee-**floks'**-ah-sin
(Tequin, Zymar)

CATEGORY AND SCHEDULE

Pregnancy Risk Category: C

Drug Class: Fluoroquinolone antiinfective

MECHANISM OF ACTION

A fluoroquinolone that inhibits two enzymes, topoisomerase II and IV, in susceptible microorganisms. ***Therapeutic Effect:*** Interferes with bacterial DNA replication. Prevents or delays resistance emergence. Bactericidal.

USES

Treatment of acute bacterial exacerbation of chronic bronchitis caused by *S. pneumoniae, H. influenzae, H. parainfluenzae, M. catarrhalis,* or *S. aureus*; acute sinusitis (*S. pneumoniae, H. influenzae*); community-acquired pneumonia (*S. pneumoniae, H. influenzae, H. para-influenzae, M. catarrhalis, M. pneumoniae, C. pneumoniae, L. pneumoniae*, or *S. aureus*); complicated or uncomplicated UTI (*E. coli, K. pneumoniae, P. mirabilis*); pyelonephritis (*E. coli*), acute uncomplicated rectal infections in women or uncomplicated urethral or cervical gonorrhea (*N. gonorrhoeae*); uncomplicated skin and skin-structure infections

PHARMACOKINETICS

Well absorbed from the GI tract after PO administration. Protein binding: 20%. Widely distributed. Metabolized in liver. Primarily excreted in urine. ***Half-life:*** 7–14 hr.

INDICATIONS AND DOSAGES

▸ **Chronic Bronchitis, Complicated UTIs, Pyelonephritis, Skin Infections**

PO, IV

Adults, Elderly. 400 mg/day for 7–10 days (5 days for chronic bronchitis).

▸ **Sinusitis**

PO, IV

Adults, Elderly. 400 mg/day for 10 days.

▸ **Pneumonia**

PO, IV

Adults, Elderly. 400 mg/day for 7–14 days.

▸ **Cystitis**

PO, IV

Adults, Elderly. 400 mg as a single dose or 200 mg/day for 3 days.

▸ **Urethral Gonorrhea in Men and Women, Endocervical and Rectal Gonorrhea in Women**

PO, IV

Adults, Elderly. 400 mg as a single dose.

▸ **Topical Treatment of Bacterial Conjunctivitis Caused by Susceptible Strains of Bacteria**

Ophthalmic

Adults, Elderly, Children 1 yr and older. 1 drop q2h while awake for 2 days, then 1 drop up to 4 times a day for days 3–7.

▸ **Dosage in Renal Impairment**

Creatinine Clearance	Dosage
40 ml/min	400 mg/day
Less than 40 ml/min	Initially, 400 mg/day, then 200 mg/day
Hemodialysis	Initially, 400 mg/day, then 200 mg/day
Peritoneal dialysis	Initially, 400 mg/day, then 200 mg/day

SIDE EFFECTS/ADVERSE REACTIONS

Occasional

Nausea, vaginitis, diarrhea, headache, dizziness tendinopathy, Ophthalmic: conjunctival irritation, increased tearing, corneal inflammation

Rare

Abdominal pain, constipation, dyspepsia, stomatitis, edema, insomnia, abnormal dreams, diaphoresis, altered taste, rash Ophthalmic: corneal swelling, dry eye, eye pain, eyelid swelling, headache, red eye, reduced visual acuity, altered taste

PRECAUTIONS AND CONTRAINDICATIONS

Hypersensitivity to quinolones

Caution:

Reduce dose with creatinine clearance less than 40 ml/min; probenecid increases half-life; children younger than 18 yr, lactation, seizure history, avoid use with class IA and III antiarrhythmics; many prolong QT interval; cross resistance with other fluoroquinolones, monitor blood glucose in diabetes

DRUG INTERACTIONS OF CONCERN TO DENTISTRY

- Use caution with erythromycin and tricyclic antidepressants (no data, risk of prolonged QT interval)
- Decreased absorption: divalent and trivalent cations, iron and zinc salts
- Increased risk of CNS stimulation and seizures: NSAIDs

SERIOUS REACTIONS

! Pseudomembranous colitis as evidenced by severe abdominal pain and cramps, severe watery diarrhea, and fever may occur.

! Superinfection manifested as genital or anal pruritus, ulceration, or changes in oral mucosa and moderate to severe diarrhea may occur.

DENTAL CONSIDERATIONS

General:

- Determine why patient is taking the drug.
- Monitor vital signs at every appointment because of cardiovascular side effects.
- Examine for oral manifestation of opportunistic infection.
- Advise patient if dental drugs prescribed have a potential for photosensitivity.
- Ruptures of the shoulder, hand, and Achilles tendons requiring surgical repair or resulting in prolonged disability have been reported with use of fluoroquinolones. Question patient about history of side effects associated with fluoroquinolone use.

Consultations:

- Physician consultation is advised in the presence of an acute dental infection requiring another antibiotic.

Teach Patient/Family to:

- Minimize exposure to sunlight and wear sunscreen if sun exposure is planned.
- Discontinue treatment and inform dentist immediately if patient experiences pain or inflammation of a tendon and to rest and refrain from exercise.

Gatifloxacin Ophthalmic

General:

- Avoid dental light in patient's eyes; offer dark glasses for patient comfort.

gefitinib

geh-**fih**′-tih-nib
(Iressa)

CATEGORY AND SCHEDULE

Pregnancy Risk Category: D

Drug Class: Antineoplastic-miscellaneous; epidermal growth factor receptor inhibitor

MECHANISM OF ACTION

Blocks the signaling pathway that binds to the epidermal growth factor receptor (EGFR) on the surface of normal and cancer cells. EGFR activates the enzyme tyrosine kinase, which sends signals instructing the cells to grow.
Therapeutic Effect: Inhibits the growth of cancer cells.

USES

Treatment of advanced/metastatic non–small-cell lung cancer in those who have not responded to platinum or docetaxel products

PHARMACOKINETICS

Slowly absorbed and extensively distributed throughout the body. Protein binding: 90%. Undergoes extensive metabolism in the liver. Excreted in the feces. ***Half-life:*** 48 hr.

INDICATIONS AND DOSAGES

▸ **Non–Small-Cell Lung Cancer**

PO

Adults, Elderly. 250 mg/day; may increase to 500 mg/day for patients receiving drugs that may decrease gefitinib blood concentrations, such as rifampin and phenytoin

SIDE EFFECTS/ADVERSE REACTIONS

Frequent
Diarrhea, rash, acne
Occasional
Dry skin, nausea, vomiting, pruritus
Rare
Anorexia, asthenia, weight loss, peripheral edema, eye pain

PRECAUTIONS AND CONTRAINDICATIONS

None known

DRUG INTERACTIONS OF CONCERN TO DENTISTRY

- Decreased plasma levels: sodium bicarbonate
- Decreased metabolism: potent inhibitors of CYP3A4 isoenzymes (ketoconazole, itraconazole, erythromycin, clarithromycin)

SERIOUS REACTIONS

! Pancreatitis and ocular hemorrhage occur rarely.
! Hypersensitivity reaction produces angioedema and urticaria.

DENTAL CONSIDERATIONS

General:

- If additional analgesia is required for dental pain, consider alternative analgesics (NSAIDs) in patients taking opioids for acute or chronic pain.
- This drug may be used in the hospital or on an outpatient basis. Confirm the patient's disease and treatment status.
- Consider semisupine chair position for patients with respiratory disease.
- Examine for oral manifestation of opportunistic infection.
- Patients may have received other chemotherapy or radiation: confirm medical and drug history.

• Caution: drug interactions with drugs used in dentistry.

Consultations:

• Medical consultation may be required to assess disease control and patient's ability to tolerate stress.

• Medical consultation may be required to assess immunologic status during cancer chemotherapy and determine safety risk, if any, posed by the required dental treatment.

Teach Patient/Family to:

• Encourage effective oral hygiene to prevent soft tissue inflammation.

• Use caution to prevent trauma when using oral hygiene aids.

• Update health and medication history if physician makes any changes in evaluation or drug regimens; include OTC, herbal, and nonherbal remedies in the update.

gemcitabine hydrochloride

jem-**cih′**-tah-bean hi-droh-**klor′**-ide

(Gemzar)

CATEGORY AND SCHEDULE

Pregnancy Risk Category: D

Drug Class: Antineoplastic-miscellaneous; nucleoside analogue

MECHANISM OF ACTION

An antimetabolite that inhibits ribonucleotide reductase, the enzyme necessary for catalyzing DNA synthesis.

Therapeutic Effect: Produces death in cells undergoing DNA synthesis.

USES

Treatment of cancer of the breast, pancreas, and lung

PHARMACOKINETICS

Not extensively distributed after IV infusion (increased with length of infusion). Protein binding: less than 10%. Excreted primarily in urine as metabolite. ***Half-life:*** 42–94 min (influenced by gender of patient and duration of infusion).

INDICATIONS AND DOSAGES

▸ Non–Small-Cell Lung Cancer (in Combination with Cisplatin)

IV

Adults, Elderly, Children. 1000 mg/m^2 on days 1, 8 and 15, repeated every 28 days; or 1250 mg/m^2 on days 1 and 8. Repeat every 21 days.

▸ Pancreatic Cancer

IV

Adults. 1000 mg/m^2 once weekly for up to 7 wk or until toxicity necessitates decreasing dosage or withholding the dose, followed by 1 wk of rest. Subsequent cycles should consist of once-weekly dose for 3 consecutive wk out of every 4 wk. For patients completing cycles at 1000 mg/m^2, increase dose to 1250 mg/m^2 as tolerated. Dose for next cycle may be increased to 1500 mg/m^2.

▸ Dosage Reduction Guidelines

Dosage adjustments should be on the basis of granulocyte count and platelet count, as follows:

Absolute Granulocyte Counts (cells/mm^3)	Platelet Count (cells/mm^3)	% of Full Dose
1000	100,000	100
500–999	50,000–99,999	75
Fewer than 500	Fewer than 50,000	Hold

SIDE EFFECTS/ADVERSE REACTIONS

Frequent

Nausea and vomiting, generalized pain, fever, mild to moderate pruritic rash, mild to moderate dyspnea, constipation, peripheral edema

Occasional

Diarrhea, petechiae, alopecia, stomatitis, infection, somnolence, paresthesia

Rare

Diaphoresis, rhinitis, insomnia, malaise

PRECAUTIONS AND CONTRAINDICATIONS

None known

DRUG INTERACTIONS OF CONCERN TO DENTISTRY

• None reported

SERIOUS REACTIONS

! Severe myelosuppression, as evidenced by anemia, thrombocytopenia, and leukopenia, is a common reaction.

DENTAL CONSIDERATIONS

General:

• Monitor vital signs at every appointment because of cardiovascular side effects.
• Consider semisupine chair position for patients with respiratory disease.
• If additional analgesia is required for dental pain, consider alternative analgesics in patients taking narcotics for acute or chronic pain.
• Examine for oral manifestation of opportunistic infection.
• Avoid products that affect platelet function, such as aspirin and NSAIDs.
• This drug may be used in the hospital or on an outpatient basis. Confirm the patient's disease and treatment status.
• Chlorhexidine mouth rinse prior to and during chemotherapy may reduce severity of mucositis.
• Patient on chronic drug therapy may rarely present with symptoms of blood dyscrasias, which can include infection, bleeding, and poor healing. If dyscrasia is present, caution patient to prevent oral tissue trauma when using oral hygiene aids.
• Palliative medication may be required for management of oral side effects.
• Short appointments and a stress-reduction protocol may be required for anxious patients.
• Patients may be at risk of bleeding; check for oral signs.
• Oral infections should be eliminated and/or treated aggressively.

Consultations:

• Medical consultation should include routine blood counts including platelet counts and bleeding time.
• Consult physician; prophylactic or therapeutic antiinfectives may be indicated if surgery or periodontal treatment is required.
• Medical consultation may be required to assess immunologic status during cancer chemotherapy and determine safety risk, if any, posed by the required dental treatment.
• Medical consultation may be required to assess disease control and patient's ability to tolerate stress.

Teach Patient/Family to:

• Be aware of oral side effects.
• Use effective, atraumatic oral hygiene to prevent soft tissue inflammation.
• Report oral lesions, soreness, or bleeding to dentist.
• Prevent trauma when using oral hygiene aids.

• Update health and medication history if physician makes any changes in evaluation or drug regimens; include OTC, herbal, and nonherbal remedies in the update.

gemfibrozil

jem-**fi**′-broe-zil

(Apo-Gemfibrozil[CAN], Ausgem[AUS], Gemfibromax[AUS], Jezil[AUS], Lipazil[AUS], Lopid, Novo-Gemfibrozil[CAN])

Do not confuse Lopid with Lorabid or Levbid.

CATEGORY AND SCHEDULE

Pregnancy Risk Category: C

Drug Class: Antihyperlipidemic

MECHANISM OF ACTION

A fibric acid derivative that inhibits lipolysis of fat in adipose tissue; decreases liver uptake of free fatty acids and reduces hepatic triglyceride production. Inhibits synthesis of very low-density lipoproteins (VLDLs) carrier apolipoprotein B.

Therapeutic Effect: Lowers serum cholesterol and triglycerides (decreases VLDL, low-density lipoproteins [LDLs]; increases high-density lipoproteins [HDLs]).

USES

Treatment of type IIb, IV, and V hyperlipidemia

PHARMACOKINETICS

Well absorbed from the GI tract. Protein binding: 99%. Metabolized in liver. Primarily excreted in urine. Not removed by hemodialysis.

Half-life: 1.5 hr.

INDICATIONS AND DOSAGES

▸ **Hyperlipidemia**

PO

Adults, Elderly. 1200 mg/day in 2 divided doses 30 min before breakfast and dinner.

SIDE EFFECTS/ADVERSE REACTIONS

Frequent

Dyspepsia

Occasional

Abdominal pain, diarrhea, nausea, vomiting, fatigue

Rare

Constipation, acute appendicitis, vertigo, headache, rash, pruritus, altered taste

PRECAUTIONS AND CONTRAINDICATIONS

Liver dysfunction (including primary biliary cirrhosis), preexisting gallbladder disease, severe renal dysfunction

Caution:

Monitor hematologic and hepatic function, lactation

DRUG INTERACTIONS OF CONCERN TO DENTISTRY

• None reported

SERIOUS REACTIONS

! Cholelithiasis, cholecystitis, acute appendicitis, pancreatitis, and malignancy occur rarely.

DENTAL CONSIDERATIONS

General:

• Patients on chronic drug therapy may rarely have symptoms of blood dyscrasias, which can include infection, bleeding, and poor healing.

Consultations:

• In a patient with symptoms of blood dyscrasias, request a medical consultation for blood studies and

postpone dental treatment until normal values are reestablished.

gemifloxacin mesylate

jem-ih-**flocks′**-ah-sin **mess′**-ah-late
(Factive)

CATEGORY AND SCHEDULE

Pregnancy Risk Category: C

Drug Class: Fluoroquinolone antiinfective

MECHANISM OF ACTION

A fluoroquinolone that inhibits the enzyme DNA gyrase in susceptible microorganisms, interfering with bacterial cell replication and repair. ***Therapeutic Effect:*** Bactericidal.

USES

Treatment of acute bacterial exacerbation of chronic bronchitis caused by susceptible strains of *S. pneumoniae, H. influenzae, H. parainfluenzae,* or *M. catarrhalis;* community-acquired pneumonia caused by susceptible strains of *S. pneumoniae* (except drug-resistant strains), *H. influenzae, M. catarrhalis, M. pneumoniae, C. pneumoniae,* or *K. pneumoniae*

PHARMACOKINETICS

Rapidly and well absorbed from the GI tract. Protein binding: 70%. Widely distributed. Penetrates well into lung tissue and fluid. Undergoes limited metabolism in the liver. Primarily excreted in feces; lesser amount eliminated in urine. Partially removed by hemodialysis. ***Half-life:*** 4–12 hr.

INDICATIONS AND DOSAGES

▸ Acute Bacterial Exacerbation of Chronic Bronchitis

PO

Adults, Elderly. 320 mg once a day for 5 days.

▸ Community-Acquired Pneumonia

PO

Adults, Elderly. 320 mg once a day for 7 days.

▸ Dosage in Renal Impairment

Dosage and frequency are modified on the basis of creatinine clearance.

Creatinine Clearance	Dosage
Greater than 40 ml/min	320 mg once a day
40 ml/min or less	160 mg once a day

SIDE EFFECTS/ADVERSE REACTION

Occasional

Diarrhea, rash, nausea

Rare

Headache, abdominal pain, dizziness, tendon ruptures

PRECAUTIONS AND CONTRAINDICATIONS

Concurrent use of amiodarone, quinidine, procainamide, or sotalol; history of prolonged QT interval; hypersensitivity to fluoroquinolones; uncorrected electrolyte disorders (such as hypokalemia and hypomagnesemia)

Caution:

Safety and efficacy in children younger than 18 yr, pregnancy and nursing not established; may prolong QT interval, risk of tendinitis and tendon rupture, epilepsy, cerebral arteriosclerosis, renal dysfunction

G

DRUG INTERACTIONS OF CONCERN TO DENTISTRY

• Decreased absorption: divalent or trivalent antacids, iron or zinc salts
• Use with caution or avoid drugs that affect QT interval: erythromycin, antipsychotics, tricyclic antidepressants

SERIOUS REACTIONS

! Antibiotic-associated colitis may result from altered bacterial balance. Hypersensitivity reactions, including photosensitivity (as evidenced by rash, pruritus, blisters, edema, and burning skin), have occurred in patients receiving fluoroquinolones.

DENTAL CONSIDERATIONS

General:
• Determine why patient is taking the drug.
• Avoid dental light in patient's eyes; offer dark glasses for patient comfort.
• Examine for oral manifestation of opportunistic infection.
• Advise patient if dental drugs prescribed have a potential for photosensitivity.
• As with other fluoroquinolones there is a risk of tendinitis and tendon rupture.
• Consider semisupine chair position for patient comfort if GI side effects occur.

Consultations:
• Consult with patient's physician if an acute dental infection occurs and another antiinfective is required.

Teach Patient/Family:
• When chronic dry mouth occurs, advise patient to:
  • Avoid mouth rinses with high alcohol content because of drying effects.
  • Use daily home fluoride products for anticaries effect.
  • Use sugarless gum, frequent sips of water, or saliva substitutes.

gentamicin sulfate

jen-ta-**mye′**-sin **suhl′**-fate
(Alcomicin[CAN], Cidomycin[CAN], Garamycin, Genoptic, Gentak, Gentacidin)

CATEGORY AND SCHEDULE

Pregnancy Risk Category: C

Drug Class: Aminoglycoside antiinfective ophthalmic

MECHANISM OF ACTION

An aminoglycoside antibiotic that irreversibly binds to the protein of bacterial ribosomes.
Therapeutic Effect: Interferes with protein synthesis of susceptible microorganisms. Bacteriostatic.

USES

Treatment of external eye infection

PHARMACOKINETICS

Rapid, complete absorption after IM administration. Protein binding: less than 30%. Widely distributed (does not cross the blood-brain barrier, low concentrations in CSF). Excreted unchanged in urine. Removed by hemodialysis. ***Half-life:*** 2–4 hr (increased in impaired renal function and neonates; decreased in cystic fibrosis and burn or febrile patients).

INDICATIONS AND DOSAGES

▸ Acute Pelvic, Bone, Intraabdominal, Joint, Respiratory Tract, Burn Wound, Postoperative and Skin or Skin-Structure Infections; Complicated UTIs; Septicemia; Meningitis

IV, IM

Adults, Elderly. Usual dosage, 3–6 mg/kg/day in divided doses q8h or 4–6.6 mg/kg once a day.

Children 5–12 yr. Usual dosage 2–2.5 mg/kg/dose q8h.

Children younger than 5 yr. Usual dosage, 2.5 mg/kg/dose q8h.

Neonates. Usual dosage 2.5–3.5 mg/kg/dose q8–12h.

▸ Hemodialysis

IV, IM

Adults, Elderly. 0.5–0.7 mg/kg/dose after dialysis.

Children. 1.25–1.75 mg/kg/dose after dialysis.

Intrathecal

Adults. 4–8 mg/day.

Children 3 mo–12 yr. 1–2 mg/day.

Neonates. 1 mg/day.

▸ Superficial Eye Infections

Ophthalmic Ointment

Adults, Elderly. Usual dosage, apply thin strip to conjunctiva 2–3 times a day.

Ophthalmic Solution

Adults, Elderly, Children. Usual dosage, 1–2 drops q2–4h up to 2 drops/hr.

▸ Superficial Skin Infections

Topical

Adults, Elderly. Usual dosage, apply 3–4 times a day.

▸ Dosage in Renal Impairment

Creatinine clearance greater than 41–60 ml/min. Dosage interval q12h.

Creatinine clearance 20–40 ml/min. Dosage interval q24h.

Creatinine clearance less than 20 ml/min. Monitor levels to determine dosage interval.

SIDE EFFECTS/ADVERSE REACTIONS

Occasional

IM: Pain, induration

IV: Phlebitis, thrombophlebitis, hypersensitivity reactions (fever, pruritus, rash, urticaria)

Ophthalmic: Burning, tearing, itching, blurred vision

Topical: Redness, itching

Rare

Alopecia, hypertension, weakness

EENT: Poor corneal wound healing, temporary visual haze, overgrowth of nonsusceptible organisms

PRECAUTIONS AND CONTRAINDICATIONS

Hypersensitivity to gentamicin, other aminoglycosides (cross-sensitivity), or their components; sulfite sensitivity may result in anaphylaxis, especially in asthmatic patients.

Caution:

Antibiotic hypersensitivity

DRUG INTERACTIONS OF CONCERN TO DENTISTRY

- Increased risk of nephrotoxicity: cephalosporins, vancomycin, enflurane
- Increased neuromuscular blockade: neuromuscular-blocking drugs

SERIOUS REACTIONS

! Nephrotoxicity (as evidenced by increased BUN and serum creatinine levels and decreased creatinine clearance) may be reversible if the drug is stopped at the first sign of symptoms.

! Irreversible ototoxicity (manifested as tinnitus, dizziness, ringing or roaring in the ears, and diminished hearing) and neurotoxicity (as evidenced by headache, dizziness, lethargy, tremors, and visual disturbances) occur occasionally. The risk of these effects increases

G

with higher dosages or prolonged therapy and when the solution is applied directly to the mucosa.

! Suprainfections, particularly with fungal infections, may result from bacterial imbalance no matter which administration route is used.

! Ophthalmic application may cause paresthesia of conjunctiva or mydriasis.

DENTAL CONSIDERATIONS

General:

- For selected infections in the hospital setting; provide emergency dental treatment only.
- Examine for oral manifestation of opportunistic infection.
- Determine why patient is taking the drug.
- Caution patient regarding allergy to medication.

Consultations:

- Medical consultation may be required to assess disease control and patient's ability to tolerate stress.

Teach Patient/Family to:

- Encourage effective oral hygiene to prevent soft tissue inflammation.
- Prevent trauma when using oral hygiene aids.
- Report oral lesions, soreness, or bleeding to dentist.

gentamicin sulfate; prednisolone acetate

jen-ta-**mye'**sin **suhl'**-feyt; pred-**nis'**-oh-lone **ass'**-eh-tayte (Pred-G, Pred-G S.O.P.)

CATEGORY AND SCHEDULE

Pregnancy Risk Category: C

Drug Class: Aminoglycoside antiinfective ophthalmic

MECHANISM OF ACTION

Gentamicin is an aminoglycoside that irreversibly binds to the protein of bacterial ribosomes. Prednisolone is an adrenal corticosteroid that inhibits accumulation of inflammatory cells at inflammation sites, phagocytosis, lysosomal enzyme release, and synthesis and release of mediators of inflammation.

Therapeutic Effect: Interferes in protein synthesis of susceptible microorganisms. Prevents or suppresses cell-mediated immune reactions; decreases or prevents tissue response to inflammatory process.

USES

Treatment of external eye infection

PHARMACOKINETICS

None reported

INDICATIONS AND DOSAGES

▸ **Treatment of Steroid Responsive Inflammatory Conditions, Superficial Ocular Infections**

Ophthalmic Ointment

Adults, Elderly. Apply ½ inch ribbon in the conjunctival sac 1–3 times a day.

Ophthalmic Suspension

Adults, Elderly. Instill 1 drop 2–4 times a day. During the initial 24–48 hr, the dosing frequency may be increased if necessary up to 1 drop/hr.

SIDE EFFECTS/ADVERSE REACTIONS

Occasional

Burning, tearing, itching, blurred vision

Rare

Delayed wound healing, secondary infection, intraocular pressure increased, glaucoma

PRECAUTIONS AND CONTRAINDICATIONS

Viral disease of the cornea and conjunctiva (including epithelia herpes simplex keratitis, vaccinia, varicella), mycobacterial or fungal infection of the eye, uncomplicated removal of a corneal foreign body, hypersensitivity to gentamicin, prednisolone, other aminoglycosides, or corticosteroids, or any component of the formulation

SERIOUS REACTIONS

! Optic nerve damage occurs rarely.

DENTAL CONSIDERATIONS

General:

• Avoid dental light in patient's eyes; offer dark glasses for patient comfort.

glatiramer

gla-**teer**′-ah-mer
(Copaxone)
Do not confuse Copaxone with Compazine.

CATEGORY AND SCHEDULE

Pregnancy Risk Category: B

Drug Class: Multiple sclerosis agent

MECHANISM OF ACTION

An immunosuppressive whose exact mechanism is unknown. May act by modifying immune processes thought to be responsible for the pathogenesis of multiple sclerosis.
Therapeutic Effect: Slows progression of multiple sclerosis.

USES

Reduction of the frequency of relapses in patients with relapsing-remitting multiple sclerosis

PHARMACOKINETICS

Substantial fraction of glatiramer is hydrolyzed locally. Some fraction of injected material enters lymphatic circulation, reaching regional lymph nodes; some may enter systemic circulation intact.

INDICATIONS AND DOSAGES

▸ **Multiple Sclerosis**

Subcutaneous

Adults, Elderly. 20 mg once a day.

SIDE EFFECTS/ADVERSE REACTIONS

Expected

Pain, erythema, inflammation, or pruritus at injection site; asthenia

Frequent

Arthralgia, vasodilation, anxiety, hypertonia, nausea, transient chest pain, dyspnea, flu-like symptoms, rash, pruritus

Occasional

Palpitations, back pain, diaphoresis, rhinitis, diarrhea, urinary urgency

Rare

Anorexia, fever, neck pain, peripheral edema, ear pain, facial edema, vertigo, vomiting

PRECAUTIONS AND CONTRAINDICATIONS

Hypersensitivity to glatiramer or mannitol

DRUG INTERACTIONS OF CONCERN TO DENTISTRY

• None reported.

SERIOUS REACTIONS

! Infection is a common effect.
! Lymphadenopathy occurs occasionally.

DENTAL CONSIDERATIONS

General:

• Monitor vital signs at every appointment because of cardiovascular side effects.
• Protect patient's eyes from accidental spatter during dental treatment.
• Avoid dental light in patient's eyes; offer dark glasses for patient comfort.
• Short appointments may be required because of effects of disease on musculature.
• Short appointments and a stress-reduction protocol may be required for anxious patients.
• Advise patient if dental drugs prescribed have a potential for photosensitivity.
• Inquire about history of disease, any physical limitations, and other drugs the patient may be taking.
• For longer dental appointments, offer patient frequent breaks.

Consultations:

• Consultation with physician may be necessary if sedation or general anesthesia is required.
• Medical consultation may be required to assess disease control and patient's ability to tolerate stress.

Teach Patient/Family to:

• Encourage effective oral hygiene to prevent soft tissue inflammation.
• Prevent trauma when using oral hygiene aids.
• Update health and medication history if physician makes any changes in evaluation or drug regimens; include OTC, herbal, and nonherbal remedies in the update.

glimepiride

gly-**mep′**-er-ide
(Amaryl)
Do not confuse glimepiride with glipizide or glyburide.

CATEGORY AND SCHEDULE

Pregnancy Risk Category: C

Drug Class: Oral antidiabetic (second generation)

MECHANISM OF ACTION

A second-generation sulfonylurea that promotes release of insulin from beta cells of the pancreas and increases insulin sensitivity at peripheral sites.
Therapeutic Effect: Lowers blood glucose concentration.

USES

Stable adult-onset diabetes mellitus (type 2); may also be used with insulin or metformin where diet and exercise are not effective in controlling hyperglycemia.

PHARMACOKINETICS

Route	Onset	Peak	Duration
PO	N/A	2–3 hr	24 hr

Completely absorbed from the GI tract. Protein binding: greater than 99%. Metabolized in the liver. Excreted in urine and eliminated in feces. ***Half-life:*** 5–9.2 hr.

INDICATIONS AND DOSAGES

▸ **Diabetes Mellitus**

PO

Adults, Elderly. Initially, 1–2 mg once a day, with breakfast or first main meal. Maintenance: 1–4 mg once a day. After dose of 2 mg is reached, dosage should be increased in increments of up to 2 mg q1–2wk, on the basis of blood glucose response. Maximum: 8 mg/day.

▸ Dosage in Renal Impairment

PO

Adults. 1 mg once a day.

SIDE EFFECTS/ADVERSE REACTIONS

Frequent

Altered taste sensation, dizziness, somnolence, weight gain, constipation, diarrhea, heartburn, nausea, vomiting, stomach fullness, headache

Occasional

Increased sensitivity of skin to sunlight, peeling of skin, itching, rash

PRECAUTIONS AND CONTRAINDICATIONS

Diabetic complications, such as ketosis, acidosis and diabetic coma; severe hepatic or renal impairment; monotherapy for type 1 diabetes mellitus; stress situations, including severe infection, trauma, and surgery

Caution:

Malnourished; adrenal, pituitary, or hepatic insufficiency; hypoglycemia recognition in elderly or in those taking β-blockers; increased risk of cardiovascular mortality has been reported in patients using oral hypoglycemics; alcohol use; lactation; children

DRUG INTERACTIONS OF CONCERN TO DENTISTRY

• Risk of potentiation of hypoglycemic effects: NSAIDs, salicylates, sulfonamides, β-adrenergic blockers, ketoconazole

SERIOUS REACTIONS

! Overdose or insufficient food intake may produce hypoglycemia, especially with increased glucose demands.

! GI hemorrhage, cholestatic hepatic jaundice, leukopenia, thrombocytopenia, pancytopenia, agranulocytosis, and aplastic or hemolytic anemia occur rarely.

G

DENTAL CONSIDERATIONS

General:

• Be prepared to manage hypoglycemia.

• Short appointments and a stress-reduction protocol may be required for anxious patients.

• Question patient about self-monitoring of drug's antidiabetic effect, including blood glucose values or finger-stick records.

• Ensure that patient is following prescribed diet and regularly takes medication.

• Patients on chronic drug therapy may rarely have symptoms of blood dyscrasias, which can include infection, bleeding, and poor healing.

• Diabetics may be more susceptible to infection and have delayed wound healing.

• Place on frequent recall to evaluate healing response.

• Advise patient if dental drugs prescribed have a potential for photosensitivity.

Consultations:

• Medical consultation may be required to assess disease control.

• In a patient with symptoms of blood dyscrasias, request a medical consultation for blood studies and postpone treatment until normal values are reestablished.

• Medical consultation may include data from patient's blood glucose monitoring, including glycosylated hemoglobin or HbA_{1c} testing.

Teach Patient/Family to:
• Encourage effective oral hygiene to prevent soft tissue inflammation.
• Use caution to prevent trauma when using oral hygiene aids.
• Update health and drug history if physician makes any changes in evaluation or drug regimens.

glipizide

glip′-ih-zide
(Glucotrol, Glucotrol XL, Melizide[AUS], Mini DiaB[AUS])
Do not confuse glipizide with glimepiride or glyburide.

CATEGORY AND SCHEDULE

Pregnancy Risk Category: C

Drug Class: Oral antidiabetic (second generation)

MECHANISM OF ACTION

A second-generation sulfonylurea that promotes the release of insulin from beta cells of the pancreas and increases insulin sensitivity at peripheral sites.
Therapeutic Effect: Lowers blood glucose concentration.

USES

Stable adult-onset diabetes mellitus (type 2)

PHARMACOKINETICS

Route	Onset	Peak	Duration
PO	15–30 min	2–3 hr	12–24 hr
Extended	2–3 hr	6–12 hr	24 hr

Well absorbed from the GI tract. Protein binding: 99%. Metabolized in the liver. Excreted in urine.
Half-life: 2–4 hr.

INDICATIONS AND DOSAGES

▸ **Diabetes Mellitus**

PO

Adults. Initially, 5 mg/day or 2.5 mg in the elderly or those with hepatic disease. Adjust dosage in 2.5- to 5-mg increments at intervals of several days. Maximum single dose: 15 mg. Maximum dose/day: 40 mg. Maintenance (extended-release tablet): 20 mg/day.
Elderly. Initially, 2.5–5 mg/day. May increase by 2.5–5 mg/day q1–2wk.

SIDE EFFECTS/ADVERSE REACTIONS

Frequent
Altered taste sensation, dizziness, somnolence, weight gain, constipation, diarrhea, heartburn, nausea, vomiting, stomach fullness, headache
Occasional
Increased sensitivity of skin to sunlight, peeling of skin, itching, rash

PRECAUTIONS AND CONTRAINDICATIONS

Diabetic ketoacidosis with or without coma, type 1 diabetes mellitus
Caution:
Elderly, cardiac disease, severe renal disease, severe hepatic disease, thyroid disease

DRUG INTERACTIONS OF CONCERN TO DENTISTRY

• Increased hypoglycemic effects: salicylates, ketoconazole
• Decreased action of glipizide: corticosteroids
• Disulfiram-like reaction: alcohol

SERIOUS REACTIONS

! Overdose or insufficient food intake may produce hypoglycemia, especially with increased glucose demands.

! GI hemorrhage, cholestatic hepatic jaundice, leukopenia, thrombocytopenia, pancytopenia, agranulocytosis, and aplastic or hemolytic anemia occurs rarely.

DENTAL CONSIDERATIONS

General:

- Be prepared to manage hypoglycemia.
- Monitor vital signs at every appointment because of cardiovascular side effects.
- Patients on chronic drug therapy may rarely have symptoms of blood dyscrasias, which can include infection, bleeding, and poor healing.
- Short appointments and a stress-reduction protocol may be required for anxious patients.
- Place on frequent recall to evaluate healing response.
- Diabetics may be more susceptible to infection and have delayed wound healing.
- Question patient about self-monitoring of drug's antidiabetic effect, including blood glucose values or finger-stick records.
- Ensure that patient is following prescribed diet and regularly takes medication.
- Avoid prescribing aspirin-containing products.

Consultations:

- In a patient with symptoms of blood dyscrasias, request a medical consultation for blood studies and postpone dental treatment until normal values are reestablished.
- Medical consultation may be required to assess disease control.
- Medical consultation may include data from patient's blood glucose monitoring, including glycosylated hemoglobin or HbA_{1c} testing.

Teach Patient/Family to:

- Encourage effective oral hygiene to prevent soft tissue inflammation.
- Use caution to prevent injury when using oral hygiene aids.
- Avoid mouth rinses with high alcohol content because of drying effects.

glucagon hydrochloride

glue′-ka-gon hi-droh-**klor**′-ide

(GlucaGen, GlucaGen Diagnostic Kit, GlucaGen[AUS], Glucagon, Glucagon Diagnostic Kit, Glucagon Emergency Kit)

Do not confuse glucagon with Glaucon.

CATEGORY AND SCHEDULE

Pregnancy Risk Category: B

Drug Class: Antihypoglycemic, hormone

MECHANISM OF ACTION

A glucose-elevating agent that promotes hepatic glycogenolysis, gluconeogenesis. Stimulates production of cyclic adenosine monophosphate (cAMP), which results in increased plasma glucose concentration, smooth muscle relaxation, and an inotropic myocardial effect.

Therapeutic Effect: Increases plasma glucose level.

USES

Severe hypoglycemia; as a diagnostic aid to facilitate in the radiologic examination of the GI tract by relaxing smooth muscle

PHARMACOKINETICS

Parenteral: Peak levels in 20 min (subcutaneous) or 13 min (IM); extensively metabolized in liver, kidney, and plasma.

INDICATIONS AND DOSAGES

▸ Hypoglycemia

IV, IM, Subcutaneous

Adults, Elderly, Children weighing more than 20 kg. 0.5–1 mg. May give 1 or 2 additional doses if response is delayed.

Children weighing 20 kg or less. 0.5 mg.

▸ Diagnostic Aid

IV, IM

Adults, Elderly. 0.25–2 mg 10 min prior to procedure.

SIDE EFFECTS/ADVERSE REACTIONS

Occasional

Nausea, vomiting

Rare

Allergic reaction, such as urticaria, respiratory distress, and hypotension

PRECAUTIONS AND CONTRAINDICATIONS

Hypersensitivity to glucagon or beef or pork proteins, known pheochromocytoma

Caution:

For hypoglycemia in type 1 diabetes give supplemental carbohydrates as soon as possible; insulinoma, starvation, glycogen depletion, adrenal insufficiency, chronic hypoglycemia, lactation

DRUG INTERACTIONS OF CONCERN TO DENTISTRY

- Patients taking β-adrenergic blockers: may be expected to have a transient but greater increase in B/P and pulse

SERIOUS REACTIONS

! Overdose may produce persistent nausea and vomiting and hypokalemia, marked by severe weakness, decreased appetite, irregular heartbeat, and muscle cramps.

DENTAL CONSIDERATIONS

General:

- Glucagon may be used as an emergency drug for severe hypoglycemia. Patients should be closely monitored and referred immediately for evaluation.
- IV glucose may be required for patients nonresponsive to glucagon.
- Unconscious patients should awaken within 15 min or less.

glyburide

glye′-byoor-ide

(Daonil[CAN], DiaBeta, Euglucon[CAN], Glimel[AUS], Glynase, Micronase, Semi-Daonil[AUS], Semi-Euglucon[AUS])

Do not confuse glyburide with glimepiride or glipizide, or Micronase with Micro-K or Micronor.

CATEGORY AND SCHEDULE

Pregnancy Risk Category: C

Drug Class: Oral antidiabetic (second-generation)

MECHANISM OF ACTION

A second-generation sulfonylurea that promotes release of insulin from beta cells of the pancreas and increases insulin sensitivity at peripheral sites.

Therapeutic Effect: Lowers blood glucose concentration.

USES

Treatment of stable adult-onset diabetes mellitus (Type 2)

PHARMACOKINETICS

Route	Onset	Peak	Duration
PO	0.25–1 hr	1–2 hr	12–24 hr

Well absorbed from the GI tract. Protein binding: 99%. Metabolized in the liver to weakly active metabolite. Primarily excreted in urine. Not removed by hemodialysis. ***Half-life:*** 1.4–1.8 hr.

INDICATIONS AND DOSAGES

▸ Diabetes Mellitus

PO

Adults. Initially, 2.5–5 mg. May increase by 2.5 mg/day at weekly intervals. Maintenance: 1.25–20 mg/day. Maximum: 20 mg/day.
Elderly. Initially, 1.25–2.5 mg/day. May increase by 1.25–2.5 mg/day at 1- to 3-wk intervals.
PO (Micronized Tablets [Glynase])
Adults, Elderly. Initially, 0.75–3 mg/day. May increase by 1.5 mg/day at weekly intervals. Maintenance: 0.75–12 mg/day as a single dose or in divided doses.

▸ Dosage in Renal Impairment

Glyburide is not recommended in patients with creatinine clearance less than 50 ml/min.

SIDE EFFECTS/ADVERSE REACTIONS

Frequent
Altered taste sensation, dizziness, somnolence, weight gain, constipation, diarrhea, heartburn, nausea, vomiting, stomach fullness, headache
Occasional
Increased sensitivity of skin to sunlight, peeling of skin, itching, rash

PRECAUTIONS AND CONTRAINDICATIONS

Diabetic ketoacidosis with or without coma, monotherapy for type 1 diabetes mellitus
Caution:
Elderly, cardiac disease, severe renal disease, severe hepatic disease, thyroid disease, severe hypoglycemia reactions

DRUG INTERACTIONS OF CONCERN TO DENTISTRY

- Increased hypoglycemic effects: NSAIDs, salicylates, ketoconazole
- Decreased action of glyburide: corticosteroids
- Disulfiram-like reaction: alcohol

SERIOUS REACTIONS

! Overdose or insufficient food intake may produce hypoglycemia, especially in patients with increased glucose demands.
! Cholestatic jaundice, leukopenia, thrombocytopenia, pancytopenia, agranulocytosis, and aplastic or hemolytic anemia occur rarely.

DENTAL CONSIDERATIONS

General:
- Be prepared to manage hypoglycemia.
- Monitor vital signs at every appointment because of cardiovascular side effects.
- Patients on chronic drug therapy may rarely have symptoms of blood dyscrasias, which can include infection, bleeding, and poor healing.
- Place on frequent recall to evaluate healing response.
- Ensure that patient is following prescribed diet and regularly takes medication.
- Short appointments and stress-reduction protocol may be required for anxious patients.
- Patients with diabetes may be more susceptible to infection and have delayed wound healing.
- Question patient about self-monitoring of drug's antidiabetic effect, including blood glucose values or finger-stick records.

• Avoid prescribing aspirin-containing products.

Consultations:

• In a patient with symptoms of blood dyscrasias, request a medical consultation for blood studies and postpone dental treatment until normal values are reestablished.

• Medical consultation may be required to assess disease control.

• Medical consultation may include data from patient's blood glucose monitoring, including glycosylated hemoglobin or HbA_{1c} testing.

Teach Patient/Family to:

• Encourage effective oral hygiene to prevent soft tissue inflammation.

• Use caution to prevent injury when using oral hygiene aids.

• Avoid mouth rinses with high alcohol content because of drying effects.

glycopyrrolate

glye-koe-**pye**′-roe-late

(Robinul, Robinul Forte, Robinul Injection[AUS])

Do not confuse Robinul with Reminyl.

CATEGORY AND SCHEDULE

Pregnancy Risk Category: B

Drug Class: Anticholinergic

MECHANISM OF ACTION

A quaternary anticholinergic that inhibits action of acetylcholine at postganglionic parasympathetic sites in smooth muscle, secretory glands, and CNS.

Therapeutic Effect: Reduces salivation and excessive secretions of respiratory tract; reduces gastric secretions and acidity.

USES

Decreased secretions before surgery, reversal of neuromuscular blockade, peptic ulcer disease, irritable bowel syndrome

PHARMACOKINETICS

Poorly and irregularly absorbed from GI tract after oral administration. Metabolized in the liver. Primarily excreted in urine. ***Half-life:*** 1.7 hr.

INDICATIONS AND DOSAGES

▸ Preoperative Inhibition of Salivation and Excessive Respiratory Tract Secretions

IM

Adults, Elderly. 4 mcg/kg 30–60 min before procedure.

Children 2 yr and older. 4 mcg/kg.

Children younger than 2 yr. 4–9 mcg/kg.

▸ To Block Effects of Anticholinesterase Agents

IV

Adults, Elderly. 0.2 mg for each 1 mg neostigmine or 5 mg pyridostigmine.

▸ Peptic Ulcer Disease, Adjunct

IV, IM

Adults, Elderly. 0.1 mg IV or IM 3–4 times a day.

PO

Adults, Elderly. 1–2 mg 2–3 times a day. Maximum: 8 mg/day.

SIDE EFFECTS/ADVERSE REACTIONS

Frequent

Dry mouth, decreased sweating, constipation

Occasional

Blurred vision, gastric bloating, urinary hesitancy, somnolence (with high dosage), headache, intolerance to light, loss of taste, nervousness, flushing, insomnia, impotence, mental confusion or excitement (particularly in the elderly and children), temporary lightheadedness (with parenteral form), local irritation (with parenteral form)

Rare

Dizziness, faintness

PRECAUTIONS AND CONTRAINDICATIONS

Acute hemorrhage, myasthenia gravis, narrow-angle glaucoma, obstructive uropathy, paralytic ileus, tachycardia, ulcerative colitis

Caution:

Elderly, lactation, prostatic hypertrophy, renal disease, CHF, pulmonary disease, hyperthyroidism

DRUG INTERACTIONS OF CONCERN TO DENTISTRY

- Increased anticholinergic effect: antihistamines, phenothiazines, meperidine, haloperidol, scopolamine, atropine
- Do not mix with diazepam, pentobarbital, in syringe or solution
- Constipation, urinary retention: opioid analgesics
- Reduced absorption of ketoconazole

SERIOUS REACTIONS

! Overdose may produce temporary paralysis of ciliary muscle; pupillary dilation; tachycardia; palpitations; hot, dry, or flushed skin; absence of bowel sounds; hyperthermia; increased respiratory rate; ECG abnormalities; nausea; vomiting; rash over face or upper trunk; CNS stimulation; and psychosis (marked by agitation, restlessness, rambling speech, visual hallucinations, paranoid behavior, and delusions, followed by depression).

DENTAL CONSIDERATIONS

General:

- May be useful to control salivation in adults during dental procedures.
- Avoid dental light in patient's eyes; offer dark glasses for patient comfort.
- Assess salivary flow as a factor in caries, periodontal disease, and candidiasis.

Consultation:

- Physician should be informed if significant xerostomic side effects occur (e.g., increased caries, sore tongue, problems eating or swallowing, difficulty wearing prosthesis) so that a medication change can be considered.

Teach Patient/Family:

- When chronic dry mouth occurs, advise patient to:
  - Avoid mouth rinses with high alcohol content because of drying effects.
  - Use daily home fluoride products for anticaries effect.
  - Use sugarless gum, frequent sips of water, or saliva substitutes.

G

goserelin acetate

gos-**er**′-ah-lin **ass**′-eh-tayte
(Zoladex, Zoladex Implant[AUS], Zoladex LA)

CATEGORY AND SCHEDULE

Pregnancy Risk Category: D (advanced breast cancer), X (endometriosis, endometrial thinning)

Drug Class: Gonadotropin-releasing hormone, antineoplastic (hormone); synthetic decapeptide analogue of LHRH

MECHANISM OF ACTION

A gonadotropin-releasing hormone analogue and antineoplastic agent that stimulates the release of luteinizing hormone (LH) and follicle-stimulating hormone (FSH) from the anterior pituitary gland. In males, increases testosterone concentrations initially, and then suppresses secretion of LH and FSH, resulting in decreased testosterone levels.

Therapeutic Effect: In females, causes a reduction in ovarian size and function, reduction in uterine and mammary gland size and regression of sex-hormone–responsive tumors. In males, produces pharmacologic castration and decreases the growth of abnormal prostate tissue.

USES

Treatment of advanced prostate cancer stage B2-C (10.8 mg), endometriosis, advanced breast cancer, endometrial thinning (3.6 mg)

PHARMACOKINETICS

Peak serum concentrations in 14–28 days. ***Half-life:*** 4.5 hr.

INDICATIONS AND DOSAGES

▸ Prostatic Carcinoma

Implant

Adults older than 18 yr, Elderly. 3.6 mg every 28 days or 10.8 mg q12wk subcutaneously into upper abdominal wall.

▸ Breast Carcinoma, Endometriosis

Implant

Adults. 3.6 mg every 28 days subcutaneously into upper abdominal wall.

▸ Endometrial Thinning

Implant

Adults. 3.6 mg subcutaneously into upper abdominal wall as a single dose or in 2 doses 4 wk apart.

SIDE EFFECTS/ADVERSE REACTIONS

Frequent

Headache, hot flashes, depression, diaphoresis, sexual dysfunction, decreased erection, lower urinary tract symptoms

Occasional

Pain, lethargy, dizziness, insomnia, anorexia, nausea, rash, upper respiratory tract infection, hirsutism, abdominal pain

Rare

Pruritus

PRECAUTIONS AND CONTRAINDICATIONS

Pregnancy

DRUG INTERACTIONS OF CONCERN TO DENTISTRY

- None reported

SERIOUS REACTIONS

! Arrhythmias, CHF and hypertension occur rarely.

! Ureteral obstruction and spinal cord compression have been observed. An immediate orchiectomy may be necessary if these conditions occur.

DENTAL CONSIDERATIONS

General:

- Monitor vital signs at every appointment because of cardiovascular side effects.
- Determine why patient is taking the drug.
- If additional analgesia is required for dental pain, consider alternative analgesics (NSAIDs) in patients taking opioids for acute or chronic pain.

- Consider semisupine chair position for patient comfort if GI side effects occur.
- Assess salivary flow as a factor in caries, periodontal disease, and candidiasis.
- If used in prostate cancer, consider urinary retention concern and avoid anticholinergic drugs that may aggravate retention.
- Patients may be taking other medications; see complete drug and herbal history.

Consultations:

- Medical consultation may be required to assess immunologic status during cancer chemotherapy and determine safety risk, if any, posed by the required dental treatment.
- Medical consultation may be required to assess disease control and patient's ability to tolerate stress.

Teach Patient/Family to:

- When chronic dry mouth occurs advise patient to:
  - Avoid mouth rinses with high alcohol content because of drying effects.
  - Use daily home fluoride products for anticaries effect.
  - Use sugarless gum, frequent sips of water, or saliva substitutes.
- Encourage effective oral hygiene to prevent soft tissue inflammation.
- Report oral lesions, soreness, or bleeding to dentist.
- Prevent trauma when using oral hygiene aids.
- Update health and medication history if physician makes any changes in evaluation or drug regimens; include OTC, herbal, and nonherbal remedies in the update.

granisetron

gra-**ni**'se-tron
(Kytril, Sancuso)

CATEGORY AND SCHEDULE

Pregnancy Risk Category: B

Drug Class: Antiemetics, 5-HT_3 receptor antagonists

MECHANISM OF ACTION

A 5-HT_3 receptor antagonist that acts centrally in the chemoreceptor trigger zone of the area postrema, in the brain, and peripherally at the vagal nerve terminals in the intestines.

***Therapeutic Effect*:** Prevents nausea and vomiting.

USES

Prevention of chemotherapy-induced nausea and vomiting
Prevention of radiation-induced nausea and vomiting
Postoperative nausea or vomiting (PONV)

PHARMACOKINETICS

Route	Onset	Peak	Duration
IV	1–3 min	N/A	24 hr
Oral	N/A	N/A	Generally up to 24 hr
Topical	N/A	48 hr	N/A

Rapidly and widely distributed to tissues. Protein binding: 65%. Metabolized in the liver to both active and inactive metabolites. Granisetron is metabolized via CYP3A4 and CYP1A1. Eliminated in urine and feces. Topical: slowly absorbed. ***Half-life:*** 6 hr (oral), 9 hr (IV), 36 hr (transdermal).

INDICATIONS AND DOSAGES

▸ Prevention of Chemotherapy-Induced Nausea and Vomiting

PO

Adults, Elderly. 1 mg 1 hr before chemotherapy, followed by second tablet 12 hr later on the days of chemotherapy or 2 mg as a single dose any time within 1 hr prior to chemotherapy.

IV

Adults, Elderly, Children 2 yr and older. 10 mcg/kg/dose (or 1 mg/dose) within 30 min before chemotherapy.

Transdermal Patch

Adults, 18 yr and older. Apply one patch to clean, dry, intact healthy skin on upper outer arm 24 to 48 hr before chemotherapy; remove at least 24 hr after chemotherapy is completed. May wear patch for up to 7 days. Do not cut patch. Each patch contains 34.3 mg of granisetron; it releases 3.1 mg of granisetron per 24 hr for up to 7 days.

▸ Prevention of Radiation-Induced Nausea and Vomiting

PO

Adults, Elderly. 2 mg once a day, given 1 hr before radiation therapy.

▸ Postoperative Nausea or Vomiting

PO

Adults, Elderly, Children 4 yr and older. 0–40 mcg/kg as a single postoperative dose.

IV

Adults, Elderly. 1 mg IV push as a single postoperative dose.

Children, 4 yr and older. 20–40 mcg/kg. Maximum: 1 mg.

SIDE EFFECTS/ADVERSE REACTIONS

Frequent

Headache, constipation, asthenia

Occasional

Diarrhea, abdominal pain, somnolence, dyspepsia, hypertension, fever, dizziness, anxiety, insomnia

Rare

Altered taste, hypersensitivity reaction, QT prolongation

PRECAUTIONS AND CONTRAINDICATIONS

Hypersensitivity to granisetron, benzyl alcohol, or any component of the formulation

Cardiac arrhythmias

Breast-feeding

Caution:

Topical: direct sun or UV light

DRUG INTERACTIONS OF CONCERN TO DENTISTRY

- CYP450 3A4 and 1A1 inducers and inhibitors: May alter granisetron concentrations.
- Apomorphine: May cause profound hypotension and altered consciousness.
- Phenobarbital: May increase plasma clearance.

SERIOUS REACTIONS

! Hypertension, hypotension, QT prolongation, arrhythmias such as sinus bradycardia, atrial fibrillation, varying degrees of A-V block, ventricular ectopy including non-sustained tachycardia, and ECG abnormalities have been observed.

! Rare cases of hypersensitivity reactions, sometimes severe (e.g., anaphylaxis, shortness of breath, hypotension, urticaria), have been reported.

DENTAL CONSIDERATIONS

General:

- Assess the patient for nausea and vomiting.

Consultations:

- Medical consultation may be required to assess disease control.

Teach Patient/Family to:

- Inform the patient that granisetron is effective shortly after administration in preventing nausea and vomiting.
- Explain to the patient that the drug may affect the sense of taste temporarily.
- Teach the patient other methods of reducing nausea and vomiting, such as lying quietly and avoiding strong odors.
- Instruct the patient not to apply transdermal patch to red, damaged, or irritated skin. The transdermal system should not be cut.

griseofulvin

griz-ee-oh-**full′**-vin
(Fulvicin P/G, Fulvicin U/F, Grifulvin V, Gris-PEG, Grisovin[AUS])

CATEGORY AND SCHEDULE

Pregnancy Risk Category: C

Drug Class: Antifungal

MECHANISM OF ACTION

An antifungal that inhibits fungal cell mitosis by disrupting mitotic spindle structure.
Therapeutic Effect: Fungistatic.

USES

Mycotic infections: tinea corporis, tinea pedis, tinea cruris, tinea barbae, tinea capitis, tinea unguium if caused by *Epidermophyton, Microsporum,* or *Trichophyton*

PHARMACOKINETICS

Variable GI absorption after oral administration; fatty meals may enhance absorption. Peak blood levels: 4 hr. Deposited in keratinized cells.

INDICATIONS AND DOSAGES

▸ Tinea Capitis, Tinea Corporis, Tinea Cruris, Tinea Pedis, Tinea Unguium

PO (Microsize Tablets, Oral Suspension)
Adults. Usual dosage, 500–1000 mg as a single dose or in divided doses.
Children 2 yr and older. Usual dosage, 10–20 mg/kg/day.
PO (Ultramicrosize Tablets)
Adults. Usual dosage, 330–750 mg/day as a single dose or in divided doses.
Children 2 yr and older. 5–10 mg/kg/day.

SIDE EFFECTS/ADVERSE REACTIONS

Occasional

Hypersensitivity reaction (including pruritus, rash and urticaria), headache, nausea, diarrhea, excessive thirst, flatulence, oral thrush, dizziness, insomnia

Rare

Paresthesia of hands or feet, proteinuria, photosensitivity reaction

PRECAUTIONS AND CONTRAINDICATIONS

Hepatocellular failure, porphyria

DRUG INTERACTIONS OF CONCERN TO DENTISTRY

- Possible decreased effects: phenobarbital

SERIOUS REACTIONS

! Granulocytopenia occurs rarely.

DENTAL CONSIDERATIONS

General:

- Determine why patient is taking the drug.
- Assess salivary flow as a factor in caries, periodontal disease, and candidiasis.

- Examine for oral manifestation of opportunistic infection.
- Advise patient if dental drugs prescribed have a potential for photosensitivity.

Teach Patient/Family to:

- Report oral lesions, soreness, or bleeding to dentist.
- Encourage effective oral hygiene to prevent soft tissue inflammation.
- Report sore throat, oral burning sensation, fever, or fatigue, any of which could indicate presence of a superinfection.
- Update health and medication history if physician makes any changes in evaluation or drug regimens; include OTC, herbal, and nonherbal remedies in the update.
- Avoid concurrent use of alcohol.
- When chronic dry mouth occurs advise patient to:
  - Avoid mouth rinses with high alcohol content because of drying effects.
  - Use daily home fluoride products for anticaries effect.
  - Use sugarless gum, frequent sips of water, or saliva substitutes.

guaifenesin

gwye-**fen′**-eh-sin

(Balminil[CAN], Benylin E[CAN], Guiatuss, Humibid LA, Mucinex, Organidin, Robitussin, Tussin)

Do not confuse guaifenesin with guanfacine.

CATEGORY AND SCHEDULE

Pregnancy Risk Category: C

OTC

Drug Class: Expectorant, glyceryl guaiacolate

MECHANISM OF ACTION

An expectorant that stimulates respiratory tract secretions by decreasing adhesiveness and viscosity of phlegm.

Therapeutic Effect: Promotes removal of viscous mucus.

USES

Treatment of dry, nonproductive cough

PHARMACOKINETICS

Well absorbed from the GI tract. Metabolized in the liver. Excreted in urine.

INDICATIONS AND DOSAGES

▸ **Expectorant**

PO

Adults, Elderly, Children older than 12 yr. 200–400 mg q4h.

Children 6–12 yr. 100–200 mg q4h. Maximum: 1.2 g/day.

Children 2–5 yr. 50–100 mg q4h.

Children younger than 2 yr. 12 mg/kg/day in 6 divided doses.

PO (Extended-Release)

Adults, Elderly, Children older than 12 yr. 600–1200 mg q12h. Maximum: 2.4 g/day.

Children 2–5 yr. 600 mg q12h. Maximum: 600 mg/day.

SIDE EFFECTS/ADVERSE REACTIONS

Rare

Dizziness, headache, rash, diarrhea, nausea, vomiting, abdominal pain

PRECAUTIONS AND CONTRAINDICATIONS

Hypersensitivity, persistent cough

SERIOUS REACTIONS

! Overdose may produce nausea and vomiting.

DENTAL CONSIDERATIONS

General:

- Consider semisupine chair position for patients with respiratory disease.
- Elective dental treatment may be precluded by significant coughing episodes.

guanabenz

gwan′-ah-benz
(Wytensin)

CATEGORY AND SCHEDULE

Pregnancy Risk Category: C

Drug Class: Centrally acting antihypertensive

MECHANISM OF ACTION

An α-adrenergic agonist that stimulates α_2-adrenergic receptors. Inhibits sympathetic CNS cardioaccelerator and vasoconstrictor center impulses to heart, kidneys, peripheral vasculature.
Therapeutic Effect: Decreases systolic, diastolic B/P. Chronic use decreases peripheral vascular resistance.

USES

Treatment of hypertension

PHARMACOKINETICS

Well absorbed from GI tract. Widely distributed. Protein binding: 90%. Metabolized in liver. Excreted in urine and feces. Not removed by hemodialysis. ***Half-life:*** 6 hr.

INDICATIONS AND DOSAGES

▸ **Hypertension**

PO

Adults. Initially, 4 mg 2 times a day. Increase by 4–8 mg at 1–2 wk intervals.

Elderly. Initially, 4 mg/day. May increase q1–2 wk. Maintenance: 8–16 mg/day. Maximum: 32 mg/day.

SIDE EFFECTS/ADVERSE REACTIONS

Frequent

Drowsiness, dry mouth, dizziness

Occasional

Weakness, headache, nausea, decreased sexual ability

Rare

Ataxia, sleep disturbances, rash, itching, diarrhea, constipation, altered taste, muscle aches

PRECAUTIONS AND CONTRAINDICATIONS

History of hypersensitivity to guanabenz or any component of the formulation

Caution:

Lactation, children younger than 12 yr, severe coronary insufficiency, recent MI, cerebrovascular disease, severe hepatic or renal failure

DRUG INTERACTIONS OF CONCERN TO DENTISTRY

- Increased CNS depression: alcohol, all CNS depressants
- Decreased hypotensive effects: NSAIDs, especially indomethacin, sympathomimetics

SERIOUS REACTIONS

! Abrupt withdrawal may result in rebound hypertension manifested as nervousness, agitation, anxiety, insomnia, hand tingling, tremors, flushing, and sweating.

! Overdosage produces hypotension, somnolence, lethargy, irritability, bradycardia, and miosis (pupillary constriction).

DENTAL CONSIDERATIONS

General:

- Monitor vital signs at every appointment because of cardiovascular side effects.
- Limit use of sodium-containing products, such as saline IV fluids, for patients with a dietary salt restriction.
- Assess salivary flow as a factor in caries, periodontal disease, and candidiasis.
- Stress from dental procedures may compromise cardiovascular function; determine patient risk.
- Short appointments and a stress-reduction protocol may be required for anxious patients.

Consultations:

- Medical consultation may be required to assess disease control and patient's ability to tolerate stress.

Teach Patient/Family:

- When chronic dry mouth occurs, advise patient to:
  - Avoid mouth rinses with high alcohol content because of drying effects.
  - Use daily home fluoride products for anticaries effect.
  - Use sugarless gum, frequent sips of water, or saliva substitutes.

guanadrel sulfate

gwahn′-ah-drel **sull′**-fate
(Hylorel)

CATEGORY AND SCHEDULE

Pregnancy Risk Category: C

Drug Class: Antihypertensive

MECHANISM OF ACTION

An adrenergic blocking agent that depletes norepinephrine from adrenergic nerve endings. Prevents release of norepinephrine normally produced by nerve stimulation.
Therapeutic Effect: Reduces B/P.

USES

Treatment of hypertension

PHARMACOKINETICS

Rapidly and well absorbed from GI tract. Widely distributed. Protein binding: 20%. Primarily excreted in urine. ***Half-life:*** 10 hr.

INDICATIONS AND DOSAGES

▸ **Hypertension**

PO

Adults. Initially, 5 mg 2 times a day. Increase at 1–4 wk intervals. Maintenance: 20–75 mg/day in 2 divided doses. Maximum: 400 mg/day.

Elderly. Initially, 5 mg/day. May gradually increase at 1–4 wk intervals. Maintenance: 20–75 mg/day in 2 divided doses.

SIDE EFFECTS/ADVERSE REACTIONS

Frequent

Fatigue, headache, faintness, drowsiness, nocturia, urinary frequency, change in weight, aching limbs, shortness of breath (resting)

Occasional

Cough, change in vision, paresthesia, confusion, indigestion, constipation, anorexia, peripheral edema, leg cramps

Rare

Depression, altered sleep, nausea, vomiting, dry mouth, throat, impotence, backache

PRECAUTIONS AND CONTRAINDICATIONS

Frank CHF, pheochromocytoma, hypersensitivity to guanadrel or any component of the formulation

Caution:

Elderly, bronchial asthma, peptic ulcer, electrolyte imbalances, vascular disease

DRUG INTERACTIONS OF CONCERN TO DENTISTRY

- Increased orthostatic hypotension: alcohol, opioid analgesics, barbiturates, phenothiazines, haloperidol
- Decreased hypotensive effect: ephedrine, sympathomimetics, NSAIDs, indomethacin, tricyclic antidepressants

SERIOUS REACTIONS

! Overdose may produce blurred vision, severe dizziness/faintness.

DENTAL CONSIDERATIONS

General:

- Monitor vital signs at every appointment because of cardiovascular side effects.
- After supine positioning, have patient sit upright for at least 2 min before standing to avoid orthostatic hypotension.
- Limit use of sodium-containing products, such as saline IV fluids, for patients with a dietary salt restriction.
- Stress from dental procedures may compromise cardiovascular function; determine patient risk.
- Short appointments and a stress-reduction protocol may be required for anxious patients.
- Assess salivary flow as a factor in caries, periodontal disease, and candidiasis.

Consultations:

- Medical consultation may be required to assess disease control and patient's ability to tolerate stress.

Teach Patient/Family:

- When chronic dry mouth occurs, advise patient to:
  - Avoid mouth rinses with high alcohol content because of drying effects.
  - Use daily home fluoride products for anticaries effect.
  - Use sugarless gum, frequent sips of water, or saliva substitutes.

G

guanethidine monosulfate

gwahn-**eth′**-ih-deen mah-no-**sull′**-fate

(Ismelin)

CATEGORY AND SCHEDULE

Pregnancy Risk Category: C

Drug Class: Antihypertensive

MECHANISM OF ACTION

An adrenergic blocker that inhibits the release of catecholamines produced by sympathetic nerve stimulation, thus suppressing peripheral sympathetic vasoconstriction.

Therapeutic Effect: Decreases B/P.

USES

Treatment of moderate-to-severe hypertension

PHARMACOKINETICS

Absorption is highly variable among patients. Protein binding: 26%. Metabolized in liver. Excreted in urine and feces. ***Half-life:*** 5–10 days.

INDICATIONS AND DOSAGES

▸ **Hypertension**

PO

Adults. Initially, 10 mg/day. May increase in 10–25 mg increments at 5–7 day intervals. Maximum: 100 mg/day. Lower initial doses are recommended for the elderly.

SIDE EFFECTS/ADVERSE REACTIONS

Frequent

Bradycardia, dizziness, blurred vision, orthostatic hypotension, fluid retention

Occasional

Impotence, inhibition of ejaculation, nasal stuffiness

Rare

Apnea, hypertension, renal dysfunction

PRECAUTIONS AND CONTRAINDICATIONS

MAOI therapy within 1 wk, overt CHF, pheochromocytoma, hypersensitivity to guanethidine or any component of the formulation

Caution:

Lactation, children; peptic ulcer, asthma, frequent orthostatic hypotension, fever, renal impairment

DRUG INTERACTIONS OF CONCERN TO DENTISTRY

- Increased orthostatic hypotension: alcohol, opioid analgesics, barbiturates, phenothiazines, haloperidol
- Decreased hypotensive effect: ephedrine, NSAIDs, indomethacin, sympathomimetics, tricyclic antidepressants

SERIOUS REACTIONS

! Arrhythmias, angina, and pulmonary edema have been reported.

! Overdosage may produce bradycardia, diarrhea, nausea, orthostatic hypotension, and shock.

DENTAL CONSIDERATIONS

General:

- Monitor vital signs at every appointment because of cardiovascular and respiratory side effects.
- Patients on chronic drug therapy may rarely have symptoms of blood dyscrasias, which can include infection, bleeding, and poor healing.
- Assess salivary flow as a factor in caries, periodontal disease, and candidiasis.
- After supine positioning, have patient sit upright for at least 2 min before standing to avoid orthostatic hypotension.
- Limit use of sodium-containing products, such as saline IV fluids, for patients with a dietary salt restriction.
- Stress from dental procedures may compromise cardiovascular function; determine patient risk.
- Short appointments and a stress-reduction protocol may be required for anxious patients.
- Use vasoconstrictors with caution, in low doses and with careful aspiration. Avoid using gingival retraction cord with epinephrine.
- Consider semisupine chair position for patients with respiratory distress.

Consultations:

- Medical consultation may be required to assess disease control and patient's ability to tolerate stress.
- In a patient with symptoms of blood dyscrasias, request a medical consultation for blood studies and postpone dental treatment until normal values are reestablished.

Teach Patient/Family to:
• Encourage effective oral hygiene to prevent soft tissue inflammation.
• Use caution to prevent injury when using oral hygiene aids.
• When chronic dry mouth occurs, advise patient to:
  • Avoid mouth rinses with high alcohol content because of drying effects.
  • Use daily home fluoride products for anticaries effect.
  • Use sugarless gum, frequent sips of water, or saliva substitutes.

guanfacine

gwan′-fa-seen
(Tenex)

CATEGORY AND SCHEDULE

Pregnancy Risk Category: B

Drug Class: Antihypertensive

MECHANISM OF ACTION

An α-adrenergic agonist that stimulates α_2-adrenergic receptors and inhibits sympathetic cardioaccelerator and vasoconstrictor center to heart, kidneys, peripheral vasculature.
Therapeutic Effect: Decreases systolic, diastolic B/P. Chronic use decreases peripheral vascular resistance.

USES

Treatment of hypertension in individual using a thiazide diuretic or other antihypertensive

PHARMACOKINETICS

Well absorbed from GI tract. Widely distributed. Protein binding: 71%. Metabolized in liver. Excreted in urine and feces. Not removed by hemodialysis. ***Half-life:*** 17 hr.

INDICATIONS AND DOSAGES

▸ **Hypertension**
PO
Adults, Elderly. Initially, 1 mg/day. Increase by 1 mg/day at intervals of 3–4 wk up to 3 mg/day in single or divided doses.

G

SIDE EFFECTS/ADVERSE REACTIONS

Frequent
Dry mouth, somnolence
Occasional
Fatigue, headache, asthenia (loss of strength, energy), dizziness

PRECAUTIONS AND CONTRAINDICATIONS

History of hypersensitivity to guanfacine or any component of the formulation

DRUG INTERACTIONS OF CONCERN TO DENTISTRY

• Possible increase in CNS depression: alcohol and all CNS depressants
• Possible reduced antihypertensive effect: NSAIDs
• Possible increase in antihypertensive effects: other antihypertensive drugs

SERIOUS REACTIONS

! Overdosage may produce difficult breathing, dizziness, faintness, severe drowsiness, bradycardia.

DENTAL CONSIDERATIONS

General:
• Monitor vital signs at every appointment because of cardiovascular side effects.

• After supine positioning, have patient sit upright for at least 2 min before standing to avoid orthostatic hypotension.
• Limit use of sodium-containing products, such as saline IV fluids, for patients with a dietary salt restriction.
• Assess salivary flow as a factor in caries, periodontal disease, and candidiasis.
• Short appointments and a stress-reduction protocol may be required for anxious patients.
• Stress from dental procedures may compromise cardiovascular function; determine patient risk.
• Use precaution if sedation or general anesthesia is required; risk of hypotensive episode.

Consultations:

• Medical consultation may be required to assess disease control and patient's ability to tolerate stress.

Teach Patient/Family to:

• Update health and medication history if physician makes any changes in evaluation or drug regimens; include OTC, herbal, and nonherbal remedies in the update.
• Use caution when driving or performing other tasks requiring mental alertness; avoid if drowsiness occurs.
• When chronic dry mouth occurs advise patient to:
  • Avoid mouth rinses with high alcohol content because of drying effects.
  • Use daily home fluoride products for anticaries effect.
  • Use sugarless gum, frequent sips of water, or saliva substitutes.

halcinonide

hal-**sin′**-oh-nide
(Halog, Halog-E)

CATEGORY AND SCHEDULE

Pregnancy Risk Category: C

Drug Class: Corticosteroid, synthetic topical

MECHANISM OF ACTION

A topical corticosteroid that has antiinflammatory, antipruritic, and vasoconstrictive properties. The exact mechanism of the antiinflammatory process is unclear. ***Therapeutic Effect:*** Reduces or prevents tissue response to the inflammatory process.

USES

Treatment of inflammation of corticosteroid-responsive dermatoses

PHARMACOKINETICS

Well absorbed systemically. Large variation in absorption among sites. Protein binding: varies. Metabolized in liver. Primarily excreted in urine.

INDICATIONS AND DOSAGES

▸ **Dermatoses**

Topical

Adults, Elderly. Apply sparingly 1–3 times a day.

SIDE EFFECTS/ADVERSE REACTIONS

Occasional

Itching, redness, irritation, burning at site of application, dryness, folliculitis, acneiform eruptions, hypopigmentation

Rare

Allergic contact dermatitis, maceration of the skin, secondary infection, skin atrophy

PRECAUTIONS AND CONTRAINDICATIONS

History of hypersensitivity to halcinonide or other corticosteroids

SERIOUS REACTIONS

! The serious reactions of long-term therapy and the addition of occlusive dressings are reversible hypothalamic-pituitary-adrenal (HPA) axis suppression, manifestations of Cushing's syndrome, hyperglycemia, and glucosuria.

DENTAL CONSIDERATIONS

General:

• Place on frequent recall to evaluate healing response when used on chronic basis.

Teach Patient/Family to:

• Encourage effective oral hygiene to prevent soft tissue inflammation.
• Return for oral evaluation if response of oral tissues has not occurred in 7–14 days.
• Apply at bedtime or after meals for maximum effect.
• Apply with cotton-tipped applicator by pressing, not rubbing, paste on lesion.
• Avoid use on oral herpetic ulcerations.

halobetasol

hal-oh-**bay′**-ta-sol
(Ultravate)

CATEGORY AND SCHEDULE

Pregnancy Risk Category: C

Drug Class: Topical corticosteroid, group VI potency

MECHANISM OF ACTION

A corticosteroid that inhibits accumulation of inflammatory cells at inflammation sites, phagocytosis, lysosomal enzyme release, and synthesis or release of mediators of inflammation.
Therapeutic Effect: Decreases or prevents tissue response to inflammatory process.

USES

Treatment of psoriasis, eczema, contact dermatitis, pruritus

PHARMACOKINETICS

Variation in absorption among individuals and sites: scrotum 36%, forehead 7%, scalp 4%, forearm 1%.

INDICATIONS AND DOSAGES

▸ Dermatoses, Corticosteroid-Unresponsive
Topical
Adults, Elderly, Children 12 yr and older. Apply 1–2 times a day. Maximum: 50 g for 2 wk.

SIDE EFFECTS/ADVERSE REACTIONS

Frequent
Burning, stinging, pruritus
Rare
Cushing's syndrome, hyperglycemia, glucosuria, hypothalamic-pituitary-adrenal axis suppression

PRECAUTIONS AND CONTRAINDICATIONS

Hypersensitivity to halobetasol or other corticosteroids
Caution:
Lactation, viral infections, bacterial infections

SERIOUS REACTIONS

! Overdosage can occur from topically applied halobetasol absorbed in sufficient amounts to produce systemic effects producing reversible adrenal suppression, manifestations of Cushing's syndrome, hyperglycemia, and glucosuria in some patients.

DENTAL CONSIDERATIONS

Teach Patient/Family to:
- Avoid use on oral herpetic ulcerations.

haloperidol

ha-loe-**per'**-ih-dole
(Apo-Haloperidol[CAN], Haldol, Haldol Decanoate, Novo-Peridol[CAN], Peridol[CAN], Serenace[AUS])
Do not confuse Haldol with Halcion, Halog or Stadol.

CATEGORY AND SCHEDULE

Pregnancy Risk Category: C

Drug Class: Antipsychotic/butyrophenone

MECHANISM OF ACTION

An antipsychotic, antiemetic, and antidyskinetic agent that competitively blocks postsynaptic dopamine receptors, interrupts nerve impulse movement, and increases turnover of dopamine in the brain. Has strong extrapyramidal and antiemetic effects; weak anticholinergic and sedative effects.
Therapeutic Effect: Produces tranquilizing effect.

USES

Treatment of psychotic disorders, control of tics and vocal utterances in Tourette's syndrome, short-term treatment of hyperactive children showing excessive motor activity

PHARMACOKINETICS

Readily absorbed from the GI tract. Protein binding: 92%. Extensively metabolized in the liver. Primarily excreted in urine. Not removed by hemodialysis. ***Half-life:*** 12–37 hr PO; 10–19 hr IV; 17–25 hr IM.

INDICATIONS AND DOSAGES

▸ **Treatment of Psychotic Disorders**

PO

Adults, Children 12 yr and older. Initially, 0.5–5 mg 2–3 times a day. Dosage gradually adjusted as needed.

Elderly. 0.5–2 mg 2–3 times a day. Dosage gradually adjusted as needed.

Children 3–12 yr or weighing 15–40 kg. Initially, 0.05 mg/kg/day in 2–3 divided doses. May increase by 0.5 mg increments at 5–7 day intervals. Maximum: 0.15 mg/kg/day in divided doses.

IM

Adults, Elderly, Children 12 yr and older. Initially, 2–5. May repeat at 1-hr intervals as needed. Maximum: 100 mg/day.

IM (Decanoate)

Adults, Elderly, Children 12 yr and older. Initially, 10–15 times previous daily oral dose up to maximum initial dose of 100 mg. Maximum: 300 mg/mo.

▸ **Treatment of Nonpsychotic Disorders, Tourette's Syndrome**

PO

Children 3–12 yr or weighing 15–40 kg. Initially, 0.05 mg/kg/day in 2–3 divided doses. May increase by 0.5 mg at 5–7 day intervals. Maximum: 0.075 mg/kg/day.

SIDE EFFECTS/ADVERSE REACTIONS

Frequent

Blurred vision, constipation, orthostatic hypotension, dry mouth, swelling or soreness of female breasts, peripheral edema

Occasional

Allergic reaction, difficulty urinating, decreased thirst, dizziness, decreased sexual function, drowsiness, nausea, vomiting, photosensitivity, lethargy

PRECAUTIONS AND CONTRAINDICATIONS

Angle-closure glaucoma, CNS depression, myelosuppression, Parkinson's disease, severe cardiac or hepatic disease

Caution:

Lactation, seizure disorders, hypertension, hepatic disease, cardiac disease

DRUG INTERACTIONS OF CONCERN TO DENTISTRY

- Increased sedation: other CNS depressants, alcohol, barbiturate anesthetics, opioid analgesics
- Hypotension, tachycardia: epinephrine
- Increased extrapyramidal effects: phenothiazines and related drugs (haloperidol, droperidol), metoclopramide
- Additive photosensitization: tetracyclines
- Increased anticholinergic effects: anticholinergics
- Suspected increase in neurologic side effects: fluconazole, itraconazole, ketoconazole

SERIOUS REACTIONS

! Extrapyramidal symptoms appear to be dose related and typically occur in the first few days of therapy. Marked drowsiness and

H

lethargy, excessive salivation, and fixed stare occur frequently.
! Less common reactions include severe akathisia (motor restlessness) and acute dystonias (such as torticollis, opisthotonos, and oculogyric crisis).
! Tardive dyskinesia (tongue protrusion, puffing of the cheeks, chewing or puckering of the mouth) may occur during long-term therapy or after discontinuing the drug and may be irreversible. Elderly female patients have a greater risk of developing this reaction.

DENTAL CONSIDERATIONS

General:

- Monitor vital signs at every appointment because of cardiovascular side effects.
- After supine positioning, have patient sit upright for at least 2 min before standing to avoid orthostatic hypotension.
- Assess salivary flow as a factor in caries, periodontal disease, and candidiasis.
- Avoid dental light in patient's eyes; offer dark glasses for patient comfort.
- Assess for presence of extrapyramidal motor symptoms, such as tardive dyskinesia and akathisia. Extrapyramidal motor activity may complicate dental treatment.
- Geriatric patients are more susceptible to drug effects; use lower dose.
- Use vasoconstrictors with caution, in low doses and with careful aspiration. Avoid use of gingival retraction cord with epinephrine.

Consultations:

- Take precautions if dental surgery is anticipated and anesthesia is required.
- Confirm patient's mental ability to give informed consent.
- Refer to physician if signs of tardive dyskinesia or akathisia are present.
- Physician should be informed if significant xerostomic side effects occur (e.g., increased caries, sore tongue, problems eating or swallowing, difficulty wearing prosthesis) so that a medication change can be considered.

Teach Patient/Family to:

- Encourage effective oral hygiene to prevent soft tissue inflammation.
- Use caution to prevent injury when using oral hygiene aids.
- Use powered tooth brush if patient has difficulty holding conventional devices.
- When chronic dry mouth occurs, advise patient to:
  - Avoid mouth rinses with high alcohol content because of drying effects.
  - Use daily home fluoride products for anticaries effect.
  - Use sugarless gum, frequent sips of water, or saliva substitutes.

histrelin

his-**trel′**-in
(Supprelin LA)

CATEGORY AND SCHEDULE

Pregnancy Risk Category: X
Controlled substance: Schedule IV

Drug Class: Gonadotropin releasing hormone agonist

MECHANISM OF ACTION

Inhibits gonadotropin secretion. It increases level of luteinizing

hormone (LH) and follicle-stimulating hormone (FSH) upon initiation of treatment but after continuous administration will decrease LH, FSH, testosterone, and estrogen.
Therapeutic Effect: Histrelin slows prostate cancer growth by lowering testosterone levels, decreasing estrogen levels in females, and decreasing testosterone levels in males.

USES

Palliative treatment of advanced prostate cancer and children with central precocious puberty (CPP).

PHARMACOKINETICS

Rapidly absorbed after injection (92%). Protein binding: 70%. Metabolism in liver via C-terminal dealkylation and hydrolysis.
Half-life: ~4 hr.

INDICATIONS AND DOSAGES

Adult. Palliative treatment of advanced prostate cancer: one 50-mg implant (releases 65 mcg per day over 12 months) inserted subcutaneously for 12 months.
Pediatric. CPP: one 50-mg implant inserted subcutaneously every 12 months. Discontinue at the appropriate time for the onset of puberty.
Safety and efficacy in children younger than 2 yr have not been established.

SIDE EFFECTS/ADVERSE REACTIONS

Frequent
Hot sweats, headache, fatigue, implant site reaction (bruising, discomfort, itching, pain, soreness, swelling, and tingling)

Occasional
Erectile dysfunction, insomnia, abdominal discomfort, constipation, weight gain, keloid scar, postprocedural pain, pain at the application site, menorrhagia

PRECAUTIONS AND CONTRAINDICATIONS

Contraindicated in patients with a history of hypersensitivity to GnRH, GnRH agonist analogs, histrelin acetate, or any component of the product; pregnancy (may cause fetal harm and spontaneous abortion). Not recommended in pediatric patients (<2 yr of age).
Initial agonistic action can occur; there is an initial transient increase of estrogen in females and testosterone in both males and females, which may temporarily worsen symptoms.

DRUG INTERACTIONS OF CONCERN TO DENTISTRY

• None reported.

SERIOUS REACTIONS

! Pituitary adenoma, pituitary apoplexy (frequently secondary to pituitary adenoma), urinary tract obstruction, and spinal cord compression may occur in rare cases.

DENTAL CONSIDERATIONS

• Avoid bright dental light directly into patient's eyes; use sunglasses for patient's comfort.
Consultations:
• Medical consultation may be required to assess disease control.
• Review patient's medical and drug history, including over the counter and herbal.
• If additional analgesia is required for dental pain, consider alternative

analgesics (NSAIDs) in patient taking opioids for acute or chronic pain.

Teach Patient/Family to:

• Encourage effective oral hygiene to prevent soft tissue inflammation.

• Use caution to prevent injury when using oral hygiene aids.

homatropine hydrobromide

hoe-**ma**′-troe-peen
high-droh-**broh**′-mide
(Isopto Homatropine, Minims Homatropine[CAN])

CATEGORY AND SCHEDULE

Pregnancy Risk Category: C

Drug Class: Mydriatic (topical)

MECHANISM OF ACTION

An ophthalmic agent that blocks response of iris sphincter muscle and the accommodative muscle of the ciliary body to cholinergic stimulation, resulting in dilation and loss of accommodation.
Therapeutic Effect: Produces cycloplegia and mydriasis for refraction.

USES

Treatment of cycloplegic refraction, uveitis, mydriatic lens opacities

PHARMACOKINETICS

Maximum mydriatic effect occurs within 10–30 min; maximum cycloplegic effect occurs within 30–90 min. Duration of mydriasis is 6 hr–4 days; duration of cycloplegia is 10–48 hr.

INDICATIONS AND DOSAGES

▸ **Mydriasis and Cycloplegia for Refraction**

Ophthalmic

Adults, Elderly. Instill 1–2 drops of 2% solution or 1 drop of 5% solution before the procedure. Repeat at 5- to 10-min intervals as needed. Maximum: 3 doses for refraction.

Children. Instill 1 drop of 2% solution immediately before the procedure. Repeat at 10-min intervals as needed.

▸ **Uveitis**

Ophthalmic

Adults, Elderly. Instill 1–2 drops of 2% or 5% solution 2–3 times a day up to every 3–4 hr as needed.

Children. Instill 1 drop of 2% solution 2–3 times a day.

SIDE EFFECTS/ADVERSE REACTIONS

Frequent

Blurred vision, photophobia

Occasional

Irritation, increased intraocular pressure, congestion

Rare

Eczematoid dermatitis, edema, exudates, follicular conjunctivitis, somnolence, vascular congestion

PRECAUTIONS AND CONTRAINDICATIONS

Narrow-angle glaucoma, acute hemorrhage, hypersensitivity to homatropine or any component of the formulation

Caution:

Children, elderly, hypertension, hyperthyroidism, diabetes

DRUG INTERACTIONS OF CONCERN TO DENTISTRY

• Avoid concurrent use with pilocarpine
• Increased anticholinergic effects with other anticholinergic drugs (when significant absorption from the eye occurs)

SERIOUS REACTIONS

! Overdosage may produce symptoms of blurred vision, urinary retention, and tachycardia.
! Anticholinergic toxicity is caused by strong binding of the drug to cholinergic receptors.

DENTAL CONSIDERATIONS

General:

• Avoid dental light in patient's eyes; offer dark glasses for patient comfort.

hydralazine hydrochloride

high-**dral′**-ah-zeen
high-droh-**klor′**-ide
(Alphapress[AUS], Apresoline, Novo-Hylazin[CAN])
Do not confuse hydralazine with hydroxyzine.

CATEGORY AND SCHEDULE

Pregnancy Risk Category: C

Drug Class: Antihypertensive, direct-acting peripheral vasodilator

MECHANISM OF ACTION

An antihypertensive with direct vasodilating effects on arterioles. ***Therapeutic Effect:*** Decreases B/P and systemic resistance.

USES

Treatment of essential hypertension; parenteral: treatment of severe essential hypertension

PHARMACOKINETICS

Route	Onset	Peak	Duration
PO	20–30 min	N/A	2–4 hr
IV	5–20 min	N/A	2–6 hr

Well absorbed from the GI tract. Widely distributed. Protein binding: 85%–90%. Metabolized in the liver to active metabolite. Primarily excreted in urine. Not removed by hemodialysis. ***Half-life:*** 3–7 hr (increased with impaired renal function).

INDICATIONS AND DOSAGES

▸ **Moderate to Severe Hypertension**

PO

Adults. Initially, 10 mg 4 times a day. May increase by 10–25 mg/dose q2–5 days. Maximum: 300 mg/day.
Children. Initially, 0.75–1 mg/kg/day in 2–4 divided doses, not to exceed 25 mg/dose. May increase over 3–4 wk. Maximum: 7.5 mg/kg/day (5 mg/kg/day in infants).

IV, IM

Adults, Elderly. Initially, 10–20 mg/dose q4–6h. May increase to 40 mg/dose.
Children. Initially, 0.1–0.2 mg/kg/dose (maximum: 20 mg) q4–6h, as needed, up to 1.7–3.5 mg/kg/day in divided doses q4–6h.

▸ **Dosage in Renal Impairment**

Dosage interval is based on creatinine clearance.

Creatinine Clearance	Dosage Interval
10–50 ml/min	q8h
Less than 10 ml/min	q8–24h

SIDE EFFECTS/ADVERSE REACTIONS

Frequent

Headache, palpitations, tachycardia (generally disappears in 7–10 days)

Occasional

GI disturbance (nausea, vomiting, diarrhea), paraesthesia, fluid retention, peripheral edema, dizziness, flushed face, nasal congestion

H

PRECAUTIONS AND CONTRAINDICATIONS

Coronary artery disease, lupus erythematosus, rheumatic heart disease

Caution:

CVA, advanced renal disease

DRUG INTERACTIONS OF CONCERN TO DENTISTRY

• Reduced effects: NSAIDs, indomethacin, sympathomimetics

SERIOUS REACTIONS

! High dosage may produce lupus erythematosus-like reaction, including fever, facial rash, muscle and joint aches and splenomegaly.

! Severe orthostatic hypotension, skin flushing, severe headache, myocardial ischemia, and cardiac arrhythmias may develop.

! Profound shock may occur with severe overdosage.

DENTAL CONSIDERATIONS

General:

• Monitor vital signs at every appointment because of cardiovascular side effects.

• Limit dose or avoid vasoconstrictor.

• Patients on chronic drug therapy may rarely have symptoms of blood dyscrasias, which can include infection, bleeding, and poor healing.

• Limit use of sodium-containing products, such as saline IV fluids, for patients with a dietary salt restriction.

• After supine positioning, have patient sit upright for at least 2 min to avoid orthostatic hypotension.

Consultations:

• In a patient with symptoms of blood dyscrasias, request a medical consultation for blood studies and postpone dental treatment until normal values are reestablished.

• Medical consultation may be required to assess disease control and patient's ability to tolerate stress.

Teach Patient/Family to:

• Encourage effective oral hygiene to prevent soft tissue inflammation.

• Use caution to prevent injury when using oral hygiene aids.

hydrochlorothiazide

high-droe-klor-oh-**thye′**-ah-zide (Apo-Hydro[CAN], Aquazide H, Dichlotride[AUS], Dithiazide[AUS], Esidrix, HydroDIURIL, Microzide, Oretic)

CATEGORY AND SCHEDULE

Pregnancy Risk Category: B (D if used in pregnancy-induced hypertension)

Drug Class: Thiazide diuretic

MECHANISM OF ACTION

A sulfonamide derivative that acts as a thiazide diuretic and antihypertensive. As a diuretic, blocks reabsorption of water, sodium, and potassium at the

cortical diluting segment of the distal tubule. As an antihypertensive reduces plasma, extracellular fluid volume, and peripheral vascular resistance by direct effect on blood vessels.
Therapeutic Effect: Promotes diuresis; reduces B/P.

USES
Treatment of edema, hypertension, diuresis, CHF

PHARMACOKINETICS

Route	Onset	Peak	Duration
PO (diuretic)	2 hr	4–6 hr	6–12 hr

Variably absorbed from the GI tract. Primarily excreted unchanged in urine. Not removed by hemodialysis. ***Half-life:*** 5.6–14.8 hr.

INDICATIONS AND DOSAGES
▸ **Edema, Hypertension**
PO
Adults. 12.5–100 mg/day. Maximum: 200 mg/day.
▸ **Usual Pediatric Dosage**
PO
Children 6 mo–12 yr. 2 mg/kg/day in 2 divided doses. Maximum: 200 mg/day.
Children younger than 6 mo. 2–4 mg/kg/day in 2 divided doses. Maximum: 37.5 mg/day.

SIDE EFFECTS/ADVERSE REACTIONS
Expected
Increase in urinary frequency and urine volume
Frequent
Potassium depletion
Occasional
Orthostatic hypotension, headache, GI disturbances, photosensitivity

PRECAUTIONS AND CONTRAINDICATIONS
Anuria, history of hypersensitivity to sulfonamides or thiazide diuretics, renal decompensation
Caution:
Hypokalemia, renal disease, hepatic disease, gout, COPD, lupus erythematosus, diabetes mellitus

DRUG INTERACTIONS OF CONCERN TO DENTISTRY
• Decreased hypotensive response: NSAIDs

SERIOUS REACTIONS
! Vigorous diuresis may lead to profound water and electrolyte depletion, resulting in hypokalemia, hyponatremia, and dehydration.
! Acute hypotensive episodes may occur.
! Hyperglycemia may occur during prolonged therapy.
! Pancreatitis, blood dyscrasias, pulmonary edema, allergic pneumonitis, and dermatologic reactions occur rarely.
! Overdose can lead to lethargy and coma without changes in electrolytes or hydration.

DENTAL CONSIDERATIONS
General:
• Monitor vital signs at every appointment because of cardiovascular side effects.
• Limit dose or avoid vasoconstrictor.
• Patients on chronic drug therapy may rarely have symptoms of blood dyscrasias, which can include infection, bleeding, and poor healing.
• After supine positioning, have patient sit upright for at least 2 min before standing to avoid orthostatic hypotension.

• Assess salivary flow as a factor in caries, periodontal disease, and candidiasis.
• Limit use of sodium-containing products, such as saline IV fluids, for patients with a dietary salt restriction.
• Stress from dental procedures may compromise cardiovascular function; determine patient risk.
• Short appointments and a stress-reduction protocol may be required for anxious patients.
• Patients taking diuretics should be monitored for serum K levels.

Consultations:

• In a patient with symptoms of blood dyscrasias, request a medical consultation for blood studies and postpone dental treatment until normal values are reestablished.
• Medical consultation may be required to assess disease control and patient's ability to tolerate stress.
• Physician should be informed if significant xerostomic side effects occur (e.g., increased caries, sore tongue, problems eating or swallowing, difficulty wearing prosthesis) so that a medication change can be considered.

Teach Patient/Family to:

• Encourage effective oral hygiene to prevent soft tissue inflammation.
• Use caution to prevent injury when using oral hygiene aids.
• When chronic dry mouth occurs, advise patient to:
  • Avoid mouth rinses with high alcohol content because of drying effects.
  • Use daily home fluoride products for anticaries effect.
  • Use sugarless gum, frequent sips of water, or saliva substitutes.

hydrocodone bitartrate

high-drough-**koe′**-doan bye-**tar′**-trate
(Hycodan[CAN], Robidone[CAN])

CATEGORY AND SCHEDULE

Pregnancy Risk Category: C
Controlled Substance: Schedule III

Drug Class: Opioid analgesic

MECHANISM OF ACTION

An opioid analgesic and antitussive that binds with opioid receptors in the CNS.

Therapeutic Effect: Alters the perception of and emotional response to pain; suppresses cough reflex.

USES

Treatment of hyperactive and nonproductive cough; mild-to-moderate pain; normally used in combination with aspirin or acetaminophen for post-treatment pain control.

PHARMACOKINETICS

Route	Onset	Peak	Duration
PO (analgesic)	10–20 min	30–60 min	4–6 hr
PO (antitussive)	N/A	N/A	4–6 hr

Well absorbed from the GI tract. Metabolized in the liver. Primarily excreted in urine. ***Half-life:*** 3.8 hr (increased in elderly).

INDICATIONS AND DOSAGES

▸ **Analgesia**

PO

Adults, Children older than 12 yr. 5–10 mg q4–6h.

Elderly. 2.5–5 mg q4–6h.

▸ **Cough**

PO

Adults. 5–10 mg q4–6h as needed. Maximum: 15 mg/dose.

Children. 0.6 mg/kg/day in 3–4 divided doses at intervals of at least 4 hr. Maximum single dose: 5 mg (children 2–12 yr), 1.25 mg (children younger than 2 yr).

PO (Extended-Release)

Adults. 10 mg q12h.

Children 6–12 yr. 5 mg q12h.

SIDE EFFECTS/ADVERSE REACTIONS

Frequent

Sedation, hypotension, diaphoresis, facial flushing, dizziness, somnolence

Occasional

Urine retention, blurred vision, constipation, dry mouth, headache, nausea, vomiting, difficult or painful urination, euphoria, dysphoria

PRECAUTIONS AND CONTRAINDICATIONS

Hypersensitivity, addiction (narcotic)

Caution:

Addictive personality, lactation, increased intracranial pressure, MI (acute), severe heart disease, respiratory depression, hepatic disease, renal disease, children younger than 18 yr

DRUG INTERACTIONS OF CONCERN TO DENTISTRY

- Increased CNS depression: alcohol, other opioids, phenothiazines, sedative/hypnotics, skeletal muscle relaxants, general anesthetics
- Contraindication: MAOIs
- Increased effects of anticholinergics

SERIOUS REACTIONS

! Overdose results in respiratory depression, skeletal muscle flaccidity, cold or clammy skin, cyanosis and extreme somnolence progressing to seizures, stupor, and coma.

! The patient who uses hydrocodone repeatedly may develop a tolerance to the drug's analgesic effect, as well as physical dependence.

! The drug may have a prolonged duration of action and cumulative effect in patients with hepatic or renal impairment.

DENTAL CONSIDERATIONS

General:

- Monitor vital signs at every appointment because of cardiovascular and respiratory side effects.
- After supine positioning, have patient sit upright for at least 2 min to avoid orthostatic hypotension.
- Psychologic and physical dependence may occur with chronic administration.
- Determine why the patient is taking the drug.

Teach Patient/Family to:

- Avoid mouth rinses with high alcohol content because of drying effects.

hydrocodone

high-droe-**koe′**-done

Hydrocodone and acetaminophen (Anexsia, Bancap HC, Ceta-Plus, Co-Gesic, Hydrocet, Hydrogesic, Ibudone, Lorcet 10/650, Lorcet-HD Lorcet Plus, Lortab, Margesic H, Maxidone, Norco, Reprexain, Stagesic, Vicodin, Vicodin ES, Vicodin HP, Zydone); hydrocodone and aspirin (Damason-P); hydrocodone and chlorpheniramine (Tussionex); hydrocodone and guaifenesin (Codiclear DH, Hycosin, Hycotuss, Kwelcof, Pneumotussin, Vicodin Tuss, Vitussin); hydrocodone and homatropine (Hycodan and Hydromet, Hydropane, Tussigon); hydrocodone and ibuprofen, (Vicoprofen); hydrocodone and pseudoephedrine (Detussin, Histussin D, P-V Tussin); hydrocodone, chlorpheniramine, phenylephrine, acetaminophen and caffeine (Hycomine Compound)

CATEGORY AND SCHEDULE

Pregnancy Risk Category: C
Controlled substance: Schedule III

Drug Class: Antitussive opioid analgesic, nonopioid analgesic

MECHANISM OF ACTION

Hydrocodone blocks pain perception in the cerebral cortex by binding to specific opiate receptors (μ and κ) at neuronal membranes of synapses. This binding results in a decreased synaptic chemical transmission throughout the CNS, thus inhibiting the flow of pain sensations into the higher centers and causing analgesia.

Therapeutic Effect: Alters perception of pain and produces analgesic effect.

USES

Treatment of hyperactive and nonproductive cough, mild pain

PHARMACOKINETICS

Well absorbed. Metabolized in liver. Excreted in urine. ***Half-life:*** 3.3–3.4 hr.

INDICATIONS AND DOSAGES

Analgesia

▸ **Hydrocodone and Acetaminophen**

PO

Adults, Children older than 13 yr or weighing more than 50 kg. 2.5–10 mg q4–6h. Maximum: 60 mg/day hydrocodone. Maximum dose of acetaminophen: 4 g/day.

Elderly. 2.5–5 mg hydrocodone q4–6h. Titrate dose to appropriate analgesic effect. Maximum: 4 g/day acetaminophen.

Children 2–13 yr or weighing less than 50 kg. 0.135 mg/kg/dose hydrocodone q4–6h. Maximum: 6 doses/day of hydrocodone or maximum recommended dose of acetaminophen.

Hydrocodone and Aspirin

PO

Adults. 2.5–10 mg q4–6h. Maximum: 60 mg/day hydrocodone.

Elderly. 2.5–5 mg hydrocodone q4–6h. Titrate dose to appropriate analgesic effect.

Children 2–13 yr or weighing less than 50 kg. 0.135 mg/kg/dose hydrocodone q4–6h.

Hydrocodone and Chlorpheniramine

Adults, Elderly, Children 12 yr and older. 5 ml q12h. Maximum: 10 ml/24h.

Children 6–12 yr. 2.5 ml q12h. Maximum: 5 ml/24h.

Hydrocodone and Guaifenesin
Adults, Elderly, Children 12 yr and older. 5 ml q4h. Maximum: 30 ml/24h.
Children 2–12 yr. 2.5 ml q4h.
Children younger than 2 yr. 0.3 mg/kg/day (hydrocodone) in 4 divided doses.
Hydrocodone and Homatropine
Adults, Elderly. 10 mg (hydrocodone) q4–6h. A single dose should not exceed 15 mg and should not be administered more frequently than q4h.
Children. 0.6 mg/kg/day (hydrocodone) in 3–4 divided doses. Do not administer more frequently than q4h.
Hydrocodone and Ibuprofen
Adults. 7.5–15 mg (hydrocodone) q4–6h as needed for pain. Maximum: 5 tablets/day.
Hydrocodone and Pseudoephedrine
Adults, Elderly. 5 ml 4 times a day.
Hydrocodone, Chlorpheniramine, Phenylephrine, Acetaminophen, and Caffeine
Adults, Elderly. 1 tablet q4h up to 4 times a day.

SIDE EFFECTS/ADVERSE REACTIONS

Frequent
Dizziness, sedation, drowsiness, bradycardia
Occasional
Anxiety, dysphoria, euphoria, fear, lethargy, light-headedness, malaise, mental clouding, mental impairment, mood changes, physiological dependence, sedation, somnolence, constipation, bradycardia, heartburn, nausea, vomiting
Rare
Hypersensitivity reaction, rash

PRECAUTIONS AND CONTRAINDICATIONS

CNS depression, severe respiratory depression, hypersensitivity to hydrocodone, or any component of the formulation

DRUG INTERACTIONS OF CONCERN TO DENTISTRY

- Increased CNS depression: alcohol, local anesthetics, other opioids, phenothiazines, sedative/hypnotics, skeletal muscle relaxants, general anesthetics
- Contraindication: MAOIs
- Increased effects of anticholinergics

SERIOUS REACTIONS

! Cardiac arrest, circulatory collapse, coma, hypotension, hypoglycemic coma, ureteral spasm, urinary retention, vesical sphincter spasm, agranulocytosis, bleeding time prolonged, hemolytic anemia, iron deficiency anemia, occult blood loss, thrombocytopenia, hepatic necrosis, hepatitis, skeletal muscle rigidity, renal toxicity, renal tubular necrosis have been reported.
! Hearing impairment or loss have been reported with chronic overdose.
! Acute airway obstruction, apnea, dyspnea, and respiratory depression occur rarely and are usually dose related.

DENTAL CONSIDERATIONS

General:
- Monitor vital signs at every appointment because of cardiovascular and respiratory side effects.
- After supine positioning, have patient sit upright for at least 2 min to avoid orthostatic hypotension.
- Psychologic and physical dependence may occur with chronic administration.

• Determine why the patient is taking the drug.
Teach Patient/Family to:
• Avoid mouth rinses with high alcohol content because of drying effects.

hydrocortisone

high-droh-**kor′**-tih-sone
(A-Hydrocort, Anusol-HC, Colifoam[AUS], Cortaid, Cortef cream[AUS], Cortic cream[AUS], Cortic DS[AUS], Cortifoam, Cortizone-5, Cortizone-10, Derm-Aid cream[AUS], Dermaide[AUS], Dermaide soft cream[AUS], Ego Cort cream[AUS], Emcort, HICOR[AUS], HICOR Eye Ointment[AUS], Hysone[AUS], Hytone, Locoid, Nupercainal Hydrocortisone Cream, Preparation H Hydrocortisone, Proctocort, Sequent HICOR[AUS], Solu-Cortef, Squibb HC[AUS], Westcort)

CATEGORY AND SCHEDULE

Pregnancy Risk Category: C
OTC (Hydrocortisone 0.5% and 1% Cream, Gel, and Ointment)

Drug Class: Corticosteroid

MECHANISM OF ACTION

An adrenocortical steroid that inhibits accumulation of inflammatory cells at inflammation sites, phagocytosis, lysosomal enzyme release, and synthesis and release of mediators of inflammation.
Therapeutic Effect: Prevents or suppresses cell-mediated immune reactions. Decreases or prevents tissue response to inflammatory process.

USES

Treatment of psoriasis, eczema, contact dermatitis, pruritus

PHARMACOKINETICS

Route	Onset	Peak	Duration
IV	N/A	4–6 hr	8–12 hr

Well absorbed after IM administration. Widely distributed. Metabolized in the liver. ***Half-life:*** Plasma, 1.5–2 hr; biologic, 8–12 hr.

INDICATIONS AND DOSAGES

▸ **Acute Adrenal Insufficiency**
IV
Adults, Elderly. 100 mg IV bolus; then 300 mg/day in divided doses q8h.
Children. 1–2 mg/kg IV bolus; then 150–250 mg/day in divided doses q6–8h.
Infants. 1–2 mg/kg/dose IV bolus; then 25–150 mg/day in divided doses q6–8h.

▸ **Antiinflammation, Immunosuppression**
IV, IM
Adults, Elderly. 15–240 mg q12h.
Children. 1–5 mg/kg/day in divided doses q12h.

▸ **Physiologic Replacement**
PO
Children. 0.5–0.75 mg/kg/day in divided doses q8h.
IM
Children. 0.25–0.35 mg/kg/day as a single dose.

▸ **Status Asthmaticus**
IV
Adults, Elderly. 100–500 mg q6h.
Children. 2 mg/kg/dose q6h.

▸ **Shock**
IV
Adults, Elderly, Children 12 yr and older. 100–500 mg q6h.
Children younger than 12 yr. 50 mg/kg. May repeat in 4 hr, then q24h as needed.

▸ **Adjunctive Treatment of Ulcerative Colitis**
Rectal
Adults, Elderly. 100 mg at bedtime for 21 nights or until clinical and proctologic remission occurs (may require 2–3 mo of therapy).
Rectal (Cortifoam)
Adults, Elderly. 1 applicator 1–2 times a day for 2–3 wk, then every second day until therapy ends.
Topical
Adults, Elderly. Apply sparingly 2–4 times a day.

SIDE EFFECTS/ADVERSE REACTIONS

Frequent
Insomnia, heartburn, nervousness, abdominal distention, diaphoresis, acne, mood swings, increased appetite, facial flushing, delayed wound healing, increased susceptibility to infection, diarrhea or constipation
Occasional
Headache, edema, change in skin color, frequent urination
Topical: Itching, redness, irritation
Rare
Tachycardia, allergic reaction (such as rash and hives), psychological changes, hallucinations, depression
Topical: Allergic contact dermatitis, purpura
Systemic: Absorption more likely with use of occlusive dressings or extensive application in young children

PRECAUTIONS AND CONTRAINDICATIONS

Fungal, tuberculosis, or viral skin lesions; serious infections
Caution:
Lactation, viral infections, bacterial infections

DRUG INTERACTIONS OF CONCERN TO DENTISTRY

• Inhibitors of CYP hepatic isoenzymes (e.g., azole antifungals, macrolide antibiotics): potential increased blood levels of hydrocortisone and increased hydrocortisone toxicity
• Aspirin, salicylates: potentially increased salicylate GI irritation and toxicity
• Anticoagulants: variable effects on coagulation levels, potentially increased bleeding

SERIOUS REACTIONS

! Long-term therapy may cause hypocalcemia, hypokalemia, muscle wasting (especially in arms and legs), osteoporosis, spontaneous fractures, amenorrhea, cataracts, glaucoma, peptic ulcer disease, and CHF.
! Abruptly withdrawing the drug after long-term therapy may cause anorexia, nausea, fever, headache, sudden severe joint pain, rebound inflammation, fatigue, weakness, lethargy, dizziness, and orthostatic hypotension.

DENTAL CONSIDERATIONS

Topical Form
General:
• Place on frequent recall to evaluate healing response if used on a chronic basis.
• Long-term use may produce adrenocortical suppression; supplementation may be required for some dental procedures.

H

Teach Patient/Family to:
- Encourage effective oral hygiene to prevent soft tissue inflammation.
- Apply at bedtime or after meals for maximum effect.
- Avoid use on oral herpetic ulcerations.
- Apply with cotton-tipped applicator by pressing, not rubbing, paste on lesion.
- Return for oral evaluation if response of oral tissues has not occurred in 7–14 days.

hydroflumethiazide

high-droh-floo-meth-**eye**′-ah-zide (Diucardin, Saluron)

CATEGORY AND SCHEDULE

Pregnancy Risk Category: C, D if used in pregnancy-induced hypertension

Drug Class: Antidiuretic, central and nephrogenic diabetes insipidus; antihypertensive; antiurolithic, calcium calculi; diuretic

MECHANISM OF ACTION

A diuretic that blocks reabsorption of water and the electrolytes sodium and potassium at cortical diluting segment of distal tubule. As an antihypertensive, it reduces plasma and extracellular fluid volume and decreases peripheral vascular resistance (PVR) by direct effect on blood vessels.
Therapeutic Effect: Promotes diuresis, reduces B/P.

USES

Treatment of high B/P (hypertension)

PHARMACOKINETICS

Rapidly but incompletely absorbed from the GI tract. Metabolized to metabolite that is extensively bound to red blood cells and has a longer half-life than parent compound. Primarily excreted in urine. Not removed by hemodialysis. ***Half-life:*** 2–17 hr.

INDICATIONS AND DOSAGES

▸ **Edema**

PO

Adults, Elderly. Initially, 50 mg 2 times a day. Maintenance: 25–200 mg/day.

▸ **Hypertension**

Adults, Elderly, Children. 1 mg/kg/day. Initially, 50 mg 2 times a day. Maintenance: 50–100 mg/day.

SIDE EFFECTS/ADVERSE REACTIONS

Expected
Increase in urine frequency and volume
Frequent
Potassium depletion
Occasional
Postural hypotension, headache, GI disturbances, photosensitivity reaction

PRECAUTIONS AND CONTRAINDICATIONS

Anuria, history of hypersensitivity to sulfonamides or thiazide diuretics, renal decompensation, pregnancy

DRUG INTERACTIONS OF CONCERN TO DENTISTRY

- Decreased hypotensive response: NSAIDs

SERIOUS REACTIONS

! Vigorous diuresis may lead to profound water loss and electrolyte depletion, resulting in hypokalemia, hyponatremia, and dehydration.
! Acute hypotensive episodes may occur.

! Hyperglycemia may be noted during prolonged therapy.
! GI upset, pancreatitis, dizziness, paresthesias, headache, blood dyscrasias, pulmonary edema, allergic pneumonitis, and dermatologic reactions occur rarely.
! Overdosage can lead to lethargy and coma without changes in electrolytes or hydration.

DENTAL CONSIDERATIONS

General:

- Monitor vital signs at every appointment due to cardiovascular side effects.
- Limit dose or avoid vasoconstrictor.
- Patient on chronic drug therapy may rarely present with symptoms of blood dyscrasias, which can include infection, bleeding, and poor healing. If dyscrasia is present, caution patient to prevent oral tissue trauma when using oral hygiene aids.
- After supine positioning, have patient sit upright for at least 2 min before standing to avoid orthostatic hypotension.
- Assess salivary flow as a factor in caries, periodontal disease, and candidiasis.
- Limit use of sodium-containing products, such as saline IV fluids, for patients with a dietary salt restriction.
- Stress from dental procedures may compromise cardiovascular function, determine patient risk.
- Patients taking diuretics should be monitored for serum K levels.

Consultations:

- In a patient with symptoms of blood dyscrasias, request a medical consultation for blood studies and postpone treatment until normal values are reestablished.
- Medical consultation may be required to assess disease control and patient's ability to tolerate stress.
- Physician should be informed if significant xerostomic side effects occur (increased caries, sore tongue, problems eating or swallowing, difficulty wearing prosthesis) so that a medication change can be considered.

Teach Patient/Family to:

- Encourage effective oral hygiene to prevent soft tissue inflammation.
- Prevent trauma when using oral hygiene aids.
- When chronic dry mouth occurs advise patient to:
  - Avoid mouth rinses with high alcohol content due to drying effects.
  - Use daily home fluoride products for anticaries effect.
  - Use sugarless gum, frequent sips of water, or saliva substitutes.
- Update health and medication history if physician makes any changes in evaluation or drug regimens; include OTC, herbal, and nonherbal remedies in the update.

hydromorphone hydrochloride

high-droe-**mor′**-fone
high-droh-**klor′**-ide
(Dilaudid, Dilaudid HP, Hydromorph Contin[CAN], Palladone)
Do not confuse with morphine or Dilantin.

CATEGORY AND SCHEDULE

Pregnancy Risk Category: C
Controlled Substance: Schedule II

Drug Class: Synthetic opioid analgesic

MECHANISM OF ACTION

An opioid agonist that binds to opioid receptors in the CNS, reducing the intensity of pain stimuli from sensory nerve endings. ***Therapeutic Effect:*** Alters the perception of and emotional response to pain; suppresses cough reflex.

USES

Treatment of moderate-to-severe pain

PHARMACOKINETICS

Route	Onset	Peak	Duration
PO	30 min	90–120 min	4 hr
IV	10–15 min	15–30 min	2–3 hr
IM	15 min	30–60 min	4–5 hr
Subcutaneous	15 min	30–90 min	4 hr
Rectal	15–30 min	N/A	N/A

Well absorbed from the GI tract after IM administration. Widely distributed. Metabolized in the liver. Excreted in urine. ***Half-life:*** 1–3 hr.

INDICATIONS AND DOSAGES

▸ Analgesia

PO

Adults, Elderly, Children weighing 50 kg and more. 2–4 mg q3–4h. Range: 2–8 mg/dose.

Children older than 6 mo and weighing less than 50 kg. 0.03–0.08 mg/kg/dose q3–4h.

PO (Extended-Release)

Adults, Elderly. 12–32 mg once a day.

IV

Adults, Elderly, Children weighing more than 50 kg. 0.2–0.6 mg q2–3h.

Children weighing 50 kg or less. 0.015 mg/kg/dose q3–6h as needed.

Rectal

Adults, Elderly. 3 mg q4–8h.

▸ Patient-Controlled Analgesia (PCA)

IV

Adults, Elderly. 0.05–0.5 mg at 5–15 min lockout. Maximum (4 hr): 4–6 mg.

Epidural

Adults, Elderly. Bolus dose of 1–1.5 mg at rate of 0.04–0.4 mg/hr. DEM and dose of 0.15 mg at 30-min lockout.

▸ Cough

PO

Adults, Elderly, Children older than 12 yr. 1 mg q3–4h.

Children 6–12 yr. 0.5 mg q3–4h.

SIDE EFFECTS/ADVERSE REACTIONS

Frequent

Somnolence, dizziness, hypotension (including orthostatic hypotension), decreased appetite

Occasional

Confusion, diaphoresis, facial flushing, urine retention, constipation, dry mouth, nausea, vomiting, headache, pain at injection site

Rare

Allergic reaction, depression

PRECAUTIONS AND CONTRAINDICATIONS

Hypersensitivity, addiction (narcotic), MAOIs

Caution:

Addictive personality, lactation, increased intracranial pressure, MI (acute), severe heart disease, respiratory depression, hepatic disease, renal disease, children younger than 18 yr

DRUG INTERACTIONS OF CONCERN TO DENTISTRY

• Effects may be increased with other CNS depressants: alcohol, narcotics, sedative/hypnotics, skeletal muscle relaxants
• Increased effects of anticholinergic drugs

SERIOUS REACTIONS

! Overdose results in respiratory depression, skeletal muscle flaccidity, cold or clammy skin, cyanosis and extreme somnolence progressing to seizures, stupor, and coma.
! The patient who uses hydromorphone repeatedly may develop a tolerance to the drug's analgesic effect, as well as physical dependence.
! This drug may have a prolonged duration of action and cumulative effect in patients with hepatic or renal impairment.

DENTAL CONSIDERATIONS

General:
• Monitor vital signs at every appointment because of cardiovascular and respiratory side effects.
• After supine positioning, have patient sit upright for at least 2 min to avoid orthostatic hypotension.
• Assess salivary flow as a factor in caries, periodontal disease, and candidiasis.
• Psychologic and physical dependence may occur with chronic administration.
• Determine why the patient is taking the drug.
• Avoid use in patients with chronic obstructive pulmonary disease.

Teach Patient/Family to:
• Avoid mouth rinses with high alcohol content because of drying effects.

hydroxychloroquine sulfate

high-drox-ee-**klor′**-oh-kwin **sull′**-fate
(Apo-Hydroxyquine[CAN], Plaquenil)
Do not confuse hydroxychloroquine with hydrocortisone or hydroxyzine.

CATEGORY AND SCHEDULE

Pregnancy Risk Category: C

Drug Class: Antimalarial

MECHANISM OF ACTION

An antimalarial and antirheumatic that concentrates in parasite acid vesicles, increasing the pH of the vesicles and interfering with parasite protein synthesis. Antirheumatic action may involve suppressing formation of antigens responsible for hypersensitivity reactions.
Therapeutic Effect: Inhibits parasite growth.

USES

Treatment of malaria caused by *P. vivax, P. malariae, P. ovale, P. falciparum* (some strains); lupus erythematosus; rheumatoid arthritis

PHARMACOKINETICS

PO: Peak 1–2 hr. ***Half-life:*** 3–5 days; metabolized in liver; excreted in urine, feces, breast milk; crosses placenta.

INDICATIONS AND DOSAGES

▸ Treatment of Acute Attack of Malaria (Dosage in mg Base)

PO

Dose	Times	Adult	Children
Initial	Day 1	620 mg	10 mg/kg
Second	6 hr later	310 mg	5 mg/kg
Third	Day 2	310 mg	5 mg/kg
Fourth	Day 3	310 mg	5 mg/kg

H

▸ Suppression of Malaria

PO

Adults. 310 mg base weekly on same day each wk, beginning 2 wk before entering an endemic area and continuing for 4–6 wk after leaving the area.

Children. 5 mg base/kg/wk, beginning 2 wk before entering an endemic area and continuing for 4–6 wk after leaving the area. If therapy is not begun before exposure, administer a loading dose of 10 mg base/kg in 2 equally divided doses 6 hr apart, followed by the usual dosage regimen.

▸ Rheumatoid Arthritis

PO

Adults. Initially, 400–600 mg (310–465 mg base) daily for 5–10 days, gradually increased to optimum response level. Maintenance (usually within 4–12 wk): Dosage decreased by 50% and then continued at maintenance dose of 200–400 mg/day. Maximum effect may not be seen for several months.

▸ Lupus Erythematosus

PO

Adults. Initially, 400 mg once or twice a day for several wk or mo. Maintenance: 200–400 mg/day.

SIDE EFFECTS/ADVERSE REACTIONS

Frequent

Mild, transient headache; anorexia; nausea; vomiting

Occasional

Visual disturbances, nervousness, fatigue, pruritus (especially of palms, soles, and scalp), irritability, personality changes, diarrhea

Rare

Stomatitis, dermatitis, impaired hearing

PRECAUTIONS AND CONTRAINDICATIONS

Long-term therapy for children, porphyria, psoriasis, retinal or visual field changes

Caution:

Blood dyscrasias, severe GI disease, neurologic disease, alcoholism, hepatic disease, G6PD deficiency, psoriasis, eczema

DRUG INTERACTIONS OF CONCERN TO DENTISTRY

• None reported

SERIOUS REACTIONS

! Ocular toxicity, especially retinopathy, may occur and may progress even after drug is discontinued.

! Prolonged therapy may result in peripheral neuritis, neuromyopathy, hypotension, ECG changes, agranulocytosis, aplastic anemia, thrombocytopenia, seizures, and psychosis.

! Overdosage may result in headache, vomiting, visual disturbances, drowsiness, seizures, and hypokalemia followed by cardiovascular collapse and death.

DENTAL CONSIDERATIONS

General:

- Patients on chronic drug therapy may rarely have symptoms of blood dyscrasias, which can include infection, bleeding, and poor healing.
- Avoid dental light in patient's eyes; offer dark glasses for patient comfort.
- Determine why the patient is taking the drug.

Consultations:

- In a patient with symptoms of blood dyscrasias, request a medical consultation for blood studies and postpone dental treatment until normal values are reestablished.

Teach Patient/Family to:

- Encourage effective oral hygiene to prevent soft tissue inflammation.
- Avoid mouth rinses with high alcohol content because of drying effects.

hydroxyurea

high-**drocks**′-ee-your-**ee**′-ah
(Droxia, Hydrea, Mylocel)

CATEGORY AND SCHEDULE

Pregnancy Risk Category: D

Drug Class: Antineoplastic

MECHANISM OF ACTION

A synthetic urea analog that inhibits DNA synthesis without interfering with RNA synthesis or protein.
Therapeutic Effect: Interferes with the normal repair process of cancer cells damaged by irradiation.

USES

Treatment of melanoma, chronic myelocytic leukemia (CML), recurrent or metastatic ovarian cancer, in combination with irradiation therapy for carcinomas of the head and neck (except the lip); sickle cell anemia

PHARMACOKINETICS

PO: Readily absorbed with PO use, peak level in 2 hr; 80% excreted in urine.

INDICATIONS AND DOSAGES

▸ **Melanoma; Recurrent, Metastatic, or Inoperable Ovarian Carcinoma**

PO

Adults, Elderly. 80 mg/kg every 3 days or 20–30 mg/kg/day as a single dose.

▸ **Control of Primary Squamous Cell Carcinoma of the Head and Neck, Excluding Lips (in Combination with Radiation Therapy)**

PO

Adults, Elderly. 80 mg/kg every 3 days, beginning at least 7 days before starting radiation therapy.

▸ **Resistant CML**

PO

Adults, Elderly. 20–30 mg/kg once a day.
Children. 10–20 mg/kg once a day.

▸ **HIV Infection**

PO

Adults, Elderly. 500 mg twice a day with didanosine.

▸ **Sickle Cell Anemia**

PO

Adults, Elderly, Children. Initially, 15 mg/kg once a day. May increase by 5 mg/kg/day. Maximum: 35 mg/kg/day.

SIDE EFFECTS/ADVERSE REACTIONS

Frequent

Nausea, vomiting, anorexia, constipation, or diarrhea

H

Occasional
Mild, reversible rash; facial flushing; pruritus; fever; chills; malaise
Rare
Alopecia, headache, drowsiness, dizziness, disorientation

PRECAUTIONS AND CONTRAINDICATIONS

WBC count less than 2500/mm^3 or platelet count less than 100,000/mm^3
Caution:
Monitor blood counts and hemoglobin, renal impairment, elderly

H

DRUG INTERACTIONS OF CONCERN TO DENTISTRY

- None reported

SERIOUS REACTIONS

! Myelosuppression may cause hematologic toxicity (manifested as leukopenia and, to a lesser extent, thrombocytopenia and anemia).

DENTAL CONSIDERATIONS

General:
- Patients receiving chemotherapy may be taking chronic opioids for pain. Consider NSAIDs for dental pain management.
- Patients receiving chemotherapy may require palliative therapy for stomatitis.
- Patients on chronic drug therapy may rarely have symptoms of blood dyscrasias, which can include infection, bleeding, and poor healing.

Consultations:
- Medical consultation may be required to assess disease control.
- In a patient with symptoms of blood dyscrasias, request a medical consultation for blood studies and postpone dental treatment until normal values are reestablished.

Teach Patient/Family to:
- See dentist immediately if secondary oral infection occurs.
- When chronic dry mouth occurs, advise patient to:
  - Avoid mouth rinses with high alcohol content because of drying effects.
  - Use sugarless gum, frequent sips of water, or saliva substitutes.
  - Use daily home fluoride products for anticaries effect.

hydroxyzine

high-**drox**′-ih-zeen
(Apo-Hydroxyzine[CAN], Atarax, Novo-Hydroxyzin[CAN], Vistaril)
Do not confuse hydroxyzine with hydralazine or hydroxyurea.

CATEGORY AND SCHEDULE

Pregnancy Risk Category: C

Drug Class: Antianxiety, antihistamine

MECHANISM OF ACTION

A piperazine derivative that competes with histamine for H_1 receptor sites in the GI tract, blood vessels, and respiratory tract. May exert CNS depressant activity in subcortical areas. Diminishes vestibular stimulation and depresses labyrinthine function.
Therapeutic Effect: Produces anxiolytic, anticholinergic, antihistaminic, and analgesic effects; relaxes skeletal muscle; controls nausea and vomiting.

USES

Treatment of anxiety, preoperatively or postoperatively to prevent nausea and vomiting, to potentiate narcotic analgesics, sedation, pruritus

PHARMACOKINETICS

Route	Onset	Peak	Duration
PO	15–30 min	N/A	4–6 hr

Well absorbed from the GI tract and after parenteral administration. Metabolized in the liver. Primarily excreted in urine. Not removed by hemodialysis. ***Half-life:*** 20–25 hr (increased in the elderly).

INDICATIONS AND DOSAGES

▸ **Anxiety**

PO

Adults, Elderly. 25–100 mg 4 times a day. Maximum: 600 mg/day.

▸ **Nausea and Vomiting**

IM

Adults, Elderly. 25–100 mg/dose q4–6h.

▸ **Pruritus**

PO

Adults, Elderly. 25 mg 3–4 times a day.

▸ **Preoperative Sedation**

PO

Adults, Elderly. 50–100 mg.

IM

Adults, Elderly. 25–100 mg.

▸ **Usual Pediatric Dosage**

PO

Children. 2 mg/kg/day in divided doses q6–8h.

IM

Children. 0.5–1 mg/kg/dose q4–6h.

SIDE EFFECTS/ADVERSE REACTIONS

Side effects are generally mild and transient.

Frequent

Somnolence, dry mouth, marked discomfort with IM injection

Occasional

Dizziness, ataxia, asthenia, slurred speech, headache, agitation, increased anxiety

Rare

Paradoxical CNS reactions, such as hyperactivity or nervousness in children and excitement or restlessness in elderly or debilitated patients (generally noted during first 2 wk of therapy, particularly in presence of uncontrolled pain)

PRECAUTIONS AND CONTRAINDICATIONS

Hypersensitivity, avoid in pregnancy

Caution:

Elderly, debilitated, hepatic disease, renal disease

DRUG INTERACTIONS OF CONCERN TO DENTISTRY

- Increased CNS depressant effect: alcohol, all CNS depressants
- Increased anticholinergic effects: other antihistamines, anticholinergics, opioid analgesics

SERIOUS REACTIONS

! A hypersensitivity reaction, including wheezing, dyspnea, and chest tightness, may occur.

DENTAL CONSIDERATIONS

General:

- Potentiates other CNS depressant drugs. When used in combination, the dose of other CNS depressants should be reduced by half.
- Assess salivary flow as a factor in caries, periodontal disease, and candidiasis.
- Geriatric patients are more susceptible to drug effects; use lower dose.
- Have someone drive patient to and from dental appointment if the drug is prescribed for sedation during dental therapy.

Teach Patient/Family:
- When chronic dry mouth occurs, advise patient to:
  - Avoid mouth rinses with high alcohol content because of drying effects.
  - Use sugarless gum, frequent sips of water, or saliva substitutes.
  - Use daily home fluoride products for anticaries effect.

hyoscyamine

high-oh-**sye**′-ah-meen
(Anaspaz, Buscopan[CAN], Cystospaz, Cystospaz-M, Hyoscine, Levbid, Levsin, Levsin S/L, Levsinex, NuLev, Spacol, Spacol T/S, Symax SL, Symax SR)
Do not confuse Anaspaz with Anaprox.

CATEGORY AND SCHEDULE

Pregnancy Risk Category: C

Drug Class: Anticholinergic

MECHANISM OF ACTION

A GI antispasmodic and anticholinergic agent that inhibits the action of acetylcholine at post-ganglionic (muscarinic) receptor sites.
Therapeutic Effect: Decreases secretions (bronchial, salivary, sweat gland) and gastric juices and reduces motility of GI and urinary tract.

USES

Treatment of peptic ulcer disease in combination with other drugs, other GI disorders, other spastic disorders such as parkinsonism, preoperatively to reduce secretions, GU disorders (cystitis, renal colic), partial heart block

PHARMACOKINETICS

PO: Duration 4–6 hr; metabolized by liver, excreted in urine. ***Half-life:*** 3.5 hr.

INDICATIONS AND DOSAGES

▸ **GI Tract Disorders**
PO
Adults, Elderly, Children 12 yr and older. 0.125–0.25 mg q4h as needed. Extended-release: 0.375–0.75 mg q12h. Maximum: 1.5 mg/day.
Children 2–11 yr. 0.0625–0.125 mg q4h as needed. Extended-release: 0.375 mg q12h. Maximum: 0.75 mg/day.
IV, IM
Adults, Elderly, Children 12 yr and older. 0.25–0.5 mg q4h for 1–4 doses.
▸ **Hypermotility of Lower Urinary Tract**
PO, Sublingual
Adults, Elderly. 0.15–0.3 mg 4 times a day; or extended-release 0.375 mg q12h.
▸ **Infant Colic**
PO
Infants. Individualized drops dosed q4h as needed.

SIDE EFFECTS/ADVERSE REACTIONS

Frequent
Dry mouth (sometimes severe), decreased sweating, constipation
Occasional
Blurred vision, bloated feeling, urinary hesitancy, somnolence (with high dosage), headache, intolerance to light, loss of taste, nervousness, flushing, insomnia, impotence, mental confusion or excitement (particularly in the elderly and children), temporary

light-headedness (with parenteral form), local irritation (with parenteral form)
Rare
Dizziness, faintness

PRECAUTIONS AND CONTRAINDICATIONS

GI or GU obstruction, myasthenia gravis, narrow-angle glaucoma, paralytic ileus, severe ulcerative colitis
Caution:
Hyperthyroidism, CAD, dysrhythmias, CHF, ulcerative colitis, hypertension, hiatal hernia, hepatic disease, renal disease, urinary retention

DRUG INTERACTIONS OF CONCERN TO DENTISTRY

- Increased anticholinergic effect: other anticholinergics, opioid analgesics
- Decreased effect of phenothiazines

SERIOUS REACTIONS

! Overdose may produce temporary paralysis of ciliary muscle; pupillary dilation; tachycardia; palpitations; hot, dry, or flushed skin; absence of bowel sounds; hyperthermia; increased respiratory rate; ECG abnormalities; nausea; vomiting; rash over face or upper trunk; CNS stimulation; and psychosis (marked by agitation, restlessness, rambling speech, visual hallucinations, paranoid behavior, and delusions, followed by depression).

DENTAL CONSIDERATIONS

General:
- After supine positioning, have patient sit upright for at least 2 min to avoid orthostatic hypotension.
- Assess salivary flow as a factor in caries, periodontal disease, and candidiasis.
- Avoid dental light in patient's eyes; offer dark glasses for patient comfort.

Consultation:
- Physician should be informed if significant xerostomic side effects occur (e.g., increased caries, sore tongue, problems eating or swallowing, difficulty wearing prosthesis) so that a medication change can be considered.

Teach Patient/Family to:
- Encourage effective oral hygiene to prevent soft tissue inflammation.
- When chronic dry mouth occurs, advise patient to:
  - Avoid mouth rinses with high alcohol content because of drying effects.
  - Use sugarless gum, frequent sips of water, or artificial saliva substitutes.
  - Use daily home fluoride products for anticaries effect.

H

ibandronate sodium

eye-**band'**-droh-nate **soe'**-dee-um
(Boniva)

CATEGORY AND SCHEDULE

Pregnancy Risk Category: C

Drug Class: Bisphosphonate; calcium regulator

I

MECHANISM OF ACTION

A bisphosphonate that binds to bone hydroxyapatite (part of the mineral matrix of bone) and inhibits osteoclast activity.
Therapeutic Effect: Reduces rate of bone turnover and bone resorption, resulting in a net gain in bone mass.

USES

Treatment and prevention of osteoporosis in postmenopausal women

PHARMACOKINETICS

Absorbed in the upper GI tract. Extent of absorption impaired by food or beverages (other than plain water). Rapidly binds to bone. Unabsorbed portion is eliminated in urine. Protein binding: 90%.
Half-life: 10–60 hr.

INDICATIONS AND DOSAGES

▸ **Osteoporosis**

PO

Adults, Elderly. 2.5 mg daily.

SIDE EFFECTS/ADVERSE REACTIONS

Frequent

Back pain; dyspepsia, including epigastric distress and heartburn; peripheral discomfort; diarrhea; headache; myalgia

Occasional

Dizziness, arthralgia, asthenia

Rare

Vomiting, hypersensitivity reaction, osteonecrosis of the jaw

PRECAUTIONS AND CONTRAINDICATIONS

Hypersensitivity to other bisphosphonates, including alendronate, etidronate, pamidronate, risedronate, and tiludronate; inability to stand or sit upright for at least 60 min; severe renal impairment with creatinine clearance less than 30 ml/min; uncorrected hypocalcemia

DRUG INTERACTIONS OF CONCERN TO DENTISTRY

- Decreased absorption: antacids containing aluminum, calcium, or magnesium salts, vitamin D
- Use with monitoring, risk of increased GI side effects: aspirin and NSAIDs

SERIOUS REACTIONS

! Upper respiratory tract infection occurs occasionally.
! Overdose causes hypocalcemia, hypophosphatemia, and significant GI disturbances.

DENTAL CONSIDERATIONS

General:

- Bisphosphonates may increase the risk for osteonecrosis of the jaw (see section on "Medically Compromised Patients" for management considerations).
- Consider semisupine chair position for patient comfort if GI side effects occur.
- Patient may need assistance in getting into and out of dental chair. Adjust chair position for patient comfort.
- Emphasize importance of caries prevention.

Consultations:
- Medical consultation may be required to assess disease control and patient's ability to tolerate stress.

Teach Patient/Family to:
- Observe regular recall schedule and practice effective oral hygiene to minimize risk of osteonecrosis of the jaw.
- Update health and medication history if physician makes any changes in evaluation or drug regimens; include OTC, herbal, and nonherbal remedies in the update.

ibuprofen

eye-byoo-**pro′**-fen
(Act-3[AUS], Advil, Apo-Ibuprofen, Brufen[AUS], Codral Period Pain[AUS], Ibudone, Motrin, Novoprofen[CAN], Nurofen[AUS], Rafen[AUS], Reprexain)

CATEGORY AND SCHEDULE

Pregnancy Risk Category: B (D if used in third trimester or near delivery)
OTC (Tablets: 200 mg, Oral Suspension: 100 mg/5 ml)

Drug Class: Nonsteroidal antiinflammatory

MECHANISM OF ACTION

An NSAID that inhibits prostaglandin synthesis. Also produces vasodilation by acting centrally on the heat-regulating center of the hypothalamus. ***Therapeutic Effect:*** Produces analgesic and antiinflammatory effects and decreases fever.

USES

Treatment of rheumatoid arthritis, osteoarthritis, primary dysmenorrhea, gout, mild to moderate pain, fever

PHARMACOKINETICS

Route	Onset	Peak	Duration
PO (analgesic)	0.5 hr	N/A	4–6 hr
PO (antirheumatic)	2 days	1–2 wk	N/A

Rapidly absorbed from the GI tract. Protein binding: greater than 90%. Metabolized in the liver. Primarily excreted in urine. Not removed by hemodialysis. ***Half-life:*** 2–4 hr.

INDICATIONS AND DOSAGES

▸ **Acute or Chronic Rheumatoid Arthritis, Osteoarthritis, Migraine Pain, Gouty Arthritis**
PO
Adults, Elderly. 400–800 mg 3–4 times a day. Maximum: 3.2 g/day.

▸ **Mild-to-Moderate Pain, Primary Dysmenorrhea**
PO
Adults, Elderly. 200–400 mg q4–6h as needed. Maximum: 1.6 g/day.

▸ **Fever, Minor Aches, or Pain**
PO
Adults, Elderly. 200–400 mg q4–6h. Maximum: 1.6 g/day.
Children. 5–10 mg/kg/dose q6–8h. Maximum: 40 mg/kg/day. OTC: 7.5 mg/kg/dose q6–8h. Maximum: 30 mg/kg/day.

▸ **Juvenile Arthritis**
PO
Children. 30–70 mg/kg/day in 3–4 divided doses. Maximum: 400 mg/day in children weighing less than 20 kg, 600 mg/day in children weighing 20–30 kg, 800 mg/day in

children weighing greater than 30–40 kg.

SIDE EFFECTS/ADVERSE REACTIONS

Occasional

Nausea with or without vomiting, dyspepsia, dizziness, rash

Rare

Diarrhea or constipation, flatulence, abdominal cramps or pain, pruritus

PRECAUTIONS AND CONTRAINDICATIONS

Active peptic ulcer, chronic inflammation of GI tract, GI bleeding disorders or ulceration, history of hypersensitivity to aspirin or NSAIDs

Possible increased risk for adverse cardiovascular events in patients at risk for thromboembolism

Caution:

Lactation, children, bleeding disorders, GI disorders, cardiac disorders, hypersensitivity to other antiinflammatory agents

DRUG INTERACTIONS OF CONCERN TO DENTISTRY

- GI ulceration, bleeding: aspirin, alcohol (three or more drinks per day), corticosteroids
- Decreased action: salicylates
- Nephrotoxicity: acetaminophen (prolonged use), methotrexate
- Possible risk of decreased renal function: cyclosporine
- SSRIs: NSAIDs increase risk of GI side effects
- When prescribed for dental pain:
  - Risk of increased effects: oral anticoagulants, oral antidiabetics, lithium, methotrexate
  - Decreased antihypertensive effects of diuretics, β-adrenergic blockers, and ACE inhibitors

SERIOUS REACTIONS

! Acute overdose may result in metabolic acidosis.

! Rare reactions with long-term use include peptic ulcer disease, GI bleeding, gastritis, a severe hepatic reaction (cholestasis, jaundice), nephrotoxicity (dysuria, hematuria, proteinuria, nephrotic syndrome), and a severe hypersensitivity reaction (particularly in patients with systemic lupus erythematosus or other collagen diseases).

DENTAL CONSIDERATIONS

General:

- Patients on chronic drug therapy may rarely have symptoms of blood dyscrasias, which can include infection, bleeding, and poor healing.
- Assess salivary flow as a factor in caries, periodontal disease, and candidiasis.
- Avoid prescribing aspirin-containing products.
- Consider semisupine chair position for patients with arthritic disease.
- Severe stomach bleeding may occur in patients who regularly use NSAIDs in recommended doses, when the patient is also taking another NSAID, anticoagulant/antiplatelet drug, or steroid drug, if the patient has GI or peptic ulcer disease, if they are 60 years or older, or when NSAIDs are taken longer than directed. Warn patients of the potential for severe stomach bleeding.

Consultations:

- In a patient with symptoms of blood dyscrasias, request a medical consultation for blood studies and postpone dental treatment until normal values are reestablished.
- Medical consultation may be required to assess disease control.

• Increased risk of adverse effects in patients with a history of thromboembolism, stroke, MI.

Teach Patient/Family to:

• Follow labeled directions for OTC products.
• Encourage effective oral hygiene to prevent soft tissue inflammation.
• Use caution to prevent injury when using oral hygiene aids.
• Warn patient of potential risks of NSAIDs.
• When chronic dry mouth occurs, advise patient to:
  • Avoid mouth rinses with high alcohol content because of drying effects.
  • Use sugarless gum, frequent sips of water, or saliva substitutes.
  • Use daily home fluoride products for anticaries effect.

ibuprofen + famotidine

eye-byoo-**proe**′-fen & fa-**moe**′-ti-deen
(Duexis)

CATEGORY AND SCHEDULE

Pregnancy Risk Category: C

Drug Class: Nonsteroidal antiinflammatory drug (NSAID), histamine H_2 antagonist

MECHANISM OF ACTION

Ibuprofen: An NSAID that inhibits prostaglandin synthesis. Also produces vasodilation by acting centrally on the heat-regulating center of the hypothalamus. Famotidine: An antiulcer agent and gastric acid secretion inhibitor that inhibits histamine action at H_2 receptors of parietal cells.
Therapeutic Effect: Treatment of symptoms of rheumatoid arthritis and osteoarthritis while minimizing risk of ulcerogenic effects.

USES

Reduction of the risk of NSAID-associated gastric ulcers in patients who require an NSAID for the treatment of rheumatoid arthritis or osteoarthritis

PHARMACOKINETICS

Ibuprofen: Rapidly absorbed from the GI tract. Protein binding: greater than 90%. Metabolized in the liver. Primarily excreted in urine.
Famotidine: Rapidly, incompletely absorbed from the GI tract. 15%–20% plasma protein bound. Partially metabolized in the liver. Primarily excreted in urine.
Half-life: Ibuprofen: 2–4 hr. Famotidine: 2.5–3.5 hr.

INDICATIONS AND DOSAGES

▸ NSAID-Associated Ulcer Prophylaxis During Treatment for Osteoarthritis/Rheumatoid Arthritis

PO

Adults. 1 tablet (800 mg ibuprofen/26.6 mg famotidine) 3 times daily.
Not recommended for use in patients with renal impairment.

SIDE EFFECTS/ADVERSE REACTIONS

Frequent

Nausea, diarrhea, upper respiratory tract infection, dyspepsia

Occasional

Hypertension, peripheral edema, headache, urinary tract infection, anemia, back pain, arthralgia, nasopharyngitis

PRECAUTIONS AND CONTRAINDICATIONS

Avoid use in patients with hypersensitivity to H_2-receptor antagonists; history of asthma, urticaria, or allergic-type reaction to aspirin or other NSAIDs; perioperative pain in the setting of coronary artery bypass graft (CABG) surgery; late stages of pregnancy (>30 wk). Use with caution in patients with hepatic impairment, hypertension, and renal impairment. May increase the risk of hyperkalemia. May cause serious adverse skin events including exfoliative dermatitis, Stevens-Johnson syndrome, and toxic epidermal necrolysis. Use is contraindicated for treatment of perioperative pain in the setting of CABG surgery. Risk of MI and stroke may be increased with use following CABG surgery.

DRUG INTERACTIONS OF CONCERN TO DENTISTRY

- NSAIDs, aspirin: increased toxicity of Duexis
- Reduced absorption of azole antifungal drugs (e.g., ketoconazole)
- Reduced antiplatelet effect of aspirin
- Aminoglycoside antibiotics: increased risk of renal failure
- Corticosteroids: increased risk of gastrointestinal ulceration and bleeding
- Reduced effectiveness of antihypertensive medications (e.g., thiazide diuretics)

SERIOUS REACTIONS

! NSAIDs are associated with an increased risk of adverse cardiovascular thrombotic events, including fatal MI and stroke. NSAIDs may increase risk of gastrointestinal irritation, inflammation, ulceration, bleeding, and perforation. These events can be fatal and may occur at any time during therapy and without warning.

DENTAL CONSIDERATIONS

General:

- Duexis is not indicated for short-term management of acute dental pain.
- Consider use of non-NSAID pain relievers (e.g., acetaminophen, opioids).
- Patients taking Duexis are at increased risk of intraoperative and postoperative bleeding.
- Administration of other NSAIDs to patients taking Duexis can result in serious NSAID toxicity, including gastrointestinal ulceration and hemorrhage, thromboembolism.
- Monitor vital signs at every appointment due to adverse cardiovascular effects.
- Increased risk of adverse effects in patients with a history of thromboembolism, stroke, MI.

Consultations:

- Consult physician to report signs and symptoms of adverse cardiovascular and gastrointestinal effects.

Teach Patient/Family to:

- Report changes in disease status and drug regimen.

ibutilide fumarate

eye-**byoo′**-ti-lide **fyoo′**-muh-reyt
(Corvert)

CATEGORY AND SCHEDULE

Pregnancy Risk Category: C

Drug Class: Antidysrhythmic

MECHANISM OF ACTION

An antiarrhythmic that prolongs both atrial and ventricular action potential duration and increases the atrial and ventricular refractory period. Activates slow, inward

current (mostly of sodium), produces mild slowing of sinus node rate and AV conduction, and causes dose-related prolongation of QT interval.
Therapeutic Effect: Converts arrhythmias to sinus rhythm.

USES

For rapid conversion of atrial fibrillation/flutter occurring within 1 wk of coronary artery bypass or valve surgery

PHARMACOKINETICS

After IV administration, highly distributed, rapidly cleared. Protein binding: 40%. Primarily excreted in urine as metabolite. ***Half-life:*** 2–12 hr (average: 6 hr).

INDICATIONS AND DOSAGES

▸ Rapid Conversion of Atrial Fibrillation or Flutter of Recent Onset to Normal Sinus Rhythm

IV Infusion

Adults, Elderly weighing 60 kg and more. One vial (1 mg) given over 10 min. If arrhythmia does not stop within 10 min after end of initial infusion, a second 1 mg/10-min infusion may be given.

Adults, Elderly weighing less than 60 kg. 0.01 mg/kg given over 10 min. If arrhythmia does not stop within 10 min after end of initial infusion, a second 0.01 mg/kg, 10-min infusion may be given.

SIDE EFFECTS/ADVERSE REACTIONS

Ibutilide is generally well tolerated.

Occasional

Ventricular extrasystoles (5.1%), ventricular tachycardia (4.9%), headache (3.6%), hypotension, orthostatic hypotension (2%)

Rare

Bundle-branch block, AV block, bradycardia, hypertension

PRECAUTIONS AND CONTRAINDICATIONS

None known

DRUG INTERACTIONS OF CONCERN TO DENTISTRY

- Potential for arrhythmia: drugs that prolong the QT interval, such as antidepressants

SERIOUS REACTIONS

! Sustained polymorphic ventricular tachycardia, occasionally with QT prolongation (torsades de pointes) occurs rarely.
! Overdose results in CNS toxicity, including CNS depression, rapid and gasping breathing, and seizures.
! Expect prolongation of repolarization may be exaggerated.
! Existing arrhythmias may worsen or new arrhythmias may develop.

DENTAL CONSIDERATIONS

General:

- Acute-use drug for use in hospitals, emergency rooms, or cardiac labs.
- Patients who have received this drug for arrhythmias may be at risk when it is combined with other drugs that prolong the QT interval.

Consultations:

- Medical consultation may be required to assess disease control and patient's ability to tolerate stress.

Teach Patient/Family to:

- Update health and medication history if physician makes any changes in evaluation or drug regimens; include OTC, herbal, and nonherbal remedies in the update.

idarubicin hydrochloride

eye-dah-**roo′**-bi-sin high-droh-**klor′**-ide
(Idamycin PFS, Zavedos)
Do not confuse idarubicin with doxorubicin, or Idamycin with Adriamycin.

CATEGORY AND SCHEDULE

Pregnancy Risk Category: D

Drug Class: Anthracycline antibiotic; antineoplastic

MECHANISM OF ACTION

An anthracycline antibiotic that inhibits nucleic acid synthesis by interacting with the enzyme topoisomerase II, which promotes DNA strand supercoiling.
Therapeutic Effect: Causes death of rapidly dividing cells.

USES

Treatment of acute myeloid leukemia (AML)

PHARMACOKINETICS

Widely distributed. Protein binding: 97%. Rapidly metabolized in the liver to active metabolite. Primarily eliminated by biliary excretion. Not removed by hemodialysis. ***Half-life:*** 4–46 hr; metabolite: 8–92 hr.

INDICATIONS AND DOSAGES

▸ AML

IV

Adults. 8–12 mg/m^2/day for 3 days in combination with Ara-C.
Children (solid tumor). 5 mg/m^2 once a day for 3 days.
Children (leukemia). 10–12 mg/m^2 once a day for 3 days.

▸ Dosage in Hepatic or Renal Impairment

Dosage is modified on the basis of serum creatinine or bilirubin level.

Serum Level	Dose Reduction
Serum creatinine 2 mg/dl or more	25%
Serum bilirubin greater than 2.5 mg/dl	50%
Serum bilirubin greater than 5 mg/dl	Do not give

SIDE EFFECTS/ADVERSE REACTIONS

Frequent

Nausea, vomiting, complete alopecia (scalp, axillary, pubic hair), abdominal cramping, diarrhea, mucositis

Occasional

Hyperpigmentation of nail beds, phalangeal and dermal creases, fever, headache

Rare

Conjunctivitis, neuropathy

PRECAUTIONS AND CONTRAINDICATIONS

Preexisting arrhythmias, cardiomyopathy, myelosuppression, pregnancy, severe CHF

DRUG INTERACTIONS OF CONCERN TO DENTISTRY

• Dental drug interactions have not been studied.

SERIOUS REACTIONS

! Myelosuppression may cause hematologic toxicity (manifested principally as leukopenia and, to a lesser extent, anemia and thrombocytopenia), usually within 10–15 days of starting therapy.
! Blood counts typically return to normal levels by the third week.

! Cardiotoxicity (either acute, manifested as transient ECG abnormalities, or chronic, manifested as CHF) may occur.

DENTAL CONSIDERATIONS

General:

• If additional analgesia is required for dental pain, consider alternative analgesics (acetaminophen) in patients taking opioids for acute or chronic pain.
• Examine for oral manifestation of opportunistic infection.
• This drug may be used in the hospital or on an outpatient basis. Confirm the patient's disease and treatment status.
• Chlorhexidine mouth rinse prior to and during chemotherapy may reduce severity of mucositis.
• Patient on chronic drug therapy may rarely present with symptoms of blood dyscrasias, which can include infection, bleeding, and poor healing. If dyscrasia is present, caution patient to prevent oral tissue trauma when using oral hygiene aids.
• Palliative medication may be required for management of oral side effects.

Consultations:

• Consult physician; prophylactic or therapeutic antiinfectives may be indicated if surgery or periodontal treatment is required.
• Medical consultation may be required to assess immunologic status during cancer chemotherapy and determine safety risk, if any, posed by the required dental treatment.
• Medical consultation may be required to assess disease control and patient's ability to tolerate stress.

Teach Patient/Family to:

• Be aware of oral side effects.
• Encourage effective oral hygiene to prevent soft tissue inflammation.
• Report oral lesions, soreness, or bleeding to dentist.
• Prevent trauma when using oral hygiene aids.
• Update health and medication history if physician makes any changes in evaluation or drug regimens; include OTC, herbal, and nonherbal remedies in the update.

idursulfase

eye-dur-**sul**′-face
(Elaprase)

CATEGORY AND SCHEDULE

Pregnancy Risk Category: C

Drug Class: Enzyme

MECHANISM OF ACTION

A recombinant form of iduronate-2-sulfatase that allows for catabolism of glycosaminoglycans. Hunter syndrome is a disease caused by insufficient levels of this lysosomal enzyme, iduronate-2-sulfate.
Therapeutic Effect: Replaces enzyme (iduronate-2-sulfatase).

USES

Treatment of Hunter syndrome

PHARMACOKINETICS

Half-life: 44–48 min.

INDICATIONS AND DOSAGES

▸ **Hunter Syndrome**

IV

Adults. 0.5 mg/kg once a wk.
Children (5 yr and older). 0.5 mg/kg once a wk.

SIDE EFFECTS/ADVERSE REACTIONS

Frequent

Fever, headache, antibody development, arthralgia, limb pain, pruritus, hypertension, malaise, visual disturbance, wheezing, musculoskeletal pain, musculoskeletal dysfunction, chest wall, urticaria, abscess, pruritic rash, skin disorder, atrial abnormality, anxiety, irritability, dyspepsia, infusion-site edema, superficial injury

Rare

Angioedema, cardiac arrhythmia, cyanosis, hypotension, infection, pulmonary embolism, respiratory distress, respiratory failure, seizure

PRECAUTIONS AND CONTRAINDICATIONS

Hypersensitivity to idursulfase or its components

Caution:

Impaired respiratory function, fever

DRUG INTERACTIONS OF CONCERN TO DENTISTRY

- None reported

SERIOUS REACTIONS

! Anaphylactic reactions have been reported.

DENTAL CONSIDERATIONS

General:

- Monitor vital signs at every appointment because of cardiovascular side effects.
- Consider semisupine chair position for patient comfort because of respiratory complications.
- Avoid aspirin and NSAIDs.
- Consider visual disturbances when presenting instructions to patients.

Consultations:

- Consult physician to determine disease control and ability of patient to tolerate dental procedures.

Teach Patient/Family to:

- Update medication/health history whenever symptoms of disease or medication regimen is changed.
- Use effective, atraumatic oral hygiene measures to reduce soft tissue inflammation.
- Use home fluoride products for anticaries effect.

ifosfamide

eye-**fos**′-fah-mide

(Holoxan[AUS], Ifex)

CATEGORY AND SCHEDULE

Pregnancy Risk Category: D

Drug Class: Alkylating agent; antineoplastic

MECHANISM OF ACTION

An alkylating agent that inhibits DNA and RNA protein synthesis by cross-linking with DNA and RNA strands, preventing cell growth. Cell cycle-phase nonspecific.

Therapeutic Effect: Interferes with DNA and RNA function.

USES

Treatment of cancer of the testicles as well as some other kinds of cancer

PHARMACOKINETICS

Metabolized in the liver to active metabolite. Crosses the blood-brain barrier (to a limited extent). Primarily excreted in urine. Removed by hemodialysis. ***Half-life:*** 15 hr.

INDICATIONS AND DOSAGES

▸ **Germ Cell Testicular Carcinoma**

IV

Adults. 700–2000 mg/m^2/day for 5 consecutive days. Repeat every 3 wk or after recovery from hematologic toxicity. Administer with mesna.

Children. 1200–1800 mg/m^2/day for 5 days every 21–28 days.

SIDE EFFECTS/ADVERSE REACTIONS

Frequent

Alopecia, nausea, vomiting

Occasional

Confusion, somnolence, hallucinations, infection

Rare

Dizziness, seizures, disorientation, fever, malaise, stomatitis

PRECAUTIONS AND CONTRAINDICATIONS

Pregnancy, severe myelosuppression

DRUG INTERACTIONS OF CONCERN TO DENTISTRY

• None reported.

SERIOUS REACTIONS

! Hemorrhagic cystitis with hematuria and dysuria occurs frequently if a protective agent (mesna) is not used.

! Myelosuppression, characterized by leukopenia and, to a lesser extent, thrombocytopenia occurs frequently.

! Pulmonary toxicity, hepatotoxicity, nephrotoxicity, cardiotoxicity, and CNS toxicity (manifested as confusion, hallucinations, somnolence, and coma) may require discontinuation of therapy.

DENTAL CONSIDERATIONS

General:

• Determine why patient is taking the drug.

• If additional analgesia is required for dental pain, consider alternative analgesics (NSAIDs) in patients taking narcotics for acute or chronic pain.

• Examine for oral manifestation of opportunistic infection.

• Avoid products that affect platelet function, such as aspirin and NSAIDs.

• This drug may be used in the hospital or on an outpatient basis. Confirm the patient's disease and treatment status.

• Chlorhexidine mouth rinse prior to and during chemotherapy may reduce severity of mucositis.

• Patient on chronic drug therapy may rarely present with symptoms of blood dyscrasias, which can include infection, bleeding, and poor healing. If dyscrasia is present, caution patient to prevent oral tissue trauma when using oral hygiene aids.

• Palliative medication may be required for management of oral side effects.

• Short appointments and a stress-reduction protocol may be required for anxious patients.

• Patients may be at risk of bleeding; check for oral signs.

• Oral infections should be eliminated and/or treated aggressively.

Consultations:

• Medical consultation should include routine blood counts including platelet counts and bleeding time.

• Consult physician; prophylactic or therapeutic antiinfectives may be indicated if surgery or periodontal treatment is required.

• Medical consultation may be required to assess immunologic status during cancer chemotherapy and determine safety risk, if any, posed by the required dental treatment.

- Medical consultation may be required to assess disease control and patient's ability to tolerate stress.

Teach Patient/Family to:

- Be aware of oral side effects.
- Encourage effective oral hygiene to prevent soft tissue inflammation.
- Report oral lesions, soreness, or bleeding to dentist.
- Prevent trauma when using oral hygiene aids.
- Update health and medication history if physician makes any changes in evaluation or drug regimens; include OTC, herbal, and nonherbal remedies in the update.

iloperidone

i-lo-**per′**-i-done
(Fanapt)

CATEGORY AND SCHEDULE

Pregnancy Risk Category: C

Drug Class: Antipsychotic agent, atypical; dopamine and serotonin antagonist

MECHANISM OF ACTION

Antagonizes dopamine Type 2 and serotonin Type 2 receptors.
Therapeutic Effect: Diminishes symptoms of schizophrenia.

USES

Schizophrenia

PHARMACOKINETICS

Well absorbed following PO administration. Bioavailability: 96%. Protein binding: 95%. Primarily metabolized by CYP2D6 and CYP3A4 to active metabolites P95 and P88. Partially excreted in urine; partially excreted in feces. ***Half-life:*** 18–37 hr; for iloperidone. P88 and P95 in CYP2D6 extensive metabolizers: 18, 26, and 23 hr, respectively; poor metabolizers: 33, 37, and 31 hr, respectively.

INDICATIONS AND DOSAGES

▸ **Schizophrenia**

PO

Adults. Initially, 1 mg twice a day. Maintenance dose: 12–24 mg a day. May titrate dose as needed according to the following dosing schedule: 2 mg twice a day on day 2; 4 mg twice a day on day 3; 6 mg twice on day 4; 8 mg twice a day on day 5; 10 mg twice a day on day 6; 12 mg twice a day on day 7. Max dose: 12 mg twice a day.

SIDE EFFECTS/ADVERSE REACTIONS

Frequent

Tachycardia, dry mouth, nausea, dizziness, somnolence

Occasional

Orthostatic hypotension, hypotension, diarrhea, abdominal discomfort, ejaculation failure, weight gain, blurred vision, nasal congestion, nasopharyngitis, upper respiratory tract infection, dyspnea, arthralgia, musculoskeletal stiffness, rash

Rare

Palpitation, erectile dysfunction, urinary incontinence, weight loss, muscle spasm, myalgia, conjunctivitis, low hematocrit

PRECAUTIONS AND CONTRAINDICATIONS

Hypersensitivity to iloperidone or its components

Caution:
Elderly with dementia-related psychosis (increased mortality)—black box warning
Hepatic impairment
Neuroleptic malignant syndrome
Tardive dyskinesia
Seizures
Leukopenia, neutropenia, agranulocytosis
Patients at risk for suicide
Cognitive and motor impairment
Hyperglycemia, diabetes, patients should be monitored for signs and symptoms of hyperglycemia
QT prolongation; electrolyte disturbances; serum potassium and magnesium should be monitored as hypokalemia and hypomagnesemia may increase the risk of QT prolongation

DRUG INTERACTIONS OF CONCERN TO DENTISTRY

- CNS depressants, alcohol: Additive CNS depressant effects
- Antihypertensive agents: May enhance the hypotensive effects
- CYP2D6 inhibitors: May increase iloperidone concentrations
- CYP3A4 inhibitors: May increase iloperidone concentrations
- QT-interval prolonging drugs: May cause additive effects

SERIOUS REACTIONS

! Prolongation of QT interval may produce torsades de pointes. Patients with bradycardia, hypokalemia, hypomagnesemia are at increased risk.

! Priapism has been reported.

! Orthostatic hypotension including dizziness, tachycardia, and syncope with standing may occur.

! Cerebrovascular accident and transient ischemic attack can occur.

! Monitor for thoughts of suicide.

DENTAL CONSIDERATIONS

General:

- Monitor vital signs at every appointment because of cardiovascular side effects.
- After supine positioning, have patient sit upright for at least 2 min before standing to avoid orthostatic hypotension.
- Assess salivary flow as a factor in caries, periodontal disease, and candidiasis.
- Assess for presence of extrapyramidal motor symptoms such as tardive dyskinesia and akathisia. Extrapyramidal motor activity may complicate dental treatment.
- Consider semisupine chair position for patient comfort if GI side effects occur.

Consultations:

- In a patient with symptoms of blood dyscrasias, request a medical consultation for blood studies and postpone treatment until normal values are reestablished.
- Medical consultation may be required to assess disease control.
- Physician should be informed if significant xerostomic side effects occur (e.g., increased caries, sore tongue, problems eating or swallowing, difficulty wearing prosthesis) so that medication change can be considered.
- Consultation with physician may be necessary if sedation or general anesthesia is required.

Teach Patient/Family to:

- Encourage effective oral hygiene to prevent soft tissue inflammation.
- Prevent trauma when using oral hygiene aids.
- When chronic dry mouth occurs, advise patient to:
  - Avoid mouth rinses with high alcohol content because of drying effects.

• Use daily home fluoride products for anticaries effect.
• Use sugarless gum, frequent sips of water, or saliva substitutes

iloprost

eye-low-prost
(Ventavis)

CATEGORY AND SCHEDULE

Pregnancy Risk Category: C

Drug Class: Agents for pulmonary hypertension

I

MECHANISM OF ACTION

A prostaglandin that dilates systemic and pulmonary arterial vascular beds, alters pulmonary vascular resistance, and suppresses vascular smooth muscle proliferation. Inhibits platelet aggregation.
Therapeutic Effect: Improves symptoms and exercise tolerance in patients with pulmonary hypertension; delays deterioration of condition.

USES

Pulmonary hypertension in patients with NYHA Class III or IV symptoms

PHARMACOKINETICS

Protein binding: 60%. Metabolized in liver; primarily by beta-oxidation of the carboxyl side chain to tetranoriloprost. Primarily excreted in urine; minimal elimination in feces. ***Half-life:*** 20–30 min.

INDICATIONS AND DOSAGES

▸ Pulmonary Hypertension in Patients with NYHA Class III or IV Symptoms
Oral Inhalation
Adults, Elderly. Initially, 2.5 mcg/dose; if tolerated, increased to 5 mcg/dose. Administer 6–9 times a day at intervals of 2 hr or longer while patient is awake. Maintenance: 5 mcg/dose. Maximum daily dose: 45 mcg.

SIDE EFFECTS/ADVERSE REACTIONS

Frequent
Increased cough, headache, flushing (vasodilation)
Occasional
Flu-like symptoms, nausea, trismus, jaw pain, hypotension
Rare
Insomnia, syncope, palpitations, vomiting, back pain, muscle cramps, GGT increased, CHF

PRECAUTIONS AND CONTRAINDICATIONS

Hypersensitivity to iloprost or any component of the formulation.
If signs of pulmonary edema occur when inhaled iloprost is administered in patients with pulmonary hypertension, treatment should be stopped immediately; may be a sign of pulmonary venous hypertension.
Caution:
Hepatic impairment
Renal impairment
Elderly
Pregnancy
Bleeding disorders
Hypotension (systolic B/P <85 mm Hg)
Respiratory disease (COPD, severe asthma, acute pulmonary infections)

DRUG INTERACTIONS OF CONCERN TO DENTISTRY

• Anticoagulants, antiplatelet agents: May increased the risk of bleeding

• Antihypertensives, other vasodilators: May increase the hypotensive effects of iloprost
• Monoamine oxidase inhibitors (MAOIs): Additive hypotensive effects

SERIOUS REACTIONS

! Hemoptysis and pneumonia occur occasionally.
! CHF, renal failure, dyspnea, and chest pain occur rarely.

DENTAL CONSIDERATIONS

General:
• Monitor vital signs at every appointment due to cardiovascular side effects.
• After supine positioning, have patient sit upright for at least 2 min before standing to avoid orthostatic hypotension.
• Assess for signs of pulmonary venous hypertension (pulmonary edema).
Consultations:
• Medical consultation may be required to assess disease control.
Teach Patient/Family to:
• Encourage effective oral hygiene to prevent soft tissue inflammation.
• Use soft tooth brush to reduce risk of bleeding.
• Immediately report any sign of infection to the dentist.

imatinib mesylate

im′-ah-tin-ib **me**′-sil-ate
(Gleevec, Glivec[AUS])

CATEGORY AND SCHEDULE

Pregnancy Risk Category: D

Drug Class: Antineoplastic

MECHANISM OF ACTION

Inhibits Bcr-Abl tyrosine kinase, an enzyme created by the Philadelphia chromosome abnormality found in patients with chronic myeloid leukemia (CML).
Therapeutic Effect: Suppresses tumor growth during the three stages of CML; blast crisis, accelerated phase, and chronic phase.

USES

Treatment of CML in blast crisis, accelerated phase or chronic phase after failure of interferon-α therapy; GI stromal tumors

PHARMACOKINETICS

Well absorbed after PO administration. Binds to plasma proteins, particularly albumin. Metabolized in the liver. Eliminated mainly in the feces as metabolites. ***Half-life:*** 18 hr.

INDICATIONS AND DOSAGES

▸ **CML**

PO

Adults, Elderly. 400 mg/day for patients in chronic-phase CML; 600 mg/day for patients in accelerated phase or blast crisis. May increase dosage from 400 to 600 mg/day for patients in chronic phase or from 600 to 800 mg (given as 300–400 mg twice a day) for patients in accelerated phase or blast crisis in the absence of a severe drug reaction or severe neutropenia or thrombocytopenia in the following circumstances: progression of the disease, failure to achieve a satisfactory hematologic response after 3 mo or more of treatment, or loss of a previously achieved hematologic response.
Children. 260 mg/m^2 a day as a single daily dose or in 2 divided doses.

SIDE EFFECTS/ADVERSE REACTIONS

Frequent

Nausea, diarrhea, vomiting, headache, fluid retention (periorbital, lower extremities), rash, musculoskeletal pain, muscle cramps, arthralgia

Occasional

Abdominal pain, cough, myalgia, fatigue, fever, anorexia, dyspepsia, constipation, night sweats, pruritus

Rare

Nasopharyngitis, petechiae, asthenia, epistaxis

PRECAUTIONS AND CONTRAINDICATIONS

Known hypersensitivity to imatinib

Caution:

Fluid retention, edema risk; neutropenia, thrombocytopenia, GI irritation, liver function abnormalities; safety in lactation or pediatric patients has not been studied

DRUG INTERACTIONS OF CONCERN TO DENTISTRY

- Increased plasma levels with CYP3A4 isoenzyme inhibitors: ketoconazole; possibly macrolide antibiotics, itraconazole, benzodiazepines
- Use acetaminophen with caution or avoid if hepatotoxicity is present
- Possible decrease in plasma concentrations: dexamethasone, carbamazepine, St. John's wort (herb)

SERIOUS REACTIONS

! Severe fluid retention (manifested as pleural effusion, pericardial effusion, pulmonary edema, and ascites) and hepatotoxicity occur rarely.

! Neutropenia and thrombocytopenia are expected responses to the drug.

! Respiratory toxicity, manifested as dyspnea and pneumonia, may occur.

DENTAL CONSIDERATIONS

General:

- Prophylactic or therapeutic antibiotics may be indicated to prevent or treat infection if surgery or periodontal debridement is required.
- Patients taking opioids for acute or chronic pain should be given alternative analgesics for dental pain.
- Short appointments and a stress reduction protocol may be required for anxious patients.
- Consider local hemostasis measures to control excessive bleeding.
- Patients on chronic drug therapy may rarely have symptoms of blood dyscrasias, which can include infection, bleeding, and poor healing.
- Consider semisupine chair position for patient comfort if GI side effects occur.

Consultations:

- In a patient with symptoms of blood dyscrasias, request a medical consultation for blood studies and postpone treatment until normal values are reestablished.
- Consultation with physician may be necessary if sedation or general anesthesia is required.
- Medical consultation should include routine blood counts, including platelet counts and bleeding time.

Teach Patient/Family to:

- Encourage effective oral hygiene to prevent soft tissue inflammation, infection.
- Inform dentist of unusual bleeding episodes following dental treatment.

imipramine

ih-**mih′**-prah-meen
(Apo-Imipramine[CAN], Melipramine[AUS], Tofranil, Tofranil-PM)
Do not confuse imipramine with desipramine.

CATEGORY AND SCHEDULE

Pregnancy Risk Category: D

Drug Class: Antidepressant (tricyclic)

MECHANISM OF ACTION

A tricyclic antidepressant, antibulimic, anticataleptic, antinarcoleptic, antineuralgic, antineuritic, and antipanic agent that blocks the reuptake of neurotransmitters, such as norepinephrine and serotonin, at presynaptic membranes, increasing their concentration at postsynaptic receptor sites.
Therapeutic Effect: Relieves depression and controls nocturnal enuresis.

USES

Treatment of depression, enuresis in children

PHARMACOKINETICS

PO: Steady state 2–5 days.
Half-life: 6–20 hr; metabolized by liver; excreted by kidneys, feces; crosses placenta; excreted in breast milk.

INDICATIONS AND DOSAGES

▸ Depression

PO

Adults. Initially, 75–100 mg/day. May gradually increase to 300 mg/day for hospitalized patients, or 200 mg/day for outpatients; then reduce dosage to effective maintenance level, 50–150 mg/day.
Elderly. Initially, 10–25 mg/day at bedtime. May increase by 10–25 mg every 3–7 days. Range: 50–150 mg/day.
Children. 1.5 mg/kg/day. May increase by 1 mg/kg every 3–4 days. Maximum: 5 mg/kg/day.

▸ Enuresis

PO

Children older than 6 yr. Initially, 10–25 mg at bedtime. May increase by 25 mg/day. Maximum: 50 mg for children older than 12 yr.

SIDE EFFECTS/ADVERSE REACTIONS

Frequent

Somnolence, fatigue, dry mouth, blurred vision, constipation, delayed micturition, orthostatic hypotension, diaphoresis, impaired concentration, increased appetite, urine retention, photosensitivity

Occasional

GI disturbances (nausea, metallic taste)

Rare

Paradoxical reactions, (agitation, restlessness, nightmares, insomnia), extrapyramidal symptoms (particularly fine hand tremors)

PRECAUTIONS AND CONTRAINDICATIONS

Acute recovery period after MI, use within 14 days of MAOIs.

Caution:

Suicidal patients, severe depression, increased intraocular pressure, narrow-angle glaucoma, urinary retention, cardiac disease, hepatic disease, hyperthyroidism, electroshock therapy, elective surgery, elderly, MAOIs

DRUG INTERACTIONS OF CONCERN TO DENTISTRY

• Increased anticholinergic effects: muscarinic blockers, antihistamines, phenothiazines
• Increased effects of direct-acting sympathomimetics (epinephrine, levonordefrin)
• Potential risk of increased CNS depression: alcohol, barbiturates, benzodiazepines, other CNS depressants
• Decreased antihypertensive effects: clonidine, guanadrel, guanethidine
• Avoid concurrent use with St. John's wort (herb)
• Suspected increased tricyclic antidepressant effects: fluconazole, ketoconazole
• Increased serum levels of carbamazepine
• Caution in using drugs metabolized by CYP2D6: increased effects

SERIOUS REACTIONS

! Overdose may produce seizures; cardiovascular effects, such as severe orthostatic hypotension, dizziness, tachycardia, palpitations, and arrhythmias; and altered temperature regulation, including hyperpyrexia or hypothermia.
! Abrupt discontinuation after prolonged therapy may produce headache, malaise, nausea, vomiting, and vivid dreams.

DENTAL CONSIDERATIONS

General:
• Monitor vital signs at every appointment because of cardiovascular side effects.
• Limit dose or avoid vasoconstrictor.
• Assess salivary flow as a factor in caries, periodontal disease, and candidiasis.
• Patients on chronic drug therapy may rarely have symptoms of blood dyscrasias, which can include infection, bleeding, and poor healing.
• After supine positioning, have patient sit upright for at least 2 min to avoid orthostatic hypotension.
• Use vasoconstrictors with caution, in low doses, and with careful aspiration. Avoid use of gingival retraction cord with epinephrine.
• Place on frequent recall because of oral side effects.
Consultations:
• In a patient with symptoms of blood dyscrasias, request a medical consultation for blood studies and postpone dental treatment until normal values are reestablished.
• Medical consultation may be required to assess disease control.
• Physician should be informed if significant xerostomic side effects occur (e.g., increased caries, sore tongue, problems eating or swallowing, difficulty wearing prosthesis) so that a medication change can be considered.
Teach Patient/Family to:
• Encourage effective oral hygiene to prevent soft tissue inflammation.
• Prevent injury when using oral hygiene aids.
• When chronic dry mouth occurs, advise patient to:
  • Avoid mouth rinses with high alcohol content because of drying effects.
  • Use sugarless gum, frequent sips of water, or saliva substitutes.
  • Use daily home fluoride products for anticaries effect.

imiquimod
im-**ick**′-wih-mod
(Aldara)

CATEGORY AND SCHEDULE
Pregnancy Risk Category: C

Drug Class: Immune response modifier

MECHANISM OF ACTION
An immune response modifier whose mechanism of action is unknown.
Therapeutic Effect: Reduces genital and perianal warts.

USES
Treatment of external genital and perianal warts, condylomata acuminata

PHARMACOKINETICS
Minimal absorption after topical administration. Minimal excretion in urine and feces.

INDICATIONS AND DOSAGES
▸ **Warts/Condyloma Acuminata**
Topical
Adults, Elderly, Children 12 yr and older. Apply 3 times a wk before normal sleeping hours; leave on skin 6–10 hr. Remove following treatment period. Continue therapy for maximum of 16 wk.

SIDE EFFECTS/ADVERSE REACTIONS
Frequent
Local skin reactions: erythema, itching, burning, erosion, excoriation/flaking, fungal infections (women)
Occasional
Pain, induration, ulceration, scabbing, soreness, headache, flu-like symptoms

PRECAUTIONS AND CONTRAINDICATIONS
History of hypersensitivity to imiquimod
Caution:
Has not been evaluated in papilloma viral diseases, cream may weaken condoms and diaphragms, external use only, lactation, children younger 18 yr

DRUG INTERACTIONS OF CONCERN TO DENTISTRY
- None reported

SERIOUS REACTIONS
! None reported

DENTAL CONSIDERATIONS
General:
- Oral manifestations of the disease may occur in the oral mucosa.
- Patient may have history of other sexually-transmitted diseases (STDs).

Consultations:
- Medical consultation may be required to assess disease control.

Teach Patient/Family to:
- Report oral lesions to the dentist.
- Update health and drug history if physician makes any changes in evaluation or drug regimens.

indacaterol
in-da-**kat**′er-ol
(Arcapta)
Do not confuse indacaterol with albuterol or formoterol.

CATEGORY AND SCHEDULE
Pregnancy Risk Category: C

Drug Class: Beta$_2$-adrenergic agonist, long-acting

MECHANISM OF ACTION

A long-acting bronchodilator that stimulates β_2-adrenergic receptors in the lungs, resulting in relaxation of bronchial smooth muscle.
Therapeutic Effect: Relieves bronchospasm, reduces airway resistance.

USES

Long-term maintenance treatment of airflow obstruction in chronic obstructive pulmonary disease (COPD) including chronic bronchitis and/or emphysema

I

PHARMACOKINETICS

Absorbed from bronchi after inhalation. 95% plasma protein bound. Hepatic metabolism via CYP3A4, CYP2D6, and CYP1A1 enzymes. Excreted in urine primarily (90%). ***Half-life:*** 40–56 hr.

INDICATIONS AND DOSAGES

▸ **COPD, Maintenance**

Oral inhalation

Adults. 1 inhalation (75 mcg/inhalation) once daily; maximum: 1 inhalation once daily.

SIDE EFFECTS/ADVERSE REACTIONS

Frequent

Nasopharyngitis, headache, cough

Occasional

Nausea, oropharyngeal pain, dizziness, tachycardia

PRECAUTIONS AND CONTRAINDICATIONS

Hypersensitivity to indacaterol or any component of the formulation. Not approved for the treatment of asthma. Use with caution in patients with cardiovascular disease, diabetes, hyperthyroidism, hypokalemia, and seizure disorders.

DRUG INTERACTIONS OF CONCERN TO DENTISTRY

• Epinephrine: possible increased risk of adverse effects
• Phenothiazines: potential interaction resulting in cardiac conduction disturbance (prolonged QT interval)

SERIOUS REACTIONS

! Long-acting β_2-agonists (LABAs) increase the risk of asthma-related deaths.

DENTAL CONSIDERATIONS

General:

• Indacaterol is not a rescue inhaler and should not be used as such in an emergency.
• Monitor vital signs at every appointment because of cardiovascular adverse effects.
• Assess salivary flow as a factor in caries, periodontal disease, and candidiasis.
• Consider semisupine chair position for patient comfort because of respiratory effects of disease.
• Short, midday appointments and a stress-reduction protocol may be required for anxious patients.
• A short-acting inhaler should be available to manage acute respiratory deterioration.
• Avoid prescribing aspirin and aspirin-containing products.

Consultations:

• Consult physician to assess disease control and patient's ability to tolerate stress.

Teach Patient/Family to:

• Gargle, rinse mouth with water and expectorate after each aerosol use.
• Avoid mouth rinses with high alcohol content because of drying effect.
• Use home fluoride products for anticaries effect.

• Use sugarless/xylitol gum, frequent sips of water, or saliva substitutes if dry mouth occurs.

indapamide

in-**dap**′-ah-mide
(Dapa-tabs[AUS], Indahexal[AUS], Insig[AUS], Lozide[CAN], Lozol, Natrilix[AUS], Natrilix SR[AUS])
Do not confuse indapamide with iodamide or iopamidol.

CATEGORY AND SCHEDULE

Pregnancy Risk Category: B (D if used in pregnancy-induced hypertension)

Drug Class: Diuretic, thiazide-like

MECHANISM OF ACTION

A thiazide-like diuretic that blocks reabsorption of water, sodium, and potassium at the cortical diluting segment of the distal tubule; also reduces plasma and extracellular fluid volume and peripheral vascular resistance by direct effect on blood vessels.
Therapeutic Effect: Promotes diuresis and reduces B/P.

USES

Treatment of edema, hypertension

PHARMACOKINETICS

PO: Onset 1–2 hr, peak 2 hr, duration up to 36 hr. ***Half-life:*** 14–18 hr; excreted in urine, feces.

INDICATIONS AND DOSAGES

▸ **Edema**

PO

Adults. Initially, 2.5 mg/day, may increase to 5 mg/day after 1 wk.

▸ **Hypertension**

PO

Adults, Elderly. Initially, 1.25 mg, may increase to 2.5 mg/day after 4 wk or 5 mg/day after additional 4 wk.

SIDE EFFECTS/ADVERSE REACTIONS

Frequent

Fatigue, numbness of extremities, tension, irritability, agitation, headache, dizziness, light-headedness, insomnia, muscle cramps

Occasional

Tingling of extremities, urinary frequency, urticaria, rhinorrhea, flushing, weight loss, orthostatic hypotension, depression, blurred vision, nausea, vomiting, diarrhea or constipation, dry mouth, impotence, rash, pruritus

PRECAUTIONS AND CONTRAINDICATIONS

Hypersensitivity, anuria

Caution:

Hypokalemia, dehydration, ascites, hepatic disease, severe renal disease

DRUG INTERACTIONS OF CONCERN TO DENTISTRY

• Decreased hypotensive response: NSAIDs

SERIOUS REACTIONS

! Vigorous diuresis may lead to profound water and electrolyte depletion, resulting in hypokalemia, hyponatremia, and dehydration.

! Acute hypotensive episodes may occur.

! Hyperglycemia may occur during prolonged therapy.

! Pancreatitis, blood dyscrasias, pulmonary edema, allergic pneumonitis, and dermatologic reactions occur rarely.

! Overdose can lead to lethargy and coma without changes in electrolytes or hydration.

DENTAL CONSIDERATIONS

General:

- Monitor vital signs at every appointment because of cardiovascular side effects.
- Patients on chronic drug therapy may rarely have symptoms of blood dyscrasias, which can include infection, bleeding, and poor healing.
- After supine positioning, have patient sit upright for at least 2 min before standing to avoid orthostatic hypotension.
- Assess salivary flow as a factor in caries, periodontal disease, and candidiasis.
- Limit use of sodium-containing products, such as saline IV fluids, for patients with a dietary salt restriction.
- Stress from dental procedures may compromise cardiovascular function; determine patient risk.
- Short appointments and a stress-reduction protocol may be required for anxious patients.
- Patients on diuretic therapy should be monitored for serum K levels.

Consultations:

- In a patient with symptoms of blood dyscrasias, request a medical consultation for blood studies and postpone dental treatment until normal values are reestablished.
- Medical consultation may be required to assess disease control and patient's ability to tolerate stress.

Teach Patient/Family to:

- Encourage effective oral hygiene to prevent soft tissue inflammation.
- Use caution to prevent injury when using oral hygiene aids.
- When chronic dry mouth occurs, advise patient to:
  - Avoid mouth rinses with high alcohol content because of drying effects.
  - Use sugarless gum, frequent sips of water, or saliva substitutes.
  - Use daily home fluoride products for anticaries effect.

indinavir

in-**din**′-ah-veer

(Crixivan)

Do not confuse indinavir with Denavir.

CATEGORY AND SCHEDULE

Pregnancy Risk Category: C

Drug Class: Antiviral

MECHANISM OF ACTION

A protease inhibitor that suppresses HIV protease, an enzyme necessary for splitting viral polyprotein precursors into mature and infectious viral particles.

Therapeutic Effect: Interrupts HIV replication, slowing the progression of HIV infection.

USES

Treatment of HIV infection; prophylaxis after needle stick with AZT and lamivudine within 2 hr of needle stick

PHARMACOKINETICS

Rapidly absorbed after PO administration. Protein binding: 60%. Metabolized in the liver. Primarily excreted in urine. Unknown if removed by hemodialysis. ***Half-life:*** 1.8 hr (increased in impaired hepatic function).

INDICATIONS AND DOSAGES

▸ HIV Infection (in Combination with Other Antiretrovirals)

PO

Adults. 800 mg (two 400-mg capsules) q8h.

▸ HIV Infection in Patients with Hepatic Insufficiency

PO

Adults. 600 mg q8h.

SIDE EFFECTS/ADVERSE REACTIONS

Frequent

Nausea, abdominal pain, headache, diarrhea

Occasional

Vomiting, asthenia, fatigue, insomnia, accumulation of fat in waist, abdomen, or back of neck

Rare

Abnormal taste sensation, heartburn, symptomatic urinary tract disease, transient renal dysfunction

PRECAUTIONS AND CONTRAINDICATIONS

Hypersensitivity to indinavir; nephrolithiasis

Caution:

Nephrolithiasis (requires adequate hydration), hyperbilirubinemia, serum transaminase elevation, hepatic impairment, dose reduction of rifabutin required, lactation, children

DRUG INTERACTIONS OF CONCERN TO DENTISTRY

- Contraindicated with triazolam, midazolam, macrolide antibiotics
- Reduce dose when given with ketoconazole

SERIOUS REACTIONS

! Nephrolithiasis (flank pain with or without hematuria) occurs in 4% of patients.

DENTAL CONSIDERATIONS

General:

- Consider semisupine chair position when GI side effects occur.
- Assess salivary flow as a factor in caries, periodontal disease, and candidiasis.
- Monitor vital signs at every appointment because of cardiovascular side effects.
- Examine for oral manifestation of opportunistic infection.
- Patients with gastroesophageal reflux may have oral symptoms, including burning mouth, secondary candidiasis, and signs of tooth erosion.

Consultations:

- Medical consultation may be required to assess disease control.

Teach Patient/Family to:

- Encourage effective oral hygiene to prevent soft tissue inflammation.
- Report oral lesions, soreness, or bleeding to dentist.
- Update health history/drug record if physician makes any changes in evaluation or drug regimens.
- When chronic dry mouth occurs, advise patient to:
  - Avoid mouth rinses with high alcohol content because of drying effects.
  - Use daily home fluoride products for anticaries effect.
  - Use sugarless gum, frequent sips of water, or saliva substitutes.

indomethacin

in-doe-**meth′**-ah-sin
(Apo-Indomethacin[CAN], Arthrexin[AUS], Indocid[CAN], Indocin, Indocin-IV, Indocin-SR, Novomethacin[CAN])
Do not confuse Indocin with Imodium or Vicodin.

CATEGORY AND SCHEDULE

Pregnancy Risk Category: B (D if used after 34 wk gestation, close to delivery, or for longer than 48 hr)

Drug Class: Nonsteroidal antiinflammatory

I

MECHANISM OF ACTION

An NSAID that produces analgesic and antiinflammatory effects by inhibiting prostaglandin synthesis. Also increases the sensitivity of the premature ductus to the dilating effects of prostaglandins.
Therapeutic Effect: Reduces the inflammatory response and intensity of pain. Closure of the patent ductus arteriosus.

USES

Treatment of rheumatoid arthritis, osteoarthritis, ankylosing rheumatoid spondylitis, acute gouty arthritis

PHARMACOKINETICS

PO: Onset 1–2 hr, peak 3 hr, duration 4–6 hr; 99% plasma-protein binding; metabolized in liver, kidneys; excreted in urine, bile, feces, breast milk; crosses placenta

INDICATIONS AND DOSAGES

▸ Moderate-to-Severe Rheumatoid Arthritis, Osteoarthritis, Ankylosing Spondylitis

PO

Adults, Elderly. Initially, 25 mg 2–3 times a day; increased by 25–50 mg/wk up to 150–200 mg/day, or 75 mg/day (extended-release) up to 75 mg twice a day.
Children. 1–2 mg/kg/day. Maximum: 150–200 mg/day.

▸ Acute Gouty Arthritis

PO

Adults, Elderly. Initially, 100 mg, then 50 mg 3 times a day.

▸ Acute Shoulder Pain

PO

Adults, Elderly. 75–150 mg/day in 3–4 divided doses.

▸ Usual Rectal Dosage

Adults, Elderly. 50 mg 4 times a day.
Children. Initially, 1.5–2.5 mg/kg/day, increased up to 4 mg/kg/day. Maximum: 150–200 mg/day.

▸ Patent Ductus Arteriosus

IV

Neonates. Initially, 0.2 mg/kg. Subsequent doses are on the basis of age, as follows:
Neonates older than 7 days. 0.25 mg/kg for second and third doses.
Neonates 2–7 days. 0.2 mg/kg for second and third doses.
Neonates less than 48 hr. 0.1 mg/kg for second and third doses.

SIDE EFFECTS/ADVERSE REACTIONS

Frequent

Headache, nausea, vomiting, dyspepsia, dizziness

Occasional

Depression, tinnitus, diaphoresis, somnolence, constipation, diarrhea, bleeding disturbances in patent ductus arteriosus

Rare
Hypertension, confusion, urticaria, pruritus, rash, blurred vision

PRECAUTIONS AND CONTRAINDICATIONS

Active GI bleeding or ulcerations; hypersensitivity to aspirin, indomethacin, or other NSAIDs; renal impairment, thrombocytopenia.

Caution:
Lactation, children, bleeding disorders, GI disorders, cardiac disorders, hypersensitivity to other antiinflammatory agents, depression

DRUG INTERACTIONS OF CONCERN TO DENTISTRY

- Increased GI bleeding, ulceration: corticosteroids, alcohol, aspirin, other NSAIDs
- Renal toxicity: acetaminophen (high doses, prolonged use)
- Possible risk of decreased renal function: cyclosporine
- When prescribed for dental pain:
  - Risk of increased effects: oral anticoagulants, oral antidiabetics, lithium, methotrexate
  - Decreased antihypertensive effects of diuretics, β-adrenergic blockers, ACE inhibitors
  - Increased toxicity of zidovudine
  - SSRIs: increased risk of GI side effects

SERIOUS REACTIONS

! Paralytic ileus and ulceration of the esophagus, stomach, duodenum, or small intestine may occur.
! Patients with impaired renal function may develop hyperkalemia and worsening of renal impairment.
! Indomethacin use may aggravate epilepsy, parkinsonism, and depression or other psychiatric disturbances.
! Nephrotoxicity, including dysuria, hematuria, proteinuria, and nephrotic syndrome, occurs rarely.
! Metabolic acidosis or alkalosis, apnea, and bradycardia occur rarely in patients with patent ductus arteriosus.

DENTAL CONSIDERATIONS

General:
- Avoid prescribing aspirin-containing products.
- Patients on chronic drug therapy may rarely have symptoms of blood dyscrasias, which can include infection, bleeding, and poor healing.
- Assess salivary flow as a factor in caries, periodontal disease, and candidiasis.
- Consider semisupine chair position for patients with arthritic disease.
- Severe stomach bleeding may occur in patients who regularly use NSAIDs in recommended doses, when the patient is also taking another NSAID, an anticoagulant/antiplatelet drug, or steroid drug, if the patient has GI or peptic ulcer disease, if they are 60 years or older, or when NSAIDs are taken longer than directed. Warn patients of the potential for severe stomach bleeding.

Consultations:
- In a patient with symptoms of blood dyscrasias, request a medical consultation for blood studies and postpone dental treatment until normal values are reestablished.
- Medical consultation may be required to assess disease control.

Teach Patient/Family to:
- Encourage effective oral hygiene to prevent soft tissue inflammation.
- Use caution to prevent injury when using oral hygiene aids.

I

• When chronic dry mouth occurs, advise patient to:
  • Avoid mouth rinses with high alcohol content because of drying effects.
  • Use sugarless gum, frequent sips of water, or saliva substitutes.
  • Use daily home fluoride products for anticaries effect.
• Warn patient of potential risks of NSAIDs.

I

infliximab

in-**flicks**′-ih-mab

(Remicade)

Do not confuse Remicade with Reminyl.

CATEGORY AND SCHEDULE

Pregnancy Risk Category: C

Drug Class: Antiinflammatory

MECHANISM OF ACTION

A monoclonal antibody that binds to tumor necrosis factor (TNF), inhibiting functional activity of TNF. Reduces infiltration of inflammatory cells.

Therapeutic Effect: Decreases inflamed areas of the intestine.

USES

Reduces signs and symptoms, progression of structural damage in rheumatoid arthritis in combination with methotrexate; improvement of physical function in moderate-to-severe rheumatoid arthritis in combination with methotrexate; reduction in signs and symptoms in patients with Crohn's disease with inadequate response to conventional therapy, long-term control of remission-level Crohn's disease; reduces and maintains fistulas in Crohn's disease

PHARMACOKINETICS

Route	Onset	Peak	Duration
IV (Crohn's disease)	1–2 wk	N/A	8–48 wk
IV (rheumatoid arthritis)	3–7 days	N/A	6–12 wk

Absorbed into the GI tissue; primarily distributed in the vascular compartment. ***Half-life:*** 9.5 days.

INDICATIONS AND DOSAGES

▸ Moderate-to-Severe Crohn's Disease

IV Infusion

Adults, Elderly. 5 mg/kg as a single IV infusion.

▸ Fistulizing Crohn's Disease

IV Infusion

Adults, Elderly. Initially, 5 mg/kg followed by additional 5-mg/kg doses at 2 and 6 wk after first infusion.

▸ Rheumatoid Arthritis

IV Infusion

Adults, Elderly. 3 mg/kg; followed by additional doses at 2 and 6 wk after first infusion. Then q8wk.

SIDE EFFECTS/ADVERSE REACTIONS

Frequent

Headache, nausea, fatigue, fever

Occasional

Fever or chills during infusion, pharyngitis, vomiting, pain, dizziness, bronchitis, rash, rhinitis, cough, pruritus, sinusitis, myalgia, back pain

Rare

Hypotension or hypertension, paresthesia, anxiety, depression, insomnia, diarrhea, urinary tract infection

PRECAUTIONS AND CONTRAINDICATIONS

Sensitivity to infliximab or murine proteins, sepsis, serious active infection

Caution:

Risk of serious infections, risk of autoimmunity, chronic use increases risk of lymphoma, do not give live vaccines to patients taking this drug, patients should be tested for tuberculosis before starting therapy, no data on lactation or pediatric use

DRUG INTERACTIONS OF CONCERN TO DENTISTRY

- No drug interaction studies conducted

SERIOUS REACTIONS

! Hypersensitivity reaction, lupus-like syndrome, and severe hepatic reactions may occur.

DENTAL CONSIDERATIONS

General:

- Determine why patient is taking the drug.
- Avoid drugs that irritate the GI tract.
- Question patient about other drugs being taken.
- Examine for oral manifestation of opportunistic infection.
- Report oral infections to patient's physician; treat infections aggressively.

Consultations:

- Medical consultation may be required to assess disease control and patient's ability to tolerate stress.

Teach Patient/Family to:

- Encourage effective oral hygiene to prevent soft tissue inflammation, infection.
- Immediately report any signs or symptoms of oral infection.

ingenol mebutate

in′-je nol **meb**′-u-tate
(Picato)

CATEGORY AND SCHEDULE

Pregnancy Risk Category: C

Drug Class: Topical skin product

MECHANISM OF ACTION

Ingenol mebutate appears to induce primary necrosis of actinic keratosis with a subsequent neutrophil-mediated inflammatory response with antibody-dependent cytotoxicity of residual disease cells; killing residual disease cells may prevent future relapse.
Therapeutic Effect: Clears signs of red, scaly skin lesions due to actinic keratosis.

USES

Topical treatment of actinic keratosis

PHARMACOKINETICS

Minimal systemic absorption with proper application. ***Half-life:*** None reported.

INDICATIONS AND DOSAGES

▸ Actinic Keratoses

Topical

Adults. Face and scalp: Apply 0.015% gel once daily to affected area for 3 consecutive days. Trunk/extremities: Apply 0.05% gel once daily to affected area for 2 consecutive days.

SIDE EFFECTS/ADVERSE REACTIONS

Frequent

Erythema, flaking/scaling, crusting, swelling, vesiculation/pustulation, erosion/ulceration, application site pain

Occasional
Headache, periorbital edema, nasopharyngitis

PRECAUTIONS AND CONTRAINDICATIONS
Severe eye pain, eyelid edema, eyelid ptosis, and periorbital edema can occur after exposure.

DRUG INTERACTIONS OF CONCERN TO DENTISTRY
- None reported

SERIOUS REACTIONS
! Severe reactions including erythema, crusting, swelling, vesiculation/pustulation, and erosion/ulceration can occur.

DENTAL CONSIDERATIONS
General:
- Avoid contacting and irritating areas on the head and neck being treated with ingenol.

Teach Patient/Family to:
- Report changes in disease status and drug regimen.

insulin
in′-su-lin
Rapid acting: Insulin Lispro (Humalog); Insulin Aspart (Novolog, NovoMix 30[AUS], Novorapid[AUS]); Regular Insulin (Actrapid[AUS], Humulin R, Novolin R, Regular Iletin II); Intermediate acting: NPH (Humulin N, Novolin N, NPH Iletin II); Lente: (Humulin L, Lente Iletin II, Monotard[AUS], Novolin L); Long acting: Insulin Glargine (Lantus)

CATEGORY AND SCHEDULE
Pregnancy Risk Category: B

Drug Class: Hormone, antidiabetic

MECHANISM OF ACTION
An exogenous insulin that facilitates passage of glucose, potassium, and magnesium across the cellular membranes of skeletal and cardiac muscle and adipose tissue. Controls storage and metabolism of carbohydrates, protein, and fats. Promotes conversion of glucose to glycogen in the liver.
Therapeutic Effect: Controls glucose levels in diabetic patients.

USES
Treatment of severe ketoacidosis, type 1 (IDDM) and type 2 (NIDDM; when diet, weight control, exercise, or oral hypoglycemics are not sufficient); hyperkalemia, hyperalimentation

PHARMACOKINETICS

Drug Form	Onset (hr)	Peak (hr)	Duration (hr)
Lispro	0.25	0.5–1.5	4–5
Insulin aspart	1/6	1–3	3–5
Regular	0.5–1	2–4	5–7
NPH	1–2	6–14	24
Lente	1–3	6–14	24
Insulin glargine	N/A	N/A	24

Long Acting: Lantus.

INDICATIONS AND DOSAGES
▸ **Treatment of Insulin-Dependent Type 1 Diabetes Mellitus and Non–Insulin-Dependent Type 2 Diabetes Mellitus When Diet or Weight Control Has Failed to Maintain Satisfactory Blood Glucose Levels or in Event of Fever, Infection, Pregnancy, Surgery, or Trauma, or Severe Endocrine, Hepatic or Renal Dysfunction; Emergency Treatment of Ketoacidosis (Regular Insulin); to**

Promote Passage of Glucose Across Cell Membrane in Hyperalimentation (Regular Insulin): to Facilitate Intracellular Shift of Potassium in Hyperkalemia (Regular Insulin)
Subcutaneous
Adults, Elderly, Children. 0.5–1 unit/kg/day.
Adolescents (during growth spurt). 0.8–1.2 unit/kg/day.

SIDE EFFECTS/ADVERSE REACTIONS

Occasional
Localized redness, swelling, and itching caused by improper injection technique or allergy to cleansing solution or insulin
Infrequent
Somogyi effect, including rebound hyperglycemia with chronically excessive insulin dosages: systemic allergic reaction, marked by rash, angioedema, and anaphylaxis; lipodystrophy or depression at injection site because of breakdown of adipose tissue; lipohypertrophy or accumulation of subcutaneous tissue at injection site because of inadequate site rotation
Rare
Insulin resistance

PRECAUTIONS AND CONTRAINDICATIONS

Hypersensitivity or insulin resistance may require change of type or species source of insulin

DRUG INTERACTIONS OF CONCERN TO DENTISTRY

• Increased hypoglycemia: salicylates, NSAIDs (large doses and chronic use), alcohol
• Hyperglycemia: corticosteroids, epinephrine

SERIOUS REACTIONS

! Severe hypoglycemia caused by hyperinsulinism may occur with insulin overdose, decrease or delay of food intake, or excessive exercise and in those with brittle diabetes.
! Diabetic ketoacidosis may result from stress, illness, omission of insulin dose, or long-term poor insulin control.

DENTAL CONSIDERATIONS

General:
• Monitor vital signs at every appointment.
• Potential for hypoglycemia.
• Place on frequent recall to evaluate healing response.
• Diabetics may be more susceptible to infection and have delayed wound healing.
• Assess salivary flow as a factor in caries, periodontal disease, and candidiasis.
• Prophylactic antibiotics may be indicated in uncontrolled diabetics to prevent infection if surgery or deep scaling is planned.
• Ensure that patient is following prescribed diet and regularly takes medication.
• Question patient about self-monitoring of drug's antidiabetic effect, including blood glucose values or finger-stick records.
• Keep a readily available source of sugar or fruit juice in case of insulin overdose.
Consultations:
• Medical consultation may be required to assess disease control and patient's ability to tolerate stress.
• Medical consultation may include data from patient's blood glucose monitoring, including glycosylated hemoglobin or HbA_{1c} testing.

Teach Patient/Family to:
• Encourage effective oral hygiene to prevent soft tissue inflammation.
• Use caution to prevent injury when using oral hygiene aids.
• Avoid mouth rinses with high alcohol content because of drying effects.

insulin glargine

in′-su-lin **glare**′-jeen
(Lantus)

CATEGORY AND SCHEDULE

Pregnancy Risk Category: C

Drug Class: Hormone, antidiabetic

I

MECHANISM OF ACTION

An exogenous insulin that facilitates passage of glucose, potassium, magnesium across cellular membranes of skeletal and cardiac muscle, adipose tissue; controls storage and metabolism of carbohydrates, protein, fats. Promotes conversion of glucose to glycogen in liver.
Therapeutic Effect: Controls glucose levels in diabetic patients.

USES

Treatment of severe ketoacidosis, Type 1 (IDDM) and Type 2 (NIDDM; when diet, weight control, exercise, or oral hypoglycemics are not sufficient); hyperkalemia, hyperalimentation

PHARMACOKINETICS

Drug Form	Onset (hr)	Peak (hr)	Duration (hr)
Insulin glargine	N/A	N/A	24

Metabolized at the carboxyl terminus of the B chain in the subcutaneous depot to form two active metabolites. Unchanged drug and degradation products are present throughout circulation.

INDICATIONS AND DOSAGES

▸ **Treatment of Insulin-Dependent Type 1 Diabetes Mellitus, Non–Insulin-Dependent Type 2 Diabetes Mellitus When Diet or Weight Control Therapy Has Failed to Maintain Satisfactory Blood Glucose Levels or in Event of Fever, Infection, Pregnancy, Severe Endocrine, Liver or Renal Dysfunction, Surgery, or Trauma, Regular Insulin Used in Emergency Treatment of Ketoacidosis, to Promote Passage of Glucose Across Cell Membrane in Hyperalimentation, to Facilitate Intracellular Shift of Potassium in Hyperkalemia**
Subcutaneous
Adults, Elderly, Children. 10 units once daily, preferably at bedtime, adjusted according to patient response.

SIDE EFFECTS/ADVERSE REACTIONS

Frequent
Hypoglycemia
Occasional
Local redness, swelling, itching, caused by improper injection technique or allergy to cleansing solution or insulin
Infrequent
Systemic allergic reaction, marked by rash, angioedema, and anaphylaxis, lipodystrophy, or depression at injection site because of breakdown of adipose tissue, lipohypertrophy, or accumulation of subcutaneous tissue at injection site

because of lack of adequate site rotation
Rare
Insulin resistance

PRECAUTIONS AND CONTRAINDICATIONS

Hypersensitivity or insulin resistance may require change of type or species source of insulin

DRUG INTERACTIONS OF CONCERN TO DENTISTRY

- Increased hypoglycemia: salicylates, NSAIDs (large doses and chronic use), alcohol
- Hyperglycemia: corticosteroids, epinephrine

SERIOUS REACTIONS

! Severe hypoglycemia caused by hyperinsulinism may occur in overdose of insulin, decrease or delay of food intake, excessive exercise, or those with brittle diabetes.
! Diabetic ketoacidosis may result from stress, illness, omission of insulin dose, or long-term poor insulin control.

DENTAL CONSIDERATIONS

General:
- Monitor vital signs at every appointment.
- Potential for hypoglycemia.
- Place on frequent recall to evaluate healing response.
- Diabetics may be more susceptible to infection and have delayed wound healing.
- Assess salivary flow as a factor in caries, periodontal disease, and candidiasis.
- Prophylactic antibiotics may be indicated in uncontrolled diabetics to prevent infection if invasive procedures are planned.
- Ensure that patient is following prescribed diet and regularly takes medication.
- Question patient about self-monitoring of drug's antidiabetic effect, including blood glucose values or finger-stick records.
- Keep a readily available source of glucose in case of insulin overdose.

Consultations:
- Medical consultation may be required to assess disease control and patient's ability to tolerate stress.
- Medical consultation may include data from patient's blood glucose monitoring, including glycosylated hemoglobin or HbA_{1c} testing.

Teach Patient/Family to:
- Encourage effective oral hygiene to prevent soft tissue inflammation.
- Use caution to prevent injury when using oral hygiene aids.
- Avoid mouth rinses with high alcohol content because of drying effects.

insulin glulisine

in′-su-lin **gluh′**-lih-seen
(Apidra)

CATEGORY AND SCHEDULE

Pregnancy Risk Category: C

Drug Class: Hormone, antidiabetic

MECHANISM OF ACTION

A recombinant, rapid-acting insulin analog that facilitates passage of glucose, potassium, magnesium across cellular membranes of skeletal and cardiac muscle, adipose tissue; controls storage and metabolism of carbohydrates, protein, fats. Promotes conversion of glucose to glycogen in liver.

Therapeutic Effect: Controls glucose levels in diabetic patients.

USES

Treatment of severe ketoacidosis, Type 1 (IDDM) and Type 2 (NIDDM; when diet, weight control, exercise, or oral hypoglycemics are not sufficient); hyperkalemia, hyperalimentation

PHARMACOKINETICS

Drug Form	Onset (hr)	Peak (min)	Duration (hr)
Insulin Glulisine	20 min	55 min	5 hr

INDICATIONS AND DOSAGES

▸ Diabetes Mellitus (Type 1 and Type 2)

Subcutaneous, Infusion Pump

Adults, Elderly, Children. Individualize per patient needs.

SIDE EFFECTS/ADVERSE REACTIONS

Occasional

Local redness, swelling, itching, caused by improper injection technique or allergy to cleansing solution or insulin

Infrequent

Somogyi effect, including rebound hyperglycemia, with chronically excessive insulin doses. Systemic allergic reaction, marked by rash, angioedema, and anaphylaxis, lipodystrophy or depression at injection site because of breakdown of adipose tissue, lipohypertrophy or accumulation of subcutaneous tissue at injection site because of lack of adequate site rotation

Rare

Insulin resistance

PRECAUTIONS AND CONTRAINDICATIONS

Current hypoglycemic episode, hypersensitivity, or insulin resistance may require change of type or species source of insulin

DRUG INTERACTIONS OF CONCERN TO DENTISTRY

- Increased hypoglycemia: salicylates, NSAIDs (large doses and chronic use), alcohol
- Hyperglycemia: corticosteroids, epinephrine

SERIOUS REACTIONS

! Severe hypoglycemia caused by hyperinsulinism may occur in overdose of insulin, decrease or delay of food intake, excessive exercise, or those with brittle diabetes.

! Diabetic ketoacidosis may result from stress, illness, omission of insulin dose, or long-term poor insulin control.

DENTAL CONSIDERATIONS

General:

- Monitor vital signs at every appointment.
- Potential for hypoglycemia.
- Place on frequent recall to evaluate healing response.
- Diabetics may be more susceptible to infection and have delayed wound healing.
- Assess salivary flow as a factor in caries, periodontal disease, and candidiasis.
- Prophylactic antibiotics may be indicated in uncontrolled diabetics to prevent infection if surgery or deep scaling is planned.
- Ensure that patient is following prescribed diet and regularly takes medication.

• Question patient about self-monitoring of drug's antidiabetic effect, including blood glucose values or finger-stick records.
• Keep a readily available source of glucose in case of insulin overdose.

Consultations:

• Medical consultation may be required to assess disease control and patient's ability to tolerate stress.
• Medical consultation may include data from patient's blood glucose monitoring, including glycosylated hemoglobin or HbA_{1c} testing.

Teach Patient/Family to:

• Encourage effective oral hygiene to prevent soft tissue inflammation.
• Use caution to prevent injury when using oral hygiene aids.
• Avoid mouth rinses with high alcohol content because of drying effects.

interferon alfa-2a

in-ter-**fear**′-on **al**′-fa
(Roferon-A)
Do not confuse interferon alfa-2a with interferon alfa-2b.

CATEGORY AND SCHEDULE

Pregnancy Risk Category: C

Drug Class: Biologic response modifier

MECHANISM OF ACTION

A biological response modifier that inhibits viral replication in virus-infected cells, suppresses cell proliferation, increases phagocytic action of macrophage, and augments specific lymphocytic cell toxicity. ***Therapeutic Effect:*** Prevents rapid growth of malignant cells; inhibits hepatitis virus.

USES

Treatment of hairy-cell leukemia in patients older than 18 yr, AIDS-related Kaposi's sarcoma (KS), chronic hepatitis C, chronic myelogenous leukemia

PHARMACOKINETICS

Well absorbed after IM and subcutaneous administration. Undergoes proteolytic degradation during reabsorption in kidneys. ***Half-life:*** 2 hr (IM); 3 hr (subcutaneous).

INDICATIONS AND DOSAGES

▸ **Hairy Cell Leukemia**

IM, Subcutaneous

Adults. Initially, 3 million units/day for 16–24 wk. Maintenance: 3 million units 3 times a wk. Do not use 36-million-unit vial.

▸ **Chronic Myelocytic Leukemia**

IM, Subcutaneous

Adults. 9 million units/day.

▸ **Melanoma**

IM, Subcutaneous

Adults, Elderly. 12 million units/m^2 3 times a wk for 3 mo.

▸ **AIDS-Related KS**

IM, Subcutaneous

Adults. Initially, 36 million units/day for 10–12 wk, may give 3 million units on day 1, 9 million units on day 2, 18 million units on day 3, then 36 million units/day for remaining 10–12 wk. Maintenance: 36 million units/day 3 times a wk.

▸ **Chronic Hepatitis C**

IM, Subcutaneous

Adults, Elderly. 6 million units 3 times a wk for 3 mo, then 3 million units 3 times a wk for 9 mo.

SIDE EFFECTS/ADVERSE REACTIONS

Frequent

Flu-like symptoms, nausea, vomiting, cough, dyspnea,

hypotension, edema, chest pain, dizziness, diarrhea, weight loss, altered taste, abdominal discomfort, confusion, paresthesia, depression, visual and sleep disturbances, diaphoresis, lethargy

Occasional

Alopecia (partial), rash, dry throat or skin, pruritus, flatulence, constipation, hypertension, palpitations, sinusitis

Rare

Hot flashes, hypermotility, Raynaud's syndrome, bronchospasm, earache, ecchymosis

PRECAUTIONS AND CONTRAINDICATIONS

Autoimmune hepatitis

Caution:

Severe hypotension, dysrhythmia, tachycardia, lactation, children younger than 18 yr, severe renal or hepatic disease, convulsion disorder, thrombophlebitis, coagulation disorders, hemophilia, GI bleeding; closely monitor patients; severe, life-threatening neuropsychiatric, autoimmune, ischemic, or infectious disorders may cause or aggravate these conditions

DRUG INTERACTIONS OF CONCERN TO DENTISTRY

- Risk of hepatotoxicity in severe liver disease: acetaminophen

SERIOUS REACTIONS

! Arrhythmias, CVA, transient ischemic attacks, CHF, pulmonary edema, and MI occur rarely.

DENTAL CONSIDERATIONS

General:

- Determine why the patient is taking the drug.
- Monitor vital signs at every appointment because of cardiovascular side effects.
- Patients on chronic drug therapy may rarely have symptoms of blood dyscrasias, which can include infection, bleeding, and poor healing.
- Palliative medication may be required for oral side effects.
- Assess salivary flow as a factor in caries, periodontal disease, and candidiasis.
- Consider semisupine chair position for patient comfort if GI side effects occur.
- Avoid elective dental procedures if severe neutropenia (more than 500 cells/mm^3) or thrombocytopenia (more than 50,000 cell/mm^3) is present.
- Antibiotic prophylaxis is indicated in severely neutropenic patients.
- Patient history should include all medications and herbal or nonherbal remedies taken by the patient.
- Severe side effects may require deferring elective dental procedures until drug therapy is completed.
- Evaluate efficacy of oral hygiene home care; preventive appointments may be necessary.

Consultations:

- Medical consultation may be required to assess disease control.
- In a patient with symptoms of blood dyscrasias, request a medical consultation for blood studies and postpone treatment until normal values are reestablished.
- Liver function tests may be required to determine chronic liver disease.

Teach Patient/Family to:

- Encourage effective oral hygiene to prevent soft tissue inflammation.
- Report oral lesions, soreness, or bleeding to dentist.
- Update medical/drug records if physician makes any changes in evaluation or drug regimens.

- When chronic dry mouth occurs, advise patient to:
  - Avoid mouth rinses with high alcohol content because of drying effects.
  - Use sugarless gum, frequent sips of water, or saliva substitutes.
  - Use daily home fluoride products for anticaries effect.

interferon alfa-2a/2b

in-ter-**fear**′-on **al**′-fa
(Roferon-A)/(Intron-A)

CATEGORY AND SCHEDULE

Pregnancy Risk Category: C

Drug Class: Biologic response modifier

MECHANISM OF ACTION

A biologic response modifier that inhibits viral replication in virus-infected cells.
Therapeutic Effect: Suppresses cell proliferation; increases phagocytic action of macrophages; augments specific lymphocytic cell toxicity.

USES

Treatment of hairy-cell leukemia, malignant melanoma, and AIDS-related Kaposi's sarcoma (KS). They are also used to treat laryngeal papillomatosis (growths in the respiratory tract) in children, genital warts, and some kinds of hepatitis.

PHARMACOKINETICS

Interferon alfa-2a
Well absorbed after IM, subcutaneous administration. Undergoes proteolytic degradation during reabsorption in kidney.
Half-life: IM: 2 hr; Subcutaneous: 3 hr.

Interferon alfa-2b
Well absorbed after IM, subcutaneous administration. Undergoes proteolytic degradation during reabsorption in kidney.
Half-life: 2–3 hr.

INDICATIONS AND DOSAGES

▸ Hairy-Cell Leukemia
Interferon alfa-2a
Subcutaneous/IM
Adults. Initially, 3 million units/day for 16–24 wk. Maintenance: 3 million units 3 times a wk. Do not use 36-million-unit vial.
Interferon alfa-2b
Subcutaneous/IM
Adults. 2 million units/m^2 3 times a wk. If severe adverse reactions occur, modify dose or temporarily discontinue.

▸ Chronic Myelocytic Leukemia (CML)
Interferon alfa-2a
Subcutaneous/IM
Adults. 9 million units daily.

▸ Condylomata Acuminate
Interferon alfa-2b
Intralesional
Adults. 1 million units/lesion 3 times a wk for 3 wk. Use only 10-million-unit vial, reconstitute with no more than 1 ml diluent. Use tuberculin (TB) syringe with 25- or 26-gauge needle. Give in evening with acetaminophen, which alleviates side effects.

▸ Melanoma
Interferon alfa-2a
Subcutaneous/IM
Adults, Elderly. 12 million units/m^2 3 times a wk for 3 mo.
Interferon alfa-2b
IV
Adults. Initially, 20 million units/m^2 5 times a wk for 4 wk. Maintenance: 10 million units IM/Subcutaneous for 48 wk.

▸ **AIDS-Related KS**
Interferon alfa-2a
Subcutaneous/IM
Adults. Initially, 36 million units/day for 10–12 wk, may give 3 million units on day 1; 9 million units on day 2; 18 million units on day 3; then begin 36 million units/day for remainder of 10–12 wk.
Maintenance: 36 million units/day 3 times a wk.
Interferon alfa-2b
Subcutaneous/IM
Adults. 30 million units/m^2 3 times a wk. Use only 50 million units vials. If severe adverse reactions occur, modify dose or temporarily discontinue.

▸ **Chronic Hepatitis B**
Interferon alfa-2b
Subcutaneous/IM
Adults. 30–35 million units/wk, 5 million units/day or 10 million units 3 times a wk.

▸ **Chronic Hepatitis C**
Interferon alfa-2a
Subcutaneous/IM
Adults. Initially, 6 million units once a day for 3 wk, then 3 million units 3 times a wk for 6 mo.
Interferon alfa-2b
Subcutaneous/IM
Adults. 3 million units 3 times a wk for up to 6 mo, for up to 18–24 mo for chronic hepatitis C.

SIDE EFFECTS/ADVERSE REACTIONS

Frequent

Interferon alfa-2a: Flu-like symptoms, including fever, fatigue, headache, aches, pains, anorexia, chills, nausea, vomiting, coughing, dyspnea, hypotension, edema, chest pain, dizziness, diarrhea, weight loss, taste change, abdominal discomfort, confusion, paresthesia, depression, visual and sleep disturbances, diaphoresis, lethargy
Interferon alfa-2b: Flu-like symptoms, including fever, fatigue, headache, aches, pains, anorexia, and chills, rash with hairy cell leukemia (KS only)
KS: All previously mentioned side effects plus depression, dyspepsia, dry mouth or thirst, alopecia, rigors

Occasional

Interferon alfa-2a: Partial alopecia, rash, dry throat or skin, pruritus, flatulence, constipation, hypertension, palpitations, sinusitis
Interferon alfa-2b: Dizziness, pruritus, dry skin, dermatitis, alteration in taste

Rare

Interferon alfa-2a: Hot flashes, hypermotility, Raynaud's syndrome, bronchospasm, earache, ecchymosis
Interferon alfa-2b: Confusion, leg cramps, back pain, gingivitis, flushing, tremors, nervousness, eye pain

PRECAUTIONS AND CONTRAINDICATIONS

Hypersensitivity to any component of the formulations

Caution:

Preexisting psoriasis and sarcoidosis, do not use in patients with platelet counts less than 50,000/mm^3, preexisting CV disease, suicidal tendency, depression, preexisting psychiatric diseases, depressed bone marrow; safety and efficacy in lactation and children younger than 18 yr have not been established

DRUG INTERACTIONS OF CONCERN TO DENTISTRY

• Risk of hepatotoxicity in severe liver disease: acetaminophen

SERIOUS REACTIONS

! Arrhythmias, stroke, transient ischemic attacks, CHF, pulmonary edema, and MI occur rarely with interferon alfa-2a.

! Hypersensitivity reaction occurs rarely with interferon alfa-2b.
! Severe adverse reactions of flu-like symptoms appear dose related with interferon alfa-2b.

DENTAL CONSIDERATIONS

General:
- Determine why the patient is taking the drug.
- Monitor vital signs at every appointment because of cardiovascular side effects.
- After supine positioning, have patient sit upright for at least 2 min to avoid orthostatic hypotension.
- Palliative medication may be required for oral side effects.
- Assess salivary flow as a factor in caries, periodontal disease, and candidiasis.
- Patients on chronic drug therapy may rarely have symptoms of blood dyscrasias, which can include infection, bleeding, and poor healing.
- Consider semisupine chair position for patient comfort if GI side effects occur.
- Avoid elective dental procedures if severe neutropenia (fewer than 500 cells/mm^3) or thrombocytopenia (fewer than 50,000 cell/mm^3) is present.
- Antibiotic prophylaxis is indicated in severely neutropenic patients.
- Patient history should include all medications and herbal or nonherbal remedies taken by the patient.
- Severe side effects may require deferring elective dental procedures until drug therapy is completed.
- Evaluate efficacy of oral hygiene home care; preventive appointments may be necessary.

Consultations:
- Medical consultation may be required to assess disease control.
- In a patient with symptoms of blood dyscrasias, request a medical consultation for blood studies and postpone treatment until normal values are reestablished.
- Liver function tests may be required to determine chronic liver disease.

Teach Patient/Family to:
- Encourage effective oral hygiene to prevent soft tissue inflammation.
- Report oral lesions, soreness, or bleeding to dentist.
- Update medical/drug records if physician makes any changes in evaluation or drug regimens.
- When chronic dry mouth occurs, advise patient to:
    - Avoid mouth rinses with high alcohol content because of drying effects.
    - Use sugarless gum, frequent sips of water, or saliva substitutes.
    - Use daily home fluoride products for anticaries effect.

interferon alfa-2b

in-ter-**fear′**-on **al′**-fa
(Intron-A)
Do not confuse interferon alfa-2b with interferon alfa-2a.

CATEGORY AND SCHEDULE

Pregnancy Risk Category: C

Drug Class: Biologic response modifier

MECHANISM OF ACTION

A biological response modifier that inhibits viral replication in virus-infected cells, suppresses cell proliferation, increases phagocytic action of macrophages, and augments specific cytotoxicity of lymphocytes for target cells.

Therapeutic Effect: Prevents rapid growth of malignant cells; inhibits hepatitis virus.

USES

Treatment of hairy-cell leukemia in patients older than 18 yr, malignant melanoma, chronic hepatitis B, follicular lymphoma, AIDS-related Kaposi's sarcoma (KS), chronic hepatitis C, condylomata acuminata

PHARMACOKINETICS

Well absorbed after IM and subcutaneous administration. Undergoes proteolytic degradation during reabsorption in kidneys. ***Half-life:*** 2–3 hr.

INDICATIONS AND DOSAGES

▸ Hairy-Cell Leukemia

IM, Subcutaneous

Adults. 2 million units/m^2 3 times a wk. If severe adverse reactions occur, modify dose or temporarily discontinue drug.

▸ Condyloma Acuminatum

Intralesional

Adults. 1 million units/lesion 3 times a wk for 3 wk. Use only 10-million-unit vial, and reconstitute with no more than 1 ml diluent.

▸ AIDS-Related KS

IM, Subcutaneous

Adults. 30 million units/m^2 3 times a wk. Use only 50-million-unit vials. If severe adverse reactions occur, modify dose or temporarily discontinue drug.

▸ Chronic Hepatitis C

IM, Subcutaneous

Adults. 3 million units 3 times a wk for up to 6 mo. For patients who tolerate therapy and whose ALT(SGPT) level normalizes within 16 wk, therapy may be extended for up to 18–24 mo.

▸ Chronic Hepatitis B

IM, Subcutaneous

Adults. 30–35 million units weekly, either as 5 million units/day or 10 million units 3 times a wk.

▸ Malignant Melanoma

IV

Adults. Initially, 20 million units/m^2 5 times a wk for 4 wk. Maintenance: 10 million units IM or subcutaneously 3 times a wk for 48 wk.

▸ Follicular Lymphoma

Subcutaneous

Adults. 5 million units 3 times a wk for up to 18 mo.

SIDE EFFECTS/ADVERSE REACTIONS

Frequent

Flu-like symptoms, rash (only in patients with hairy-cell leukemia KS)

Patients with KS: All previously mentioned side effects and depression, dyspepsia, dry mouth or thirst, alopecia, rigors

Occasional

Dizziness, pruritus, dry skin, dermatitis, altered taste

Rare

Confusion, leg cramps, back pain, gingivitis, flushing, tremors, nervousness, eye pain

PRECAUTIONS AND CONTRAINDICATIONS

Hypersensitivity

DRUG INTERACTIONS OF CONCERN TO DENTISTRY

• Risk of hepatotoxicity in severe liver disease: acetaminophen

SERIOUS REACTIONS

! Hypersensitivity reactions occur rarely.

! Severe flu-like symptoms may occur at higher doses.

DENTAL CONSIDERATIONS

General:

- Determine why the patient is taking the drug.
- Monitor vital signs at every appointment because of cardiovascular side effects.
- Palliative medication may be required for oral side effects.
- Assess salivary flow as a factor in caries, periodontal disease, and candidiasis.
- Patients on chronic drug therapy may rarely have symptoms of blood dyscrasias, which can include infection, bleeding, and poor healing.
- Consider semisupine chair position for patient comfort if GI side effects occur.
- Avoid elective dental procedures if severe neutropenia (more than 500 cells/mm^3) or thrombocytopenia (more than 50,000 cell/mm^3) is present.
- Antibiotic prophylaxis is indicated in severely neutropenic patients.
- Patient history should include all medications and herbal or nonherbal remedies taken by the patient.
- Severe side effects may require deferring elective dental procedures until drug therapy is completed.
- Evaluate efficacy of oral hygiene home care; preventive appointments may be necessary.

Consultations:

- Medical consultation may be required to assess disease control.
- In a patient with symptoms of blood dyscrasias, request a medical consultation for blood studies and postpone treatment until normal values are reestablished.
- Liver function tests may be required to determine chronic liver disease.

Teach Patient/Family to:

- Encourage effective oral hygiene to prevent soft tissue inflammation.
- Report oral lesions, soreness, or bleeding to dentist.
- Update medical/drug records if physician makes any changes in evaluation or drug regimens.
- When chronic dry mouth occurs, advise patient to:
    - Avoid mouth rinses with high alcohol content because of drying effects.
    - Use sugarless gum, frequent sips of water, or saliva substitutes.
    - Use daily home fluoride products for anticaries effect.

interferon alfa-n3

in-ter-**fear**′-on **al**′-fa
(Alferon N)

CATEGORY AND SCHEDULE

Pregnancy Risk Category: C

Drug Class: Biologic response modifier

MECHANISM OF ACTION

A biological response modifier that inhibits viral replication in virus-infected cells, suppresses cell proliferation, increases phagocytic action of macrophages, and augments specific cytotoxicity of lymphocytes for target cells.
Therapeutic Effect: Inhibits viral growth in condylomata acuminatum.

USES

Intralesional treatment of refractory or recurring external condylomata acuminata in patients 18 yr or older

PHARMACOKINETICS

Plasma levels below detectable limits.

INDICATIONS AND DOSAGES

▸ **Condyloma Acuminatum**

Intralesional

Adults, Children 18 yr and older. 0.05 ml (250,000 international units) per wart twice a wk up to 8 wk. Maximum dose/treatment session: 0.5 ml (2.5 million international units). Do not repeat for 3 mo after initial 8 wk course unless warts enlarge or new warts appear.

SIDE EFFECTS/ADVERSE REACTIONS

Frequent

Flu-like symptoms

Occasional

Dizziness, pruritus, dry skin, dermatitis, altered taste

Rare

Confusion, leg cramps, back pain, gingivitis, flushing, tremor, nervousness, eye pain

PRECAUTIONS AND CONTRAINDICATIONS

Previous history of anaphylactic reaction to egg protein, mouse immunoglobulin, or neomycin

Caution:

CV disease, unstable angina, uncontrolled CHF, severe pulmonary disease, diabetes mellitus with ketoacidosis, coagulation disorders, severe myelosuppression, seizure disorders, risk of transmitting blood-borne infectious disease, lactation, use in children younger than 18 yr has not been established

DRUG INTERACTIONS OF CONCERN TO DENTISTRY

- None reported

SERIOUS REACTIONS

! Hypersensitivity reaction occurs rarely.

! Severe flu-like symptoms may occur at higher doses.

DENTAL CONSIDERATIONS

General:

- Determine why the patient is taking the drug.
- Following injection, advise patient to take acetaminophen (if there are no contraindications for its use) in PM to ease flu-like symptoms.
- Advise patient if dental drugs prescribed have a potential for photosensitivity.
- Consider semisupine chair position for patient comfort if GI side effects occur.

Consultations:

- Medical consultation may be required to assess disease control.

Teach Patient/Family to:

- Update medical/drug records if physician makes any changes in evaluation or drug regimens.

interferon gamma-1b

in-ter-**fear**′-on **gamm**′-ah

(Actimmune, Imukin[AUS])

CATEGORY AND SCHEDULE

Pregnancy Risk Category: C

Drug Class: Biologic response modifier

MECHANISM OF ACTION

A biological response modifier that induces activation of macrophages in blood monocytes to phagocytes, which is necessary in the body's cellular immune response to intracellular and extracellular pathogens. Enhances phagocytic function and antimicrobial activity of monocytes.

Therapeutic Effect: Decreases signs and symptoms of serious infections in chronic granulomatous disease.

USES
Reduces the severity and frequency of infections associated with chronic granulomatous disease; delays disease progression in patients with severe, malignant osteoporosis

PHARMACOKINETICS
Slowly absorbed after subcutaneous administration.

INDICATIONS AND DOSAGES
▸ Chronic Granulomatous Disease; Severe, Malignant Osteoporosis

Subcutaneous

Adults, Children older than 1 yr.
50 mcg/m^2 (1.5 million units/m^2) in patients with body surface area (BSA) greater than 0.5 m^2; 1.5 mcg/kg/dose in patients with BSA 0.5 m^2 or less. Give 3 times a wk.

SIDE EFFECTS/ADVERSE REACTIONS
Frequent

Fever, headache, rash, chills, fatigue, diarrhea

Occasional

Vomiting, nausea

Rare

Weight loss, myalgia, anorexia

PRECAUTIONS AND CONTRAINDICATIONS
Hypersensitivity to *E. coli*–derived products

Caution:

Cardiac disease, seizure disorders, CNS disorders, myelosuppression, lactation, children younger than 1 yr; monitor hematologic values q3mo

DRUG INTERACTIONS OF CONCERN TO DENTISTRY
• None reported

SERIOUS REACTIONS
! Interferon gamma-1b may exacerbate preexisting CNS disturbances, including decreased mental status, gait disturbance, and dizziness, as well as cardiac disorders.

DENTAL CONSIDERATIONS
General:

• Determine why the patient is taking the drug.
• Patients on chronic drug therapy may rarely have symptoms of blood dyscrasias, which can include infection, bleeding, and poor healing.
• Ask patient about side effects associated with drug use (abnormal hematologic values).
• Consider semisupine chair position for patient comfort if GI side effects occur.
• Place on frequent recall to evaluate healing response.
• Severe side effects may require deferring elective dental procedures until drug therapy is completed.
• Antibiotic prophylaxis is indicated in severely neutropenic patients.
• Avoid elective dental procedures if severe neutropenia (fewer than 500 cells/mm^3) or thrombocytopenia (fewer than 50,000 cell/mm^3) is present.

Consultations:

• In a patient with symptoms of blood dyscrasias, request a medical consultation for blood studies and postpone dental treatment until normal values are reestablished.
• Medical consultation may be required to assess disease control and patient's ability to tolerate stress.

Teach Patient/Family to:

• Encourage effective oral hygiene to prevent soft tissue inflammation.
• Use caution to prevent trauma when using oral hygiene aids.
• Update medical history and drug records if physician makes any

changes in evaluation or drug regimens.

ipratropium bromide

eye-pra-**troep′**-ee-um **broh′**-mide (Apo-Ipravent[CAN], Aproven[AUS], Atrovent, Atrovent Aerosol[AUS], Atrovent Nasal[AUS], Atrovent NPH, Novo-Ipramide[CAN], Nu-Ipratropium[CAN], PMS-Ipratropium[CAN])

Do not confuse Atrovent with Alupent.

CATEGORY AND SCHEDULE

Pregnancy Risk Category: B

Drug Class: Anticholinergic bronchodilator

MECHANISM OF ACTION

An anticholinergic that blocks the action of acetylcholine at parasympathetic sites in bronchial smooth muscle.

Therapeutic Effect: Causes bronchodilation and inhibits nasal secretions.

USES

Treatment of bronchodilation during bronchospasm in those with COPD, bronchitis, emphysema, asthma; not for rapid bronchodilation, maintenance treatment only; rhinorrhea, rhinorrhea associated with allergic and nonallergic perennial rhinitis in children age 6–11 yr, rhinorrhea associated with common cold

PHARMACOKINETICS

Route	Onset	Peak	Duration
Inhalation	1–3 min	1–2 hr	4–6 hr

Minimal systemic absorption after inhalation. Metabolized in the liver (systemic absorption). Primarily eliminated in feces. ***Half-life:*** 1.5–4 hr.

INDICATIONS AND DOSAGES

▸ **Bronchospasm, Acute Treatment**

Inhalation

Adults, Elderly, Children. 4–8 puffs as needed.

Nebulization

Adults, Elderly, Children 12 yr and older. 500 mcg q30min for 3 doses, then q2–4h as needed.

Children younger than 12 yr. 250 mcg q20min for 3 doses, then q2–4h as needed.

▸ **Bronchospasm, Maintenance Treatment**

Inhalation

Adults, Elderly, Children 12 yr and older. 2–3 puffs q6h.

Children younger than 12 yr. 1–2 puffs q6h.

Nebulization

Adults, Elderly, Children 12 yr and older. 500 mcg q6h.

Children younger than 12 yr. 250–500 mcg q6h.

▸ **Rhinorrhea**

Intranasal

Adults, Children older than 5 yr. 2 sprays of 0.06% solution 3–4 times a day.

Adults, Children older than 6 yr. 2 sprays of (0.03%) solution 2–3 times a day.

SIDE EFFECTS/ADVERSE REACTIONS

Frequent

Inhalation: Cough, dry mouth, headache, nausea

Nasal: Dry nose and mouth, headache, nasal irritation

Occasional

Inhalation: Dizziness, transient increased bronchospasm

Rare
Inhalation: Hypotension, insomnia, metallic or unpleasant taste, palpitations, urine retention
Nasal: Diarrhea or constipation, dry throat, abdominal pain, stuffy nose

PRECAUTIONS AND CONTRAINDICATIONS

History of hypersensitivity to atropine
Caution:
Lactation, children younger than 12 yr, narrow-angle glaucoma, prostatic hypertrophy, bladder neck obstruction

DRUG INTERACTIONS OF CONCERN TO DENTISTRY

• Increased effects of anticholinergic drugs

SERIOUS REACTIONS

! Worsening of angle-closure glaucoma, acute eye pain, and hypotension occur rarely.

DENTAL CONSIDERATIONS

General:
• Monitor vital signs at every appointment because of cardiovascular and respiratory side effects.
• Assess salivary flow as a factor in caries, periodontal disease, and candidiasis.
• Acute asthmatic episodes may be precipitated in the dental office. Sympathomimetic inhalants should be available for emergency use.
• Consider semisupine chair position for patients with respiratory disease.
• Place on frequent recall because of oral side effects.
Consultations:
• Medical consultation may be required to assess disease control and patient's ability to tolerate stress.
Teach Patient/Family to:
• Rinse mouth with water after each inhaled dose to prevent dryness.
• When chronic dry mouth occurs, advise patient to:
  • Avoid mouth rinses with high alcohol content because of drying effects.
  • Use sugarless gum, frequent sips of water, or saliva substitutes.
  • Use daily home fluoride products for anticaries effect.

irbesartan

erb-ah-**sar′**-tan
(Avapro, Karvea[AUS])

CATEGORY AND SCHEDULE

Pregnancy Risk Category: C (D if used in second or third trimester)

Drug Class: Angiotensin II receptor antagonist, antihypertensive

MECHANISM OF ACTION

An angiotensin II receptor, type AT1, antagonist that blocks the vasoconstrictor and aldosterone-secreting effects of angiotensin II, inhibiting the binding of angiotensin II to the AT1 receptors.
Therapeutic Effect: Causes vasodilation, decreases peripheral resistance, and decreases B/P.

USES

Treatment of hypertension alone or in combination with other antihypertensive drugs; nephropathy in type 2 diabetes

PHARMACOKINETICS

Rapidly and completely absorbed after PO administration. Protein binding: 90%. Undergoes hepatic metabolism to inactive metabolite. Recovered primarily in feces and, to a lesser extent, in urine. Not removed by hemodialysis. ***Half-life:*** 11–15 hr.

INDICATIONS AND DOSAGES

▸ Hypertension Alone or in Combination with Other Antihypertensives

PO

Adults, Elderly, Children 13 yr and older. Initially, 75–150 mg/day. May increase to 300 mg/day.
Children 6–12 yr. Initially, 75 mg/day. May increase to 150 mg/day.

▸ Nephropathy

PO

Adults, Elderly. Target dose of 300 mg/day.

SIDE EFFECTS/ADVERSE REACTIONS

Occasional

Upper respiratory tract infection, fatigue, diarrhea, cough

Rare

Heartburn, dizziness, headache, nausea, rash

PRECAUTIONS AND CONTRAINDICATIONS

Bilateral renal artery stenosis, biliary cirrhosis or obstruction, primary hyperaldosteronism, severe hepatic insufficiency

Caution:

Hypersensitivity to other angiotensin II receptor antagonists, volume- or salt-depleted patients, renal impairment, lactation, children

DRUG INTERACTIONS OF CONCERN TO DENTISTRY

- None reported

SERIOUS REACTIONS

! Overdosage may manifest as hypotension and tachycardia. Bradycardia occurs less often.

DENTAL CONSIDERATIONS

General:

- Monitor vital signs at every appointment because of cardiovascular side effects.
- Limit dose or avoid vasoconstrictor.
- Limit use of sodium-containing products, such as saline IV fluids, for those patients with a dietary salt restriction.
- Stress from dental procedures may compromise cardiovascular function; determine patient risk.
- Short appointments and a stress-reduction protocol may be required for anxious patients.
- Use precaution if sedation or general anesthesia is required; risk of hypotensive episode.
- After supine positioning, have patient sit upright for at least 2 min before standing to avoid orthostatic hypotension.
- Consider semisupine chair position for patient comfort if GI side effects occur.

Consultations:

- Consultation with physician may be necessary if sedation or general anesthesia is required.
- Medical consultation may be required to assess disease control and patient's ability to tolerate stress; risk of hypotensive episode.

Teach Patient/Family to:

- Update health and drug history if physician makes any changes in evaluation or drug regimens.

isocarboxazid

eye-soe-kar-**box**′-ah-zid
(Marplan)

CATEGORY AND SCHEDULE

Pregnancy Risk Category: C

Drug Class: Antidepressant-monoamine oxidase inhibitor

MECHANISM OF ACTION

An antidepressant that inhibits the MAO enzyme system at CNS storage sites. The reduced MAO activity causes an increased concentration in epinephrine, norepinephrine, serotonin, and dopamine at neuron receptor sites. ***Therapeutic Effect:*** Produces antidepressant effect.

USES

Treatment of depression

PHARMACOKINETICS

PO: Good absorption; maximum MAO inhibition 5–10 days, duration up to 2 wk; metabolized by liver; excreted by kidneys.

INDICATIONS AND DOSAGES

▸ Depression Refractory to Other Antidepressants or Electroconvulsive Therapy

PO

Adults, Elderly. Initially, 10 mg 3 times a day. May increase to 60 mg/day.

SIDE EFFECTS/ADVERSE REACTIONS

Frequent

Postural hypotension, drowsiness, decreased sexual ability, weakness, trembling, visual disturbances

Occasional

Tachycardia, peripheral edema, nervousness, chills, diarrhea, anorexia, constipation, xerostomia

Rare

Hepatitis, leukopenia, parkinsonian syndrome

PRECAUTIONS AND CONTRAINDICATIONS

Cardiovascular disease (CVD), cerebrovascular disease, liver impairment, pheochromocytoma, liver impairment

Caution:

Suicidal patients, concurrent use with other antidepressants (patients must stop taking MAOI 14 days before initiating therapy with other antidepressants), general anesthesia, severe depression, schizophrenia, diabetes mellitus, lactation, children younger than 16 yr

DRUG INTERACTIONS OF CONCERN TO DENTISTRY

- Increased pressor effects: indirect-acting sympathomimetics (ephedrine)
- Hyperpyretic crisis, convulsions, hypertensive episode: meperidine, possibly other opioids, carbamazepine
- Increased anticholinergic effects: anticholinergics, antihistamines
- Increased effects of alcohol, barbiturates, benzodiazepines, CNS depressants, SSRIs, tricyclic antidepressants, cyclobenzaprine, bupropion, buspirone, dextromethorphan, antihypertensive

SERIOUS REACTIONS

! Hypertensive crisis, marked by severe hypertension, occipital headache radiating frontally, neck stiffness or soreness, nausea, vomiting, sweating, fever or chilliness, clammy skin, dilated pupils, palpitations, tachycardia or bradycardia, and constricting chest pain.

DENTAL CONSIDERATIONS

General:

- Monitor vital signs at every appointment because of cardiovascular side effects.
- After supine positioning, have patient sit upright for at least 2 min to avoid orthostatic hypotension.
- Patients on chronic drug therapy may rarely have symptoms of blood

dyscrasias, which can include infection, bleeding, and poor healing.
- Consider semisupine chair position for patient comfort if GI side effects occur.
- Assess salivary flow as a factor in caries, periodontal disease, and candidiasis.
- Hypertensive episodes are possible even though there are no specific contraindications to vasoconstrictor use in local anesthetics.
- Short appointments and a stress-reduction protocol may be required for anxious patients.

Consultations:
- Medical consultation may be required to assess disease control and patient's ability to tolerate stress.
- In a patient with symptoms of blood dyscrasias, request a medical consultation for blood studies and postpone treatment until normal values are reestablished.

Teach Patient/Family:
- When chronic dry mouth occurs, advise patient to:
  - Avoid mouth rinses with high alcohol content because of drying effects.
  - Use daily home fluoride products for anticaries effect.
  - Use sugarless gum, frequent sips of water, or saliva substitutes.

isoetharine hydrochloride

eye-soe-**eth′**-ah-reen high-droh-**klor′**-ide
(Beta-2, Bronkometer, Bronkosol, Dey-Lute)

CATEGORY AND SCHEDULE

Pregnancy Risk Category: C

Drug Class: Adrenergic β_2-agonist

MECHANISM OF ACTION

A sympathomimetic (adrenergic) agonist that stimulates β_2-adrenergic receptors in the lungs, resulting in relaxation of bronchial smooth muscle.

Therapeutic Effect: Relieves bronchospasm, reduces airway resistance.

USES

Treatment of bronchospasm, asthma

PHARMACOKINETICS

Rapidly, well absorbed from the GI tract. Extensive metabolism in GI tract. Unknown extent metabolized in liver and lungs. Excreted in urine. ***Half-life:*** 4 hr.

INDICATIONS AND DOSAGES

▸ **Bronchospasm**

Hand-Bulb Nebulizer

Adults, Elderly. 4 inhalations (range: 3–7 inhalations) undiluted. May be repeated up to 5 times a day.

Metered Dose Inhalation

Adults, Elderly. 1–2 inhalations q4h. Wait 1 min before administering second inhalation.

IPPB, Oxygen Aerolization

Adults, Elderly. 0.5–1 ml of a 0.5% or 0.5 ml of a 1% solution diluted 1:3.

SIDE EFFECTS/ADVERSE REACTIONS

Occasional

Tremor, nausea, nervousness, palpitations, tachycardia, peripheral vasodilation, dryness of mouth, throat, dizziness, vomiting, headache, increased B/P, insomnia

PRECAUTIONS AND CONTRAINDICATIONS

History of hypersensitivity to sympathomimetics

Caution:
Cardiac disorders, hyperthyroidism, diabetes mellitus, prostatic hypertrophy

DRUG INTERACTIONS OF CONCERN TO DENTISTRY

- Increased effects of both drugs: other sympathomimetics
- Increased dysrhythmia: halogenated hydrocarbon anesthetics

SERIOUS REACTIONS

! Excessive sympathomimetic stimulation may produce palpitations, extrasystoles, tachycardia, chest pain, slight increase in B/P followed by a substantial decrease, chills, sweating, and blanching of skin.
! Too frequent or excessive use may lead to loss of bronchodilating effectiveness and severe and paradoxical bronchoconstriction.

DENTAL CONSIDERATIONS

General:

- Assess salivary flow as a factor in caries, periodontal disease, and candidiasis.
- Consider semisupine chair position for patients with respiratory disease.
- Acute asthmatic episodes may be precipitated in the dental office. Sympathomimetic inhalants should be available for emergency use.

Consultations:

- Medical consultation may be required to assess disease control and patient's ability to tolerate stress.

Teach Patient/Family to:

- Rinse mouth with water after each inhaled dose to prevent dryness.
- When chronic dry mouth occurs, advise patient to:
  - Avoid mouth rinses with high alcohol content because of drying effects.
  - Use sugarless gum, frequent sips of water, or saliva substitutes.
  - Use daily home fluoride products for anticaries effect.

isoniazid

eye-soe-**nye**′-ah-zid
(INH, Isotamine[CAN], Nydrazid, PMS Isoniazid[CAN])

CATEGORY AND SCHEDULE

Pregnancy Risk Category: C

Drug Class: Antitubercular

MECHANISM OF ACTION

An isonicotinic acid derivative that inhibits mycolic acid synthesis and causes disruption of the bacterial cell wall and loss of acid-fast properties in susceptible mycobacteria. Active only during bacterial cell division.
Therapeutic Effect: Bactericidal against actively growing intracellular and extracellular susceptible mycobacteria.

USES

Treatment and prevention of tuberculosis (TB)

PHARMACOKINETICS

Readily absorbed from the GI tract. Protein binding: 10%–15%. Widely distributed (including to CSF). Metabolized in the liver. Primarily excreted in urine. Removed by hemodialysis. ***Half-life:*** 0.5–5 hr.

INDICATIONS AND DOSAGES

▸ **TB (in Combination with One or More Antituberculars)**
PO, IM
Adults, Elderly. 5 mg/kg/day as a single dose. Maximum 300 mg/day.

I

Children. 10–15 mg/kg/day as a single dose. Maximum 300 mg/day.

▸ **Prevention of TB**

PO, IM

Adults, Elderly. 300 mg/day as a single dose.

Children. 10 mg/kg/day as a single dose. Maximum 300 mg/day.

SIDE EFFECTS/ADVERSE REACTIONS

Frequent

Nausea, vomiting, diarrhea, abdominal pain

Rare

Pain at injection site, hypersensitivity reaction

PRECAUTIONS AND CONTRAINDICATIONS

Acute hepatic disease, history of hypersensitivity reactions or hepatic injury with previous isoniazid therapy

Caution:

Renal disease; diabetic retinopathy cataracts; ocular defects; hepatic disease; fatal hepatitis, especially in black women and Hispanic women; children younger than 13 yr, monitor liver function

DRUG INTERACTIONS OF CONCERN TO DENTISTRY

- Increased hepatotoxicity: alcohol, acetaminophen, carbamazepine
- Decreased effectiveness: glucocorticoids, especially prednisolone
- Increased plasma concentration: benzodiazepines, alfentanil
- Decreased effect of ketoconazole, miconazole

SERIOUS REACTIONS

! Rare reactions include neurotoxicity (as evidenced by ataxia and paraesthesia), optic neuritis, and hepatotoxicity.

DENTAL CONSIDERATIONS

General:

- Patients on chronic drug therapy may rarely have symptoms of blood dyscrasias, which can include infection, bleeding, and poor healing.
- Patients with active TB should not be treated.
- Medical consultation may be required to assess disease control.
- Examine for evidence of oral signs of disease.
- Do not treat patients with active tuberculosis.

Consultations:

- In a patient with symptoms of blood dyscrasias, request a medical consultation for blood studies and postpone dental treatment until normal values are reestablished.

Teach Patient/Family to:

- Use caution to prevent injury when using oral hygiene aids.

isosorbide

eye-soe-**sor′**-bide

isosorbide dinitrate (Apo-ISDN[CAN], Cedocard[CAN], Dilatrate, Isogen[AUS], Isordil, Sorbidin[AUS]); isosorbide mononitrate (Duride[AUS], Imdur, Imtrate[AUS], ISMO, Monodur Durules[AUS], Monoket)

Do not confuse with Inderal, Isuprel, K-Dur, or Plendil.

CATEGORY AND SCHEDULE

Pregnancy Risk Category: C

Drug Class: Nitrate antianginal

MECHANISM OF ACTION

A nitrate that stimulates intracellular cyclic guanosine monophosphate (cGMP).

Therapeutic Effect: Relaxes vascular smooth muscle of both arterial and venous vasculature. Decreases preload and afterload.

USES

Treatment of chronic stable angina pectoris

PHARMACOKINETICS

Route	Onset	Peak	Duration
Sublingual	2–10 min	N/A	1–2 days
Chewable	3 min	N/A	0.5–2 hr
PO	45–60 min	N/A	4–6 hr
Sustained-release	30 min	N/A	6–12 hr

Mononitrate well absorbed after PO administration. Dinitrate poorly absorbed and metabolized in the liver to its activate metabolite isosorbide mononitrate. Excreted in urine and feces. ***Half-life:*** 1–4 hr, dinitrate; 4 hr, mononitrate.

INDICATIONS AND DOSAGES

▸ Acute Angina, Prophylactic Management in Situations Likely to Provoke Attack

Sublingual

Adults, Elderly. Initially, 2.5–5 mg. Repeat at 5–10 min intervals. No more than 3 doses in 15–30 min period.

▸ Acute Prophylactic Management of Angina

Sublingual

Adults, Elderly. 5–10 mg q2–3h.

▸ Long-Term Prophylaxis of Angina

PO

Adults, Elderly. Initially, 5–20 mg 3–4 times a day. Maintenance: 10–40 mg q6h. Consider 2–3 times a day, last dose no later than 7 PM to minimize intolerance.

PO (Mononitrate)

Adults, Elderly. 20 mg 2 times a day, 7 hr apart. First dose upon awakening in morning.

PO (Extended Release)

Adults, Elderly. Initially, 40 mg. Maintenance: 40–80 mg 2–3 times a day. Consider 1–2 times a day, last dose at 2 PM to minimize intolerance.

PO (Imdur)

Adults, Elderly. 60–120 mg/day as single dose.

▸ CHF

PO (Chewable)

Adults, Elderly. 5–10 mg every 2–3 hr.

SIDE EFFECTS/ADVERSE REACTIONS

Frequent

Burning and tingling at oral point of dissolution (sublingual), headache (may be severe) occurs mostly in early therapy, diminishes rapidly in intensity, usually disappears during continued treatment; transient flushing of face and neck, dizziness (especially if patient is standing immobile or is in a warm environment), weakness, postural hypotension, nausea, vomiting, restlessness

Occasional

GI upset, blurred vision, dry mouth

PRECAUTIONS AND CONTRAINDICATIONS

Closed-angle glaucoma, GI hypermotility or malabsorption (extended-release tablets), head trauma, hypersensitivity to nitrates, increased intracranial pressure, postural hypotension, severe anemia (extended-release tablets)

Caution:

Postural hypotension, lactation, children

DRUG INTERACTIONS OF CONCERN TO DENTISTRY

• Increased effects: alcohol, other vasodilator-type drugs
• Severe hypotension: sildenafil, vardenafil, tadalafil

SERIOUS REACTIONS

! Blurred vision or dry mouth may occur (drug should be discontinued).
! Severe postural hypotension manifested by fainting, pulselessness, cold or clammy skin, and diaphoresis may occur.
! Tolerance may occur with repeated, prolonged therapy (minor tolerance with intermittent use of sublingual tablets). Tolerance may not occur with extended-release form.
! High dose tends to produce severe headache.

DENTAL CONSIDERATIONS

General:

• Monitor vital signs at every appointment because of cardiovascular side effects.
• After supine positioning, have patient sit upright for at least 2 min before standing to avoid orthostatic hypotension.
• Stress from dental procedures may compromise cardiovascular function; determine patient risk.
• Assess salivary flow as a factor in caries, periodontal disease, and candidiasis.
• Short appointments and a stress-reduction protocol may be required for anxious patients.
• Consider semisupine chair position for patients with respiratory distress.
• Use vasoconstrictors with caution, in low doses, and with careful aspiration. Avoid use of gingival retraction cord with epinephrine.
• Nitroglycerin should be available in case of an acute anginal episode.

Consultations:

• Medical consultation may be required to assess disease control and patient's ability to tolerate stress.

Teach Patient/Family:

• When chronic dry mouth occurs, advise patient to:
  • Avoid mouth rinses with high alcohol content because of drying effects.
  • Use sugarless gum, frequent sips of water, or saliva substitutes.
  • Use daily home fluoride products for anticaries effect.

isosorbide dinitrate/ isosorbide mononitrate

ahy-suh-**sawr**′-bayd
dye-**nye**′-trate
isosorbide dinitrate (Apo-ISDN[CAN], Cedocard[CAN], Dilatrate, Isogen[AUS], Isordil, Sorbidin[AUS]); isosorbide mononitrate (Duride[AUS], Imdur, Imdur Durules[AUS], Imtrate[AUS], ISMO, Monodur Durules[AUS], Monoket)
Do not confuse Isordil with Isuprel or Plendil, or Imdur with Inderal or K-Dur.

CATEGORY AND SCHEDULE

Pregnancy Risk Category: C

Drug Class: Nitrate antianginal

MECHANISM OF ACTION

A nitrate that stimulates intracellular cyclic guanosine monophosphate.
Therapeutic Effect: Relaxes vascular smooth muscle of both arterial and venous vasculature. Decreases preload and afterload.

USES

Treatment of chronic stable angina pectoris

PHARMACOKINETICS

Route	Onset	Peak	Duration
Dinitrate	2–5 min	N/A	1–2 hr
Sublingual oral (chewable)	2–5 min	N/A	1–2 hr
Oral	15–40 min	N/A	4–6 hr
Oral sustained (release)	30 min	N/A	12 hr
Mononitrate oral (extended release)	60 min	N/A	N/A

Dinitrate poorly absorbed and metabolized in the liver to its active metabolite isosorbide mononitrate. Mononitrate well absorbed after PO administration. Excreted in urine and feces. ***Half-life:*** Dinitrate, 1–4 hr; mononitrate, 4 hr.

INDICATIONS AND DOSAGES

▸ Angina

PO (Isosorbide Dinitrate)

Adults, Elderly. 5–40 mg 4 times a day. Sustained-release: 40 mg q8–12h.

PO (Isosorbide Mononitrate)

Adults, Elderly. 5–10 mg twice a day given 7 hr apart. Sustained-release: Initially, 30–60 mg/day in morning as a single dose. May increase dose at 3-day intervals. Maximum: 240 mg/day.

SIDE EFFECTS/ADVERSE REACTIONS

Frequent

Burning and tingling at oral point of dissolution (sublingual), headache (possibly severe) occurs mostly in early therapy, diminishes rapidly in intensity, and usually disappears during continued treatment, transient flushing of face and neck, dizziness (especially if patient is standing immobile or is in a warm environment), weakness, orthostatic hypotension, nausea, vomiting, restlessness

Occasional

GI upset, blurred vision, dry mouth

PRECAUTIONS AND CONTRAINDICATIONS

Closed-angle glaucoma, GI hypermotility or malabsorption (extended-release tablets), head trauma, hypersensitivity to nitrates, increased intracranial pressure, orthostatic hypotension, severe anemia (extended-release tablets)

DRUG INTERACTIONS OF CONCERN TO DENTISTRY

- Increased effects: alcohol and other drugs that can lower B/P
- Severe hypotension: sildenafil, vardenafil, tadalafil

SERIOUS REACTIONS

! Blurred vision or dry mouth may occur (drug should be discontinued).

! Isosorbide administration may cause severe orthostatic hypotension manifested by fainting, pulselessness, cold or clammy skin, and diaphoresis.

! Tolerance may occur with repeated, prolonged therapy, but may not occur with the extended-release form. Minor tolerance may be seen with intermittent use of sublingual tablets.

! High dosage tends to produce severe headache.

DENTAL CONSIDERATIONS

General:

- Monitor vital signs at every appointment because of cardiovascular side effects.
- After supine positioning, have patient sit upright for at least 2 min before standing to avoid orthostatic hypotension.

I

• Assess salivary flow as a factor in caries, periodontal disease, and candidiasis.
• Stress from dental procedures may compromise cardiovascular function; determine patient risk.
• Use vasoconstrictors with caution, in low doses, and with careful aspiration. Avoid use of gingival retraction cord with epinephrine.
• Short appointments and a stress-reduction protocol may be required for anxious patients.
• Nitroglycerin should be available in case of acute anginal episode.

Consultations:

• Medical consultation may be required to assess disease control and patient's ability to tolerate stress.

Teach Patient/Family to:

• Encourage effective oral hygiene to prevent soft tissue inflammation.
• When chronic dry mouth occurs, advise patient to:
  • Avoid mouth rinses with high alcohol content because of drying effects.
  • Use sugarless gum, frequent sips of water, or saliva substitutes.
  • Use daily home fluoride products for anticaries effect.

isoxsuprine hydrochloride

eye-**sox**′-soo-preen high-droh-**klor**′-ide (Vasodilan)

CATEGORY AND SCHEDULE

Pregnancy Risk Category: C

Drug Class: Peripheral vasodilator

MECHANISM OF ACTION

The mechanism of action of isoxsuprine hydrochloride is not fully understood. Increases muscle blood flow. May have a direct action on vascular smooth muscle. β-adrenergic stimulation of the uterus.

Therapeutic Effect: Relieves symptoms associated with cerebral vascular insufficiency. Inhibits preterm labor.

USES

Treatment of symptoms of cerebrovascular insufficiency; peripheral vascular disease, including arteriosclerosis obliterans, thromboangiitis obliterans, Raynaud's disease

PHARMACOKINETICS

The pharmacokinetics of isoxsuprine hydrochloride is not fully understood. ***Half-life:*** Unknown.

INDICATIONS AND DOSAGES

▸ **Raynaud's Syndrome**

IV Infusion

Adults, Elderly. 10–20 mg 3–4 times a day.

SIDE EFFECTS/ADVERSE REACTIONS

Rare

Hypotension, tachyarrhythmia, rash, abdominal discomfort, nausea, dizziness

PRECAUTIONS AND CONTRAINDICATIONS

Arterial bleeding (recent), immediately postpartum

Caution:

Tachycardia

DRUG INTERACTIONS OF CONCERN TO DENTISTRY

• Increased effects: alcohol and drugs that also lower B/P

SERIOUS REACTIONS

! Pulmonary edema occurs rarely.

DENTAL CONSIDERATIONS

General:

• Monitor vital signs at every appointment because of cardiovascular and respiratory side effects.
• After supine positioning, have patient sit upright for at least 2 min before standing to avoid orthostatic hypotension.
• Short appointments and a stress-reduction protocol may be required for anxious patients.
• Drugs used for conscious sedation that lower B/P may potentiate the hypotensive effects.
• Use vasoconstrictors with caution, in low doses, and with careful aspiration. Avoid use of gingival retraction cord with epinephrine.

Consultations:

• Medical consultation may be required to assess disease control and patient's ability to tolerate stress.

isradipine

is-**rad**′-ih-peen
(DynaCirc, DynaCirc CR)
Do not confuse DynaCirc with Dynabac or Dynacin.

CATEGORY AND SCHEDULE

Pregnancy Risk Category: C

Drug Class: Calcium channel blocker

MECHANISM OF ACTION

An antihypertensive that inhibits calcium movement across cardiac and vascular smooth-muscle cell membranes. Potent peripheral vasodilator that does not depress SA or AV nodes.
Therapeutic Effect: Produces relaxation of coronary vascular smooth muscle and coronary vasodilation. Increases myocardial oxygen delivery to those with vasospastic angina.

USES

Treatment of essential hypertension, alone or with a thiazide diuretic; unapproved: angina, Raynaud's disease

PHARMACOKINETICS

Route	Onset	Peak	Duration
PO	2–3 hr	2–4 wk (with multiple doses) 8–16 hr (with single dose)	N/A
PO (controlled-release)	2 hr	8–10 hr	N/A

Well absorbed from the GI tract. Protein binding: 95%. Metabolized in the liver (undergoes first-pass effect). Primarily excreted in urine. Not removed by hemodialysis.
Half-life: 8 hr.

INDICATIONS AND DOSAGES

▸ **Hypertension**

PO

Adults, Elderly. Initially 2.5 mg twice a day. May increase by 2.5 mg at 2- to 4-wk intervals. Range: 5–20 mg/day

SIDE EFFECTS/ADVERSE REACTIONS

Frequent
Peripheral edema, palpitations (higher frequency in females)
Occasional
Facial flushing, cough, gingival enlargement
Rare
Angina, tachycardia, rash, pruritus

PRECAUTIONS AND CONTRAINDICATIONS

Cardiogenic shock, CHF, heart block, hypotension, sinus bradycardia, ventricular tachycardia
Caution:
CHF, hypotension, hepatic disease, lactation, children, renal disease, elderly

DRUG INTERACTIONS OF CONCERN TO DENTISTRY

• Decreased effect: indomethacin, possibly other NSAIDs, phenobarbital
• Increased effect: parenteral and inhalational general anesthetics, other drugs with hypotensive actions, itraconazole
• Increased effects of carbamazepine

SERIOUS REACTIONS

! Overdose produces nausea, drowsiness, confusion, and slurred speech.
! CHF occurs rarely.

DENTAL CONSIDERATIONS

General:
• Monitor cardiac status; take vital signs at each appointment because of cardiovascular side effects. Consider a stress-reduction protocol to prevent stress-induced angina during the dental appointment.
• After supine positioning, have patient sit upright for at least 2 min before standing to avoid orthostatic hypotension.
• Place on frequent recall to monitor for possible gingival enlargement.
• Limit use of sodium-containing products, such as saline IV fluids, for patients with a dietary salt restriction.
• Assess salivary flow as a factor in caries, periodontal disease, and candidiasis.
• Use vasoconstrictors with caution, in low doses, and with careful aspiration. Avoid use of gingival retraction cord with epinephrine.
• Patients on chronic drug therapy may rarely have symptoms of blood dyscrasias, which can include infection, bleeding, and poor healing.
Consultations:
• In a patient with symptoms of blood dyscrasias, request a medical consultation for blood studies and postpone dental treatment until normal values are reestablished.
• Medical consultation may be required to assess disease control and patient's ability to tolerate stress.
Teach Patient/Family to:
• Encourage effective oral hygiene to prevent soft tissue inflammation and minimize gingival enlargement.
• Schedule frequent oral prophylaxis.
• When chronic dry mouth occurs, advise patient to:
  • Avoid mouth rinses with high alcohol content because of drying effects.
  • Use sugarless gum, frequent sips of water, or saliva substitutes.
  • Use daily home fluoride products for anticaries effect.

itraconazole

it-ra-**con**′-ah-zoll
(Sporanox)
Do not confuse Sporanox with Suprax.

CATEGORY AND SCHEDULE

Pregnancy Risk Category: C

Drug Class: Antifungal, systemic (triazole)

MECHANISM OF ACTION

A fungistatic antifungal that inhibits the synthesis of ergosterol, a vital component of fungal cell formation. ***Therapeutic Effect:*** Damages the fungal cell membrane, altering its function.

USES

Treatment of aspergillosis, blastomycosis, histoplasmosis (pulmonary and extrapulmonary); fungal infections of nails (onychomycosis); *Candida* infections of esophagus or mouth (oral sol only)

PHARMACOKINETICS

Moderately absorbed from the GI tract. Absorption is increased if the drug is taken with food. Protein binding: 99%. Widely distributed, primarily in the fatty tissue, liver, and kidneys. Metabolized in the liver to active metabolite. Primarily excreted in urine. Not removed by hemodialysis. ***Half-life:*** 21 hr; metabolite, 12 hr.

INDICATIONS AND DOSAGES

▸ **Blastomycosis, Histoplasmosis**

PO

Adults, Elderly. Initially, 200 mg once a day. Maximum: 400 mg/day in 2 divided doses.

IV

Adults, Elderly. 200 mg twice a day for 4 doses, then 200 mg once a day.

▸ **Aspergillosis**

PO

Adults, Elderly. 600 mg/day in 3 divided doses for 3–4 days, then 200–400 mg/day in 2 divided doses.

IV

Adults, Elderly. 200 mg twice a day for 4 doses, then 200 mg once a day.

▸ **Esophageal Candidiasis**

PO

Adults, Elderly. Swish 10 ml in mouth for several seconds, then swallow. Maximum: 200 mg/day.

▸ **Oropharyngeal Candidiasis**

PO

Adults, Elderly. Vigorously swish 10 ml in mouth for several seconds (20 ml total daily dose) once a day.

SIDE EFFECTS/ADVERSE REACTIONS

Frequent

Nausea, rash

Occasional

Vomiting, headache, diarrhea, hypertension, peripheral edema, fatigue, fever

Rare

Abdominal pain, dizziness, anorexia, pruritus

PRECAUTIONS AND CONTRAINDICATIONS

Hypersensitivity to itraconazole, fluconazole, ketoconazole, or miconazole

Caution:

Lactation, liver toxicity, oral anticoagulants (monitor patient), strong inhibitor of CYP3A4 isoenzymes—note drug interactions

DRUG INTERACTIONS OF CONCERN TO DENTISTRY

• Increased risk of rhabdomyolysis: lovastatin, simvastatin

• Increased risk of hypoglycemia: oral antidiabetics
• Increased metabolism: phenobarbital, carbamazepine
• May increase plasma levels of cyclosporine
• Increased CNS depression with triazolam, midazolam (inhibits metabolism of certain benzodiazepines: (e.g., midazolam, triazolam), buspirone, allopurinol (Zyloprim), felodipine)
• Decreased effects: didanosine
• Increased plasma levels: saquinavir, nisoldipine, haloperidol, carbamazepine, erythromycin, clarithromycin
• Avoid itraconazole use with HMG-CoA reductase inhibitors (statins) or lower their dose
• May inhibit warfarin metabolism
• Suspected increase in plasma levels: cola beverages
• Decrease in plasma levels: grapefruit juice
• Decreased effects: didanosine (take 2 hr before didanosine tabs)
• May increase levels and side effects of HMG-CoA reductase inhibitors (statins)
• Increased plasma levels of alfentanil, buspirone, carbamazepine, corticosteroids, zolpidem
• Suspected decrease in oral contractive effectiveness; suggest alternative method of contraception

SERIOUS REACTIONS

! Hepatitis (as evidenced by anorexia, abdominal pain, unusual fatigue or weakness, jaundiced skin or sclera, and dark urine) occurs rarely.

DENTAL CONSIDERATIONS

General:
• Monitor vital signs at every appointment because of cardiovascular side effects.
• Determine why the patient is taking the drug.
• Consider semisupine chair position for patient comfort because of GI effects of drug.
Consultations:
• Medical consultation may be required to assess patient's ability to tolerate stress.

ivacaftor

eye-va-**kaf'**-tor
(Kalydeco)

CATEGORY AND SCHEDULE

Pregnancy Risk Category: B

Drug Class: Cystic fibrosis transmembrane conductance regulator potentiator

MECHANISM OF ACTION

Potentiates epithelial cell chloride ion transport of defective (G551D mutant) cell-surface CFTR protein, thereby improving the regulation of salt and water absorption and secretion in various tissues (e.g., lung, gastrointestinal tract).
Therapeutic Effect: Targets the genetic defect that causes cystic fibrosis.

USES

Treatment of cystic fibrosis (CF) in patients who have a G551D mutation in the cystic fibrosis transmembrane conductance regulator (CFTR) gene

PHARMACOKINETICS

Variable absorption after oral administration; increased (by two- to fourfold) with fatty foods. 99% plasma protein bound. Extensive hepatic metabolism via CYP3A4 to active and inactive metabolites. Excreted primarily via feces (88%). *Half-life:* 12 hr.

INDICATIONS AND DOSAGES

▸ Cystic Fibrosis

Oral

Adults. 150 mg every 12 hr. Administer with high-fat-containing foods.

Children older than 6 yr. 150 mg every 12 hr.

▸ Dosage in Hepatic Impairment

Moderate impairment (Child-Pugh class B): 150 mg once daily.

Severe impairment (Child-Pugh class C): Not recommended for use.

SIDE EFFECTS/ADVERSE REACTIONS

Frequent

Headache, nasal congestion, nasopharyngitis, rash, abdominal pain, diarrhea, nausea, upper respiratory tract infection, nasal congestion

Occasional

Dizziness, acne, hyperglycemia, arthralgia, pharyngeal erythema

PRECAUTIONS AND CONTRAINDICATIONS

Avoid use in patients with severe hepatic and renal impairment.

DRUG INTERACTIONS OF CONCERN TO DENTISTRY

- CYP3A4 inhibitors (e.g., macrolide antibiotics, azole antifungals): increased risk of adverse effects of ivacaftor
- CYP3A4 inducers (e.g., rifampin, St. John's wort): reduced effectiveness of ivacaftor

SERIOUS REACTIONS

! None known

DENTAL CONSIDERATIONS

General:

- Adverse effects include dizziness; precautions should be taken when seating and dismissing the patient.
- Patients taking ivacaftor may experience oropharyngeal pain, nasopharyngitis, nasal congestion, and upper respiratory tract infections, and this should be considered in the diagnosis of oropharyngeal pain and infections and positioning patient for comfort.
- Avoid prescribing drugs associated with nausea and respiratory depression (e.g., opioids).

Consultations:

- Consult physician to determine disease status and ability of patient to tolerate dental procedures.

Teach Patient/Family to:

- Report changes in disease status and medication regimen.

ivermectin

eye-ver-mek-tin

(Sklice)

CATEGORY AND SCHEDULE

Pregnancy Risk Category: C

Drug Class: Antiparasitic agent, topical; pediculocide

MECHANISM OF ACTION

Ivermectin is a semisynthetic anthelminthic agent that binds selectively to glutamate-gated chloride ion channels. This increases permeability of cell membranes to chloride ions, then hyperpolarization of the nerve or muscle cell, and finally death of the parasite.

Therapeutic Effect: Pediculicidal

USES
Topical treatment of head lice (*Pediculus capitis*) infestation

PHARMACOKINETICS
Minimal systemic absorption with proper application. ***Half-life:*** None reported.

INDICATIONS AND DOSAGES
▸ **Head Lice**

Topical

Adults, Children older than 6 mo. Apply sufficient amount (up to 1 tube) to completely cover dry scalp and hair; for single-dose use only.

SIDE EFFECTS/ADVERSE REACTIONS
Frequent

Burning sensation on skin

Occasional

Conjunctivitis, dandruff, dry skin, eye irritation, ocular hyperemia

PRECAUTIONS AND CONTRAINDICATIONS
None reported

DRUG INTERACTIONS OF CONCERN TO DENTISTRY
• None reported

SERIOUS REACTIONS
! None known

DENTAL CONSIDERATIONS
General:

• Avoid contact with and irritation of areas being treated.

Teach Patient/Family to:

• Report changes in disease status and medication regimen.

ixabepilone
ix-ab-**ep′**-i-lone

(Ixempra)

CATEGORY AND SCHEDULE
Pregnancy Risk Category: D

Drug Class: Antineoplastic agent, antimicrotubular, epothilone B analog

MECHANISM OF ACTION
Semisynthetic analog of epothilone B. Inhibits microtubules, stops cell division in the G2-M phase and results in subsequent cell death. Suppresses the dynamic instability of beta-tubulin subunits (alpha-beta-II and alpha-beta-III).

USES
Breast cancer, metastatic or locally advanced, as monotherapy in patients whose tumors are resistant or refractory to anthracyclines, taxanes, and capecitabine

Breast cancer, metastatic or locally advanced, in combination with capecitabine in patients who are resistant to treatment with an anthracycline and a taxane, or whose cancer is taxane resistant and for whom further anthracycline therapy is contraindicated

PHARMACOKINETICS
Protein binding: 67% to 77%. Extensively metabolized in liver via CYP3A4. At least 30 identified metabolites (inactive). Primarily excreted in feces (65%); urine (21%). ***Half-life:*** 52 hr.

INDICATIONS AND DOSAGES
Adult. Breast cancer as monotherapy or combination with capecitabine: 40 mg/m^2 IV over 3 hr every 3 wk.

Note: All patients must premedicate with an oral H_1-antagonist (e.g., diphenhydramine 50 mg) and an oral H_2-antagonist (e.g., ranitidine 150–300 mg) 1 hr prior to infusion. Patients with a history of hypersensitivity should premedicate with corticosteroids (e.g., dexamethasone 20 mg) intravenously 30 min prior to infusion or orally 60 min prior to infusion. Body surface area (BSA) is capped at a maximum of 2.2 m^2.
Pediatric. Safety and efficacy have not been established in pediatric patients.

DOSE ADJUSTMENT

Avoid concurrent use of CYP3A4 inhibitors. If concomitant use is necessary, reduce ixabepilone dose to 20 mg/m^2. When a CYP3A4 inhibitor is discontinued, allow a 1-wk washout prior to increasing dose of ixabepilone.
Hepatic impairment (bilirubin greater than 1.5 times upper limit of normal [ULN] and up to 3 times ULN and AST/ALT of up to 10 times ULN), when used as monotherapy: starting dose of 20 mg/m^2; may escalate dose up to 30 mg/m^2 maximum in subsequent cycles.
Febrile neutropenia: reduce dose by 20% when given either as monotherapy or in combination with capecitabine.

SIDE EFFECTS/ADVERSE REACTIONS

Frequent
Alopecia, nail changes, abdominal pain, constipation, diarrhea, nausea, stomatitis, vomiting
Occasional
Edema, hot flush, chest pain, fever, pain, dizziness, insomnia

PRECAUTIONS AND CONTRAINDICATIONS

Contraindicated in combination with capecitabine in patients with AST or ALT greater than 2.5 times ULN or bilirubin greater than 1 time ULN because of increased risk of toxicity and neutropenia-related death
Hypersensitivity reaction to Cremophor El or its derivatives
Contraindicated in patients with neutrophil count less than 1500 cells/mm^3
Contraindicated in patients with platelet count less than 100,000 cells/mm^3
Use with caution in patients with cardiovascular diseases, diabetes (increased risk of severe neuropathy), and in patients taking alcohol-containing products, CYP450 3A4 inhibitors, and inducers. Ixabepilone can cause myelosuppression, peripheral neuropathy (especially during the first 3 cycles of treatment), and cognitive impairment.
Alcohol-containing product (39.8% dehydrated alcohol)

DRUG INTERACTIONS OF CONCERN TO DENTISTRY

- CYP3A4 inhibitors (e.g., erythromycin): May increase levels and adverse effects of ixabepilone

SERIOUS REACTIONS

! Patients with liver impairment may have an increase in the risk of hepatic toxicity and neutropenia-related death.
! Left ventricular dysfunction, myocardial ischemia, myelosuppression, and peripheral neuropathy may occur.

I

DENTAL CONSIDERATIONS

General:

- If additional analgesia is required for dental pain, consider alternative analgesics (acetaminophen) in patient taking opioids for acute or chronic pain.
- Avoid alcohol-containing products (elixirs, mouth rinses) to assist maintenance of alcohol abstinence.
- Stomatitis, mucositis, and dysgeusia may occur and complicate dental treatment.

Consultations:

- Medical consultation may be required to assess disease control and patient's ability to tolerate stress.

Teach Patient/Family to:

- Encourage effective oral hygiene to prevent soft tissue inflammation.
- Prevent trauma when using oral hygiene aids.
- Avoid mouth rinses with high alcohol content because of drying effect.
- Update health and medication history if physician makes any changes in evaluation or drug regimens; include OTC, herbal, and nonherbal remedies in the update.
- Be alert for the possibility of stomatitis, mucositis, and taste alterations and the need to see dentist immediately if signs of inflammation occur.

kanamycin sulfate

kan-ah-**mye′**-sin **suhl′**-feyt
(Kantrex)

CATEGORY AND SCHEDULE

Pregnancy Risk Category: Unavailable for irrigating solution

Drug Class: Aminoglycoside; antibiotic

MECHANISM OF ACTION

An aminoglycoside antibiotic that irreversibly binds to protein on bacterial ribosomes.
Therapeutic Effect: Interferes with protein synthesis of susceptible microorganisms, bacteriostatic.

USES

Treatment of wound, surgical site irrigation

INDICATIONS AND DOSAGES

Wound and Surgical Site Irrigation
Adults, Elderly. 0.25% solution to irrigate pleural space, ventricular or abscess cavities, wounds, or surgical sites.

SIDE EFFECTS/ADVERSE REACTIONS

Occasional
Hypersensitivity reactions (fever, pruritus, rash, urticaria)
Rare
Headache

PRECAUTIONS AND CONTRAINDICATIONS

Hypersensitivity to kanamycin, other aminoglycosides (cross-sensitivity), or their components

DRUG INTERACTIONS OF CONCERN TO DENTISTRY

- Increased risk of nephrotoxicity, ototoxicity and neuromuscular blockade: concurrent use with other aminoglycosides
- Risk of inactivation: β-lactam antiinfectives

SERIOUS REACTIONS

! None known

DENTAL CONSIDERATIONS

General:
- For selected infections in the hospital setting, provide palliative emergency dental treatment only.
- Examine for oral manifestation of opportunistic infection.
- Determine why patient is taking the drug.
- Caution regarding allergy to medication.

Consultations:
- Medical consultation may be required to assess disease control.

Teach Patient/Family to:
- Encourage effective oral hygiene to prevent soft tissue inflammation.
- Report oral lesions, soreness, or bleeding to dentist.
- Prevent trauma when using oral hygiene aids.

ketamine

key′-tah-meen
(Ketalar)

CATEGORY AND SCHEDULE

Pregnancy Risk Category: B

Drug Class: Anesthetic, general

MECHANISM OF ACTION
A rapidly acting general anesthetic that selectively blocks afferent impulses and interacts with CNS transmitter systems.
Therapeutic Effect: Produces an anesthetic state characterized by profound analgesia and normal pharyngeal-laryngeal reflexes.

USES
Production of loss of consciousness before and during surgery

PHARMACOKINETICS

Route	Onset	Peak	Duration
IM (anesthetic)	3–4 min	N/A	12–25 min
IM (analgesic)	30 min	N/A	15–30 min
IV (anesthetic)	30 sec	N/A	5–10 min
IV (analgesic)	10–15 min	N/A	N/A

Rapidly distributed. Metabolized in the liver. Primarily excreted in urine. ***Half-life:*** Distribution: 10–15 min, elimination: 2–3 hr.

INDICATIONS AND DOSAGES
▸ Sole Anesthetic for Short Diagnostic and Surgical Procedures That Do Not Require Skeletal Muscle Relaxation, Induction of Anesthesia Before Administering Other General Anesthetics, Supplement to Low-Potency Agents
IV
Adults, Elderly. 1–4.5 mg/kg.
Children. 0.5–2 mg/kg.
IM
Adults, Elderly. 3–8 mg/kg.
Children. 3–7 mg/kg.

SIDE EFFECTS/ADVERSE REACTIONS
Frequent
Increased B/P and pulse rate; emergence reaction (marked by dreamlike state, delirium, hallucinations, and vivid imagery and occasionally accompanied by confusion, excitement, and irrational behavior; lasts from a few hr to 24 hr after ketamine administration)
Occasional
Pain at injection site
Rare
Rash

PRECAUTIONS AND CONTRAINDICATIONS
Aneurysms, angina, CHF, elevated intracranial pressure, hypertension, psychotic disorders, thyrotoxicosis

DRUG INTERACTIONS OF CONCERN TO DENTISTRY
- Increased risk of hypotension and respiratory depression: all CNS depressants

SERIOUS REACTIONS
! Continuous or repeated intermittent infusion may result in extreme somnolence and circulatory or respiratory depression.
! Too-rapid IV administration of ketamine may produce severe hypotension, respiratory depression, and irregular muscle movements.
! Prolonged respiratory depression: nondepolarizing muscle relaxants.

DENTAL CONSIDERATIONS
General:
- Warning: Ketamine should be administered by persons trained in the administration of general anesthesia. Patients must be continually monitored, and facilities for maintenance of a patent airway,

ventilatory support, oxygen supplementation, and circulatory resuscitation must be immediately available. Strict aseptic technique must be followed in handling ketamine.
• Monitor for increased B/P and pulse rate; emergence reactions including hallucinations, delirium, dreamlike states, vivid imagery often accompanied by confusion, excitement, and irrational behavior.
• Responsible person must drive the patient home after recovery.
• Use safety measures: side rails, night light, and call bell within reach.

Consultations:
• Consultation with physician may be necessary if sedation or general anesthesia is required.

Teach Patient/Family to:
• Avoid performing tasks that require mental alertness or motor skills for 24 hr after anesthesia has been discontinued.

ketoconazole

kee-toe-**kon**′-ah-zole
(Apo-Ketocomazole[CAN], Nizoral, Nizoral AD, Sebizole[AUS])
Do not confuse Nizoral with Nasarel.

CATEGORY AND SCHEDULE

Pregnancy Risk Category: C
OTC (1% shampoo only)

Drug Class: Imidazole antifungal

MECHANISM OF ACTION

A fungistatic antifungal that inhibits the synthesis of ergosterol, a vital component of fungal cell formation.
Therapeutic Effect: Damages the fungal cell membrane, altering its function.

USES

Treatment of systemic candidiasis, chronic mucocutaneous candidiasis, cutaneous candidiasis, candiduria, coccidioidomycosis, histoplasmosis, chromomycosis, para-coccidioidomycosis, severe recalcitrant cutaneous dermatophyte infections

PHARMACOKINETICS

PO: Peak 1–2 hr. ***Half-life:*** 2 hr, terminal 8 hr; highly protein bound; metabolized in liver; excreted in bile, feces; requires acid pH for absorption; distributed poorly to CSF.

INDICATIONS AND DOSAGES

▸ **Histoplasmosis, Blastomycosis, Systemic Candidiasis, Chronic Mucocutaneous Candidiasis, Coccidioidomycosis, Paracoccidioidomycosis, Chromomycosis, Seborrheic Dermatitis, *Tinea Corporis, Tinea Capitis, Tinea Manus, Tinea Cruris, Tinea Pedis, Tinea Unguium* (Onychomycosis), Oral Thrush, Candiduria**

PO
Adults, Elderly. 200–400 mg/day.
Children. 3.3–6.6 mg/kg/day. Maximum: 800 mg/day in 2 divided doses.

Topical
Adults, Elderly. Apply to affected area 1–2 times a day for 2–4 wk.

Shampoo
Adults, Elderly. Use twice a wk for 4 wk, allowing at least 3 days between shampooing. Use intermittently to maintain control.

K

SIDE EFFECTS/ADVERSE REACTIONS

Occasional
Nausea, vomiting
Rare
Abdominal pain, diarrhea, headache, dizziness, photophobia, pruritus
Topical: itching, burning, irritation

PRECAUTIONS AND CONTRAINDICATIONS

Hypersensitivity, lactation, fungal meningitis, loratadine, triazolam, dofetilide
Caution:
Renal disease, hepatic disease, drug-induced achlorhydria, potent inhibitor of CYP3A4 isoenzymes

K

DRUG INTERACTIONS OF CONCERN TO DENTISTRY

- Hepatotoxicity: alcohol, high-dose long-term use, acetaminophen, carbamazepine, sulfonamides
- Decreased absorption: antacids (take 2 hr after ketoconazole), proton pump inhibitors
- Leukocyte disorders: tacrolimus
- Contraindicated with triazolam, lovastatin, dofetilide
- Inhibits the metabolism of benzodiazepines (e.g., midazolam, triazolam)
- May inhibit metabolism of warfarin
- Decreased effects: didanosine (take 2 hr before didanosine tabs)
- May increase plasma levels and side effects of HMG-CoA reductase inhibitors (statins), cyclosporine
- Increased serum levels of indinavir, saquinavir, ritonavir, nisoldipine, haloperidol, carbamazepine, tricyclic antidepressants, buspirone, zolpidem, corticosteroids
- Suspected decrease in oral contraceptive effectiveness; may need to suggest additional contraception

SERIOUS REACTIONS

! Hematologic toxicity (as evidenced by thrombocytopenia, hemolytic anemia, and leukopenia) occurs occasionally.
! Hepatotoxicity may occur within 1 wk to several mo after starting therapy.
! Anaphylaxis occurs rarely.

DENTAL CONSIDERATIONS

General:
- To prevent reinoculation of *Candida* infection, dispose of tooth brush or other contaminated oral hygiene devices used during period of infection.
- Determine if medication controls disease.
- Place on frequent recall to evaluate healing response.
- Assess salivary flow as a factor in caries, periodontal disease, and candidiasis.

Teach Patient/Family to:
- Avoid mouth rinses with high alcohol content because of drying effects.

ketoprofen

kee-toe-**proe′**-fen
(Apo-Keto[CAN], Novo-Keto-EC, Orudis[AUS], Orudis KT[CAN], Orudis SR[AUS], Oruvail, Oruvail SR[AUS], Rhodis[CAN])

CATEGORY AND SCHEDULE

Pregnancy Risk Category: B (D if used in third trimester or near delivery)
OTC (tablets)

Drug Class: Nonsteroidal antiinflammatory

MECHANISM OF ACTION

An NSAID that produces analgesic and antiinflammatory effects by inhibiting prostaglandin synthesis. ***Therapeutic Effect:*** Reduces the inflammatory response and intensity of pain.

USES

Treatment of osteoarthritis, rheumatoid arthritis, dysmenorrhea; OTC: minor aches and pains

PHARMACOKINETICS

PO: Peak 2 hr. ***Half-life:*** 3–3.5 hr; 99% plasma-protein binding; metabolized in liver; excreted in urine (metabolites), breast milk

INDICATIONS AND DOSAGES

▸ Acute or Chronic Rheumatoid Arthritis and Osteoarthritis

PO

Adults. Initially, 75 mg 3 times a day or 50 mg 4 times a day.

Elderly. Initially, 25–50 mg 3–4 times a day. Maintenance: 150–300 mg/day in 3–4 divided doses.

PO (Extended Release)

Adults, Elderly. 100–200 mg once a day.

▸ Mild-to-Moderate Pain, Dysmenorrhea

PO

Adults, Elderly. 25–50 mg q6–8h. Maximum: 300 mg/day.

▸ OTC Dosage

PO

Adults, Elderly. 12.5 mg q4–6h. Maximum: 6 tabs/day.

▸ Dosage in Renal Impairment

Mild. 150 mg/day maximum.

Severe. 100 mg/day maximum.

SIDE EFFECTS/ADVERSE REACTIONS

Frequent

Dyspepsia

Occasional

Nausea, diarrhea or constipation, flatulence, abdominal cramps, headache

Rare

Anorexia, vomiting, visual disturbances, fluid retention

PRECAUTIONS AND CONTRAINDICATIONS

Active peptic ulcer disease, chronic inflammation of the GI tract, GI bleeding or ulceration, history of hypersensitivity to aspirin or NSAIDs

Caution:

Lactation, children, bleeding disorders, GI disorders, cardiac disorders, hypersensitivity to other antiinflammatory agents, elderly, children younger than 16 yr

Potential for increased adverse cardiovascular events in patients at risk for thromboembolism

DRUG INTERACTIONS OF CONCERN TO DENTISTRY

- GI ulceration, bleeding: aspirin, other NSAIDs, alcohol, corticosteroids
- Nephrotoxicity: acetaminophen (prolonged use)
- Possible risk of decreased renal function: cyclosporine
- Increased photosensitizing effect: tetracycline
- SSRIs: NSAIDs increase risk of GI side effects
- When prescribed for dental pain:
  - Risk of increased effects: oral anticoagulants, oral antidiabetics, lithium, methotrexate
  - Decreased effects of diuretics

SERIOUS REACTIONS

! Rare reactions with long-term use include peptic ulcer disease, GI bleeding, gastritis, severe hepatic reactions (cholestasis, jaundice), nephrotoxicity (dysuria, hematuria, proteinuria, nephrotic syndrome), and severe hypersensitivity reaction (bronchospasm, angioedema).

DENTAL CONSIDERATIONS

General:

- Increased risk of adverse effects in patients at risk of thromboembolism, history of stroke, MI.
- Patients on chronic drug therapy may rarely have symptoms of blood dyscrasias, which can include infection, bleeding, and poor healing.
- Assess salivary flow as a factor in caries, periodontal disease, and candidiasis.
- Avoid prescribing for dental use in pregnancy.
- Avoid prescribing aspirin-containing products or giving to patient taking aspirin.
- Consider semisupine chair position for patients with arthritic disease.
- Severe stomach bleeding may occur in patients who regularly use NSAIDs in recommended doses, when the patient is also taking another NSAID, a blood thinning, or steroid drug, if the patient has GI or peptic ulcer disease, if they are 60 yr or older, or when NSAIDs are taken longer than directed. Warn patients of the potential for severe stomach bleeding.

Consultations:

- In a patient with symptoms of blood dyscrasias, request a medical consultation for blood studies and postpone dental treatment until normal values are reestablished.
- Medical consultation may be required to assess disease control.

Teach Patient/Family to:

- Encourage effective oral hygiene to prevent soft tissue inflammation.
- Use caution to prevent injury when using oral hygiene aids.
  - Warn patient of potential risks of NSAIDs.
- When chronic dry mouth occurs, advise patient to:
  - Avoid mouth rinses with high alcohol content because of drying effects.
  - Use sugarless gum, frequent sips of water, or saliva substitutes.
  - Use daily home fluoride products for anticaries effect.

ketorolac tromethamine

kee-**tor′**-oh-lak
tro-**meth′**-ay-meen
(Acular, Acular LS, Acular PF, Toradol)
Do not confuse Acular with Acthar or Ocular.

CATEGORY AND SCHEDULE

Pregnancy Risk Category: C (D if used in third trimester)

Drug Class: Nonsteroidal antiinflammatory

MECHANISM OF ACTION

An NSAID that inhibits prostaglandin synthesis and reduces prostaglandin levels in the aqueous humor.

Therapeutic Effect: Relieves pain stimulus and reduces intraocular inflammation.

USES

Short-term treatment of acute mild-to-moderate pain

PHARMACOKINETICS

Route	Onset	Peak	Duration
PO	30–60 min	1.5–4 hr	4–6 hr
IV/IM	30 min	1–2 hr	4–6 hr

Readily absorbed from the GI tract, after IM administration. Protein binding: 99%. Largely metabolized in the liver. Primarily excreted in urine. Not removed by hemodialysis. ***Half-life:*** 3.8–6.3 hr (increased with impaired renal function and in the elderly).

INDICATIONS AND DOSAGES

▸ Short-Term Relief of Mild-to-Moderate Pain (Multiple Doses)

PO

Adults, Elderly. 10 mg q4–6h. Maximum: 40 mg/24 hr.

IV, IM

Adults younger than 65 yr. 30 mg q6h. Maximum: 120 mg/24 hr.

Adults 65 yr and older, those with renal impairment, those weighing less than 50 kg. 15 mg q6h. Maximum: 60 mg/24 hr.

Children 2–16 yr. 0.5 mg/kg q6h.

▸ Short-Term Relief of Mild-to-Moderate Pain (Single Dose)

IV

Adults younger than 65 yr, Children 17 yr and older weighing more than 50 kg. 30 mg.

Adults 65 yr and older, with renal impairment, weighing less than 50 kg. 15 mg.

Children 2–16 yr. 0.5 mg/kg. Maximum: 15 mg.

IM

Adults younger than 65 yr, Children 17 yr and older, weighing more than 50 kg. 60 mg.

Adults 65 yr and older, with renal impairment, weighing less than 50 kg. 30 mg.

Children 2–16 yr. 1 mg/kg. Maximum: 15 kg.

▸ Allergic Conjunctivitis

Ophthalmic

Adults, Elderly, Children 3 yr and older. 1 drop 4 times a day.

▸ Cataract Extraction

Ophthalmic

Adults, Elderly. 1 drop 4 times a day. Begin 24 hr after surgery and continue for 2 wk.

▸ Refractive Surgery

Ophthalmic

Adults, Elderly. 1 drop 4 times a day for 3 days.

SIDE EFFECTS/ADVERSE REACTIONS

Frequent

Headache, nausea, abdominal cramps or pain, dyspepsia, oral lichenoid reaction

Occasional

Diarrhea

Ophthalmic: Transient stinging and burning

Rare

Constipation, vomiting, flatulence, stomatitis, dizziness

Ophthalmic: Ocular irritation, allergic reactions, superficial ocular infection, keratitis

PRECAUTIONS AND CONTRAINDICATIONS

Active peptic ulcer disease, chronic inflammation of GI tract, GI bleeding or ulceration, history of hypersensitivity to aspirin or NSAIDs

Caution:

Children, GI disorders, cardiac disorders, hypersensitivity to other antiinflammatory agents

Increased potential for adverse cardiovascular events in patients at risk for thromboembolism

DRUG INTERACTIONS OF CONCERN TO DENTISTRY

- GI ulceration, bleeding: aspirin, alcohol, corticosteroids
- Contraindicated with probenecid
- Possible risk of decreased renal function: cyclosporine

• SSRIs: NSAIDs increase risk of GI side effects
• When prescribed for dental pain:
  • Risk of increased effects: oral anticoagulants, oral antidiabetics, lithium, methotrexate
  • Decreased antihypertensive effects of diuretics, β-blockers, ACE inhibitors

SERIOUS REACTIONS

! Rare reactions with long-term use include peptic ulcer disease, GI bleeding, gastritis, severe hepatic reactions (cholestasis, jaundice), nephrotoxicity (glomerular nephritis, interstitial nephritis, nephrotic syndrome), and an acute hypersensitivity reaction (including fever, chills, and joint pain).

DENTAL CONSIDERATIONS

General:
• Increased risk of adverse effects in patients at risk of thromboembolism, history of stroke, MI.
• Assess salivary flow as a factor in caries, periodontal disease, and candidiasis.
• Avoid prescribing in pregnancy.
• Avoid prescribing aspirin or other NSAIDs.
• Avoid long-term use for chronic pain syndromes; combined use of IV or IM and oral doses must not exceed 5 days.

Consultations:
• Medical consultation may be required to assess disease control.

Teach Patient/Family to:
• Avoid mouth rinses with high alcohol content because of drying effects.

▸ **Ketorolac Tromethamine (Ocular)**

General:
• Determine why patient is taking the drug.
• Avoid dental light in patient's eyes; offer dark glasses for patient comfort.

ketotifen fumarate

kee-toe-**tye′**-fen **fyoo′**-mah-rate
(Apo-Ketotifen[CAN], Novo-Ketotifen[CAN], Zaditen[CAN], Zaditor)

CATEGORY AND SCHEDULE

Pregnancy Risk Category: C

Drug Class: Antihistamine

MECHANISM OF ACTION

Selective histamine H_1-antagonist and mast cell stabilizer, suppresses release of mediators from cells involved in hypersensitivity reactions, and decreases chemotaxis and activation of eosinophils.
Therapeutic Effect: Reduces symptoms of allergic conjunctivitis.

USES

Temporary prevention of itching of the eyes caused by allergic conjunctivitis

PHARMACOKINETICS

None reported

INDICATIONS AND DOSAGES

▸ **Allergic Conjunctivitis**

Ophthalmic

Adults, Elderly, Children 3 yr or older. 1 drop into affected eye q8–12h.

SIDE EFFECTS/ADVERSE REACTIONS

Frequent

Conjunctival infection, headache, rhinitis

Occasional

Allergic reaction, burning, stinging, eyelid disorder, flu-like syndrome, keratitis, mydriasis, ocular discharge or pain, pharyngitis, photophobia, rash

PRECAUTIONS AND CONTRAINDICATIONS

Hypersensitivity to ketotifen or any component of the formulation (the preservative is benzalkonium chloride)

Caution:

Prevent contamination of ophthalmic solution by careful use, do not wear contact lens if eyes are red, delay inserting contacts up to 10 min after drops are placed in eyes; lactation, children younger than 3 yr

DRUG INTERACTIONS OF CONCERN TO DENTISTRY

• None reported

SERIOUS REACTIONS

! No serious signs and symptoms have been seen after ingestion up to 20 mg.

DENTAL CONSIDERATIONS

General:

• Avoid dental light in patient's eyes; offer dark glasses for patient comfort.

labetalol hydrochloride

la-**bet'**-ah-lole high-droh-**klor'**-ide
(Normodyne, Presolol[AUS], Trandate)
Do not confuse Trandate with tramadol or Trental.

CATEGORY AND SCHEDULE

Pregnancy Risk Category: C (D if used in second or third trimester)

Drug Class: Nonselective adrenergic β-blocker and selective α_1-blocker; antihypertensive

MECHANISM OF ACTION

An antihypertensive that blocks α_1-, β_1-, and β_2 (large doses)-adrenergic receptor sites. Large doses increase airway resistance.
Therapeutic Effect: Slows sinus heart rate; decreases peripheral vascular resistance, cardiac output, and B/P.

USES

Treatment of mild-to-severe hypertension

PHARMACOKINETICS

Route	Onset	Peak	Duration
PO	0.5–2 hr	2–4 hr	8–12 hr
IV	2.5 min	5–15 min	2–4 hr

Completely absorbed from the GI tract. Protein binding: 50%. Undergoes first-pass metabolism. Metabolized in the liver. Primarily excreted in urine. Not removed by hemodialysis. ***Half-life:*** PO, 6–8 hr; IV, 5.5 hr.

INDICATIONS AND DOSAGES

▸ Hypertension

PO

Adults. Initially, 100 mg twice a day adjusted in increments of 100 mg twice a day q2–3 days. Maintenance: 200–400 mg twice a day. Maximum: 2.4 g/day.
Elderly. Initially, 100 mg 1–2 times a day. May increase as needed.

▸ Severe Hypertension, Hypertensive Emergency

IV

Adults. Initially, 20 mg. Additional doses of 20–80 mg may be given at 10-min intervals, up to a total dose of 300 mg.

IV Infusion

Adults. Initially, 2 mg/min up to total dose of 300 mg.

PO (after IV therapy)

Adults. Initially, 200 mg; then, 200–400 mg in 6–12 hr. Increase dose at 1-day intervals to desired level.

SIDE EFFECTS/ADVERSE REACTIONS

Frequent
Drowsiness, difficulty sleeping, unusual fatigue or weakness, diminished sexual ability, transient scalp tingling
Occasional
Dizziness, dyspnea, peripheral edema, depression, anxiety, constipation, diarrhea, nasal congestion, nausea, vomiting, abdominal discomfort
Rare
Altered taste, dry eyes, increased urination, paresthesia

PRECAUTIONS AND CONTRAINDICATIONS

Bronchial asthma, cardiogenic shock, second- or third-degree heart block, severe bradycardia, uncontrolled CHF

Caution:
Major surgery, lactation, diabetes mellitus, renal disease, thyroid disease, COPD, well-compensated heart failure, CAD, nonallergic bronchospasm

DRUG INTERACTIONS OF CONCERN TO DENTISTRY

- Decreased metabolism: lidocaine
- Decreased effect: sympathomimetics
- Decreased hypotensive effects: indomethacin and other NSAIDs
- Increased hypotension, myocardial depression: hydrocarbon-inhalation anesthetics
- Increased plasma levels: diphenhydramine

SERIOUS REACTIONS

! Labetalol administration may precipitate or aggravate CHF because of decreased myocardial stimulation.

! Abrupt withdrawal may precipitate ischemic heart disease, producing sweating, palpitations, headache, and tremors.

! May mask signs and symptoms of acute hypoglycemia (tachycardia, B/P changes) in patients with diabetes.

DENTAL CONSIDERATIONS

General:

- Monitor vital signs at every appointment because of cardiovascular side effects.
- Patients on chronic drug therapy may rarely have symptoms of blood dyscrasias, which can include infection, bleeding, and poor healing.
- Assess salivary flow as a factor in caries, periodontal disease, and candidiasis.
- Limit dose of vasoconstrictors, or avoid use of vasoconstriction.
- After supine positioning, have patient sit upright for at least 2 min before standing to avoid orthostatic hypotension.
- Limit use of sodium-containing products, such as saline IV fluids, for patients with a dietary salt restriction.
- Stress from dental procedures may compromise cardiovascular function; determine patient risk.
- Short appointments and a stress-reduction protocol may be required for anxious patients.

Consultations:

- Medical consultation may be required to assess disease control and patient's ability to tolerate stress.
- In a patient with symptoms of blood dyscrasias, request a medical consultation for blood studies and postpone dental treatment until normal values are reestablished.

Teach Patient/Family to:

- When chronic dry mouth occurs, advise patient to:
  - Avoid mouth rinses with high alcohol content because of drying effects.
  - Use sugarless gum, frequent sips of water, or saliva substitutes.
  - Use daily home fluoride products for anticaries effect.

L

lacosamide

lah-**kose**′-a-mide
(Vimpat)
Do not confuse with lamisil, lanoxin.

CATEGORY AND SCHEDULE

Pregnancy Risk Category: C

Drug Class: Anticonvulsant

MECHANISM OF ACTION

An anticonvulsant and antineuralgic agent whose exact mechanism is unknown but may be related to enhancement of sodium channel inactivation and modulation of collapsing response mediator protein-2 (CRMP-2). Lacosamide decreases the availability of voltage-gated sodium channels.

USES

Adjunctive therapy of partial-onset seizures in patients 17 yr and older

PHARMACOKINETICS

Completely absorbed following oral administration (100%), can be taken with food. Peak plasma concentrations reached in 1–5 hr, widely distributed. Protein binding <15%. Undergoes hepatic metabolism (CYP2C19). ***Half-life:*** 13 hr. Excreted primarily by the kidneys.

INDICATIONS AND DOSAGES

▸ Partial-Onset Seizures

Adult. PO 50 mg twice daily. May be increased at weekly intervals by 100 mg/day given as 2 divided doses, up to 200–400 mg/day, based on response and tolerability (intravenous form also available when oral administration not feasible).

SIDE EFFECTS/ADVERSE REACTIONS

Frequent

Dizziness, diplopia, blurred vision, headache, nausea

Occasional

Abnormal vision, ataxia, fatigue, nystagmus, somnolence, tremor, vomiting

PRECAUTIONS AND CONTRAINDICATIONS

Hypersensitivity to lacosamide or any of its ingredients, hepatic impairment. Safety in children not established

DRUG INTERACTIONS OF CONCERN TO DENTISTRY

• None reported

SERIOUS REACTIONS

! Hypersensitivity

DENTAL CONSIDERATIONS

General:

• Assess salivary flow as a factor in caries, periodontal disease, and candidiasis.

• Morning appointments and stress-reduction protocol may be needed for anxious patients.

• Be prepared to manage seizures and/or nausea.

• After supine positioning, allow patient to sit upright for 2 minutes to avoid occurrence of dizziness.

Consultations:

Consult with physician to determine seizure control and ability to tolerate dental procedures.

Teach Patient/Family to:

• Avoid mouth rinses with high alcohol content because of drying effect.

• Use home fluoride products for anticaries effect.

• Use sugarless/xylitol gum, frequent sips of water, or saliva substitutes if dry mouth occurs.

lamivudine

la-**miv**′-yoo-deen
(Epivir, Epivir-HBV, Heptovir[CAN], Zeffix[AUS])
Do not confuse lamivudine with lamotrigine.

CATEGORY AND SCHEDULE

Pregnancy Risk Category: C

Drug Class: Antiviral, nucleoside analogue

MECHANISM OF ACTION

An antiviral that inhibits HIV reverse transcriptase by viral DNA chain termination. Also inhibits RNA- and DNA-dependent DNA polymerase, an enzyme necessary for HIV replication.
Therapeutic Effect: Interrupts HIV replication, slowing the progression of HIV infection.

USES

Used in combination with zidovudine for the treatment of HIV infection and to reduce disease progression and death in AIDS; HBV dose form: chronic hepatitis B associated with evidence of hepatitis B viral replication and liver inflammation

PHARMACOKINETICS

Rapidly and completely absorbed from the GI tract. Protein binding: less than 36%. Widely distributed (crosses the blood-brain barrier). Primarily excreted unchanged in urine. Not removed by hemodialysis or peritoneal dialysis. ***Half-life:*** 11–15 hr (intracellular), 2–11 hr (serum, adults), 1.7–2 hr (serum, children) (increased in impaired renal function).

INDICATIONS AND DOSAGES

▸ HIV Infection (in Combination with Other Antiretrovirals)

PO

Adults, Children 12–16 yr, weighing 50 kg (100 lb) or more. 150 mg twice a day or 300 mg once a day.
Adults weighing less than 50 kg. 2 mg/kg twice a day.
Children 3 mo–11 yr. 4 mg/kg twice a day (up to 150 mg/dose).

▸ Chronic Hepatitis B

PO

Adults, Children 17 yr and older. 100 mg/day.
Children younger than 17 yr. 3 mg/kg/day. Maximum: 100 mg/day.

▸ Dosage in Renal Impairment

Dosage and frequency are modified on the basis of creatinine clearance.

Creatinine Clearance	Dosage
50 ml/min or higher	150 mg twice a day
30–49 ml/min	150 mg once a day
15–29 ml/min	150 mg first dose, then
100 mg once a day	5–14 ml/min
150 mg first dose, then	50 mg once a day
Less than 5 ml/min	50 mg first dose, then 25 mg once a day

SIDE EFFECTS/ADVERSE REACTIONS

Frequent

Headache, nausea, malaise and fatigue, nasal disturbances, diarrhea, cough, musculoskeletal pain, neuropathy, insomnia, anorexia, dizziness, fever or chills

Occasional

Depression, myalgia, abdominal cramps, dyspepsia, arthralgia

PRECAUTIONS AND CONTRAINDICATIONS

Hypersensitivity, history of pancreatitis as child

Caution:
Reduce dose in renal disease, lactation

DRUG INTERACTIONS OF CONCERN TO DENTISTRY

• None reported

SERIOUS REACTIONS

! Pancreatitis occurs in 13% of pediatric patients.
! Anemia, neutropenia, and thrombocytopenia occur rarely.

DENTAL CONSIDERATIONS

General:
• Patients on chronic drug therapy may rarely have symptoms of blood dyscrasias, which can include infection, bleeding, and poor healing.
• Examine for oral manifestation of opportunistic infections.
Consultations:
• In a patient with symptoms of blood dyscrasias, request a medical consultation for blood studies and postpone dental treatment until normal values are reestablished.
• Medical consultation may be required to assess disease control and patient's ability to tolerate stress.
Teach Patient/Family to:
• Encourage effective oral hygiene to prevent soft tissue inflammation.
• Use caution to prevent trauma when using oral hygiene aids.
• See dentist immediately if secondary oral infection occurs.

L

lamotrigine

la-**moe**′-trih-jeen
(Apo-Lamotrigine[CAN], Lamictal, Lamictal CD)
Do not confuse lamotrigine with lamivudine.

CATEGORY AND SCHEDULE

Pregnancy Risk Category: C

Drug Class: Antiepileptic

MECHANISM OF ACTION

An anticonvulsant whose exact mechanism is unknown. May block voltage-gated sodium channels, thus stabilizing neuronal membranes and regulating presynaptic transmitter release of excitatory amino acids.
Therapeutic Effect: Reduces seizure activity.

USES

Adjunctive treatment of refractive partial seizures in adults and adjunctive treatment for Lennox-Gastaut syndrome in pediatric and adult patients; long-term maintenance of bipolar 1 disorder

PHARMACOKINETICS

Rapidly absorbed from the GI tract. Protein binding: 55%. Metabolized primarily by glucuronic acid conjugation. Excreted in the urine.
Half-life: 13–30 hr.

INDICATIONS AND DOSAGES

▸ **Seizure Control in Patients Receiving Enzyme-Inducing Antiepileptic Drug (EIAEDS), But Not Valproic Acid**
PO
Adults, Elderly, Children older than 12 yr: Recommended as add-on therapy: 50 mg once a day for 2 wk, followed by 100 mg/day in 2 divided

doses for 2 wk. Maintenance: Dosage may be increased by 100 mg/day every wk, up to 300–500 mg/day in 2 divided doses. *Children 2–12 yr.* 0.6 mg/kg/day in 2 divided doses for 2 wk, then 1.2 mg/kg/day in 2 divided doses for wk 3 and 4. Maintenance: 5–15 mg/kg/day. Maximum: 400 mg/day.

▸ Seizure Control in Patients Receiving Combination Therapy of EIAEDS and Valproic Acid

PO

Adults, Elderly, Children older than 12 yr. 25 mg every other day for 2 wk, followed by 25 mg once a day for 2 wk. Maintenance: Dosage may be increased by 25–50 mg/day q1–2wk, up to 150 mg/day in 2 divided doses.

Children 2–12 yr. 0.15 mg/kg/day in 2 divided doses for 2 wk, then 0.3 mg/kg/day in 2 divided doses for wk 3 and 4. Maintenance: 1–5 mg/kg/day in 2 divided doses. Maximum: 200 mg/day.

▸ Conversion to Monotherapy for Patients Receiving EIAED

PO

Adults, Elderly, Children 16 yr and older. 500 mg/day in 2 divided doses. Titrate to desired dose while maintaining EIAED at fixed level, then withdraw EIAED by 20% each week over a 4-wk period.

▸ Conversion to Monotherapy for Patients Receiving Valproic Acid

PO

Adults, Elderly, Children 16 yr and older. Titrate lamotrigine to 200 mg/day, maintaining valproic acid dose. Maintain lamotrigine dose and decrease valproic acid to 500 mg/day, no greater than 500 mg/day/wk, then maintain 500 mg/day for 1 wk. Increase lamotrigine to 300 mg/day and decrease valproic acid to 250 mg/day. Maintain for 1 wk, then discontinue valproic acid and increase lamotrigine by 100 mg/day each wk until maintenance dose of 500 mg/day reached.

▸ Bipolar Disorder in Patients Receiving EIAED

PO

Adults, Elderly. 50 mg/day for 2 wk, then 100 mg/day for 2 wk, then 200 mg/day for 1 wk, then 300 mg/day for 1 wk, then up to usual maintenance dose 400 mg/day in divided doses.

▸ Bipolar Disorder in Patients Receiving Valproic Acid

PO

Adults, Elderly. 25 mg/day every other day for 2 wk, then 25 mg/day for 2 wk, then 50 mg/day for 1 wk, then 100 mg/day. Usual maintenance dose with valproic acid: 100 mg/day.

▸ Discontinuation Therapy

Adults, Children older than 12 yr. A dosage reduction of approximately 50% per week over at least 2 wk is recommended.

SIDE EFFECTS/ADVERSE REACTIONS

Frequent

Dizziness, diplopia, headache, ataxia, nausea, blurred vision, somnolence, rhinitis, dry mouth, halitosis

Occasional

Rash, pharyngitis, vomiting, cough, flu-like symptoms, diarrhea, dysmenorrhea, fever, insomnia, dyspepsia

Rare

Constipation, tremors, anxiety, pruritus, vaginitis, hypersensitivity reaction

PRECAUTIONS AND CONTRAINDICATIONS

Hypersensitivity

Caution:

Elderly, children younger than 16 yr, dose adjustment with other anticonvulsants, seizure risk with drug withdrawal, renal or hepatic impairment; can cause Stevens-Johnson syndrome, toxic epidermal necrolysis

DRUG INTERACTIONS OF CONCERN TO DENTISTRY

- Increased excretion: chronic, high-dose acetaminophen, but significance is unclear
- Increased blood levels of carbamazepine

SERIOUS REACTIONS

! Abrupt withdrawal may increase seizure frequency.

! Serious rashes, including Stevens-Johnson syndrome, requiring hospitalization and discontinuation of treatment have been reported.

L

DENTAL CONSIDERATIONS

General:

- Morning appointments and a stress-reduction protocol may be required for anxious patients.
- Determine type of epilepsy, seizure frequency, and quality of seizure control.
- Evaluate respiration characteristics and rate.
- Assess salivary flow as factor in caries, periodontal disease, and candidiasis.
- Patients on chronic drug therapy may rarely have symptoms of blood dyscrasias, which can include infection, bleeding, and poor healing.
- Place on frequent recall because of oral side effects.

Consultations:

- Medical consultation may be required to assess disease control and the patient's ability to tolerate stress.
- In a patient with symptoms of blood dyscrasias, request a medical consultation for blood studies and postpone dental treatment until normal values are reestablished.

Teach Patient/Family to:

- Encourage effective oral hygiene to prevent soft tissue inflammation.
- Use powered tooth brush if patient has difficulty holding conventional devices.
- When chronic dry mouth occurs, advise patient to:
  - Avoid mouth rinses with high alcohol content because of drying effects.
  - Use daily home fluoride products for anticaries effect.
  - Use sugarless gum, frequent sips of water, or saliva substitutes.

lanreotide

lan-**ree**′-oh-tide

(Somatuline Depot)

CATEGORY AND SCHEDULE

Pregnancy Risk Category: C

Drug Class: Somatostatin

MECHANISM OF ACTION

Octapeptide somatostatin analog that inhibits insulin-like growth factor-1 (IGF-1) and growth hormone. High affinity for somatostatin type 2 (SSTR2) and 5 (SSTR5) receptors in pituitary gland, pancreas, and growth hormone (GH) secreting neoplasms of pituitary gland. Lesser affinity for somatostatin receptors 1, 3, and 4 (SSTR1, SSTR3 and SSTR4).

USES

Acromegaly (long-term therapy in patients who have had inadequate response to surgery and/or radiotherapy; or when surgery and/ or radiotherapy is not an option)
For long-term treatment of acromegaly in patients who fail to respond to surgery and radiotherapy.

PHARMACOKINETICS

Protein binding: 79%–83%. Extensive metabolism in GI tract after biliary excretion. Bioavailability: 69%–83%. Less than 5% of lanreotide excreted in urine; less than 0.5% recovered unchanged in feces, indicative of some biliary excretion. ***Half-life***: 23–36 days.

INDICATIONS AND DOSAGES

SC Injection
Adult. Acromegaly: 90 mg deep SC injection every 4 wk for 3 months. After 3 months adjust dose based on clinical response:
GH >1 to = 2.5 ng/mL, IGF-1 normal and clinical symptoms controlled: maintain dose at 90 mg every 4 wk
GH > 2.5 ng/mL, IGF-1 elevated and/or clinical symptoms uncontrolled, increase dose to 120 mg every 4 wk
GH = 1 ng/mL, IGF-1 normal and clinical symptoms controlled: reduce dose to 60 mg every 4 wk
Dose Adjustments
Renal impairment: 60 mg deep SC injection every 4 wk.
Hepatic impairment: 60 mg deep SC injection every 4 wk.
Geriatric: no dosage adjustment necessary.
Pediatric: Safety and effectiveness in pediatric patients have not been established.

SIDE EFFECTS/ADVERSE REACTIONS

Frequent
Injection site reaction, abdominal pain, diarrhea, nausea, bradycardia, and cholelithiasis

PRECAUTIONS AND CONTRAINDICATIONS

There are no contraindications listed in the manufacturer's labeling.
Use caution in patients with cardiac disease, diabetes mellitus, gallbladder disease, hypothyroidism, renal impairment, and hepatic impairment.

DRUG INTERACTIONS OF CONCERN TO DENTISTRY

- None reported

SERIOUS REACTIONS

! Bradycardia, hypo- and hyperglycemia, gallstones, decreases in thyroid function, renal impairment, and hepatic impairment have occurred.

DENTAL CONSIDERATIONS

General:
- Patient may need assistance in getting into and out of dental chair.
- Adjust chair position for patient comfort.
- Consider semisupine chair position for patient comfort if GI side effects occur.

Consultations:
- Medical consultation may be required to assess disease control and patient's ability to tolerate stress.
- Consultation with physician may be necessary if sedation or general anesthesia is required.

L

Teach Patient/Family to:

- Update health and medication history if physician makes any changes in evaluation or drug regimens; include OTC, herbal, and nonherbal remedies in the update.
- Use effective oral hygiene to prevent soft tissue inflammation.
- Use caution to prevent injury when using oral hygiene aids.

lansoprazole

lan-**soe**′-pra-zole

(Prevacid, Prevacid IV, Prevacid Solu-Tab, Zoton[AUS])

Do not confuse Prevacid with Pepcid, Pravachol, or Prevpac.

CATEGORY AND SCHEDULE

Pregnancy Risk Category: B

Drug Class: Antisecretory, proton pump inhibitor

MECHANISM OF ACTION

A proton pump inhibitor that selectively inhibits the parietal cell membrane enzyme system (hydrogen-potassium adenosine triphosphatase) or proton pump. ***Therapeutic Effect:*** Suppresses gastric acid secretion.

USES

Short-term treatment for healing and symptomatic relief of active duodenal ulcer and benign gastric ulcer, erosive esophagitis, and gastroesophageal reflux disease (GERD); maintenance of healing of duodenal ulcers; long-term treatment of pathologic hypersecretory syndromes; NSAID-associated gastric ulcers in patients who continue NSAID use; short-term treatment of symptomatic GERD

PHARMACOKINETICS

Route	Onset	Peak	Duration
PO (15 mg)	2–3 hr	N/A	8–24 hr
PO (30 mg)	1–2 hr	N/A	Longer than 24 hr

Rapid and complete absorption (food may decrease absorption) once drug has left stomach. Protein binding: 97%. Distributed primarily to gastric parietal cells and converted to two active metabolites. Extensively metabolized in the liver. Eliminated in bile and urine. Not removed by hemodialysis. ***Half-life:*** 1.5 hr (increased in the elderly and in those with hepatic impairment).

INDICATIONS AND DOSAGES

▸ **Duodenal Ulcer**

PO

Adults, Elderly. 15 mg/day, before eating, preferably in the morning, for up to 4 wk.

▸ **Erosive Esophagitis**

PO

Adults, Elderly. 30 mg/day, before eating, for up to 8 wk. If healing does not occur within 8 wk (in 5%–10% of cases), may give for additional 8 wk. Maintenance: 15 mg/day.

IV

Adults, Elderly. 30 mg once a day for up to 7 days. Switch to oral lansoprazole therapy as soon as patient can tolerate oral route.

▸ **Gastric Ulcer**

PO

Adults. 30 mg/day for up to 8 wk.

▸ **NSAID Gastric Ulcer**

PO

Adults, Elderly. (Healing): 30 mg/day for up to 8 wk. (Prevention): 15 mg/day for up to 12 wk.

▸ **Healed Duodenal Ulcer, GERD**
PO
Adults. 15 mg/day.
▸ **Usual Pediatric Dosage**
Children 3 mo–14 yr, weighing more than 20 kg. 30 mg once daily.
Children 3 mo–14 yr, weighing 10–20 kg. 15 mg once daily.
Children 3 mo–14 yr, weighing less than 10 kg. 7.5 mg once daily.
▸ ***Helicobacter pylori* Infection**
PO
Adults. 30 mg twice a day for 10 days (with amoxicillin and clarithromycin).
▸ **Pathologic Hypersecretory Conditions (Including Zollinger-Ellison Syndrome)**
PO
Adults, Elderly. 60 mg/day. Individualize dosage according to patient needs and for as long as clinically indicated. Administer up to 120 mg/day in divided doses.

SIDE EFFECTS/ADVERSE REACTIONS

Occasional
Diarrhea, abdominal pain, rash, pruritus, altered appetite
Rare
Nausea, headache

PRECAUTIONS AND CONTRAINDICATIONS

Hypersensitivity
Caution:
Children younger than 18 yr, elderly (limit doses to 30 mg/day), severe hepatic disease

DRUG INTERACTIONS OF CONCERN TO DENTISTRY

• Drug interactions not established but potentially can interfere with absorption of amoxicillin, ketoconazole

SERIOUS REACTIONS

! Bilirubinemia, eosinophilia, and hyperlipemia occur rarely.

DENTAL CONSIDERATIONS

General:
• Consider semisupine chair position for patient comfort because of GI effects of disease.
• Question the patient about tolerance of NSAIDs or aspirin related to GI problem.
• Patients with GERD may have oral symptoms, including burning mouth, secondary candidiasis, and oral signs of dental erosion.
• Assess salivary flow as factor in caries, periodontal disease, and candidiasis.
Teach Patient/Family to:
• When chronic dry mouth occurs, advise patient to:
  • Avoid mouth rinses with high alcohol content because of drying effects.
  • Use daily home fluoride products for anticaries effect.
  • Use sugarless gum, frequent sips of water, or saliva substitutes.

L

lanthanum carbonate

lan′-tha-num **kar′**-boh-nate
(Fosrenol)

CATEGORY AND SCHEDULE

Pregnancy Risk Category: C

Drug Class: Phosphate binder

MECHANISM OF ACTION

A phosphate regulator that dissociates in the acidic environment of the upper GI tract to lanthanum ions, which bind to dietary phosphate released from food during digestion, forming highly insoluble lanthanum phosphate complexes. ***Therapeutic Effect:*** Reduces phosphate absorption.

USES

Treatment of end-stage renal disease

PHARMACOKINETICS

Phosphate complexes are eliminated in feces.

INDICATIONS AND DOSAGES

▸ Reduce Serum Phosphate in End-Stage Renal Disease

PO

Adults, Elderly. 750–1500 mg in divided doses, taken with or immediately after a meal. Dosage may be titrated in 750-mg increments q2–3wk on the basis of serum phosphate levels.

L

SIDE EFFECTS/ADVERSE REACTIONS

Frequent

Nausea, vomiting, dialysis graft occlusion, abdominal pain

PRECAUTIONS AND CONTRAINDICATIONS

None known

DRUG INTERACTIONS OF CONCERN TO DENTISTRY

• None reported

SERIOUS REACTIONS

! None known

DENTAL CONSIDERATIONS

General:

• Question patient about renal dialysis history and use of other medications.

• Dental drugs known to interact with antacid products should not be taken within 2 hr of lanthanum carbonate.

• Dental procedures must be scheduled to appropriately sequence with dialysis regimen.

• Question patient about coexisting cardiovascular disease, related medications, and any bleeding problems.

• Avoid nephrotoxic drugs; dose adjustment may be required for renal-excreted drugs.

• Oral infections should be eliminated and/or treated aggressively.

• Patient may have AV shunt in place.

• Monitor and record vital signs.

• Consider semisupine chair position for patient comfort if GI side effects occur.

• Question patient about tolerance of NSAIDS or aspirin related to GI disease.

• After supine positioning, have patient sit upright for at least 2 min before standing to avoid orthostatic hypotension.

• Antiinfective prophylaxis may be indicated for patient on dialysis; consult physician.

Consultations:

• Consultation with physician may be necessary if sedation or general anesthesia is required.

• Medical consultation may be required to assess disease control and patient's ability to tolerate stress.

Teach Patient/Family to:

• Encourage effective oral hygiene to prevent soft tissue inflammation.

• Prevent trauma when using oral hygiene aids.

• Update health and medication history if physician makes any changes in evaluation/drug regimens; include OTC, herbal, and nonherbal drugs in the update.

lapatinib

lah-**pah'**-ti-nib
(Tykerb)

CATEGORY AND SCHEDULE

Pregnancy Risk Category: D

Drug Class: Antineoplastic agent, tyrosine kinase inhibitor; epidermal growth factor receptor (EGFR) inhibitor

MECHANISM OF ACTION

Lapatinib is a 4-anilinoquinazoline kinase inhibitor that inhibits EGFR (ErbB1) and human epidermal receptor type 2 (HER2 [ErbB2]) by reversibly binding to tyrosine kinase, blocking phosphorylation and activation of downstream second messenger (Erk1/2 and Akt), and regulating cellular proliferation and survival in ErbB-expressing tumors.

USES

Combination with capecitabine for patients with advanced or metastatic breast cancer whose tumors overexpress HER2 and for those who have taken an anthracycline, a taxane, and trastuzumab

PHARMACOKINETICS

Incomplete and variable absorption. Protein binding: >99% to albumin and α_1-acid glycoprotein. Metabolized in the liver extensively via CYP3A4 and 3A5 and less extensively via CYP2C19 and 2C8. ***Half-life***: about 24 hr. Time to peak in the plasma: 3–6 hr. Excreted unchanged in the feces (27%) and urine (<2%).

INDICATIONS AND DOSAGES

▸ **Breast Cancer**

PO

Adults. 250 mg once daily (in combination with capecitabine).
Dosage adjustment for concomitant use with 3A4 inhibitors: 500 mg once daily with careful monitoring.
Dosage adjustment for concomitant use with 3A4 inducers: titrate up to 4500 mg/day with careful monitoring.
Dosage in hepatic impairment: 750 mg once daily.
Dosage adjustment for cardiac toxicity: discontinue for decreased left ventricular ejection fraction (LVEF) ≥ grade 2 or LVEF < LLN; consider restarting 1000 mg once daily after 2 wk if normal LVEF and patient experiences no symptoms.
Other toxicities: Discontinue with any toxicity if ≥ grade 2. May restart after if toxicity resolves to = grade 1. 1000 mg once daily for persistent toxicity.

SIDE EFFECTS/ADVERSE REACTIONS

Frequent

Fatigue, palmar-plantar erythrodysesthesia (hand-and-foot syndrome), rash, diarrhea, nausea, vomiting, abdominal pain, mucosal inflammation, stomatitis, dyspepsia, anemia, neutropenia, thrombocytopenia, AST increased, total bilirubin increased, ALT increased, limb pain, back pain, dyspnea

Occasional

Decreased LVEF, insomnia, dry skin

PRECAUTIONS AND CONTRAINDICATIONS

Hypersensitivity to lapatinib or any component of the formulation.

Lapatinib is a hazardous agent. Handle and dispose of with caution.
Avoid use in pregnancy and lactation.
Use with caution in patients with a history of use of anthracyclines and chest wall irradiation for the treatment of left ventricular dysfunction.
Use with caution in patients with hepatic impairment. Hepatotoxicity (ALT or AST > 3 times upper limit of normal [ULN] and total bilirubin >1.5 times ULN) has been documented, may be severe and/or fatal.
Caution with CYP 3A4 inhibitors (e.g., erythromycin) and grapefruit; dose adjustments may be needed.

L

DRUG INTERACTIONS OF CONCERN TO DENTISTRY

• Use with caution when in combination with vasoconstrictors (epinephrine, levonordefrin) in local anesthetic because of the possible risk of QT prolongation (torsade de pointes).
• CYP3A4 inhibitors: Concomitant use with CYP3A4 inhibitors (e.g., erythromycin) may result in increased lapatinib concentrations.

SERIOUS REACTIONS

! Hepatotoxicity adverse effect (ALT or AST >3 times ULN and total bilirubin >1.5 times ULN) has been documented; may be severe and/or fatal.
! Interstitial lung disease has been reported.
! Decrease in LVEF may occur.
! QTc prolongation may occur.
! Administration during pregnancy or lactation may cause fatal harm.

DENTAL CONSIDERATIONS

General:
• Stomatitis may complicate dental treatment.
• Consider semisupine chair position for patient comfort if GI side effects occur.
Consultations:
• Medical consultation may be required to assess disease control and ability of patient to tolerate dental treatment.
Teach Patient/Family to:
• Use good oral hygiene to prevent soft tissue inflammation.
• Use oral hygiene aids with caution to prevent injury.
• Alert for the possibility of stomatitis and the need to see dentist immediately if signs of inflammation occur.

latanoprost

la-**ta′**-noe-prost
(Xalatan)
Do not confuse with Xanax.

CATEGORY AND SCHEDULE

Pregnancy Risk Category: C

Drug Class: Prostaglandin F_{2a} analogue

MECHANISM OF ACTION

An ophthalmic agent that is a prostanoid-selective FP receptor agonist.
Therapeutic Effect: Reduces intraocular pressure (IOP) by reducing aqueous humor production.

USES

Treatment of open-angle glaucoma and ocular hypertension in patients intolerant to other IOP-lowering drugs

PHARMACOKINETICS

Absorbed through the cornea where the isopropyl ester prodrug is hydrolyzed to acid form to become biologically active. Highly lipophilic. The acid of latanoprost can be measured in the aqueous humor during the first 4 hr and in the plasma only during the first hr after local administration. In the cornea, latanoprost is hydrolyzed to the biologically active acid. Metabolized in liver if it reaches systemic circulation. Metabolized to 1,2-dinor metabolite and 1,2,3,4-tetranor metabolite. Primarily eliminated by the kidneys. ***Half-life:*** 17 min.

INDICATIONS AND DOSAGES

▸ **Glaucoma, Ocular Hypertension**

Ophthalmic

Adults, Elderly. 1 drop (1.5 mcg) in affected eye(s) once daily, in the evening.

SIDE EFFECTS/ADVERSE REACTIONS

Frequent

Blurred vision

Occasional

Eyelash changes, eyelid skin darkening, iris pigmentation

Rare

Macular edema

PRECAUTIONS AND CONTRAINDICATIONS

Hypersensitivity to latanoprost or benzalkonium chloride, or any other component of the formulation

Caution:

Gradual change in eye color, avoid contamination of sterile solution, renal or hepatic impairment, remove contact lens before using, administer at least 5 min apart if other ophthalmic drug is also used, nursing, pediatrics

DRUG INTERACTIONS OF CONCERN TO DENTISTRY

• None reported at this time

SERIOUS REACTIONS

! Pigmentation is expected to increase as long as latanoprost is administered but after discontinuation, pigmentation of the iris is likely to be permanent while pigmentation of the periorbital tissue and eyelash changes has been reported as reversible.

! Inflammation (iritis/uveitis) and macular edema, including cystoid macular edema, have been reported.

DENTAL CONSIDERATIONS

General:

• Avoid use of anticholinergic drugs, atropine-like drugs, propantheline, and diazepam (benzodiazepines) in patient with glaucoma.

• Check compliance of patient with prescribed drug regimen for glaucoma.

• Avoid dental light in patient's eyes; offer dark glasses for patient comfort.

Consultations:

• Medical consultation may be required to assess disease control.

leflunomide

le-**flu**′-na-mide

(Arava)

CATEGORY AND SCHEDULE

Pregnancy Risk Category: X

Drug Class: Antiarthritic, immunosuppressive

MECHANISM OF ACTION
An immunomodulatory agent that inhibits dihydroorotate dehydrogenase, the enzyme involved in autoimmune process that leads to rheumatoid arthritis.
Therapeutic Effect: Reduces signs and symptoms of rheumatoid arthritis and slows structural damage.

USES
Reduction of signs and symptoms and to retard structural damage in active rheumatoid arthritis as demonstrated by x-ray erosion and joint space narrowing

PHARMACOKINETICS
Well absorbed after PO administration. Protein binding: greater than 99%. Metabolized to active metabolite in the GI wall and liver. Excreted through both renal and biliary systems. Not removed by hemodialysis. ***Half-life:*** 16 days.

L

INDICATIONS AND DOSAGES
▸ Rheumatoid Arthritis

PO

Adults, Elderly. Initially, 100 mg/day for 3 days, then 10–20 mg/day.

SIDE EFFECTS/ADVERSE REACTIONS
Frequent

Diarrhea, respiratory tract infection, alopecia, rash, nausea

PRECAUTIONS AND CONTRAINDICATIONS
Pregnancy or plans to become pregnant, chronic renal or hepatic insufficiency, rifampin

Caution:

Chronic renal or hepatic insufficiency, rifampin, children younger than 18 yr

DRUG INTERACTIONS OF CONCERN TO DENTISTRY
• None reported.

SERIOUS REACTIONS
! Transient thrombocytopenia and leukopenia occur rarely.

DENTAL CONSIDERATIONS
General:

• Monitor vital signs at every appointment because of cardiovascular side effects.
• Consider semisupine chair position for patient comfort if GI side effects occur.
• Examine for oral manifestation of opportunistic infection.
• If acute oral infection occurs, inform physician.
• Assess salivary flow as a factor in caries, periodontal disease, and candidiasis.

Consultations:

• Consult the patient's family if needed.

Teach Patient/Family to:

• Encourage effective oral hygiene to prevent soft tissue inflammation.
• Use powered tooth brush if patient has difficulty holding conventional devices.
• When chronic dry mouth occurs, advise patient to:
  • Avoid mouth rinses with high alcohol content because of drying effects.
  • Use daily home fluoride products for anticaries effect.
  • Use sugarless gum, frequent sips of water, or saliva substitutes.

letrozole

leh′-troe-zoll
(Femara)
Do not confuse Femara with Femhrt.

CATEGORY AND SCHEDULE

Pregnancy Risk Category: D

Drug Class: Antineoplastic

MECHANISM OF ACTION

Decreases the level of circulating estrogen by inhibiting aromatase, an enzyme that catalyzes the final step in estrogen production.
Therapeutic Effect: Inhibits the growth of breast cancers that are stimulated by estrogens.

USES

Treatment of locally advanced or metastatic breast cancer in postmenopausal women either hormone receptor positive or hormone receptor unknown; advanced breast cancer in postmenopausal women with disease progression following antiestrogen therapy

PHARMACOKINETICS

Rapidly and completely absorbed. Metabolized in the liver. Primarily eliminated by the kidneys. Unknown if removed by hemodialysis.
Half-life: Approximately 2 days.

INDICATIONS AND DOSAGES

▸ Breast Cancer

PO

Adults, Elderly. 2.5 mg/day. Continue until tumor progression is evident.

SIDE EFFECTS/ADVERSE REACTIONS

Frequent

Musculoskeletal pain (back, arm, leg), nausea, headache

Occasional

Constipation, arthralgia, fatigue, vomiting, hot flashes, diarrhea, abdominal pain, cough, rash, anorexia, hypertension, peripheral edema

Rare

Asthenia, somnolence, dyspepsia, weight gain, pruritus

PRECAUTIONS AND CONTRAINDICATIONS

Hypersensitivity

Caution:

Lactation, children (no studies), for postmenopausal women only, thrombocytopenia and decreased lymphocyte counts, liver impairment

DRUG INTERACTIONS OF CONCERN TO DENTISTRY

- None reported

SERIOUS REACTIONS

! None known

DENTAL CONSIDERATIONS

General:

- Patients taking opioids for acute or chronic pain should be given alternative analgesics for dental pain.
- Patients on chronic drug therapy may rarely have symptoms of blood dyscrasias, which can include infection, bleeding, and poor healing.
- Palliative medication may be required for management of oral side effects.
- Examine for oral manifestation of opportunistic infection.

• Consider semisupine chair position for patient comfort if GI side effects occur.
• Monitor vital signs at every appointment because of cardiovascular and respiratory side effects.

Consultations:

• In a patient with symptoms of blood dyscrasias, request a medical consultation for blood studies and postpone treatment until normal values are reestablished.

Teach Patient/Family to:

• Encourage effective oral hygiene to prevent soft tissue inflammation.
• Be aware of the possibility of secondary oral infection and the need to see dentist immediately if signs of infection occur.

L

leucovorin calcium (folinic acid, citrovorum factor)

loo-koe-**vor**′-in **kal**′-see-um
(Calcium Leucovorin[AUS], Wellcovorin)
Do not confuse Wellcovorin with Wellbutrin or Wellferon.

CATEGORY AND SCHEDULE

Pregnancy Risk Category: C

Drug Class: Folic acid antagonist antidote, antineoplastic adjunct

MECHANISM OF ACTION

An antidote to folic acid antagonists that may limit methotrexate action on normal cells by competing with methotrexate for the same transport processes into the cells.
Therapeutic Effect: Reverses toxic effects of folic acid antagonists. Reverses folic acid deficiency.

USES

Treatment of megaloblastic or macrocytic anemia caused by folic acid deficiency, overdose of folic acid antagonist, methotrexate toxicity, toxicity caused by pyrimethamine or trimethoprim; used with fluorouracil in colorectal cancer

PHARMACOKINETICS

Readily absorbed from the GI tract. Widely distributed. Primarily concentrated in the liver. Metabolized in the liver and intestinal mucosa to active metabolite. Primarily excreted in urine. ***Half-life:*** 15 min; metabolite, 30–35 min.

INDICATIONS AND DOSAGES

▸ **Conventional Rescue Dosage in Methotrexate Rescue**
PO, IV, IM
Adults, Elderly, Children. 10 mg/m^2 IM or IV one time, then PO q6h until serum methotrexate level is less than 0.05 micromolar (μM). If 24-hr serum creatinine level increases by 50% or greater over baseline or methotrexate level exceeds 50 micromolar at 24 hr or 5 micromolar at 48-hr, increase to 100 mg/m^2 IV q3h until methotrexate level is less than 0.05 micromolar.

▸ **Folic Acid Antagonist Overdose**
PO
Adults, Elderly, Children. 2–15 mg/day for 3 days or 5 mg every 3 days.

▸ **Megaloblastic Anemia**
IM
Adults, Elderly, Children. 3–6 mg/day.

▸ **Megaloblastic Anemia Secondary to Folate Deficiency**
IM
Adults, Elderly, Children. 1 mg/day.

▸ **Prevention of Hematologic Toxicity (for Toxoplasmosis), with Sulfadiazine**
PO, IV
Adults, Elderly, Children. 5–10 mg/day, repeat every 3 days.
▸ **Prevention of Hematologic Toxicity with Pyrimethamine, PCP**
PO, IV
Adults, Children. 25 mg once a wk.

SIDE EFFECTS/ADVERSE REACTIONS

Frequent
When combined with chemotherapeutic agents: Diarrhea, stomatitis, nausea, vomiting, lethargy or malaise or fatigue, alopecia, anorexia
Occasional
Urticaria, dermatitis

PRECAUTIONS AND CONTRAINDICATIONS

Pernicious anemia, other megaloblastic anemias secondary to vitamin B_{12} deficiency

DRUG INTERACTIONS OF CONCERN TO DENTISTRY

• None reported

SERIOUS REACTIONS

! Excessive dosage may negate chemotherapeutic effects of folic acid antagonists.
! Anaphylaxis occurs rarely.
! Diarrhea may cause rapid clinical deterioration.

DENTAL CONSIDERATIONS

General:
• Signs of folate deficiency may appear in oral tissues.
• Determine why the patient is taking the drug.
• Patients with severe anemia or cancer or those receiving cancer chemotherapy may have oral complaints. Palliative therapy may be required.
Consultations:
• Medical consultation may be required to assess disease control.
Teach Patient/Family to:
• Encourage effective oral hygiene to prevent soft tissue inflammation.
• Use caution to prevent trauma when using oral hygiene aids.
• Report oral lesions, soreness, or bleeding to dentist.
• See dentist immediately if secondary oral infection occurs.
• Update medical/drug records if physician makes any changes in evaluation or drug regimens; include OTC, herbal, and nonherbal drugs in the update.

L

leuprolide acetate

loo′-proe-lide **ass′**-eh-tayte
(Eligard, Lucrin[AUS], Lucrin Depot Inj[AUS], Lupron, Lupron Depot, Lupron Depot Ped, Viadur)
Do not confuse leuprolide or Lupron with Lopurin or Nuprin.

CATEGORY AND SCHEDULE

Pregnancy Risk Category: X

Drug Class: Antineoplastic hormone; gonadotropin-releasing hormone

MECHANISM OF ACTION

A gonadotropin-releasing hormone analog and antineoplastic agent that stimulates the release of luteinizing hormone (LH) and follicle-stimulating hormone (FSH) from the anterior pituitary gland.
Therapeutic Effect: Produces pharmacologic castration and decreases the growth of abnormal

prostate tissue in males; causes endometrial tissue to become inactive and atrophic in females; and decreases the rate of pubertal development in children with central precocious puberty.

USES

Treatment of metastatic prostate cancer, management of endometriosis, central precocious puberty

PHARMACOKINETICS

Rapidly and well absorbed after subcutaneous administration. Absorbed slowly after IM administration. Protein binding: 43%–49%. ***Half-life:*** 3–4 hr.

INDICATIONS AND DOSAGES

▸ Advanced Prostatic Carcinoma

IM (Lupron Depot)
Adults, Elderly. 7.5 mg every mo or 22.5 mg q3mo or 30 mg q4mo.
Subcutaneous (Eligard)
Adults, Elderly. 7.5 mg every mo or 22.5 mg q3mo or 30 mg q4mo.
Subcutaneous (Lupron)
Adults, Elderly. 1 mg/day.
Subcutaneous (Viadur)
Adults, Elderly. 65 mg implanted q12mo.

▸ Endometriosis

IM (Lupron Depot)
Adults, Elderly. 3.75 mg/mo for up to 6 mo or 11.25 mg q3mo for up to 2 doses.

▸ Uterine Leiomyomata

IM (with Iron [Lupron Depot])
Adults, Elderly. 3.75 mg/mo for up to 3 mo or 11.25 mg as a single injection.

▸ Precocious Puberty

IM (Lupron Depot)
Children. 0.3 mg/kg/dose every 28 days. Minimum: 7.5 mg. If down-regulation is not achieved, titrate upward in 3.75-mg increments q4wk.
Subcutaneous (Lupron)
Children. 20–45 mcg/kg/day. Titrate upward by 10 mcg/kg/day if down-regulation is not achieved.

SIDE EFFECTS/ADVERSE REACTIONS

Frequent
Hot flashes (ranging from mild flushing to diaphoresis)
Females: Amenorrhea, spotting
Occasional
Arrhythmias; palpitations; blurred vision; dizziness; edema; headache; burning, itching, or swelling at injection site; nausea; insomnia; weight gain
Females: Deepening voice, hirsutism, decreased libido, increased breast tenderness, vaginitis, altered mood
Males: Constipation, decreased testicle size, gynecomastia, impotence, decreased appetite, angina
Rare
Males: Thrombophlebitis

PRECAUTIONS AND CONTRAINDICATIONS

Pernicious anemia, pregnancy

DRUG INTERACTIONS OF CONCERN TO DENTISTRY

• None reported

SERIOUS REACTIONS

! Signs and symptoms of metastatic prostatic carcinoma (such as bone pain, dysuria or hematuria, and weakness or paresthesia of the lower extremities) occasionally worsen 1 to 2 wk after the initial dose but then subside with continued therapy.
! Pulmonary embolism and MI occur rarely.

DENTAL CONSIDERATIONS

General:

- If additional analgesia is required for dental pain, consider alternative analgesics (NSAIDs) in patients taking narcotics for acute or chronic pain.
- Monitor and record vital signs.
- Assess salivary flow as a factor in caries, periodontal disease, and candidiasis.
- This drug may be used in the hospital or on an outpatient basis. Confirm the patient's disease and treatment status.
- Consider semisupine chair position for patient comfort if GI side effects occur.
- Question patient about tolerance of NSAIDS or aspirin related to GI disease.
- Patient on chronic drug therapy may rarely present with symptoms of blood dyscrasias, which can include infection, bleeding, and poor healing. If dyscrasia is present, caution patient to prevent oral tissue trauma when using oral hygiene aids.
- Examine for oral manifestation of opportunistic infection.

Consultations:

- Medical consultation may be required to assess immunologic status during cancer chemotherapy and determine safety risk, if any, posed by the required dental treatment.
- Consider consulting with physician before prescribing drugs that may cause constipation (opioids).
- Medical consultation may be required to assess disease control and patient's ability to tolerate stress.
- In a patient with symptoms of blood dyscrasias, request a medical consultation for blood studies and postpone treatment until normal values are reestablished.

Teach Patient/Family to:

- When chronic dry mouth occurs advise patient to:
  - Avoid mouth rinses with high alcohol content because of drying effects.
  - Use daily home fluoride products for anticaries effect.
  - Use sugarless gum, frequent sips of water, or saliva substitutes.
- Prevent trauma when using oral hygiene aids.
- Report oral lesions, soreness, or bleeding to dentist.
- Update health and medication history if physician makes any changes in evaluation or drug regimens; include OTC, herbal, and nonherbal drugs in the update.

L

levalbuterol

lee-val-**byoot′**-err-all

(Xopenex)

Do not confuse Xopenex with Xanax.

CATEGORY AND SCHEDULE

Pregnancy Risk Category: C

Drug Class: Bronchodilator

MECHANISM OF ACTION

A sympathomimetic that stimulates β_2-adrenergic receptors in the lungs resulting in relaxation of bronchial smooth muscle.

Therapeutic Effect: Relieves bronchospasm and reduces airway resistance.

USES

Treatment or prevention of bronchospasm in adults and children older than 6 yr with reversible obstructive airway disease

PHARMACOKINETICS

Route	Onset	Peak	Duration
Inhalation	10–17 min	1.5 hr	5–6 hr

Metabolized in the liver to inactive metabolite. ***Half-life:*** 3.3–4 hr.

INDICATIONS AND DOSAGES

▸ Treatment and Prevention of Bronchospasm

Nebulization

Adults, Elderly, Children 12 yr and older. Initially, 0.63 mg 3 times a day 6–8 hr apart. May increase to 1.25 mg 3 times a day with dose monitoring.

Children 3–11 yr. Initially 0.31 mg 3 times a day. Maximum: 0.63 mg 3 times a day.

SIDE EFFECTS/ADVERSE REACTIONS

Frequent

Tremors, nervousness, headache, throat dryness and irritation

Occasional

Cough, bronchial irritation

Rare

Somnolence, diarrhea, dry mouth, flushing, diaphoresis, anorexia

PRECAUTIONS AND CONTRAINDICATIONS

History of hypersensitivity to sympathomimetics

Caution:

Paradoxic bronchospasm, cardiovascular disorders, seizures, diabetes, hyperthyroidism, coronary insufficiency, cardiac arrhythmias, hypertension, not to exceed recommended dose, β-adrenergic blockers, MAOIs, tricyclic antidepressants, lactation, children younger than 12 yr

DRUG INTERACTIONS OF CONCERN TO DENTISTRY

- None reported.

SERIOUS REACTIONS

! Excessive sympathomimetic stimulation may produce palpitations, extrasystoles, tachycardia, chest pain, a slight increase in B/P followed by a substantial decrease, chills, diaphoresis, and blanching of skin.

! Too-frequent or excessive use may lead to decreased bronchodilating effectiveness and severe, paradoxical bronchoconstriction.

DENTAL CONSIDERATIONS

General:

- Monitor vital signs at every appointment because of cardiovascular side effects.
- Assess salivary flow as a factor in caries, periodontal disease, and candidiasis.
- Consider semisupine chair position for patients with respiratory disease.
- Short midday appointments and a stress-reduction protocol may be required for anxious patients.
- Be aware that aspirin or sulfite preservatives in vasoconstrictor-containing products can exacerbate asthma.
- Acute asthmatic episodes may be precipitated in the dental office. Rapid-acting sympathomimetic inhalants should be available for emergency use. A stress-reduction protocol may be required.

Consultations:
• Medical consultation may be required to assess disease control and patient's ability to tolerate stress.
Teach Patient/Family to:
• Rinse mouth with water after each dose of inhalation dosage forms to prevent dryness.
• When chronic dry mouth occurs, advise patient to:
  • Avoid mouth rinses with high alcohol content because of drying effects.
  • Use daily home fluoride products for anticaries effect.
  • Use sugarless gum, frequent sips of water, or saliva substitutes.

levetiracetam

leva-tir-**ass**′-eh-tam
(Keppra)
Do not confuse Keppra with Kaletra.

CATEGORY AND SCHEDULE

Pregnancy Risk Category: C

Drug Class: Antiepileptic

MECHANISM OF ACTION

An anticonvulsant that inhibits burst firing without affecting normal neuronal excitability.
Therapeutic Effect: Prevents seizure activity.

USES

Adjunctive therapy in adults with partial-onset seizures

PHARMACOKINETICS

PO: Bioavailability 100%, onset 1 hr, peak plasma levels 20 min–2 hr. ***Half-life:*** 6–8 hr, less than 10% plasma protein bound, limited hepatic metabolism, renal excretion (66%).

INDICATIONS AND DOSAGES

▸ **Partial-Onset Seizures**

PO

Adults, Elderly. Initially, 500 mg q12h. May increase by 1000 mg/day q2wk. Maximum: 3000 mg/day.
Children 4–16 yr. 10–20 mg/kg/day in 2 divided doses. May increase at weekly intervals by 10–20 mg/kg. Maximum: 60 mg/kg.

▸ **Dosage in Renal Impairment**

Dosage is modified on the basis of creatinine clearance.

Creatinine Clearance (ml/min)	Dosage
Higher than 80 ml/min	500–1500 mg q12h
50–80 ml/min	500–1000 mg q12h
30–50 ml/min	250–750 mg q12h
Less than 30 ml/min	250–500 mg q12h
End-stage renal disease using dialysis	500–1000 mg q12h, after dialysis, a 250- to 500-mg supplemental dose is recommended

SIDE EFFECTS/ADVERSE REACTIONS

Frequent
Somnolence, asthenia, headache, infection
Occasional
Dizziness, pharyngitis, pain, depression, nervousness, vertigo, rhinitis, anorexia

Rare
Amnesia, anxiety, emotional lability, cough, sinusitis, anorexia, diplopia

PRECAUTIONS AND CONTRAINDICATIONS

Hypersensitivity reaction
Caution:
Lactation, children, blood dyscrasias

DRUG INTERACTIONS OF CONCERN TO DENTISTRY

• None reported

SERIOUS REACTIONS

! None known

DENTAL CONSIDERATIONS

General:
• Short appointments and a stress-reduction protocol may be required for anxious patients.
• Ask patient about type of epilepsy, seizure frequency, and quality of seizure control.
Consultation:
• Medical consultation may be required to assess disease control and patient's ability to tolerate stress.
• In patients with symptoms of blood dyscrasias, request a medical consultation for blood studies and postpone treatment until normal values are reestablished.
Teach Patient/Family to:
• Update health and drug history if physician makes changes in evaluation or drug regimens; include OTC, herbal, and nonherbal drugs in the update.

levobetaxolol hydrochloride

le-vo-bay-**tax′**-oh-lol
high-droh-**klor′**-ide
(Betaxon)
Do not confuse with levobunolol.

CATEGORY AND SCHEDULE

Pregnancy Risk Category: C

Drug Class: Antiglaucoma agent (ophthalmic)

MECHANISM OF ACTION

An antiglaucoma agent that blocks β_1-adrenergic receptors. Reduces aqueous humor production.
Therapeutic Effect: Reduces intraocular pressure (IOP).

USES

Treatment of certain types of glaucoma

PHARMACOKINETICS

Route	Onset	Peak	Duration
Eye drops	30 min	2 hr	12 hr

INDICATIONS AND DOSAGES

▸ **Glaucoma, Ocular Hypertension**
Ophthalmic
Adults, Elderly. Instill 1 drop 2 times a day.

SIDE EFFECTS/ADVERSE REACTIONS

Frequent
Ocular discomfort
Occasional
Blurred vision
Rare
Anxiety, dizziness, vertigo, headache

PRECAUTIONS AND CONTRAINDICATIONS

Sinus bradycardia, second- or third-degree atrioventricular (AV) block, cardiogenic shock, overt heart failure, hypersensitivity to betaxolol, levobetaxolol or any component of levobetaxolol formulations

DRUG INTERACTIONS OF CONCERN TO DENTISTRY

- None reported

SERIOUS REACTIONS

! Diabetes, hypothyroidism, bradycardia, tachycardia, hypertension, hypotension, heart block, alopecia, dermatitis, psoriasis, arthritis, tendonitis, dyspnea and other respiratory symptoms (e.g., bronchitis, pneumonia, rhinitis, sinusitis, pharyngitis) occur rarely.
! Ophthalmic overdosage may produce bradycardia, hypotension, bronchospasm, and acute cardiac failure.

DENTAL CONSIDERATIONS

General:
- Determine why patient is taking the drug.
- Avoid drugs with anticholinergic activity, such as antihistamines, opioids, benzodiazepines, propantheline, atropine, and scopolamine.
- Avoid dental light in patient's eyes; offer dark glasses for patient comfort.
- Question glaucoma patient about compliance with prescribed drug regimen.

Consultations:
- Medical consultation may be required to assess disease control.

Teach Patient/Family to:
- Update health and medication history if physician makes any changes in evaluation or drug regimens; include OTC, herbal, and nonherbal drugs in the update.

levobunolol hydrochloride

lee-vo-**byoo′**-no-lol high-droh-**klor′**-ide
(AK-Beta, Betagan, Novo-Levobunolol[CAN], Optho-Bunolol[CAN], PMS-Levobunolol[CAN])
Do not confuse with levobetaxolol.

CATEGORY AND SCHEDULE

Pregnancy Risk Category: C

Drug Class: Antiglaucoma agent (ophthalmic)

L

MECHANISM OF ACTION

A nonselective β-blocker that blocks β_1- and β_2-adrenergic receptors.
Therapeutic Effect: Reduces intraocular pressure (IOP). Decreases production of aqueous humor.

USES

Treatment of certain types of glaucoma

PHARMACOKINETICS

Well absorbed after administration. Metabolized in liver. Primarily excreted in urine. ***Half-life:*** 6.1 hr.

INDICATIONS AND DOSAGES

▸ **Glaucoma, Ocular Hypertension**
Ophthalmic
Adults, Elderly. Instill 1–2 drops in affected eye(s) once daily.

SIDE EFFECTS/ ADVERSE REACTIONS

Frequent

Burning/stinging, eye irritation, visual disturbances

Occasional

Increased light sensitivity, watering of eye

Rare

Dry eye, conjunctivitis, eye pain, diarrhea, dyspepsia

PRECAUTIONS AND CONTRAINDICATIONS

Cardiogenic shock, overt cardiac failure, second- or third-degree heart block, sinus bradycardia, hypersensitivity to levobunolol or any component of the formulation

DRUG INTERACTIONS OF CONCERN TO DENTISTRY

• Patient with glaucoma: avoid use of anticholinergic drugs, atropine-like drugs, propantheline, and diazepam (benzodiazepines)

SERIOUS REACTIONS

! Abrupt withdrawal may result in sweating, headache, and fatigue.

! Ophthalmic overdosage may produce bradycardia, hypotension, bronchospasm, and acute cardiac failure.

DENTAL CONSIDERATIONS

General:

• Check compliance of patient with prescribed drug regimen for glaucoma.

• Avoid dental light in patient's eyes; offer dark glasses for patient comfort.

Consultations:

• Consultation with physician may be necessary if sedation or anesthesia is required.

levocabastine

lev-oh-**kab′**-ah-steen

(Livostin)

CATEGORY AND SCHEDULE

Pregnancy Risk Category: C

Drug Class: Antihistamine, H_1-receptor antagonist

MECHANISM OF ACTION

An antiallergic agent that selectively antagonizes H_1 receptor.

Therapeutic Effect: Blocks histamine-associated symptoms of seasonal allergic conjunctivitis.

USES

Temporary relief of seasonal allergic conjunctivitis

PHARMACOKINETICS

Duration of action is about 2 hr. Minimal systemic absorption.

INDICATIONS AND DOSAGES

▸ **Allergic Conjunctivitis**

Ophthalmic

Adults, Elderly, Children 12 yr or older. 1 drop 4 times a day, for up to 2 wk.

SIDE EFFECTS/ADVERSE REACTIONS

Frequent

Transient stinging, burning, discomfort, headache

Occasional

Dry mouth, fatigue, eye dryness, lacrimation and discharge, eyelid edema

Rare

Rash, erythema, nausea, dyspnea

PRECAUTIONS AND CONTRAINDICATIONS

Wearing of soft contact lenses (product contains benzalkonium chloride), hypersensitivity to levocabastine or any component of the formulation
Caution:
Lactation, children younger than 12 yr

DRUG INTERACTIONS OF CONCERN TO DENTISTRY

• None reported

SERIOUS REACTIONS

! None reported

DENTAL CONSIDERATIONS

General:
• Question patient about history of allergy to avoid using other potential allergens.
• Avoid dental light in patient's eyes; offer dark glasses for patient comfort.
• Evaluate respiration characteristics and rate.
• Use for less than 2 wk should not present a problem with dry mouth.
Teach Patient/Family to:
• When chronic dry mouth occurs, advise patient to:
  • Avoid mouth rinses with high alcohol content because of drying effects.
  • Use daily home fluoride products for anticaries effect.
  • Use sugarless gum, frequent sips of water, or saliva substitutes.

levocetirizine

lee-vo-seh-**teer′**-ah-zeen
(Xyzal [U.S.], Xuzal, Xusal, Xozal, Vozet [intl.])

CATEGORY AND SCHEDULE

Pregnancy Risk Category: B

Drug Class: Nonsedating antihistamine, blocks H_1 receptors

MECHANISM OF ACTION

Active enantiomer of cetirizine, blocks peripheral H_1 histamine receptors, reduces signs and symptoms related to mild allergies.
Therapeutic Effect: Blockade of peripheral actions of histamines results in reduction of bronchial constriction and respiratory and exocrine secretions related to allergy.

USES

Seasonal allergic rhinitis, chronic idiopathic urticaria

PHARMACOKINETICS

Rapidly and extensively absorbed after oral administration, protein binding: 91%. Metabolized in the liver by CYP3A4 (14%) and taurine conjugation; metabolites primarily excreted in urine (85%) and feces (13%). ***Half-life***: 8–9 hr.

INDICATIONS AND DOSAGES

▸ Seasonal Rhinitis

Adults and Children 12 yr. PO 5 mg (tablet) or 2 tsp (10 ml oral solution) once daily in the evening
Children 6 to 11 yr. PO 2.5 mg (one-half tablet) or 1 tsp (5 ml oral solution) once daily in the evening

SIDE EFFECTS/ADVERSE REACTIONS

Frequent
Somnolence, nasopharyngitis, fatigue, dry mouth, pharyngitis
Occasional
Pyrexia, cough, nosebleed
Rare
Palpitations, fatigue

PRECAUTIONS AND CONTRAINDICATIONS

Activities requiring mental alertness
Nursing
Geriatric patients
Renal impairment
Contraindicated by hypersensitivity to levocetirizine, end-stage renal disease, pediatric patients with impaired renal function

L

DRUG INTERACTIONS OF CONCERN TO DENTISTRY

• Theoretical potentiation of CNS depressants (e.g., sedatives) in susceptible individuals

SERIOUS REACTIONS

! Hypersensitivity
! Hallucinations, suicidal ideation, orofacial dyskinesia, hypotension
! Cholestasis, glomerulonephritis, still birth

DENTAL CONSIDERATIONS

General:
• Assess salivary flow as a factor in caries, periodontal disease, and candidiasis.
• After supine positioning, allow patient to sit upright for 2 minutes to avoid occurrence of dizziness.
• Consider levocetirizine as an etiologic factor in oral inflammation (pharyngitis).

Consultations:
• Consult with physician to determine disease control and ability to tolerate dental procedures.

Teach Patient/Family to:
• If dry mouth occurs:
  • Avoid mouth rinses with high alcohol content because of drying effect.
  • Use home fluoride products for anticaries effect.
  • Use sugarless/xylitol gum, frequent sips of water, or saliva substitutes.

levodopa

lev-oh-**dope**′-ah
(Dopar, Larodopa)

CATEGORY AND SCHEDULE

Pregnancy Risk Category: C

Drug Class: Antiparkinson agent

MECHANISM OF ACTION

A dopamine prodrug that is converted to dopamine in basal ganglia. Increases dopamine concentrations in the brain, inhibiting hyperactive cholinergic activity.
Therapeutic Effect: Decreases signs and symptoms of Parkinson's disease.

USES

Treatment of Parkinsonism of various causes

PHARMACOKINETICS

About 30% absorbed. May be reduced with high-protein meal. Protein binding: minimal. Crosses blood-brain barrier. Converted to dopamine. Eliminated primarily in urine and to a lesser amount in feces and expired air. Not removed by hemodialysis. ***Half-life:*** 0.75–1.5 hr.

INDICATIONS AND DOSAGES

▸ Parkinsonism

PO

Adults, Elderly. Initially, 0.5–1 g 2–4 times a day. May increase in increments not exceeding 0.75 g every 3–7 days, up to a maximum of 8 g/day.

SIDE EFFECTS/ADVERSE REACTIONS

Frequent

Uncontrolled body movements of the face, tongue, arms, and upper body; nausea and vomiting; anorexia

Occasional

Depression, anxiety, confusion, nervousness, difficulty urinating, irregular heartbeats, hiccoughs, dizziness, light-headedness, decreased appetite, blurred vision, constipation, dry mouth, flushed skin, headache, insomnia, diarrhea, unusual tiredness, darkening of urine, discolored sweat

Rare

Hypertension, ulcer, hemolytic anemia, marked by tiredness or weakness

PRECAUTIONS AND CONTRAINDICATIONS

Nonselective MAOI therapy, hypersensitivity to levodopa or any component of its formulation

Caution:

Renal disease, cardiac disease, hepatic disease, respiratory disease, MI with dysrhythmia, convulsions, peptic ulcer, asthma, endocrine disease, affective disorders, psychosis, lactation, children younger than 12 yr

DRUG INTERACTIONS OF CONCERN TO DENTISTRY

- Decreased absorption: anticholinergics
- Decreased therapeutic effect: benzodiazepines, pyridoxine (vitamin B_6), tricyclic antidepressants

SERIOUS REACTIONS

! High incidence of involuntary dystonic and dyskinetic movements may be noted in patients on long-term therapy.

! Mental changes, such as paranoid ideation, psychotic episodes, and depression, may be noted.

! Numerous mild-to-severe CNS psychiatric disturbances may include reduced attention span, anxiety, nightmares, daytime somnolence, euphoria, fatigue, paranoia, and hallucinations.

DENTAL CONSIDERATIONS

General:

- Patients on chronic drug therapy may rarely have symptoms of blood dyscrasias, which can include infection, bleeding, and poor healing.
- Assess salivary flow as a factor in caries, periodontal disease, and candidiasis.
- After supine positioning, have patient sit upright for at least 2 min before standing to avoid orthostatic hypotension.
- Avoid dental light in patient's eyes; offer dark glasses for patient comfort.

Consultations:

- In a patient with symptoms of blood dyscrasias, request a medical consultation for blood studies and postpone dental treatment until normal values are reestablished.

• Take precautions if dental surgery is anticipated and anesthesia is required.
• Medical consultation may be required to assess disease control.

Teach Patient/Family to:

• Use powered tooth brush if patient has difficulty holding conventional devices.
• When chronic dry mouth occurs, advise patient to:
  • Avoid mouth rinses with high alcohol content because of drying effects.
  • Use sugarless gum, frequent sips of water, or saliva substitutes.
  • Use daily home fluoride products for anticaries effect.

L

levofloxacin

lev-oh-**flox′**-ah-sin
(Iquix, Levaquin, Quixin)

CATEGORY AND SCHEDULE

Pregnancy Risk Category: C

Drug Class: Fluoroquinolone antiinfective

MECHANISM OF ACTION

A fluoroquinolone that inhibits the enzyme DNA gyrase in susceptible microorganisms, interfering with bacterial cell replication and repair. ***Therapeutic Effect:*** Bactericidal.

USES

Treatment of acute infections caused by susceptible bacterial strains causing acute maxillary sinusitis, acute bacterial exacerbation of chronic bronchitis, community-acquired pneumonia, nosocomial pneumonia, complicated and uncomplicated skin and skin-structure infections, uncomplicated UTI, and acute pyelonephritis; nosocomial pneumonia; chronic bacterial prostatitis

PHARMACOKINETICS

Well absorbed after both PO and IV administration. Protein binding: 8%–24%. Penetrates rapidly and extensively into leukocytes, epithelial cells, and macrophages. Lung concentrations are 2–5 times higher than those of plasma. Eliminated unchanged in the urine. Partially removed by hemodialysis. ***Half-life:*** 8 hr.

INDICATIONS AND DOSAGES

▸ **Bronchitis**

PO, IV

Adults, Elderly. 500 mg q24h for 7 days.

▸ **Community-Acquired Pneumonia**

PO

Adults, Elderly. 750 mg/day for 5 days.

▸ **Pneumonia**

PO, IV

Adults, Elderly. 500 mg q24h for 7–14 days.

▸ **Acute Maxillary Sinusitis**

PO, IV

Adults, Elderly. 500 mg q24h for 10–14 days.

▸ **Skin and Skin-Structure Infections**

PO, IV

Adults, Elderly. 500 mg q24h for 7–10 days.

▸ **UTIs, Acute Pyelonephritis**

PO, IV

Adults, Elderly. 250 mg q24h for 10 days.

▸ **Bacterial Conjunctivitis**

Ophthalmic

Adults, Elderly, Children 1 yr and older. 1–2 drops q2h for 2 days (up to 8 times a day), then 1–2 drops q4h for 5 days.

▸ **Corneal Ulcer**
Ophthalmic
Adults, Elderly, Children older than 5 yr: Days 1–3: Instill 1–2 drops q30min to 2 hr while awake and 4–6 hr after retiring. Days 4 through completion: 1–2 drops q1–4h while awake.

▸ **Dosage in Renal Impairment**
For bronchitis, pneumonia, sinusitis, and skin and skin-structure infections, dosage and frequency are modified on the basis of creatinine clearance.

Creatinine Clearance	Dosage
50–80 ml/min	No change
20–49 ml/min	500 mg initially, then 250 mg q24h
10–19 ml/min	500 mg initially, then 250 mg q48h
Dialysis	500 mg initially, then 250 mg q48h

For UTIs and pyelonephritis, dosage and frequency are modified on the basis of creatinine clearance.

Creatinine Clearance	Dosage
20 ml/min	No change
10–19 ml/min	250 mg initially, then 250 mg q48h

SIDE EFFECTS/ADVERSE REACTIONS

Occasional
Diarrhea, nausea, abdominal pain, dizziness, drowsiness, headache, light-headedness
Ophthalmic: Local burning or discomfort, margin crusting, crystals or scales, foreign body sensation, ocular itching, altered taste

Rare
Flatulence; altered taste; pain; inflammation or swelling in calves, hands, or shoulder; chest pain; difficulty breathing; palpitations; edema; tendon pain; rupture of Achilles tendon
Ophthalmic: Corneal staining, keratitis, allergic reaction, eyelid swelling, tearing, reduced visual acuity

PRECAUTIONS AND CONTRAINDICATIONS

Hypersensitivity to levofloxacin, other fluoroquinolones, or nalidixic acid

Caution:
Children younger than 18 yr; seizure disorders, renal insufficiency, excessive exposure to sunlight, alterations in blood glucose (diabetes), lactation, drink fluids liberally; tendon rupture of shoulder, hand, and Achilles tendon, monitor blood glucose

DRUG INTERACTIONS OF CONCERN TO DENTISTRY

- Interference with absorption: solutions with multivalent cations (e.g., magnesium)
- Increased seizure risk: NSAIDs
- May increase effects of warfarin (monitor bleeding)

SERIOUS REACTIONS

! Antibiotic-associated colitis and other superinfections may occur from altered bacterial balance.
! Hypersensitivity reactions, including photosensitivity (as evidenced by rash, pruritus, blisters, edema, and burning skin), have occurred in patients receiving fluoroquinolones.

DENTAL CONSIDERATIONS

General:
- Determine why patient is taking the drug.

L

• If prescribed for dental condition, advise patient of potential for photosensitivity.

Consultations:

• Consult with patient's physician if an acute dental infection occurs and another antiinfective is required.

Teach Patient/Family to:

• Minimize exposure to sunlight and wear sunscreen if sun exposure is planned.

• Discontinue treatment and inform dentist immediately if patient experiences pain or inflammation of a tendon, and to rest and refrain from exercise.

L

levothyroxine

lev-oh-thye-**rox**′-een

(Droxine[AUS], Eltroxin[CAN], Eutroxsig[AUS], Levothroid, Levoxyl, Novothyrox[CAN], Oroxine[AUS], Synthroid, Unithroid)

Do not confuse levothyroxine with liothyronine.

CATEGORY AND SCHEDULE

Pregnancy Risk Category: A

Drug Class: Thyroid hormone

MECHANISM OF ACTION

A synthetic isomer of thyroxine involved in normal metabolism, growth, and development, especially of the CNS in infants. Possesses catabolic and anabolic effects.

Therapeutic Effect: Increases basal metabolic rate, enhances gluconeogenesis, and stimulates protein synthesis.

USES

Treatment of hypothyroidism, myxedema coma, thyroid hormone replacement, cretinism, chronic thyroiditis, euthyroid goiters, management of thyroid cancer

PHARMACOKINETICS

Variable, incomplete absorption from the GI tract. Protein binding: greater than 99%. Widely distributed. Deiodinated in peripheral tissues, minimal metabolism in the liver. Eliminated by biliary excretion. ***Half-life:*** 6–7 days.

INDICATIONS AND DOSAGES

▸ Hypothyroidism

PO

Adults, Elderly. Initially, 12.5–50 mcg. May increase by 25–50 mcg/day q2-4wk. Maintenance: 100–200 mcg/day.

Children 13 yr and older. 150 mcg/day.

Children 6–12 yr. 100–125 mcg/day.

Children 1–5 yr. 75–100 mcg/day.

Children 7–11 mo. 50–75 mcg/day.

Children 3–6 mo. 25–50 mcg/day.

Children 3 mo and younger. 10–15 mcg/day.

▸ Thyroid Suppression Therapy

PO

Adults, Elderly. 2–6 mcg/kg/day for 7–10 days.

▸ Thyroid-Stimulating Hormone Suppression in Thyroid Cancer, Nodules, Euthyroid Goiters

PO

Adults, Elderly. 2–6 mcg/kg/day for 7–10 days.

IV

Adults, Elderly, Children. Initial dosage approximately half the previously established oral dosage.

SIDE EFFECTS/ADVERSE REACTIONS

Occasional

Reversible hair loss at the start of therapy (in children)

Rare
Dry skin, GI intolerance, rash, hives, pseudotumor cerebri or severe headache in children

PRECAUTIONS AND CONTRAINDICATIONS

Hypersensitivity to tablet components, such as tartrazine; allergy to aspirin; lactose intolerance; MI and thyrotoxicosis uncomplicated by hypothyroidism; treatment of obesity
Caution:
Elderly, angina pectoris, hypertension, ischemia, cardiac disease, lactation

DRUG INTERACTIONS OF CONCERN TO DENTISTRY

• Increased effects of sympathomimetics when thyroid doses are not carefully monitored or in patients with coronary artery disease

SERIOUS REACTIONS

! Excessive dosage produces signs and symptoms of hyperthyroidism, including weight loss, palpitations, increased appetite, tremors, nervousness, tachycardia, hypertension, headache, insomnia, and menstrual irregularities.
! Cardiac arrhythmias occur rarely.

DENTAL CONSIDERATIONS

General:
• Uncontrolled hypothyroid patients may be more responsive to CNS depressants.
• Increased nervousness, excitability, sweating, or tachycardia may indicate a patient with uncontrolled hyperthyroidism or a dose of medication that is too high.
• Uncontrolled patients should be referred for medical treatment.
• Observe appropriate limitations of vasoconstrictor doses.
• Monitor vital signs at every appointment because of CV side effects.
Consultations:
• Medical consultation may be required to assess disease control.

lidocaine hydrochloride

lye′-doe-kane high-droh-**klor′**-ide
(Lidoderm, Lignocaine Gel[AUS], Xylocaine, Xylocaine Aerosol[AUS], Xylocaine Ointment[AUS], Oraqix[US], Xylocaine Viscous Topical Solution[AUS], Xylocard[CAN], Zilactin-L[CAN], Zingo)

CATEGORY AND SCHEDULE

Pregnancy Risk Category: B

Drug Class: Antidysrhythmic (class IB)

MECHANISM OF ACTION

An amide anesthetic that blocks conduction of nerve impulses.
Therapeutic Effect: Causes temporary loss of feeling and sensation. Also an antiarrhythmic that decreases depolarization, automaticity, excitability of the ventricle during diastole by direct action. Inhibits ventricular arrhythmias.

USES

Ventricular tachycardia, ventricular dysrhythmias during cardiac surgery, MI, digitalis toxicity, cardiac catheterization; for acute management only, local pain control

L

PHARMACOKINETICS

Route	Onset	Peak	Duration
IV	30–90 sec	N/A	10–20 min
Local Anesthetic	2.5 min	N/A	30–60 min

Completely absorbed after IM administration. Protein binding: 60%–80%. Widely distributed. Metabolized in the liver. Primarily excreted in urine. Minimally removed by hemodialysis. ***Half-life:*** 1–2 hr.

INDICATIONS AND DOSAGES

▸ Rapid Control of Acute Ventricular Arrhythmias after an MI, Cardiac Catheterization, Cardiac Surgery, or Digitalis-Induced Ventricular Arrhythmias

L

IM

Adults, Elderly. 300 mg (or 4.3 mg/kg). May repeat in 60–90 min.

IV

Adults, Elderly. Initially, 50–100 mg (1 mg/kg) IV bolus at rate of 25–50 mg/min. May repeat in 5 min. Give no more than 200–300 mg in 1 hr. Maintenance: 20–50 mcg/kg/min (1–4 mg/min) as IV Infusion

Children, Infants. Initially, 0.5–1 mg/kg IV bolus; may repeat but total dose not to exceed 3–5 mg/kg. Maintenance: 10–50 mcg/kg/min as IV infusion.

▸ Dental or Surgical Procedures, Childbirth

Infiltration or Nerve Block

Adults. Local anesthetic dosage varies with procedure, degree of anesthesia, vascularity, duration. Maximum dose: 7 (500 mg absolute with epinephrine), 4.5 mg/kg (300 mg absolute without epinephrine). Do not repeat within 2 hr.

▸ Local Skin Disorders (Minor Burns, Insect Bites, Prickly Heat, Skin Manifestations of Chickenpox, Abrasions), and Mucous Membrane Disorders (Local Anesthesia of Oral, Nasal, and Laryngeal Mucous Membranes; Local Anesthesia of Respiratory, Urinary Tract; Relief of Discomfort of Pruritus Ani, Hemorrhoids, Pruritus Vulvae)

Topical

Adults, Elderly. Apply to affected areas as needed.

▸ Treatment of Shingles-Related Skin Pain

Topical (Dermal Patch)

Adults, Elderly. Apply to intact skin over most painful area (up to 3 applications once for up to 12 hr in a 24-hr period).

SIDE EFFECTS/ADVERSE REACTIONS

CNS effects are generally dose related and of short duration

Occasional

IM: Pain at injection site

Topical: Burning, stinging, tenderness at application site

Rare

Generally with high dose: Drowsiness; dizziness; disorientation; light-headedness; tremors; apprehension; euphoria; sensation of heat, cold, or numbness; blurred or double vision; ringing or roaring in ears (tinnitus); nausea; seizures, post-seizure depression with cardiorespiratory arrest

PRECAUTIONS AND CONTRAINDICATIONS

Adams-Stokes syndrome, hypersensitivity to amide-type local anesthetics, septicemia (spinal anesthesia), supraventricular arrhythmias, Wolff-Parkinson-White syndrome

Caution:
Lactation, children, renal disease, liver disease, CHF, respiratory depression, malignant hyperthermia (questionable), elderly; need to monitor ECG

DRUG INTERACTIONS OF CONCERN TO DENTISTRY

Patch Form
- None reported

Injectable Form
- Potentiation of other CNS depressants

SERIOUS REACTIONS

! Although serious adverse reactions to lidocaine are uncommon, high dosage by any route may produce cardiovascular depression, bradycardia, hypotension, arrhythmias, heart block, cardiovascular collapse, and cardiac arrest.

! CNS toxicity may occur, especially with regional anesthesia use, progressing rapidly from mild side effects to tremors, somnolence, seizures, vomiting, and respiratory depression.

! Methemoglobinemia (evidenced by cyanosis) has occurred following topical application of lidocaine for teething discomfort and laryngeal anesthetic spray.

DENTAL CONSIDERATIONS

▸ Patch Form

General:
- Use no more than one patch per area, remove after 15 min to avoid toxicity.

Teach Patient/Family to:
- Prevent injury while numbness is present and to refrain from gum chewing and eating after dental treatment.
- Report unresolved oral lesions to dentist.

lidocaine transoral delivery system

lye′-doe-kane
(DentiPatch)

CATEGORY AND SCHEDULE

Pregnancy Risk Category: B

Drug Class: Amide local anesthetic

MECHANISM OF ACTION

Inhibits nerve impulses from sensory nerves, which produces anesthesia.

USES

Mild topical anesthesia of mucous membranes of the mouth before superficial dental procedures

PHARMACOKINETICS

Topical: Onset 2.5 min, duration of approximately 30 min after removal; blood levels less than 0.1 ng/ml limited absorption; hepatic metabolism, urinary excretion.

INDICATIONS AND DOSAGES

Topical
Adult. Apply one patch to area of application after drying with gauze; leave in place until local anesthesia is produced but no longer than 15 min.

SIDE EFFECTS/ADVERSE REACTIONS

Oral: Taste alteration, stomatitis, erythema, mucosa irritation
CNS: Headache, excitatory or depressor actions, dizziness, nervousness, confusion, tinnitus, twitching, tremors (associated with excessive systemic absorption)

CV: Bradycardia, hypotension, cardiovascular collapse (with excessive systemic absorption)
GI: Nausea
Misc: Allergic reactions to this agent or to other ingredients in the formulation (rare)

PRECAUTIONS AND CONTRAINDICATIONS

Hypersensitivity to amide-type local anesthetics

Caution:

Local anesthetic toxicity, no pediatric (children younger than 12 yr) or geriatric studies have been made, liver dysfunction, onset longer for maxilla, lactation, contains phenylalanine (caution phenylketonurics)

DRUG INTERACTIONS OF CONCERN TO DENTISTRY

- None reported

SERIOUS REACTIONS

! CNS excitation and depression, potential respiratory depression (at high blood levels).
! Bradycardia, hypotension, cardiovascular collapse, cardiac arrest (at high blood levels).
! Serious allergic reactions (rare).

DENTAL CONSIDERATIONS

General:

- Use no more than one patch per area, remove after 15 min to avoid toxicity.

Teach Patient/Family to:

- Prevent injury while numbness is present and to refrain from gum chewing and eating after dental treatment.
- Report unresolved oral lesions to dentist.

linagliptin + metformin hydrochloride

lin′-a-**glip**′-tin & met-**for**′-min
(Jentadueto)
Do not confuse with sitagliptin and metformin.

CATEGORY AND SCHEDULE

Pregnancy Risk Category: B

Drug Class: Antidiabetic agent, biguanide; antidiabetic agent, dipeptidyl peptidase IV (DPP-IV) inhibitor

MECHANISM OF ACTION

Linagliptin: Increases and prolongs active incretin levels, thereby increasing insulin release and decreasing glucagon levels in the circulation in a glucose-dependent manner. Metformin: An antihyperglycemic that decreases hepatic production of glucose. Decreases absorption of glucose and improves insulin sensitivity.
Therapeutic Effect: Lowers blood glucose concentrations by increasing insulin release, and decreasing insulin resistance.

USES

Management of type 2 diabetes mellitus (noninsulin dependent, NIDDM) as an adjunct to diet and exercise in patients not adequately controlled on metformin or linagliptin monotherapy

PHARMACOKINETICS

Linagliptin: Moderately absorbed after oral administration. 99% plasma protein bound. Minor hepatic metabolism. Primarily excreted unchanged in the feces (85%). Metformin: Slowly, incompletely absorbed after oral administration. Food delays or decreases the extent of absorption. Negligible plasma protein binding. Negligible hepatic metabolism. Primarily distributed to intestinal mucosa and salivary glands. Primarily excreted unchanged in urine (90%). ***Half-life:*** Linagliptin: 12 hr. Metformin: 3–6 hr.

INDICATIONS AND DOSAGES

▸ Type 2 Diabetes Mellitus

PO

Adults. Initial doses should be based on current dose of linagliptin and metformin.
Patients inadequately controlled on metformin alone: Initial dose: Linagliptin 5 mg/day plus current daily dose of metformin given in 2 equally divided doses; maximum: linagliptin 5 mg/metformin 2000 mg daily.
Patients inadequately controlled on linagliptin alone: Initial dose: Metformin 1000 mg/day plus linagliptin 5 mg/day given in 2 equally divided doses.
Dosing adjustments: Metformin component may be gradually increased up to the maximum dose. Maximum dose: Linagliptin 5 mg/ metformin 2000 mg daily.
Elderly. Do not use in patients ≥80 yr of age unless normal renal function has been established. Avoid use in patients with hepatic and renal impairment.

SIDE EFFECTS/ADVERSE REACTIONS

Frequent

Hypoglycemia, nasopharyngitis, upper respiratory tract infection, headache, GI disturbances (including diarrhea, nausea, vomiting, abdominal bloating, flatulence, and anorexia)

Occasional

Abdominal pain, nausea, diarrhea, anaphylaxis, angioedema, rash, urticaria, exfoliative skin reactions, unpleasant or metallic taste

PRECAUTIONS AND CONTRAINDICATIONS

Hypersensitivity to linagliptin, metformin, or any component of the formulation, Avoid use in hepatic and renal dysfunction. Anaphylaxis, angioedema, and Stevens-Johnson syndrome may occur. Use with caution in patients with cardiovascular and respiratory disease.

DRUG INTERACTIONS OF CONCERN TO DENTISTRY

• CYP3A4 and P-glycoprotein inducers (e.g., carbamazepine, barbiturates): potentially reduced efficacy of Jentadueto

SERIOUS REACTIONS

! Lactic acidosis is a rare but potentially severe consequence of therapy with metformin.

DENTAL CONSIDERATIONS

General:

• Be prepared to manage episodes of hypoglycemia.
• Short appointments and a stress-reduction protocol may be needed for anxious patients.
• Nasopharyngitis and diarrhea may affect diagnoses and need for treatment interruptions.
• Question patient about self-monitoring of blood glucose levels.
• Some diabetics may be more susceptible to infection and have delayed wound healing.
• Place on frequent recall to monitor healing response and maintain good oral hygiene.

Consultations:
• Consult physician to determine disease control and patient's ability to tolerate dental procedures.
• Notify physician immediately if symptoms of lactic acidosis are observed (malaise, myalgia, respiratory distress, somnolence, or abdominal distress).
• Medical consultation may include data from patient's blood glucose monitoring, including glycosylated hemoglobin or HbA1c tests.
• Oral and maxillofacial surgical procedures associated with significantly restricted food intake require a medical consultation and temporary cessation of Jentadueto.

Teach Patient/Family to:
• Report changes in disease status and medication regimen.
• Use effective oral hygiene to prevent soft tissue inflammation.

lincomycin HCl

lin-koe-**my**′-sin
(Bactramycin, Lincocin, Lincomycin)

CATEGORY AND SCHEDULE

Pregnancy Risk Category: B

Drug Class: Antibacterial

MECHANISM OF ACTION

A lincosamide antibiotic that specifically binds on the 50S subunit and affects the process of peptide chain initiation.
Therapeutic Effect: Bacteriostatic.

USES

Infections caused by group A β-hemolytic streptococci, pneumococci, staphylococci (respiratory tract, skin, soft tissue, UTIs; osteomyelitis; septicemia), and anaerobes

PHARMACOKINETICS

Rapidly absorbed from the GI tract. Protein binding: Unknown. Metabolized in liver. Primarily excreted in urine. Not removed by hemodialysis. ***Half-life:*** 5.4 hr (prolonged with renal or hepatic impairment).

INDICATIONS AND DOSAGES

▸ **Serious Infection Caused by Susceptible Strains of Streptococci, Pneumococci, and Staphylococci**

PO

Adults. 500 mg 3 times a day (500 mg approximately q8h).
Children older than 1 mo. 30 mg/kg/day (15 mg/lb/day) divided into 3 or 4 equal doses.

▸ **More Severe Infection Caused by Susceptible Strains of Streptococci, Pneumococci, and Staphylococci**

PO

Adults. 500 mg or more 4 times a day (500 mg or more approximately q6h).
Children older than 1 mo. 60 mg/kg/day (30 mg/lb/day) divided into 3 or 4 equal doses.

▸ **Serious Infection Caused by Susceptible Strains of Streptococci, Pneumococci, and Staphylococci**

IM

Adults. 600 mg (2 ml) q24h.
Children older than 1 mo. One injection of 10 mg/kg (5 mg/lb) q24h.

▸ **More Severe Infection Caused by Susceptible Strains of Streptococci, Pneumococci, and Staphylococci**

IM

Adults. 600 mg (2 ml) q12h or more often.

Children older than 1 mo. One injection of 10 mg/kg (5 mg/lb) q12h or more often.

▸ **Serious Infection Caused by Susceptible Strains of Streptococci, Pneumococci, and Staphylococci**

IV

Adults. 600 mg (2 ml) to 1 g q8–12h.

Children older than 1 mo. One injection of 10 mg/kg (5 mg/lb) q12h or more often. Depending on the severity of the infection, 10–20 mg/kg/day (5–10 mg/lb/day) can be infused in divided doses as described for adults.

▸ **More Severe Infection Caused by Susceptible Strains of Streptococci, Pneumococci, and Staphylococci**

IV

Adults. 600 mg (2 ml) to 1 g q8–12h. Maximum: 8 g/day. Intravenous doses are given on the basis of 1 g lincomycin diluted in not less than 100 ml of appropriate solution and infused over a period of not less than 1 hr.

▸ **Subconjunctival Injection**

Adults. Inject 0.25 ml (75 mg).

▸ **Dosage in Renal Impairment**

An appropriate dose is 25%–30% of that recommended for patients with normally functioning kidneys.

SIDE EFFECTS/ADVERSE REACTIONS

Frequent

Abdominal pain, nausea, vomiting, diarrhea

Occasional

Phlebitis, thrombophlebitis with IV administration, pain, induration at IM injection site, allergic reaction, urticaria, pruritus, tinnitus, vertigo

Rare

Dermatitis

PRECAUTIONS AND CONTRAINDICATIONS

History of hypersensitivity to clindamycin or lincomycin

Caution:

Renal disease, liver disease, GI disease, elderly, lactation

DRUG INTERACTIONS OF CONCERN TO DENTISTRY

- Decreased action of erythromycin

SERIOUS REACTIONS

Alert

! Antibiotic-associated colitis, as evidenced by severe abdominal pain and tenderness, fever, and watery and severe diarrhea, may occur during and several weeks after lincomycin therapy.

! Cardiopulmonary arrest and hypotension have been reported.

L

DENTAL CONSIDERATIONS

General:

- Determine why the patient is taking the drug.

Consultations:

- Medical consultation may be required to assess disease control.

Teach Patient/Family to:

- Encourage effective oral hygiene to prevent soft tissue inflammation.
- Use caution to prevent injury when using oral hygiene aids.
- Notify dentist if diarrhea occurs.
- When used for dental infection, advise patient to:
  - Report sore throat, oral burning sensation, fever, fatigue, any of which could indicate superinfection.
  - Take at prescribed intervals and complete dosage regimen.
  - Immediately notify the dentist if signs or symptoms of infection increase.

linezolid

lin-**ez**′-oh-lid
(Zyvox, Zyvoxam)
Do not confuse Zyvox with Zovirax.

CATEGORY AND SCHEDULE

Pregnancy Risk Category: C

Drug Class: Antibiotic, oxazolidinone derivative

MECHANISM OF ACTION

An oxalodinone antiinfective that binds to a site on bacterial 23S ribosomal RNA, preventing the formation of a complex that is essential for bacterial translation. ***Therapeutic Effect:*** Bacteriostatic against enterococci and staphylococci; bactericidal against streptococci.

L

USES

Treatment of vancomycin-resistant *E. faecium* infections; nosocomial pneumonia caused by *S. aureus* (methicillin resistant and susceptible) and *S. pneumoniae* (penicillin susceptible); complicated skin and skin-structure infections caused by *S. aureus* (methicillin resistant and susceptible), *S. pyogenes*, or *S. agalactiae;* uncomplicated skin and skin-structure infections caused by *S. aureus* (methicillin susceptible); community-acquired pneumonia caused by *S. pneumoniae* (penicillin susceptible) or *S. aureus* (methicillin susceptible); and diabetic foot infections without osteomyelitis caused by gram-positive bacteria

PHARMACOKINETICS

Rapidly and extensively absorbed after PO administration. Protein binding: 31%. Metabolized in the liver by oxidation. Excreted in urine. ***Half-life:*** 4–5.4 hr.

INDICATIONS AND DOSAGES

▸ **Vancomycin-Resistant Infections**

PO, IV

Adults, Elderly, Children older than 11 yr. 600 mg q12h for 14–28 days.

▸ **Pneumonia, Complicated Skin, and Skin-Structure Infections**

PO, IV

Adults, Elderly, Children older than 11 yr. 600 mg q12h for 10–14 days.

▸ **Uncomplicated Skin and Skin-Structure Infections**

PO

Adults, Elderly. 400 mg q12h for 10–14 days.

Children older than 11 yr. 600 mg q12h for 10–14 days.

Children 5–11 yr. 10 mg/kg/dose q12h for 10–14 days.

▸ **Usual Neonate Dosage**

PO, IV

Neonates. 10 mg/kg/dose q8–12h.

SIDE EFFECTS/ADVERSE REACTIONS

Occasional

Diarrhea, nausea, headache

Rare

Altered taste, vaginal candidiasis, fungal infection, dizziness, tongue discoloration

PRECAUTIONS AND CONTRAINDICATIONS

Hypersensitivity

Caution:

May promote overgrowth of nonsusceptible bacterial strains, monitor platelet counts in patients at risk for bleeding, lactation, pediatric doses not established, use longer than 28 days, selectively inhibits monoamine oxidase enzymes, potentiation of serotonergic drugs, hepatic disease, hemodialysis patients; risk of myelosuppression, monitor CBC counts, avoid tyramine-containing foods

DRUG INTERACTIONS OF CONCERN TO DENTISTRY

- Potential to increase pressor effects of indirect-action sympathomimetic drugs and vasopressors, such as dopaminergic drugs, phenylephrine, phenylpropanolamine, and pseudoephedrine
- Interactions with vasoconstrictors in local anesthetics has not been studied

SERIOUS REACTIONS

! Thrombocytopenia and myelosuppression occur rarely.

! Antibiotic-associated colitis and other superinfections may result from altered bacterial balance.

DENTAL CONSIDERATIONS

General:

- Determine why patient is taking the drug.
- Use vasoconstrictor with caution, in low doses, and with careful aspiration. Avoid using gingival retraction cord containing epinephrine.
- Patients on chronic drug therapy may rarely have symptoms of blood dyscrasias, which can include infection, bleeding, and poor healing.
- Examine for oral manifestation of opportunistic infection.
- Consider semisupine chair position for patient comfort if GI side effects occur.

Consultations:

- In a patient with symptoms of blood dyscrasias, request a medical consultation for blood studies and postpone treatment until normal values are reestablished.
- Medical consultation may be required to assess disease control and patient's ability to tolerate stress.
- Physician consultation is advised in the presence of an acute dental infection requiring another antibiotic.

Teach Patient/Family to:

- See dentist immediately if secondary oral infection occurs.
- Report sore throat, oral burning sensation, fever, fatigue, any of which could indicate presence of a superinfection.

liothyronine (T3)

lye-oh-**thye**′-roe-neen

(Cytomel, Tertroxin[AUS], Triostat)

Do not confuse liothyronine with levothyroxine.

CATEGORY AND SCHEDULE

Pregnancy Risk Category: A

Drug Class: Thyroid hormone

MECHANISM OF ACTION

A synthetic form of triiodothyronine (T3), a thyroid hormone involved in normal metabolism, growth, and development, especially of the CNS in infants. Possesses catabolic and anabolic effects.

Therapeutic Effect: Increases basal metabolic rate, enhances gluconeogenesis, and stimulates protein synthesis.

USES

Treatment of hypothyroidism, myxedema coma, thyroid hormone replacement, cretinism, nontoxic goiter, T3 suppression test; thyroiditis, euthyroid goiter

PHARMACOKINETICS

PO: Peak 12–48 hr. ***Half-life:*** 0.6–1.4 days.

INDICATIONS AND DOSAGES

▸ Hypothyroidism

PO

Adults, Elderly. Initially, 25 mcg/day. May increase in increments of 12.5–25 mcg/day q1–2wk. Maximum 100 mcg/day.
Children. Initially, 5 mcg/day. May increase by 5 mcg/day q3–4wk. Maintenance: 100 mcg/day (children older than 3 yr); 50 mcg/day (children 1–3 yr); 20 mcg/day (infants).

▸ Myxedema

PO

Adults, Elderly. Initially, 5 mcg/day. Increase by 5–10 mcg q1–2wk (after 25 mcg/day has been reached, may increase in 12.5-mcg increments). Maintenance: 50–100 mcg/day.

▸ Nontoxic Goiter

PO

Adults, Elderly. Initially, 5 mcg/day. Increase by 5–10 mcg/day q1–2wk. When 25 mcg/day has been reached, may increase by 12.5–25 mcg/day q1–2wk. Maintenance: 75 mcg/day.
Children. 5 mcg/day. May increase by 5 mcg q1–2wk. Maintenance: 15–20 mcg/day.

▸ Congenital Hypothyroidism

PO

Children. Initially, 5 mcg/day. Increase by 5 mcg/day q3–4 days. Maintenance: Full adult dosage (children older than 3 yr); 50 mcg/day (children 1–3 yr); 20 mcg/day (infants).

▸ T3 Suppression Test

PO

Adults, Elderly. 75–100 mcg/day for 7 days; then repeat I131 thyroid uptake test.

▸ Myxedema Coma, Precoma

IV

Adults, Elderly. Initially, 25–50 mcg (10–20 mcg in patients with cardiovascular disease). Total dose at least 65 mcg/day.

SIDE EFFECTS/ADVERSE REACTIONS

Occasional

Reversible hair loss at start of therapy (in children)

Rare

Dry skin, GI intolerance, rash, hives, pseudotumor cerebri or severe headache in children

PRECAUTIONS AND CONTRAINDICATIONS

MI and thyrotoxicosis uncomplicated by hypothyroidism; obesity

Caution:

Elderly, angina pectoris, hypertension, ischemia, cardiac disease, lactation

DRUG INTERACTIONS OF CONCERN TO DENTISTRY

- Hypertension, tachycardia: ketamine
- Increased effects of sympathomimetics when thyroid doses are not carefully monitored or in patients with coronary artery disease

SERIOUS REACTIONS

! Excessive dosage produces signs and symptoms of hyperthyroidism, including weight loss, palpitations, increased appetite, tremors, nervousness, tachycardia, hypertension, headache, insomnia, and menstrual irregularities.

! Cardiac arrhythmias occur rarely.

L

DENTAL CONSIDERATIONS

General:

• Patients with uncontrolled hypothyroidism may be more responsive to CNS depressants.

• Increased nervousness, excitability, sweating, or tachycardia may indicate a patient with uncontrolled hyperthyroidism or a dose of medication that is too high. Uncontrolled patients should be referred for medical treatment.

Consultations:

• Medical consultation may be required to assess disease control.

• Observe appropriate limitations of vasoconstrictor doses.

liraglutide

lir-a-**gloo'**-tide
(Victoza)

CATEGORY AND SCHEDULE

Pregnancy Risk Category: C

Drug Class: Antidiabetic agent, glucagon-like peptide-1 (GLP-1) receptor agonist

MECHANISM OF ACTION

Liraglutide is a long-acting analogue of human glucagon-like peptide-1 (GLP-1) (an incretin hormone) that increases glucose-dependent insulin secretion, decreases inappropriate glucagon secretion, increases B-cell growth/replication, slows gastric emptying, and decreases food intake.
Therapeutic Effect: Lowers blood glucose concentration and HbA1c.

USES

Treatment of type 2 diabetes mellitus (noninsulin dependent, NIDDM) to improve glycemic control

PHARMACOKINETICS

Following subcutaneous injection, bioavailability is 55%. Endogenously metabolized by dipeptidyl peptidase IV (DPP-IV) and endogenous endopeptidases. Excreted via urine and feces. ***Half-life:*** 13 hr.

INDICATIONS AND DOSAGES

▸ **Treatment of Type 2 Diabetes**

Subcutaneous injection

Adults. Initially, 0.6 mg once daily for 1 wk, then increase to 1.2 mg once daily; may increase further to 1.8 mg once daily if optimal glycemic response not achieved with 1.2 mg/day.

SIDE EFFECTS/ADVERSE REACTIONS

Frequent

Nausea, diarrhea, vomiting

Occasional

Injection site reactions, headache, constipation

PRECAUTIONS AND CONTRAINDICATIONS

Hypersensitivity to liraglutide or any component of the formulation; history of or family history of medullary thyroid carcinoma (MTC); patients with multiple endocrine neoplasia syndrome type 2 (MEN2). May cause pancreatitis. Avoid use in patients with moderate-to-severe renal impairment. Use with caution in patients with hepatic impairment.

DRUG INTERACTIONS OF CONCERN TO DENTISTRY

• Reduced absorption of orally administered drugs (e.g., preoperative antibiotics, sedatives).

SERIOUS REACTIONS

! Dose- and duration-dependent thyroid C-cell tumors have

developed in animal studies with liraglutide therapy; relevance in humans unknown.

DENTAL CONSIDERATIONS

General:

- Be prepared to manage episodes of hypoglycemia.
- Short appointments and a stress-reduction protocol may be needed for anxious patients.
- Headache, nausea, and diarrhea may require treatment interruptions.
- Question patient about self-monitoring of blood glucose levels.
- Some diabetics may be more susceptible to infection and have delayed wound healing.
- Place on frequent recall to monitor healing response and maintain good oral hygiene.

Consultations:

- Consult physician to determine disease control and patient's ability to tolerate dental procedures.
- Notify physician immediately if symptoms of lactic acidosis are observed (malaise, myalgia, respiratory distress, somnolence, or abdominal distress).
- Medical consultation may include data from patient's blood glucose monitoring, including glycosylated hemoglobin or HbA1c tests.
- Oral and maxillofacial surgical procedures associated with significantly restricted food intake require a medical consultation and temporary cessation of Jentadueto.

Teach Patient/Family to:

- Report changes in disease status and medication regimen.
- Use effective oral hygiene to prevent soft tissue inflammation.

liotrix

lye′-oh-trix
(Thyrolar, Thyrolar-1, Thyrolar-1/2, Thyrolar-1/4, Thyrolar-2, Thyrolar-3)

CATEGORY AND SCHEDULE

Pregnancy Risk Category: A

Drug Class: Thyroid hormone

MECHANISM OF ACTION

A synthetic form of levothyroxine (T4) and triiodothyronine (T3) involved in normal metabolism, growth, and development, especially the CNS of infants. Possesses catabolic and anabolic effects.
Therapeutic Effect: Increases basal metabolic rate, enhances gluconeogenesis, stimulates protein synthesis.

USES

Treatment of hypothyroidism, thyroid hormone replacement, thyroiditis, euthyroid goiter

PHARMACOKINETICS

T4 is partially absorbed from the GI tract. T3 is almost completely absorbed. Widely distributed. Deiodinated in peripheral tissues, minimal metabolism in the liver.
Half-life: Unknown.

INDICATIONS AND DOSAGES

▸ **Hypothyroidism**

PO

Adults, Elderly. Initially, 50 mcg (0.05 mg) levothyroxine and 12.5 mcg (0.0125 mg) liothyronine per day, with increments of a like amount at monthly intervals until the desired result is obtained. Maintenance: 50–100 mcg (0.05–0.1 mg) levothyroxine and

12.5–25 mcg (0.0125–0.025 mg) liothyronine per day.

▸ **Congenital Hypothyroidism**

PO

Children older than 12 yr. More than 150 mcg of levothyroxine per day.

Children 6–12 yr. 100–150 mcg of levothyroxine per day.

Children 1–5 yr. 75–100 mcg of levothyroxine per day.

Children 6–12 mo. 50–75 mcg of levothyroxine per day.

Children 0–6 mo. 25–50 mcg of levothyroxine per day.

▸ **Myxedema**

PO

Adults, Elderly. Initially, 12.5 mcg (0.0125 mg) levothyroxine and 3.1 mcg (0.0031 mg) liothyronine per day, with increments of a like amount q2–3wk until the desired result is obtained. Maintenance: 50–100 mcg (0.05–0.1 mg) levothyroxine and 12.5–25 mcg (0.0125–0.025 mg) liothyronine per day.

▸ **Thyroid Cancer**

PO

Adults, Elderly. Larger amounts of thyroid hormone than those used for replacement therapy are required.

▸ **Thyroid Suppression Therapy**

PO

Adults, Elderly. Usual dosage of levothyroxine 2.6 mcg/kg/day for 7–10 days.

SIDE EFFECTS/ADVERSE REACTIONS

Occasional

Reversible hair loss at the start of therapy (in children)

Rare

Dry skin, GI intolerance, rash, hives, pseudotumor cerebri or severe headache in children

PRECAUTIONS AND CONTRAINDICATIONS

Uncorrected adrenal cortical insufficiency, untreated thyrotoxicosis, or hypersensitivity to any of active constituents

Caution:

Elderly, angina pectoris, hypertension, ischemia, cardiac disease, lactation

DRUG INTERACTIONS OF CONCERN TO DENTISTRY

• Hypertension, tachycardia: ketamine

• Increased effects of sympathomimetics when thyroid doses are not carefully monitored or in patients with coronary artery disease

SERIOUS REACTIONS

! Excessive dosage produces signs and symptoms of hyperthyroidism, including weight loss, palpitations, increased appetite, tremors, nervousness, tachycardia, hypertension, headache, insomnia, menstrual irregularities.

! Cardiac arrhythmias occur rarely.

DENTAL CONSIDERATIONS

General:

• Patients with uncontrolled hypothyroidism may be more responsive to CNS depressants.

• Increased nervousness, excitability, sweating, or tachycardia may indicate a patient with uncontrolled hyperthyroidism or a dose of medication that is too high. Uncontrolled patients should be referred for medical treatment.

• Observe appropriate limitations of vasoconstrictor doses.

Consultations:

• Medical consultation may be required to assess disease control.

Teach Patient/Family to:
- Encourage effective oral hygiene to prevent soft tissue inflammation.
- Avoid mouth rinses with high alcohol content because of drying effects.

lisdexamfetamine dimesylate

liz-dex-am-**fet′**-a-meen
(Vyvanase)

CATEGORY AND SCHEDULE

Pregnancy Risk Category: C
Controlled substance: Schedule II

Drug Class: CNS stimulant, amphetamine

L

MECHANISM OF ACTION

The actual mechanism for attention-deficit/hyperactivity disorder (ADHD) is not known. Prodrug of dextroamphetamine thought to block the neuronal reuptake of norepinephrine and dopamine.

USES

Used for treatment of ADHD.

PHARMACOKINETICS

Rapid absorption. Dextroamphetamine active metabolite. Mean CSF concentrations are 80% those of plasma. ***Half-life***: lisdexamfetamine <1 hr and dextroamphetamine 10–13 hr. Metabolized into dextroamphetamine and l-lysine through non–CYP-mediated hepatic or intestinal metabolism. Excreted primarily in the urine (96%), and small amount in feces.

INDICATIONS AND DOSAGES

▸ **ADHD**

PO

Adults. 30 mg once daily in the morning. May increase in increments of 10 mg or 20 mg/day at weekly intervals until optimal response. Maximum 70 mg/day.
Children (6–12 yr). 30 mg once daily in the morning. May increase in increments of 10 mg or 20 mg/day at weekly intervals until optimal response. Maximum 70 mg/day.

SIDE EFFECTS/ADVERSE REACTIONS

Adult

Frequent

Insomnia, decreased appetite, xerostomia

Occasional

Increase blood pressure, increased heart rate, anxiety, jitteriness, agitation, restlessness, hyperhidrosis, diarrhea, nausea, anorexia, tremor, dyspnea

▸ **Children**

Frequent

Headache, insomnia, decreased appetite, xerostomia, abdominal pain

Occasional

Irritability, dizziness, affects lability, fever, somnolence, tic, vomiting, weight loss, nausea

PRECAUTIONS AND CONTRAINDICATIONS

Hypersensitivity to lisdexamfetamine, sympathomimetic amines, or its components.
Avoid in patients with pre-existing structural cardiac abnormalities or other heart conditions because serious cardiovascular events including sudden death have been reported.
Avoid in patients with history of ethanol or drug abuse since prolonged drug use may lead to dependency.

Avoid in patients with moderate to severe hypertension, arteriosclerosis, hyperthyroidism, or symptomatic cardiovascular diseases.
Use with caution in patients with hypertension and other cardiovascular conditions that might exacerbate increases in blood pressure and/ or heart rate.
Use with caution in patients with history of or pre-existing psychosis, bipolar disorder, aggressive behavior, seizure disorder, and Tourette's syndrome.
Abrupt discontinuation following high doses or for prolonged period may lead to withdrawal syndrome.

DRUG INTERACTIONS OF CONCERN TO DENTISTRY

• Blood pressure should be monitored prior to administering local anesthetic with vasoconstrictors since dextroamphetamine is known to increase blood pressure.
• Tricyclic antidepressants: may potentiate the anticholinergic effects of tricyclic antidepressants.

SERIOUS REACTIONS

! Serious cardiovascular events, including sudden death, may occur in patients with pre-existing structural cardiac abnormalities or other heart conditions.
! Potential for drug dependency may occur with prolonged use.
! Prolonged administration to children with ADHD may produce a temporary suppression of normal weight and height patterns.

DENTAL CONSIDERATIONS

General:
• Monitor vital signs at every appointment because of cardiovascular side effects.
• Observe appropriate limitations of vasoconstrictor doses.
• Assess salivary flow as a factor in caries, periodontal disease, and candidiasis.
• Consider semisupine chair position for patient comfort because of respiratory effects of disease.

Teach Patient/Family to:
• When chronic dry mouth occurs, advise patient to:
  • Avoid mouth rinses with high alcohol content because of drying effects.
  • Use sugarless gum, frequent sips of water, or saliva substitutes.
  • Use daily home fluoride products for anticaries effect.

L

lisinopril

lye-**sin**′-oh-pril
(Apo-Lisinopril[CAN], Fibsol[AUS], Lisodur[AUS], Prinivil, Zestril)
Do not confuse lisinopril with fosinopril; Prinivil with Desyrel, Plendil, Proventil, or Restoril; Fibsol with Lioresal; or Zestril with Zostrix. Do not confuse lisinopril's combination form Zestoretic with Prilosec.

CATEGORY AND SCHEDULE

Pregnancy Risk Category: C (D if used in second or third trimester)

Drug Class: Angiotensin-converting enzyme (ACE) inhibitor

MECHANISM OF ACTION

This ACE inhibitor suppresses the renin-angiotensin-aldosterone system and prevents conversion of angiotensin I to angiotensin II, a potent vasoconstrictor; may also

inhibit angiotensin II at local vascular and renal sites. Decreases plasma angiotensin II, increases plasma renin activity, and decreases aldosterone secretion.
Therapeutic Effect: Reduces peripheral arterial resistance, B/P, afterload, pulmonary capillary wedge pressure (preload), and pulmonary vascular resistance. In those with heart failure, also decreases heart size, increases cardiac output, and exercise tolerance time.

USES

Treatment of mild-to-moderate hypertension, post-MI if hemodynamically stable, heart failure

L

PHARMACOKINETICS

Route	Onset	Peak	Duration
PO	1 hr	6 hr	24 hr

Incompletely absorbed from the GI tract. Protein binding: 25%. Primarily excreted unchanged in urine. Removed by hemodialysis.
Half-life: 12 hr (half-life is prolonged in those with impaired renal function).

INDICATIONS AND DOSAGES

▸ Hypertension (Used Alone)
PO
Adults. Initially, 10 mg/day. May increase by 5–10 mcg/day at 1- to 2-wk intervals. Maximum: 40 mg/day.
Elderly. Initially, 2.5–5 mg/day. May increase by 2.5–5 mg/day at 1- to 2-wk intervals. Maximum: 40 mg/day.

▸ Hypertension (Used in Combination with Other Antihypertensives)
PO
Adults. Initially, 2.5–5 mg/day titrated to patient's needs.

▸ Adjunctive Therapy for Management of Heart Failure
PO
Adults, Elderly. Initially, 2.5–5 mg/day. May increase by no more than 10 mg/day at intervals of at least 2 wk. Maintenance: 5–40 mg/day.

▸ Improve Survival in Patients after an MI
PO
Adults, Elderly. Initially, 5 mg, then 5 mg after 24 hr, 10 mg after 48 hr, then 10 mg/day for 6 wk. For patients with low systolic B/P, give 2.5 mg/day for 3 days, then 2.5–5 mg/day.

▸ Dosage in Renal Impairment
Titrate to patient's needs after giving the following initial dose:

Creatinine Clearance	% Normal Dose
10–50 ml/min	50–75
Less than 10 ml/min	25–50

SIDE EFFECTS/ADVERSE REACTIONS

Frequent
Headache, dizziness, postural hypotension
Occasional
Chest discomfort, fatigue, rash, abdominal pain, nausea, diarrhea, upper respiratory infection
Rare
Palpitations, tachycardia, peripheral edema, insomnia, paresthesia, confusion, constipation, dry mouth, muscle cramps

PRECAUTIONS AND CONTRAINDICATIONS

History of angioedema from previous treatment with ACE inhibitors

Caution:
Lactation, renal disease, hyperkalemia

DRUG INTERACTIONS OF CONCERN TO DENTISTRY

- Increased hypotension: alcohol, phenothiazines
- Decreased hypotensive effects: indomethacin and possibly other NSAIDs, sympathomimetics
- Suspected reduction in the antihypertensive and vasodilator effects by salicylates; monitor B/P if used concurrently

SERIOUS REACTIONS

! Excessive hypotension ("first-dose syncope") may occur in patients with CHF and severe salt and volume depletion.
! Angioedema (swelling of face and lips) and hyperkalemia occurs rarely.
! Agranulocytosis and neutropenia may be noted in patients with collagen vascular disease, including scleroderma and systemic lupus erythematosus, and impaired renal function.
! Nephrotic syndrome may be noted in patients with history of renal disease.

DENTAL CONSIDERATIONS

General:

- Monitor vital signs at every appointment because of cardiovascular and respiratory side effects.
- After supine positioning, have patient sit upright for at least 2 min before standing to avoid orthostatic hypotension.
- Patients on chronic drug therapy may rarely have symptoms of blood dyscrasias, which can include infection, bleeding, and poor healing.
- Assess salivary flow as a factor in caries, periodontal disease, and candidiasis.
- Limit use of sodium-containing products, such as saline IV fluids, for patients with a dietary salt restriction.
- Use vasoconstrictors with caution, in low doses, and with careful aspiration.
- Short appointments and a stress-reduction protocol may be required for anxious patients.

Consultations:

- Medical consultation may be required to assess disease control and patient's ability to tolerate stress.
- In a patient with symptoms of blood dyscrasias, request a medical consultation for blood studies and postpone dental treatment until normal values are reestablished.
- Take precautions if dental surgery is anticipated and sedation or general anesthesia is required; risk of hypotensive episode.

Teach Patient/Family to:

- Encourage effective oral hygiene to prevent soft tissue inflammation.
- Use caution to prevent injury when using oral hygiene aids.
- When chronic dry mouth occurs, advise patient to:
  - Avoid mouth rinses with high alcohol content because of drying effects.
  - Use sugarless gum, frequent sips of water, or saliva substitutes.
  - Use daily home fluoride products for anticaries effect.

lithium carbonate/ lithium citrate

lith′-ee-um
kahr′-buh-neyt/**sit′**-rayte
lithium carbonate (Duralith[CAN], Eskalith, Lithi.carb[AUS], Lithobid, Quilonum SR[AUS]), lithium citrate (Cibalith-S)
Do not confuse Lithobid with Levbid, Lithostat, or Lithotabs.

CATEGORY AND SCHEDULE

Pregnancy Risk Category: D

Drug Class: Antimanic, inorganic salt

MECHANISM OF ACTION

A psychotherapeutic agent that affects the storage, release, and reuptake of neurotransmitters. Antimanic effect may result from increased norepinephrine reuptake and serotonin receptor sensitivity. ***Therapeutic Effect:*** Produces antimanic and antidepressant effects.

USES

Treatment of manic-depressive illness (manic phase), prevention of bipolar manic-depressive psychosis

PHARMACOKINETICS

Rapidly and completely absorbed from the GI tract. Primarily excreted unchanged in urine. Removed by hemodialysis. ***Half-life:*** 18–24 hr (increased in elderly).

INDICATIONS AND DOSAGES

Alert
During acute phase, a therapeutic serum lithium concentration of 1–1.4 mEq/L is required. For long-term control, the desired level is 0.5–1.3 mEq/L. Monitor serum drug concentration and clinical response.

▸ **Prevention or Treatment of Acute Mania, Manic Phase of Bipolar Disorder (Manic-Depressive Illness)**
PO
Adults. 300 mg 3–4 times a day or 450–900 mg slow-release form twice a day. Maximum: 2.4 g/day.
Elderly. 300 mg twice a day. May increase by 300 mg/day q1wk. Maintenance: 900–1200 mg/day.
Children 12 yr and older. 600–1800 mg/day in 3–4 divided doses (2 doses/day for slow-release).
Children younger than 12 yr. 15–60 mg/kg/day in 3–4 divided doses.

SIDE EFFECTS/ADVERSE REACTIONS

Occasional
Fine hand tremor, polydipsia, polyuria, mild nausea, dry mouth
Rare
Weight gain, bradycardia or tachycardia, acne, rash, muscle twitching, cold and cyanotic extremities, pseudotumor cerebri (eye pain, headache, tinnitus, vision disturbances)

PRECAUTIONS AND CONTRAINDICATIONS

Debilitated patients, severe cardiovascular disease, severe dehydration, severe renal disease, severe sodium depletion
Caution:
Elderly, thyroid disease, seizure disorders, diabetes mellitus, systemic infection, urinary retention

DRUG INTERACTIONS OF CONCERN TO DENTISTRY

• Increased toxicity: aspirin, indomethacin, other NSAIDs, haloperidol, metronidazole, carbamazepine

• Increased effects of neuromuscular blocking agents

SERIOUS REACTIONS

! A lithium serum concentration of 1.5–2.0 mEq/L may produce vomiting, diarrhea, drowsiness, confusion, incoordination, coarse hand tremor, muscle twitching, and T-wave depression on ECG.
! A lithium serum concentration of 2.0–2.5 mEq/L may result in ataxia, giddiness, tinnitus, blurred vision, clonic movements, and severe hypotension.
! Acute toxicity may be characterized by seizures, oliguria, circulatory failure, coma, and death.

DENTAL CONSIDERATIONS

General:
• Assess salivary flow as a factor in caries, periodontal disease, and candidiasis.
• After supine positioning, have patient sit upright for at least 2 min before standing to avoid orthostatic hypotension.
Consultations:
• Medical consultation may be required to assess disease control.
Teach Patient/Family to:
• Encourage effective oral hygiene to prevent soft tissue inflammation.
• Use caution to prevent injury when using oral hygiene aids.
• When chronic dry mouth occurs, advise patient to:
  • Avoid mouth rinses with high alcohol content because of drying effects.
  • Use sugarless gum, frequent sips of water, or saliva substitutes.
  • Use daily home fluoride products for anticaries effect.

lodoxamide

loe-**dox**′-ah-mide
(Alomide)

CATEGORY AND SCHEDULE

Pregnancy Risk Category: B

Drug Class: Mast cell stabilizer

MECHANISM OF ACTION

A mast cell stabilizer that prevents increase in cutaneous vascular permeability, antigen-stimulated histamine release, and may prevent calcium influx into mast cells. ***Therapeutic Effect:*** Inhibits sensitivity reaction.

USES

Treatment of vernal keratoconjunctivitis, vernal conjunctivitis, keratitis

PHARMACOKINETICS

Nondetectable absorption. ***Half-life:*** 8.5 hr.

INDICATIONS AND DOSAGES

▸ Treatment of Vernal Keratoconjunctivitis, Conjunctivitis, and Keratitis
Ophthalmic
Adults, Elderly, Children 2 yr or older: 1–2 drops 4 times a day, for up to 3 mo.

SIDE EFFECTS/ADVERSE REACTIONS

Frequent
Transient stinging, burning, instillation discomfort
Occasional
Ocular itching, blurred vision, dry eye, tearing/discharge/foreign body sensation, headache, dry mouth

L

Rare
Scales on lid/lash, ocular swelling, sticky sensation, dizziness, somnolence, nausea, sneezing, dry nose, rash

PRECAUTIONS AND CONTRAINDICATIONS

Wearing soft contact lenses (product contains benzalkonium chloride), hypersensitivity to lodoxamide tromethamine or any component of the formulation
Caution:
Children younger than 2 yr, lactation

DRUG INTERACTIONS OF CONCERN TO DENTISTRY

- None reported

SERIOUS REACTIONS

! None reported

DENTAL CONSIDERATIONS

General:
- Question patient about history of allergy to avoid use of other potential allergens.
- Avoid dental light in patient's eyes; offer dark glasses for patient comfort.
- Use for less than 2 wk should not present a problem with dry mouth.

Teach Patient/Family to:
- When chronic dry mouth occurs advise patient to:
  - Avoid mouth rinses with high alcohol content because of drying effects.
  - Use daily home fluoride products for anticaries effect.
  - Use sugarless gum, frequent sips of water, or saliva substitutes.

lomefloxacin hydrochloride

low-meh-**flocks**′-ah-sin high-droh-**klor**′-ide
(Maxaquin)

CATEGORY AND SCHEDULE

Pregnancy Risk Category: C

Drug Class: Fluoroquinolone antiinfective

MECHANISM OF ACTION

A quinolone that inhibits the enzyme DNA gyrase in susceptible microorganisms, interfering with bacterial cell replication and repair. ***Therapeutic Effect:*** Bactericidal.

USES

Treatment of lower respiratory tract infections (pneumonia, bronchitis); GU infections (prostatitis, UTIs); preoperatively to reduce UTIs in transurethral and transrectal surgical procedures caused by susceptible gram-negative organisms

PHARMACOKINETICS

Well absorbed from the GI tract. Protein binding: 10%. Widely distributed. Metabolized in the liver. Primarily excreted in urine. Not removed by hemodialysis. ***Half-life:*** 4–6 hr (increased with impaired renal function and in the elderly).

INDICATIONS AND DOSAGES

▸ **Complicated UTIs**
PO
Adults, Elderly. 400 mg/day for 10–14 days.

▸ **Uncomplicated UTIs**
PO
Adults (Females). 400 mg/day for 3 days.

▸ **Lower Respiratory Tract Infections**
PO
Adults, Elderly. 400 mg/day for 10 days.
▸ **Surgical Prophylaxis**
PO
Adults, Elderly. 400 mg 2–6 hr before surgery.
▸ **Dosage in Renal Impairment**
Dosage and frequency are modified on the basis of creatinine clearance.

Creatinine Clearance	Dosage
41 ml/min and higher	No change
10–40 ml/min	400 mg initially, then 200 mg/day for 10–14 days

SIDE EFFECTS/ADVERSE REACTIONS

Occasional
Nausea, headache, photosensitivity, dizziness
Rare
Diarrhea

PRECAUTIONS AND CONTRAINDICATIONS

Hypersensitivity to quinolones
Caution:
Lactation, children, elderly, renal disease, seizure disorders, excessive sunlight; tendon rupture in shoulder, hand, and Achilles tendons

DRUG INTERACTIONS OF CONCERN TO DENTISTRY

- Decreased effects: antacids
- Increased levels of cyclosporine, caffeine

SERIOUS REACTIONS

! Antibiotic-associated colitis and other superinfections may result from altered bacterial balance.
! Hypersensitivity reactions, including photosensitivity (as evidenced by rash, pruritus, blisters, edema, and burning skin), have occurred in patients receiving fluoroquinolones.
! Arthropathy may occur if the drug is given to children younger than 18 yr.

DENTAL CONSIDERATIONS

General:
- Because of drug interactions, do not use ingestible sodium bicarbonate products, such as the Prophy-Jet air polishing system, until 2 hr after drug use.
- Use caution in prescribing caffeine-containing analgesics.
- Determine why the patient is taking the drug.
- Avoid dental light in patient's eyes; offer dark glasses for patient comfort.
- Ruptures of the shoulder, hand, and Achilles tendons that required surgical repair or resulted in prolonged disability have been reported with this drug.

Consultations:
- Consult with patient's physician if an acute dental infection occurs and another antiinfective is required.

Teach Patient/Family to:
- Use caution to prevent injury when using oral hygiene aids.
- Avoid mouth rinses with high alcohol content because of drying effects.
- Minimize exposure to sunlight and wear sunscreen if sun exposure is planned.
- Discontinue treatment and inform dentist immediately if patient experiences pain or inflammation of a tendon, and to rest and refrain from exercise.

lomustine

low-**mew′**-steen
(CeeNU)

CATEGORY AND SCHEDULE

Pregnancy Risk Category: D

Drug Class: Antineoplastic alkylating agent

MECHANISM OF ACTION

An alkylating agent and nitrosourea that inhibits DNA and RNA protein synthesis by cross-linking with DNA and RNA strands, preventing cell division. Cell cycle–phase nonspecific.

Therapeutic Effect: Interferes with DNA and RNA function.

L

USES

Treatment of Hodgkin's disease; lymphomas; melanomas; multiple myeloma; brain, lung, bladder, kidney, colon cancer

PHARMACOKINETICS

PO: Well absorbed. ***Half-life:*** 16–48 hr; 50% protein bound; metabolized in liver; excreted in urine; crosses blood-brain barrier; excreted in breast milk.

INDICATIONS AND DOSAGES

▸ Disseminated Hodgkin's Disease, Primary and Metastatic Brain Tumors

PO

Adults, Elderly. 100–130 mg/m^2 as single dose. Repeat dose at intervals of at least 6 wk but not until circulating blood elements have returned to acceptable levels. Adjust dose on the basis of hematologic response to previous dose.

Children. 75–150 mg/m^2 as a single dose every 6 wk.

SIDE EFFECTS/ADVERSE REACTIONS

Frequent

Nausea, vomiting (occurring 45 min–6 hr after dose and lasting 12–24 hr); anorexia (often follows for 2–3 days)

Occasional

Neurotoxicity (confusion, slurred speech), stomatitis, darkening of skin, diarrhea, rash, pruritus, alopecia

PRECAUTIONS AND CONTRAINDICATIONS

Pregnancy

Caution:

Radiation therapy, geriatric patient, lactation

DRUG INTERACTIONS OF CONCERN TO DENTISTRY

• This drug depresses bone marrow function, which may increase risk of bleeding; avoid drugs that can increase bleeding, such as aspirin, NSAIDs

SERIOUS REACTIONS

! Myelosuppression may result in hematologic toxicity, manifested principally as leukopenia, mild anemia, and thrombocytopenia. Leukopenia occurs about 6 wk after a dose, thrombocytopenia about 4 wk after a dose; both persist for 1–2 wk.

! Refractory anemia and thrombocytopenia occur commonly if lomustine therapy continues for more than 1 yr.

! Hepatotoxicity occurs infrequently.

! Large cumulative doses of lomustine may result in renal damage.

DENTAL CONSIDERATIONS

General:

- Patients on chronic drug therapy may rarely have symptoms of blood dyscrasias, which can include infection, bleeding, and poor healing.
- Consider semisupine chair position for patient comfort if GI side effects occur.
- Palliative medication may be required for oral side effects.
- Consider local hemostasis measures to prevent excessive bleeding.
- Prophylactic antibiotics may be indicated to prevent infection if surgery or deep scaling is planned.
- Patients taking opioids for acute or chronic pain should be given alternative analgesics for dental pain.
- Avoid prescribing aspirin-containing products.

Consultations:

- In a patient with symptoms of blood dyscrasias, request a medical consultation for blood studies and postpone dental treatment until normal values are reestablished.
- Patients on cancer chemotherapy should have an adequate WBC count before completing dental procedures that may produce a wound. Consult to determine blood count before appointment.

Teach Patient/Family to:

- Encourage effective oral hygiene to prevent soft tissue inflammation.
- Use caution to prevent trauma when using oral hygiene aids.
- See dentist immediately if secondary oral infection occurs.
- Report oral lesions, soreness, or bleeding to dentist.
- Avoid mouth rinses with high alcohol content because of drying and irritating effects.
- Update medical/drug records if physician makes any changes in evaluation or drug regimens; include OTC, herbal, and nonherbal drugs in the update.

loperamide hydrochloride

loe-**per′**-ah-mide
high-droh-**klor′**-ide
(Apo-Loperamide[CAN], Gastro-Stop[AUS], Imodium, Imodium A-D, Loperacap[CAN], Novo-Loperamide[CAN])
Do not confuse Imodium with Indocin or Ionamin.

CATEGORY AND SCHEDULE

Pregnancy Risk Category: B
OTC liquid, tablets

Drug Class: Antidiarrheal (opioid)

MECHANISM OF ACTION

An antidiarrheal that directly inhibits the intestinal wall smooth muscles. ***Therapeutic Effect:*** Slows intestinal motility and prolongs transit time of intestinal contents by reducing fecal volume, diminishing loss of fluid and electrolytes, and increasing viscosity and bulk of stool.

USES

Treatment of diarrhea (cause undetermined), chronic diarrhea, ileostomy discharge

PHARMACOKINETICS

Poorly absorbed from the GI tract. Protein binding: 97%. Metabolized in the liver. Eliminated in feces and excreted in urine. Not removed by hemodialysis. ***Half-life:*** 9.1–14.4 hr.

INDICATIONS AND DOSAGES

▸ Acute Diarrhea

PO (Capsules)

Adults, Elderly. Initially, 4 mg; then 2 mg after each unformed stool. Maximum: 16 mg/day.

Children 9–12 yr, weighing more than 30 kg. Initially, 2 mg 3 times a day for 24 hr.

Children 6–8 yr, weighing 20–30 kg. Initially, 2 mg twice a day for 24 hr.

Children 2–5 yr, weighing 13–20 kg. Initially, 1 mg 3 times a day for 24 hr. Maintenance: 1 mg/10 kg only after loose stool.

▸ Chronic Diarrhea

PO

Adults, Elderly. Initially, 4 mg; then 2 mg after each unformed stool until diarrhea is controlled.

Children. 0.08–0.24 mg/kg/day in 2–3 divided doses. Maximum: 2 mg/dose.

▸ Traveler's Diarrhea

PO

Adults, Elderly. Initially, 4 mg; then 2 mg after each loose bowel movement (LBM). Maximum: 8 mg/day for 2 days.

Children 9–11 yr. Initially, 2 mg; then 1 mg after each LBM. Maximum: 6 mg/day for 2 days.

Children 6–8 yr. Initially, 1 mg; then 1 mg after each LBM. Maximum: 4 mg/day for 2 days.

SIDE EFFECTS/ADVERSE REACTIONS

Frequent

Dry mouth

Rare

Somnolence, abdominal discomfort, allergic reaction (such as rash and itching)

PRECAUTIONS AND CONTRAINDICATIONS

Acute ulcerative colitis (may produce toxic megacolon), diarrhea associated with pseudomembranous enterocolitis caused by broad-spectrum antibiotics or to organisms that invade intestinal mucosa (such as *Escherichia coli, Shigella,* and *Salmonella*), patients who must avoid constipation

Caution:

Lactation, children younger than 2 yr, liver disease, dehydration, bacterial disease

DRUG INTERACTIONS OF CONCERN TO DENTISTRY

- Increased action: opioid analgesics

SERIOUS REACTIONS

! Toxicity results in constipation, GI irritation, including nausea and vomiting, and CNS depression. Activated charcoal is used to treat loperamide toxicity.

DENTAL CONSIDERATIONS

General:

- Assess salivary flow as a factor in caries, periodontal disease, and candidiasis.
- Evaluate respiration characteristics and rate.
- Consider semisupine chair position for patient comfort because of GI effects of drug.
- This drug product is normally used only for a few doses for acute problems; however, some patients may have to take it for longer time periods as dictated by contributing disease.

Teach Patient/Family to:

- When chronic dry mouth occurs, advise patient to:
  - Avoid mouth rinses with high alcohol content because of drying effects.
  - Use sugarless gum, frequent sips of water, or saliva substitutes.

• Use daily home fluoride products for anticaries effect.

loracarbef

lor-ah-**kar′**-bef
(Lorabid)
Do not confuse loracarbef or Lorabid with Lortab.

CATEGORY AND SCHEDULE

Pregnancy Risk Category: B

Drug Class: Antibiotic, second-generation cephalosporin

MECHANISM OF ACTION

A second-generation cephalosporin that binds to bacterial cell membranes and inhibits cell wall synthesis.
Therapeutic Effect: Bactericidal.

USES

Treatment of gram-negative organisms: *H. influenzae, E. coli, P. mirabilis, Klebsiella*; gram-positive organisms: *S. pneumoniae, S. pyogenes, S. aureus;* upper/lower respiratory tract infection, acute maxillary sinusitis, pharyngitis, tonsillitis; urinary tract and skin infections; otitis media; some in vitro activity against anaerobes

PHARMACOKINETICS

Peak 1 hr. ***Half-life:*** 1 hr; excreted in urine as unchanged drug.

INDICATIONS AND DOSAGES

▸ **Bronchitis**
PO
Adults, Elderly, Children 12 yr and older. 200–400 mg q12h for 7 days.

▸ **Pharyngitis**
PO
Adults, Elderly, Children 12 yr and older. 200 mg q12h for 10 days.
Children 6 mo–11 yr. 7.5 mg/kg q12h for 10 days.

▸ **Pneumonia**
PO
Adults, Elderly, Children 12 yr and older. 400 mg q12h for 14 days.

▸ **Sinusitis**
PO
Adults, Elderly, Children 12 yr and older. 400 mg q12h for 10 days.
Children 6 mo–11 yr. 15 mg/kg q12h for 10 days.

▸ **Skin and Soft-Tissue Infections**
PO
Adults, Elderly, Children 12 yr and older. 200 mg q12h for 7 days.
Children 6 mo–11 yr. 7.5 mg/kg q12h for 7 days.

▸ **UTIs**
PO
Adults, Elderly, Children 6 mo–12 yr. 200–400 mg q12h for 7–14 days.

▸ **Otitis Media**
PO
Children 6 mo–12 yr. 15 mg/kg q12h for 10 days.

SIDE EFFECTS/ADVERSE REACTIONS

Frequent
Abdominal pain, anorexia, nausea, vomiting, diarrhea
Occasional
Rash, pruritus
Rare
Dizziness, headache, vaginitis

PRECAUTIONS AND CONTRAINDICATIONS

History of anaphylactic reaction to penicillins or hypersensitivity to cephalosporins
Caution:
Lactation, children, renal disease

DRUG INTERACTIONS OF CONCERN TO DENTISTRY

• Decreased effects: tetracyclines, erythromycins, lincomycins

SERIOUS REACTIONS

! Antibiotic-associated colitis and other superinfections may result from altered bacterial balance.
! Hypersensitivity reactions (ranging from rash, urticaria, and fever to anaphylaxis) occur in less than 5% of patients—most commonly in patients with a history of drug allergies, especially to penicillins.

DENTAL CONSIDERATIONS

General:
• Take precautions regarding allergy to medication.
• Determine why the patient is taking the drug.
• Examine for evidence of oral manifestations of blood dyscrasias (infection, bleeding, poor healing).
Consultations:
• Medical consultation may be required to assess disease control.
• Medical consultation for blood studies (CBC); leukopenic or thrombocytopenic side effects may result in infection, delayed healing, and excessive bleeding. Postpone elective dental treatment until normal values are maintained.
Teach Patient/Family to:
• Encourage effective oral hygiene to prevent soft tissue inflammation.

loratadine

lore-**at**′-ah-deen
(Alavert, Claratyne[AUS], Claritin, Claritin RediTab, Dimetapp, Tavist ND)

CATEGORY AND SCHEDULE

Pregnancy Risk Category: B

Drug Class: Antihistamine, H_1 histamine antagonist

MECHANISM OF ACTION

A long-acting antihistamine that competes with histamine for H_1 receptor sites on effector cells.
Therapeutic Effect: Prevents allergic responses mediated by histamine, such as rhinitis, urticaria, and pruritus.

USES

Treatment of seasonal allergic rhinitis, idiopathic chronic urticaria

PHARMACOKINETICS

Route	Onset	Peak	Duration
PO	1–3 hr	8–12 hr	Longer than 24 hr

Rapidly and almost completely absorbed from the GI tract. Protein binding: 97%; metabolite, 73%–77%. Distributed mainly to the liver, lungs, GI tract, and bile. Metabolized in the liver to active metabolite; undergoes extensive first-pass metabolism. Eliminated in urine and feces. Not removed by hemodialysis. ***Half-life:*** 8.4 hr; metabolite, 28 hr (increased in elderly and hepatic impairment).

INDICATIONS AND DOSAGES

▸ **Allergic Rhinitis, Urticaria**

PO

Adults, Elderly, Children 6 yr and older: 10 mg once a day.
Children 2–5 yr: 5 mg once a day.

▸ **Dosage in Hepatic Impairment**

For adults, elderly, and children 6 yr and older dosage is reduced to 10 mg every other day.

SIDE EFFECTS/ADVERSE REACTIONS

Frequent
Headache, fatigue, somnolence
Occasional
Dry mouth, nose, or throat
Rare
Photosensitivity

PRECAUTIONS AND CONTRAINDICATIONS

Hypersensitivity to loratadine or its ingredients
Caution:
Increased intraocular pressure, bronchial asthma, patients at risk for syncope or drowsiness, reduce dose in renal impairment to every other day

DRUG INTERACTIONS OF CONCERN TO DENTISTRY

- Increased CNS depression: all CNS depressants, alcohol
- Increased anticholinergic effect: anticholinergics, antihistamines, antiparkinsonian drugs
- Increased plasma concentration: ketoconazole

SERIOUS REACTIONS

! None known

DENTAL CONSIDERATIONS

General:

- Assess salivary flow as a factor in caries, periodontal disease, and candidiasis.
- Consider semisupine chair position for patients with respiratory disease.
- Conscious sedation drugs may produce synergistic, sedative action.

Teach Patient/Family to:

- Encourage effective oral hygiene to prevent soft tissue inflammation.
- When chronic dry mouth occurs, advise patient to:
  - Avoid mouth rinses with high alcohol content because of drying effects.
  - Use sugarless gum, frequent sips of water, or saliva substitutes.
  - Use daily home fluoride products for anticaries effect.

L

lorazepam

lor-**ah**′-zeh-pam
(Apo-Lorazepam[CAN], Ativan, Lorazepam Intensol, Novolorazepam[CAN])
Do not confuse lorazepam with Alprazolam.

CATEGORY AND SCHEDULE

Pregnancy Risk Category: D
Controlled Substance Schedule: IV

Drug Class: Benzodiazepine, antianxiety

MECHANISM OF ACTION

A benzodiazepine that enhances the action of the inhibitory neurotransmitter gamma-aminobutyric acid in the CNS, affecting memory, as well as motor, sensory, and cognitive function.
Therapeutic Effect: Produces anxiolytic, anticonvulsant, sedative, muscle relaxant, and antiemetic effects.

USES

Treatment of anxiety, preoperatively in sedation, acute alcohol withdrawal symptoms, muscle spasm

PHARMACOKINETICS

Route	Onset	Peak	Duration
PO	60 min	N/A	8–12 hr
IV	15–30 min	N/A	8–12 hr
IM	30–60 min	N/A	8–12 hr

Well absorbed after PO and IM administration. Protein binding: 85%. Widely distributed. Metabolized in the liver. Primarily excreted in urine. Not removed by hemodialysis. ***Half-life:*** 10–20 hr.

INDICATIONS AND DOSAGES

▸ Anxiety

PO

Adults. 1–10 mg/day in 2–3 divided doses. Average: 2–6 mg/day.
Elderly. Initially, 0.5–1 mg/day. May increase gradually. Range: 0.5–4 mg.

IV

Adults, Elderly. 0.02–0.06 mg/kg q2–6h.

IV Infusion

Adults, Elderly. 0.01–0.1 mg/kg/hr.

PO, IV

Children. 0.05 mg/kg/dose q4–8h. Range: 0.02–0.1 mg/kg. Maximum: 2 mg/dose.

▸ Insomnia Caused by Anxiety

PO

Adults. 2–4 mg at bedtime.
Elderly. 0.5–1 mg at bedtime.

▸ Preoperative Sedation

IV

Adults, Elderly. 0.044 mg/kg 15–20 min before surgery. Maximum total dose: 2 mg.

IM

Adults, Elderly. 0.05 mg/kg 2 hr before procedure. Maximum total dose: 4 mg.

▸ Status Epilepticus

IV

Adults, Elderly. 4 mg over 2–5 min. May repeat in 10–15 min. Maximum: 8 mg in 12-hr period.
Children. 0.1 mg/kg over 2–5 min. May give second dose of 0.05 mg/kg in 15–20 min. Maximum: 4 mg.
Neonates. 0.05 mg/kg. May repeat in 10–15 min.

SIDE EFFECTS/ADVERSE REACTIONS

Frequent

Somnolence (initially in the morning), ataxia, confusion

Occasional

Blurred vision, slurred speech, hypotension, headache

Rare

Paradoxical CNS restlessness or excitement in elderly or debilitated

PRECAUTIONS AND CONTRAINDICATIONS

Angle-closure glaucoma; preexisting CNS depression; severe hypotension; severe uncontrolled pain

Caution:

Elderly, debilitated, hepatic disease, renal disease, myasthenia gravis

DRUG INTERACTIONS OF CONCERN TO DENTISTRY

- Increased effects: alcohol, all CNS depressants, probenecid
- Increased sedation, hallucination: scopolamine
- Possible increase in CNS side effects of kava kava (herb)

SERIOUS REACTIONS

! Abrupt or too-rapid withdrawal may result in pronounced restlessness, irritability, insomnia, hand tremors, abdominal or muscle cramps, diaphoresis, vomiting, and seizures.
! Overdose results in somnolence, confusion, diminished reflexes, and coma.

DENTAL CONSIDERATIONS

General:
• After supine positioning, have patient sit upright for at least 2 min before standing to avoid orthostatic hypotension.
• Elderly persons are more prone to orthostatic hypotension and have increased sensitivity to anticholinergic and sedative effects; use lower dose.
• When administered with opioid analgesic, reduce dose of opioid by one-third.
• Psychologic and physical dependence may occur with chronic administration.
• Have someone drive patient to and from dental office when drug used for conscious sedation.
Consultations:
• Medical consultation may be required to assess disease control.
Teach Patient/Family to:
• Encourage effective oral hygiene to prevent soft tissue inflammation.
• Avoid mouth rinses with high alcohol content because of drying effects.

losartan

lo-**sar′**-tan
(Cozaar)
Do not confuse Cozaar with Zocor.

CATEGORY AND SCHEDULE

Pregnancy Risk Category: C (D if used in second or third trimesters)

Drug Class: Angiotensin II receptor antagonist

MECHANISM OF ACTION

An angiotensin II receptor, type AT1, antagonist that blocks vasoconstrictor and aldosterone-secreting effects of angiotensin II, inhibiting the binding of angiotensin II to the AT1 receptors.
Therapeutic Effect: Causes vasodilation, decreases peripheral resistance, and decreases B/P.

USES

Treatment of hypertension, as a single drug or in combination with other antihypertensives; for reduction of stroke risk in patients with hypertension and left ventricular hypertrophy; nephropathy in Type 2 diabetes mellitus

PHARMACOKINETICS

Route	Onset	Peak	Duration
PO	N/A	6 hr	24 hr

Well absorbed after PO administration. Protein binding: 98%. Undergoes first-pass metabolism in the liver to active metabolites. Excreted in urine and via the biliary system. Not removed by hemodialysis. ***Half-life:*** 2 hr, metabolite: 6–9 hr.

L

INDICATIONS AND DOSAGES

▸ **Hypertension**

PO

Adults, Elderly. Initially, 50 mg once a day. Maximum: May be given once or twice a day, with total daily doses ranging from 25–100 mg.

▸ **Nephropathy**

PO

Adults, Elderly. Initially, 50 mg/day. May increase to 100 mg/day based on B/P response.

▸ **Stroke Reduction**

PO

Adults, Elderly. 50 mg/day. Maximum: 100 mg/day.

▸ **Hypertension in Patients with Impaired Hepatic Function**

PO

Adults, Elderly. Initially, 25 mg/day.

SIDE EFFECTS/ADVERSE REACTIONS

Frequent

Upper respiratory tract infection

Occasional

Dizziness, diarrhea, cough

Rare

Insomnia, dyspepsia, heartburn, back and leg pain, muscle cramps, myalgia, nasal congestion, sinusitis

PRECAUTIONS AND CONTRAINDICATIONS

Hypersensitivity, second or third trimester of pregnancy

Caution:

Lactation, children, sodium- and volume-depleted patients, renal impairment.

DRUG INTERACTIONS OF CONCERN TO DENTISTRY

- Potential for increased hypotensive effects with other hypotensive drugs and sedatives
- Suspected increase in antihypertensive effects: fluconazole, ketoconazole; monitor B/P if used concurrently

SERIOUS REACTIONS

! Overdosage may manifest as hypotension and tachycardia. Bradycardia occurs less often.

DENTAL CONSIDERATIONS

General:

- Monitor vital signs at every appointment because of cardiovascular effects.
- Limit use of sodium-containing products, such as saline IV fluids, for patients with a dietary salt restriction.
- Stress from dental procedures may compromise cardiovascular function; determine patient risk.
- Assess salivary flow as a factor in caries, periodontal disease, and candidiasis.
- Short appointments and a stress-reduction protocol may be required for anxious patients.
- Consider semisupine chair position for patient comfort because of respiratory side effects of drug.
- Use precaution if sedation or general anesthesia is required; risk of hypotensive episode.

Consultations:

- Medical consultation may be required to assess disease control and patient's ability to tolerate stress.

Teach Patient/Family to:

- Update health and drug history if physician makes any changes in evaluation or drug regimens; include OTC, herbal, and nonherbal drugs in the update.
- When chronic dry mouth occurs, advise patient to:
    - Avoid mouth rinses with high alcohol content because of drying effects.

• Use daily home fluoride products for anticaries effect.
• Use sugarless gum, frequent sips of water, or saliva substitutes.

loteprednol

loh-teh-**pred′**-nol
(Alrex, Lotemax)

CATEGORY AND SCHEDULE

Pregnancy Risk Category: C

Drug Class: Topical glucocorticoid

MECHANISM OF ACTION

A glucocorticoid that inhibits accumulation of inflammatory cells at inflammation sites, phagocytosis, lysosomal enzyme release and synthesis and/or release of mediators of inflammation.
Therapeutic Effect: Prevents and suppresses cell and tissue immune reactions, inflammatory process.

USES

Treatment of steroid-responsive inflammation of the conjunctiva, cornea, and anterior segments of the globe associated with allergic conjunctivitis, acne rosacea, iritis, superficial punctate keratitis, and so on when topical steroid use is acceptable to reduce inflammation and edema, postoperative inflammation after ocular surgery (Lotemax 0.5%); temporary relief of symptoms of seasonal allergic conjunctivitis (Alrex 0.2%)

PHARMACOKINETICS

Metabolized by enzymes in the eye, minimizing systemic adverse effects.

INDICATIONS AND DOSAGES

▸ **Treatment of Seasonal Allergic Conjunctivitis, Giant Papillary Conjunctivitis, Uritis**
Ophthalmic
Adults, Elderly. Instill 1 drop 4 times a day for 4–6 wk.

SIDE EFFECTS/ADVERSE REACTIONS

Frequent
Blurred vision
Occasional
Decreased vision, watering of eyes, eye pain, nausea, vomiting, burning, stinging, redness of eyes

PRECAUTIONS AND CONTRAINDICATIONS

Acute epithelial herpes simplex keratitis, fungal diseases of ocular structures, vaccinia, varicella, ocular tuberculosis, hypersensitivity, after removal of corneal foreign body, mycobacterial eye infection, acute, purulent, untreated eye infection
Caution:
Prolonged use may result in glaucoma, increased risk of secondary ocular infections, delayed healing after cataract surgery; avoid contamination of sterile container; lactation, safety in children not established; possible adrenocortical suppression.

DRUG INTERACTIONS OF CONCERN TO DENTISTRY

• None reported

SERIOUS REACTIONS

! Glaucoma with optic nerve damage, cataract formation, and secondary ocular infection occur rarely.

DENTAL CONSIDERATIONS

General:

- Avoid dental light in patient's eyes; offer dark glasses for patient comfort.
- Determine why patient is taking the drug.
- Determine possible need for supplementation for some dental procedures.

loteprednol etabonate; tobramycin

loe-te-**pred′**-nol eh-tah-**bone′**-ayte; toe-bra-**mye′**-sin
(Zylet)

L

CATEGORY AND SCHEDULE

Pregnancy Risk Category: C

Drug Class: Corticosteroid, ophthalmic; antiinflammatory, steroidal, ophthalmic

MECHANISM OF ACTION

A combination ophthalmic product of an aminoglycoside and a glucocorticoid. Loteprednol is a glucocorticoid that inhibits accumulation of inflammatory cells at inflammation sites, phagocytosis, lysosomal enzyme release and synthesis, and/or release of mediators of inflammation. Tobramycin is an antibiotic that irreversibly binds to protein on bacterial ribosomes.

Therapeutic Effect: Prevents and suppresses cell and tissue immune reactions and inflammatory process. Interferes with protein synthesis of susceptible microorganisms.

USES

Treatment of inflammation of the eye, which may occur with certain eye problems or following eye surgery.

PHARMACOKINETICS

Limited systemic absorption.

INDICATIONS AND DOSAGES

▸ **Steroid-Responsive Inflammatory Ocular Conditions for Which a Corticosteroid is Indicated and Where Superficial Bacterial Ocular Infection or a Risk of Bacterial Ocular Infection Exists**

Ophthalmic

Adults, Elderly. Apply 1 or 2 drops into the affected eye(s) q4–6h. During the initial 24–48 hr, the dosing may be increased to every 1–2 hr. Gradually decrease by improvement in clinical signs.

SIDE EFFECTS/ADVERSE REACTIONS

Frequent

Blurred vision

Occasional

Tearing, burning, itching, redness, swelling of eyelid, decreased vision, eye pain

Rare

Nausea, vomiting

PRECAUTIONS AND CONTRAINDICATIONS

Viral diseases of the cornea and conjunctiva including epithelial herpes simplex keratitis (dendritic keratitis), vaccinia, varicella, and mycobacterial infection of the eye and fungal diseases of ocular structures, hypersensitivity to any of loteprednol, tobramycin or any component of the formulation and to other corticosteroids

DRUG INTERACTIONS OF CONCERN TO DENTISTRY

- None reported

SERIOUS REACTIONS

! Glaucoma with optic nerve damage, cataract formation, and

secondary ocular infection occurs rarely.
! Secondary infection, especially fungal infections of the cornea, may occur after use of this medication. These infections are more frequent with long-term applications.

DENTAL CONSIDERATIONS

General:

- Avoid dental light in patient's eyes; offer dark glasses for patient comfort.
- Determine why patient is taking the drug.
- Determine possible need for supplementation for some dental procedures.

lovastatin

lo′-va-sta-tin
(Altoprev, Lotrel, Mevacor)
Do not confuse lovastatin with Leustatin or Livostin, or Mevacor with Mivacron.

CATEGORY AND SCHEDULE

Pregnancy Risk Category: X

Drug Class: Cholesterol-lowering agent

MECHANISM OF ACTION

An antihyperlipidemic that inhibits HMG-CoA reductase, the enzyme that catalyzes the early step in cholesterol synthesis.
Therapeutic Effect: Decreases low-density lipoprotein (LDL) cholesterol, very low-density lipoprotein (VLDL) cholesterol, plasma triglycerides; increases high-density lipoprotein (HDL) cholesterol.

USES

As an adjunct in homozygous familial hypercholesterolemia, mixed hyperlipidemia, elevated serum triglyceride levels, and type IV hyperproteinemia; also reduces total cholesterol LDL-C, apoB, and triglyceride levels; patient should first be placed on cholesterol-lowering diet; primary prevention of CHD and to slow CHD progression

PHARMACOKINETICS

Route	Onset	Peak	Duration
PO	3 days	4–6 wk	N/A

Incompletely absorbed from the GI tract (increased on empty stomach). Protein binding: 95%. Hydrolyzed in the liver to active metabolite. Primarily eliminated in feces. Not removed by hemodialysis. ***Half-life:*** 1.1–1.7 hr.

INDICATIONS AND DOSAGES

▸ Hyperlipoproteinemia, Primary Prevention of Coronary Artery Disease

PO

Adults, Elderly. Initially, 20–40 mg/day with evening meal. Increase at 4-wk intervals up to maximum of 80 mg/day. Maintenance: 20–80 mg/day in single or divided doses.

PO (Extended-Release)

Adults, Elderly. Initially, 20 mg/day. May increase at 4-wk intervals up to 60 mg/day.

Children 10–17 yr. 10–40 mg/day with evening meal.

▸ Heterozygous Familial Hypercholesterolemia

PO

Children 10–17 yr. Initially, 10 mg/day. May increase to 20 mg/day after 8 wk and 40 mg/day after 16 wk if needed.

L

SIDE EFFECTS/ADVERSE REACTIONS

Generally well tolerated. Side effects usually mild and transient.

Frequent
Headache, flatulence, diarrhea, abdominal pain or cramps, rash, and pruritus

Occasional
Nausea, vomiting, constipation, dyspepsia

Rare
Dizziness, heartburn, myalgia, blurred vision, eye irritation

PRECAUTIONS AND CONTRAINDICATIONS

Active liver disease, pregnancy, unexplained elevated liver function tests

Caution:
Past liver disease, alcoholics, severe acute infections, trauma, hypotension, uncontrolled seizure disorders, severe metabolic disorders, electrolyte imbalances

DRUG INTERACTIONS OF CONCERN TO DENTISTRY

- Increased myalgia, rhabdomyolysis: macrolide antibiotics (erythromycin), cyclosporine
- Contraindicated with itraconazole, ketoconazole, erythromycin

SERIOUS REACTIONS

! There is a potential for cataract development.

DENTAL CONSIDERATIONS

General:
- Consider semisupine chair position for patient comfort because of GI side effects.

Teach Patient/Family to:
- Avoid mouth rinses with high alcohol content because of drying effects.

loxapine

lox′-ah-peen
(Apo-Loxapine[CAN], Loxapac[CAN], Loxitane)

CATEGORY AND SCHEDULE

Pregnancy Risk Category: C

Drug Class: Antipsychotic

MECHANISM OF ACTION

A dibenzodiazepine derivative that interferes with the binding of dopamine at postsynaptic receptor sites in brain. Strong anticholinergic effects.
Therapeutic Effect: Suppresses locomotor activity, produces tranquilization.

USES

Treatment of psychotic disorders

PHARMACOKINETICS

Onset of action occurs within 1 hr. Metabolized to active metabolites 8-hydroxyloxapine, 7-hydroxyloxapine, and 8-hydroxyamoxapine. Excreted in urine. ***Half-life:*** 4 hr.

INDICATIONS AND DOSAGES

▸ Psychotic Disorders

PO
Adults. 10 mg 2 times a day. Increase dosage rapidly during first wk to 50 mg, if needed. Usual therapeutic, maintenance range: 60–100 mg daily in 2–4 divided doses. Maximum: 250 mg/day.

SIDE EFFECTS/ADVERSE REACTIONS

Frequent

Blurred vision, confusion, drowsiness, dry mouth, dizziness, light-headedness

Occasional

Allergic reaction (rash, itching), decreased urination, constipation, decreased sexual ability, enlarged breasts, headache, photosensitivity, nausea, vomiting, insomnia, weight gain

PRECAUTIONS AND CONTRAINDICATIONS

Severe CNS depression, comatose states, hypersensitivity to loxapine or any component of the formulation

Caution:

Lactation, seizure disorders, hepatic disease, cardiac disease, prostatic hypertrophy, cardiac conditions, children younger than 16 yr

DRUG INTERACTIONS OF CONCERN TO DENTISTRY

- Increased effects of both drugs: anticholinergics
- Increased CNS depression: alcohol, all CNS depressants
- Decreased effects of sympathomimetics, carbamazepine

SERIOUS REACTIONS

! Extrapyramidal symptoms frequently noted are akathisia (motor restlessness, anxiety). Less frequently noted are akinesia (rigidity, tremors, salivation, mask-like facial expression, reduced voluntary movements). Infrequently noted dystonias: torticollis (neck muscle spasm), opisthotonos (rigidity of back muscles), and oculogyric crisis (rolling back of eyes). Tardive dyskinesia (protrusion of tongue, puffing of cheeks, chewing/puckering of mouth) occurs rarely but may be irreversible. Risk is greater in female elderly patients.

DENTAL CONSIDERATIONS

General:

- Patients on chronic drug therapy may rarely have symptoms of blood dyscrasias, which can include infection, bleeding, and poor healing.
- Assess salivary flow as a factor in caries, periodontal disease, and candidiasis.
- Assess for presence of extrapyramidal motor symptoms, such as tardive dyskinesia and akathisia. Extrapyramidal motor activity may complicate dental treatment.
- After supine positioning, have patient sit upright for at least 2 min before standing to avoid orthostatic hypotension.

Consultations:

- In a patient with symptoms of blood dyscrasias, request a medical consultation for blood studies and postpone dental treatment until normal values are reestablished.
- If signs of tardive dyskinesia or akathisia are present, refer to physician.
- Physician should be informed if significant xerostomic side effects occur (e.g., increased caries, sore tongue, problems eating or swallowing, difficulty wearing prosthesis) so that a medication change can be considered.

Teach Patient/Family to:

- Encourage effective oral hygiene to prevent soft tissue inflammation.

• Use caution to prevent injury when using oral hygiene aids.
• Use powered tooth brush if patient has difficulty holding conventional devices.
• When chronic dry mouth occurs, advise patient to:
  • Avoid mouth rinses with high alcohol content because of drying effects.
  • Use sugarless gum, frequent sips of water, or saliva substitutes.
  • Use daily home fluoride products for anticaries effect.

lucinactant

loo-sin-**ak′**-tant
(Surfaxin)

L

CATEGORY AND SCHEDULE

Pregnancy Risk Category: None

Drug Class: Lung surfactant

MECHANISM OF ACTION

Lucinactant is a synthetic surfactant. Surfactant administration replaces deficient or ineffective endogenous lung surfactant in neonates at risk of developing RDS. Surfactant prevents the alveoli from collapsing during expiration by lowering surface tension between air and alveolar surfaces.
Therapeutic Effect: Improves lung compliance and respiratory gas exchange.

USES

Prevention of respiratory distress syndrome (RDS) in premature infants at high risk for RDS

PHARMACOKINETICS

Minimal systemic absorption.
Half-life: None reported.

INDICATIONS AND DOSAGES

▸ **Respiratory Distress Prophylaxis**
Endotracheal
Premature infants. 5.8 ml/kg birth weight; up to 3 subsequent doses (total of 4 doses) may be administered at ≥6-hr intervals within the first 48 hr of life.

SIDE EFFECTS/ADVERSE REACTIONS

Frequent
Endotracheal tube reflux, obstruction, oxygen desaturation
Occasional
Bradycardia

PRECAUTIONS AND CONTRAINDICATIONS

None reported

DRUG INTERACTIONS OF CONCERN TO DENTISTRY

• None reported

SERIOUS REACTIONS

! None known

DENTAL CONSIDERATIONS

General:
• Monitor vital signs for possible cardiovascular adverse effects.
• Children taking lucinactant are susceptible to respiratory dysfunction and must be monitored accordingly.
• Adults who may have been treated with lucinactant are subject to severe adverse effects, including multiorgan failure, sepsis, renal failure, hypoxia, encephalopathy, hypotension, and pulmonary embolism.

Consultations:
• Consult physician prior to any dental procedures due to severe nature of underlying disease and adverse effects of drug.

lurasidone

loo-**ras**′-i-done
(Latuda)
Do not confuse with Lantus.

CATEGORY AND SCHEDULE

Pregnancy Risk Category: B

Drug Class: Antipsychotic agent, atypical

MECHANISM OF ACTION

Lurasidone is an atypical antipsychotic with mixed serotonin-dopamine antagonist activity. The addition of serotonin antagonism to dopamine antagonism is thought to improve symptoms of psychoses and reduce extrapyramidal side effects as compared to typical antipsychotics.
Therapeutic Effect: Diminishes manifestations of schizophrenia.

USES

Treatment of schizophrenia

PHARMACOKINETICS

Rapidly absorbed after oral administration. 99% plasma protein bound. Hepatic metabolism via CYP3A4 to two active metabolites. Primarily excreted unchanged in the feces (80%). ***Half-life:*** 18 hr.

INDICATIONS AND DOSAGES

▸ **Schizophrenia**

PO

Adults. Initially, 40 mg once daily; titration is not required; maximum recommended dose: 160 mg daily with a meal.

▸ **Dosage in Renal Impairment**

Cl_{cr} <50 ml/min: Initially, 20 mg daily; maximum: 80 mg daily.

▸ **Dosage in Hepatic Impairment**

Moderate impairment (Child-Pugh class B): Initially, 20 mg daily; maximum: 80 mg daily.
Severe impairment (Child-Pugh class C): Initially, 20 mg daily; maximum: 40 mg daily.

SIDE EFFECTS/ADVERSE REACTIONS

Frequent
Somnolence, akathisia, nausea, extrapyramidal symptoms
Occasional
Tachycardia , insomnia, agitation, anxiety, dizziness, dystonia, fatigue, restlessness, dyspepsia, vomiting, weight gain, salivary hypersecretion, abdominal pain, diarrhea, back pain, blurred vision

PRECAUTIONS AND CONTRAINDICATIONS

Hypersensitivity to lurasidone or any component of the formulation. May cause altered cardiac conduction, blood dyscrasias, cerebrovascular events, dyslipidemia, esophageal dysmotility, extrapyramidal symptoms (EPS), hyperglycemia, neuroleptic malignant syndrome, orthostatic hypotension, sedation, suicidal ideation, weight gain, impaired temperature regulation. Use with caution in patients with cardiovascular disease, Parkinson's disease, seizures.

DRUG INTERACTIONS OF CONCERN TO DENTISTRY

• CYP3A4 inhibitors (e.g., macrolide antibiotics, azole antifungals): increased likelihood of adverse effects

• CYP3A4 inducers (e.g., carbamazepine, barbiturates): reduced efficacy of lurasidone

SERIOUS REACTIONS

! Elderly patients with dementia-related psychosis treated with antipsychotics are at an increased risk of death compared to placebo.

DENTAL CONSIDERATIONS

General:

• After supine positioning, allow patient to sit upright for at least 2 min before standing to avoid orthostatic hypotension.
• Monitor vital signs for possible cardiovascular adverse effects.
• Monitor patients for symptoms of hyperglycemia and diabetes mellitus, including excessive thirst, hunger and frequent urination and weakness.
• Monitor for signs and symptoms of agranulocytosis, neutropenia, and leukopenia (e.g., infection).
• Avoid hypoxia and use conservative doses of local anesthetic due to decreased seizure threshold.
• Use caution when seating and dismissing patient due to motor impairment and somnolence.

Consultations:

• Consult physician to determine status of disease and ability of patient to tolerate dental procedures.

Teach Patient/Family to:

• Report changes in disease and drug regimen.

mafenide

ma′-fe-nide
(Sulfamylon)

CATEGORY AND SCHEDULE

Pregnancy Risk Category: C

Drug Class: Antibacterial, topical; antifungal, topical

MECHANISM OF ACTION

A topical antiinfective that decreases the number of bacteria in avascular tissue of second- and third-degree burns.
Therapeutic Effect: Bacteriostatic. Promotes spontaneous healing of deep partial-thickness burns.

USES

Prevention and treatment of bacterial or fungal infections

PHARMACOKINETICS

Absorbed through devascularized areas into systemic circulation following topical administration. Excreted in the form of its metabolite rhocarboxybenzenes sulfonamide.

INDICATIONS AND DOSAGES

▸ Burns

Topical
Adults, Elderly, Children. Apply 1–2 times a day.

SIDE EFFECTS/ADVERSE REACTIONS

Difficult to distinguish side effects and effects of severe burn
Frequent
Pain, burning upon application
Occasional
Allergic reaction (usually 10–14 days after initiation): itching, rash, facial edema, swelling; unexplained syndrome of marked hyperventilation with respiratory alkalosis
Rare
Delay in eschar separation, excoriation of new skin

PRECAUTIONS AND CONTRAINDICATIONS

Hypersensitivity to mafenide or sulfite or any other component of the formulation

DRUG INTERACTIONS OF CONCERN TO DENTISTRY

- None reported

SERIOUS REACTIONS

! Hemolytic anemia, porphyria, bone marrow depression, superinfections (especially with fungi), metabolic acidosis occurs rarely.

M

DENTAL CONSIDERATIONS

General:
- Dental management depends on extent and severity of burns and patient's ability to cooperate; above all use aseptic techniques.
- Provide palliative dental care for dental emergencies only.
- Monitor and record vital signs.

Consultations:
- Medical consultation may be required to assess disease control and patient's ability to tolerate stress.
- Consult patient's physician if an acute dental infection occurs and another antiinfective is required.

Teach Patient/Family to:
- Encourage effective oral hygiene to prevent soft tissue inflammation.
- Prevent trauma when using oral hygiene aids.

magaldrate

mag′-ahl-drate
(Iosopan Plus, Lowsium Plus, Riopan Plus)

CATEGORY AND SCHEDULE

Pregnancy Risk Category: C

Drug Class: Antacid/aluminum/magnesium hydroxide

MECHANISM OF ACTION

An antacid that causes fewer hydrogen ions to be available for diffusion through the GI mucosa. ***Therapeutic Effect:*** Reduces and neutralizes gastric acid.

USES

An antacid for hyperacidity

M

PHARMACOKINETICS

Onset 10–15 min, duration longer than 3 hr.

INDICATIONS AND DOSAGES

▸ **Hyperacidity and Gas**

PO

Adults, Elderly. 540–1080 mg between meals and at bedtime.

SIDE EFFECTS/ADVERSE REACTIONS

Rare

Constipation, diarrhea, fluid retention, dizziness or lightheadedness, continuing discomfort, irregular heartbeat, loss of appetite, mood or mental changes, muscle weakness, unusual tiredness or weakness, weight loss, chalky taste

PRECAUTIONS AND CONTRAINDICATIONS

Hypersensitivity to magaldrate, colostomy or ileostomy, appendicitis, ulcerative colitis, diverticulitis

Caution:

Elderly, fluid restriction, decreased GI motility, GI obstruction, dehydration, renal disease, sodium-restricted diets, colitis, gastric outlet obstruction syndrome, colostomy

DRUG INTERACTIONS OF CONCERN TO DENTISTRY

- Decreased absorption of anticholinergics, corticosteroids, sodium fluoride, tetracycline, ketoconazole, chlordiazepoxide, ciprofloxacin, metronidazole

SERIOUS REACTIONS

! None known

DENTAL CONSIDERATIONS

General:

- If prescribing oral form of a drug for which risk of decreased absorption is reported, advise taking doses at least 2 hr after or before antacid use.
- Avoid drugs that could exacerbate upper GI distress (aspirin and NSAIDs).
- Consider semisupine chair position for patient comfort because of GI effects of disease.

maprotiline

mah-**pro**′-tih-leen
(Ludiomil)

CATEGORY AND SCHEDULE

Pregnancy Risk Category: B

Drug Class: Tetracyclic antidepressant

MECHANISM OF ACTION

A tetracyclic compound that blocks reuptake norepinephrine by CNS presynaptic neuronal membranes, increasing availability at postsynaptic neuronal receptor sites, and enhances synaptic activity. ***Therapeutic Effect:*** Produces antidepressant effect, with prominent sedative effects and low anticholinergic activity.

USES

Treatment of depression, depression with anxiety, manic depression

PHARMACOKINETICS

Slowly and completely absorbed after PO administration. Protein binding: 88%. Metabolized in liver by hydroxylation and oxidative modification. Excreted in urine. Unknown if removed by hemodialysis. ***Half-life:*** 27–58 hr.

INDICATIONS AND DOSAGES

▸ Mild-to-Moderate Depression

PO

Adults. 75 mg/day to start, in 1–4 divided doses.

Elderly. 50–75 mg/day. In 2 wk, increase dosage gradually in 25 mg increments until therapeutic response is achieved. Reduce to lowest effective maintenance level.

▸ Severe Depression

PO

Adults. 100–150 mg/day in 1–4 divided doses. May increase gradually to maximum 225 mg/day.

▸ Usual Elderly Dosage

PO

Initially, 25 mg at bedtime. May increase by 25 mg q3–7 days. Maintenance: 50–75 mg/day.

SIDE EFFECTS/ADVERSE REACTIONS

Frequent

Drowsiness, fatigue, dry mouth, blurred vision, constipation, delayed micturition, postural hypotension, excessive sweating, disturbed concentration, increased appetite, urinary retention

Occasional

GI disturbances (nausea, GI distress, metallic taste sensation), photosensitivity

Rare

Paradoxical reaction (agitation, restlessness, nightmares, insomnia), extrapyramidal symptoms (particularly fine hand tremors)

PRECAUTIONS AND CONTRAINDICATIONS

Acute recovery period following MI, within 14 days of MAOI ingestion, known or suspected seizure disorder, hypersensitivity to maprotiline or any component of the formulation

Caution:

Suicidal patients, severe depression, increased intraocular pressure, narrow-angle glaucoma, urinary retention, cardiac disease, hepatic or renal disease, hypothyroidism, hyperthyroidism, electroshock therapy, elective surgery, elderly, lactation, prostate hypertrophy, schizophrenia, MAOIs

DRUG INTERACTIONS OF CONCERN TO DENTISTRY

- Increased effects of direct-acting sympathomimetics (epinephrine)
- Potential risk of increased CNS depression: alcohol, and all CNS depressants
- Decreased antihypertensive effect: clonidine, guanadrel, guanethidine

SERIOUS REACTIONS

! Higher incidence of seizures than with tricyclic antidepressants, especially in those with no previous history of seizures.

! High dosage may produce cardiovascular effects, such as severe postural hypotension,

dizziness, tachycardia, palpitations, and arrhythmias.
! May also result in altered temperature regulation (hyperpyrexia or hypothermia).
! Abrupt withdrawal from prolonged therapy may produce headache, malaise, nausea, vomiting, and vivid dreams.

DENTAL CONSIDERATIONS

General:
• Monitor vital signs at every appointment because of cardiovascular side effects.
• Patients on chronic drug therapy may rarely have symptoms of blood dyscrasias, which can include infection, bleeding, and poor healing.
• Assess salivary flow as a factor in caries, periodontal disease, and candidiasis.
• After supine positioning, have patient sit upright for at least 2 min before standing to avoid orthostatic hypotension.
• Use of epinephrine in gingival retraction cord is contraindicated.
  • Use vasoconstrictors with caution, in low doses, and with careful aspiration.

Consultations:
• In a patient with symptoms of blood dyscrasias, request a medical consultation for blood studies and postpone dental treatment until normal values are reestablished.
• Take precautions if dental surgery is anticipated and anesthesia is required.
• Medical consultation may be required to assess disease control.
• Physician should be informed if significant xerostomic side effects occur (e.g., increased caries, sore tongue, problems eating or swallowing, difficulty wearing prosthesis) so that a medication change can be considered.

Teach Patient/Family to:
• Encourage effective oral hygiene to prevent soft tissue inflammation.
• Use caution to prevent injury when using oral hygiene aids.
• When chronic dry mouth occurs, advise patient to:
  • Avoid mouth rinses with high alcohol content because of drying effects.
  • Use sugarless gum, frequent sips of water, or saliva substitutes.
  • Use daily home fluoride products for anticaries effect.

mebendazole

meh-**ben′**-dah-zole
(Vermox)

CATEGORY AND SCHEDULE

Pregnancy Risk Category: C

Drug Class: Anthelmintic; carbamate

MECHANISM OF ACTION

A synthetic benzimidazole derivative that degrades parasite cytoplasmic microtubules and irreversibly blocks glucose uptake in helminths and larvae. Vermicidal.
Therapeutic Effect: Depletes glycogen, decreases ATP, causes helminth death.

USES

Treatment of pinworms, roundworms, hookworms, whipworms, thread-worms, pork tapeworms, dwarf tapeworms, beef tapeworms, hydatid cyst

PHARMACOKINETICS
Poorly absorbed from GI tract (absorption increases with food). Metabolized in liver. Primarily eliminated in feces. ***Half-life:*** 2.5–9 hr (half-life increased with impaired renal function).

INDICATIONS AND DOSAGES
▸ **Trichuriasis, Ascariasis, Hookworm**

PO

Adults, Elderly, Children older than 2 yr. 1 tablet in morning and at bedtime for 3 days.

▸ **Enterobiasis**

PO

Adults, Elderly, Children older than 2 yr. 1 tablet one time.

SIDE EFFECTS/ADVERSE REACTIONS
Occasional

Nausea, vomiting, headache, dizziness, transient abdominal pain, diarrhea with massive infection and expulsion of helminths

Rare

Fever

PRECAUTIONS AND CONTRAINDICATIONS
Hypersensitivity to mebendazole or any component of the formulation

DRUG INTERACTIONS OF CONCERN TO DENTISTRY
• Decreased plasma levels: carbamazepine

SERIOUS REACTIONS
! High dosage may produce reversible myelosuppression (granulocytopenia, leukopenia, neutropenia).

DENTAL CONSIDERATIONS
General:

• Determine why patient is taking the drug.

• Patient on chronic drug therapy may rarely present with symptoms of blood dyscrasias, which can include infection, bleeding, and poor healing. If dyscrasia is present, caution patient to prevent oral tissue trauma when using oral hygiene aids.

• Question patient about other drugs he or she is taking.

Consultations:

• In a patient with symptoms of blood dyscrasias, request a medical consultation for blood studies and postpone treatment until normal values are reestablished.

mecasermin
mek-ah-**sir′**-men

(Increlex)

CATEGORY AND SCHEDULE
Pregnancy Risk Category: C

Drug Class: Growth hormone

MECHANISM OF ACTION
An insulin-like growth factor-1 (IGF-1) that stimulates the uptake of glucose, fatty acids, and amino acids so that metabolism supports growing tissues.

Therapeutic Effect: Promotes effects of growth hormone.

USES
Treatment for growth failure in children with severe primary IGF-1 deficiency

PHARMACOKINETICS

Absorption has not been determined. Protein binding: greater than 80% bound to IGFBP-3 and acid-labile subunit. Metabolized in liver and kidney. ***Half-life:*** 5.8 hr.

INDICATIONS AND DOSAGES

▸ Primary IGF-1 Deficiency (Severe)

SC

Children. Initially, 0.04–0.08 mg/kg twice a day. Maintenance: May increase by 0.04 mg/kg per dose. Maximum: 0.12 mg/kg twice a day. The drug should be given shortly before or after (20 min) a meal or snack—do not administer when the meal or snack is omitted. Intravenous administration is contraindicated.

SIDE EFFECTS/ADVERSE REACTIONS

Occasional

Hyper/hypoglycemia, headache, snoring, tonsillar hypertrophy, heart murmur, convulsion, dizziness, vomiting, arthralgia, bone pain, extremity pain, muscular atrophy, injection site reactions, papilledema, ear pain, hypoacusis, middle ear fluid, otitis media, serous otitis media, tympanometry abnormal, hematuria, lymphadenopathy, iron-deficiency anemia, ovarian cysts, thymus hypertrophy, thyromegaly, increased liver enzymes

Rare

Hypoglycemic seizure, loss of consciousness secondary to hypoglycemia, intracranial hypertension

PRECAUTIONS AND CONTRAINDICATIONS

Hypersensitivity to mecasermin or its components

Caution:

Avoid in patients with closed epiphyses, active or suspected neoplasia, driving or operating machinery because of hypoglycemic effects

DRUG INTERACTIONS OF CONCERN TO DENTISTRY

- None reported

SERIOUS REACTIONS

! Lymphoid tissue (e.g., tonsillar) hypertrophy associated with complications, such as snoring, sleep apnea, and chronic middle ear effusions have been reported.
! Intracranial hypertension with papilledema, visual changes, headache, nausea and/or vomiting have been reported.
! Local or systemic allergic reactions may occur.

DENTAL CONSIDERATIONS

General:

- Potential acute hypoglycemia

meclizine

mek′-lih-zeen

(Antivert, Bonamine[CAN], Bonine)

Do not confuse Antivert with Axert.

CATEGORY AND SCHEDULE

Pregnancy Risk Category: B

Drug Class: Antihistamine

MECHANISM OF ACTION

An anticholinergic that reduces labyrinthine excitability and diminishes vestibular stimulation of the labyrinth, affecting the chemoreceptor trigger zone.

Therapeutic Effect: Reduces nausea, vomiting, and vertigo.

USES

Treatment of vertigo, motion sickness

PHARMACOKINETICS

Route	Onset	Peak	Duration
PO	30–60 min	N/A	12–24 hr

Well absorbed from the GI tract. Widely distributed. Metabolized in the liver. Primarily excreted in urine. ***Half-life:*** 6 hr.

INDICATIONS AND DOSAGES

▸ **Motion Sickness**

PO

Adults, Elderly, Children 12 yr and older: 12.5–25 mg 1 hr before travel. May repeat q12–24h. May require a dose of 50 mg.

▸ **Vertigo**

PO

Adults, Elderly, Children 12 yr and older: 25–100 mg/day in divided doses, as needed.

SIDE EFFECTS/ADVERSE REACTIONS

Frequent

Drowsiness

Occasional

Blurred vision; dry mouth, nose, or throat

PRECAUTIONS AND CONTRAINDICATIONS

Hypersensitivity to cyclizines

Caution:

Children, narrow-angle glaucoma, urinary retention, lactation, prostatic hypertrophy, elderly, asthma, hypersensitivity to cyclizines

DRUG INTERACTIONS OF CONCERN TO DENTISTRY

- Increased effect of alcohol, other CNS depressants, anticholinergics

SERIOUS REACTIONS

! A hypersensitivity reaction, marked by eczema, pruritus, rash, cardiac disturbances, and photosensitivity, may occur.

! Overdose may produce CNS depression (manifested as sedation, apnea, cardiovascular collapse, or death) or severe paradoxical reactions (such as hallucinations, tremor, and seizures).

! Children may experience paradoxical reactions, including restlessness, insomnia, euphoria, nervousness, and tremors.

! Overdose in children may result in hallucinations, seizures, and death.

DENTAL CONSIDERATIONS

General:

- Assess salivary flow as a factor in caries, periodontal disease, and candidiasis.

Teach Patient/Family to:

- When chronic dry mouth occurs, advise patient to:
  - Avoid mouth rinses with high alcohol content because of drying effects.
  - Use daily home fluoride products for anticaries effect.
  - Use sugarless gum, frequent sips of water, or saliva substitutes.

meclofenamate sodium

me-kloe-**fen**′-a-mate **soe**′-dee-um
(Meclomen[CAN])
Do not confuse with meclizine.

CATEGORY AND SCHEDULE

Pregnancy Risk Category: B (D if used in third trimester or near delivery)

Drug Class: Nonsteroidal antiinflammatory

MECHANISM OF ACTION

A nonsteroidal antiinflammatory drug that inhibits prostaglandin synthesis by decreasing activity of the enzyme, cyclooxygenase, which results in decreased formation of prostaglandin precursors.
Therapeutic Effect: Reduces inflammatory response and intensity of pain stimulus reaching sensory nerve endings.

USES

Treatment of mild-to-moderate pain, osteoarthritis, rheumatoid arthritis, dysmenorrhea

PHARMACOKINETICS

PO route, onset 15 min, peak 0.5–1.5 hr, duration 2–4 hr. Completely absorbed from the GI tract. Widely distributed. Protein binding: greater than 99%. Metabolized in liver. Primarily excreted in urine and feces as metabolites. Not removed by hemodialysis. ***Half-life:*** 2–3.3 hr.

INDICATIONS AND DOSAGES

▸ **Mild-to-Moderate Pain**
PO
Adults, Elderly. 50 mg q4–6h as needed.

▸ **Excessive Menstrual Blood Loss and Primary Dysmenorrhea**
PO
Adults, Elderly. 100 mg 3 times a day for 6 days, starting at the onset of menstrual flow.

▸ **Rheumatoid Arthritis, Osteoarthritis**
PO
Adults, Elderly. 200–400 mg 3–4 times a day.

SIDE EFFECTS/ADVERSE REACTIONS

Frequent
Diarrhea, nausea, abdominal cramping/pain, dyspepsia (heartburn, indigestion, epigastric pain), oral lichenoid reaction
Occasional
Flatulence, rash, dizziness
Rare
Constipation, anorexia, stomatitis, headache, ringing in the ears, rash

PRECAUTIONS AND CONTRAINDICATIONS

Active peptic ulcer disease, chronic inflammation of GI tract, GI bleeding disorders, GI ulceration, history of hypersensitivity to aspirin or NSAIDs
Caution:
Lactation, children younger than 14 yr, bleeding disorders, upper GI disorders, cardiac disorders, hypersensitivity to other antiinflammatory agents

DRUG INTERACTIONS OF CONCERN TO DENTISTRY

- GI ulceration, bleeding: aspirin, alcohol, corticosteroids, bisphosphonates
- Nephrotoxicity: acetaminophen (prolonged use)
- Possible risk of decreased renal function: cyclosporine

• SSRIs: NSAIDs increase risk of GI side effects
• When prescribed for dental pain:
  • Risk of increased effects: oral anticoagulants, oral antidiabetics, lithium, methotrexate
  • Decreased effects of diuretics, β-adrenergic blockers

SERIOUS REACTIONS

! Overdosage may result in headache, seizure, vomiting, and cerebral edema.

! Peptic ulcer disease, GI bleeding, gastritis, severe hepatic reactions, such as jaundice, nephrotoxicity, marked by hematuria, dysuria, proteinuria, and severe hypersensitivity reaction, including bronchospasm, and facial edema occur rarely.

DENTAL CONSIDERATIONS

General:

• Increased potential for adverse cardiovascular events in patients at risk for thromboembolism.
• Patients on chronic drug therapy may rarely have symptoms of blood dyscrasias, which can include infection, bleeding, and poor healing.
• Assess salivary flow as a factor in caries, periodontal disease, and candidiasis.
• Avoid prescribing for dental use in pregnancy.
• Avoid prescribing aspirin-containing products.
• Consider semisupine chair position for patients with rheumatic disease.
• Severe stomach bleeding may occur in patients who regularly use NSAIDs in recommended doses, when the patient is also taking another NSAID, a blood thinning, or steroid drug, if the patient has GI or peptic ulcer disease, if they are 60 yr or older, or when NSAIDs are taken longer than directed. Warn patients of the potential for severe stomach bleeding.

Consultations:

• In a patient with symptoms of blood dyscrasias, request a medical consultation for blood studies and postpone dental treatment until normal values are reestablished.
• Medical consultation may be required to assess disease control.

Teach Patient/Family to:

• Encourage effective oral hygiene to prevent soft tissue inflammation.
• Use caution to prevent injury when using oral hygiene aids.
• Warn patient of potential risks of NSAIDs.
• When chronic dry mouth occurs, advise patient to:
  • Avoid mouth rinses with high alcohol content because of drying effects.
  • Use sugarless gum, frequent sips of water, or saliva substitutes.
  • Use daily home fluoride products for anticaries effect.

medroxyprogesterone acetate

me-**drox**′-ee-proe-**jess**′-te-rone **ass**′-ih-tate

(Depo-Provera, Depo-Provera Contraceptive, Novo-Medrone[CAN], Provera, Ralovera[AUS])

Do not confuse medroxyprogesterone with hydroxyprogesterone, methylprednisolone, or methyltestosterone.

CATEGORY AND SCHEDULE

Pregnancy Risk Category: X

Drug Class: Progestogen

MECHANISM OF ACTION

A hormone that transforms endometrium from proliferative to secretory in an estrogen-primed endometrium. Inhibits secretion of pituitary gonadotropins.
Therapeutic Effect: Prevents follicular maturation and ovulation. Stimulates growth of mammary alveolar tissue and relaxes uterine smooth muscle. Corrects hormonal imbalance.

USES

Treatment of uterine bleeding (abnormal), secondary amenorrhea, endometrial cancer, metastatic renal cancer, contraceptive; with estrogens to reduce incidence of endometrial hyperplasia, cancer

M

PHARMACOKINETICS

Slowly absorbed after IM administration. Protein binding: 90%. Metabolized in the liver. Primarily excreted in urine.
Half-life: 30 days.

INDICATIONS AND DOSAGES

▸ **Endometrial Hyperplasia**
PO
Adults. 2.5–10 mg/day for 14 days.

▸ **Secondary Amenorrhea**
PO
Adults. 5–10 mg/day for 5–10 days, beginning at any time during menstrual cycle or 2.5 mg/day.

▸ **Abnormal Uterine Bleeding**
PO
Adults. 5–10 mg/day for 5–10 days, beginning on calculated day 16 or day 21 of menstrual cycle.

▸ **Endometrial, Renal Carcinoma**
IM
Adults, Elderly. Initially, 400–1000 mg; repeat at 1-wk intervals. If improvement occurs and disease is stabilized, begin maintenance with as little as 400 mg/mo.

▸ **Prevention of Pregnancy**
IM
Adults. 150 mg q3mo.

SIDE EFFECTS/ADVERSE REACTIONS

Frequent
Transient menstrual abnormalities (including spotting, change in menstrual flow or cervical secretions, and amenorrhea) at initiation of therapy
Occasional
Edema, weight change, breast tenderness, nervousness, insomnia, fatigue, dizziness
Rare
Alopecia, depression, dermatologic changes, headache, fever, nausea

PRECAUTIONS AND CONTRAINDICATIONS

Carcinoma of breast; estrogen-dependent neoplasm; history of or active thrombotic disorders, such as cerebral apoplexy, thrombophlebitis, or thromboembolic disorders; hypersensitivity to progestins; known or suspected pregnancy; missed abortion; severe hepatic dysfunction; undiagnosed abnormal genital bleeding; use as pregnancy test
Caution:
Lactation, hypertension, asthma, blood dyscrasias, gallbladder disease, CHF, diabetes mellitus, bone disease, depression, migraine headache, convulsive disorders, hepatic disease, renal disease, family history of cancer of breast or reproductive tract

SERIOUS REACTIONS

! Thrombophlebitis, pulmonary or cerebral embolism, and retinal thrombosis occur rarely.

DENTAL CONSIDERATIONS

General:
• Place on frequent recall to evaluate inflammatory and healing response.
Teach Patient/Family to:
• Encourage effective oral hygiene to prevent soft tissue inflammation.

medrysone

meh′-dri-sone
(HMS Liquifilm)

CATEGORY AND SCHEDULE

Pregnancy Risk Category: C

Drug Class: Antiinflammatory, steroidal, ophthalmic; corticosteroid, ophthalmic

MECHANISM OF ACTION

A topical synthetic corticosteroid that inhibits accumulation of inflammatory cells at inflammation sites.
Therapeutic Effect: Inhibits inflammatory process.

USES

Prevention of permanent damage to the eye, which may occur with certain eye problems. Also provides relief from redness, irritation, and other discomfort.

PHARMACOKINETICS

Absorbed through aqueous humor. Metabolized in liver if absorbed. Excreted in urine and feces.

INDICATIONS AND DOSAGES

▸ **Ophthalmic Disorders**
Ophthalmic
Adults, Elderly, Children 3 yr and older: Instill 1 drop up to every 4 hr.

SIDE EFFECTS/ADVERSE REACTIONS

Frequent
Blurred vision
Occasional
Decreased vision, watering of eyes, eye pain, burning, stinging, redness of eyes, nausea, vomiting

PRECAUTIONS AND CONTRAINDICATIONS

Active superficial herpes simplex, conjunctival or corneal viral disease, fungal diseases of the eye, ocular tuberculosis, hypersensitivity to medrysone or any component of the formulation

DRUG INTERACTIONS OF CONCERN TO DENTISTRY

• None reported

SERIOUS REACTIONS

! Systemic absorption may occur with topical application.
! Cataracts, corneal thinning, corneal ulcers, delayed wound healing, optic nerve damage, and glaucoma have been reported.

DENTAL CONSIDERATIONS

General:
• Determine why patient is taking the drug.
• Avoid dental light in patient's eyes; offer dark glasses for patient comfort.
• Chronic use may result in adrenocorticoid suppression. Consider possible need for supplementation for some dental procedures.

mefenamic acid

meh-feh-**nam′**-ik
(Apo-Mefenamic[CAN], Nu-Mefenamic[CAN], PMS-Mefenamic Acid[CAN], Ponstan[CAN], Ponstel)

CATEGORY AND SCHEDULE

Pregnancy Risk Category: C (D if used in third trimester or near delivery)

Drug Class: Nonsteroidal antiinflammatory

MECHANISM OF ACTION

A nonsteroidal antiinflammatory that produces analgesic and antiinflammatory effect by inhibiting prostaglandin synthesis.
Therapeutic Effect: Reduces inflammatory response and intensity of pain stimulus reaching sensory nerve endings.

USES

Treatment of mild-to-moderate pain, dysmenorrhea, inflammatory disease

PHARMACOKINETICS

Rapidly absorbed from the GI tract. Protein binding: high. Metabolized in liver. Partially excreted in urine and partially in the feces. Not removed by hemodialysis. ***Half-life:*** 3.5 hr.

INDICATIONS AND DOSAGES

▸ **Mild-to-Moderate Pain, Lower Back Pain, Dysmenorrhea**

PO

Adults, Elderly, Children 14 yr and older. Initially, 500 mg to start, then 250 mg q4h as needed. Maximum: 1 wk of therapy.

SIDE EFFECTS/ADVERSE REACTIONS

Occasional

Dyspepsia, including heartburn, indigestion, flatulence, abdominal cramping, constipation, nausea, diarrhea, epigastric pain, vomiting, headache, nervousness, dizziness, bleeding, elevated liver function tests, tinnitus, oral lichenoid reaction

Rare

Fluid retention, arrhythmias, tachycardia, confusion, drowsiness, rash, dry eyes, blurred vision, hot flashes

PRECAUTIONS AND CONTRAINDICATIONS

History of hypersensitivity to aspirin or NSAIDs, pregnancy

Caution:

Lactation, children, bleeding disorders, GI disorders, cardiac disorders, hypersensitivity to other antiinflammatory agents

DRUG INTERACTIONS OF CONCERN TO DENTISTRY

- GI bleeding, ulceration: aspirin, alcohol, corticosteroids
- Nephrotoxicity: acetaminophen (prolonged use and high doses)
- Possible risk of decreased renal function: cyclosporine
- SSRIs: NSAIDs increase risk of GI side effects
- When prescribed for dental pain:
  - Risk of increased effects of oral anticoagulants, oral antidiabetics, lithium, methotrexate
  - Decreased effects of diuretics

SERIOUS REACTIONS

! Peptic ulcer, GI bleeding, gastritis, and severe hepatic reaction, such as cholestasis and jaundice, occur rarely.

M

! Nephrotoxicity, including dysuria, hematuria, proteinuria, and nephrotic syndrome and severe hypersensitivity reaction, marked by bronchospasm, and angioedema occur rarely.

DENTAL CONSIDERATIONS

General:

- Avoid prescribing for dental use in pregnancy.
- Avoid prescribing aspirin-containing products.
- Potential for increased adverse cardiovascular events in patients at risk for thromboembolism.
- Severe stomach bleeding may occur in patients who regularly use NSAIDs in recommended doses, when the patient is also taking another NSAID, a blood thinning, or steroid drug, if the patient has GI or peptic ulcer disease, if they are 60 yr or older, or when NSAIDs are taken longer than directed. Warn patients of the potential for severe stomach bleeding.

Consultations:

- Medical consultation may be required to assess disease control.

Teach Patient/Family to:

- Warn patient of potential risks of NSAIDs.

mefloquine

meh′-flow-quine

(Lariam)

Do not confuse with Librium.

CATEGORY AND SCHEDULE

Pregnancy Risk Category: C

Drug Class: Antimalarial

MECHANISM OF ACTION

A quinolone-methanol compound structurally similar to quinine that destroys the asexual blood forms of malarial pathogens, *Plasmodium falciparum, P. vivax, P. malariae, P. ovale.*

Therapeutic Effect: Inhibits parasite growth.

USES

Prevention or treatment of malaria, a red blood cell infection transmitted by the bite of a mosquito

PHARMACOKINETICS

Well absorbed from the GI tract. Protein binding: 98%. Widely distributed, including CSF. Metabolized in liver. Primarily excreted in urine. ***Half-life:*** 21–22 days.

INDICATIONS AND DOSAGES

▸ **Suppression of Malaria**

PO

Adults. 250 mg base weekly starting 1 wk before travel, continuing weekly during travel and for 4 wk after leaving endemic area.

Children more than 45 kg. 250 mg weekly starting 1 wk before travel, continuing weekly during travel and for 4 wk after leaving endemic area.

Children 30–45 kg. 187.5 mg (¾ tablet) weekly starting 1 wk before travel, continuing weekly during travel and for 4 wk after leaving endemic area.

Children 20–30 kg. 125 mg (½ tablet) weekly starting 1 wk before travel, continuing weekly during travel and for 4 wk after leaving endemic area.

Children 10–20 kg. 62.5 mg (¼ tablet) weekly starting 1 wk before travel, continuing weekly during travel and for 4 wk after leaving endemic area.

M

▸ **Treatment of Malaria**
PO
Adults. 1250 mg as a single dose.
Children. 15–25 mg/kg in a single dose. Maximum: 1250 mg.

SIDE EFFECTS/ADVERSE REACTIONS

Occasional
Mild transient headache, difficulty concentrating, insomnia, lightheadedness, vertigo, diarrhea, nausea, vomiting, visual disturbances, tinnitus
Rare
Aggressive behavior, anxiety, bradycardia, depression, hallucinations, hypotension, panic attacks, paranoia, psychosis, syncope, tremors

PRECAUTIONS AND CONTRAINDICATIONS

Cardiac abnormalities, severe psychiatric disorders, epilepsy, history of hypersensitivity to mefloquine

DRUG INTERACTIONS OF CONCERN TO DENTISTRY

- None reported

SERIOUS REACTIONS

! Prolonged therapy may result in peripheral neuritis, neuromyopathy, hypotension, ECG changes, agranulocytosis, aplastic anemia, thrombocytopenia, seizures, and psychosis.
! Overdosage may result in headache, vomiting, visual disturbance, drowsiness, and seizures.

DENTAL CONSIDERATIONS

General:
- Consider semisupine chair position for patient comfort if GI side effects occur.
- Question patient about tolerance of NSAIDs or aspirin related to GI disease.
- Determine why patient is taking the drug.
- Be aware of patient's disease, its severity and frequency of NSAIDs or aspirin related to GI disease.
- Monitor and record vital signs.

Consultations:
- Medical consultation may be required to assess disease control and patient's ability to tolerate stress.

Teach Patient/Family to:
- Prevent trauma when using oral hygiene aids.
- Avoid performing tasks that require mental alertness.

megestrol acetate

meh-**jess**′-trole **ass**′-eh-tayte
(Apo-Megestrol[CAN], Megace, Megostat[AUS])

CATEGORY AND SCHEDULE

Pregnancy Risk Category: X (for suspension), D (for tablets)

Drug Class: Progestin

MECHANISM OF ACTION

A hormone and antineoplastic agent that suppresses the release of luteinizing hormone from the anterior pituitary gland by inhibiting pituitary function.
Therapeutic Effect: Shrinks tumors. Also increases appetite by an unknown mechanism.

USES

Treatment of breast, endometrial cancer, renal cell cancer; AIDS wasting syndrome

PHARMACOKINETICS

Well absorbed from the GI tract. Metabolized in the liver; excreted in urine.

INDICATIONS AND DOSAGES

▸ **Palliative Treatment of Advanced Breast Cancer**

PO

Adults, Elderly. 160 mg/day in 4 equally divided doses.

▸ **Palliative Treatment of Advanced Endometrial Carcinoma**

PO

Adults, Elderly. 40–320 mg/day in divided doses. Maximum: 800 mg/day in 1–4 divided doses.

▸ **Anorexia, Cachexia, Weight Loss**

PO

Adults, Elderly. 800 mg (20 ml)/day.

SIDE EFFECTS/ADVERSE REACTIONS

Frequent

Weight gain secondary to increased appetite

Occasional

Nausea, breakthrough bleeding, backache, headache, breast tenderness, carpal tunnel syndrome

Rare

Feelings of coldness

PRECAUTIONS AND CONTRAINDICATIONS

Hypersensitivity

SERIOUS REACTIONS

! Thrombophlebitis and pulmonary embolism occur rarely.

DENTAL CONSIDERATIONS

General:

- Place on frequent recall to evaluate inflammatory and healing response.
- Patients receiving chemotherapy may require palliative treatment for stomatitis.

Teach Patient/Family to:

- Encourage effective oral hygiene to prevent soft tissue inflammation.

meloxicam

mel-**oks′**-ih-kam

(Mobic)

CATEGORY AND SCHEDULE

Pregnancy Risk Category: C (D if used in third trimester or near delivery)

Drug Class: Nonsteroidal antiinflammatory

MECHANISM OF ACTION

An NSAID that produces analgesic and antiinflammatory effects by inhibiting prostaglandin synthesis. ***Therapeutic Effect:*** Reduces the inflammatory response and intensity of pain.

USES

Relief of signs and symptoms of osteoarthritis

PHARMACOKINETICS

Route	Onset	Peak	Duration
PO (analgesic)	30 min	4–5 hr	N/A

Well absorbed after PO administration. Protein binding: 99%. Metabolized in the liver. Eliminated in urine and feces. Not removed by hemodialysis. ***Half-life:*** 15–20 hr.

INDICATIONS AND DOSAGES

▸ **Osteoarthritis, Rheumatoid Arthritis**

PO

Adults. Initially, 7.5 mg/day. Maximum: 15 mg/day.

SIDE EFFECTS/ADVERSE REACTIONS

Frequent
Dyspepsia, headache, diarrhea, nausea
Occasional
Dizziness, insomnia, rash, pruritus, flatulence, constipation, vomiting
Rare
Somnolence, urticaria, photosensitivity, tinnitus

PRECAUTIONS AND CONTRAINDICATIONS

Aspirin-induced nasal polyps associated with bronchospasm
Caution:
Preexisting asthma, anaphylactic reactions to NSAIDs, serious GI side effects may occur, GI ulcer or GI bleeding; avoid in late pregnancy, liver dysfunction, dehydration, long-term use, edema, heart failure, hypertension, ACE inhibitors, lactation, elderly

DRUG INTERACTIONS OF CONCERN TO DENTISTRY

- Increased risk of GI side effects: long-duration NSAIDs, aspirin (except low-dose form), oral glucocorticoids, alcoholism, smoking, older age, and generally poor health
- Increased blood levels: lithium
- Reduced natriuretic effect: furosemide and other loop diuretics
- SSRIs: NSAIDs increase risk of GI side effects

SERIOUS REACTIONS

! Rare reactions with long-term use include peptic ulcer disease, GI bleeding, gastritis, severe hepatic reaction (jaundice), nephrotoxicity (hematuria, dysuria, proteinuria), and a severe hypersensitivity reaction (bronchospasm, angioedema).

DENTAL CONSIDERATIONS

General:
- Potential for increased adverse cardiovascular events in patients at risk for thromboembolism.
- Assess salivary flow as a factor in caries, periodontal disease, and candidiasis.
- Avoid prescribing for dental use in pregnancy.
- Patients on chronic drug therapy may rarely have symptoms of blood dyscrasias, which can include infection, bleeding, and poor healing.
- Consider semisupine chair position for patient comfort if GI side effects occur.
- Severe stomach bleeding may occur in patients who regularly use NSAIDs in recommended doses, when the patient is also taking another NSAID, a blood thinning, or steroid drug, if the patient has GI or peptic ulcer disease, if they are 60 yr or older, or when NSAIDs are taken longer than directed. Warn patients of the potential for severe stomach bleeding.

Consultations:
- In a patient with symptoms of blood dyscrasias, request a medical consultation for blood studies and postpone treatment until normal values are reestablished.

Teach Patient/Family to:
- Use powered tooth brush if patient has difficulty holding conventional devices.
- Update health and drug history if physician makes any changes in evaluation or drug regimens; include OTC, herbal, and nonherbal drugs in the update.
- Encourage effective oral hygiene to prevent soft tissue inflammation.

M

• Prevent trauma when using oral hygiene aids.
• Warn patient of potential risks of NSAIDs.
• When chronic dry mouth occurs, advise patient to:
  • Avoid mouth rinses with high alcohol content because of drying effects.
  • Use daily home fluoride products for anticaries effect.
  • Use sugarless gum, frequent sips of water, or saliva substitutes.

melphalan

mel′-fah-lan
(Alkeran)
Do not confuse Alkeran with Leukeran, or melphalan with Mephyton or Myleran.

CATEGORY AND SCHEDULE

Pregnancy Risk Category: D

Drug Class: Antineoplastic

MECHANISM OF ACTION

An alkylating agent that inhibits protein synthesis primarily by cross-linking with strands of DNA and RNA, producing cell death. Cell cycle–phase nonspecific.
Therapeutic Effect: Disrupts nucleic acid function.

USES

Palliative treatment of multiple myeloma and nonresectable epithelial carcinoma of the ovary

PHARMACOKINETICS

Half-life: 1.5 hr; first-pass hepatic metabolism; plasma levels vary; metabolites excreted in urine.

INDICATIONS AND DOSAGES

▸ Ovarian Carcinoma

PO
Adults, Elderly. 0.2 mg/kg/day for 5 successive days. Repeat at 4- to 6-wk intervals.

▸ Multiple Myeloma

PO
Adults. Initially, 6 mg once a day, adjusted as indicated; or 0.15 mg/kg/day for 7 days or 0.25 mg/kg/day for 4 days. Repeat at 4- to 6-wk intervals.
IV
Adults. 16 mg/m^2/dose every 2 wk for 4 doses, then repeated monthly according to protocol.

▸ Dosage in Renal Impairment

PO, IV
BUN level greater than 30 mg/dl. Decrease melphalan dosage by 50%. Serum creatinine level greater than 1.5 mg/dl. Decrease the melphalan dosage by 50%.

SIDE EFFECTS/ADVERSE REACTIONS

Frequent
Nausea, vomiting (may be severe with large dose)
Occasional
Diarrhea, stomatitis, rash, pruritus, alopecia

PRECAUTIONS AND CONTRAINDICATIONS

Pregnancy, severe myelosuppression
Caution:
Severe bone marrow depression risk, renal impairment

DRUG INTERACTIONS OF CONCERN TO DENTISTRY

• Increased toxicity: antineoplastics, radiation

SERIOUS REACTIONS

! Myelosuppression may cause hematologic toxicity, manifested

principally as leukopenia and thrombocytopenia and, to lesser extent, anemia, pancytopenia, and agranulocytosis. Leukopenia may occur as early as 5 days after drug initiation.
! WBC and platelet counts return to normal levels during the fifth week of therapy, but leukopenia and thrombocytopenia may last more than 6 wk after the drug is discontinued.
! Hyperuricemia, marked by hematuria, crystalluria, and flank pain, may occur.

DENTAL CONSIDERATIONS

General:
- Patients receiving chemotherapy may be taking chronic opioids for pain. Consider NSAIDs for dental pain management.
- Patients receiving chemotherapy may require palliative therapy for stomatitis.
- Patients on chronic drug therapy may rarely have symptoms of blood dyscrasias, which can include infection, bleeding, and poor healing.

Consultations:
- Medical consultation may be required to assess disease control.
- In a patient with symptoms of blood dyscrasias, request a medical consultation for blood studies and postpone dental treatment until normal values are reestablished.

Teach Patient/Family to:
- See dentist immediately if secondary oral infection occurs.
- When chronic dry mouth occurs, advise patient to:
  - Avoid mouth rinses with high alcohol content because of drying effects.
  - Use sugarless gum, frequent sips of water, or saliva substitutes.
  - Use daily home fluoride products for anticaries effect.

M

memantine hydrochloride

meh-**man′**-teen
high-droh-**klor′**-ide
(Ebixa[AUS], Namenda)

CATEGORY AND SCHEDULE

Pregnancy Risk Category: B

Drug Class: NMDA receptor antagonist

MECHANISM OF ACTION

A neurotransmitter inhibitor that decreases the effects of glutamate, the principal excitatory neurotransmitter in the brain. Persistent CNS excitation by glutamate is thought to cause the symptoms of Alzheimer's disease.
Therapeutic Effect: May reduce clinical deterioration in moderate to severe Alzheimer's disease.

USES

Treatment of moderate-to-severe dementia of Alzheimer's disease

PHARMACOKINETICS

Rapidly and completely absorbed after PO administration. Protein binding: 45%. Undergoes little metabolism; most of the dose is excreted unchanged in urine.
Half-life: 60–80 hr.

INDICATIONS AND DOSAGES

▸ Alzheimer's Disease

PO

Adults, Elderly. Initially, 5 mg once a day. May increase dosage at intervals of at least 1 wk in 5-mg increments to 10 mg/day (5 mg twice a day), then 15 mg/day (5 mg and 10 mg as separate doses), and finally 20 mg/day (10 mg twice a day). Target dose: 20 mg/day.

SIDE EFFECTS/ADVERSE REACTIONS

Occasional

Dizziness, headache, confusion, constipation, hypertension, cough

Rare

Back pain, nausea, fatigue, anxiety, peripheral edema, arthralgia, insomnia

PRECAUTIONS AND CONTRAINDICATIONS

Severe renal impairment

Caution:

Moderate to severe renal impairment, alkaline urine pH, safety and efficacy in nursing mothers and pediatric patients have not been established

DRUG INTERACTIONS OF CONCERN TO DENTISTRY

- None reported

SERIOUS REACTIONS

! None known

DENTAL CONSIDERATIONS

General:

- Monitor vital signs at every appointment because of cardiovascular side effects.
- Patients with Alzheimer's disease may be taking other drugs; get a complete drug history.
- Drug may be used late in disease process; ensure caregiver or responsible person understands informed consent.
- Place on frequent recall to evaluate oral health.

Consultations:

- Consultation with physician may be necessary if sedation or general anesthesia is required.

Teach Patient/Family to:

- Use powered tooth brush if patient has difficulty holding conventional devices.
- Encourage effective oral hygiene to prevent soft tissue inflammation/infection.
- Prevent trauma when using oral hygiene aids.
- Update health and drug history and reporting changes in health status, drug regimen, or disease/treatment status; include OTC, herbal, and nonherbal drugs in the update.

meperidine hydrochloride

me-**per′**-ih-deen

high-droh-**klor′**-ide

(Demerol, Pethidine Injection[AUS])

Do not confuse with Demulen or Dymelor.

CATEGORY AND SCHEDULE

Pregnancy Risk Category: B (D if used for prolonged periods or at high dosages at term)

Controlled Substance: Schedule II

Drug Class: Synthetic opioid analgesic

MECHANISM OF ACTION

An opioid agonist that binds to opioid receptors in the CNS. ***Therapeutic Effect:*** Alters the perception of and emotional response to pain.

USES

Treatment of moderate-to-severe pain, preoperatively in sedation techniques

PHARMACOKINETICS

Route	Onset	Peak	Duration
PO	15 min	60 min	2–4 hr
IV	Less than 5 min	5–7 min	2–3 hr
IM	10–15 min	30–50 min	2–4 hr
SC	10–15 min	30–50 min	2–4 hr

M

Variably absorbed from the GI tract; well absorbed after IM administration. Protein binding: 60%–80%. Widely distributed. Metabolized in the liver to active metabolite. Primarily excreted in urine. Not removed by hemodialysis. ***Half-life:*** 2.4–4 hr; metabolite 8–16 hr (increased in hepatic impairment and disease).

INDICATIONS AND DOSAGES

▸ Analgesia

PO, IM, Subcutaneous

Adults, Elderly. 50–150 mg q3–4h.
Children. 1.1–1.5 mg/kg q3–4h. Don't exceed single dose of 100 mg.

▸ Patient-Controlled Analgesia

IV

Adults. Loading dose: 50–100 mg. Intermittent bolus: 5–30 mg. Lockout interval: 10–20 min. Continuous infusion: 5–40 mg/hr. Maximum (4-hr): 200–300 mg.

▸ Dosage in Renal Impairment

Dosage is based on creatinine clearance.

Creatinine Clearance	Dosage
10–50 ml/min	75% of usual dose
Less than 10 ml/min	50% of usual dose

SIDE EFFECTS/ADVERSE REACTIONS

Frequent

Sedation, hypotension (including orthostatic hypotension), diaphoresis, facial flushing, dizziness, nausea, vomiting, constipation

Occasional

Confusion, arrhythmias, tremors, urine retention, abdominal pain, dry mouth, headache, irritation at injection site, euphoria, dysphoria

Rare

Allergic reaction (rash, pruritus), insomnia

PRECAUTIONS AND CONTRAINDICATIONS

Delivery of premature infant, diarrhea because of poisoning, use within 14 days of MAOIs

Caution:

Addictive personality, lactation, increased intracranial pressure, MI (acute), severe heart disease, respiratory depression, hepatic disease, renal disease, children younger than 18 yr

DRUG INTERACTIONS OF CONCERN TO DENTISTRY

- Increased effects with all CNS depressants, neuromuscular blocking agents
- Contraindication: MAOIs, sibutramine
- Increased effects of anticholinergics
- Suspected increase in normeperidine levels: ritonavir
- Increased risk of hypotension: antihypertensive drugs

SERIOUS REACTIONS

! Overdose results in respiratory depression, skeletal muscle flaccidity, cold or clammy skin, cyanosis, and extreme somnolence progressing to seizures, stupor, and coma. The antidote is 0.4 mg naloxone.
! The patient who uses meperidine repeatedly may develop a tolerance to the drug's analgesic effect and physical dependence.

DENTAL CONSIDERATIONS

General:
- Avoid prescribing for dental use in pregnancy.
- After supine positioning, have patient sit upright for at least 2 min before standing to avoid orthostatic hypotension.
- Psychologic and physical dependence may occur with chronic administration.

Teach Patient/Family to:
- Avoid mouth rinses with high alcohol content because of drying effects.

mephentermine sulfate

meh-**fen′**-ter-meen **sull′**-fate
(Wyamine Sulfate)

CATEGORY AND SCHEDULE

Pregnancy Risk Category: C

Drug Class: Sympathomimetic

MECHANISM OF ACTION

A sympathomimetic amine that acts indirectly by releasing norepinephrine and directly by exerting a slight effect on α and β_1 receptors and a moderate effect on β_2 receptors mediating vasodilation. ***Therapeutic Effect:*** Produces cardiac stimulation.

USES

Treatment of hypotension because of anesthesia, ganglionic blockade, or hemorrhage

PHARMACOKINETICS

Onset of action occurs immediately and persists 15–30 min. Metabolized in liver. Excreted in urine. ***Half-life:*** 17–18 hr.

INDICATIONS AND DOSAGES

▸ **Hypotension (Secondary to Spinal Anesthesia)**

IM/IV

Adults. 30–45 mg as a single injection.

▸ **Prophylaxis of Hypotension in Spinal Anesthesia**

IM/IV

Adults. 30–45 mg 10–20 min before anesthesia.

SIDE EFFECTS/ADVERSE REACTIONS

Occasional

Anxiety, nervousness, cardiac arrhythmias, increased B/P

PRECAUTIONS AND CONTRAINDICATIONS

Concurrent use or within 14 days of discontinuation of MAOI therapy, hypotension induced by chlorpromazine, hypersensitivity to mephentermine or sympathomimetic amines

DRUG INTERACTIONS OF CONCERN TO DENTISTRY

- Increased risk of arrhythmia: halogenated hydrocarbon anesthetics

SERIOUS REACTIONS

! Mephentermine may produce arrhythmias, including transient extrasystoles, AV block, and hypertension.

M

! CNS effects, including hyperexcitability, prolonged wakefulness, weeping, incoherence, convulsions, flushing, tremors, and hallucinations, may occur with large doses of mephentermine.

DENTAL CONSIDERATIONS

General:

- For use in hospitals or emergencies for selected hypotensive episodes.

mephobarbital

me′-foe-**bar′**-bi-tal

(Mebaral)

CATEGORY AND SCHEDULE

Pregnancy Risk Category: D

Controlled substance: Schedule IV

Drug Class: Barbiturate anticonvulsant

MECHANISM OF ACTION

A barbiturate that increases seizure threshold in the motor cortex.

Therapeutic Effect: Depresses monosynaptic and polysynaptic transmission in the CNS.

USES

Treatment of generalized tonic-clonic (grand mal) or absence (petit mal) seizures, sedation

PHARMACOKINETICS

PO route onset 20–60 min, peak N/A, duration 6–8 hr. Well absorbed after PO administration. Widely distributed. Metabolized in liver to active metabolite, a form of phenobarbital. Minimally excreted in urine. Removed by hemodialysis. ***Half-life:*** 34 hr.

INDICATIONS AND DOSAGES

▸ Epilepsy

PO

Adults, Elderly. 400–600 mg/day in divided doses or at bedtime.

Children older than 5 yr. 32–64 mg 3 or 4 times a day.

Children younger than 5 yr. 16–32 mg 3 or 4 times a day.

▸ Sedation

PO

Adults, Elderly. 32–100 mg/day in 3–4 divided doses.

Children. 16–32 mg in 3–4 divided doses.

SIDE EFFECTS/ADVERSE REACTIONS

Frequent

Dizziness, light-headedness, somnolence

Occasional

Confusion, headache, insomnia, mental depression, nervousness, nightmares, unusual excitement

Rare

Rash, paradoxical CNS hyperactivity or nervousness in children, excitement or restlessness in elderly, generally noted during first 2 wk of therapy, particularly noted in presence of uncontrolled pain

PRECAUTIONS AND CONTRAINDICATIONS

Porphyria, history of hypersensitivity to mephobarbital or other barbiturates

Caution:

Hepatic disease, renal disease, lactation, alcoholism, drug abuse, hyperthyroidism

DRUG INTERACTIONS OF CONCERN TO DENTISTRY

- Increased effects: alcohol, all CNS depressants

M

- Decreased effects of corticosteroids, doxycycline, carbamazepine

SERIOUS REACTIONS

! Abrupt withdrawal after prolonged therapy may produce effects including markedly increased dreaming, nightmares or insomnia, tremors, sweating, vomiting, to hallucinations, delirium, seizures, and status epilepticus.
! Skin eruptions appear as hypersensitivity reaction.
! Blood dyscrasias, liver disease, and hypocalcemia occur rarely.
! Overdosage produces cold or clammy skin, hypothermia, severe CNS depression, cyanosis, rapid pulse, and Cheyne-Stokes respirations.
! Toxicity may result in severe renal impairment.

DENTAL CONSIDERATIONS

General:

- Determine type of epilepsy, seizure frequency, and quality of seizure control. A stress-reduction protocol may be required.
- Avoid use in pregnancy.
- Monitor vital signs at every appointment because of cardiovascular and respiratory side effects.
- Patients on chronic drug therapy may rarely have symptoms of blood dyscrasias, which can include infection, bleeding, and poor healing.
- Barbiturates induce liver microsomal enzymes, which alters the metabolism of other drugs.
- Avoid drugs that may lower seizure threshold (phenothiazines).
- Be sure patient is regularly taking medication.

Consultations:

- In a patient with symptoms of blood dyscrasias, request a medical consultation for blood studies and postpone dental treatment until normal values are reestablished.
- Medical consultation may be required to assess disease control and patient's ability to tolerate stress.

Teach Patient/Family to:

- Encourage effective oral hygiene to prevent soft tissue inflammation.
- Use caution to prevent injury when using oral hygiene aids.
- Avoid mouth rinses with high alcohol content because of drying effects.

mepivacaine HCl

me-**piv′**-ah-kane
high-droh-**klor′**-ide
(Carbocaine Caudal 1.5%[AUS], Carbocaine HCl, Polocaine, Polocaine-MPF)

CATEGORY AND SCHEDULE

Pregnancy Risk Category: C

Drug Class: Amide local anesthetic

MECHANISM OF ACTION

An amide anesthetic that blocks conduction of nerve impulses. ***Therapeutic Effect:*** Causes temporary loss of feeling and sensation.

USES

Local dental anesthesia, nerve block, caudal anesthesia, epidural, pain relief, paracervical block, transvaginal block or infiltration

M

PHARMACOKINETICS

Onset	Peak	Duration
3–20 min	N/A	2–2.5 hr

Protein binding: 75%. Rapidly metabolized in liver. Small amount is excreted in urine. ***Half-life:*** 1.9–3.2 hr; 8.7–9 hr (neonates).

INDICATIONS AND DOSAGES

▸ Regional Anesthesia

Children: Maximum dose of mepivacaine should not exceed 4.4 mg/kg.

Adult: 6.6 mg/kg not to exceed a total aggregate dose of 400 mg (MRD).

SIDE EFFECTS/ADVERSE REACTIONS

M

CNS and cardiovascular effects are generally dose related and of short duration

Occasional

Burning, stinging, tenderness

Rare

Generally with high dose: Drowsiness, dizziness, disorientation, light-headedness, tremors, apprehension, euphoria, blurred or double vision, ringing or roaring in ears (tinnitus), nausea, sensation of heat, cold, numbness

PRECAUTIONS AND CONTRAINDICATIONS

Hypersensitivity to any local anesthetic agent of the amide-type or to other components of solutions of mepivacaine

Caution:

Elderly, severe drug allergies

DRUG INTERACTIONS OF CONCERN TO DENTISTRY

- CNS depressants: may see increased risk of CNS depression with all CNS depressants, especially in children and when larger doses are used.
- Avoid placing dental cartridges in disinfectant solutions.
- Avoid excessive exposure of dental cartridges to light or heat, which hastens deterioration of vasoconstrictor; observe for color change in local anesthetic solution.
- Risk of cardiovascular side effects: rapid intravascular administration of local anesthetic containing vasoconstrictor, either alone or in patients taking tricyclic antidepressants, MAOIs, digitalis drugs, cocaine, phenothiazines, β-blockers, and in the presence of halogenated-hydrocarbon general anesthetics; use lowest effective vasoconstrictor dose and careful aspiration techniques.
- Avoid use of vasoconstrictors in patients with uncontrolled hyperthyroidism, diabetes, angina, or hypertension; refer these patients for medical treatment before elective dental procedures.

SERIOUS REACTIONS

! CNS toxicity may occur, especially with regional anesthesia use, progressing rapidly from mild side effects to tremors, somnolence, seizures, vomiting, and respiratory depression.

! Allergic reactions, bradyarrhythmia, cardiac arrest, fetal bradycardia, heart block, hypotension, seizure, and ventricular arrhythmia have been reported.

! Allergic reactions occur rarely.

DENTAL CONSIDERATIONS

General:

• Drug is often used with a vasoconstrictor for increased duration of action.
• Monitor vital signs at every appointment because of cardiovascular and respiratory side effects.

Teach Patient/Family to:

• Use care to prevent injury while numbness exists and to refrain from chewing gum and eating following dental anesthesia.
• Report any signs of infection, muscle pain, or fever to dentist when feeling returns.
• Report any unusual soft tissue reactions.

meprobamate

meh-proe-**ba′**-mate
(Miltown, Novo-Mepro[CAN])

CATEGORY AND SCHEDULE

Pregnancy Risk Category: D
Schedule IV

Drug Class: Sedative-hypnotic, anxiolytic

MECHANISM OF ACTION

A carbamate derivative that affects the thalamus and limbic system. Appears to inhibit multi-neuronal spinal reflexes.
Therapeutic Effect: Relieves pain or muscle spasms.

USES

Treatment of anxiety disorders

PHARMACOKINETICS

Slowly absorbed from the GI tract. Protein binding: 0%–30%. Metabolized in liver. Excreted in urine and feces. Moderately dialyzable. ***Half-life:*** 10 hr.

INDICATIONS AND DOSAGES

▸ Anxiety Disorders

PO

Adults, Children 12 yr and older. 400 mg 3–4 times. Maximum: 2400 mg/day.
Children 6–12 yr. 100–200 mg 2–3 times a day.
Elderly. Use lowest effective dose. 200 mg 2–3 times a day.

▸ Dosage in Renal Impairment

Creatinine Clearance	Dosage Interval
10–50 ml/min	Every 9–12 hr
Less than 10 ml/min	Every 12–18 hr

SIDE EFFECTS/ADVERSE REACTIONS

Frequent

Drowsiness, dizziness

Occasional

Tachycardia, palpitations, headache, light-headedness, dermatitis, diarrhea, nausea, vomiting, dyspnea, rash, weakness, blurred vision, wheezing

PRECAUTIONS AND CONTRAINDICATIONS

Acute intermittent porphyria, hypersensitivity to meprobamate or related compounds

Caution:

Suicidal patients, severe depression, renal disease, hepatic disease, elderly

DRUG INTERACTIONS OF CONCERN TO DENTISTRY

• Increased effects: CNS depressants, alcohol

SERIOUS REACTIONS

! Agranulocytosis, aplastic anemia, leucopenia, anaphylaxis, cardiac arrhythmias, hypotensive crisis, syncope, Stevens-Johnson syndrome and bullous dermatitis have been reported.
! Overdose may cause CNS depression, ataxia, coma, shock, hypotension, and death.

DENTAL CONSIDERATIONS

General:

• Monitor vital signs at every appointment because of cardiovascular side effects.
• Avoid use in pregnancy.
• Patients on chronic drug therapy may rarely have symptoms of blood dyscrasias, which can include infection, bleeding, and poor healing.
• Assess salivary flow as a factor in caries, periodontal disease, and candidiasis.
• Avoid dental light in patient's eyes; offer dark glasses for patient comfort.
• Determine why the patient is taking the drug.
• Psychologic and physical dependence may occur with chronic administration.

Consultations:

• In a patient with symptoms of blood dyscrasias, request a medical consultation for blood studies and postpone dental treatment until normal values are reestablished.
• Medical consultation may be required to assess disease control.

Teach Patient/Family to:

• Encourage effective oral hygiene to prevent soft tissue inflammation.
• Use caution to prevent injury when using oral hygiene aids.
• When chronic dry mouth occurs, advise patient to:
  • Avoid mouth rinses with high alcohol content because of drying effects.
  • Use sugarless gum, frequent sips of water, or saliva substitutes.
  • Use daily home fluoride products for anticaries effect.

mercaptopurine (6-MP)

mur-cap-tow-**pure′**-een
(Purinethol)

CATEGORY AND SCHEDULE

Pregnancy Risk Category: D

Drug Class:
Antineoplastic-antimetabolite

MECHANISM OF ACTION

An antimetabolite that is incorporated into RNA and DNA, blocks purine synthesis, and inhibits DNA and RNA synthesis.
Therapeutic Effect: Causes death of cancer cells.

USES

Treatment of acute lymphatic leukemia (ALL), acute myelogenous leukemia (AML)

PHARMACOKINETICS

Incompletely absorbed when taken orally; metabolized in liver; excreted in urine.

INDICATIONS AND DOSAGES

▸ ALL

PO

Adults, Elderly, Children. 2.5–5 mg/kg once a day as induction dose. Maintenance: 1.5–2.5 mg/kg/day.

▸ **Dosage in Renal Impairment**
Creatinine clearance less than 50 ml/min. Administer usual dose q48h.

SIDE EFFECTS/ADVERSE REACTIONS

Frequent
Myelosuppression (leading to leukopenia, thrombocytopenia, anemia), intrahepatic cholestasis, hepatic necrosis
Occasional
Drug fever, hyperpigmentation, rash, hyperuricemia, nausea, vomiting, diarrhea, stomatitis, anorexia, abdominal pain, mucositis

PRECAUTIONS AND CONTRAINDICATIONS

Pregnancy, severe myelosuppression or hepatic disease
Caution:
Renal disease

DRUG INTERACTIONS OF CONCERN TO DENTISTRY

- Increased risk of hepatotoxicity: hepatotoxic drugs

SERIOUS REACTIONS

! Myelosuppression, hepatic necrosis, and gastroenteritis may occur.

DENTAL CONSIDERATIONS

General:
- Patients on chronic drug therapy may rarely have symptoms of blood dyscrasias, which can include infection, bleeding, and poor healing.
- Avoid prescribing aspirin-containing products.
- Prophylactic antibiotics may be indicated to prevent infection if surgery or deep scaling is planned.
- Patients receiving chemotherapy may require palliative treatment for stomatitis.

Consultations:
- In a patient with symptoms of blood dyscrasias, request a medical consultation for blood studies and postpone dental treatment until normal values are reestablished.

Teach Patient/Family to:
- Encourage effective oral hygiene to prevent soft tissue inflammation.
- Use caution to prevent injury when using oral hygiene aids.
- Avoid mouth rinses with high alcohol content.

meropenem

mare-oh-**peh′**-nem
(Merrem IV)

CATEGORY AND SCHEDULE

Pregnancy Risk Category: B

Drug Class: Antiinfective, miscellaneous; carbapenem

MECHANISM OF ACTION

A carbapenem that binds to penicillin-binding proteins and inhibits bacterial cell wall synthesis. ***Therapeutic Effect:*** Bactericidal.

USES

Treatment of infections caused by bacteria

PHARMACOKINETICS

After IV administration, widely distributed into tissues and body fluids, including CSF. Protein binding: 2%. Primarily excreted unchanged in urine. Removed by hemodialysis. ***Half-life:*** 1 hr.

INDICATIONS AND DOSAGES

▸ Mild-to-Moderate Infections

IV

Adults, Elderly. 0.5–1 g q8h.
Children 3 mo and older. 20 mg/kg/dose q8h.
Children younger than 3 mo. 20 mg/kg/dose q8–12h.

▸ Meningitis

IV

Adults, Elderly, Children weighing 50 kg or more. 2 g q8h.
Children 3 mo and older weighing less than 50 kg. 40 mg/kg q8h. Maximum: 2 g/dose.

▸ Dosage in Renal Impairment

Dosage and frequency are modified on the basis of creatinine clearance.

Creatinine Clearance	Dosage	Interval
26–49 ml/min	Recommended dose (1000 mg)	q12h
10–25 ml/min	½ of recommended dose	q12h
Less than 10 ml/min	½ of recommended dose	q24h

SIDE EFFECTS/ADVERSE REACTIONS

Frequent

Diarrhea, nausea, vomiting, headache, inflammation at injection site

Occasional

Oral candidiasis, rash, pruritus

Rare

Constipation, glossitis

PRECAUTIONS AND CONTRAINDICATIONS

None known

DRUG INTERACTIONS OF CONCERN TO DENTISTRY

- Increased or prolonged plasma levels: probenecid

SERIOUS REACTIONS

! Antibiotic-associated colitis and other superinfections may occur.
! Anaphylactic reactions have been reported.
! Seizures may occur in those with CNS disorders (including brain lesions and a history of seizures), bacterial meningitis, or impaired renal function.

DENTAL CONSIDERATIONS

General:

- For selected infections in the hospital setting: provide emergency dental treatment only.
- Examine for oral manifestation of opportunistic infection.
- Determine why patient is taking the drug.
- Caution regarding allergy to medication.

Consultations:

- Consult patient's physician if an acute dental infection occurs and another antiinfective is required.
- Medical consultation may be required to assess disease control.

Teach Patient/Family to:

- Encourage effective oral hygiene to prevent soft tissue inflammation.
- Report oral lesions, soreness, or bleeding to dentist.
- Prevent trauma when using oral hygiene aids.

mesalamine/ 5-aminosalicylic acid (5-ASA)

mez-**al**′-a-meen/
ah-mee-no-sal-i-**sill**′-ik
(Apriso, Asacol, Asacol HD, Canasa, FIV-ASA, Lialda, Mesasal[CAN], Pentasa, Rowasa, Salofalk[CAN])

CATEGORY AND SCHEDULE

Pregnancy Risk Category: B; C (Asacol and Asacol HD)

Drug Class: Gastrointestinals, salicylates, antiinflammatory

MECHANISM OF ACTION

A salicylic acid derivative that locally inhibits arachidonic acid metabolite production, thus inhibiting cyclooxygenase, which is increased in patients with chronic inflammatory bowel disease. Interferes with leukotriene synthesis.
Therapeutic Effect: Blocks prostaglandin and leukotriene production and reduces inflammation in the colon.

USES

Ulcerative colitis
Proctosigmoiditis
Proctitis

PHARMACOKINETICS

Poorly absorbed from the colon. Moderately absorbed from the GI tract. Bioavailability: 20%–30% (oral); 10%–35% (rectal). Metabolized in the liver to active metabolite. Unabsorbed portion eliminated in feces; absorbed portion excreted in urine. Unknown if removed by hemodialysis.
Half-life: oral: 0.5–10 hr; metabolite, 2–15 hr; extended release: 9–10 hr; 12–14 hr, metabolite; rectal: 5–7 hr; metabolite, 6–7 hr.

INDICATIONS AND DOSAGES

▸ Ulcerative Colitis (Induction of Remission), Proctosigmoiditis, Proctitis

PO (Asacol)
Adults, Elderly. 800 mg 3 times a day (total daily dose of 2.4 g) for 6 wk.
PO (Pentasa)
Adults, Elderly. 1 g (4 Pentasa 250 mg capsules or 2 Pentasa 500 mg capsules) 4 times a day for 8 wk.
PO (Lialda)
Adults. Two to four tablets (1.2 g) once daily with food; total daily dose of 2.4 g or 4.8 g; treatment duration up to 8 wk.
Rectal (Rectal Suspension, Rowasa)
Adults, Elderly. 60 ml (4 g) at bedtime; retain overnight (about 8 hr) for 3–6 wk or if remission is achieved.
Rectal (Suppository, Canasa)
Adults. 1 suppository (1 g), once daily at bedtime. Retain for 1–3 hr or longer to achieve maximum benefit.

▸ To Maintain Remission in Ulcerative Colitis

PO (Asacol)
Adults, Elderly. 1.6 g/day in divided doses.
PO (Pentasa)
Adults, Elderly. 1 g 4 times a day
PO (Apriso)
Adults, Elderly. Four capsules (1.5 g/day) in the morning with or without food.

M

SIDE EFFECTS/ADVERSE REACTIONS

Mesalamine is generally well tolerated, with only mild and transient effects.

Frequent

PO: Abdominal cramps or pain, diarrhea, dizziness, headache, nausea, vomiting, rhinitis, unusual fatigue, flu-like symptoms, nasopharyngitis, sinusitis

Rectal: Abdominal or stomach cramps, flatulence, headache, nausea

Occasional

PO: Hair loss, decreased appetite, back or joint pain, flatulence, acne

Rectal: Hair loss

Rare

PO: Renal impairment, pericarditis, pancreatitis, rectal hemorrhaging, hematologic disorders, hepatitis, hepatotoxicity

Rectal: Anal irritation

M

PRECAUTIONS AND CONTRAINDICATIONS

Hypersensitivity to mesalamine, any other components of this medication, or salicylates

Rectal suppository: Hypersensitivity to mesalamine (5-aminosalicylic acid) or to the suppository vehicle [saturated vegetable fatty acid esters (hard fat)]; sulfite sensitivity in those using Rowasa

Caution:

Renal disease

Liver disease

Children (safety and efficacy not determined)

DRUG INTERACTIONS OF CONCERN TO DENTISTRY

- Anticoagulants (e.g., low molecular weight heparin, warfarin): May decrease anticoagulant effects
- Varicella virus vaccine: May result in enhanced risk of developing Reye's syndrome

Apriso

- Antacids: May dissolve the coating of the granules of Apriso capsules thereby altering bioavailability

SERIOUS REACTIONS

! Sulfite sensitivity may occur in susceptible patients (with Rowasa), manifested by cramping, headache, diarrhea, fever, rash, hives, itching, and wheezing. Discontinue drug immediately.

! Hepatitis, pancreatitis, pericarditis, and renal impairment occur rarely with oral forms.

DENTAL CONSIDERATIONS

General:

- Determine if the patient has an allergy to sulfa-based products.
- Determine why the patient is using this medication.
- Determine if the patient is pregnant.

Consultations:

- Medical consultation may be required to assess disease control.
- Laboratory tests may be ordered to assess kidney and liver function.

Teach Patient/Family to:

- Report oral lesions, soreness, or bleeding to dentist.
- When chronic dry mouth occurs, advise patient to:
  - Avoid mouth rinses with high alcohol content because of drying effects.
  - Use daily home fluoride products for anticaries effect.
  - Use sugarless gum, frequent sips of water, or saliva substitutes.

mesna

mez′-na
(Mesnex, Uromitexan[CAN])

CATEGORY AND SCHEDULE

Pregnancy Risk Category: B

Drug Class: Cytoprotective agent; antineoplastic adjunct, antidote

MECHANISM OF ACTION

An antineoplastic adjunct and cytoprotective agent that binds with and detoxifies urotoxic metabolites of ifosfamide and cyclophosphamide.

Therapeutic Effect: Inhibits ifosfamide- and cyclophosphamide-induced hemorrhagic cystitis.

USES

Detoxifying agent used as a protectant against hemorrhagic cystitis induced by ifosfamide, cyclophosphamide

PHARMACOKINETICS

Rapidly metabolized after IV administration to mesna disulfide, which is reduced to mesna in kidney. Excreted in urine. ***Half-life:*** 24 min.

INDICATIONS AND DOSAGES

▸ Prevention of Hemorrhagic Cystitis in Patients Receiving Ifosfamide

IV

Adults, Elderly. 20% of ifosfamide dose at time of ifosfamide administration and 4 and 8 hr after each dose of ifosfamide. Total dose: 60% of ifosfamide dosage. Range: 60%–160% of the daily ifosfamide dose.

▸ Prevention of Hemorrhagic Cystitis in Patients Receiving Cyclophosphamide

PO

Adults, Elderly. 40% of cyclophosphamide dose q4h for 3 doses.

IV

Adults, Elderly. 20% of cyclophosphamide dose at time of cyclophosphamide administration and q3h for 3–4 doses.

SIDE EFFECTS/ADVERSE REACTIONS

Frequent

Bad taste, soft stools

Large doses: Diarrhea, myalgia, headache, fatigue, nausea, hypotension, allergic reaction

PRECAUTIONS AND CONTRAINDICATIONS

None known

DRUG INTERACTIONS OF CONCERN TO DENTISTRY

- None reported

SERIOUS REACTIONS

! Hematuria occurs rarely.

DENTAL CONSIDERATIONS

General:

- Patient will be taking ifosfamide or cyclophosphamide; determine use and disease.
- Question patient about other diseases and medications taken.
- Note side effects and precautions associated with chemotherapeutic drugs.

Consultations:

- Medical consultation should include routine blood counts including platelet counts and bleeding time.

• Consult physician; prophylactic or therapeutic antiinfectives may be indicated if surgery or periodontal treatment is required.
• Medical consultation may be required to assess immunologic status during cancer chemotherapy and determine safety risk, if any, posed by the required dental treatment.
• Medical consultation may be required to assess disease control and patient's ability to tolerate stress.

Teach Patient/Family to:
• Encourage effective oral hygiene to prevent soft tissue inflammation.
• Prevent trauma when using oral hygiene aids.
• Report oral lesions, soreness, or bleeding to dentist.
• Update health and medication history if physician makes any changes in evaluation or drug regimens; include OTC, herbal, and nonherbal drugs in the update.

mesoridazine besylate

mez-oh-**rid**′-ah-zeen **bes**′-il-ayte
(Serentil)
Do not confuse Serentil with Proventil, Serevent, or sertraline.

CATEGORY AND SCHEDULE

Pregnancy Risk Category: C

Drug Class: Phenothiazine antipsychotic

MECHANISM OF ACTION

A phenothiazine that blocks dopamine at postsynaptic receptor sites in the brain.

Therapeutic Effect: Diminishes schizophrenic behavior. Also has anticholinergic and sedative effects.

USES

Treatment of psychotic disorders, schizophrenia when inadequate response with other antipsychotic drugs

PHARMACOKINETICS

PO: Onset erratic, peak 2 hr, duration 4–6 hr.
IM: Onset 15–30 min, peak 30 min, duration 6–8 hr. Metabolized by liver, excreted in urine, crosses placenta, excreted in breast milk.

INDICATIONS AND DOSAGES

▸ Schizophrenia

PO
Adults, Elderly. 25–50 mg 3 times a day. Maximum: 400 mg/day.
IM
Adults, Elderly. Initially, 25 mg. May repeat in 30–60 min. Range: 25–200 mg.

▸ Severe Behavioral Problems (Combativeness or Explosive, Hyperexcitable Behavior) Associated with Neurologic Diseases

PO
Elderly. Initially, 10 mg once or twice a day. May increase at 4–7 day intervals. Maximum: 250 mg.
IM
Adults, Elderly. Initially, 25 mg. May repeat in 30–60 min. Range: 25–200 mg.

SIDE EFFECTS/ADVERSE REACTIONS

Frequent
Orthostatic hypotension, dizziness, syncope (occur frequently after first injection, occasionally after subsequent injections, and rarely with oral form)

Occasional
Somnolence (during early therapy), dry mouth, blurred vision, lethargy, constipation or diarrhea, nasal congestion, peripheral edema, urine retention
Rare
Ocular changes, altered skin pigmentation (in those taking high doses for prolonged periods), darkening of urine

PRECAUTIONS AND CONTRAINDICATIONS

Coma, myelosuppression, severe cardiovascular disease, severe CNS depression, subcortical brain damage
Caution:
Lactation, seizure disorders, hypertension, hepatic disease, cardiac disease, prostatic hypertrophy, intestinal obstruction, respiratory conditions, dose-related prolongation of QTc interval

DRUG INTERACTIONS OF CONCERN TO DENTISTRY

• Increased sedation: other CNS depressants, alcohol, barbiturate anesthetics, opioid analgesics
• Hypotension, tachycardia: epinephrine
• Increased extrapyramidal effects: phenothiazines and related drugs (haloperidol, droperidol), metoclopramide
• Additive photosensitization: tetracyclines
• Increased anticholinergic effects: anticholinergics

SERIOUS REACTIONS

! Abrupt withdrawal after long-term therapy may precipitate nausea, vomiting, gastritis, dizziness, and tremors.
! Blood dyscrasias, particularly agranulocytosis and mild leukopenia, may occur.
! Mesoridazine use may lower the seizure threshold.

DENTAL CONSIDERATIONS

General:
• Monitor vital signs at every appointment because of cardiovascular side effects.
• Patients on chronic drug therapy may rarely have symptoms of blood dyscrasias, which can include infection, bleeding, and poor healing.
• After supine positioning, have patient sit upright for at least 2 min before standing to avoid orthostatic hypotension.
• Assess salivary flow as a factor in caries, periodontal disease, and candidiasis.
• Avoid dental light in patient's eyes; offer dark glasses for patient comfort.
• Assess for presence of extrapyramidal motor symptoms, such as tardive dyskinesia and akathisia. Extrapyramidal motor activity may complicate dental treatment.
• Geriatric patients are more susceptible to drug effects; use lower dose.
• Use vasoconstrictors with caution, in low doses, and with careful aspiration. Avoid use of gingival retraction cord with epinephrine.
Consultations:
• In a patient with symptoms of blood dyscrasias, request a medical consultation for blood studies and postpone dental treatment until normal values are reestablished.
• Take precautions if dental surgery is anticipated and anesthesia is required.
• Refer to physician if signs of tardive dyskinesia or akathisia are present.

• Physician should be informed if significant xerostomic side effects occur (e.g., increased caries, sore tongue, problems eating or swallowing, difficulty wearing prosthesis) so that a medication change can be considered.

Teach Patient/Family to:

• Encourage effective oral hygiene to prevent soft tissue inflammation.
• Use caution to prevent injury when using oral hygiene aids.
• Use powered tooth brush if patient has difficulty holding conventional devices.
• When chronic dry mouth occurs, advise patient to:
  • Avoid mouth rinses with high alcohol content because of drying effects.
  • Use sugarless gum, frequent sips of water, or saliva substitutes.
  • Use daily home fluoride products for anticaries effect.

M

metaproterenol sulfate

met-ah-proe-**ter′**-eh-nole **suhl′**-feyt
(Alupent)
Do not confuse metaproterenol with metipranolol or metoprolol, or Alupent with Atrovent.

CATEGORY AND SCHEDULE

Pregnancy Risk Category: C

Drug Class: Selective β_2-agonist

MECHANISM OF ACTION

A sympathomimetic that stimulates β_2-adrenergic receptors, resulting in relaxation of bronchial smooth muscle.

Therapeutic Effect: Relieves bronchospasm and reduces airway resistance.

USES

Treatment of bronchial asthma, bronchospasm

PHARMACOKINETICS

3% absorbed through lungs after inhalation. Primarily metabolized in the GI tract. Duration 1–5 hr following a single dose (reduced to 1–2.5 hr after repetitive dosing).

INDICATIONS AND DOSAGES

▸ Treatment of Bronchospasm

PO

Adults, Children 10 yr and older. 20 mg 3–4 times a day.
Elderly. 10 mg 3–4 times a day. May increase to 20 mg/dose.
Children 6–9 yr. 10 mg 3–4 times a day.
Children 2–5 yr. 1.3–2.6 mg/kg/day in 3–4 divided doses.
Children younger than 2 yr. 0.4 mg/kg 3–4 times a day.

Inhalation

Adults, Elderly, Children 12 yr and older. 2–3 inhalations q3–4h. Maximum: 12 inhalations/24 hr.

Nebulization

Adults, Elderly, Children 12 yr and older. 10–15 mg (0.2–0.3 ml) of 5% q4–6h.
Children younger than 12 yr, Infants. 0.5–1 mg/kg (0.01–0.02 ml/kg) of 5% q4–6h.

SIDE EFFECTS/ADVERSE REACTIONS

Frequent

Rigors, tremors, anxiety, nausea, dry mouth

Occasional

Dizziness, vertigo, asthenia, headache, GI distress, vomiting, cough, dry throat

Rare
Somnolence, diarrhea, altered taste

PRECAUTIONS AND CONTRAINDICATIONS

Angle-closure glaucoma, preexisting arrhythmias associated with tachycardia
Caution:
Cardiac disorders, hyperthyroidism, diabetes mellitus, prostatic hypertrophy

DRUG INTERACTIONS OF CONCERN TO DENTISTRY

• Increased effects of both drugs: other sympathomimetics, CNS stimulants
• Increased dysrhythmias: halogenated hydrocarbon anesthetics

SERIOUS REACTIONS

! Excessive sympathomimetic stimulation may cause palpitations, extrasystoles, tachycardia, chest pain, a slight increase in B/P followed by a substantial decrease, chills, diaphoresis, and blanching of skin.
! Too-frequent or excessive use may lead to decreased drug effectiveness and severe, paradoxical bronchoconstriction.

DENTAL CONSIDERATIONS

General:
• Assess salivary flow as a factor in caries, periodontal disease, and candidiasis.
• Consider semisupine chair position for patients with respiratory disease.
• Short appointments and a stress-reduction protocol may be required for anxious patients.
• Be aware that NSAIDs or sulfite preservatives in vasoconstrictor-containing products can exacerbate asthma.
• Acute asthmatic episodes may be precipitated in the dental office. Sympathomimetic inhalants should be available for emergency use.
Consultations:
• Medical consultation may be required to assess disease control and patient's ability to tolerate stress.
Teach Patient/Family to:
• Rinse mouth with water after each inhaled dose to prevent dryness.
• When chronic dry mouth occurs, advise patient to:
  • Avoid mouth rinses with high alcohol content because of drying effects.
  • Use sugarless gum, frequent sips of water, or saliva substitutes.
  • Use daily home fluoride products for anticaries effect.

metaraminol

met-ar-**am′**-ih-nol
(Aramine)

CATEGORY AND SCHEDULE

Pregnancy Risk Category: D

Drug Class: Adrenergic agonists

MECHANISM OF ACTION

An α-adrenergic receptor agonist that causes vasoconstriction, reflex bradycardia, inhibits GI smooth muscle and vascular smooth muscle supplying skeletal muscle and increases heart rate and force of heart muscle contraction.
Therapeutic Effect: Increases both systolic and diastolic pressure.

USES

Treatment and prevention of hypotension because of hemorrhage, spinal anesthesia, and shock associated with brain damage

PHARMACOKINETICS

Route	Onset	Peak	Duration
IM (Pressor Effect)	10 min	N/A	20–60 min
IV	1–2 min	N/A	
SC	5–20 min	N/A	

Metabolized in the liver. Excreted in the urine and the bile.

INDICATIONS AND DOSAGES

▸ Prevention of Hypotension

IM/Subcutaneous

Adults, Elderly. 2–10 mg as a single dose.

Children. 0.01 mg/kg as a single dose.

▸ Adjunctive Treatment of Hypotension

IV

Adults, Elderly. 15–100 mg IV infusion, administered at a rate to maintain the desired B/P.

▸ Severe Shock

IV

Adults, Elderly. 0.5–5 mg direct IV injection followed by 15–100 mg IV infusion in 250–500 ml fluid for control of B/P.

SIDE EFFECTS/ADVERSE REACTIONS

Occasional

Tachycardia, hypertension, cardiac arrhythmias, flushing, palpitations, hypotension, angina, tremors, nervousness, headache, dizziness, weakness, sloughing of skin, nausea, abscess formation, diaphoresis

PRECAUTIONS AND CONTRAINDICATIONS

Cyclopropane or halothane anesthesia, use of MAOIs, pregnancy, hypersensitivity to metaraminol

DRUG INTERACTIONS OF CONCERN TO DENTISTRY

• Increased risk of arrhythmia: halogenated hydrocarbon anesthetics

SERIOUS REACTIONS

! Overdosage produces hypertension, cerebral hemorrhage, cardiac arrest, and seizures.

DENTAL CONSIDERATIONS

General:

• Acute-use drug for use in hospitals or emergency rooms for selected hypotensive episodes.

metaxalone

me-**tax**′-ah-lone

(Skelaxin)

CATEGORY AND SCHEDULE

Pregnancy Risk Category: C

Drug Class: Muscle relaxant

MECHANISM OF ACTION

A central depressant whose exact mechanism is unknown. Many effects because of its central depressant actions.

Therapeutic Effect: Relieves pain of muscle spasms.

USES

Adjunct to rest, physical therapy, and other measures for relief of discomfort associated with acute, painful musculoskeletal conditions

PHARMACOKINETICS

PO route onset 1 hr, peak 3 hr, duration 4–6 hr. Well absorbed from

the GI tract. Metabolized in liver. Primarily excreted in urine.
Half-life: 9 hr.

INDICATIONS AND DOSAGES

▸ **Muscle Relaxant**

PO

Adults, Elderly, Children older than 12 yr. 800 mg 3–4 times a day.

SIDE EFFECTS/ADVERSE REACTIONS

Occasional

Drowsiness, headache, light-headedness, dermatitis, nausea, vomiting, stomach cramps, dyspnea

PRECAUTIONS AND CONTRAINDICATIONS

Impaired renal or hepatic function, history of drug-induced hemolytic anemias or other anemias, history of hypersensitivity to metaxalone

Caution:

Preexisting hepatic impairment, lactation, children younger than 12 yr, alcohol use

DRUG INTERACTIONS OF CONCERN TO DENTISTRY

• No data reported; however, this drug can cause CNS depression: monitor patients if other CNS depressants are used.

SERIOUS REACTIONS

! Overdose may cause CNS depression, coma, shock, and respiratory depression.

DENTAL CONSIDERATIONS

General:

• Determine why patient is taking the drug.

• Patients on chronic drug therapy may rarely have symptoms of blood dyscrasias, which can include infection, bleeding, and poor healing.

• Consider semisupine chair position for patient comfort if GI side effects occur.

Consultations:

• In a patient with symptoms of blood dyscrasias, request a medical consultation for blood studies and postpone treatment until normal values are reestablished.

Teach Patient/Family to:

• Update health and drug history if physician makes any changes in evaluation or drug regimens; include OTC, herbal, and nonherbal drugs in the update.

metformin hydrochloride

met-**for′**-min high-droh-**klor′**-ide
(Diabex[AUS], Diaformin[AUS], Fortamet, Glucohexal[AUS], Glucomet[AUS], Glucophage, Glucophage XL, Glycon[CAN], Novo-Metformin[CAN], Riomet)

CATEGORY AND SCHEDULE

Pregnancy Risk Category: B

Drug Class: Oral hypoglycemic, biguanide derivative

MECHANISM OF ACTION

An antihyperglycemic that decreases hepatic production of glucose. Decreases absorption of glucose and improves insulin sensitivity.
Therapeutic Effect: Improves glycemic control, stabilizes or decreases body weight, and improves lipid profile.

USES

Treatment of Type 2 diabetes mellitus

PHARMACOKINETICS

Slowly, incompletely absorbed after oral administration. Food delays or decreases the extent of absorption. Protein binding: Negligible. Primarily distributed to intestinal mucosa and salivary glands. Primarily excreted unchanged in urine. Removed by hemodialysis. ***Half-life:*** 3–6 hr.

INDICATIONS AND DOSAGES

▸ **Diabetes Mellitus**

PO (500-mg, 1000-mg Tablet)

Adults, Elderly. Initially, 500 mg twice a day, with morning and evening meals. May increase in 500-mg increments every wk, in divided doses. May give twice a day up to 2000 mg/day (e.g., 1000 mg twice a day [with morning and evening meals]). If 2500 mg/day are required, give 3 times a day with meals. Maximum: 2500 mg/day.

Children 10–16 yr. Initially, 500 mg twice a day. May increase by 500 mg/day at weekly intervals. Maximum: 2000 mg/day.

PO (850-mg Tablet)

Adults, Elderly. Initially, 850-mg/day, with morning meal. May increase dosage in 850-mg increments every other week, in divided doses. Maintenance: 850 mg twice a day, with morning and evening meals. Maximum: 2550 mg/day (850 mg 3 times a day).

PO (Extended-Release Tablets)

Adults, Elderly. Initially, 500 mg once a day. May increase by 500 mg/day at weekly intervals. Maximum: 2000 mg once a day.

▸ **Adjunct to Insulin Therapy**

PO

Adults, Elderly. Initially, 500 mg/day. May increase by 500 mg at 7-day intervals. Maximum: 2500 mg/day (2000 mg/day for extended-release form).

SIDE EFFECTS/ADVERSE REACTIONS

Occasional

GI disturbances (including diarrhea, nausea, vomiting, abdominal bloating, flatulence, and anorexia) that are transient and resolve spontaneously during therapy

Rare

Unpleasant or metallic taste that resolves spontaneously during therapy

PRECAUTIONS AND CONTRAINDICATIONS

Acute CHF, MI, cardiovascular collapse, renal disease or dysfunction, respiratory failure, septicemia

Caution:

Elderly, lactation, children, interferes with vitamin B_{12} absorption; avoid alcohol use

DRUG INTERACTIONS OF CONCERN TO DENTISTRY

- None reported

SERIOUS REACTIONS

! Lactic acidosis occurs rarely but is a fatal complication in 50% of cases. Lactic acidosis is characterized by an increase in blood lactate levels (higher than 5 mmol/L), a decrease in blood pH, and electrolyte disturbances. Signs and symptoms of lactic acidosis include unexplained hyperventilation, myalgia, malaise, and somnolence, which may advance to cardiovascular collapse (shock), acute CHF, acute MI, and prerenal azotemia.

DENTAL CONSIDERATIONS

General:

- Short appointments and a stress-reduction protocol may be required for anxious patients.

• Consider semisupine chair position for patient comfort if GI side effects occur.
• Question patient about self-monitoring of drug's antidiabetic effect, including blood glucose values or finger-stick records.
• Ensure that patient is following prescribed diet and regularly takes medication.
• Diabetics may be more susceptible to infection and have delayed wound healing.
• Place on frequent recall to evaluate healing response.

Consultations:
• Medical consultation may be required to assess disease control and patient's ability to tolerate stress.
• Notify physician immediately if symptoms of lactic acidosis are observed (myalgia, respiratory distress, weakness, diarrhea, malaise, muscle cramps, somnolence).
• Medical consultation may include data from patient's blood glucose monitoring, including glycosylated hemoglobin or HbA_{1c} testing.
• Oral and maxillofacial surgical procedures associated with significantly restricted food intake require a medical consultation and temporary cessation of metformin use.

Teach Patient/Family to:
• Encourage effective oral hygiene to prevent soft-tissue inflammation.
• Understand that alteration of taste may be because of drug side effects.

methadone hydrochloride

meth'-ah-done
high-droh-**klor'**-ide
(Dolophine, Metadol[CAN], Methadone Intensol, Methadose, Physeptone[AUS])

CATEGORY AND SCHEDULE

Pregnancy Risk Category: B (D if used for prolonged periods or at high dosages at term)
Controlled Substance: Schedule II

Drug Class: Synthetic opioid analgesic

MECHANISM OF ACTION

An opioid agonist that binds with opioid receptors in the CNS.
Therapeutic Effect: Alters the perception of and emotional response to pain; reduces withdrawal symptoms from other opioid drugs.

USES

Treatment of severe pain, opioid withdrawal program

PHARMACOKINETICS

Route	Onset	Peak	Duration
Oral	0.5–1 hr	1.5–2 hr	6–8 hr
IM	10–20 min	N/A	4–5 hr
IV	N/A	15–30 min	3–4 hr

Well absorbed after IM injection. Protein binding: 80%–85%. Metabolized in the liver. Primarily excreted in urine. Not removed by hemodialysis. ***Half-life:*** 15–25 hr.

INDICATIONS AND DOSAGES

▸ **Analgesia**

PO

Adults, Elderly. Initially, 5–10 mg q3–4h.

M

Children. 0.1–0.2 mg/kg q6h as needed. Maximum: 10 mg/dose.
IV, IM, Subcutaneous
Adults, Elderly. Initially, 2.5–10 mg q3–4h.

▸ **Opioid Addiction**
IM, PO
Adults, Elderly. 15–40 mg once daily or as needed. Reduce dose at 1–2 day intervals based on patient response. Maintenance: Individualized.

SIDE EFFECTS/ADVERSE REACTIONS

Frequent
Sedation, decreased B/P (including orthostatic hypotension), diaphoresis, facial flushing, constipation, dizziness, nausea, vomiting
Occasional
Confusion, urine retention, palpitations, abdominal cramps, visual changes, dry mouth, headache, decreased appetite, anxiety, insomnia
Rare
Allergic reaction (rash, pruritus)

PRECAUTIONS AND CONTRAINDICATIONS

Delivery of premature infant, diarrhea because of poisoning, hypersensitivity to narcotics, labor
Caution:
Addictive personality, lactation, increased intracranial pressure, MI (acute), severe heart disease, respiratory depression, hepatic disease, renal disease, children younger than 18 yr

DRUG INTERACTIONS OF CONCERN TO DENTISTRY

- Increased CNS depression: alcohol, narcotics, sedative-hypnotics, skeletal muscle relaxants, benzodiazepines, and other CNS depressants
- Increased effects of anticholinergics

SERIOUS REACTIONS

! Overdose results in respiratory depression, skeletal muscle flaccidity, cold or clammy skin, cyanosis, and extreme somnolence progressing to seizures, stupor, and coma. The antidote is 0.4 mg naloxone.
! The patient who uses methadone long-term may develop a tolerance to the drug's analgesic effect and physical dependence.

DENTAL CONSIDERATIONS

General:
- Assess salivary flow as a factor in caries, periodontal disease, and candidiasis.
- Psychologic and physical dependence may occur with chronic administration.
- Determine why the patient is taking the drug.
- Be aware of the special needs of patients who are in recovery from substance abuse.
- In an opioid-dependent patient, NSAIDs are the drugs of choice for posttreatment pain control.

Consultations:
- Patients in the methadone maintenance program should not receive additional opioids or other controlled substances without a consultation.

Teach Patient/Family:
- When chronic dry mouth occurs, advise patient to:
    - Avoid mouth rinses with high alcohol content because of drying effects.

• Use sugarless gum, frequent sips of water, or saliva substitutes.
• Use daily home fluoride products for anticaries effect.

methamphetamine

meth-am-**fet′**-ah-meen
(Desoxyn, Gradumet)
Do not confuse with Dextran, dextromethorphan, or Excedrin.

CATEGORY AND SCHEDULE

Pregnancy Risk Category: C
Controlled substance: Schedule II

Drug Class: Amphetamine

MECHANISM OF ACTION

A sympathomimetic amine related to amphetamine and ephedrine that enhances CNS stimulant activity. Peripheral actions include elevation of systolic and diastolic B/P and weak bronchodilator and respiratory stimulant action.
Therapeutic Effect: Increases motor activity, mental alertness; decreases drowsiness, fatigue.

USES

Treatment of exogenous obesity, minimal brain dysfunction, attention-deficit/hyperactivity disorder (ADHD)

PHARMACOKINETICS

Rapidly absorbed from the GI tract. Metabolized in liver. Primarily excreted in the urine. Unknown if removed by hemodialysis. ***Half-life:*** 4–5 hr.

INDICATIONS AND DOSAGES

▸ **ADHD**
PO
Adults, Children 6 yr and older. Initially, 2.5–5 mg 1–2 times a day. Increase by 5 mg/day at weekly intervals until therapeutic response achieved.

▸ **Appetite Suppressant**
PO
Adults, Children 12 yr and older. 5 mg daily, given 30 min before meals. Extended-release 10–15 mg in the morning.

SIDE EFFECTS/ADVERSE REACTIONS

Frequent
Irregular pulse, increased motor activity, talkativeness, nervousness, mild euphoria, insomnia
Occasional
Headache, chills, dry mouth, GI distress, worsening depression in patients who are clinically depressed, tachycardia, palpitations, chest pain

PRECAUTIONS AND CONTRAINDICATIONS

Advanced arteriosclerosis, agitated states, glaucoma, history of drug abuse, history of hypersensitivity to sympathomimetic amines, hyperthyroidism, moderate to severe hypertension, symptomatic cardiovascular disease, within 14 days following discontinuation of an MAOI
Caution:
Gilles de la Tourette's syndrome, lactation, children younger than 6 yr

DRUG INTERACTIONS OF CONCERN TO DENTISTRY

• Increased effect of methamphetamine: CNS stimulants, sympathomimetics

• Decreased effects of both drugs: haloperidol, sedative-hypnotics
• Ventricular dysrhythmia: inhalation anesthetics

SERIOUS REACTIONS

! Overdose may produce skin pallor, flushing, arrhythmias, and psychosis.
! Abrupt withdrawal following prolonged administration of high dosage may produce lethargy which may last for weeks.
! Prolonged administration to children with ADHD may produce a temporary suppression of normal weight and height patterns.

DENTAL CONSIDERATIONS

General:
• Monitor vital signs at every appointment due to cardiovascular side effects.
• Assess salivary flow as a factor in caries, periodontal disease, and candidiasis.
Consultations:
• Physician should be informed if significant xerostomic side effects occur (e.g., increased caries, sore tongue, problems eating or swallowing, difficulty wearing prosthesis) so that a medication change can be considered.
Teach Patient/Family to:
• When chronic dry mouth occurs, advise patient to:
  • Avoid mouth rinses with high alcohol content because of drying effects.
  • Use sugarless gum, frequent sips of water, or saliva substitutes.
  • Use daily home fluoride products for anticaries effect.

methazolamide

meth-ah-**zole**′-ah-mide
(Apo-Methazolamide[CAN], GlaucTabs, Neptazane)
Do not confuse with nefazodone.

CATEGORY AND SCHEDULE

Pregnancy Risk Category: C

Drug Class: Carbonic anhydrase inhibitor

MECHANISM OF ACTION

A noncompetitive inhibitor of carbonic anhydrase that inhibits the enzyme at the luminal border of cells of the proximal tubule. Increases urine volume and changes to an alkaline pH with subsequent decreases in the excretion of titratable acid and ammonia.
Therapeutic Effect: Produces a diuretic and antiglaucoma effect.

USES

Treatment of open-angle glaucoma or preoperatively in narrow-angle glaucoma; can be used with miotic, osmotic agents

PHARMACOKINETICS

PO route onset 2–4 hr, peak 6–8 hr, duration 10–18 hr. Well absorbed slowly from the GI tract. Protein binding: 55%. Distributed into the tissues (including CSF). Metabolized slowly from the GI tract. Partially excreted in urine. Not removed by hemodialysis. ***Half-life:*** 14 hr.

INDICATIONS AND DOSAGES

▸ **Glaucoma**
PO
Adults, Elderly. 50–100 mg/day 2–3 times a day.

SIDE EFFECTS/ADVERSE REACTIONS

Occasional

Paresthesias, hearing dysfunction or tinnitus, fatigue, malaise, loss of appetite, taste alteration, nausea, vomiting, diarrhea, polyuria, drowsiness, confusion, hypokalemia

Rare

Metabolic acidosis, electrolyte imbalance, transient myopia, urticaria, melena, hematuria, glycosuria, hepatic insufficiency, flaccid paralysis, photosensitivity, convulsions, and rarely, crystalluria, renal calculi

PRECAUTIONS AND CONTRAINDICATIONS

Kidney or liver dysfunction, severe pulmonary obstruction, hypersensitivity to methazolamide or any component of the formulation

Caution:

Hypercalciuria, lactation, children

DRUG INTERACTIONS OF CONCERN TO DENTISTRY

Methazolamide (Neptazane, GlaucTabs)

• Toxicity: salicylates (high doses)

• Hypokalemia: corticosteroids (systemic use)

SERIOUS REACTIONS

! Malaise and complaints of tiredness and myalgia are signs of excessive dosing and acidosis in the elderly.

! Stevens-Johnson syndrome, toxic epidermal necrolysis, fulminant hepatic necrosis, agranulocytosis, aplastic anemia, and other blood dyscrasias have been reported and have caused fatalities.

DENTAL CONSIDERATIONS

General:

• Avoid dental light in patient's eyes; offer dark glasses for patient comfort.

• Avoid prescribing aspirin-containing products.

• Consider semisupine chair position for patient comfort if GI side effects occur.

• Question patient about tolerance of NSAIDs or aspirin related to GI disease.

• Patient on chronic drug therapy may rarely present with symptoms of blood dyscrasias, which can include infection, bleeding, and poor healing.

• Caution patient to prevent oral tissue trauma when using oral hygiene aids.

Consultations:

• In a patient with symptoms of blood dyscrasias, request a medical consultation for blood studies and postpone treatment until normal values are reestablished.

Teach Patient/Family to:

• Encourage effective oral hygiene to prevent soft tissue inflammation.

• Prevent trauma when using oral hygiene aids.

• Update health and medication history if physician makes any changes in evaluation or drug regimens; include OTC, herbal, and nonherbal drugs in the update.

methenamine

meh-**theh**′-nah-meen
(Dehydral[CAN], Hiprex, Hip-Rex[CAN], Mandelamine, Urasal[CAN], Urex)

CATEGORY AND SCHEDULE

Pregnancy Risk Category: C

Drug Class: Urinary antiinfective

MECHANISM OF ACTION

A hippuric acid salt that hydrolyzes to formaldehyde and ammonia in acidic urine.
Therapeutic Effect: Formaldehyde has antibacterial action. Bactericidal.

M

USES

Prophylaxis and treatment of uncomplicated UTIs

PHARMACOKINETICS

Readily absorbed from the GI tract. Partially metabolized by hydrolysis (unless protected by enteric coating) and partially by the liver. Primarily excreted in urine. ***Half-life:*** 3–6 hr.

INDICATIONS AND DOSAGES

▸ UTI

PO

Adults, Elderly. 1 g 2 times/day (as hippurate). 1 g 4 times/day (as mandelate).
Children 6–12 yr. 25–0 mg/kg/day q12h (as hippurate). 50–75 mg/kg/day q6h (as mandelate).

SIDE EFFECTS/ADVERSE REACTIONS

Occasional
Rash, nausea, dyspepsia, difficulty urinating
Rare
Bladder irritation, increased liver enzymes

PRECAUTIONS AND CONTRAINDICATIONS

Moderate to severe renal impairment, hepatic impairment (hippurate salt), tartrazine sensitivity (Hiprex contains tartrazine), hypersensitivity to methenamine or any of its components
Caution:
Renal disease, lactation

DRUG INTERACTIONS OF CONCERN TO DENTISTRY

- None reported

SERIOUS REACTIONS

! Crystalluria can occur when methenamine is given in large doses.

DENTAL CONSIDERATIONS

General:

- Determine why the patient is taking the drug.
- Antibiotics for dental infections are not contraindicated, but a physician consultation may be advisable.
- Palliative treatment may be required for oral side effects.
- Consider semisupine chair position for patient comfort because of GI effects of drug.

methimazole

meth-**im**′-ah-zole
(Tapazole)

CATEGORY AND SCHEDULE

Pregnancy Risk Category: D

Drug Class: Thyroid hormone antagonist

MECHANISM OF ACTION

A thiomidazole derivative that inhibits synthesis of thyroid hormone by interfering with the incorporation of iodine into tyrosyl residues.

Therapeutic Effect: Effectively treats hyperthyroidism by decreasing thyroid hormone levels.

USES

Treatment of hyperthyroidism

PHARMACOKINETICS

PO: Onset 30–40 min, duration 2–4 hr. ***Half-life:*** 1–2 hr; excreted in urine, bile, breast milk; crosses placenta.

INDICATIONS AND DOSAGES

▸ Hyperthyroidism

PO

Adults, Elderly. Initially, 15–60 mg/day in 3 divided doses. Maintenance: 5–15 mg/day.

Children. Initially, 0.4 mg/kg/day in 3 divided doses. Maintenance: ½ the initial dose.

SIDE EFFECTS/ADVERSE REACTIONS

Frequent

Fever, rash, pruritus

Occasional

Dizziness, loss of taste, nausea, vomiting, stomach pain, peripheral neuropathy or numbness in fingers, toes, face

Rare

Swollen lymph nodes or salivary glands

PRECAUTIONS AND CONTRAINDICATIONS

Hypersensitivity, infection, bone marrow depression, hepatic disease, pregnancy (first or second trimester)

Caution:

Infection, bone marrow depression, hepatic disease

DRUG INTERACTIONS OF CONCERN TO DENTISTRY

- Increased cardiovascular side effects in uncontrolled patients: anticholinergics and sympathomimetics
- Patients with uncontrolled hyperthyroidism are at risk when vasoconstrictors are used
- Patients with uncontrolled hypothyroidism may be more responsive to CNS depressants

SERIOUS REACTIONS

! Agranulocytosis as long as 4 mo after therapy, pancytopenia, and hepatitis have occurred.

M

DENTAL CONSIDERATIONS

General:

- Monitor vital signs at every appointment because of cardiovascular effects of disease.
- Patients on chronic drug therapy may rarely have symptoms of blood dyscrasias; examine for evidence of oral manifestations of blood dyscrasias (infection, bleeding, poor healing).
- Evaluate for clotting ability during periodontal instrumentation.
- Evaluate for control of hyperthyroidism. Patients with uncontrolled condition should not be treated in the dental office until thyroid values are normalized.
- Patients with uncontrolled condition should be referred for medical evaluation and treatment.

Consultations:

- Medical consultation may be required to assess disease control.
- Medical consultation for blood studies (CBC); leukopenic or

thrombocytopenic side effects may result in infection, delayed healing, and excessive bleeding. Postpone elective dental treatment until normal values are maintained.

Teach Patient/Family to:

- Encourage effective oral hygiene to prevent soft tissue inflammation.
- Use caution in use of oral hygiene aids to prevent injury.

methocarbamol

meth-oh-**kar′**-ba-mole
(Carbacot, Robaxin)

CATEGORY AND SCHEDULE

Pregnancy Risk Category: C

Drug Class: Skeletal muscle relaxant

MECHANISM OF ACTION

A carbamate derivative of guaifenesin that causes skeletal muscle relaxation by general CNS depression.

Therapeutic Effect: Relieves muscle spasticity.

USES

Adjunct for relief in painful musculoskeletal conditions

PHARMACOKINETICS

Rapidly and almost completely absorbed from the GI tract. Protein binding: 46%–50%. Metabolized in liver by dealkylation and hydroxylation. Primarily excreted in urine as metabolites. ***Half-life:*** 1–2 hr.

INDICATIONS AND DOSAGES

▸ **Musculoskeletal Spasm**

IM/IV

Adults, Children 16 yr and older. 1 g q8h for no more than 3 consecutive days. May repeat course of therapy after a drug-free interval of 48 hr.

PO

Adults, Children 16 yr and older. 1.5 g 4 times a day for 2–3 days (up to 8 g/day may be given in severe conditions). Decrease to 4–4.5 g/day in 3–6 divided doses.

Elderly. Initially, 500 mg 4 times a day. May gradually increase dosage.

▸ **Tetanus Spasm**

IV

Adults. 1–3 g q6h until oral dosing is possible. Injection should be used no more than 3 consecutive days.

Children. 15 mg/kg/dose or 500 mg/m^2/dose q6h as needed. Maximum: 1.8 g/m^2/day for 3 days only.

SIDE EFFECTS/ADVERSE REACTIONS

Frequent

Transient drowsiness, weakness, dizziness, light-headedness, nausea, vomiting

Occasional

Headache, constipation, anorexia, hypotension, confusion, blurred vision, vertigo, facial flushing, rash

Rare

Paradoxical CNS excitement and restlessness, slurred speech, tremors, dry mouth, diarrhea, nocturia, impotence, bradycardia, hypotension, syncope

PRECAUTIONS AND CONTRAINDICATIONS

Hypersensitivity to methocarbamol or any component of the

formulation, renal impairment (injection formulation)
Caution:
Renal disease, hepatic disease, addictive personalities, myasthenia gravis, epilepsy

DRUG INTERACTIONS OF CONCERN TO DENTISTRY

- Increased CNS depression: alcohol, narcotics, sedative-hypnotics

SERIOUS REACTIONS

! Anaphylactoid reactions, leukopenia, and seizures (intravenous form) have been reported.
! Methocarbamol overdosage results in cardiac arrhythmias, nausea, vomiting, drowsiness, and coma.

DENTAL CONSIDERATIONS

General:
- Determine why the patient is taking the drug.
- Consider semisupine chair position for patient comfort if back is involved.

Teach Patient/Family to:
- Encourage effective oral hygiene to prevent soft tissue inflammation.
- Use caution to prevent injury when using oral hygiene aids.
- Avoid mouth rinses with high alcohol content because of drying effects.

methotrexate sodium

meth-oh-**trex**′-ate **soe**′-dee-um
(Apo-Methotrexate[CAN], Ledertrexate[AUS], Methoblastin[AUS], Rheumatrex, Trexall)
Do not confuse Trexall with Trexan.

CATEGORY AND SCHEDULE

Pregnancy Risk Category: D (X for patients with psoriasis or rheumatoid arthritis)

Drug Class: Folic acid antagonist, antineoplastic

MECHANISM OF ACTION

An antimetabolite that competes with enzymes necessary to reduce folic acid to tetrahydrofolic acid, a component essential to DNA, RNA, and protein synthesis. This action inhibits DNA, RNA, and protein synthesis.
Therapeutic Effect: Causes death of cancer cells.

USES

Treatment of acute lymphocytic leukemia (ALL), non-Hodgkin's lymphoma; in combination with other drugs for breast, lung, head, neck cancer; lymphosarcoma; psoriasis; gestational choriocarcinoma; hydatidiform mole; rheumatoid arthritis

PHARMACOKINETICS

Variably absorbed from the GI tract. Completely absorbed after IM administration. Protein binding: 50%–60%. Widely distributed. Metabolized intracellularly in the liver. Primarily excreted in urine. Removed by hemodialysis but not by peritoneal dialysis. ***Half-life:*** 8–12 hr (large doses, 8–15 hr).

INDICATIONS AND DOSAGES

▸ Trophoblastic Neoplasms
PO, IM
Adults, Elderly. 15–30 mg/day for 5 days; repeat in 7 days for 3–5 courses.

▸ Head and Neck Cancer
PO, IV, IM
Adults, Elderly. 25–50 mg/m^2 once weekly.

▸ Choriocarcinoma, Chorioadenoma Destruens, Hydatidiform Mole
PO, IM
Adults, Elderly. 15–30 mg/day for 5 days; repeat 3–5 times with 1–2 wk between courses.

▸ Breast Cancer
IV
Adults, Elderly. 30–60 mg/m^2 days 1 and 8 q3–4wk.

▸ ALL
PO, IV, IM
Adults, Elderly. Induction: 3.3 mg/m^2/day in combination with other chemotherapeutic agents.
Maintenance: 30 mg/m^2/wk PO or IM in divided doses or 2.5 mg/kg IV every 14 days.

▸ Burkitt's Lymphoma
PO
Adults. 10–25 mg/day for 4–8 days; repeat with 7- to 10-day rest between courses.

▸ Lymphosarcoma
PO
Adults, Elderly. 0.625–2.5 mg/kg/day.

▸ Mycosis Fungoides
PO
Adults, Elderly. 2.5–10 mg/day.
IM
Adults, Elderly. 50 mg/wk or 25 mg twice a wk.

▸ Rheumatoid Arthritis
PO
Adults, Elderly. 7.5 mg once a wk or 2.5 mg q12h for 3 doses once a wk. Maximum: 20 mg/wk.

▸ Juvenile Rheumatoid Arthritis
PO, IM, Subcutaneous
Children. 5–15 mg/m^2/wk as a single dose or in 3 divided doses given q12h.

▸ Psoriasis
PO
Adults, Elderly. 10–25 mg once a wk or 2.5–5 mg q12h for 3 doses once a wk.
IM
Adults, Elderly. 10–25 mg once a wk.

▸ Antineoplastic Dosage for Children
PO, IM
Children. 7.5–30 mg/m^2/wk or q2wk.
IV
Children. 10–33,000 mg/m^2 bolus or continuous infusion over 6–42 hr.

▸ Dosage in Renal Impairment
Creatinine clearance 61–80 ml/min. Reduce dose by 25%.
Creatinine clearance 51–60 ml/min. Reduce dose by 33%.
Creatinine clearance 10–50 ml/min. Reduce dose by 50%–70%.

SIDE EFFECTS/ADVERSE REACTIONS

Frequent
Nausea, vomiting, stomatitis; burning and erythema at psoriatic site (in patients with psoriasis)

Occasional
Diarrhea, rash, dermatitis, pruritus, alopecia, dizziness, anorexia, malaise, headache, drowsiness, blurred vision

PRECAUTIONS AND CONTRAINDICATIONS

Preexisting myelosuppression, severe hepatic or renal impairment

Caution:

Renal disease, lactation, drugs with potential for hepatotoxicity, monitor for hepatic toxicity, methotrexate-induced lung disease

DRUG INTERACTIONS OF CONCERN TO DENTISTRY

- Increased toxicity: aspirin, alcohol, NSAIDs
- Possible fatal interactions: NSAIDs, high-dose IV methotrexate
- Suspected increase in methotrexate toxicity: amoxicillin, tetracycline, doxycycline

SERIOUS REACTIONS

! GI toxicity may produce gingivitis, glossitis, pharyngitis, stomatitis, enteritis, and hematemesis.

! Hepatotoxicity is more likely to occur with frequent small doses than with large intermittent doses.

! Pulmonary toxicity may be characterized by interstitial pneumonitis.

! Hematologic toxicity, which may develop rapidly from marked myelosuppression, may be manifested as leukopenia, thrombocytopenia, anemia, and hemorrhage.

! Dermatologic toxicity may produce a rash, pruritus, urticaria, pigmentation, photosensitivity, petechiae, ecchymosis, and pustules.

! Severe nephrotoxicity may produce azotemia, hematuria, and renal failure.

DENTAL CONSIDERATIONS

General:

- Patients on chronic drug therapy may rarely have symptoms of blood dyscrasias, which can include infection, bleeding, and poor healing.
- Avoid prescribing aspirin- or NSAID-containing products.
- Place on frequent recall because of increased risk for infection and to evaluate healing response.
- Determine why the patient is taking the drug.
- Palliative treatment may be necessary if stomatitis or oral desquamative lesions occur.

Consultations:

- Monitor for development of opportunistic infections.
- In a patient with symptoms of blood dyscrasias, request a medical consultation for blood studies and postpone dental treatment until normal values are reestablished.
- Medical consultation may be required to assess disease control.

Teach Patient/Family to:

- Encourage effective oral hygiene to prevent soft tissue inflammation.
- Use caution to prevent injury when using oral hygiene aids.
- Use palliative therapy for sore mouth.
- Avoid mouth rinses with high alcohol content because of drying effects.

methoxy polyethylene glycol-epoetin beta

meth-**ox**′-ee-pol-ee-**eth**′-il-een-**glye**′-kol-eh-**poe**′-ee-tin-bay-ta (Mircera)

CATEGORY AND SCHEDULE

Pregnancy Risk Category: C

Drug Class: Anti-anemia agent, continuous erythropoietin receptor activator (CERA)

MECHANISM OF ACTION

Methoxy polyethylene glycol polymer, found in methoxy polyethylene glycol-epoetin beta, attaches to recombinant human erythropoietin in order to remain in the circulation much longer. Methoxy polyethylene glycol-epoetin beta slowly binds to the erythropoietin-receptor and quickly dissociates, which helps prevent internalization and degradation of the molecule. This way it remains biologically active.

USES

Used in treatment of anemia in patients with chronic renal failure (CRF).

PHARMACOKINETICS

Completely absorbed after SC administration. Bioavailability for SC administration is 62%. ***Half-life:*** 134 ± 65 hr after IV administration and 139 ± 67 hr after SC administration.

INDICATIONS AND DOSAGES

▸ Patients Not Currently Treated with an Erythropoiesis Stimulating Agent (ESA)

IV or SC

Adults. Starting 0.6 mcg/kg body weight once every 2 weeks to achieve Hb level >11 g/dl. Dose may be increased by ~25% if Hb increasing rate is <1.0 g/dl over a month. If Hb increase rate is >2 g/dl in a month or if Hb is increasing and approaching 12 g/dl, consider reducing by ~25%. If Hb continues to increase, stop therapy until Hb begins to decrease. If Hb level is >11g/dl, consider maintaining therapy once monthly using the dose equal to twice the previous once every 2-wk dose.

▸ Patients Currently Treated with an ESA

IV or SC

Patients currently on an ESA can be directly converted to methoxy polyethylene glycol-epoetin beta once a month. Monthly starting dose is 120 mcg/month, 200 mcg/month, or 360 mcg/month depends on the previous darbepoetin alfa or epoetin (table).

Previous Weekly Starting Dose Darbepoetin Alfa IV or SC Dose (mcg/week)	Previous Weekly Epoetin Alfa IV or SC Dose (IU/week)	Monthly Mircera IV or SC Dose (mcg/once monthly)
<40	<8000	120
40–80	8000–16000	200
>80	>16000	360

If a dose adjustment is required to achieve Hb level >11 g/dl, consider increase monthly dose by ~25%.

SIDE EFFECTS/ADVERSE REACTIONS

▸ Adult

Frequent

Hypertension

Occasional

Headache, thrombocytopenia, decreased average platelet count, diarrhea, muscle spasm, procedural hypotension, edema, back pain

PRECAUTIONS AND CONTRAINDICATIONS

Hypersensitivity to the active substance or any of the components. Contraindicated in patients with uncontrolled hypertension, hypertensive encephalopathy, and seizures.

Supplemental iron therapy is recommended for all patients with serum ferritin below 100 mcg/L or transferrin saturation <20%.

Patients with anti-erythropoietin antibodies should not be placed on methoxy polyethylene glycol-epoetin beta because of the risk of pure red cell aplasia.

Methoxy polyethylene glycol-epoetin beta has been studied to have effect on tumor growth and should not be used in patients with any type of malignancy.

Blood pressure should be closely monitored before, during, and after therapy.

DRUG INTERACTIONS OF CONCERN TO DENTISTRY

- None reported

SERIOUS REACTIONS

! Hypertension, hypertensive encephalopathy, and seizures have occurred.

DENTAL CONSIDERATIONS

General:

- Patient's disease, treatment history, and use of other drugs will affect patient evaluation and management.
- Determine why patient is taking the drug.
- Monitor vital signs at every appointment because of cardiovascular side effects.
- Take precautions if dental surgery is anticipated and general anesthesia is required.
- Consider semisupine chair position for patient comfort if GI side effects occur.

Consultations:

- Medical consultation may be required to assess disease control.
- Review patient's medical and drug history.

Teach Patient/Family to:

- Encourage effective oral hygiene to prevent soft tissue inflammation.
- Use caution to prevent injury when using oral hygiene aids.

methsuximide

meth-**sux′**-ih-mide

(Celontin)

Do not confuse with methoxsalen.

CATEGORY AND SCHEDULE

Pregnancy Risk Category: C

Drug Class: Anticonvulsant

MECHANISM OF ACTION

An anticonvulsant agent that increases the seizure threshold, suppresses paroxysmal spike-and-wave pattern in absence seizures, and depresses nerve transmission in the motor cortex.

Therapeutic Effect: Controls absence (petit mal) seizures.

USES

Treatment of refractory absence seizures (petit mal)

PHARMACOKINETICS

Rapidly metabolized in liver to active metabolite, *N*-desmethylmethsuximide. Primarily excreted in urine. Unknown if removed by hemodialysis. ***Half-life:*** 1.4 hr.

INDICATIONS AND DOSAGES

▸ Absence Seizures

PO

Adults, Elderly. Initially, 300 mg/day for the first wk. Increase dosage by 300 mg/day at weekly intervals until response is attained. Maintenance: 1200 mg/day at 2–4 times a day. Do not exceed 1000 mg/day in children

12–15 yr, 1200 mg/day in patients older than 15 yr.
Children. Initially, 10–15 mg/kg/day 3–4 times a day. Increase at weekly intervals. Maximum: 30 mg/kg/day.

SIDE EFFECTS/ADVERSE REACTIONS

Frequent
Drowsiness, dizziness, nausea, vomiting
Occasional
Visual abnormalities, such as spots before eyes, difficulty focusing, blurred vision, dry mouth or pharynx, tongue irritation, nervousness, insomnia, headache, constipation or diarrhea, rash, weight loss, proteinuria, edema

PRECAUTIONS AND CONTRAINDICATIONS

Hypersensitivity to succinimides or any component of the formulation
Caution:
Hepatic disease, renal disease, lactation

DRUG INTERACTIONS OF CONCERN TO DENTISTRY

- Enhanced CNS depression: alcohol, CNS depressants
- Decreased effects: phenothiazines, thioxanthenes, barbiturates
- Changes in seizure pattern, frequency: haloperidol

SERIOUS REACTIONS

! Toxic reactions appear as blood dyscrasias, including aplastic anemia, agranulocytosis, thrombocytopenia, leukopenia, leukocytosis, eosinophilia, cardiovascular disturbances, such as CHF, hypotension or hypertension, thrombophlebitis, arrhythmias, and dermatologic effects, such as rash, urticaria, pruritus, photosensitivity.

! Abrupt withdrawal may precipitate status epilepticus.

DENTAL CONSIDERATIONS

General:
- Patients on chronic drug therapy may rarely have symptoms of blood dyscrasias, which can include infection, bleeding, and poor healing.
- Avoid dental light in patient's eyes; offer dark glasses for patient comfort.
- Determine type of epilepsy, seizure frequency, and quality of seizure control. A stress-reduction protocol may be required.
- Place on frequent recall to monitor gingival condition.

Consultations:
- In a patient with symptoms of blood dyscrasias, request a medical consultation for blood studies and postpone dental treatment until normal values are reestablished.
- Take precautions if dental surgery is anticipated and anesthesia is required.
- Medical consultation may be required to assess disease control.

Teach Patient/Family to:
- Encourage effective oral hygiene to prevent soft tissue inflammation.
- Use caution to prevent injury when using oral hygiene aids.
- Avoid mouth rinses with high alcohol content if oral side effects occur.

methyldopa/ methyldopate

meth-ill-**doe**′-pa/
meth-ill-**doe**′-payte
(Aldomet, Apo-Methyldopa[CAN], Hydopa[AUS], Novomedopa[CAN], Nudopa[AUS])
Do not confuse Aldomet with Anzemet.

CATEGORY AND SCHEDULE

Pregnancy Risk Category: B

Drug Class: Centrally acting antihypertensive

MECHANISM OF ACTION

An antihypertensive agent that stimulates central inhibitory α-adrenergic receptors, lowers arterial pressure, and reduces plasma renin activity.
Therapeutic Effect: Reduces B/P.

USES

Treatment of hypertension

PHARMACOKINETICS

PO: Peak 4–6 hr, duration 12–24 hr.
IV: Peak 2 hr, duration 10–16 hr
Metabolized by liver, excreted in urine.

INDICATIONS AND DOSAGES

▸ **Moderate-to-Severe Hypertension**

PO

Adults. Initially, 250 mg 2–3 times a day for 2 days. Adjust dosage at intervals of 2 days (minimum).
Elderly. Initially, 125 mg 1–2 times a day. May increase by 125 mg q2–3 days. Maintenance: 500 mg–2 g/day in 2–4 divided doses.
Children. Initially, 10 mg/kg/day in 2–4 divided doses. Adjust dosage at intervals of 2 days (minimum). Maximum: 65 mg/kg/day or 3 g/day, whichever is less.

IV

Adults. 250–1000 mg q6–8h. Maximum: 4 g/day.
Children. Initially, 2–4 mg/kg/dose. May increase to 5–10 mg/kg/dose in 4–6 hr if no response. Maximum: 65 mg/kg/day or 3 g/day, whichever is less.

SIDE EFFECTS/ADVERSE REACTIONS

Frequent
Peripheral edema, somnolence, headache, dry mouth
Occasional
Mental changes (such as anxiety, depression), decreased sexual function or libido, diarrhea, swelling of breasts, nausea, vomiting, light-headedness, paraesthesia, rhinitis

PRECAUTIONS AND CONTRAINDICATIONS

Hepatic disease, pheochromocytoma
Caution:
Liver disease, eclampsia, severe cardiac disease

DRUG INTERACTIONS OF CONCERN TO DENTISTRY

- Decreased effects: indomethacin and other NSAIDs
- Increased pressor response: epinephrine and other sympathomimetics
- Increased sedation: haloperidol, alcohol, CNS depressants
- Increased hypotensive action of general anesthetics

SERIOUS REACTIONS

! Hepatotoxicity (abnormal liver function test results, jaundice, hepatitis), hemolytic anemia, unexplained fever and flu-like symptoms may occur. If these

M

conditions appear, discontinue the medication and contact the physician.

DENTAL CONSIDERATIONS

General:

- Monitor vital signs at every appointment because of cardiovascular side effects.
- Patients on chronic drug therapy may rarely have symptoms of blood dyscrasias, which can include infection, bleeding, and poor healing.
- Assess salivary flow as a factor in caries, periodontal disease, and candidiasis.
- Limit use of sodium-containing products, such as saline IV fluids, for patients with a dietary salt restriction.
- After supine positioning, have patient sit upright for at least 2 min before standing to avoid orthostatic hypotension.
- Stress from dental procedures may compromise cardiovascular function; determine patient risk and consider use of stress-reduction protocol.

Consultations:

- In a patient with symptoms of blood dyscrasias, request a medical consultation for blood studies and postpone dental treatment until normal values are reestablished.
- Medical consultation may be required to assess disease control and patient's ability to tolerate stress.

Teach Patient/Family to:

- Encourage effective oral hygiene to prevent soft tissue inflammation.
- Use caution to prevent injury when using oral hygiene aids.
- When chronic dry mouth occurs, advise patient to:
  - Avoid mouth rinses with high alcohol content because of drying effects.
  - Use sugarless gum, frequent sips of water, or saliva substitutes.
  - Use daily home fluoride products for anticaries effect.

methylergonovine

meth-ill-er-**gon′**-oh-veen
(Methergine)

CATEGORY AND SCHEDULE

Pregnancy Risk Category: C

Drug Class: Oxytocic

MECHANISM OF ACTION

An ergot alkaloid that stimulates α-adrenergic and serotonin receptors, producing arterial vasoconstriction. Causes vasospasm of coronary arteries and directly stimulates uterine muscle.

Therapeutic Effect: Increases strength and frequency of uterine contractions. Decreases uterine bleeding.

USES

Treatment of hemorrhage postpartum or postabortion, uterine contractions

PHARMACOKINETICS

Route	Onset	Peak	Duration
PO	5–10 min	N/A	N/A
IV	Immediate	N/A	3 hr
IM	2–5 min	N/A	N/A

Rapidly absorbed from the GI tract after IM administration. Distributed rapidly to plasma, extracellular fluid, and tissues. Metabolized in the liver

and undergoes first-pass effect. Primarily excreted in urine.
Half-life: IV (alpha phase), 2–3 min or less; IV (beta phase), 20–30 min or longer.

INDICATIONS AND DOSAGES

▸ **Prevention and Treatment of Postpartum and Postabortion Hemorrhage Caused by Atony or Involution**

PO
Adults. 0.2 mg 3–4 times a day. Continue for up to 7 days.
IV, IM
Adults. Initially, 0.2 mg. May repeat q2–4h for no more than a total of 5 doses.

SIDE EFFECTS/ADVERSE REACTIONS

Frequent
Nausea, uterine cramping, vomiting
Occasional
Abdominal pain, diarrhea, dizziness, diaphoresis, tinnitus, bradycardia, chest pain
Rare
Allergic reaction, such as rash and itching; dyspnea; severe or sudden hypertension

PRECAUTIONS AND CONTRAINDICATIONS

Hypertension, pregnancy, toxemia, untreated hypocalcemia

DRUG INTERACTIONS OF CONCERN TO DENTISTRY

- Increased effects: sympathomimetics

SERIOUS REACTIONS

! Severe hypertensive episodes may result in CVA, serious arrhythmias, and seizures.
! Hypertensive effects are more frequent with patient susceptibility, rapid IV administration, and concurrent use of regional anesthesia or vasoconstrictors.
! Peripheral ischemia may lead to gangrene.

DENTAL CONSIDERATIONS

General:
- Acute-use drug normally given in the hospital; provide palliative dental care for dental emergencies only.

Teach Patient/Family to:
- Follow up with definitive dental care at an opportune date.

methylphenidate hydrochloride

meth-ill-**fen**′-ih-date high-droh-**klor**′-ide
(Attenta[AUS], Concerta, Metadate CD, Metadate ER, Methylin, Methylin ER, PMS-Methylphenidate[CAN], Riphenidate[CAN], Ritalin, Ritalin LA, Ritalin SR)
Do not confuse Ritalin with Rifadin.

CATEGORY AND SCHEDULE

Pregnancy Risk Category: C
Controlled Substance: Schedule II

Drug Class: CNS stimulant, related to amphetamines

MECHANISM OF ACTION

A CNS stimulant that blocks the reuptake of norepinephrine and dopamine into presynaptic neurons.
Therapeutic Effect: Decreases motor restlessness and fatigue; increases motor activity, attention span, and mental alertness; produces mild euphoria.

USES

Treatment of attention-deficit/hyperactivity disorder (ADHD), narcolepsy

PHARMACOKINETICS

Onset	Peak	Duration
Immediate release	2 hr	3–5 hr
Sustained release	4–7 hr	3–8 hr
Extended release	N/A	8–12 hr

Slowly and incompletely absorbed from the GI tract. Protein binding: 15%. Metabolized in the liver. Eliminated in urine and in feces by biliary system. Unknown if removed by hemodialysis. ***Half-life:*** 2–4 hr.

INDICATIONS AND DOSAGES

▸ ADHD

PO

Children 6 yr and older. Immediate release: Initially, 2.5–5 mg before breakfast and lunch. May increase by 5–10 mg/day at weekly intervals. Maximum: 60 mg/day.

PO (Concerta)

Children 6 yr and older. Initially, 18 mg once a day; may increase by 18 mg/day at weekly intervals. Maximum: 72 mg/day.

PO (Metadate CD)

Children 6 yr and older. Initially, 20 mg/day. May increase by 20 mg/day at weekly intervals. Maximum: 60 mg/day.

PO (Ritalin LA)

Children 6 yr and older. Initially, 20 mg/day. May increase by 10 mg/day at weekly intervals. Maximum: 60 mg/day.

PO (Metadate ER, Methylin ER, Ritalin SR)

Children 6 yr and older. May replace regular tablets after daily dose is titrated and 8-hr dosage corresponds to sustained-release or extended-release tablet size.

▸ Narcolepsy

PO

Adults, Elderly. 10 mg 2–3 times a day. Range: 10–60 mg/day.

SIDE EFFECTS/ADVERSE REACTIONS

Frequent

Anxiety, insomnia, anorexia

Occasional

Dizziness, drowsiness, headache, nausea, abdominal pain, fever, rash, arthralgia, vomiting

Rare

Blurred vision, Tourette's syndrome (marked by uncontrolled vocal outbursts, repetitive body movements, and tics), palpitations

PRECAUTIONS AND CONTRAINDICATIONS

Avoid use within 14 days of MAOIs

Caution:

Hypertension, depression, seizures, lactation, drug abuse

DRUG INTERACTIONS OF CONCERN TO DENTISTRY

- Increased effects of CNS stimulants, tricyclic antidepressants, SSRIs, sympathomimetics

SERIOUS REACTIONS

! Prolonged administration to children with ADHD may delay growth.

! Overdose may produce tachycardia, palpitations, arrhythmias, chest pain, psychotic episode, seizures, and coma.

! Hypersensitivity reactions and blood dyscrasias occur rarely.

DENTAL CONSIDERATIONS

General:

- Monitor vital signs at every appointment because of cardiovascular side effects.
- Patients on chronic drug therapy may rarely have symptoms of blood dyscrasias, which can include infection, bleeding, and poor healing.
- Assess salivary flow as a factor in caries, periodontal disease, and candidiasis.
- Use vasoconstrictors with caution, in low doses.
- Determine why the patient is taking the drug.

Consultations:

- In a patient with symptoms of blood dyscrasias, request a medical consultation for blood studies and postpone dental treatment until normal values are reestablished.
- Medical consultation may be required to assess disease control.

Teach Patient/Family to:

- Encourage effective oral hygiene to prevent soft tissue inflammation.
- Use caution to prevent injury when using oral hygiene aids.
- When chronic dry mouth occurs, advise patient to:
  - Avoid mouth rinses with high alcohol content because of drying effects.
  - Use sugarless gum, frequent sips of water, or saliva substitutes.
  - Use daily home fluoride products for anticaries effect.

methylprednisolone

meth-il-pred-**niss′**-oh-lone
methylprednisolone (Medrol)
methylprednisolone acetate (Depo-Medrol, Depo-Nisolone[AUS])
methylprednisolone sodium succinate (A-Methapred, Solu-Medrol)
Do not confuse methylprednisolone with medroxyprogesterone or Medrol with Mebaral.

CATEGORY AND SCHEDULE

Pregnancy Risk Category: C

Drug Class: Glucocorticoid, immediate acting

M

MECHANISM OF ACTION

An adrenocortical steroid that suppresses migration of polymorphonuclear leukocytes and reverses increased capillary permeability.
Therapeutic Effect: Decreases inflammation.

USES

Treatment of severe inflammation, shock, adrenal insufficiency, collagen disorders

PHARMACOKINETICS

Route	Onset	Peak	Duration
PO	N/A	1–2 hr	30–36 hr
IM	N/A	4–8 days	1–4 wk

Well absorbed from the GI tract after IM administration. Widely distributed. Metabolized in the liver. Excreted in urine. Removed by hemodialysis. ***Half-life:*** 3.5 hr.

INDICATIONS AND DOSAGES

▸ Substitution Therapy for Deficiency States: Acute or Chronic Adrenal Insufficiency, Adrenal Insufficiency Secondary to Pituitary Insufficiency, and Congenital Adrenal Hyperplasia; Nonendocrine Disorders: Allergic, Collagen, Hepatic, Intestinal Tract, Ocular, Renal, and Skin Diseases; Arthritis; Bronchial Asthma; Cerebral Edema; Malignancies; and Rheumatic Carditis

PO

Adults, Elderly. Initially, 4–48 mg/day.

IV (Methylprednisolone Sodium Succinate)

Adults, Elderly. 40–250 mg q4–6h. High dosage: 30 mg/kg over at least 30 min. Repeat q4–6h for 48–72 hr.

M

▸ Spinal Cord Injury

IV Bolus

Adults, Elderly. 30 mg/kg over 15 min. Maintenance dose: 5.4 mg/kg/h over 23 hr, to be given within 45 min of bolus dose.

IM (Methylprednisolone Acetate)

Adults, Elderly. 10–80 mg/day.

Intraarticular, Intralesional

Adults, Elderly. 4–40 mg, up to 80 mg q1–5wk.

▸ Antiinflammatory/Immunosuppressant

PO/IM/IV

Pediatric. 0.5–1.7 mg/kg/day or 5–25 mg/m^2/day in 2–4 divided doses.

SIDE EFFECTS/ADVERSE REACTIONS

Frequent

Insomnia, heartburn, anxiety, abdominal distention, diaphoresis, acne, mood swings, increased appetite, facial flushing, GI distress, delayed wound healing, increased susceptibility to infection, diarrhea or constipation

Occasional

Headache, edema, tachycardia, change in skin color, frequent urination, depression

Rare

Psychosis, increased blood coagulability, hallucinations

PRECAUTIONS AND CONTRAINDICATIONS

Administration of live virus vaccines, systemic fungal infection

Caution:

Diabetes mellitus, glaucoma, osteoporosis, seizure disorders, ulcerative colitis, CHF, myasthenia gravis, renal disease, esophagitis, peptic ulcer, rifampin

DRUG INTERACTIONS OF CONCERN TO DENTISTRY

- Decreased action: barbiturates, rifampin, rifabutin
- Increased GI side effects: alcohol, salicylates, NSAIDs
- Increased action: ketoconazole, macrolide antibiotics
- Hepatotoxicity: acetaminophen (chronic, high doses)

SERIOUS REACTIONS

! Long-term therapy may cause hypocalcemia, hypokalemia, muscle wasting (especially in arms and legs), osteoporosis, spontaneous fractures, amenorrhea, cataracts, glaucoma, peptic ulcer disease, and CHF.

! Abruptly withdrawing the drug after long-term therapy may cause anorexia, nausea, fever, headache, sudden severe myalgia, rebound inflammation, fatigue, weakness, lethargy, dizziness, and orthostatic hypotension.

DENTAL CONSIDERATIONS

General:

- Patients on chronic drug therapy may rarely have symptoms of blood dyscrasias, which can include infection, bleeding, and poor healing.
- Assess salivary flow as a factor in caries, periodontal disease, and candidiasis.
- Symptoms of oral infections may be masked.
- Place on frequent recall to evaluate healing response.
- Prophylactic antibiotics may be indicated to prevent infection if surgery or deep scaling is planned.
- Avoid prescribing NSAID-containing products.
- Determine dose and duration of steroid therapy for each patient to assess risk for stress tolerance and immunosuppression.
- Patients who have been or are currently on chronic steroid therapy (longer than 2 wk) may require supplemental steroids for dental treatment.

Consultations:

- In a patient with symptoms of blood dyscrasias, request a medical consultation for blood studies and postpone dental treatment until normal values are reestablished.
- Medical consultation may be required to assess disease control.
- Consultation may be required to confirm steroid dose and duration of use.

Teach Patient/Family to:

- Encourage effective oral hygiene to prevent soft tissue inflammation.
- Use caution to prevent injury when using oral hygiene aids because of reduced healing response.
- When chronic dry mouth occurs, advise patient to:
  - Avoid mouth rinses with high alcohol content because of drying effects.
  - Use sugarless gum, frequent sips of water, or saliva substitutes.
  - Use daily home fluoride products for anticaries effect.

methyltestosterone

meth-il-tes-**tos**′-te-rone
(Android, Android-10, Android-25, Oreton Methyl, Testred, Virilon)
Do not confuse with methylprednisolone.

CATEGORY AND SCHEDULE

Pregnancy Risk Category: X
Controlled substance: Schedule III

Drug Class: Androgens, hormones/hormone modifiers

MECHANISM OF ACTION

A synthetic testosterone derivative with androgen activity that promotes growth and development of male sex organs and maintains secondary sex characteristics in androgen-deficient males.

Therapeutic Effect: Treats hypogonadism and delayed puberty in males.

USES

Replacement of the hormone when the body is unable to produce enough on its own; to stimulate the beginning of puberty in certain boys who are late starting puberty naturally; to treat certain types of breast cancer in females.

M

PHARMACOKINETICS

Well absorbed from the GI tract. Protein binding: 98%. Metabolized in liver. Primarily excreted in urine. Unknown if removed by hemodialysis. ***Half-life:*** 10–100 min.

INDICATIONS AND DOSAGES

▸ **Breast Cancer**

PO

Adults, Elderly. 50–200 mg/day.

▸ **Delayed Puberty**

PO

Adults. 10–50 mg/day.

Adults, Elderly. 50–200 mg/day.

▸ **Hypogonadism**

PO

Adults. 10–50 mg/day.

SIDE EFFECTS/ADVERSE REACTIONS

Frequent

Gynecomastia, acne, amenorrhea or other menstrual irregularities

Females: Hirsutism, deepening of voice, clitoral enlargement that may not be reversible when drug is discontinued

Occasional

Edema, nausea, insomnia, oligospermia, priapism, male pattern of baldness, bladder irritability, hypercalcemia in immobilized patients or those with breast cancer, hypercholesterolemia

Rare

Polycythemia

PRECAUTIONS AND CONTRAINDICATIONS

Pregnancy, prostatic or breast cancer in males, hypersensitivity to methyltestosterone or any other component of its formulation

DRUG INTERACTIONS OF CONCERN TO DENTISTRY

• Edema: ACTH, corticosteroids

SERIOUS REACTIONS

! Cholestatic jaundice, hepatocellular neoplasms, peliosis hepatitis, edema with or without CHF and suppression of clotting factors II, V, VII, and X have been reported.

DENTAL CONSIDERATIONS

General:

• Determine why patient is taking the drug.

• Short appointments and a stress-reduction protocol may be required for anxious patients.

• Possible risk of bleeding when used concurrently with oral anticoagulants and aspirin.

Consultations:

• Medical consultation may be required to assess disease control.

Teach Patient/Family to:

• Encourage effective oral hygiene to prevent soft tissue inflammation.

• Update health and medication history if physician makes any changes in evaluation or drug regimens; include OTC, herbal, and nonherbal drugs in the update.

metipranolol hydrochloride

met-ee-**pran**′-oh-lol

high-droh-**klor**′-ide

(OptiPranolol)

Do not confuse with metoprolol or propranolol.

CATEGORY AND SCHEDULE

Pregnancy Risk Category: C

Drug Class: Antiglaucoma agent (ophthalmic)

MECHANISM OF ACTION

An antiglaucoma agent that non-selectively blocks β-adrenergic receptors. Reduces aqueous humor production.

Therapeutic Effect: Reduces intraocular pressure (IOP).

USES

Treatment of certain types of glaucoma

PHARMACOKINETICS

Route	Onset	Peak	Duration
Eye drops	0.5–3 hr	2–7 hr	24 hr or more

Systemic absorption may occur.

INDICATIONS AND DOSAGES

▸ **Glaucoma, Ocular Hypertension**

Ophthalmic

Adults, Elderly. Instill 1 drop 2 times a day.

SIDE EFFECTS/ADVERSE REACTIONS

Frequent

Eye burning/stinging, hyperemia, blurred vision, headache, fatigue

Occasional

Sensitivity to light, dizziness, hypotension

Rare

Dry eye, conjunctivitis, eye pain, rash, muscle pain

PRECAUTIONS AND CONTRAINDICATIONS

Bronchial asthma or chronic obstructive pulmonary disease, cardiogenic shock, overt cardiac failure, second- or third-degree heart AV block, severe sinus bradycardia, hypersensitivity to metipranolol or any component of the formulation

DRUG INTERACTIONS OF CONCERN TO DENTISTRY

- Avoid or use with caution: drugs with anticholinergic effects

SERIOUS REACTIONS

! Ophthalmic overdosage may produce bradycardia, hypotension, bronchospasm, and acute cardiac failure.

! Arrhythmias and myocardial infarction have been reported.

DENTAL CONSIDERATIONS

General:

- Determine why patient is taking the drug.
- Avoid drugs with anticholinergic activity, such as antihistamines, opioids, benzodiazepines, propantheline, atropine, and scopolamine.
- Avoid dental light in patient's eyes; offer dark glasses for patient comfort.
- Question glaucoma patient about compliance with prescribed drug regimen.

Consultations:

- Medical consultation may be required to assess disease control.

Teach Patient/Family to:

- Update health and medication history if physician makes any changes in evaluation or drug regimens; include OTC, herbal, and nonherbal drugs in the update.

metoclopramide

met-oh-kloe-**pra′**-mide
(Apo-Metoclop[CAN], Maxolon[AUS], Pramin[AUS], Reglan)
Do not confuse Reglan with Renagel.

CATEGORY AND SCHEDULE

Pregnancy Risk Category: B

Drug Class: Central dopamine receptor antagonist

MECHANISM OF ACTION

A dopamine receptor antagonist that stimulates motility of the upper GI tract and decreases reflux into the esophagus. Also raises the threshold of activity in the chemoreceptor trigger zone.
Therapeutic Effect: Accelerates intestinal transit and gastric emptying; relieves nausea and vomiting.

M

USES

Prevention of nausea, vomiting induced by chemotherapy, radiation, delayed gastric emptying, gastroesophageal reflux, diabetic gastroparesis

PHARMACOKINETICS

Route	Onset	Peak	Duration
PO	30–60 min	N/A	N/A
IV	1–3 min	N/A	N/A
IM	10–15 min	N/A	N/A

Well absorbed from the GI tract. Metabolized in the liver. Protein binding: 30%. Primarily excreted in urine. Not removed by hemodialysis.
Half-life: 4–6 hr.

INDICATIONS AND DOSAGES

▸ Prevention of Chemotherapy-Induced Nausea and Vomiting

IV

Adults, Elderly, Children. 1–2 mg/kg 30 min before chemotherapy; repeat q2h for 2 doses, then q3h as needed.

▸ Postoperative Nausea and Vomiting

IV

Adults, Elderly, Children 15 yr and older. 10 mg; repeat q6–8h as needed.
Children 14 yr and younger. 0.1–0.2 mg/kg/dose; repeat q6–8h as needed.

▸ Diabetic Gastroparesis

PO, IV

Adults. 10 mg 30 min before meals and at bedtime for 2–8 wk.

PO

Elderly. Initially, 5 mg 30 min before meals and at bedtime. May increase to 10 mg.

IV

Elderly. 5 mg over 1–2 min. May increase to 10 mg.

▸ Symptomatic Gastroesophageal Reflux

PO

Adults. 10–15 mg up to 4 times a day, or single doses up to 20 mg as needed.
Elderly. Initially, 5 mg 4 times a day. May increase to 10 mg.
Children. 0.4–0.8 mg/kg/day in 4 divided doses.

▸ To Facilitate Small Bowel Intubation (Single Dose)

IV

Adults, Elderly. 10 mg as a single dose.
Children 6–14 yr. 2.5–5 mg as a single dose.
Children younger than 6 yr. 0.1 mg/kg as a single dose.

▸ Dosage in Renal Impairment

Dosage is modified on the basis of creatinine clearance.

Creatinine Clearance	% of Normal Dose
40–50 ml/min	75
10–40 ml/min	50
Less than 10 ml/min	25–50

SIDE EFFECTS/ADVERSE REACTIONS

Frequent

Somnolence, restlessness, fatigue, lethargy

Occasional

Dizziness, anxiety, headache, insomnia, breast tenderness, altered menstruation, constipation, rash, dry mouth, galactorrhea, gynecomastia

Rare

Hypotension or hypertension, tachycardia

PRECAUTIONS AND CONTRAINDICATIONS

Concurrent use of medications likely to produce extrapyramidal reactions, GI hemorrhage, GI obstruction or perforation, history of seizure disorders, pheochromocytoma

Caution:

Lactation, GI hemorrhage, CHF, asthma, hypertension, renal failure; extrapyramidal diseases, depression, concurrently with or within 14 days of discontinuing MAOIs

DRUG INTERACTIONS OF CONCERN TO DENTISTRY

• Decreased GI action: anticholinergics, opioids
• Increased sedation: alcohol, other CNS depressants
• Increased effects of succinylcholine

SERIOUS REACTIONS

! Extrapyramidal reactions occur most commonly in children and young adults (18–30 yr) receiving large doses (2 mg/kg) during chemotherapy and are usually limited to akathisia (involuntary limb movement and facial grimacing).

DENTAL CONSIDERATIONS

General:

• Assess salivary flow as a factor in caries, periodontal disease, and candidiasis.
• Assess for presence of extrapyramidal motor symptoms, such as tardive dyskinesia and akathisia. Extrapyramidal motor activity may complicate dental treatment.
• Determine why the patient is taking the drug.
• Consider semisupine chair position for patient comfort because of GI effects of disease.

Teach Patient/Family to:

• When chronic dry mouth occurs, advise patient to:
  • Avoid mouth rinses with high alcohol content because of drying effects.
  • Use sugarless gum, frequent sips of water, or saliva substitutes.
  • Use daily home fluoride products for anticaries effect.

metolazone

met-**tole**′-ah-zone
(Mykrox, Zaroxolyn)
Do not confuse metolazone with methazolamide or metoprolol, or Zaroxolyn with Zarontin.

CATEGORY AND SCHEDULE

Pregnancy Risk Category: B (D if used in pregnancy-induced hypertension)

Drug Class: Diuretic with thiazide-like effects

MECHANISM OF ACTION

A thiazide-like diuretic and antihypertensive. As a diuretic, blocks reabsorption of sodium, potassium, and chloride at the distal convoluted tubule, increasing renal excretion of sodium and water. As an antihypertensive, reduces plasma and extracellular fluid volume and peripheral vascular resistance.
Therapeutic Effect: Promotes diuresis and reduces B/P.

USES

Treatment of edema, hypertension, CHF

PHARMACOKINETICS

Route	Onset	Peak	Duration
PO (diuretic)	1 hr	2 hr	12–24 hr

M

Incompletely absorbed from the GI tract. Protein binding: 95%. Primarily excreted unchanged in urine. Not removed by hemodialysis.
Half-life: 14 hr.

INDICATIONS AND DOSAGES

▸ **Edema**

PO (Zaroxolyn)
Adults, Elderly. 5–10 mg/day. May increase to 20 mg/day in edema associated with renal disease or heart failure.
Children. 0.2–0.4 mg/kg/day in 1–2 divided doses.

▸ **Hypertension**

PO (Zaroxolyn)
Adults, Elderly. 2.5–5 mg/day.
PO (Mydrox)
Adults, Elderly. Initially, 0.5 mg/day. May increase up to 1 mg/day.

SIDE EFFECTS/ADVERSE REACTIONS

Expected
Increase in urinary frequency and urine volume
Frequent
Dizziness, light-headedness, headache
Occasional
Muscle cramps and spasm, fatigue, lethargy
Rare
Asthenia, palpitations, depression, nausea, vomiting, abdominal bloating, constipation, diarrhea, urticaria

PRECAUTIONS AND CONTRAINDICATIONS

Anuria, hepatic coma or precoma, history of hypersensitivity to sulfonamides or thiazide diuretics, renal decompensation
Caution:
Hypokalemia, renal disease, hepatic disease, gout, COPD, lupus erythematosus, diabetes mellitus

DRUG INTERACTIONS OF CONCERN TO DENTISTRY

- Increased photosensitization: tetracycline
- Decreased hypotensive response: indomethacin and other NSAIDs

SERIOUS REACTIONS

! Vigorous diuresis may lead to profound water and electrolyte depletion, resulting in hypokalemia, hyponatremia, and dehydration.
! Acute hypotensive episodes may occur.
! Hyperglycemia may occur during prolonged therapy.
! Pancreatitis, paresthesia, blood dyscrasias, pulmonary edema, allergic pneumonitis, and dermatologic reactions occur rarely.

! Overdose can lead to lethargy and coma without changes in electrolytes or hydration.

DENTAL CONSIDERATIONS

General:

- Patients on chronic drug therapy may rarely have symptoms of blood dyscrasias, which can include infection, bleeding, and poor healing.
- Assess salivary flow as a factor in caries, periodontal disease, and candidiasis.
- After supine positioning, have patient sit upright for at least 2 min before standing to avoid orthostatic hypotension.
- Short appointments and a stress-reduction protocol may be required for anxious patients.
- Limit use of sodium-containing products, such as saline IV fluids, for patients with a dietary salt restriction.
- Stress from dental procedures may compromise cardiovascular function; determine patient risk.

Consultations:

- In a patient with symptoms of blood dyscrasias, request a medical consultation for blood studies and postpone dental treatment until normal values are reestablished.
- Medical consultation may be required to assess disease control and patient's ability to tolerate stress.

Teach Patient/Family to:

- Encourage effective oral hygiene to prevent soft tissue inflammation.
- Use caution to prevent injury when using oral hygiene aids.
- When chronic dry mouth occurs, advise patient to:
  - Avoid mouth rinses with high alcohol content because of drying effects.
  - Use sugarless gum, frequent sips of water, or saliva substitutes.
  - Use daily home fluoride products for anticaries effect.

metoprolol tartrate

me-**toe′**-pro-lole **tahr′**-treyt (Apo-Metoprolol[CAN], Betaloc[CAN], Lopresor[AUS], Lopressor, Metohexal[AUS], Metolol[AUS], Minax[AUS], Nu-Metop[CAN], PMS-Metoprolol[CAN], Toprol XL)

Do not confuse metoprolol with metaproterenol or metolazone.

CATEGORY AND SCHEDULE

Pregnancy Risk Category: C (D if used in second or third trimester)

Drug Class: Antihypertensive, selective β_1-blocker

M

MECHANISM OF ACTION

An antianginal, antihypertensive, and MI adjunct that selectively blocks β_1-adrenergic receptors; high dosages may block β_2-adrenergic receptors. Decreases oxygen requirements. Large doses increase airway resistance.

Therapeutic Effect: Slows sinus node heart rate, decreases cardiac output, and reduces B/P. Also decreases myocardial ischemia severity.

USES

Treatment of mild-to-moderate hypertension, acute MI to reduce risk of cardiovascular mortality, angina pectoris, mild-to-moderate heart failure

PHARMACOKINETICS

Route	Onset	Peak	Duration
PO	10–15 min	N/A	6 hr
PO (extended release)	N/A	6–12 hr	5–8 hr
IV	Immediate	20 min	5–8 hr

Well absorbed from the GI tract. Protein binding: 12%. Widely distributed. Metabolized in the liver (undergoes significant first-pass metabolism). Primarily excreted in urine. Removed by hemodialysis. ***Half-life:*** 3–7 hr.

INDICATIONS AND DOSAGES

▸ Mild-to-Moderate Hypertension

PO

Adults. Initially, 100 mg/day as single or divided dose. Increase at weekly (or longer) intervals. Maintenance: 100–450 mg/day.

Elderly. Initially, 25 mg/day. Range: 25–300 mg/day.

PO (Extended-Release)

Adults. 50–100 mg/day as single dose. May increase at least at weekly intervals until optimal B/P attained. Maximum: 200 mg/day.

Elderly. Initially, 25–50 mg/day as a single dose. May increase at 1- to 2-wk intervals.

▸ Chronic, Stable Angina Pectoris

PO

Adults. Initially, 100 mg/day as single or divided dose. Increase at weekly (or longer) intervals. Maintenance: 100–450 mg/day.

PO (Extended-Release)

Adults. Initially, 100 mg/day as single dose. May increase at least at weekly intervals until optimal clinical response achieved. Maximum: 200 mg/day.

▸ CHF

PO (Extended-Release)

Adults. Initially, 25 mg/day. May double dose q2wk. Maximum: 200 mg/day.

▸ Early Treatment of MI

IV

Adults. 5 mg q2min for 3 doses, followed by 50 mg orally q6h for 48 hr. Begin oral dose 15 min after last IV dose. Or, in patients who do not tolerate full IV dose, give 25–50 mg orally q6h, 15 min after last IV dose.

▸ Late Treatment and Maintenance after an MI

PO

Adults. 100 mg twice a day for at least 3 mo.

SIDE EFFECTS/ADVERSE REACTIONS

Metoprolol is generally well tolerated, with transient and mild side effects

Frequent

Diminished sexual function, drowsiness, insomnia, unusual fatigue or weakness

Occasional

Anxiety, nervousness, diarrhea, constipation, nausea, vomiting, nasal congestion, abdominal discomfort, dizziness, difficulty breathing, cold hands or feet

Rare

Altered taste, dry eyes, nightmares, paraesthesia, allergic reaction (rash, pruritus)

PRECAUTIONS AND CONTRAINDICATIONS

Cardiogenic shock, MI with a heart rate less than 45 beats/min or systolic B/P less than 100 mm Hg, overt heart failure, second- or third-degree heart block, sinus bradycardia

Caution:
Major surgery, lactation, diabetes mellitus, renal disease, thyroid disease, COPD, heart failure, CAD, nonallergic bronchospasm, hepatic disease, asthma

DRUG INTERACTIONS OF CONCERN TO DENTISTRY

• Increased hypotension, bradycardia: fentanyl derivatives, inhalation anesthetics
• Decreased antihypertensive effects: NSAIDs, sympathomimetics
• May slow metabolism of lidocaine
• Decreased β-blocking effects (or decreased β-adrenergic effects) of epinephrine, levonordefrin, isoproterenol, and other sympathomimetics
• Increased plasma concentrations: diphenhydramine

SERIOUS REACTIONS

! Overdose may produce profound bradycardia, hypotension, and bronchospasm.
! Abrupt withdrawal of metoprolol may result in diaphoresis, palpitations, headache, tremulousness, exacerbation of angina, MI, and ventricular arrhythmias.
! Metoprolol administration may precipitate CHF and MI in patients with heart disease, thyroid storm in those with thyrotoxicosis, and peripheral ischemia in those with existing peripheral vascular disease.
! Hypoglycemia may occur in patients with previously controlled diabetes mellitus.

DENTAL CONSIDERATIONS

General:
• Monitor vital signs at every appointment because of cardiovascular and respiratory side effects.
• After supine positioning, have patient sit upright for at least 2 min before standing to avoid orthostatic hypotension.
• Patients on chronic drug therapy may rarely have symptoms of blood dyscrasias, which can include infection, bleeding, and poor healing.
• Assess salivary flow as a factor in caries, periodontal disease, and candidiasis.
• Stress from dental procedures may compromise cardiovascular function; determine patient risk.
• Short appointments and a stress-reduction protocol may be required for anxious patients.
• Use vasoconstrictors with caution, in low doses, and with careful aspiration. Avoid use of gingival retraction cord with epinephrine.
• Determine why patient is taking the drug.

Consultations:
• In a patient with symptoms of blood dyscrasias, request a medical consultation for blood studies and postpone dental treatment until normal values are reestablished.
• Medical consultation may be required to assess disease control and patient's ability to tolerate stress.
• Take precautions if general anesthesia is required for dental surgery.

Teach Patient/Family to:
• Encourage effective oral hygiene to prevent soft tissue inflammation.
• Use caution to prevent injury when using oral hygiene aids.

• When chronic dry mouth occurs, advise patient to:
  • Avoid mouth rinses with high alcohol content because of drying effects.
  • Use sugarless gum, frequent sips of water, or saliva substitutes.
  • Use daily home fluoride products for anticaries effect.

metronidazole hydrochloride

me-troe-**ni′**-da-zole high-droh-**klor′**-ide
(Apo-Metronidazole[CAN], Flagyl, Flagyl ER, MetroCream, MetroGel, Metrogyl[AUS], MetroLotion, Metronidazole IV[AUS], Metronide[AUS], NidaGel[CAN], Noritate, Novonidazol[CAN], Rozex[AUS])

CATEGORY AND SCHEDULE
Pregnancy Risk Category: B

Drug Class: Trichomonacide, amebicide, antiinfective

M

MECHANISM OF ACTION
A nitroimidazole derivative that disrupts bacterial and protozoal DNA, inhibiting nucleic acid synthesis.
Therapeutic Effect: Produces bactericidal, antiprotozoal, amebicidal, and trichomonacidal effects. Produces antiinflammatory and immunosuppressive effects when applied topically.

USES
Treatment of intestinal amebiasis, amebic abscess, trichomoniasis, refractory trichomoniasis, bacterial anaerobic infections, giardiasis

PHARMACOKINETICS
Well absorbed from the GI tract; minimally absorbed after topical application. Protein binding: less than 20%. Widely distributed; crosses blood-brain barrier. Metabolized in the liver to active metabolite. Primarily excreted in urine; partially eliminated in feces. Removed by hemodialysis. ***Half-life:*** 8 hr (increased in alcoholic hepatic disease and in neonates).

INDICATIONS AND DOSAGES
▸ **Amebiasis**
PO
Adults, Elderly. 500–750 mg q8h.
Children. 35–50 mg/kg/day in divided doses q8h.
▸ **Trichomoniasis**
PO
Adults, Elderly. 250 mg q8h or 2 g as a single dose.
Children. 15–30 mg/kg/day in divided doses q8h.
▸ **Anaerobic Skin and Skin-Structure, CNS, Lower Respiratory Tract, Bone, Joint, Intraabdominal, and Gynecologic Infections; Endocarditis; Septicemia**
PO, IV
Adults, Elderly, Children. 30 mg/kg/day in divided doses q6h.
Maximum: 4 g/day.
▸ **Antibiotic-Associated Pseudomembranous Colitis**
PO
Adults, Elderly. 250–500 mg 3–4 times a day for 10–14 days.
Children. 30 mg/kg/day in divided doses q6h for 7–10 days.
▸ ***Helicobacter Pylori*** **Infections**
PO
Adults, Elderly. 250–500 mg 3 times a day (in combination).
Children. 15–20 mg/kg/day in 2 divided doses.

▸ **Bacterial Vaginosis**
PO
Adults. 750 mg at bedtime for 7 days.
Intravaginal
Adults. One applicatorful twice a day or once a day at bedtime for 5 days.
▸ **Rosacea**
Topical
Adults. Apply thin layer of lotion to affected area twice a day or cream once a day.

SIDE EFFECTS/ADVERSE REACTIONS

Frequent
Systemic: Anorexia, nausea, dry mouth, metallic taste
Vaginal: Symptomatic cervicitis and vaginitis, abdominal cramps, uterine pain
Occasional
Systemic: Diarrhea or constipation, vomiting, dizziness, erythematous rash, urticaria, reddish brown urine
Topical: Transient erythema, mild dryness, burning, irritation, stinging, tearing when applied too close to eyes
Vaginal: Vaginal, perineal, or vulvar itching; vulvar swelling
Rare
Mild, transient leukopenia; thrombophlebitis with IV therapy

PRECAUTIONS AND CONTRAINDICATIONS

Hypersensitivity to metronidazole or other nitroimidazole derivatives (also parabens with topical application)
Caution:
Candida infections; avoid unnecessary use because shown to be carcinogenic in rodents

DRUG INTERACTIONS OF CONCERN TO DENTISTRY

- Disulfiram-like reaction: alcohol, alcohol-containing products
- Decreased action: phenobarbital
- Possible increase in blood levels of tacrolimus
- Enhanced effects of warfarin, carbamazepine

SERIOUS REACTIONS

! Oral therapy may result in furry tongue, glossitis, cystitis, dysuria, pancreatitis, and flattening of T waves on ECG readings.
! Peripheral neuropathy, manifested as numbness and tingling in hands or feet, is usually reversible if treatment is stopped immediately after neurologic symptoms appear.
! Seizures occur occasionally.

DENTAL CONSIDERATIONS

General:
- Patients on chronic drug therapy may rarely have symptoms of blood dyscrasias, which can include infection, bleeding, and poor healing.
- Assess salivary flow as a factor in caries, periodontal disease, and candidiasis.
- Determine why the patient is taking the drug.

Consultations:
- In a patient with symptoms of blood dyscrasias, request a medical consultation for blood studies and postpone dental treatment until normal values are reestablished.
- Medical consultation may be required to assess disease control.

Teach Patient/Family to:
- Avoid alcoholic beverages and mouth rinses.
- Report taste alterations.
- Encourage effective oral hygiene to prevent soft tissue inflammation.

- Use caution to prevent injury when using oral hygiene aids.
- When chronic dry mouth occurs, advise patient to:
  - Avoid mouth rinses with high alcohol content because of drying effects.
  - Use sugarless gum, frequent sips of water, or saliva substitutes.
  - Use daily home fluoride products for anticaries effect.

metyrosine

me-**tye**′-roe-seen
(Demser)

CATEGORY AND SCHEDULE

Pregnancy Risk Category: C

Drug Class: Antihypertensives

MECHANISM OF ACTION

A tyrosine hydroxylase inhibitor that blocks conversion of tyrosine to dihydroxyphenylalanine, the rate-limiting step in the biosynthetic pathway of catecholamines.
Therapeutic Effect: Reduces levels of endogenous catecholamines, reduces B/P.

USES

Treatment of high B/P (hypertension) caused by a disease called pheochromocytoma (a noncancerous tumor of the adrenal gland)

PHARMACOKINETICS

Well absorbed from the GI tract. Metabolized in the liver. Excreted primarily in the urine. ***Half-life:*** 7.2 hr.

INDICATIONS AND DOSAGES

▸ **Pheochromocytoma (Preoperative)**
PO
Adults, Elderly. Initially, 250 mg 4 times a day. Increase by 250–500 mg/day up to 4 g/day. Maintenance: 2–4 g/day in 4 divided doses for 5–7 days.

SIDE EFFECTS/ADVERSE REACTIONS

Frequent
Drowsiness, extrapyramidal symptoms, diarrhea
Occasional
Galactorrhea, edema of the breasts, nausea, vomiting, dry mouth, impotence, nasal congestion
Rare
Lower extremity edema, urinary problems, urticaria, anemia, depression, disorientation

PRECAUTIONS AND CONTRAINDICATIONS

Hypertension of unknown etiology, hypersensitivity to metyrosine or any component of the formulation

DRUG INTERACTIONS OF CONCERN TO DENTISTRY

- Increased CNS depression with CNS depressants
- NSAIDs may antagonize hypotensive effect

SERIOUS REACTIONS

! Serious or life-threatening allergic reaction characterized by hallucinations, hematuria, hyperstimulation after withdrawal, severe lower extremity edema, and parkinsonism.

DENTAL CONSIDERATIONS

General:

- Medication may be used in anticipation of surgery to remove the adrenal tumor.

- Hypertension may preclude all dental care except for palliative emergency treatment.
- Question patient about compliance with drug therapy.
- Risk of increased CNS depression when other CNS depressants are used.
- Use stress-reduction protocol.
- Trismus may be a symptom of excessive doses of this drug.
- Determine why patient is taking the drug.
- Monitor and record vital signs.
- Use vasoconstrictor with caution, in low doses, and with careful aspiration. Avoid using gingival retraction cord containing epinephrine.
- Assess for presence of extrapyramidal motor symptoms, such as tardive dyskinesia and akathisia; extrapyramidal motor activity may complicate dental treatment. Advise seeing physician if tardive dyskinesia or akathisia is present.

Consultations:

- Medical consultation may be required to assess disease control and patient's ability to tolerate stress.

Teach Patient/Family to:

- Encourage effective oral hygiene to prevent soft tissue inflammation.
- Not drive or perform other tasks requiring mental alertness.

mexiletine hydrochloride

mex-**il′**-eh-teen
high-droh-**klor′**-ide
(Mexitil)

CATEGORY AND SCHEDULE

Pregnancy Risk Category: C

Drug Class: Antidysrhythmic (class IB, lidocaine analog)

MECHANISM OF ACTION

An antiarrhythmic that shortens duration of action potential and decreases effective refractory period in the His-Purkinje system of the myocardium by blocking sodium transport across myocardial cell membranes.

Therapeutic Effect: Suppresses ventricular arrhythmias.

USES

Treatment of documented life-threatening ventricular dysrhythmias

PHARMACOKINETICS

PO: Peak 2–3 hr. ***Half-life:*** 12 hr; metabolized by liver; excreted unchanged by kidneys (10%); excreted in breast milk.

INDICATIONS AND DOSAGES

▸ **Arrhythmia**

PO

Adults, Elderly. Initially, 200 mg q8h. Adjust dosage by 50–100 mg at 2- to 3-day intervals. Maximum: 1200 mg/day.

SIDE EFFECTS/ADVERSE REACTIONS

Frequent

GI distress, including nausea, vomiting, and heartburn; dizziness; light-headedness; tremors

M

Occasional
Nervousness, change in sleep habits, headache, visual disturbances, paresthesia, diarrhea or constipation, palpitations, chest pain, rash, respiratory difficulty, edema

PRECAUTIONS AND CONTRAINDICATIONS
Cardiogenic shock, preexisting second- or third-degree AV block, right bundle-branch block without presence of pacemaker
Caution:
Lactation, children, renal disease, liver disease, CHF, respiratory depression, myasthenia gravis

DRUG INTERACTIONS OF CONCERN TO DENTISTRY
- No specific interactions are reported with dental drugs; however, any drug that could affect the cardiac action of mexiletine should be used in the least effective dose, such as other local anesthetics, vasoconstrictors, and anticholinergics.

SERIOUS REACTIONS
! Mexiletine has the ability to worsen existing arrhythmias or produce new ones.
! CHF may occur, and existing CHF may worsen.

DENTAL CONSIDERATIONS
General:
- Monitor vital signs at every appointment because of cardiovascular side effects.
- Patients on chronic drug therapy may rarely have symptoms of blood dyscrasias, which can include infection, bleeding, and poor healing.
- Assess salivary flow as a factor in caries, periodontal disease, and candidiasis.
- Stress from dental procedures may compromise cardiovascular function; determine patient risk and use stress-reduction protocol.

Consultations:
- In a patient with symptoms of blood dyscrasias, request a medical consultation for blood studies and postpone dental treatment until normal values are reestablished.
- Medical consultation should be made to assess disease control.
- Medical consultation may be required to assess patient's ability to tolerate stress.

Teach Patient/Family to:
- Encourage effective oral hygiene to prevent soft tissue inflammation.
- Use caution to prevent injury when using oral hygiene aids.
- When chronic dry mouth occurs, advise patient to:
  - Avoid mouth rinses with high alcohol content because of drying effects.
  - Use sugarless gum, frequent sips of water, or saliva substitutes.
  - Use daily home fluoride products for anticaries effect.

miconazole
mih-**kon′**-ah-zole
(Femizol-M, Micatin, Micozole[CAN], Monistat[CAN], Monistat-3, Monistat-7, Monistat-Derm)

CATEGORY AND SCHEDULE
Pregnancy Risk Category: C

Drug Class: Antifungal

MECHANISM OF ACTION

An imidazole derivative that inhibits synthesis of ergosterol (vital component of fungal cell formation), damaging cell membrane.
Therapeutic Effect: Fungistatic; may be fungicidal, depending on concentration.

USES

Treatment of tinea pedis, tinea cruris, tinea corporis, tinea versicolor, vaginal or vulval *Candida albicans*

PHARMACOKINETICS

Parenteral: Widely distributed in tissues. Metabolized in liver. Primarily excreted in urine. ***Half-life:*** 24 hr. Topical: No systemic absorption following application to intact skin. Intravaginally: Small amount absorbed systemically.

INDICATIONS AND DOSAGES

▸ **Coccidioidomycosis**

IV

Adults, Elderly. 1.8–3.6 g/day for 3–20 wk or longer.

▸ **Cryptococcosis**

IV

Adults, Elderly. 1.2–2.4 g/day for 3–12 wk or longer.

▸ **Petriellidiosis**

IV

Adults, Elderly. 0.6–3.0 g/day for 5–20 wk or longer.

▸ **Candidiasis**

IV

Adults, Elderly. 0.6–1.8 g/day for 1–20 wk or longer.

▸ **Paracoccidioidomycosis**

IV

Adults, Elderly. 0.2–1.2 g/day for 2–16 wk or longer.

▸ **Usual Dosage for Children**

IV

20–40 mg/kg/day in 3 divided doses. (Do not exceed 15 mg/kg for any 1 infusion.)

▸ **Vulvovaginal Candidiasis**

Intravaginally

Adults, Elderly. One 200 mg suppository at bedtime for 3 days; one 100 mg suppository or one applicatorful at bedtime for 7 days.

▸ **Topical Fungal Infections, Cutaneous Candidiasis**

Topical

Adults, Elderly, Children 2 yr and older. Apply liberally 2 times a day, morning and evening.

SIDE EFFECTS/ADVERSE REACTIONS

Frequent

Phlebitis, fever, chills, rash, itching, nausea, vomiting

Occasional

Dizziness, drowsiness, headache, flushed face, abdominal pain, constipation, diarrhea, decreased appetite

Topical: Itching, burning, stinging, erythema, urticaria

Vaginal: Vulvovaginal burning, itching, irritation, headache, skin rash

PRECAUTIONS AND CONTRAINDICATIONS

Children younger than 1 yr, hypersensitivity to miconazole or any component of the formulation

Topically: Children younger than 2 yr

Caution:

Lactation

DRUG INTERACTIONS OF CONCERN TO DENTISTRY

• Warfarin anticoagulants: potential for increased bleeding

• Drugs metabolized by CYP hepatic isoenzyme system: potential increased blood levels of metabolized drugs (e.g., benzodiazepines, phenytoin, anesthetics)

SERIOUS REACTIONS

! Anemia, thrombocytopenia, and liver toxicity occur rarely.

DENTAL CONSIDERATIONS

General:

• Examine oral mucous membranes for signs of fungal infection.

• Broad-spectrum antibiotics may evoke vaginal yeast infections.

Teach Patient/Family to:

• Prevent reinoculation of *Candida* infection by disposing of tooth brush or other contaminated oral hygiene devices used during period of infection.

M

midazolam hydrochloride

mid-**az**′-zoe-lam high-droh-**klor**′-ide
(Apo-Midazolam[CAN], Hypnovel[AUS], Versed)
Do not confuse Versed with VePesid.

CATEGORY AND SCHEDULE

Pregnancy Risk Category: D
Controlled substance: Schedule IV

Drug Class: Benzodiazepine, sedative, anesthesia adjunct

MECHANISM OF ACTION

A benzodiazepine that enhances the action of gamma-aminobutyric acid, one of the major inhibitory neurotransmitters in the brain.

Therapeutic Effect: Produces anxiolytic, hypnotic, anticonvulsant, muscle relaxant, and amnestic effects.

USES

Conscious sedation, general anesthesia induction, sedation for diagnostic endoscopic procedures, intubation, preoperative sedation, amnesia

PHARMACOKINETICS

Route	Onset	Peak	Duration
PO	10–20 min	N/A	N/A
IV	1–5 min	5–7 min	20–30 min
IM	5–15 min	15–60 min	2–6 hr

Well absorbed after IM administration. Protein binding: 97%. Metabolized in the liver to active metabolite. Primarily excreted in urine. Not removed by hemodialysis. ***Half-life:*** 1–5 hr.

INDICATIONS AND DOSAGES

▸ **Preoperative Sedation**

PO

Children. 0.25–0.5 mg/kg. Maximum: 20 mg.

IV

Children 6–12 yr. 0.025–0.05 mg/kg.
Children 6 mo–5 yr. 0.05–0.1 mg/kg.

IM

Adults, Elderly. 0.07–0.08 mg/kg 30–60 min before surgery.
Children. 0.1–0.15 mg/kg 30–60 min before surgery. Maximum: 10 mg.

▸ **Conscious Sedation for Diagnostic, Therapeutic, and Endoscopic Procedures**

IV

Adults, Elderly. 1–2.5 mg over 2 min. Titrate as needed. Maximum total dose: 2.5–5 mg.

▸ **Conscious Sedation During Mechanical Ventilation**
IV
Adults, Elderly. 0.01–0.05 mg/kg; may repeat q10–15min until adequately sedated. Then continuous infusion at initial rate of 0.02–0.1 mg/kg/hr (1–7 mg/hr).
Children older than 32 wk. Initially, 1 mcg/kg/min as continuous infusion.
Children 32 wk and younger. Initially, 0.5 mcg/kg/min as continuous infusion.

▸ **Status Epilepticus**
IV
Children older than 2 mo. Loading dose of 0.15 mg/kg followed by continuous infusion of 1 mcg/kg/min. Titrate as needed. Range: 1–18 mcg/kg/min.

SIDE EFFECTS/ADVERSE REACTIONS

Frequent
Decreased respiratory rate, tenderness at IM or IV injection site, pain during injection, oxygen desaturation, hiccups
Occasional
Hypotension, paradoxical CNS reaction
Rare
Nausea, vomiting, headache, coughing

PRECAUTIONS AND CONTRAINDICATIONS

Acute alcohol intoxication, acute angle-closure glaucoma, coma, shock
Caution:
COPD, CHF, chronic renal failure, chills, elderly, debilitated, children younger than 18 yr; to be used only by health care professionals skilled in airway maintenance and ventilation and resuscitation techniques

DRUG INTERACTIONS OF CONCERN TO DENTISTRY

- Prolonged respiratory depression: all CNS depressants, including alcohol, barbiturates, narcotics. All doses of midazolam must be reduced when used in combination with any CNS depressant. Serious respiratory and cardiovascular depression, including death, has occurred when midazolam is used in combination with other CNS depressants or given too rapidly. Medically compromised and elderly patients are at greater risk.
- Increased serum levels and prolonged effect of benzodiazepines: erythromycin, clarithromycin, ketoconazole, itraconazole, fluconazole, miconazole (systemic), diltiazem, fluvoxamine.
- Contraindicated with nelfinavir, ritonavir, indinavir, saquinavir.
- Possible increase in CNS side effects: kava kava (herb).
- Suspected increase in midazolam effects when used in general anesthesia: atorvastatin.

SERIOUS REACTIONS

! Inadequate or excessive dosage or improper administration may result in cerebral hypoxia, agitation, involuntary movements, hyperactivity, and combativeness.
! A too-rapid IV rate, excessive doses, or a single large dose increases the risk of respiratory depression or arrest.
! Respiratory depression or apnea may produce hypoxia and cardiac arrest.

DENTAL CONSIDERATIONS

General:
- Monitor vital signs every 5 min during general anesthesia because of cardiovascular and respiratory side

effects. Monitor vital signs at regular intervals during recovery.
- Degree of CNS depression is dose dependent; titrate all doses.
- Drug produces amnesia, especially in the elderly patient.
- Longer recovery period could be observed in an obese patient because half-life may be extended.
- Assist patient with ambulation until drowsy period has passed.

Teach Patient/Family to:
- Avoid driving or potentially hazardous activities until drowsiness or weakness subsides.
- Be aware of anterograde amnesia; events may not be remembered.
- Treat overdose: O_2, vasopressors, flumazenil, resuscitation measures as required.

M

midodrine

mid′-oh-drin

(Amatine, ProAmatine)

Do not confuse Amatine or ProAmatine with amantadine or protamine.

CATEGORY AND SCHEDULE

Pregnancy Risk Category: C

Drug Class: Vasopressor; orthostatic hypotension adjunct

MECHANISM OF ACTION

A vasopressor that forms the active metabolite desglymidodrine, an α_1-agonist, activating α receptors of the arteriolar and venous vasculature.

Therapeutic Effect: Increases vascular tone and B/P.

USES

Treatment of symptomatic orthostatic; hypotension

PHARMACOKINETICS

Peak 1–2 hr. ***Half-life:*** 3–4 hr, bioavailability 90%.

INDICATIONS AND DOSAGES

▸ Orthostatic Hypotension

PO

Adults, Elderly. 10 mg 3 times a day. Give during the day when patient is upright, such as upon arising, midday, and late afternoon. Do not give later than 6 PM.

▸ Dosage in Renal Impairment

Adults, Elderly. Give 2.5 mg 3 times a day; increase gradually, as tolerated.

SIDE EFFECTS/ADVERSE REACTIONS

Frequent

Paresthesia, piloerection, pruritus, dysuria, supine hypertension

Occasional

Pain, rash, chills, headache, facial flushing, confusion, dry mouth, anxiety

PRECAUTIONS AND CONTRAINDICATIONS

Acute renal function impairment, persistent hypertension, pheochromocytoma, severe cardiac disease, thyrotoxicosis, urine retention

DRUG INTERACTIONS OF CONCERN TO DENTISTRY

- Risk of increased pressor effects: α-adrenergic agonists

SERIOUS REACTIONS

! None known

DENTAL CONSIDERATIONS

General:
- Carefully review patient's medical and drug history.

• Supine hypotension is a serious side effect; a more upright chair position is highly desirable.
• Determine why patient is taking the drug.
• Monitor and record vital signs at every appointment.
• Use vasoconstrictor with caution, in low doses, and with careful aspiration. Avoid using gingival retraction cord containing epinephrine.
• Examine for oral manifestation of opportunistic infection.
• Assess salivary flow as a factor in caries, periodontal disease, and candidiasis.
• Be aware of patient's disease, its severity, and frequency when known.
• Short appointments and a stress-reduction protocol may be required for anxious patients.
• Precaution if dental surgery is anticipated or general anesthesia is required.

Consultations:
• Medical consultation may be required to assess disease control and patient's ability to tolerate stress.

Teach Patient/Family to:
• Use OTC medications, such as cough, cold, and diet preparations, cautiously because they may affect B/P.
• When chronic dry mouth occurs advise patient to:
  • Avoid mouth rinses with high alcohol content because of drying effects.
  • Use daily home fluoride products for anticaries effect.
  • Use sugarless gum, frequent sips of water, or saliva substitutes.

mifepristone

mi-fe-**pris'**-tone
(Korlym)
Do not confuse with Mirapex or misoprostol.

CATEGORY AND SCHEDULE

Pregnancy Risk Category: X

Drug Class: Abortifacient; antineoplastic agent, hormone antagonist; antiprogestin; cortisol receptor blocker

MECHANISM OF ACTION

Mifepristone is a synthetic steroid that blocks the effect of cortisol at the glucocorticoid receptor (antagonizes the effects of cortisol on glucose metabolism) while at the same time increasing circulating cortisol concentrations.
Therapeutic Effect: Treats high blood sugar caused by high cortisol levels in patents with Cushing's syndrome.

USES

To control hyperglycemia occurring secondary to hypercortisolism in patients with endogenous Cushing's syndrome who have type 2 diabetes mellitus or glucose intolerance and who failed surgery or who are not surgical candidates

PHARMACOKINETICS

Rapid absorption following oral administration. 98% plasma protein bound. Hepatic metabolism via CYP3A4 to three active metabolites. Excreted primarily via the feces (83%). ***Half-life:*** 18 hr following a slower phase where 50% eliminated between 12 and 72 hr; multiple doses (600 mg/day): 85 hr.

INDICATIONS AND DOSAGES

▸ Hyperglycemia in Patients with Cushing's Syndrome

PO

Adults. Initial dose: 300 mg once daily. Dose may be increased in 300-mg increments at intervals of ≥2–4 wk based on tolerability and symptom control. Maximum dose: 1200 mg once daily, not to exceed 20 mg/kg/day. If treatment is interrupted, reinitiate at 300 mg/day or a dose lower than the dose that caused the treatment to be stopped if interruption due to adverse reactions.

Dosage adjustment with concurrent use of strong CYP450 inhibitor therapy (e.g., ketoconazole): Maximum dose 300 mg/day.

Dosage in Renal Impairment. Maximum dose 600 mg/day. Note: Following doses of 1200 mg/day for 7 days in patients with severe renal impairment (Cl_{cr} <30 ml/min), exposure to mifepristone and its metabolites was increased and a large variability in exposure was observed.

Dosage in Hepatic Impairment. Mild-to-moderate impairment: Maximum dose 600 mg/day.

Not recommended for use in patients with severe hepatic impairment.

M

SIDE EFFECTS/ADVERSE REACTIONS

Frequent

Peripheral edema, hypertension, fatigue, headache, dizziness, pain, hypokalemia, endometrial hypertrophy, nausea, vomiting, xerostomia, diarrhea, bleeding, arthralgia, myalgia, dyspnea, sinusitis, nasopharyngitis

Occasional

Edema, anxiety, somnolence, insomnia, constipation, abdominal pain, weakness

PRECAUTIONS AND CONTRAINDICATIONS

Hypersensitivity to mifepristone or any component of the formulation. Avoid use in women with a history of unexplained vaginal bleeding, or endometrial hyperplasia with atypia or endometrial carcinoma; pregnancy. May cause adrenal insufficiency. Avoid use in patients with prolonged QT interval, congenital QT syndrome, or history of torsades de pointes. Avoid concurrent use with drugs that prolong the QT interval.

DRUG INTERACTIONS OF CONCERN TO DENTISTRY

- CYP3A4 substrates (e.g., macrolide antibiotics, azole antifungals, triazolam): mifepristone competes with CYP3A4 and increases bioavailability of such drugs
- CYP3A4 inhibitors (e.g., macrolide antibiotics, azole antifungals): increased toxicity of mifepristone
- CYP3A4 inducers (e.g., carbamazepine, barbiturates): avoid in patients taking mifepristone
- Drugs metabolized by CYP2C8/2C9 (e.g., NSAIDs): increased toxicity if administered with mifepristone
- Drugs metabolized by CYP2B6 (e.g., bupropion): increased toxicity of mifepristone
- Contraindicated with long-term corticosteroid use

SERIOUS REACTIONS

! Use of mifepristone will result in termination of pregnancy.

DENTAL CONSIDERATIONS

General:

- Monitor patient for signs and symptoms of adrenal insufficiency, especially during stressful procedures.
- Monitor patient for signs and symptoms of hyperglycemia.
- Be prepared to manage hypoglycemia.
- Monitor vital signs at every appointment due to adverse cardiovascular effects.
- Increased potential for intraoperative and postoperative bleeding.
- Precaution recommended when seating and dismissing patient due to dizziness.
- Increased potential for nausea and vomiting (e.g., during sedation).

Consultations:

- Consult physician to determine patient's disease status and ability to tolerate dental procedures.
- Consult physician to determine need for supplemental drug dosing or modification of medication regimen.

Teach Patient/Family to:

- Report changes in disease status and drug regimen.

miglitol

mig′-lee-tole
(Glyset)

CATEGORY AND SCHEDULE

Pregnancy Risk Category: B

Drug Class: Oligosaccharide, glucosidase enzyme inhibitor

MECHANISM OF ACTION

An α-glucosidase inhibitor that delays the digestion of ingested carbohydrates into simple sugars such as glucose.

Therapeutic Effect: Produces smaller rise in blood glucose concentration after meals.

USES

Treatment of type 2 diabetes when diet control is ineffective in controlling blood glucose levels, used as single agent or in combination with other oral hypoglycemics

PHARMACOKINETICS

PO: Peak plasma levels 2–3 hr; negligible plasma protein binding, not metabolized, urinary excretion.

INDICATIONS AND DOSAGES

▸ Diabetes Mellitus

PO

Adults, Elderly. Initially, 25 mg 3 times a day with first bite of each main meal. Maintenance: 50 mg 3 times a day. Maximum: 100 mg 3 times a day.

SIDE EFFECTS/ADVERSE REACTIONS

Frequent

Flatulence, loose stools, diarrhea, abdominal pain

Occasional

Rash

PRECAUTIONS AND CONTRAINDICATIONS

Colonic ulceration, diabetic ketoacidosis, hypersensitivity to miglitol, inflammatory bowel disease, partial intestinal obstruction

Caution:

Renal impairment, hypoglycemia, lactation, children

DRUG INTERACTIONS OF CONCERN TO DENTISTRY

- None reported

DENTAL CONSIDERATIONS

General:

- Ensure that patient is following prescribed diet and regularly takes medication.
- Type 2 patients may also be using insulin. Should symptomatic hypoglycemia occur while taking this drug, use glucose rather than sucrose because of interference with sucrose metabolism.
- Place on frequent recall to evaluate healing response.
- Short appointments and a stress-reduction protocol may be required for anxious patients.
- Diabetics may be more susceptible to infection and have delayed wound healing.
- Consider semisupine chair position for patient comfort if GI side effects occur.
- Question patient about self-monitoring of drug's antidiabetic effect, including blood glucose values or finger-stick records.
- Examine for oral manifestation of opportunistic infection.

Consultations:

- Medical consultation may be required to assess disease control and patient's ability to tolerate stress.
- Medical consultation may include data from patient's blood glucose monitoring, including glycosylated hemoglobin or HbA_{1c} testing.

Teach Patient/Family to:

- Update health and drug history if physician makes any changes in evaluation or drug regimens; include OTC, herbal, and nonherbal drugs in update.
- Encourage effective oral hygiene to prevent soft tissue inflammation.

M

miglustat

mig′-lew-stat
(Zavesca)

CATEGORY AND SCHEDULE

Pregnancy Risk Category: X

Drug Class: Enzyme inhibitor

MECHANISM OF ACTION

A Gaucher's disease agent that inhibits the enzyme, glucosylceramide synthase, reducing the rate of synthesis of most glycosphingolipids. Allows the residual activity of the deficient enzyme, glucocerebrosidase, to be more effective in degrading lysosomal storage within tissues.
Therapeutic Effect: Minimizes conditions associated with Gaucher's disease, such as anemia and bone disease.

USES

Treatment of adult patients with mild to moderate Type 1 Gaucher's disease for whom enzyme replacement therapy is not an option

PHARMACOKINETICS

PO: Maximum plasma levels 2–2.5 hr. ***Half-life:*** about 6–7 hr; oral bioavailability 97%, no plasma protein binding, excreted unchanged in urine.

INDICATIONS AND DOSAGES

▸ **Gaucher's Disease**

PO

Adults, Elderly. One 100-mg capsule 3 times a day at regular intervals.

▸ **Dosage in Renal Impairment**

Patients with creatinine clearance of 50–70 ml/min. Dosage is reduced to 100 mg twice a day.

Patients with creatinine clearance of 30–49 ml/min. Dosage is 100 mg once a day.

SIDE EFFECTS/ADVERSE REACTIONS

Expected

Diarrhea, weight loss, dry mouth

Frequent

Hand tremors, flatulence, headache, abdominal pain, nausea

Occasional

Paresthesia, anorexia, dyspepsia, leg cramps, vomiting

PRECAUTIONS AND CONTRAINDICATIONS

Women who are or may become pregnant

Caution:

Efficacy and safety not evaluated in patients younger than 18 yr or older than 65 yr, renal impairment, women of reproductive age, provide pretreatment neurologic evaluation, lactation

DRUG INTERACTIONS OF CONCERN TO DENTISTRY

- None reported

SERIOUS REACTIONS

! Thrombocytopenia occurs in 7% of patients.

! Overdose produces dizziness and neutropenia.

DENTAL CONSIDERATIONS

General:

- Ask patient about disease control.
- Question patient about nosebleeds or other bleeding events.
- Short appointments and a stress-reduction protocol may be required for anxious patients.
- Avoid products that affect platelet function, such as aspirin and NSAIDs.
- Patients on chronic drug therapy may rarely have symptoms of blood dyscrasias, which can include infection, bleeding, and poor healing.
- Assess salivary flow as a factor in caries, periodontal disease, and candidiasis.
- Consider semisupine chair position for patient comfort as needed.
- Place on frequent recall to evaluate healing response.

Consultations:

- Medical consultation may be required to assess disease control and patient's ability to tolerate stress.
- Medical consultation should include routine blood counts, including platelet counts and bleeding time.
- In a patient with symptoms of blood dyscrasias, request a medical consultation for blood studies and postpone treatment until normal values are reestablished.

Teach Patient/Family to:

- Inform dentist of unusual bleeding episodes following dental treatment.
- Encourage effective oral hygiene to prevent soft tissue inflammation/infection.
- Use powered tooth brush if patient has difficulty holding conventional devices.

milnacipran

(mil-nah-**sip**-ran)

(Savella)

Do not confuse with minocycline or Miltown.

CATEGORY AND SCHEDULE

Pregnancy Risk Category: C

Drug Class: Fibromyalgia agent

MECHANISM OF ACTION

Central inhibition of norepinephrine and serotonin reuptake (SNRI). ***Therapeutic Effect:*** Reduces perception of pain in CNS.

USES

Fibromyalgia pain

PHARMACOKINETICS

Well absorbed orally, 85%–90% bioavailability. Widely distributed, protein binding 13%. Partially metabolized in the liver, ***Half-life:*** 6–8 hr. Excreted by the kidneys, 55% as unchanged drug.

INDICATIONS AND DOSAGES

▸ Fibromyalgia

PO

Adults, Elderly. 50 mg twice daily, beginning with 12.5 mg total dose on first day of therapy, 12.5 mg twice daily on second and third days of therapy, 25 mg twice daily on days 4 through 7.

SIDE EFFECTS/ADVERSE REACTIONS

Frequent

Anorexia, constipation, dizziness, flushing, headache, hyperhidrosis, hypertension, insomnia, nausea, palpitations, tachycardia, vomiting, dry mouth

Occasional

Blurred vision, chills, disorder of ejaculation, dysuria, migraine, rash, tremors, weight loss

Rare

Abdominal pain and cramps, abnormal liver function tests, delirium, diarrhea, drowsiness, dysgeusia, dyspepsia, dyspnea, ecchymosis, epistaxis, erectile dysfunction, fatigue, fever, hemorrhage, hepatitis, hyperprolactinemia, irritability, leucopenia, changes in libido, pupil dilation, neuroleptic malignant syndrome, night sweats, peripheral edema, muscle pain/rhabdomyolysis, seizures, serotonin syndrome, SIADH syndrome, Stevens-Johnson syndrome, suicidal thoughts, thrombocytopenia, urinary retention

PRECAUTIONS AND CONTRAINDICATIONS

Hypersensitivity milnacipran hydrochloride or its ingredients, children younger than 18 yr, narrow-angle glaucoma, seizure disorder, alcoholism, liver disease, serotonin syndrome, severe renal disease, suicidal patients

Caution:

Children (possible suicide), renal function impairment, pregnancy/lactation

DRUG INTERACTIONS OF CONCERN TO DENTISTRY

- Increased risk of CNS depression: all CNS depressants, alcohol. May potentiate mental impairment and somnolence, postural hypotension, avoid alcohol
- Epinephrine: possible hypertension, cardiac dysrhythmias
- MAOIs: increased risk of serotonin syndrome
- Tramadol, tapentadol: increased risk of serotonin syndrome
- Selective serotonin reuptake inhibitors (SSRIs) (e.g., fluoxetine): potentially life-threatening serotonin syndrome

SERIOUS REACTIONS

! Serotonin syndrome (agitation, coma, autonomic instability including tachycardia, neuromuscular abnormalities, diarrhea, nausea, vomiting)

! Increased risk of suicide (children, patients with suicidal tendencies)

DENTAL CONSIDERATIONS

General:
- Avoid postural hypotension.
- Monitor vital signs for possible cardiovascular adverse effects.
- Assess salivary flow as a factor in caries, periodontal disease, and candidiasis.
- Avoid or limit doses of vasoconstrictor in local anesthetic.
- Avoid in patients taking MAOIs or SSRIs.

Teach Patient/Family to:
- Avoid mouth rinses with high alcohol content because of drying effect.
- Use home fluoride products for anticaries effect.
- Use sugarless/xylitol gum, frequent sips of water, or saliva substitutes if dry mouth occurs.

minocycline hydrochloride

mi-noe-**sye**′-kleen
high-droh-**klor**′-ide
(Akamin[AUS], Arrestin[US], Dynacin, Minocin, Periostat Minomycin[AUS], Myrac, Novo Minocycline[CAN])
Do not confuse Dynacin with Dynabac or Minocin with Mithracin or niacin.

CATEGORY AND SCHEDULE

Pregnancy Risk Category: D

Drug Class: Tetracycline antiinfective

MECHANISM OF ACTION

A tetracycline antibiotic that inhibits bacterial protein synthesis by binding to ribosomes.
Therapeutic Effect: Bacteriostatic.

USES

Treatment of syphilis, *C. trachomatis* infection, gonorrhea, lymphogranuloma venereum, rickettsial infections, inflammatory acne, *M. marinum, Neisseria meningitidis* carriers, actinomycosis, anthrax, acute necrotizing ulcerative gingivitis, AA-induced periodontitis, and other susceptible infections; dental product is an adjunct to scaling and root planing in adult periodontitis

PHARMACOKINETICS

PO: Peak 2–3 hr. ***Half-life:*** 11–17 hr; 55%–88% protein bound; excreted in urine, feces, breast milk; crosses placenta.

INDICATIONS AND DOSAGES

▸ **Mild, Moderate, or Severe Prostate, Urinary Tract, and CNS Infections (excluding meningitis); Uncomplicated Gonorrhea; Inflammatory Acne; Brucellosis; Skin Granulomas; Cholera; Trachoma; Nocardiasis; Yaws; and Syphilis When Penicillins Are Contraindicated**

PO

Adults, Elderly. Initially, 100–200 mg, then 100 mg q12h or 50 mg q6h.

IV

Adults, Elderly. Initially, 200 mg, then 100 mg q12h up to 400 mg/day.

PO, IV

Children older than 8 yr. Initially, 4 mg/kg, then 2 mg/kg q12h.

SIDE EFFECTS/ADVERSE REACTIONS

Frequent

Dizziness, light-headedness, diarrhea, nausea, vomiting, abdominal cramps, possibly severe photosensitivity, drowsiness, vertigo

M

Occasional
Altered pigmentation of skin or mucous membranes, rectal or genital pruritus, stomatitis

PRECAUTIONS AND CONTRAINDICATIONS

Children younger than 8 yr, hypersensitivity to tetracyclines, last half of pregnancy
The use of tetracycline drugs during tooth development (last half of pregnancy, infancy, and childhood up to the age of 8 may cause permanent discoloration of the teeth (yellow-gray-brown). Enamel hypoplasia has also been reported. May also cause retardation of skeletal development and deformations.
Caution:
Hepatic disease, lactation

DRUG INTERACTIONS OF CONCERN TO DENTISTRY

- Decreased effect: antacids, milk, or other calcium- and aluminum-containing products
- Decreased effect of penicillins
- Oral contraceptives: advise patient of a potential risk for decreased contraceptive action, to maintain compliance with oral contraceptive use while using antibiotics, and to consider the use of additional nonhormonal contraception
- Contraindicated with isotretinoin (Accutane)
- Drug interactions of concern to dentistry minocycline HCl (microspheres)

SERIOUS REACTIONS

! Superinfection (especially fungal), anaphylaxis, and benign intracranial hypertension may occur.
! Bulging fontanelles occur rarely in infants.

DENTAL CONSIDERATIONS

General:
- Avoid prescribing during pregnancy.
- This drug is reported to cause intrinsic staining in erupted permanent teeth not associated with the calcification stage.
- The drug readily distributes to gingival crevicular fluid.
- Do not prescribe drug during pregnancy or in patients younger than 8 yr because of tooth discoloration.
- Advise patient if dental drugs prescribed have a potential for photosensitivity.
- Do not use ingestible sodium bicarbonate products, such as the Prophy-Jet air polishing system, at the same time dose is taken; take minocycline 2 hr later.
- Determine why the patient is taking the drug.
- Dental staining or enamel hypoplasia may be associated with exposure to this drug before birth or up to the age of 8. Tetracycline stains may be extremely resistant to ordinary tooth-whitening procedures.

Consultations:
- Medical consultation may be required to assess disease control.

Teach Patient/Family to:
- Encourage effective oral hygiene to prevent soft tissue inflammation.
- Use caution to prevent injury when using oral hygiene aids.
- Avoid mouth rinses with high alcohol content because of drying effects.
- When used for dental infection, advise patient to:
    - Report sore throat, oral burning sensation, fever, fatigue, any of which could indicate superinfection.
    - Take at prescribed intervals and complete dosage regimen.

• Immediately notify the dentist if signs or symptoms of infection increase.

▸ **Microspheres**

General:

• Follow all general precautions when using tetracyclines.

Teach Patient/Family to:

• Avoid eating hard, crunchy foods for 1 wk.

• Postpone tooth brushing for 12 hr.

• Postpone use of interproximal cleaning devices for 10 days.

• Notify dentist immediately if pain, swelling, or other unexpected symptoms occur.

minoxidil

mih-**nox′**-ih-dill

(Apo-Gain[CAN], Loniten, Milnox[CAN], Regaine[AUS], Rogaine, Rogaine Extra Strength)

Do not confuse Loniten with Lotensin.

CATEGORY AND SCHEDULE

Pregnancy Risk Category: C

OTC (topical solution)

Drug Class: Antihypertensive

MECHANISM OF ACTION

An antihypertensive and hair growth stimulant that has direct action on vascular smooth muscle, producing vasodilation of arterioles.

Therapeutic Effect: Decreases peripheral vascular resistance and B/P; increases cutaneous blood flow; stimulates hair follicle epithelium and hair follicle growth.

USES

Treatment of severe hypertension not responsive to other therapy (used with a diuretic and α-adrenergic antagonist); topically to treat androgenic alopecia

PHARMACOKINETICS

Route	Onset	Peak	Duration
PO	0.5 hr	2–8 hr	2–5 days

Well absorbed from the GI tract; minimal absorption after topical application. Protein binding: None. Widely distributed. Metabolized in the liver to active metabolite. Primarily excreted in urine. Removed by hemodialysis. ***Half-life:*** 4.2 hr.

INDICATIONS AND DOSAGES

▸ **Severe Symptomatic Hypertension, Hypertension Associated with Organ Damage, Hypertension That Has Failed to Respond to Maximal Therapeutic Dosages of a Diuretic or Two Other Antihypertensives**

PO

Adults. Initially, 5 mg/day. Increase with at least 3-day intervals to 10 mg, then 20 mg, then up to 40 mg/day in 1–2 doses.

Elderly. Initially, 2.5 mg/day. May increase gradually. Maintenance: 10–40 mg/day. Maximum: 100 mg/day.

Children. Initially, 0.1–0.2 mg/kg (5 mg maximum) daily. Gradually increase at a minimum of 3-day intervals. Maintenance: 0.25–1 mg/kg/day in 1–2 doses. Maximum: 50 mg/day.

▸ **Hair Regrowth**

Topical

Adults. 1 ml to affected areas of scalp 2 times a day. Total daily dose not to exceed 2 ml.

SIDE EFFECTS/ADVERSE REACTIONS

Frequent

PO: Edema with concurrent weight gain, hypertrichosis (elongation, thickening, increased pigmentation of fine body hair; develops in 80% of patients within 3–6 wk after beginning therapy)

Occasional

PO: T-wave changes (usually revert to pretreatment state with continued therapy or drug withdrawal)

Topical: Pruritus, rash, dry or flaking skin, erythema

Rare

PO: Breast tenderness, headache, photosensitivity reaction

Topical: Allergic reaction, alopecia, burning sensation at scalp, soreness at hair root, headache, visual disturbances

PRECAUTIONS AND CONTRAINDICATIONS

Pheochromocytoma

Caution:

Lactation, children, renal disease, CAD, CHF

DRUG INTERACTIONS OF CONCERN TO DENTISTRY

• Decreased effects: NSAIDs, indomethacin, sympathomimetics

• Increased hypotension: CNS depressant drug used in conscious sedation technique may also lower B/P

SERIOUS REACTIONS

! Tachycardia and angina pectoris may occur because of increased oxygen demands associated with increased heart rate and cardiac output.

! Fluid and electrolyte imbalance and CHF may occur, especially if a diuretic is not given concurrently with minoxidil.

! Too rapid reduction in B/P may result in syncope, CVA, MI, and ocular or vestibular ischemia.

! Pericardial effusion and tamponade may be seen in patients with impaired renal function who are not on dialysis.

DENTAL CONSIDERATIONS

General:

• Monitor vital signs at every appointment because of cardiovascular side effects.

• Patients on chronic drug therapy may rarely have symptoms of blood dyscrasias, which can include infection, bleeding, and poor healing.

• Limit use of sodium-containing products, such as saline IV fluids, for patients with a dietary salt restriction.

• Short appointments and a stress-reduction protocol may be required for anxious patients.

• After supine positioning, have patient sit upright for at least 2 min before standing to avoid orthostatic hypotension.

Consultations:

• In a patient with symptoms of blood dyscrasias, request a medical consultation for blood studies and postpone dental treatment until normal values are reestablished.

• Medical consultation may be required to assess disease control and patient's ability to tolerate stress.

mirtazapine

mir-**taz'**-ah-peen
(Avanza[AUS], Mirtazon[AUS], Remeron, Remeron Soltab)
Do not confuse Remeron with Premarin.

CATEGORY AND SCHEDULE

Pregnancy Risk Category: C

Drug Class: Tetracyclic antidepressant

MECHANISM OF ACTION

A tetracyclic compound that acts as an antagonist at presynaptic α_2-adrenergic receptors, increasing both norepinephrine and serotonin neurotransmission. Has low anticholinergic activity.
Therapeutic Effect: Relieves depression and produces sedative effects.

USES

Treatment of depression

PHARMACOKINETICS

Rapidly and completely absorbed after PO administration; absorption not affected by food. Protein binding: 85%. Metabolized in the liver. Primarily excreted in urine. Unknown if removed by hemodialysis. ***Half-life:*** 20–40 hr (longer in males [37 hr] than females [26 hr]).

INDICATIONS AND DOSAGES

▸ **Depression**

PO

Adults. Initially, 15 mg at bedtime. May increase by 15 mg/day q1–2wk. Maximum: 45 mg/day.
Elderly. Initially, 7.5 mg at bedtime. May increase by 7.5–15 mg/day q1–2wk. Maximum: 45 mg/day.

SIDE EFFECTS/ADVERSE REACTIONS

Frequent
Somnolence, dry mouth, increased appetite, constipation, weight gain
Occasional
Asthenia, dizziness, flu-like symptoms, abnormal dreams
Rare
Abdominal discomfort, vasodilation, paresthesia, acne, dry skin, thirst, arthralgia

PRECAUTIONS AND CONTRAINDICATIONS

Use within 14 days of MAOIs
Caution:
Hepatic impairment, renal impairment, elderly, nursing, pediatric, suicidal ideation, cardiovascular or cerebrovascular disease aggravated by hypotension, avoid alcohol use

DRUG INTERACTIONS OF CONCERN TO DENTISTRY

• Impairment of cognitive and motor performance with diazepam or other drugs used in conscious sedation
• Use opioid analgesics with caution because of impairment of cognitive or motor performance; NSAIDs or acetaminophen may be a more appropriate choice

SERIOUS REACTIONS

! Mirtazapine poses a higher risk of seizures than tricyclic antidepressants, especially in those with no previous history of seizures.
! Overdose may produce cardiovascular effects, such as severe orthostatic hypotension, dizziness, tachycardia, palpitations, and arrhythmias.
! Abrupt discontinuation after prolonged therapy may produce

headache, malaise, nausea, vomiting, and vivid dreams.
! Agranulocytosis occurs rarely.

DENTAL CONSIDERATIONS

General:
• Patients on chronic drug therapy may rarely have symptoms of blood dyscrasias, which can include infection, bleeding, and poor healing.
• Assess salivary flow as a factor in caries, periodontal disease, and candidiasis.
• Monitor vital signs at every appointment because of cardiovascular side effects.
• Consider semisupine chair position for patient comfort if GI or MS side effects occur.
• Place on frequent recall if oral side effects are a problem.

M

Consultations:
• In a patient with symptoms of blood dyscrasias, request a medical consultation for blood studies and postpone dental treatment until normal values are reestablished.
• Take precaution if dental surgery is anticipated and sedation or general anesthesia is required; risk of hypotensive episode.
• Medical consultation may be required to assess disease control.
• Physician should be informed if significant xerostomic side effects occur (e.g., increased caries, sore tongue, problems eating or swallowing, difficulty wearing prosthesis) so that a medication change can be considered.

Teach Patient/Family to:
• Encourage effective oral hygiene to prevent soft tissue inflammation.
• Use caution to prevent soft tissue trauma when using oral hygiene aids.
• Update health history/drug record if physician makes any changes in evaluation or drug regimens; include OTC, herbal, and nonherbal drugs in update.
• Not drive or perform other tasks requiring alertness.
• When chronic dry mouth occurs, advise patient to:
  • Avoid mouth rinses with high alcohol content because of drying effects.
  • Use daily home fluoride products for anticaries effect.
  • Use sugarless gum, frequent sips of water, or saliva substitutes.

misoprostol

mis-oh-**pros′**-toll
(Cytotec)
Do not confuse with Cytomel.

CATEGORY AND SCHEDULE

Pregnancy Risk Category: X

Drug Class: Gastric mucosa protectant

MECHANISM OF ACTION

A prostaglandin that inhibits basal, nocturnal gastric acid secretion via direct action on parietal cells.
Therapeutic Effect: Increases production of protective gastric mucus.

USES

Prevention of NSAID-induced gastric ulcers

PHARMACOKINETICS

Rapidly absorbed from GI tract. Rapidly converted to active metabolite. Primarily excreted in urine. ***Half-life:*** 20–40 min.

INDICATIONS AND DOSAGES

▸ Prevention of NSAID-Induced Gastric Ulcer

PO

Adults. 200 mcg 4 times a day with food (last dose at bedtime). Continue for duration of NSAID therapy. May reduce dosage to 100 mcg if 200 mcg dose is not tolerable.

Elderly. 100–200 mcg 4 times a day with food.

SIDE EFFECTS/ADVERSE REACTIONS

Frequent

Abdominal pain, diarrhea

Occasional

Nausea, flatulence, dyspepsia, headache

Rare

Vomiting, constipation

PRECAUTIONS AND CONTRAINDICATIONS

Pregnancy (produces uterine contractions), hypersensitivity to misoprostol or any component of the formulation

Caution:

Lactation, children, elderly, renal disease

SERIOUS REACTIONS

! Overdosage may produce sedation, tremors, convulsions, dyspnea, palpitations, hypotension, and bradycardia.

DENTAL CONSIDERATIONS

General:

- Avoid NSAIDs and salicylates in patients with active upper GI disease; acetaminophen/opioids are more appropriate for pain control in these patients.

Consultations:

- Medical consultation may be required to assess disease control.

mitotane

my′-tow-tane

(Lysodren)

CATEGORY AND SCHEDULE

Pregnancy Risk Category: C

Drug Class: Antineoplastic

MECHANISM OF ACTION

A hormonal agent that inhibits activity of the adrenal cortex.

Therapeutic Effect: Suppresses functional and nonfunctional adrenocortical neoplasms by direct cytoxic effect.

USES

Treatment of adrenocortical carcinoma

M

PHARMACOKINETICS

Adequately absorbed orally (40%). ***Half-life:*** 18–159 days; hepatic metabolism; excreted in urine, bile.

INDICATIONS AND DOSAGES

▸ Adrenocortical Carcinomas

PO

Adults, Elderly. Initially, 2–6 g/day in 3–4 divided doses. Increase by 2–4 g/day every 3–7 days up to 9–10 g/day. Range: 2–16 g/day.

SIDE EFFECTS/ADVERSE REACTIONS

Frequent

Anorexia, nausea, vomiting, diarrhea, lethargy, somnolence, adrenocortical insufficiency, dizziness, vertigo, maculopapular rash, hypouricemia

Occasional

Blurred or double vision, retinopathy, hearing loss, excessive salivation, urine abnormalities (hematuria, cystitis, albuminuria), hypertension, orthostatic hypotension, flushing, wheezing, dyspnea, generalized aching, fever

PRECAUTIONS AND CONTRAINDICATIONS

Known hypersensitivity to mitotane
Caution:
Lactation, hepatic disease, infection; avoid use or discontinue if adrenal cortical suppression occurs

DRUG INTERACTIONS OF CONCERN TO DENTISTRY

- Increased CNS depression: all CNS depressants
- Decreased effects of corticosteroids; if glucocorticoid replacement is necessary, use hydrocortisone

SERIOUS REACTIONS

! Brain damage and functional impairment may occur with long-term, high-dosage therapy.

DENTAL CONSIDERATIONS

General:
- Evaluate respiration characteristics and rate.
- Drug may cause adrenal hypofunction, especially under conditions of stress such as surgery, trauma, or acute illness. Patients should be carefully monitored and given hydrocortisone or mineralocorticoid as needed.
- Consider semisupine chair position for patient comfort if GI side effects occur.
- Patients taking opioids for acute or chronic pain should be given alternative analgesics for dental pain.

Consultations:
- Medical consultation may be required to assess disease control and patient's ability to tolerate stress.

Teach Patient/Family to:
- See dentist immediately if secondary oral infection occurs.
- Report oral lesions, soreness, or bleeding to dentist.
- Update medical/drug records if physician makes any changes in evaluation or drug regimens; include OTC, herbal, and nonherbal drugs in update.

mitoxantrone

my-toe-**zan′**-trone
(Novantrone, Onkotrone[AUS])

CATEGORY AND SCHEDULE

Pregnancy Risk Category: D

Drug Class: Antineoplastic, antiinfective, immunomodulator; synthetic anthraquinone

MECHANISM OF ACTION

An anthracenedione that inhibits B-cell, T-cell, and macrophage proliferation and DNA and RNA synthesis. Active throughout the entire cell cycle.
Therapeutic Effect: Causes cell death.

PHARMACOKINETICS

Protein binding: 78%. Widely distributed. Metabolized in the liver. Primarily eliminated in feces by the biliary system. Not removed by hemodialysis. ***Half-life:*** 2.3–13 days.

USES

Treatment of some kinds of cancer. It is also used to treat some forms of multiple sclerosis.

PHARMACOKINETICS

Highly bound to plasma proteins, metabolized in liver, excreted via renal, hepatobiliary systems.
Half-life: 24–72 hr.

INDICATIONS AND DOSAGES

▸ **Leukemias**

IV

Adults, Elderly, Children 2 yr and older. 12 mg/m^2 once a day for 2–3 days.

Children younger than 2 yr. 0.4 mg/kg once a day for 3–5 days.

▸ **Acute Leukemia in Relapse**

IV

Adults, Elderly, Children older than 2 yr. 8–12 mg/m^2 once a day for 4–5 days.

▸ **Acute Nonlymphocytic Leukemia**

IV

Adults, Elderly, Children older than 2 yr. 10 mg/m^2 once a day for 3–5 days.

▸ **Solid Tumors**

IV

Adults, Elderly. 12–14 mg/m^2 once q3–4wk.

Children. 18–20 mg/m^2 once q3–4wk.

▸ **Prostate Cancer**

IV

Adults, Elderly. 12–14 mg/m^2 every 21 days.

▸ **Multiple Sclerosis**

IV

Adults, Elderly. 12 mg/m^2/dose q3mo.

SIDE EFFECTS/ADVERSE REACTIONS

Frequent

Nausea, vomiting, diarrhea, cough, headache, stomatitis, abdominal discomfort, fever, alopecia

Occasional

Ecchymosis, fungal infection, conjunctivitis, UTI

Rare

Arrhythmias

PRECAUTIONS AND CONTRAINDICATIONS

Baseline left ventricular ejection fraction less than 50%, cumulative lifetime mitoxantrone dose of 140 mg/m^2 or more, multiple sclerosis with hepatic impairment

DRUG INTERACTIONS OF CONCERN TO DENTISTRY

• None reported

SERIOUS REACTIONS

! Myelosuppression may be severe, resulting in GI bleeding, hematologic toxicity, sepsis, and pneumonia.

! Renal failure, seizures, jaundice, and CHF may occur.

! Cardiotoxicity has been reported during therapy.

DENTAL CONSIDERATIONS

General:

• Monitor and record vital signs.

• If additional analgesia is required for dental pain, consider alternative analgesics in patients taking opioids for acute or chronic pain.

• Examine for oral manifestation of opportunistic infection.

• Avoid products that affect platelet function, such as NSAIDs.

• This drug may be used in the hospital or on an outpatient basis. Confirm the patient's disease and treatment status.

• Chlorhexidine mouth rinse prior to and during chemotherapy may reduce severity of mucositis.

• Patient on chronic drug therapy may rarely present with symptoms of blood dyscrasias, which can include infection, bleeding, and poor healing. If dyscrasia is present,

caution patient to prevent oral tissue trauma when using oral hygiene aids.
• Palliative medication may be required for management of oral side effects.
• Short appointments and a stress-reduction protocol may be required for anxious patients.
• Provide emergency dental care only during drug use.
• Patients may be at risk of bleeding; check for oral signs.
• Oral infections should be eliminated and treated aggressively.
• Patients may have received other chemotherapy or radiation; confirm medical and drug history.
• Place on frequent recall because of oral side effects.

Consultations:
• Medical consultation should include routine blood counts including platelet counts and bleeding time.
• Consult physician; prophylactic or therapeutic antiinfectives may be indicated if surgery or periodontal treatment is required.
• Medical consultation may be required to assess immunologic status during cancer chemotherapy and determine safety risk, if any, posed by the required dental treatment.
• Medical consultation may be required to assess disease control and patient's ability to tolerate stress.

Teach Patient/Family to:
• See dentist immediately if secondary oral infection occurs.
• Be aware of oral side effects.
• Encourage effective oral hygiene to prevent soft tissue inflammation.
• Report oral lesions, soreness, or bleeding to dentist.
• Prevent trauma when using oral hygiene aids.
• Update health and medication history if physician makes any changes in evaluation or drug regimens; include OTC, herbal, and nonherbal drugs in the update.

modafinil

moe-**da'f**-in-nill
(Alertec[CAN], Modavigil[AUS], Provigil)

CATEGORY AND SCHEDULE

Pregnancy Risk Category: C

Drug Class: CNS stimulant

MECHANISM OF ACTION

An α_1-agonist that may bind to dopamine reuptake carrier sites, increasing α activity and decreasing θ and β brain wave activity.
Therapeutic Effect: Reduces the number of sleep episodes and total daytime sleep.

USES

Improvement of wakefulness in narcolepsy, obstructive sleep apnea, shift work sleep disorder

PHARMACOKINETICS

Well absorbed. Protein binding: 60%. Widely distributed. Metabolized in the liver. Excreted by the kidneys. Unknown if removed by hemodialysis. ***Half-life:*** 8–10 hr.

INDICATIONS AND DOSAGES

▸ **Narcolepsy, Other Sleep Disorders**
PO
Adults, Elderly. 200–400 mg/day.

SIDE EFFECTS/ADVERSE REACTIONS

Frequent
Anxiety, insomnia, nausea
Occasional
Anorexia, diarrhea, dizziness, dry mouth or skin, muscle stiffness, polydipsia, rhinitis, paresthesia, tremor, headache, vomiting

PRECAUTIONS AND CONTRAINDICATIONS

Hypersensitivity
Caution:
Ischemic heart disease, left ventricular hypertrophy, mitral valve prolapse, recent MI, unstable angina, renal impairment, hepatic impairment, lactation, children younger than 16 yr, drug abuse

DRUG INTERACTIONS OF CONCERN TO DENTISTRY

- No documented dental drug interactions reported; however, because it induces cytochrome P-450 isoenzymes, other P-450 isoenzyme inducers or inhibitors (antifungal agents, erythromycin) could result in a drug interaction.

SERIOUS REACTIONS

! Agitation, excitation, hypertension, and insomnia may occur.

DENTAL CONSIDERATIONS

General:
- Monitor vital signs at every appointment because of cardiovascular side effects.
- Assess salivary flow as a factor in caries, periodontal disease, and candidiasis.
- Consider semisupine chair position for patient comfort because of GI side effects of drug.
- Short appointments and a stress-reduction protocol may be required for anxious patients.

Teach Patient/Family to:
- Prevent trauma when using oral hygiene aids.
- When chronic dry mouth occurs, advise patient to:
  - Avoid mouth rinses with high alcohol content because of drying effects.
  - Use daily home fluoride products for anticaries effect.
  - Use sugarless gum, frequent sips of water, or saliva substitutes.

moexipril hydrochloride

moe-**ex**′-ah-pril
high-droh-**klor**′-ide
(Univasc)

CATEGORY AND SCHEDULE

Pregnancy Risk Category: C (D if used in second or third trimesters)

Drug Class: Angiotensin-converting enzyme (ACE) inhibitor

M

MECHANISM OF ACTION

An ACE inhibitor that suppresses the renin-angiotensin-aldosterone system and prevents conversion of angiotensin I to angiotensin II, a potent vasoconstrictor; may also inhibit angiotensin II at local vascular and renal sites.
Therapeutic Effect: Reduces peripheral arterial resistance and lowers B/P.

USES

Treatment of hypertension as a single drug or in combination with a thiazide diuretic

PHARMACOKINETICS

Route	Onset	Peak	Duration
PO	1 hr	3–6 hr	24 hr

Incompletely absorbed from the GI tract. Food decreases drug absorption. Rapidly converted to active metabolite. Protein binding: 50%. Primarily recovered in feces, partially excreted in urine. Unknown if removed by dialysis. ***Half-life:*** 1 hr, metabolite 2–9 hr.

INDICATIONS AND DOSAGES

▸ **Hypertension**

PO

Adults, Elderly. For patients not receiving diuretics, initial dose is 7.5 mg once a day 1 hr before meals. Adjust according to B/P effect. Maintenance: 7.5–30 mg a day in 1–2 divided doses 1 hr before meals.

▸ **Hypertension in Patients with Impaired Renal Function**

PO

Adults, Elderly. 3.75 mg once a day in patients with creatinine clearance of 40 ml/min. Maximum: May titrate up to 15 mg/day.

SIDE EFFECTS/ADVERSE REACTIONS

Occasional

Cough, headache, dizziness, fatigue

Rare

Flushing, rash, myalgia, nausea, vomiting

PRECAUTIONS AND CONTRAINDICATIONS

History of angioedema from previous treatment with ACE inhibitors

Caution:

Food retards absorption, renal or hepatic impairment, CHF, SLE, scleroderma, renal artery stenosis, lactation, children

DRUG INTERACTIONS OF CONCERN TO DENTISTRY

- IV fluids containing potassium: risk of hyperkalemia
- Increased hypotension: other hypotensive drugs, alcohol, phenothiazines
- Decreased hypotensive effects: indomethacin, possibly other NSAIDs, sympathomimetics
- Suspected reduction in the antihypertensive and vasodilator effects by salicylates; monitor B/P if used concurrently

SERIOUS REACTIONS

! Excessive hypotension ("first-dose syncope") may occur in patients with CHF and in those who are severely salt or volume depleted.

! Angioedema (swelling of face and lips) and hyperkalemia occur rarely.

! Agranulocytosis and neutropenia may be noted in those with collagen vascular disease, including scleroderma and systemic lupus erythematosus, and impaired renal function.

! Nephrotic syndrome may be noted in those with history of renal disease.

DENTAL CONSIDERATIONS

General:

- Monitor vital signs at every appointment because of cardiovascular side effects.

• After supine positioning, have patient sit upright for at least 2 min before standing to avoid orthostatic hypotension.
• Take precautions if dental surgery is anticipated and general anesthesia is required.
• Patients on chronic drug therapy may rarely have symptoms of blood dyscrasias, which can include infection, bleeding, and poor healing.
• Stress from dental procedures may compromise cardiovascular function; determine patient risk.
• Assess salivary flow as a factor in caries, periodontal disease, and candidiasis.
• Short appointments and a stress-reduction protocol may be required for anxious patients.

Consultations:

• Medical consultation may be required to assess disease control and patient's ability to tolerate stress.
• In a patient with symptoms of blood dyscrasias, request a medical consultation for blood studies and postpone dental treatment until normal values are reestablished.

Teach Patient/Family to:

• Encourage effective oral hygiene to prevent soft tissue inflammation.
• Use caution to prevent trauma when using oral hygiene aids.
• Report oral lesions, soreness, or bleeding to dentist.
• When chronic dry mouth occurs, advise patient to:
  • Avoid mouth rinses with high alcohol content because of drying effects.
  • Use daily home fluoride products for anticaries effect.
  • Use sugarless gum, frequent sips of water, or saliva substitutes.

molindone

moe-**lin**′-done
(Moban)
Do not confuse with Mobic.

CATEGORY AND SCHEDULE

Pregnancy Risk Category: C

Drug Class: Antipsychotic

MECHANISM OF ACTION

An indole derivative of dihydroindolone compounds that reduces spontaneous locomotion and aggressiveness.
Therapeutic Effect: Suppresses behavioral response in psychosis.

USES

Treatment of psychotic disorders

M

PHARMACOKINETICS

Rapidly absorbed from the GI tract. Metabolized in liver. Excreted in feces, and a small amount excreted via lungs as carbon dioxide. Not removed by dialysis. ***Half-life:*** unknown.

INDICATIONS AND DOSAGES

▸ **Schizophrenia**

PO

Adults, Children 12 yr and older. Initially, 50–75 mg/day, increased to 100 mg/day in 3–4 days. Maintenance: 5–15 mg 3–4 times a day (mild psychosis). Maintenance: 10–25 mg 3–4 times a day (moderate psychosis). Maintenance: 225 mg/day maximum in divided doses (severe psychosis).
Elderly. Start at a lower dose.

SIDE EFFECTS/ADVERSE REACTIONS

Frequent

Blurred vision, constipation, drowsiness, headache, extrapyramidal symptoms

Occasional

Mental depression

Rare

Skin rash, hot and dry skin, inability to sweat, muscle weakness, confusion, jaundice, convulsions

PRECAUTIONS AND CONTRAINDICATIONS

Severe CNS depression, hypersensitivity to molindone or any component of the formulation

Caution:

Lactation, hypertension, hepatic disease, cardiac disease, Parkinson's disease, brain tumor, glaucoma, urinary retention, diabetes mellitus, respiratory disease, prostatic hypertrophy

DRUG INTERACTIONS OF CONCERN TO DENTISTRY

- Increased sedation: alcohol, other CNS depressants
- Increased anticholinergic effect: anticholinergics, antihistamines

SERIOUS REACTIONS

! Neuroleptic malignant syndrome or tardive dyskinesia has been reported.

DENTAL CONSIDERATIONS

General:

- Patients on chronic drug therapy may rarely have symptoms of blood dyscrasias, which can include infection, bleeding, and poor healing.
- Assess salivary flow as a factor in caries, periodontal disease, and candidiasis.
- After supine positioning, have patient sit upright for at least 2 min before standing to avoid orthostatic hypotension.
- Assess for presence of extrapyramidal motor symptoms, such as tardive dyskinesia and akathisia. Extrapyramidal motor activity may complicate dental treatment.
- Use vasoconstrictors with caution, in low doses, and with careful aspiration.

Consultations:

- In a patient with symptoms of blood dyscrasias, request a medical consultation for blood studies and postpone dental treatment until normal values are reestablished.
- Medical consultation may be required to assess disease control.

Teach Patient/Family to:

- Encourage effective oral hygiene to prevent soft tissue inflammation.
- Use caution to prevent injury when using oral hygiene aids.
- When chronic dry mouth occurs, advise patient to:
  - Avoid mouth rinses with high alcohol content because of drying effects.
  - Use sugarless gum, frequent sips of water, or saliva substitutes.
  - Use daily home fluoride products for anticaries effect.

mometasone furoate monohydrate

mo-**met**′-ah-sone
(Allermax Aqueous[AUS], Asmanex Twisthaler, Elocon Cream[AUS], Elocon Ointment[AUS], Nasonex, Nasonex Nasal Spray[AUS], Novasone Cream[AUS], Novasone Lotion[AUS], Novasone Ointment[AUS])

CATEGORY AND SCHEDULE

Pregnancy Risk Category: C

Drug Class: Synthetic corticosteroid

MECHANISM OF ACTION

An adrenocorticosteroid that inhibits the release of inflammatory cells into nasal tissue, preventing early activation of the allergic reaction. ***Therapeutic Effect:*** Decreases response to seasonal and perennial rhinitis.

USES

Treatment of nasal symptoms of seasonal and perennial allergic rhinitis; prophylaxis of nasal symptoms of seasonal allergic rhinitis

PHARMACOKINETICS

Undetectable in plasma. Protein binding: 98%–99%. The swallowed portion undergoes extensive metabolism. Excreted primarily through bile and, to a lesser extent, urine. ***Half-life:*** 5.8 hr (nasal).

INDICATIONS AND DOSAGES

▸ **Allergic Rhinitis**

Nasal Spray

Adults, Elderly, Children 12 yr and older. 2 sprays in each nostril once a day.

Children 2–11 yr. 1 spray in each nostril once a day.

▸ **Asthma**

Inhalation

Adults, Elderly, Children 12 yr and older. Initially, inhale 220 mcg (1 puff) once a day. Maximum: 880 mcg once a day.

▸ **Skin Disease**

Topical

Adults, Elderly, Children 12 yr and older. Apply cream, lotion, or ointment to affected area once a day.

▸ **Nasal Polyp**

Nasal Spray

Adults, Elderly. 2 sprays in each nostril twice a day.

SIDE EFFECTS/ADVERSE REACTIONS

Occasional

Inhalation: Headache, allergic rhinitis, upper respiratory infection, muscle pain, fatigue

Nasal: Nasal irritation, stinging

Topical: Burning

Rare

Inhalation: Abdominal pain, dyspepsia, nausea

Nasal: Nasal or pharyngeal candidiasis

Topical: Pruritus

PRECAUTIONS AND CONTRAINDICATIONS

Hypersensitivity to any corticosteroid, persistently positive sputum cultures for *Candida albicans,* status asthmaticus (inhalation), systemic fungal infections, untreated localized infection involving nasal mucosa

Caution:

Caution in transferring patient from systemic to inhalation steroids;

M

active or quiescent tuberculosis, untreated fungal, bacterial, or viral infections, lactation, safety and efficacy in children younger than 12 yr not established

DRUG INTERACTIONS OF CONCERN TO DENTISTRY

- None reported

SERIOUS REACTIONS

! An acute hypersensitivity reaction, including urticaria, angioedema, and severe bronchospasm, occurs rarely.

! Transfer from systemic to local steroid therapy may unmask previously suppressed bronchial asthma condition.

DENTAL CONSIDERATIONS

General:

- Allergic rhinitis may be a factor in mouth breathing and drying of oral tissues.
- Examine for oral manifestation of opportunistic infection.

Teach Patient/Family to:

- Gargle, rinse mouth with water, and expectorate after each aerosol dose.

mometasone furoate + formoterol fumarate

moe-**met′**-a-sone **fur′**-oh-ate & for-**moh**-te-rol

(Dulera)

CATEGORY AND SCHEDULE

Pregnancy Risk Category: C

Drug Class: Beta$_2$-adrenergic agonist, long-acting; corticosteroid, inhalant (oral)

MECHANISM OF ACTION

A long-acting bronchodilator that stimulates β_2-adrenergic receptors in the lungs, resulting in relaxation of bronchial smooth muscle.

Therapeutic Effect: Stabilizes asthma and relieves bronchospasm, reduces airway resistance.

USES

Maintenance treatment of asthma where combination therapy is indicated

PHARMACOKINETICS

Mometasone: Minimal systemic absorption. 99% plasma protein bound. Hepatic metabolism via CYP3A4 enzymes. Excreted via urine and feces. Formoterol: Rapid absorption after inhalation. 64% plasma protein bound. Hepatic metabolism via direct glucuronidation and O-demethylation. Excreted via urine. ***Half-life:*** Mometasone: 5 hr. Formoterol: 10–14 hr.

INDICATIONS AND DOSAGES

▸ **Asthma**

Oral Inhalation

Adults, Children 12 yr and older. Previous therapy included inhaled medium-dose corticosteroids: Mometasone 100 mcg/formoterol 5 mcg: Two inhalations twice daily. Consider the higher dose combination for patients not adequately controlled on the lower combination following 1–2 wk of therapy. Maximum daily dose: 4 inhalations.

Previous therapy included inhaled high-dose corticosteroids: Mometasone 200 mcg/formoterol 5 mcg: Two inhalations twice daily. Maximum daily dose: 4 inhalations.

SIDE EFFECTS/ADVERSE REACTIONS

Frequent
Headache, nasopharyngitis, sinusitis
Occasional
Anaphylactoid reactions, angioedema, oral candidiasis

PRECAUTIONS AND CONTRAINDICATIONS

Hypersensitivity to mometasone, formoterol, or any component of the formulation; need for acute bronchodilation (including status asthmaticus). Not for treatment of acute asthma symptoms. May cause adrenal suppression, decreased bone density, immunosuppression, and oral candidiasis. Use with caution in patients with cardiovascular disease, diabetes, hypokalemia, cataracts, glaucoma, osteoporosis, seizure disorders, and thyroid disease. Avoid use in patients with prolonged QT interval, congenital QT syndrome, or history of torsades de pointes.

DRUG INTERACTIONS OF CONCERN TO DENTISTRY

• CYP3A4 substrates (e.g., macrolide antibiotics, azole antifungals): increased toxicity of Dulera
• Epinephrine, tricyclic antidepressants: increased risk of sympathomimetic effects, possible hypertension, cardiac dysrhythmias
• Aspirin and aspirin-containing products: avoid due to possible increased GI bleeding and increased airway resistance

SERIOUS REACTIONS

! Long-acting beta$_2$-agonists (LABAs), such as formoterol, increase the risk of asthma-related deaths. LABAs may increase the risk of asthma-related hospitalization in pediatric and adolescent patients.

DENTAL CONSIDERATIONS

General:
• Be prepared to manage acute airway distress; do not use aerosol as rescue inhaler.
• Monitor vital signs at every appointment because of adverse cardiovascular effects.
• Assess allergic rhinitis as a factor in mouth breathing and drying of oral tissues; assess salivary flow as a factor in caries, periodontal disease, and candidiasis.
• Avoid or limit doses of epinephrine in local anesthetic.
• Short, midday appointments and a stress-reduction protocol may be necessary for anxious patients.
• Examine for oral manifestations of opportunistic infections.
• Long-term use may result in adrenocortical suppression. Possible need for supplementation for some dental procedures.
Consultations:
• Consult physician to determine disease status and ability of patient to tolerate dental procedures.
Teach Patient/Family to:
• Gargle, rinse mouth with water and expectorate after each aerosol dose.
• When dry mouth occurs, avoid mouth rinses with high alcohol content; use daily home fluoride products for anticaries effect; and use sugarless gum, frequent sips of water, or saliva substitutes.

montelukast

mon-te-**loo**′-kast
(Singulair)

CATEGORY AND SCHEDULE

Pregnancy Risk Category: B

Drug Class: Selective leukotriene receptor antagonist

MECHANISM OF ACTION

An antiasthmatic that binds to cysteinyl leukotriene receptors, inhibiting the effects of leukotrienes on bronchial smooth muscle. ***Therapeutic Effect:*** Decreases bronchoconstriction, vascular permeability, mucosal edema, and mucus production.

USES

Prophylaxis and chronic treatment of asthma, seasonal allergic rhinitis

PHARMACOKINETICS

Route	Onset	Peak	Duration
PO	N/A	N/A	24 hr
PO (chewable)	N/A	N/A	24 hr

Rapidly absorbed from the GI tract. Protein binding: 99%. Extensively metabolized in the liver. Excreted almost exclusively in feces. ***Half-life:*** 2.7–5.5 hr (slightly longer in the elderly).

INDICATIONS AND DOSAGES

▸ Bronchial Asthma

PO

Adults, Elderly, Adolescents older than 14 yr. One 10-mg tablet a day, taken in the evening.

Children 6–14 yr. One 5-mg chewable tablet a day, taken in the evening.

Children 1–5 yr. One 4-mg chewable tablet a day, taken in the evening.

SIDE EFFECTS/ADVERSE REACTIONS

Adults, Adolescents 15 yr and older

Frequent

Headache

Occasional

Influenza

Rare

Abdominal pain, cough, dyspepsia, dizziness, fatigue, dental pain

Children 6–14 yr

Rare

Diarrhea, laryngitis, pharyngitis, nausea, otitis media, sinusitis, viral infection

PRECAUTIONS AND CONTRAINDICATIONS

Hypersensitivity

Caution:

Not for acute asthma attacks, not for treatment of exercise-induced bronchospasm or ASA-induced bronchospasm, chewable tablets contain aspartame, lactation; monitor patients when potent CYP3A4 isoenzyme inducers are used

DRUG INTERACTIONS OF CONCERN TO DENTISTRY

• None reported; however, monitor patients when inhibitors of CYP3A4 or CYP2C9 are prescribed.

SERIOUS REACTIONS

! None known

DENTAL CONSIDERATIONS

General:

• Midday appointments and a stress-reduction protocol may be required for anxious patients.

• Avoid prescribing NSAID-containing products.

• Acute asthmatic episodes may be precipitated in the dental office. Rapid-acting sympathomimetic inhalants should be available for emergency use.

• Be aware that aspirin or sulfite preservatives in vasoconstrictor-containing products can exacerbate asthma.

• Consider semisupine chair position for patients with respiratory disease or if GI side effects occur.
Consultations:
• Medical consultation may be required to assess disease control.
Teach Patient/Family to:
• Update health and drug history if physician makes any changes in evaluation or drug regimens; include OTC, herbal, and nonherbal drugs in the update.

moricizine hydrochloride

mor-**iss**′-ih-zeen
high-droh-**klor**′-ide
(Ethmozine)

CATEGORY AND SCHEDULE

Pregnancy Risk Category: B

Drug Class: Antidysrhythmic, type I

MECHANISM OF ACTION

An antiarrhythmic that prevents sodium current across myocardial cell membranes. Has potent local anesthetic activity and membrane stabilizing effects. Slows AV and His-Purkinje conduction and decreases action potential duration and effective refractory period.
Therapeutic Effect: Suppresses ventricular arrhythmias.

USES

Treatment of documented life-threatening dysrhythmias

PHARMACOKINETICS

Peak 0.5–2.2 hr. ***Half-life:*** 1.5–3.5 hr; protein binding greater than 90%; metabolized by the liver; metabolites excreted in feces, urine.

INDICATIONS AND DOSAGES

▸ **Arrhythmias**

PO
Adults, Elderly. 200–300 mg q8h. May increase by 150 mg/day at no less than 3-day intervals.

SIDE EFFECTS/ADVERSE REACTIONS

Frequent
Dizziness, nausea, headache, fatigue, dyspnea
Occasional
Nervousness, paraesthesia, sleep disturbances, dyspepsia, vomiting, diarrhea, dry mouth

PRECAUTIONS AND CONTRAINDICATIONS

Cardiogenic shock, preexisting second- or third-degree AV block or right bundle-branch block without pacemaker
Caution:
CHF, hypokalemia, hyperkalemia, sick sinus syndrome, lactation, children, impaired hepatic and renal function, cardiac dysfunction

DRUG INTERACTIONS OF CONCERN TO DENTISTRY

• No specific interactions are reported with dental drugs; however, any drug that could affect the cardiac action of moricizine (e.g., other local anesthetics, vasoconstrictors, anticholinergics) should be used in the lowest effective dose.

SERIOUS REACTIONS

! Moricizine may worsen existing arrhythmias or produce new ones.
! Jaundice with hepatitis occurs rarely.
! Overdosage produces vomiting, lethargy, syncope, hypotension, conduction disturbances,

M

exacerbation of CHF, MI, and sinus arrest.

DENTAL CONSIDERATIONS

General:

- Monitor vital signs at every appointment because of cardiovascular side effects.
- Assess salivary flow as a factor in caries, periodontal disease, and candidiasis.
- Stress from dental procedures may compromise cardiovascular function; determine patient risk.

Consultations:

- Medical consultation should be made to assess disease control and patient's ability to tolerate stress.

Teach Patient/Family to:

- Encourage effective oral hygiene to prevent soft tissue inflammation.
- Use caution to prevent injury when using oral hygiene aids.
- When chronic dry mouth occurs, advise patient to:
  - Avoid mouth rinses with high alcohol content because of drying effects.
  - Use sugarless gum, frequent sips of water, or saliva substitutes.
  - Use daily home fluoride products for anticaries effect.

M

morphine sulfate

mor′-feen **sull′**-fate

(Anamorph[AUS], Astramorph, Avinza, DepoDur, Duramorph, Infumorph, Kadian, Kapanol[AUS], M-Eslon, Morphine Mixtures[AUS], MS Contin, MSIR, MS Mono[AUS], Oramorph SR, RMS, Roxanol, Statex[CAN])

Do not confuse morphine with hydromorphone, or Roxanol with Roxicet.

CATEGORY AND SCHEDULE

Pregnancy Risk Category: C (D if used for prolonged periods or at high dosages at term)

Controlled Substance: Schedule II

Drug Class: Analgesic, opioid

MECHANISM OF ACTION

An opioid agonist that binds with opioid receptors in the CNS.

Therapeutic Effect: Alters the perception of and emotional response to pain; produces generalized CNS depression.

USES

Treatment of severe pain

PHARMACOKINETICS

Route	Onset	Peak	Duration
Oral solution	N/A	1 hr	3–5 hr
Tablets	N/A	1 hr	3–5 hr
Tablets (ER)	N/A	3–4 hr	8–12 hr
IV	Rapid	0.3 hr	3–5 hr
IM	5–30 min	0.5–1 hr	3–5 hr
Epidural	N/A	1 hr	12–20 hr
Subcutaneous	N/A	1.1–5 hr	3–5 hr
Rectal	N/A	0.5–1 hr	3–7 hr

Variably absorbed from the GI tract. Readily absorbed after IM or subcutaneous administration. Protein binding: 20%–35%. Widely distributed. Metabolized in the liver. Primarily excreted in urine. Removed by hemodialysis. ***Half-life:*** 2–3 hr (increased in patients with hepatic disease).

INDICATIONS AND DOSAGES

▸ **Alert**

Dosage should be titrated to desired effect.

▸ **Analgesia**

PO (Prompt Release)

Adults, Elderly. 10–30 mg q3–4h as needed.

Children. 0.2–0.5 mg/kg q3–4h as needed.

▸ **Alert**

For the Avinza dosage below, be aware that this drug is to be administered once a day only.

▸ **Alert**

For the Kadian dosage information below, be aware that this drug is to be administered q12h or once a day only.

▸ **Alert**

Be aware that pediatric dosages of extended-release preparations Kadian and Avinza have not been established.

▸ **Alert**

For the MSContin and Oramorph SR dosage information below, be aware that the daily dosage is divided and given q8h or q12h.

PO (Extended-Release [Avinza])

Adults, Elderly. Dosage requirement should be established using prompt-release formulations and is based on total daily dose. Avinza is given once a day only.

PO (Extended-Release [Kadian])

Adults, Elderly. Dosage requirement should be established using prompt-release formulations and is based on total daily dose. Dose is given once a day or divided and given q12h.

PO (Extended-Release [MSContin, Oramorph SR])

Adults, Elderly. Dosage requirement should be established using prompt-release formulations and is based on total daily dose. Daily dose is divided and given q8h or q12h.

Children. 0.3–0.6 mg/kg/dose q12h.

IV

Adults, Elderly. 2.5–5 mg q3–4h as needed. Note: Repeated doses (e.g., 1–2 mg) may be given more frequently (e.g., every hour) if needed.

Children. 0.05–0.1 mg/kg q3–4h as needed.

IV Continuous Infusion

Adults, Elderly. 0.8–10 mg/hr. Range: Up to 80 mg/hr.

Children. 10–30 mcg/kg/hr.

IM

Adults, Elderly. 5–10 mg q3–4h as needed.

Children. 0.1 mg/kg q3–4h as needed.

Epidural

Adults, Elderly. Initially, 1–6 mg bolus, infusion rate: 0.1–1 mg/hr. Maximum: 10 mg/24 hr.

Intrathecal

Adults, Elderly. One-tenth of the epidural dose: 0.2–1 mg/dose.

▸ **PCA**

IV

Adults, Elderly. Loading dose: 5–10 mg. Intermittent bolus: 0.5–3 mg. Lockout interval: 5–12 min. Continuous infusion: 1–10 mg/hr. 4-hr limit: 20–30 mg.

SIDE EFFECTS/ADVERSE REACTIONS

Frequent

Sedation, decreased B/P (including orthostatic hypotension), diaphoresis, facial flushing, constipation, dizziness, somnolence, nausea, vomiting

Occasional

Allergic reaction (rash, pruritus), dyspnea, confusion, palpitations, tremors, urine retention, abdominal cramps, vision changes, dry mouth, headache, decreased appetite, pain or burning at injection site

Rare

Paralytic ileus

PRECAUTIONS AND CONTRAINDICATIONS

Acute or severe asthma, GI obstruction, severe hepatic or renal impairment, severe respiratory depression, asthma, severe liver or renal impairment

Caution:

Addictive personality, lactation, MI (acute), severe heart disease, elderly, respiratory depression, hepatic disease, renal disease, children younger than 18 yr

DRUG INTERACTIONS OF CONCERN TO DENTISTRY

- Increased CNS depression: alcohol, all CNS depressants
- Contraindication: MAOIs
- Increased effects of anticholinergics
- Avoid drugs with opioid antagonist properties (e.g., pentazocine)

SERIOUS REACTIONS

! Overdose results in respiratory depression, skeletal muscle flaccidity, cold or clammy skin, cyanosis, and extreme somnolence progressing to seizures, stupor, and coma.

! The patient who uses morphine repeatedly may develop a tolerance to the drug's analgesic effect and physical dependence.

! The drug may have a prolonged duration of action and cumulative effect in those with hepatic and renal impairment.

DENTAL CONSIDERATIONS

General:

- Monitor vital signs at every appointment because of cardiovascular and respiratory side effects.
- Assess salivary flow as a factor in caries, periodontal disease, and candidiasis.
- After supine positioning, have patient sit upright for at least 2 min before standing to avoid orthostatic hypotension.
- Psychologic and physical dependence may occur with chronic administration.
- Determine why the patient is taking the drug.
- Consider the use of NSAIDs or acetaminophen when additional analgesia is required.

Teach Patient/Family to:

- When chronic dry mouth occurs, advise patient to:
  - Use daily home fluoride products for anticaries effect.
  - Avoid mouth rinses with high alcohol content because of drying effects.
  - Use sugarless gum, frequent sips of water, or saliva substitutes.

M

moxifloxacin hydrochloride

moks-ih-**floks′**-ah-sin high-dro-**klor′**-ide
(Avelox, Avelox IV, Vigamox)
Do not confuse Avelox with Avonex.

CATEGORY AND SCHEDULE

Pregnancy Risk Category: C

Drug Class: Fluoroquinolone antiinfective

MECHANISM OF ACTION

A fluoroquinolone that inhibits two enzymes, topoisomerase II and IV, in susceptible microorganisms. ***Therapeutic Effect:*** Interferes with bacterial DNA replication. Prevents or delays emergence of resistant organisms. Bactericidal.

USES

Treatment of acute bacterial sinusitis (*S. pneumoniae, H. influenzae,* or *M. catarrhalis*); acute bacterial exacerbation of chronic bronchitis (*S. pneumoniae, H. influenzae, H. parainfluenzae, K. pneumoniae, M. catarrhalis,* or *S. aureus*); community-acquired pneumonia (*S. pneumoniae, H. influenzae, M. catarrhalis, M. pneumoniae,* or *C. pneumoniae*); bacterial conjunctivitis caused by susceptible bacterial strains including selected aerobic gram-positive species, selected aerobic gram-negative species, and *C. trachomatis*

PHARMACOKINETICS

Well absorbed from the GI tract after PO administration. Protein binding: 50%. Widely distributed throughout body with tissue concentration often exceeding plasma concentration. Metabolized in liver. Primarily excreted in urine with a lesser amount in feces. ***Half-life:*** 10.7–13.3 hr.

INDICATIONS AND DOSAGES

▸ **Acute Bacterial Sinusitis, Community-Acquired Pneumonia**
PO, IV
Adults, Elderly. 400 mg q24h for 10 days.

▸ **Acute Bacterial Exacerbation of Chronic Bronchitis**
PO, IV
Adults, Elderly. 400 mg q24h for 5 days.

▸ **Skin and Skin–Structure Infection**
PO, IV
Adults, Elderly. 400 mg once a day for 7 days.

▸ **Topical Treatment of Bacterial Conjunctivitis Caused by Susceptible Strains of Bacteria**
Ophthalmic
Adults, Elderly, Children older than 1 yr. 1 drop 3 times a day for 7 days.

SIDE EFFECTS/ADVERSE REACTIONS

Frequent
Nausea, diarrhea
Occasional
Dizziness, headache, abdominal pain, vomiting
Ophthalmic: conjunctival irritation, reduced visual acuity, dry eye, keratitis, eye pain, ocular itching, swelling of tissue around cornea, eye discharge, fever, cough, pharyngitis, rash, rhinitis
Rare
Change in sense of taste, dyspepsia (heartburn, indigestion), photosensitivity; tendon rupture

PRECAUTIONS AND CONTRAINDICATIONS

Hypersensitivity to quinolones

Caution:
Divalent cations, retard absorption, not for use with class 1A and III antiarrhythmics, use in children not studied, cross resistance with other fluoroquinolones, may prolong QT interval in some patients, seizures, use with NSAIDs, children younger than 18 yr, lactation

DRUG INTERACTIONS OF CONCERN TO DENTISTRY

- Increased risk of CNS stimulation and seizures: NSAIDs
- Decreased absorption: divalent and trivalent antacids, iron and zinc salts
- Caution when using erythromycin, tricyclic antidepressants (no data, risk of QT interval)
- Increased risk of life-threatening arrhythmias: procainamide

SERIOUS REACTIONS

! Pseudomembranous colitis as evidenced by fever, severe abdominal cramps or pain, and severe watery diarrhea may occur.
! Superinfection manifested as anal or genital pruritus, moderate to severe diarrhea, and stomatitis may occur.

DENTAL CONSIDERATIONS

General:
- Determine why patient is taking the drug.
- Examine for oral manifestation of opportunistic infection.
- Advise patient if dental drugs prescribed have a potential for photosensitivity.
- Ruptures of the shoulder, hand, and Achilles tendons that required surgical repair or resulted in prolonged disability have been reported with the use of fluoroquinolones. Question patient about history of side effects associated with fluoroquinolone use.
- Monitor vital signs at every appointment because of cardiovascular side effects.
- Patients on chronic drug therapy may rarely have symptoms of blood dyscrasias, which can include infection, bleeding, and poor healing.
- Consider semisupine chair position for patient comfort if GI side effects occur.

Consultations:
- In a patient with symptoms of blood dyscrasias, request a medical consultation for blood studies and postpone treatment until normal values are reestablished.
- Physician consultation is advised in the presence of an acute dental infection requiring another antibiotic.

Teach Patient/Family to:
- If used for dental infection to:
  - Minimize exposure to sunlight and wear sunscreen if sun exposure is planned.
  - Discontinue treatment and inform dentist immediately if patient experiences pain or inflammation of a tendon, and to rest and refrain from exercise.

mupirocin

mew-**peer′**-oh-sin
(Bactroban)
Do not confuse with Bactrim or Bacitracin.

CATEGORY AND SCHEDULE

Pregnancy Risk Category: B

Drug Class: Topical antiinfective, pseudomonic acid A

MECHANISM OF ACTION
An antibacterial agent that inhibits bacterial protein, RNA synthesis. Less effective on DNA synthesis. Nasal: Eradicates nasal colonization of MRSA.
Therapeutic Effect: Prevents bacterial growth and replication. Bacteriostatic.

USES
Treatment of impetigo caused by *S. aureus,* ß-hemolytic streptococci, *S. pyogenes;* nasal membranes: *S. aureus*

PHARMACOKINETICS
Metabolized in skin to inactive metabolite. Transported to skin surface; removed by normal skin desquamation.

INDICATIONS AND DOSAGES
▸ Impetigo, Infected Traumatic Skin Lesions
Topical
Adults, Elderly, Children. Apply 3 times a day (may cover with gauze).
▸ Nasal Colonization of Resistant *Staphylococcus Aureus*
Intranasal
Adults, Elderly, Children 12 yr and older. Apply 2 times a day for 5 days.

SIDE EFFECTS/ADVERSE REACTIONS
Frequent
Nasal: Headache, rhinitis, upper respiratory congestion, pharyngitis, altered taste
Occasional
Nasal: Burning, stinging, cough
Topical: Pain, burning, stinging, itching
Rare
Nasal: Pruritus, diarrhea, dry mouth, epistaxis, nausea, rash
Topical: Rash, nausea, dry skin, contact dermatitis

PRECAUTIONS AND CONTRAINDICATIONS
Hypersensitivity to mupirocin or any component of the formulation
Caution:
Lactation

DRUG INTERACTIONS OF CONCERN TO DENTISTRY
- None reported

SERIOUS REACTIONS
! Superinfection may result in bacterial or fungal infections, especially with prolonged or repeated therapy.

DENTAL CONSIDERATIONS
General:
- The dentist may choose to postpone elective dental treatment if the infected site may be affected by dental treatment.

mycophenolate mofetil
my-co-**fen′**-oh-late
(CellCept)

CATEGORY AND SCHEDULE
Pregnancy Risk Category: C

Drug Class: Immunosuppressant

MECHANISM OF ACTION
An immunologic agent that suppresses the immunologically mediated inflammatory response by inhibiting inosine monophosphate dehydrogenase, an enzyme that deprives lymphocytes of nucleotides necessary for DNA and RNA

synthesis, thus inhibiting the proliferation of T and B lymphocytes.
Therapeutic Effect: Prevents transplant rejection.

USES

Prophylaxis of organ rejection in patients receiving allogenic renal or hepatic transplants, cardiac transplants (in combination with cyclosporine and corticosteroids)

PHARMACOKINETICS

Rapidly and extensively absorbed after PO administration (food decreases drug plasma concentration but doesn't affect absorption). Protein binding: 97%. Completely hydrolyzed to active metabolite mycophenolic acid. Primarily excreted in urine. Not removed by hemodialysis. ***Half-life:*** 17.9 hr.

M

INDICATIONS AND DOSAGES

▸ Prevention of Renal Transplant Rejection
PO, IV
Adults, Elderly. 1 g twice a day.
▸ Prevention of Heart Transplant Rejection
PO, IV
Adults, Elderly. 1.5 g twice a day.
▸ Prevention of Liver Transplant Rejection
PO
Adults, Elderly. 1.5 g twice a day.
IV
Adults, Elderly. 1 g twice a day.
▸ Usual Pediatric Dosage
PO
Children. 600 mg/m^2/dose twice a day. Maximum: 2 g/day.

SIDE EFFECTS/ADVERSE REACTIONS

Frequent
UTI, hypertension, peripheral edema, diarrhea, constipation, fever, headache, nausea
Occasional
Dyspepsia; dyspnea; cough; hematuria; asthenia; vomiting; edema; tremors; abdominal, chest, or back pain; oral candidiasis; acne
Rare
Insomnia, respiratory tract infection, rash, dizziness

PRECAUTIONS AND CONTRAINDICATIONS

Hypersensitivity to mycophenolic acid
Caution:
Active GI diseases, lactation, reduce dose in severe chronic renal impairment, increased risk of development of lymphomas or other malignancies and susceptibility to infection

DRUG INTERACTIONS OF CONCERN TO DENTISTRY

- Increased plasma concentration: acyclovir, ganciclovir
- Decreased availability of MPA: drugs that alter the GI flora

SERIOUS REACTIONS

! Significant anemia, leukopenia, thrombocytopenia, neutropenia, and leukocytosis may occur, particularly in those undergoing renal transplant rejection.
! Sepsis and infection occur occasionally.
! GI tract hemorrhage occurs rarely.
! Patients receiving mycophenolate have an increased risk of developing neoplasms.

DENTAL CONSIDERATIONS

General:

- Determine why the patient is taking the drug.
- Short appointments and a stress-reduction protocol may be required for anxious patients.
- Patients who have been or are currently on chronic steroid therapy (longer than 2 wk) may require supplemental steroids for dental treatment.
- Patients on chronic drug therapy may rarely have symptoms of blood dyscrasias, which can include infection, bleeding, and poor healing.
- Place on frequent recall because of oral side effects.
- Determine dose and duration of steroid for patient to assess risk for stress tolerance and immunosuppression.
- Examine for oral manifestations of opportunistic infections.
- Monitor vital signs at every appointment because of cardiovascular and respiratory side effects.
- Consider semisupine chair position for patient comfort if GI side effects occur.
- Antibiotic prophylaxis is usually recommended in patients with organ transplants and immunosuppression.
- Monitor time since organ/tissue transplant; note duration of transplant and status of renal function.
- Place on frequent recall because of possible blood dyscrasias and oral side effects.

Consultations:

- Medical consultation may be required to assess disease control and patient's ability to tolerate stress.
- In a patient with symptoms of blood dyscrasias, request a medical consultation for blood studies and postpone dental treatment until normal values are reestablished.
- Request baseline B/P in renal transplant patients for patient evaluation before dental treatment.

Teach Patient/Family to:

- See dentist immediately if secondary oral infection occurs.
- Encourage effective oral hygiene to prevent soft tissue inflammation.
- Return to dentist frequently because of possible blood dyscrasias and oral side effects.
- Report oral lesions, soreness, or bleeding to dentist.

nabumetone

na-**byu′**-meh-tone
(Apo-Nabumetone, Relafen)

CATEGORY AND SCHEDULE

Pregnancy Risk Category: C (D if used in third trimester or near delivery)

Drug Class: Nonsteroidal antiinflammatory

MECHANISM OF ACTION

An NSAID that produces analgesic and antiinflammatory effects by inhibiting prostaglandin synthesis.
Therapeutic Effect: Reduces the inflammatory response and intensity of pain.

USES

Treatment of osteoarthritis, rheumatoid arthritis, acute or chronic treatment

N

PHARMACOKINETICS

Readily absorbed from the GI tract. Protein binding: 99%. Widely distributed. Metabolized in the liver to active metabolite. Primarily excreted in urine. Not removed by hemodialysis. ***Half-life:*** 22–30 hr.

INDICATIONS AND DOSAGES

▸ **Acute or Chronic Rheumatoid Arthritis and Osteoarthritis**

PO

Adults, Elderly. Initially, 1000 mg as a single dose or in 2 divided doses. May increase up to 2000 mg/day as a single or in 2 divided doses.

SIDE EFFECTS/ADVERSE REACTIONS

Frequent

Diarrhea, abdominal cramps or pain, dyspepsia, oral lichenoid reaction

Occasional

Nausea, constipation, flatulence, dizziness, headache

Rare

Vomiting, stomatitis, confusion

PRECAUTIONS AND CONTRAINDICATIONS

Active peptic ulcer disease, chronic inflammation of GI tract, GI bleeding or ulceration, history of hypersensitivity to aspirin or NSAIDs, history of significant renal impairment

Caution:

Lactation, children, bleeding disorders, GI disorders, cardiac disorders, renal disorders, hepatic dysfunction, elderly

DRUG INTERACTIONS OF CONCERN TO DENTISTRY

- GI ulceration, bleeding: aspirin, alcohol, corticosteroids
- May decrease effects of nabumetone: salicylates
- Nephrotoxicity: acetaminophen (prolonged use and high doses)
- Possible risk of decreased renal function: cyclosporine
- SSRIs: NSAIDs increase risk of GI side effects

SERIOUS REACTIONS

! Overdose may result in acute hypotension and tachycardia.
! Rare reactions with long-term use include peptic ulcer disease.
! GI bleeding, gastritis, nephrotoxicity (dysuria, cystitis, hematuria, proteinuria, nephrotic syndrome), severe hepatic reactions (cholestasis, jaundice), and severe hypersensitivity reactions (bronchospasm, angioedema).

DENTAL CONSIDERATIONS

General:

- Potential increase of adverse cardiovascular events in patients at risk for thromboembolism.
- Patients on chronic drug therapy may rarely have symptoms of blood dyscrasias, which can include infection, bleeding, and poor healing.
- Assess salivary flow as a factor in caries, periodontal disease, and candidiasis.
- Avoid prescribing in pregnancy.
- Avoid prescribing aspirin-containing products.
- Consider semisupine chair position for patients with arthritic disease.
- Severe stomach bleeding may occur in patients who regularly use NSAIDs in recommended doses, when the patient is also taking another NSAID, a blood thinning, or steroid drug, if the patient has GI or peptic ulcer disease, if they are 60 yr or older, or when NSAIDs are taken longer than directed. Warn patients of the potential for severe stomach bleeding.

Consultations:

- In patients with symptoms of blood dyscrasias, request a medical consultation for blood studies and postpone dental treatment until normal values are reestablished.
- Medical consultation may be required to assess disease control.

Teach Patient/Family to:

- Encourage effective oral hygiene to prevent soft tissue inflammation.
- Use caution to prevent injury when using oral hygiene aids.
- Warn patient of potential risks of NSAIDs.
- When chronic dry mouth occurs, advise patient to:
  - Avoid mouth rinses with high alcohol content because of drying effects.
  - Use daily home fluoride products for anticaries effect.
  - Use sugarless gum, frequent sips of water, or saliva substitutes.

nadolol

nay′-doe-lole
(Apo-Nadol[CAN], Corgard, Novo-Nadolol[CAN])

CATEGORY AND SCHEDULE

Pregnancy Risk Category: C (D if used in second or third trimester)

Drug Class: Nonselective β-adrenergic blocker

N

MECHANISM OF ACTION

A nonselective β-blocker that blocks β_1- and β_2-adrenergenic receptors. Large doses increase airway resistance.

Therapeutic Effect: Slows sinus heart rate, decreases cardiac output and B/P. Decreases myocardial ischemia severity by decreasing oxygen requirements.

USES

Treatment of chronic stable angina pectoris, mild-to-moderate hypertension; unapproved: dysrhythmias, MI prophylaxis, vascular headache, mild-to-moderate heart failure

PHARMACOKINETICS

PO: Onset variable, peak 3–4 hr, duration 17–24 hr. ***Half-life:*** 16–20 hr; not metabolized; excreted in urine (unchanged), bile, breast milk.

INDICATIONS AND DOSAGES

▸ **Mild-to-Moderate Hypertension, Angina**

PO

Adults. Initially, 40 mg/day. May increase by 40–80 mg at 3- to 7-day intervals. Maximum: 240–360 mg/day.

Elderly. Initially, 20 mg/day. May increase gradually. Range: 20–240 mg/day.

▸ **Dosage in Renal Impairment**

Dosage is modified on the basis of creatinine clearance.

Creatinine Clearance	% of Usual Dosage
10–50 ml/min	50
Less than 10 ml/min	25

SIDE EFFECTS/ADVERSE REACTIONS

Nadolol is generally well tolerated, with transient and mild side effects

Frequent

Diminished sexual ability, drowsiness, unusual fatigue, or weakness

Occasional

Bradycardia, difficulty breathing, depression, cold hands or feet, diarrhea, constipation, anxiety, nasal congestion, nausea, vomiting

Rare

Altered taste, dry eyes, itching

PRECAUTIONS AND CONTRAINDICATIONS

Bronchial asthma, cardiogenic shock, CHF secondary to tachyarrhythmias, COPD, patients receiving MAOI therapy, second- or third-degree heart block, sinus bradycardia, uncontrolled cardiac failure

Caution:

Diabetes mellitus, renal disease, lactation, hyperthyroidism, peripheral vascular disease, myasthenia gravis

DRUG INTERACTIONS OF CONCERN TO DENTISTRY

- Sympathomimetics (epinephrine, norepinephrine, isoproterenol): elevated systolic blood pressure, bradycardia or cardiac arrest (limit or avoid vasoconstrictors)
- Slows metabolism of nadolol: lidocaine
- Increased hypotension, myocardial depression: fentanyl derivatives, hydrocarbon inhalation anesthetics
- Decreased hypotensive effect: indomethacin and other NSAIDs

SERIOUS REACTIONS

! Overdose may produce profound bradycardia and hypotension.

! Abrupt withdrawal of nadolol may result in diaphoresis, palpitations, headache, tremors, exacerbation of angina, MI, and ventricular arrhythmias.

! Nadolol administration may precipitate CHF and MI in patients with cardiac disease; thyroid storm in those with thyrotoxicosis; and peripheral ischemia in those with existing peripheral vascular disease.

! Hypoglycemia may occur in patients with previously controlled diabetes.

DENTAL CONSIDERATIONS

General:

- Monitor vital signs at every appointment because of cardiovascular side effects.
- Patients on chronic drug therapy may rarely have symptoms of blood dyscrasias, which can include infection, bleeding, and poor healing.
- After supine positioning, have patient sit upright for at least 2 min

before standing to avoid orthostatic hypotension.

- Limit use of sodium-containing products, such as saline IV fluids, for patients with a dietary salt restriction.
- Assess salivary flow as a factor in caries, periodontal disease, and candidiasis.
- Stress from dental procedures may compromise cardiovascular function; determine patient risk. Short appointments and a stress-reduction protocol may be required for anxious patients.
- Consider semisupine chair position for patients with respiratory distress.

Consultations:

- In patients with symptoms of blood dyscrasias, request a medical consultation for blood studies and postpone dental treatment until normal values are reestablished.
- Take precautions if dental surgery is anticipated and anesthesia is required.
- Medical consultation may be required to assess disease control and patient's ability to tolerate stress.

Teach Patient/Family to:

- Encourage effective oral hygiene to prevent soft tissue inflammation.
- Use caution to prevent injury when using oral hygiene aids.
- When chronic dry mouth occurs, advise patient to:
  - Avoid mouth rinses with high alcohol content because of drying effects.
  - Use daily home fluoride products for anticaries effect.
  - Use sugarless gum, frequent sips of water, or saliva substitutes.

nafarelin

naf-**ah**′-rell-in
(Synarel)

CATEGORY AND SCHEDULE

Pregnancy Risk Category: X

Drug Class: Gonadotropin; analog of gonadotropin-releasing hormone

MECHANISM OF ACTION

A gonadotropin inhibitor that initially stimulates the release of the pituitary gonadotropins, luteinizing hormone and follicle-stimulating hormone, then decreases secretion of gonadal steroids.

Therapeutic Effect: Temporarily increases ovarian steroidogenesis, abolishes the stimulatory effect on the pituitary gland, decreases secretion of gonadal steroids.

USES

Treatment of endometriosis, gonadotropin-dependent precocious puberty

PHARMACOKINETICS

Rapidly absorbed after nasal administration. Protein binding: 78%–84%, binds primarily to albumin. Metabolism: unknown. Excreted in urine. ***Half-life:*** 3 hr.

INDICATIONS AND DOSAGES

▸ **Endometriosis**

Intranasal

Adults. 400 mcg/day: 200 mcg (1 spray) into 1 nostril in morning, 1 spray into other nostril in evening. For patients with persistent regular menstruation after months of treatment, increase dose to 800 mcg/

day (1 spray into each nostril in morning and evening).

▸ **Central Precocious Puberty**

Intranasal

Children. 1600 mcg/day: 400 mcg (2 sprays into each nostril in morning and evening; total 8 sprays).

SIDE EFFECTS/ADVERSE REACTIONS

Frequent

Hot flashes, muscle pain, decreased breast size, myalgia

Occasional

Nasal irritation, decreased libido, vaginal dryness, headache, emotional lability, acne

Rare

Insomnia, edema, weight gain, seborrhea, depression

PRECAUTIONS AND CONTRAINDICATIONS

Pregnancy, other agonist analogues, undiagnosed abnormal vaginal bleeding, hypersensitivity to nafarelin or any component of the formulation

DRUG INTERACTIONS OF CONCERN TO DENTISTRY

- None reported

SERIOUS REACTIONS

! None reported

DENTAL CONSIDERATIONS

General:

- Determine why patient is taking the drug.

naftifine

naf′-ti-feen

(Naftin)

Do not confuse with nafcillin or nafarelin.

CATEGORY AND SCHEDULE

Pregnancy Risk Category: B

Drug Class: Topical antifungal

MECHANISM OF ACTION

An antifungal that selectively inhibits the enzyme squalene epoxidase in a dose-dependent manner, which results in the primary sterol, ergosterol, within the fungal membrane not being synthesized.

Therapeutic Effect: Results in fungal cell death. Fungistatic and fungicidal.

USES

Treatment of tinea cruris, tinea corporis, tinea pedis

PHARMACOKINETICS

Minimal systemic absorption. Metabolized in the liver. Excreted in the urine, as well as the feces and bile. ***Half-life:*** 48–72 hr.

INDICATIONS AND DOSAGES

▸ **Tinea Pedis, Tinea Cruris, Tinea Corporis**

Topical

Adults, Elderly, Children 12 yr and older. Apply cream 1 time a day for 4 wk or until signs and symptoms significantly improve. Apply gel 2 times a day for 4 wk or until signs and symptoms significantly improve.

SIDE EFFECTS/ADVERSE REACTIONS

Frequent

Burning, stinging

Occasional
Erythema, itching, dryness, irritation

PRECAUTIONS AND CONTRAINDICATIONS

Hypersensitivity to naftifine or any of its components
Caution:
Lactation, children

DRUG INTERACTIONS OF CONCERN TO DENTISTRY

- None reported

SERIOUS REACTIONS

! Excessive irritation may indicate hypersensitivity reaction.

nalbuphine hydrochloride

nal-**byoo**′-feen high-droh-**klor**′-ide
(Nubain)
Do not confuse Nubain with Navane.

CATEGORY AND SCHEDULE

Pregnancy Risk Category: B (D if used for prolonged periods or at high dosages at term)

Drug Class: Opioid agonist, antagonist; opioid analgesic

MECHANISM OF ACTION

An opioid agonist-antagonist that binds with opioid receptors in the CNS. May displace opioid agonists and competitively inhibit their action; may precipitate withdrawal symptoms.
Therapeutic Effect: Alters the perception of and emotional response to pain.

USES

Relief of moderate-to-severe pain, preoperative sedation, obstetric analgesia, adjunct to anesthesia

PHARMACOKINETICS

Route	Onset	Peak	Duration
IV	2–3 min	30 min	3–6 hr
IM	Less than 15 min	60 min	3–6 hr
Subcutaneous	Less than 15 min	N/A	3–6 hr

Well absorbed after IM or subcutaneous administration. Protein binding: 50%. Metabolized in the liver. Primarily eliminated in feces by biliary secretion. ***Half-life:*** 3.5–5 hr.

INDICATIONS AND DOSAGES

▸ **Analgesia**
IV, IM, Subcutaneous
Adults, Elderly. 10 mg q3–6h as needed. Don't exceed maximum single dose of 20 mg or daily dose of 160 mg. For patients receiving long-term narcotic analgesics of similar duration of action, give 25% of usual dose.
Children. 0.1–0.15 mg/kg q3–6h as needed.
▸ **Supplement to Anesthesia**
IV
Adults, Elderly. Induction: 0.3–3 mg/kg over 10–15 min. Maintenance: 0.25–0.5 mg/kg as needed.

SIDE EFFECTS/ADVERSE REACTIONS

Frequent
Sedation
Occasional
Diaphoresis, cold and clammy skin, nausea, vomiting, dizziness, vertigo, dry mouth, headache

N

Rare
Restlessness, emotional lability, paresthesia, flushing, paradoxical reaction

PRECAUTIONS AND CONTRAINDICATIONS

Respiratory rate less than 12 breaths/min

DRUG INTERACTIONS OF CONCERN TO DENTISTRY

- Increased CNS and respiratory depression: all CNS depressants
- Contraindicated with MAOIs
- Avoid use in opioid-dependent persons; risk of withdrawal reactions
- Increased risk of constipation: anticholinergics
- Increased risk of orthostatic hypotension: antihypertensive medications

N

SERIOUS REACTIONS

! Abrupt withdrawal after prolonged use may produce symptoms of narcotic withdrawal, such as abdominal cramping, rhinorrhea, lacrimation, anxiety, fever, and piloerection (goose bumps).
! Overdose results in severe respiratory depression, skeletal muscle flaccidity, cyanosis, and extreme somnolence progressing to seizures, stupor, and coma.
! Repeated use may result in drug tolerance and physical dependence.

DENTAL CONSIDERATIONS

General:
- Avoid use in an opioid-dependent patient.
- Acute-use drug; question patient about use for pain.
- If additional analgesia is required for dental pain, consider alternative analgesics (NSAIDs) in patients taking opioids for acute or chronic pain.
- Monitor and record vital signs.
- Assess salivary flow as a factor in caries, periodontal disease, and candidiasis.

Consultations:
- Medical consultation may be required to assess disease control.

Teach Patient/Family to:
- Encourage effective oral hygiene to prevent soft tissue inflammation.
- Prevent trauma when using oral hygiene aids.
- Avoid driving or other activities requiring mental alertness.
- Avoid alcohol ingestion or CNS depressants; serious CNS depression may result.
- Avoid OTC preparations that contain CNS depressants (antihistamines, cold remedies).
- When chronic dry mouth occurs advise patient to:
  - Avoid mouth rinses with high alcohol content due to drying effects.
  - Use daily home fluoride products for anticaries effect.
  - Use sugarless gum, frequent sips of water, or saliva substitutes.

nalmefene hydrochloride

nal′-meh-feen high-droh-**klor**′-ide
(Revex)

CATEGORY AND SCHEDULE

Pregnancy Risk Category: B

Drug Class: Opioid antagonist

MECHANISM OF ACTION
Reverses the effects of opioids by competitive antagonism of opioid receptors.

USES
Management of opioid overdose and complete or partial reversal of opioid drug effects, including respiratory depression

PHARMACOKINETICS
IV: Onset 2 min, peak plasma concentration 1.1–2.3 hr; can also be given IM or subcutaneously; hepatic metabolism; excreted in urine.

INDICATIONS AND DOSAGES
▸ Reversal of Opioid Depression
IV
Adult. (100 mcg/ml strength) initial dose 0.25 mcg/kg followed by 0.25 mcg/kg, incremental dose at 2–5 min intervals; cumulative doses over 1.0 mcg/kg do not provide additional therapeutic effect; titrate all doses.

Body weight (kg)	ml of 100 mcg/ml Solution
50	0.125
60	0.150
70	0.175
80	0.200
90	0.225
100	0.250

▸ Known or Suspected Opioid Overdose
IV
Adult. (1 mg/ml strength) initial 0.5 mg/70 kg; if needed, a second dose of 1.0 mg/70 kg, 2–5 min later; doses over 1.5 mg/70 kg are unlikely to be beneficial.

SIDE EFFECTS/ADVERSE REACTIONS
Oral: Dry mouth
CNS: Dizziness, headache, dysphoria, perception of pain, nervousness
CV: Tachycardia, hypertension, dysrhythmia, hypotension
GI: Nausea, abdominal cramps, vomiting, diarrhea
Resp: Pharyngitis, pulmonary edema
GU: Urinary retention
Integ: Pruritus
MS: Myalgia, joint pain
Misc: Chills

PRECAUTIONS AND CONTRAINDICATIONS
Hypersensitivity
Caution:
Nursing mothers, children, withdrawal symptoms in opioid addicts, renal impairment

DRUG INTERACTIONS OF CONCERN TO DENTISTRY
- None reported

SERIOUS REACTIONS
! Precipitation of acute withdrawal syndrome in opioid-dependent individuals.
! Tachycardia, hypertension.

DENTAL CONSIDERATIONS
General:
- This drug is intended for acute use only.
- Risk of seizures reported in animal studies; be aware of this potential.
- Serious cardiovascular events have been associated with opioid reversal in postoperative patients; doses should be carefully titrated to reduce these events.
- Buprenorphine depression may not be completely reversed.
- In all cases, the establishment of a patent airway, ventilatory assistance,

oxygen administration, and circulatory access should complement or precede opioid antagonist use.

- Significant opioid depression occurring in the dental office may require relocation of the patient to a medical facility for comprehensive management.
- Patients discharged from the office or emergency facility should be carefully observed for the return of opioid-induced depression.

naloxone hydrochloride

nal-**oks**′-one high-droh-**klor**′-ide

(Narcan)

Do not confuse naltrexone or Narcan with Norcuron.

CATEGORY AND SCHEDULE

Pregnancy Risk Category: B

Drug Class: Narcotic antagonist

MECHANISM OF ACTION

An opioid antagonist that displaces opioids at opioid-occupied receptor sites in the CNS.

Therapeutic Effect: Reverses opioid-induced sleep or sedation, increases respiratory rate, raises B/P to normal range.

USES

Treatment of respiratory depression induced by opioids, to reverse postoperative opioid depression

PHARMACOKINETICS

Route	Onset	Peak	Duration
IV	1–2 min	N/A	20–60 min
IM	2–5 min	N/A	20–60 min
Subcutaneous	2–5 min	N/A	20–60 min

Well absorbed after IM or subcutaneous administration. Metabolized in the liver. Primarily excreted in urine. ***Half-life:*** 1–1.7hr.

INDICATIONS AND DOSAGES

▸ Opioid Toxicity

IV, IM, Subcutaneous

Adults, Elderly. 0.4–2 mg q2–3min as needed. May repeat q20–60min.

Children 5 yr and older and weighing 22 kg or more. 2 mg/dose; if no response, may repeat q2–3min. May need to repeat q20–60min.

Children younger than 5 yr and weighing less than 22 kg. 0.1 mg/kg; if no response, repeat q2–3min. May need to repeat q20–60min.

▸ Postanesthesia Narcotic Reversal

IV

Children. 0.01 mg/kg; may repeat q2–3min.

▸ Neonatal Opioid-Induced Depression

IV

Neonates. May repeat q2–3min as needed. May need to repeat q1–2h.

SIDE EFFECTS/ADVERSE REACTIONS

None known; little or no pharmacologic effect in absence of narcotics

PRECAUTIONS AND CONTRAINDICATIONS

Respiratory depression due to nonopioid drugs

Caution:

Opioid dependence

DRUG INTERACTIONS OF CONCERN TO DENTISTRY

• Antagonizes effects of opioid agonists and mixed agonists/antagonists.

SERIOUS REACTIONS

! Too-rapid reversal of opioid-induced respiratory depression may result in nausea, vomiting, tremors, increased B/P, and tachycardia.
! Excessive dosage in postoperative patients may produce significant excitement, tremors, and reversal of analgesia.
! Patients with cardiovascular disease may experience hypotension or hypertension, ventricular tachycardia and fibrillation, and pulmonary edema.

DENTAL CONSIDERATIONS

General:

• This drug is indicated for acute use only.
• Risk of seizures reported in animal studies; be aware of this potential.
• Serious cardiovascular events have been associated with opioid reversal in postoperative patients; doses should be carefully titrated to reduce these events.
• Buprenorphine depression may not be completely reversed.
• In all cases, the establishment of a patent airway, ventilatory assistance, oxygen administration, and circulatory access should complement or precede opioid antagonist use.
• Significant opioid depression occurring in the dental office may require relocation of the patient to a medical facility for comprehensive management.
• Patients discharged from the office/emergency facility should be carefully observed for the return of opioid-induced depression.

naltrexone hydrochloride

nal-**trex**′-one high-droh-**klor**′-ide
(ReVia)

CATEGORY AND SCHEDULE

Pregnancy Risk Category: C

Drug Class: Opioid antagonist

MECHANISM OF ACTION

An opioid antagonist that displaces opioids at opioid-occupied receptor sites in the CNS.
Therapeutic Effect: Blocks physical effects of opioid analgesics; decreases craving for alcohol and relapse rate in alcoholism.

N

USES

Treatment of opioid addiction following detoxification, alcoholism

PHARMACOKINETICS

PO: Onset 15–30 min, peak 1–2 hr, duration is dose dependent.
Half-life: 4 hr; extensive first-pass metabolism; metabolized by liver; excreted by kidneys; crosses placenta; excreted in breast milk.

INDICATIONS AND DOSAGES

▸ **Naloxone Challenge Test to Determine if Patient is Opioid Dependent**

ALERT

Expect to perform the naloxone challenge test if there is any question that the patient is opioid dependent. Do not administer naltrexone until the naloxone challenge test is negative.

IV
Adults, Elderly. Draw 2 ml (0.8 mg) of naloxone into syringe. Inject 0.5 ml (0.2 mg); while needle is still in vein, observe patient for 30 sec for withdrawal signs or symptoms. If no evidence of withdrawal, inject remaining 1.5 ml (0.6 mg); observe patient for additional 20 min for withdrawal signs or symptoms.
Subcutaneous
Adults, Elderly. Inject 2 ml (0.8 mg) of naloxone; observe patient for 45 min for withdrawal signs or symptoms.

▸ **Treatment of Opioid Dependence in Patients Who Have Been Opioid Free for at Least 7–10 Days**
PO
Adults, Elderly. Initially, 25 mg. Observe patient for 1 hr. If no withdrawal signs or symptoms appear, give another 25 mg. May be given as 100 mg every other day or 150 mg every 3 days.

▸ **Adjunctive Treatment of Alcohol Dependence**
PO
Adults, Elderly. 50 mg once a day.

SIDE EFFECTS/ADVERSE REACTIONS

Frequent
Alcoholism: Nausea, headache, depression
Opioid addiction: Insomnia, anxiety, nervousness, headache, low energy, abdominal cramps, nausea, vomiting, arthralgia, myalgia
Occasional
Alcoholism: Dizziness, nervousness, fatigue, insomnia, vomiting, anxiety, suicidal ideation
Narcotic addiction: Irritability, increased energy, dizziness, anorexia, diarrhea or constipation, rash, chills, increased thirst

PRECAUTIONS AND CONTRAINDICATIONS

Acute hepatitis, acute opioid withdrawal, failed naloxone challenge test, hepatic failure, history of hypersensitivity to naltrexone, opioid dependence, positive urine screen for opioids

DRUG INTERACTIONS OF CONCERN TO DENTISTRY

• Decreased effects of opioid narcotics

SERIOUS REACTIONS

! Signs and symptoms of opioid withdrawal include stuffy or runny nose, tearing, yawning, diaphoresis, tremors, vomiting, piloerection, feeling of temperature change, bone pain, arthralgia, myalgia, abdominal cramps, and feeling of skin crawling.
! Accidental naltrexone overdose produces withdrawal symptoms within 5 min of ingestion that may last for up to 48 hr. Symptoms include confusion, visual hallucinations, somnolence, and significant vomiting and diarrhea.
! Hepatocellular injury may occur with large doses.

DENTAL CONSIDERATIONS

General:
• Monitor vital signs at every appointment because of cardiovascular and respiratory side effects.
• Patients on chronic drug therapy may rarely have symptoms of blood dyscrasias, which can include infection, bleeding, and poor healing.
• Patients should not be given opioid analgesics for dental pain management. Substitute with acetaminophen or NSAIDs.

• The dental professional must be aware of the patient's disease, and the patient must be active in treatment for chemical dependency.

Consultations:

• In patients with symptoms of blood dyscrasias, request a medical consultation for blood studies and postpone dental treatment until normal values are reestablished.

• Medical consultation may be required to assess disease control.

• Inform aftercare provider or counselor if sedative medications are required for proper management.

Teach Patient/Family to:

• Encourage effective oral hygiene to prevent soft tissue inflammation.

• Use caution to prevent injury when using oral hygiene aids.

naphazoline

naf-**az′**-oh-leen

(AK-Con, Albalon Liquifilm[AUS], Clear Eyes[AUS], Naphcon, Naphcon Forte[AUS], Privine, Vasocon)

CATEGORY AND SCHEDULE

Pregnancy Risk Category: C

Drug Class: Ophthalmic vasoconstrictor

MECHANISM OF ACTION

A sympathomimetic that directly acts on α-adrenergic receptors in conjunctival arterioles and nasal blood vessels.

Therapeutic Effect: Causes vasoconstriction, resulting in decreased congestion.

USES

Relief of hyperemia, irritation in superficial corneal vascularity

PHARMACOKINETICS

Instillation: Duration 2–3 hr.

INDICATIONS AND DOSAGES

▸ Nasal Congestion Resulting from Acute or Chronic Rhinitis, Common Cold, Hay Fever, or Other Allergies

Intranasal

Adults, Elderly, Children older than 12 yr. 1–2 drops or sprays in each nostril q3–6h.

Children 6–12 yr. 1 spray or drop in each nostril q6h as needed.

▸ Control of Hyperemia in Patients with Superficial Corneal Vascularity; Relief of Congestion and Inflammation; for Use During Ocular Diagnostic Procedures

Ophthalmic

Adults, Elderly, Children older than 6 yr. 1–2 drops in affected eye q3–4h for 3–4 days.

SIDE EFFECTS/ADVERSE REACTIONS

Occasional

Nasal: Burning, stinging, or drying of nasal mucosa; sneezing; rebound congestion

Ophthalmic: Blurred vision, dilated pupils, increased eye irritation

PRECAUTIONS AND CONTRAINDICATIONS

Angle-closure glaucoma, before peripheral iridectomy, patients with a narrow angle who do not have glaucoma

Caution:

Hypertension, hyperthyroidism, elderly, severe arteriosclerosis, cardiac disease

DRUG INTERACTIONS OF CONCERN TO DENTISTRY

• Increased pressor effects: tricyclic antidepressants

N

SERIOUS REACTIONS

! If naphazoline is systemically absorbed, the patient may experience tachycardia, palpitations, headache, insomnia, light-headedness, nausea, nervousness, and tremors.
! Large doses may produce tachycardia, palpitations, light-headedness, nausea, and vomiting.
! Overdose in patients older than 60 yr may produce hallucinations, CNS depression, and seizures.

DENTAL CONSIDERATIONS

General:

- Monitor vital signs at every appointment because of cardiovascular side effects.
- Avoid dental light in patient's eyes; offer dark glasses for patient comfort.

N

naproxen/naproxen sodium

na-**prox**′-en **soe**′-dee-um

naproxen: (Crysanal[AUS], EC-Naprosyn, Inza[AUS], Naprelan, Naprosyn) naproxen sodium: (Aleve, Anaprox, Anaprox DS, Apo-Naprosyn[CAN], Naprogesic[AUS], Novo-Naprox[CAN], Nu-Naprox[CAN], Pamprin)

Do not confuse Aleve with Alesse or Anaprox with Anaspaz.

CATEGORY AND SCHEDULE

Pregnancy Risk Category: B (D if used in third trimester or near delivery)

OTC (220 mg gelcaps, 220 mg tablets)

Drug Class: Nonsteroidal antiinflammatory

MECHANISM OF ACTION

An NSAID that produces analgesic and antiinflammatory effects by inhibiting prostaglandin synthesis. ***Therapeutic Effect:*** Reduces the inflammatory response and intensity of pain.

USES

Treatment of mild-to-moderate pain, osteoarthritis, rheumatoid, juvenile, gouty arthritis, ankylosing spondylitis, primary dysmenorrhea; unapproved: migraine, PMS, fever

PHARMACOKINETICS

Route	Onset	Peak	Duration
PO (analgesic)	Less than 1 hr	N/A	7 hr or less
PO (anti-rheumatic)	Less than 14 days	2–4 wk	N/A

Completely absorbed from the GI tract. Protein binding: 99%. Metabolized in the liver. Primarily excreted in urine. Not removed by hemodialysis. ***Half-life:*** 13 hr.

INDICATIONS AND DOSAGES

▸ Rheumatoid Arthritis, Osteoarthritis, Ankylosing Spondylitis

PO

Adults, Elderly. 250–500 mg naproxen (275–550 mg naproxen sodium) twice a day or 250 mg naproxen (275 mg naproxen sodium) in morning and 500 mg naproxen (550 mg naproxen sodium) in evening. Naprelan: 750–1000 mg once a day.

▸ Acute Gouty Arthritis

PO

Adults, Elderly. Initially, 750 mg naproxen (825 mg naproxen sodium), then 250 mg naproxen (275 mg naproxen sodium) q8h until attack subsides. Naprelan: Initially, 1000–1500 mg, then 1000 mg once a day until attack subsides.

▸ **Mild-to-Moderate Pain, Dysmenorrhea, Bursitis, Tendinitis**

PO

Adults, Elderly. Initially, 500 mg naproxen (550 mg naproxen sodium), then 250 mg naproxen (275 mg naproxen sodium) q6–8h as needed. Maximum: 1.25 g/day naproxen (1.375 g/day naproxen sodium). Naprelan: 1000 mg once a day.

▸ **Juvenile Rheumatoid Arthritis**

PO (Naproxen Only)

Children. 10–15 mg/kg/day in 2 divided doses. Maximum: 1000 mg/day.

SIDE EFFECTS/ADVERSE REACTIONS

Frequent

Nausea, constipation, abdominal cramps or pain, heartburn, dizziness, headache, somnolence, oral lichenoid reaction

Occasional

Stomatitis, diarrhea, indigestion

Rare

Vomiting, confusion

PRECAUTIONS AND CONTRAINDICATIONS

Hypersensitivity to aspirin, naproxen, or other NSAIDs

Caution:

Lactation, children, bleeding disorders, GI disorders, cardiac disorders, hypersensitivity to other antiinflammatory agents, elderly, more than 2 alcohol drinks daily

DRUG INTERACTIONS OF CONCERN TO DENTISTRY

- GI ulceration, bleeding: aspirin, alcohol, corticosteroids
- Nephrotoxicity: acetaminophen (chronic use and high doses)
- Possible risk of decreased renal function: cyclosporine
- Increased photosensitization: tetracycline
- Increased plasma levels: probenecid
- SSRIs: NSAIDs increase risk of GI side effects
- When prescribed for dental pain:
  - Risk of increased effects: oral anticoagulants, oral antidiabetics, trium, methotrexate
  - Decreased antihypertensive effects of diuretics, β-adrenergic blockers, and ACE inhibitors

SERIOUS REACTIONS

! Rare reactions with long-term use include peptic ulcer disease.

! GI bleeding, gastritis, severe hepatic reactions (cholestasis, jaundice), nephrotoxicity (dysuria, hematuria, proteinuria, nephrotic syndrome), and a severe hypersensitivity reaction (fever, chills, bronchospasm).

N

DENTAL CONSIDERATIONS

General:

- Possible increased adverse cardiovascular events in patients at risk for thromboembolism.
- Patients on chronic drug therapy may rarely have symptoms of blood dyscrasias, which can include infection, bleeding, and poor healing.
- Assess salivary flow as a factor in caries, periodontal disease, and candidiasis.
- Avoid prescribing for dental use in pregnancy.
- Avoid prescribing aspirin-containing products.
- Consider semisupine chair position for patients with arthritic disease.
- Severe stomach bleeding may occur in patients who regularly use NSAIDs in recommended doses,

when the patient is also taking another NSAID, a blood thinning, or steroid drug, if the patient has GI or peptic ulcer disease, if they are 60 yr or older, or when NSAIDs are taken longer than directed. Warn patients of the potential for severe stomach bleeding.

Consultations:

- In patients with symptoms of blood dyscrasias, request a medical consultation for blood studies and postpone dental treatment until normal values are reestablished.
- Medical consultation may be required to assess disease control.

Teach Patient/Family to:

- Encourage effective oral hygiene to prevent soft tissue inflammation.
- Use caution to prevent injury when using oral hygiene aids.
- Warn patient of potential risks of NSAIDs.
- When chronic dry mouth occurs, advise patient to:
  - Avoid mouth rinses with high alcohol content because of drying effects.
  - Use daily home fluoride products for anticaries effect.
  - Use sugarless gum, frequent sips of water, or saliva substitutes.

naproxen + esomeprazole

na-**prox**′-en & es-oh-**me**′-pray-zole (Vimovo)

Do not confuse Vimovo with Vimpat.

CATEGORY AND SCHEDULE

Pregnancy Risk Category: C (D if used after 30 wk gestation)

Drug Class: Nonsteroidal antiinflammatory, oral; proton pump inhibitor

MECHANISM OF ACTION

Naproxen: Reversibly inhibits cyclooxygenase-1 and -2 (COX-1 and COX-2) enzymes, which results in decreased formation of prostaglandin precursors; has antipyretic, analgesic, and antiinflammatory properties. Esomeprazole: Proton pump inhibitor that decreases acid secretion in gastric parietal cells.

Therapeutic Effect: Treatment of symptoms of rheumatoid arthritis and osteoarthritis while minimizing risk of ulcerogenic effects

USES

Reduction of the risk of NSAID-associated gastric ulcers in patients at risk of developing gastric ulcers who require an NSAID for the treatment of rheumatoid arthritis, osteoarthritis, and ankylosing spondylitis

PHARMACOKINETICS

Naproxen: Completely absorbed from the GI tract. 99% plasma protein bound. Hepatic metabolism. Excreted primarily in urine. Esomeprazole: Well absorbed from the GI tract. 97% plasma protein bound. Hepatic metabolism. Excreted primarily in urine.

Half-life: Naproxen: 13 hr. Esomeprazole: 1–1.5 hr.

INDICATIONS AND DOSAGES

▸ Reduce NSAID-Associated Gastric Ulcers During Treatment for Arthritis

PO

Adults. 1 tablet (375 mg naproxen/20 mg esomeprazole or 500 mg naproxen/20 mg esomeprazole) twice daily; maximum daily esomeprazole dose: 40 mg.

SIDE EFFECTS/ADVERSE REACTIONS

Frequent

Nausea, constipation, abdominal cramps or pain, heartburn, dizziness, headache, somnolence, oral lichenoid reaction, stomatitis, diarrhea, abdominal pain, xerostomia

Occasional

Vomiting, confusion

PRECAUTIONS AND CONTRAINDICATIONS

Hypersensitivity to esomeprazole and other proton pump inhibitors, naproxen, aspirin, and other NSAIDs, or any component of the formulation; perioperative pain in the setting of coronary artery bypass graft (CABG) surgery; late stages of pregnancy. Avoid use in patients with severe hepatic and renal impairment. Avoid concomitant use with clopidogrel since proton pump inhibitors may diminish the therapeutic effect of clopidogrel (due to reduced formation of the active metabolite of clopidogrel)

DRUG INTERACTIONS OF CONCERN TO DENTISTRY

- Increased risk of GI ulceration, bleeding: NSAIDs, aspirin, aspirin-containing products, corticosteroids
- Acetaminophen: chronic use and high doses may lead to nephrotoxicity and hepatotoxicity
- Tetracyclines: increased risk of photosensitivity
- SSRIs (e.g., fluoxetine): increased risk of NSAID-related GI adverse effects
- Antihypertensive drugs (e.g., thiazide diuretics): reduced efficacy
- Absorption of drugs: esomeprazole can elevate GI pH, which can reduce the absorption of azole antifungals, fluoroquinolones, and ampicillin

SERIOUS REACTIONS

! NSAIDs are associated with an increased risk of adverse cardiovascular thrombotic events, including MI and stroke. NSAIDs may increase risk of gastrointestinal irritation, inflammation, ulceration, bleeding, and perforation. Risk of MI and stroke may be increased with use of NSAIDs following CABG surgery. NSAIDs may cause anaphylactoid reactions, atrophic gastritis, increased incidence of osteoporosis-related bone fractures, and serious adverse skin events including exfoliative dermatitis, Stevens-Johnson syndrome (SJS), and toxic epidermal necrolysis (TEN).

DENTAL CONSIDERATIONS

General:

- Possible increased adverse cardiovascular events in patients at risk for thromboembolism.
- Increased risk of intraoperative and postoperative bleeding.
- Patients on chronic drug therapy may rarely have symptoms of blood dyscrasias, which can include infection, bleeding, and poor healing.
- Assess salivary flow as a factor in caries, periodontal disease, and candidiasis.
- Avoid prescribing Vimovo and any NSAID during pregnancy.
- Consider semisupine chair position for patients with adverse GI effects.

Consultations:

- In patients with symptoms of blood dyscrasias, request a medical consultation for blood studies and postpone dental treatment until normal values are reestablished.

• Medical consultation may be required to assess disease control.

Teach Patient/Family to:

• Use effective oral hygiene to prevent soft tissue inflammation.
• Use special oral hygiene aids if arthritic disease limits ability of patient to hold ordinary appliances.
• Use caution to prevent injury when using oral hygiene aids.
• When chronic dry mouth occurs, advise patient to:
  • Avoid mouth rinses with high alcohol content because of drying effect.
  • Use home fluoride products for anticaries effect.
  • Use sugarless/xylitol gum, frequent sips of water, or saliva substitutes.

N

naratriptan

nare-ah-**trip′**-tan
(Amerge, Naramig[AUS])
Do not confuse Amerge with Amaryl.

CATEGORY AND SCHEDULE

Pregnancy Risk Category: C

Drug Class: Serotonin agonist

MECHANISM OF ACTION

A serotonin receptor agonist that binds selectively to vascular receptors, producing a vasoconstrictive effect on cranial blood vessels.
Therapeutic Effect: Relieves migraine headache.

USES

Acute treatment of migraine attacks with or without aura in adults

PHARMACOKINETICS

Well absorbed after PO administration. Protein binding: 28%–31%. Metabolized by the liver to inactive metabolite. Eliminated primarily in urine and, to a lesser extent, in feces. ***Half-life:*** 6 hr (increased in hepatic or renal impairment).

INDICATIONS AND DOSAGES

▸ **Acute Migraine Attack**

PO

Adults. 1 mg or 2.5 mg. If headache improves but then returns, dose may be repeated after 4 hr. Maximum: 5 mg/24 hr.

▸ **Dosage in Mild-to-Moderate Hepatic or Renal Impairment**

A lower starting dose is recommended. Do not exceed 2.5 mg/24 hr.

SIDE EFFECTS/ADVERSE REACTIONS

Occasional

Nausea

Rare

Paresthesia; dizziness; fatigue; somnolence; jaw, neck, or throat pressure

PRECAUTIONS AND CONTRAINDICATIONS

Basilar or hemiplegic migraine, cerebrovascular or peripheral vascular disease, coronary artery disease, ischemic heart disease (including angina pectoris, history of MI, silent ischemia, and Prinzmetal's angina), severe hepatic impairment (Child-Pugh class C), severe renal impairment (serum creatinine less than 15 ml/min), uncontrolled hypertension, use within 24 hr of ergotamine-containing preparations or another serotonin receptor agonist, use within 14 days of MAOIs

Caution:

Risk of serious cardiovascular events, including ischemia and MI; renal/hepatic dysfunction, SSRI antidepressants, lactation, use in children not established, not recommended in elderly

DRUG INTERACTIONS OF CONCERN TO DENTISTRY

• No specific interactions with dental drugs reported.

• Should not be used within 24 hr of another 5-HT1 agonist.

SERIOUS REACTIONS

! Corneal opacities and other ocular defects may occur.

! Cardiac reactions (including ischemia, coronary artery vasospasm, and MI) and noncardiac vasospasm-related reactions (such as hemorrhage and CVA), occur rarely, particularly in patients with hypertension, diabetes, or a strong family history of coronary artery disease; obese patients; smokers; males older than 40 yr; and postmenopausal women.

DENTAL CONSIDERATIONS

General:

• This is an acute-use drug; it is doubtful that patients will come to the office if acute migraine is present.

• Be aware of patient's disease, its severity, and its frequency when known.

Consultations:

• If treating chronic orofacial pain, consult with physician of record.

• Medical consultation may be required to assess disease control and patient's ability to tolerate stress.

Teach Patient/Family to:

• Update health and drug history if physician makes any changes in evaluation or drug regimens; include OTC, herbal, and nonherbal drugs in update.

• Avoid mouth rinses with high alcohol content because of additional drying effects.

nateglinide

na-**teg**′-lin-ide

(Starlix)

CATEGORY AND SCHEDULE

Pregnancy Risk Category: C

Drug Class: Oral antidiabetic, meglitinide class

N

MECHANISM OF ACTION

An antihyperglycemic that stimulates release of insulin from β cells of the pancreas by depolarizing β cells, leading to an opening of calcium channels. Resulting calcium influx induces insulin secretion.

Therapeutic Effect: Lowers blood glucose concentration.

USES

Treatment of type 2 diabetes mellitus when hyperglycemia cannot be controlled by diet and exercise, can be used in combination with metformin, not for patients who have been chronically treated with other antidiabetic drugs

PHARMACOKINETICS

PO: Rapid absorption, peak plasma levels 1 hr, bioavailability 73%, plasma protein binding 98%, hepatic metabolism (CYP450 2C9 isoenzyme [70%] and CYP450 3A4 isoenzyme [30%]); excretion renal (83%), feces (10%).

INDICATIONS AND DOSAGES

▸ Diabetes Mellitus

PO

Adult, Elderly. 120 mg 3 times a day before meals. Initially, 60 mg may be given.

SIDE EFFECTS/ADVERSE REACTIONS

Frequent

Upper respiratory tract infection

Occasional

Back pain, flu symptoms, dizziness, arthropathy, diarrhea

Rare

Bronchitis, cough

PRECAUTIONS AND CONTRAINDICATIONS

Diabetic ketoacidosis, type 1 Diabetes mellitus

Caution:

Hypoglycemia (geriatric, malnourished, adrenal insufficiency or pituitary insufficiency more susceptible to hypoglycemia), β-blocker may mask hypoglycemia, administer before meals, infection, hepatic dysfunction, lactation, children

DRUG INTERACTIONS OF CONCERN TO DENTISTRY

- Most drug interactions not clearly identified; may act as an inhibitor of CYP450 2C9 enzymes but not CYP450 3A4. Does not appear to interact with highly protein-bound drugs
- Potentiation of hypoglycemic effects: NSAIDs, salicylates, nonselective β-blockers

SERIOUS REACTIONS

! Hypoglycemia occurs in less than 2% of patients.

DENTAL CONSIDERATIONS

General:

- If dentist prescribes any of the drugs listed in the drug interaction section, monitor patient's blood sugar levels.
- Consider semisupine chair position for patient comfort if GI side effects occur.
- Ensure that patient is following prescribed diet and regularly takes medication.
- Place on frequent recall to evaluate healing response.
- Short appointments and a stress-reduction protocol may be required.
- Diabetics may be more susceptible to infection and have delayed wound healing.

Consultations:

- Medical consultation may include data from patient's blood glucose monitoring, including glycosylated hemoglobin or HbA_{1c} testing.
- Medical consultation may be required to assess disease control and patient's ability to tolerate stress.

Teach Patient/Family to:

- Prevent trauma when using oral hygiene aids.
- Update health and drug history if physician makes any changes in evaluation or drug regimens.

nebivolol

ne-**biv**-oh-lole

(Bystolic)

CATEGORY AND SCHEDULE

Pregnancy Risk Category: C

Drug Class: Antihypertensive, β-adrenergic blocker (selective)

MECHANISM OF ACTION

An antihypertensive that possesses selective β_1 blocking activity, but loses selectivity at higher doses. Causes vasodilation through nitric oxide (NO)-production, potentiating its actions, and reducing total peripheral vascular resistance. ***Therapeutic Effect***: Decreases B/P, heart rate, and myocardial contractility; suppresses renin activity.

USES

Hypertension

PHARMACOKINETICS

Rapidly absorbed. Bioavailability of approximately 12% (extensive metabolizers) to 96% (poor metabolizers). Protein binding: 98%, mostly albumin. Extensively metabolized in the liver to active metabolites by glucuronidation and CYP450 2D6. Excreted in urine (38% in extensive metabolizers; 67% in poor metabolizers) and in feces (44% in extensive metabolizers; 13% in poor metabolizers). ***Half-life:*** 12–19 hr; 10–12 hr in extensive metabolizers and 19–32 hr in poor metabolizers.

INDICATIONS AND DOSAGES

▸ Hypertension

PO

Adults, Elderly. 5–40 mg/day. Initially, 5 mg/day. May increase at 2-wk intervals. Maximum: 40 mg/day.

▸ Dosage in Renal Impairment

Adults (creatinine clearance less than 30 ml/min). Initially, 2.5 mg/day.

Increase with caution.

▸ Dosage in Hepatic Impairment (Moderate)

Adults. 2.5 mg/day.

Increase with caution.

Not recommended in patients with severe hepatic impairment

SIDE EFFECTS/ADVERSE REACTIONS

Adults

Frequent

Fatigue, dizziness, headache

Occasional

Nausea, diarrhea, somnolence, pain, peripheral edema

Rare

Bradycardia, dyspnea, chest pain, rash, acute renal failure, erectile dysfunction, Raynaud's phenomenon, syncope, bronchospasm, acute pulmonary edema

PRECAUTIONS AND CONTRAINDICATIONS

Hypersensitivity to nebivolol or any component of the formulation
Severe bradycardia
Heart block >first degree
Cardiogenic shock
Decompensated HF
Bronchospastic disease

Caution:

Sick sinus syndrome (unless a permanent pacemaker is in place)
Severe hepatic impairment (Child Pugh >B)
Abrupt cessation of therapy
Cardiac failure, angina, acute MI
Diabetes (hypoglycemia)
Thyrotoxicosis
Peripheral vascular disease
Concurrent use with CYP2D6 inhibitors
Impaired renal or hepatic function
Anesthesia/surgery
Concomitant use with other β-blockers
Pheochromocytoma

DRUG INTERACTIONS OF CONCERN TO DENTISTRY

• Diuretics, other antihypertensives: May increase hypotensive effect of nebivolol.
• Sympathomimetics, xanthines: Increased systolic BP, bradycardia. May antagonize the effects and reduce bronchodilation.
• CYP450 2D6 inhibitors: May increase concentrations of nebivolol.
• Oral hypoglycemics and insulin: May mask symptoms of hypoglycemia and prolong hypoglycemic effect of insulin and oral hypoglycemics.
• NSAIDs: May reduce the antihypertensive effect of nebivolol.
• Digoxin: May cause serious bradycardia.
• Calcium channel blockers (verapamil, diltiazem): May cause hypotension and bradycardia.

SERIOUS REACTIONS

! Second- and third-degree atrioventricular block has been reported.
! Abrupt withdrawal may result in rebound or withdrawal hypertension, severe exacerbation of angina, myocardial infarction, and ventricular arrhythmia.
! Nebivolol administration may precipitate CHF and MI in patients with heart disease, thyroid storm in those with thyrotoxicosis, and peripheral ischemia in those with existing peripheral vascular disease.
! Hypoglycemia may occur in patients with previously controlled diabetes.

DENTAL CONSIDERATIONS

General:
• Monitor vital signs at every appointment because of cardiovascular side effects.
• Avoid vasoconstrictors or limit doses.
• After supine positioning, have patient sit upright for at least 2 min before standing to avoid orthostatic hypotension.
• Assess salivary flow as a factor in caries, periodontal disease, and candidiasis.
• Limit use of sodium-containing products, such as saline IV fluids, for those patients with dietary salt restriction.
• Stress from dental procedures may compromise cardiovascular function; determine patient risk.
• Short appointments and a stress-reduction protocol may be required for anxious patients.

Consultations:
• Medical consultation may be required to assess disease control.

Teach Patient/Family to:
• Report oral lesions, soreness, or bleeding to dentist.
• When chronic dry mouth occurs, advise patient to:
  • Avoid mouth rinses with high alcohol content because of drying effects.
  • Use daily home fluoride products for anticaries effect.
  • Use sugarless gum, frequent sips of water, or saliva substitutes.

nedocromil sodium

ned-oh-**crow′**-mil **soe′**-dee-um
(Alocril, Mireze[CAN], Tilade, Tilade CFC Free[AUS])

CATEGORY AND SCHEDULE

Pregnancy Risk Category: B

Drug Class: Antiasthmatic, mast cell stabilizer

MECHANISM OF ACTION

A mast cell stabilizer that prevents the activation and release of inflammatory mediators, such as histamine, leukotrienes, mast cells, eosinophils, and monocytes. ***Therapeutic Effect:*** Prevents both early and late asthmatic responses.

USES

Maintenance therapy in mild-to-moderate asthma; ophthalmic solution for allergic conjunctivitis

PHARMACOKINETICS

Inhalation: Peak 15 min, duration 4–6 hr. ***Half-life:*** 80 min; excreted unchanged in feces.

INDICATIONS AND DOSAGES

▸ Mild-to-Moderate Asthma

Oral Inhalation

Adults, Elderly, Children 6 yr and older. 2 inhalations 4 times a day. May decrease to 3 times a day then twice a day as asthma becomes controlled.

▸ Allergic Conjunctivitis

Ophthalmic

Adults, Elderly, Children 3 yr and older. 1–2 drops in each eye twice a day.

SIDE EFFECTS/ADVERSE REACTIONS

Frequent

Cough, pharyngitis, bronchospasm, headache, altered taste

Occasional

Rhinitis, upper respiratory tract infection, abdominal pain, fatigue

Rare

Diarrhea, dizziness

PRECAUTIONS AND CONTRAINDICATIONS

Hypersensitivity to this drug or lactose, status asthmaticus

Caution:

Lactation, renal disease, hepatic disease, safety and efficacy of inhalation in children younger than 6 yr or ophthalmic solution in children younger than 3 yr not established

DRUG INTERACTIONS OF CONCERN TO DENTISTRY

• None reported

SERIOUS REACTIONS

! None known

DENTAL CONSIDERATIONS

Nedocromil Sodium (Alocril)

General:

• Determine why patient is taking the drug.
• Avoid dental light in patient's eyes; offer dark glasses for patient comfort.
• Users may report unpleasant taste while using this product.

Nedocromil Sodium

General:

• Assess salivary flow as a factor in caries, periodontal disease, and candidiasis.
• Consider semisupine chair position for patients with respiratory disease.
• Short appointments and a stress-reduction protocol may be required for anxious patients.
• Be aware that aspirin or sulfite preservatives in vasoconstrictor-containing products can exacerbate asthma.

Consultations:

• Medical consultation may be required to assess disease control.

Teach Patient/Family to:

• Avoid mouth rinses with high alcohol content because of drying effects.
• Rinse mouth with water after each inhaled dose to prevent dryness.

nefazodone hydrochloride

neh-**faz′**-oh-doan
high-droh-**klor′**-ide
(Serzone)

CATEGORY AND SCHEDULE

Pregnancy Risk Category: C

Drug Class: Antidepressant

MECHANISM OF ACTION

Exact mechanism is unknown. Appears to inhibit neuronal uptake of serotonin and norepinephrine and to antagonize α_1-adrenergic receptors.

Therapeutic Effect: Relieves depression.

USES

Treatment of major depressive disorders

N

PHARMACOKINETICS

Rapidly and completely absorbed from the GI tract; food delays absorption. Protein binding: 99%. Widely distributed in body tissues, including CNS. Extensively metabolized to active metabolites. Excreted in urine and eliminated in feces. Unknown if removed by hemodialysis. ***Half-life:*** 2–4 hr.

INDICATIONS AND DOSAGES

▸ Depression, Prevention of Relapse of Acute Depressive Episode

PO

Adults. Initially, 200 mg/day in 2 divided doses. Gradually increase by 100–200 mg/day at intervals of at least 1 wk. Range: 300–600 mg/day.

Elderly. Initially, 100 mg/day in 2 divided doses. Subsequent dosage titration based on clinical response. Range: 200–400 mg/day.

Children. 300–400 mg/day.

SIDE EFFECTS/ADVERSE REACTIONS

Frequent

Headache, dry mouth, somnolence, nausea, dizziness, constipation, insomnia, asthenia, light-headedness

Occasional

Dyspepsia, blurred vision, diarrhea, infection, confusion, abnormal vision, pharyngitis, increased appetite, orthostatic hypotension, flushing, feeling of warmth, peripheral edema, cough, flu-like symptoms

PRECAUTIONS AND CONTRAINDICATIONS

Use within 14 days of MAOIs

Caution:

Mania, hypomania, suicidal tendencies, seizures, history of MI or unstable heart conditions, hepatic impairment, lactation, children younger than 18 yr, elderly (requires dose adjustment), priapism history, alcohol use; risk in operating auto or hazardous machinery

DRUG INTERACTIONS OF CONCERN TO DENTISTRY

- Must not be used concurrently with or within 14 days of discontinuing MAOI
- Risk of significant adverse drug interaction with triazolam, alprazolam, alcohol-containing products
- Increased sedation: St. John's wort (herb)
- Acts as an inhibitor of CYP3A4 isoenzymes: risk of interaction with drugs metabolized by CYP3A4

SERIOUS REACTIONS

! Serious reactions, such as hyperthermia, rigidity, myoclonus, extreme agitation, delirium, and coma, will occur if the patient takes an MAOI concurrently or fails to let enough time elapse when switching from an MAOI to nefazodone or vice versa.

DENTAL CONSIDERATIONS

General:

• Assess salivary flow as a factor in caries, periodontal disease, and candidiasis.
• Take vital signs at every appointment because of cardiovascular side effects.
• After supine positioning, have patient sit upright for at least 2 min before standing to avoid postural hypotension.
• Advise patient if dental drugs prescribed have a potential for photosensitivity.

Consultations:

• Medical consultation may be required to assess disease control.
• Physician should be informed if significant xerostomic side effects occur (e.g., increased caries, sore tongue, problems eating or swallowing, difficulty wearing prosthesis) so that a medication change can be considered.
• Because there is no experience with the use of conscious sedation or general anesthesia in patients taking this drug, a medical consultation is recommended for risk evaluation.
• Patients showing anorexia, jaundice, GI complaints, or malaise should be referred for medical evaluation before treatment.

Teach Patient/Family to:

• When chronic dry mouth occurs, advise patient to:
  • Avoid mouth rinses with high alcohol content because of drying effects.
  • Use daily home fluoride products for anticaries effect.
  • Use sugarless gum, frequent sips of water, or saliva substitutes.

nelarabine

nel-**ay**′-reh-been
(Arranon)

CATEGORY AND SCHEDULE

Pregnancy Risk Category: D

Drug Class: Antineoplastic

MECHANISM OF ACTION

A prodrug of deoxyguanosine analogue 9-β-D-arabinofuranosylguanine (ara-G) that disrupts DNA synthesis.
Therapeutic Effect: Induces cellular apoptosis.

USES

Treatment of relapsed or refractory T-cell acute lymphoblastic leukemia (ALL) and T-cell lymphoblastic lymphoma

PHARMACOKINETICS

Protein binding: less than 25%. Metabolized in liver to ara-G (active); also hydrolyzed to methyl guanine. Excreted in urine.
Half-life: 30 min (nelarabine); 3 hr (ara-G).

INDICATIONS AND DOSAGES

▸ T-cell ALL (Relapsed or Refractory)

IV

Adults. 1500 mg/m^2 delivered as a 2-hr infusion on days 1, 3, and 5 of a 21-day treatment cycle. Treatment cycles should be repeated until evidence of disease progression is observed.

Children. 650 mg/m^2 delivered as a 1-hr infusion daily for days 1–5 of a 21-day treatment cycle. Treatment cycles should be repeated until evidence of disease progression is observed.

▸ T-cell Lymphoblastic Lymphoma (Relapsed or Refractory)

IV

Adults. 1500 mg/m^2 delivered as a 2-hr infusion on days 1, 3, and 5 of a 21-day treatment cycle. Treatment cycles should be repeated until evidence of disease progression is observed.

Children. 650 mg/m^2 delivered as a 1-hr infusion daily for days 1–5 of a 21-day treatment cycle. Treatment cycles should be repeated until evidence of disease progression is observed.

SIDE EFFECTS/ADVERSE REACTIONS

Frequent

Anemia, neutropenia, thrombocytopenia, fatigue, nausea, leukopenia, cough, fever, diarrhea, vomiting, somnolence, dizziness, constipation, peripheral neuropathy, dyspnea, headache, hypoesthesia, weakness, peripheral edema, febrile neutropenia, hypokalemia, petechiae, edema, pain, albumin decreased, bilirubin increased, pleural effusion

Occasional

Abdominal pain, anorexia, arthralgia, infection, ataxia, back pain, muscle weakness, rigors, stomatitis, hypotension, tachycardia, hypocalcemia, confusion, epistaxis, pneumonia, sinusitis, insomnia, dehydration, limb pain, abnormal gait, depressed level of consciousness, hypomagnesemia, depression, seizure, hyper-/hypoglycemia, abdominal distension, AST increased, creatinine increased, noncardiac chest pain, wheezing, chest pain, tremor, blurred vision, motor dysfunction, taste perversion, amnesia, balance disorder, nerve paralysis, sensory loss

Rare

Aphasia, cerebral hemorrhage, coma, encephalopathy, hemiparesis, hydrocephalus, lethargy, leukoencephalopathy, loss of consciousness, mental impairment, neuropathic pain, nerve palsy, nystagmus, paralysis, sciatica, sensory disturbance, speech disorder, demyelination, ascending peripheral neuropathy, dysarthria, hyporeflexia, hypertonia, incoordination, sinus headache (1%)

PRECAUTIONS AND CONTRAINDICATIONS

Hypersensitivity to nelarabine or its components

Caution:

Do not breast-feed, compromised bone marrow reserve, chickenpox, herpes zoster, history of gout, infection

DRUG INTERACTIONS OF CONCERN TO DENTISTRY

- None reported

SERIOUS REACTIONS

! Severe neurologic events have been reported with the use of nelarabine including altered mental states, severe somnolence, convulsions, peripheral neuropathy ranging from numbness and paresthesias to motor weakness and paralysis.

! Demyelination and ascending peripheral neuropathies similar in appearance to Guillain-Barré syndrome have been reported.

! Leukopenia, anemia, neutropenia, and thrombocytopenia have been associated with nelarabine therapy.

DENTAL CONSIDERATIONS

General:

- Monitor vital signs at every appointment because of cardiovascular and respiratory adverse effects.
- Avoid aspirin and NSAIDs to prevent gastrointestinal irritation and excessive bleeding.
- Examine patient carefully for oral manifestations of opportunistic infections, blood dyscrasias, and stomatitis and mucositis.
- Confirm patient's disease status and treatment regimen.
- Chlorhexidine mouth rinse prior to and during chemotherapy may reduce severity of mucositis.
- Palliative medication may be required for management of oral adverse effects of drug.
- Patient may be taking prophylactic antiinfective drug.
- Place patient on frequent recall due to adverse oral effects of drug.

Consultations:

- Consult physician to determine control of disease and ability of patient to tolerate dental procedures.
- Consult physician to determine need for prophylactic or therapeutic antiinfective medications if oral surgery or periodontal treatment is required.
- Consult physician to assess patient's immunologic and coagulation status and determine safety risk, if any, posed by the required dental treatment.

Teach Patient/Family to:

- Be aware of oral adverse effects of drug.
- Use atraumatic, effective oral hygiene measures to prevent or minimize soft tissue inflammation.
- Report oral lesions, soreness, or bleeding to dentist.
- Update health and medication history if physician makes any changes in evaluation or drug regimen; include OTC, herbal, and nonherbal drug in update.

nelfinavir

nel-**fin**′-eh-veer

(Viracept)

CATEGORY AND SCHEDULE

Pregnancy Risk Category: B

Drug Class: Antiviral

MECHANISM OF ACTION

Inhibits the activity of HIV-1 protease, the enzyme necessary for the formation of infectious HIV. ***Therapeutic Effect:*** Formation of immature noninfectious viral particles rather than HIV replication.

USES

Treatment of HIV infection when indicated by surrogate marker changes in patients receiving nelfinavir in combination with nucleoside analogues or alone for up to 24 wk

PHARMACOKINETICS

Well absorbed after PO administration (absorption increased with food). Protein binding: 98%.

Metabolized in the liver. Highly bound to plasma proteins. Eliminated primarily in feces. Unknown if removed by hemodialysis. ***Half-life:*** 3.5–5 hr.

INDICATIONS AND DOSAGES

▸ HIV Infection

PO

Adults. 750 mg (three 250-mg tablets) 3 times a day or 1250 mg twice a day in combination with nucleoside analogs (enhances antiviral activity).

Children 2–13 yr. 0–30 mg/kg/dose 3 times a day. Maximum: 750 mg q8h.

SIDE EFFECTS/ADVERSE REACTIONS

Frequent

Diarrhea

Occasional

Nausea, rash

Rare

Flatulence, asthenia

PRECAUTIONS AND CONTRAINDICATIONS

Concurrent administration with midazolam, rifampin, or triazolam

Caution:

Pediatric use, phenylketonuria (powder contains phenylalanine), diabetes mellitus, hyperglycemia, hepatic impairment, development of resistance, hemophilia, lactation, children younger than 2 yr, an inhibitor of CYP3A4 isoenzymes; use with caution with drugs that are inducers of CYP3A4 or CYP2C19 isoenzymes

DRUG INTERACTIONS OF CONCERN TO DENTISTRY

• Contraindicated with triazolam, midazolam, and other drugs dependent on CYP3A4 for metabolism

• Increased plasma levels: azithromycin, ketoconazole

• Increased plasma concentrations of fentanyl

SERIOUS REACTIONS

• None known

DENTAL CONSIDERATIONS

General:

• Examine for oral manifestation of opportunistic infection.

• Patients on chronic drug therapy may rarely have symptoms of blood dyscrasias, which can include infection, bleeding, and poor healing.

• Palliative medication may be required for management of oral side effects.

Consultations:

• In a patient with symptoms of blood dyscrasias, request a medical consultation for blood studies and postpone treatment until normal values are reestablished.

• Medical consultation may be required to assess disease control.

Teach Patient/Family to:

• Encourage effective oral hygiene to prevent soft tissue inflammation.

• Use caution to prevent trauma when using oral hygiene aids.

• Update health and drug history if physician makes any changes in evaluation or drug regimens; include OTC, herbal, and nonherbal drugs in the update.

• See dentist immediately if secondary oral infection occurs.

neostigmine

nee-oh-**stig′**-meen
(Prostigmin)
Do not confuse neostigmine with physostigmine.

CATEGORY AND SCHEDULE

Pregnancy Risk Category: C

Drug Class: Cholinesterase inhibitor

MECHANISM OF ACTION

A cholinergic that prevents destruction of acetylcholine by inhibiting the enzyme acetylcholinesterase, thus enhancing impulse transmission across the myoneural junction.
Therapeutic Effect: Improves intestinal and skeletal muscle tone; stimulates salivary and sweat gland secretions.

USES

Myasthenia gravis, nondepolarizing neuromuscular blocker, antagonist, bladder distention, postoperative ileus

PHARMACOKINETICS

PO: Onset 45–75 min, duration 2.5–4 hr.
IM/Subcutaneous: Onset 10–30 min, duration 2.5–4 hr.
IV: Onset 4–8 min, duration 2–4 hr
Metabolized in liver, excreted in urine.

INDICATIONS AND DOSAGES

▸ Myasthenia Gravis

PO

Adults, Elderly. Initially, 15–30 mg 3–4 times a day. Increase as necessary. Maintenance: 150 mg/day (range of 15–375 mg).
Children. 2 mg/kg/day or 60 mg/m^2/day divided q3–4h.

IV, IM, Subcutaneous

Adults. 0.5–2.5 mg as needed.
Children. 0.01–0.04 mg/kg q2–4h.

▸ Diagnosis of Myasthenia Gravis

IM

Adults, Elderly. 0.022 mg/kg. If cholinergic reaction occurs, discontinue tests and administer 0.4–0.6 mg or more atropine sulfate IV.
Children. 0.025–0.04 mg/kg preceded by atropine sulfate 0.011 mg/kg subcutaneously.

▸ Prevention of Postoperative Urinary Retention

IM, Subcutaneous

Adults, Elderly. 0.25 mg q4–6h for 2–3 days.

▸ Postoperative Abdominal Distention and Urine Retention

IM, Subcutaneous

Adults, Elderly. 0.5–1 mg. Catheterize patient if voiding does not occur within 1 hr. After voiding, administer 0.5 mg q3h for 5 injections.

▸ Reversal of Neuromuscular Blockade

IV

Adults, Elderly. 0.5–2.5 mg given slowly.
Children. 0.025–0.08 mg/kg/dose.
Infants. 0.025–0.1 mg/kg/dose.

SIDE EFFECTS/ADVERSE REACTIONS

Frequent

Muscarinic effects (diarrhea, diaphoresis, increased salivation, nausea, vomiting, abdominal cramps or pain)

Occasional

Muscarinic effects (urinary urgency or frequency, increased bronchial secretions, miosis, lacrimation)

PRECAUTIONS AND CONTRAINDICATIONS

GI or GU obstruction, peritonitis
Caution:
Bradycardia, hypotension, seizure disorders, bronchial asthma, coronary occlusion, hyperthyroidism, dysrhythmias, peptic ulcer, megacolon, poor GI motility, lactation, children

DRUG INTERACTIONS OF CONCERN TO DENTISTRY

- Decreased action: hydrocarbon inhalation anesthetics, corticosteroids
- Decreased action of anticholinergics (may be contraindicated)
- Increased action of succinylcholine
- Increased toxicity of ester-type local anesthetics

SERIOUS REACTIONS

! Overdose produces a cholinergic crisis manifested as abdominal discomfort or cramps, nausea, vomiting, diarrhea, flushing, facial warmth, excessive salivation, diaphoresis, lacrimation, pallor, bradycardia or tachycardia, hypotension, bronchospasm, urinary urgency, blurred vision, miosis, and fasciculation (involuntary muscular contractions visible under the skin).

DENTAL CONSIDERATIONS

General:
- Monitor vital signs at every appointment because of cardiovascular and respiratory side effects.
- Early-morning and brief appointments are preferred because of effects of disease on oral musculature.

Consultations:
- Take precautions if dental surgery is anticipated and anesthesia is required.
- Medical consultation may be required to assess disease control and patient's tolerance for stress.

nevirapine

neh-**veer′**-ah-peen
(Viramune)

CATEGORY AND SCHEDULE

Pregnancy Risk Category: C

Drug Class: Antiviral

MECHANISM OF ACTION

A nonnucleoside reverse transcriptase inhibitor that binds directly to HIV-1 reverse transcriptase, thus changing the shape of this enzyme and blocking RNA- and DNA-dependent polymerase activity.
Therapeutic Effect: Interferes with HIV replication, slowing the progression of HIV infection.

USES

Treatment in combination with nucleoside analogues for HIV-1 infection in adults who have demonstrated clinical or immunologic deterioration

PHARMACOKINETICS

Readily absorbed after PO administration. Protein binding: 60%. Widely distributed. Extensively metabolized in the liver. Excreted primarily in urine. ***Half-life:*** 45 hr (single dose), 25–30 hr (multiple doses).

INDICATIONS AND DOSAGES

▸ **HIV Infection**

PO

Adults. 200 mg once a day for 14 days (to reduce the risk of rash). Maintenance: 200 mg twice a day in combination with nucleoside analogs.

Children older than 8 yr. 4 mg/kg once a day for 14 days; then 4 mg/kg twice a day. Maximum: 400 mg/day.

Children 2 mo–8 yr. 4 mg/kg once a day for 14 days; then 7 mg/kg twice a day.

SIDE EFFECTS/ADVERSE REACTIONS

Frequent

Rash, fever, headache, nausea, granulocytopenia (more common in children)

Occasional

Stomatitis (burning, erythema, or ulceration of the oral mucosa; dysphagia)

Rare

Paresthesia, myalgia, abdominal pain

PRECAUTIONS AND CONTRAINDICATIONS

Hypersensitivity, protease inhibitors

Caution:

Severe life-threatening skin reactions (Stevens-Johnson syndrome), fatal hepatotoxicity has occurred, renal dysfunction, lactation, children

DRUG INTERACTIONS OF CONCERN TO DENTISTRY

• Should not be given with ketoconazole; monitor patients when other CYP3A4 isoenzyme inhibitors are used.

SERIOUS REACTIONS

! Hepatitis and rash may become severe and life threatening.

DENTAL CONSIDERATIONS

General:

• Determine why patient is taking the drug.

• Examine for oral manifestation of opportunistic infection.

Consultations:

• Medical consultation may be required to assess disease control.

Teach Patient/Family to:

• Encourage effective oral hygiene to prevent soft tissue inflammation.

• Report oral lesions, soreness, or bleeding to dentist.

• Update health history/drug record if physician makes any changes in evaluation or drug regimens; include OTC, herbal, and nonherbal drugs in the update.

• See dentist immediately if secondary oral infection occurs.

niacin, nicotinic acid

nye′-ah-sin, nih-**koh′**-tin-ik **ass′**-id

(Niacor, Niaspan, Nicotinex, Slo-Niacin)

Do not confuse niacin, Niacor, or Niaspan with Minocin or nitro-bid.

CATEGORY AND SCHEDULE

Pregnancy Risk Category: A (C if used at dosages above the recommended daily allowance)

OTC

Drug Class: Vitamin B_3

MECHANISM OF ACTION

An antihyperlipidemic, water-soluble vitamin that is a component of 2 coenzymes needed for tissue

respiration, lipid metabolism, and glycogenolysis. Inhibits synthesis of very low-density lipoproteins (VLDLs).
Therapeutic Effect: Reduces total, low-density lipoprotein (LDL), and VLDL cholesterol levels and triglyceride levels; increases high-density lipoprotein (HDL) cholesterol concentration.

USES

Treatment of pellagra, hyperlipidemias (niacin), peripheral vascular disease (niacin)

PHARMACOKINETICS

Readily absorbed from the GI tract. Widely distributed. Metabolized in the liver. Primarily excreted in urine. ***Half-life:*** 45 min.

INDICATIONS AND DOSAGES

▸ **Hyperlipidemia**

PO (Immediate-Release)
Adults, Elderly. Initially, 50–100 mg twice a day for 7 days. Increase gradually by doubling dose every wk up to 1–1.5 g/day in 2–3 doses. Maximum: 3 g/day.
Children. Initially, 100–250 mg/day (maximum: 10 mg/kg/day) in 3 divided doses. May increase by 100 mg/wk or 250 mg q2–3wk. Maximum: 2250 mg/day.
PO (Timed-Release)
Adults, Elderly. Initially, 500 mg/day in 2 divided doses for 1 wk; then increase to 500 mg twice a day. Maintenance: 2 g/day.

▸ **Nutritional Supplement**

PO
Adults, Elderly. 10–20 mg/day. Maximum: 100 mg/day.

▸ **Pellagra**

PO
Adults, Elderly. 50–100 mg 3–4 times a day. Maximum: 500 mg/day.
Children. 50–100 mg 3 times a day.

SIDE EFFECTS/ADVERSE REACTIONS

Frequent
Flushing (especially of the face and neck) occurring within 20 min of drug administration and lasting for up to 30–60 min, GI upset, pruritus
Occasional
Dizziness, hypotension, headache, blurred vision, burning or tingling of skin, flatulence, nausea, vomiting, diarrhea
Rare
Hyperglycemia, glycosuria, rash, hyperpigmentation, dry skin

PRECAUTIONS AND CONTRAINDICATIONS

Active peptic ulcer disease, arterial hemorrhaging, hepatic dysfunction, hypersensitivity to niacin or tartrazine (frequently seen in patients sensitive to aspirin), severe hypotension.
Caution:
Glaucoma, cardiovascular disease, CAD, diabetes mellitus, gout, schizophrenia

DRUG INTERACTIONS OF CONCERN TO DENTISTRY

• None reported

SERIOUS REACTIONS

! Arrhythmias occur rarely.

DENTAL CONSIDERATIONS

General:
• Take vital signs at every appointment because of cardiovascular side effects.
• After supine positioning, have patient sit upright for at least 2 min before standing to avoid postural hypotension.
• Assess salivary flow as a factor in caries, periodontal disease, and candidiasis.

Teach Patient/Family to:

- When chronic dry mouth occurs, advise patient to:
  - Avoid mouth rinses with high alcohol content because of drying effects.
  - Use daily home fluoride products for anticaries effect.
  - Use sugarless gum, frequent sips of water, or saliva substitutes.

nicardipine hydrochloride

nye-**card'**-ih-peen
high-droh-**klor'**-ide
(Cardene, Cardene IV, Cardene SR)
Do not confuse nicardipine with nifedipine, Cardene with codeine, or Cardene SR with Cardizem SR or codeine.

CATEGORY AND SCHEDULE

Pregnancy Risk Category: C

Drug Class: Calcium channel blocker

MECHANISM OF ACTION

An antianginal and antihypertensive agent that inhibits calcium ion movement across cell membranes, depressing contraction of cardiac and vascular smooth muscle.
Therapeutic Effect: Increases heart rate and cardiac output. Decreases systemic vascular resistance and B/P.

USES

Treatment of chronic stable angina pectoris, hypertension

PHARMACOKINETICS

Route	Onset	Peak	Duration
PO	N/A	1–2 hr	8 hr

Rapidly, completely absorbed from the GI tract. Protein binding: 95%. Undergoes first-pass metabolism in the liver. Primarily excreted in urine. Not removed by hemodialysis.
Half-life: 2–4 hr.

INDICATIONS AND DOSAGES

▸ **Chronic Stable (Effort-Associated) Angina**

PO

Adults, Elderly. Initially, 20 mg 3 times a day. Range: 20–40 mg 3 times a day.

▸ **Essential Hypertension**

PO

Adults, Elderly. Initially, 20 mg 3 times a day. Range: 20–40 mg 3 times a day.

PO (Sustained-Release)

Adults, Elderly. Initially, 30 mg twice a day. Range: 30–60 mg twice a day.

▸ **Short-Term Treatment of Hypertension When Oral Therapy Is Not Feasible or Desirable (Substitute for Oral Nicardipine)**

IV

Adults, Elderly. 0.5 mg/hr (for patient receiving 20 mg PO q8h); 1.2 mg/hr (for patient receiving 30 mg PO q8h); 2.2 mg/hr (for patient receiving 40 mg PO q8h).

▸ **Patients Not Already Receiving Nicardipine**

IV

Adults, Elderly (gradual B/P decrease). Initially, 5 mg/hr. May increase by 2.5 mg/hr q15min. After B/P goal is achieved, decrease rate to 3 mg/hr.

Adults, Elderly (rapid B/P decrease). Initially, 5 mg/hr. May increase by

2.5 mg/hr q5min. Maximum: 15 mg/hr until desired B/P attained. After B/P goal achieved, decrease rate to 3 mg/hr.

▸ Changing From IV to Oral Antihypertensive Therapy

Adults, Elderly. Begin antihypertensives other than nicardipine when IV has been discontinued; for nicardipine, give first dose 1 hr before discontinuing IV.

▸ Dosage in Hepatic Impairment

Adults, Elderly. Initially give 20 mg twice a day; then titrate.

▸ Dosage in Renal Impairment

Adults, Elderly. Initially give 20 mg q8h (30 mg twice a day [sustained-release capsules]); then titrate.

SIDE EFFECTS/ADVERSE REACTIONS

Frequent

Headache, facial flushing, peripheral edema, light-headedness, dizziness

Occasional

Asthenia (loss of strength, energy), palpitations, angina, tachycardia

Rare

Nausea, abdominal cramps, dyspepsia, dry mouth, rash

PRECAUTIONS AND CONTRAINDICATIONS

Atrial fibrillation or flutter associated with accessory conduction pathways, cardiogenic shock, CHF, second- or third-degree heart block, severe hypotension, sinus bradycardia, ventricular tachycardia, within several hr of IV β-blocker therapy

Caution:

CHF, hypotension, hepatic injury, lactation, children, renal disease, elderly

DRUG INTERACTIONS OF CONCERN TO DENTISTRY

- Decreased effect: indomethacin, possibly other NSAIDs, phenobarbital, St. John's wort (herb)
- Increased effect: parenteral and inhalational general anesthetics or other drugs with hypotensive actions
- Possible risk of increased plasma level, monitor patient: erythromycin, ketoconazole, other CYP3A4 inhibitors
- Increased effects of nondepolarizing muscle relaxants
- Increased effects of carbamazepine

SERIOUS REACTIONS

! Overdose produces confusion, slurred speech, somnolence, marked hypotension, and bradycardia.

DENTAL CONSIDERATIONS

General:

- Monitor cardiac status; take vital signs at each appointment because of CV side effects. Consider a stress-reduction protocol to prevent stress-induced angina during the dental appointment.
- After supine positioning, have patient sit upright for at least 2 min before standing to avoid orthostatic hypotension.
- Place on frequent recall to monitor possible gingival enlargement.
- Limit use of sodium-containing products, such as saline IV fluids, for patients with a dietary salt restriction.
- Assess salivary flow as a factor in caries, periodontal disease, and candidiasis.
- Use vasoconstrictors with caution, in low doses, and with careful aspiration. Avoid use of gingival retraction cord with epinephrine.

Consultations:

- Medical consultation may be required to assess disease control and tolerance for stress.

Teach Patient/Family to:

- Encourage effective oral hygiene to prevent soft tissue inflammation and minimize gingival enlargement.
- Schedule frequent oral prophylaxis if hyperplasia occurs.
- When chronic dry mouth occurs, advise patient to:
  - Avoid mouth rinses with high alcohol content because of drying effects.
  - Use daily home fluoride products for anticaries effect.
  - Use sugarless gum, frequent sips of water, or saliva substitutes.

nicotine

nik'-oh-teen

(Commit, Habitrol[CAN], Nicabate[AUS], Nicabate CQ Clear[AUS], Nicabate CQ Lozenges[AUS], NicoDerm[CAN], NicoDerm CQ, Nicorette, Nicorette Plus[CAN], Nicotinell[AUS], Nicotrol, Nicotrol NS, Nicotrol Patch[CAN])

Do not confuse NicoDerm with Nitroderm.

CATEGORY AND SCHEDULE

Pregnancy Risk Category: D (transdermal)

OTC (NicoDerm transdermal patch, Nicotrol transdermal patch, Nicorette chewing gum)

Drug Class: Smoking deterrent

MECHANISM OF ACTION

A cholinergic-receptor agonist binds to acetylcholine receptors, producing both stimulating and depressant effects on the peripheral and central nervous systems.

Therapeutic Effect: Provides a source of nicotine during nicotine withdrawal and reduces withdrawal symptoms.

USES

Adjunct to smoking-cessation program

PHARMACOKINETICS

Absorbed slowly after transdermal administration. Protein binding: 5%. Metabolized in the liver. Excreted primarily in urine. ***Half-life:*** 4 hr.

INDICATIONS AND DOSAGES

▸ Smoking Cessation Aid to Relieve Nicotine Withdrawal Symptoms

PO (Chewing Gum)

Adults, Elderly. Usually, 10–12 pieces/day. Maximum: 30 pieces/day.

PO (Lozenge)

Adults, Elderly. One 4-mg or 2-mg lozenge q1–2h for the first 6 wk; 1 lozenge q2–4h for wk 7–9; and 1 lozenge q4–8h for wk 10–12. Maximum: 1 lozenge at a time, 5 lozenges/6 hr, 20 lozenges/day.

Transdermal

Adults, Elderly who smoke 10 cigarettes or more per day. Follow the guidelines below.

Step 1: 21 mg/day for 4–6 wk.
Step 2: 14 mg/day for 2 wk.
Step 3: 7 mg/day for 2 wk.

Adults, Elderly who smoke fewer than 10 cigarettes per day. Follow the guidelines below.

Step 1: 14 mg/day for 6 wk.
Step 2: 7 mg/day for 2 wk.

Patients weighing less than 100 lb, patients with a history of

cardiovascular disease. Initially, 14 mg/day for 4–6 wk, then 7 mg/day for 2–4 wk.
Transdermal (Nicotrol)
Adults, Elderly. 1 patch a day for 6 wk.
Nasal
Adults, Elderly. 1–2 doses/hr (1 dose = 2 sprays [1 in each nostril] = 1 mg). Maximum: 5 doses (5 mg)/hr; 40 doses (40 mg)/day.
Inhaler (Nicotrol)
Adults, Elderly. Puff on nicotine cartridge mouthpiece for about 20 min as needed.

SIDE EFFECTS/ADVERSE REACTIONS

Frequent
All forms: Hiccups, nausea
Gum: Mouth or throat soreness, nausea, hiccups
Transdermal: Erythema, pruritus, or burning at application site
Occasional
All forms: Eructation, GI upset, dry mouth, insomnia, diaphoresis, irritability
Gum: Hiccups, hoarseness
Inhaler: Mouth or throat irritation, cough
Rare
All forms: Dizziness, myalgia, arthralgia

PRECAUTIONS AND CONTRAINDICATIONS

Immediate post-MI period, life-threatening arrhythmias, severe or worsening angina
Caution:
Skin disease, angina pectoris, MI, renal or hepatic insufficiency, peptic ulcer, serious cardiac dysrhythmias, hyperthyroidism, pheochromocytoma, insulin-dependent diabetes, elderly

DRUG INTERACTIONS OF CONCERN TO DENTISTRY

- Decreased dose at cessation of smoking: acetaminophen, caffeine, oxazepam, pentazocine
- Decreased metabolism of propoxyphene (increased blood levels)

SERIOUS REACTIONS

! Overdose produces palpitations, tachyarrhythmias, seizures, depression, confusion, diaphoresis, hypotension, rapid or weak pulse, and dyspnea. Lethal dose for adults is 40–60 mg. Death results from respiratory paralysis.

DENTAL CONSIDERATIONS

General:
- Assess salivary flow as a factor in caries, periodontal disease, and candidiasis.

Teach Patient/Family to:
- When chronic dry mouth occurs, advise patient to:
  - Avoid mouth rinses with high alcohol content because of drying effects.
  - Use daily home fluoride products to prevent caries.
  - Use sugarless gum, frequent sips of water, or saliva substitutes.
- When used in conjunction with a smoking cessation program in the dental office, teach:
  - All aspects of product drug; give package insert to patient and explain:
  - That patch is to be used only to deter smoking.
  - Not to use during pregnancy; birth defects may occur.
  - To keep used and unused system out of reach of children and pets; potentially toxic if chewed or swallowed.

- To apply once per day to a non-hairy, clean, dry area of skin on upper body or upper outer arm.
- To stop smoking immediately when beginning treatment with patch.
- To apply promptly after removing from protective covering; system may lose strength.

Nicotine Polacrilex

General:

- Take vital signs at every appointment because of cardiovascular side effects.
- Temporomandibular joint (TMJ) disorder may be aggravated by chewing because of heavier viscosity of gum.

Teach Patient/Family to:

- Encourage effective oral hygiene to prevent periodontal inflammation.
- When chronic dry mouth occurs, advise patient to:
  - Avoid mouth rinses with high alcohol content because of drying effects.
  - Use daily home fluoride products for anticaries effect.
  - Use sugarless gum, frequent sips of water, or saliva substitutes.
- When used in conjunction with a smoking cessation program in the dental office, teach:
  - All aspects of product use; give package insert to patient and explain:
  - That gum is to be used only to deter smoking.
  - To avoid use in pregnancy; birth defects may occur.
  - To stop smoking when beginning treatment with gum.
  - To dispose of gum carefully because nicotine will still be present; to protect from children and pets.

nifedipine

nye-**fed′**-ih-peen

(Adalat 5[AUS], Adalat 10[AUS], Adalat 20[AUS], Adalat CC, Adalat Oros[AUS], Apo-Nifed[CAN], Nifecard[AUS], Nifedicol XL, Nifehexal[AUS], Novo-Nifedin[CAN], Nyefax[AUS], Procardia, Procardia XL)

Do not confuse nifedipine with nicardipine or nimodipine.

CATEGORY AND SCHEDULE

Pregnancy Risk Category: C

Drug Class: Calcium channel blocker

MECHANISM OF ACTION

An antianginal and antihypertensive agent that inhibits calcium ion movement across cell membranes, depressing contraction of cardiac and vascular smooth muscle.

Therapeutic Effect: Increases heart rate and cardiac output. Decreases systemic vascular resistance and B/P.

USES

Treatment of chronic stable angina pectoris, vasospastic angina, hypertension (sustained release only)

PHARMACOKINETICS

Route	Onset	Peak	Duration
Sublingual	1–5 min	N/A	N/A
PO	20–30 min	N/A	4–8 hr
PO (extended release)	2 hr	N/A	24 hr

Rapidly, completely absorbed from the GI tract. Protein binding: 92%–98%. Undergoes first-pass metabolism in the liver. Primarily excreted in urine. Not removed by hemodialysis. ***Half-life:*** 2–5 hr.

INDICATIONS AND DOSAGES

▸ Prinzmetal's Variant Angina, Chronic Stable (Effort-Associated) Angina

PO

Adults, Elderly. Initially, 10 mg 3 times a day. Increase at 7- to 14-day intervals. Maintenance: 10 mg 3 times a day up to 30 mg 4 times a day.

PO (Extended-Release)

Adults, Elderly. Initially, 30–60 mg/day. Maintenance: Up to 120 mg/day.

▸ Essential Hypertension

PO (Extended-Release)

Adults, Elderly. Initially, 30–60 mg/day. Maintenance: Up to 120 mg/day.

N

SIDE EFFECTS/ADVERSE REACTIONS

Frequent

Peripheral edema, headache, flushed skin, dizziness

Occasional

Nausea, shakiness, muscle cramps and pain, somnolence, palpitations, nasal congestion, cough, dyspnea, wheezing, oral gingival enlargement

Rare

Hypotension, rash, pruritus, urticaria, constipation, abdominal discomfort, flatulence, sexual difficulties

PRECAUTIONS AND CONTRAINDICATIONS

Advanced aortic stenosis, severe hypotension

Caution:

CHF, hypotension, sick sinus syndrome, second- or third-degree heart block, hypotension less than 90 mm Hg systolic, hepatic injury, lactation, children, renal disease

DRUG INTERACTIONS OF CONCERN TO DENTISTRY

- Decreased effect: indomethacin, possibly other NSAIDs, phenobarbital
- Increased effect: parenteral and inhalational general anesthetics or other drugs with hypotensive actions
- Possible increase in effects, monitor patients: inhibitors of CYP3A4 isoenzyme
- Increased effects of nondepolarizing muscle relaxants
- Increased effects of carbamazepine

SERIOUS REACTIONS

! Nifedipine may precipitate CHF and MI in patients with cardiac disease and peripheral ischemia.

! Overdose produces nausea, somnolence, confusion, and slurred speech.

DENTAL CONSIDERATIONS

General:

- Monitor cardiac status; take vital signs at each appointment because of cardiovascular side effects. Consider a stress-reduction protocol to prevent stress-induced angina during the dental appointment.
- After supine positioning, have patient sit upright for at least 2 min before standing to avoid orthostatic hypotension at dismissal.
- Place on frequent recall to monitor possible gingival enlargement.
- Limit use of sodium-containing products, such as saline IV fluids, for patients with a dietary salt restriction.
- Assess salivary flow as a factor in caries, periodontal disease, and candidiasis.
- Use vasoconstrictors with caution, in low doses, and with careful aspiration. Avoid use of gingival retraction cord with epinephrine.

Consultations:

- Medical consultation may be required to assess disease control and stress tolerance.

Teach Patient/Family to:

- Encourage effective oral hygiene to prevent soft tissue inflammation and minimize gingival overgrowth.
- Schedule frequent oral prophylaxis if gingival enlargement occurs.
- When chronic dry mouth occurs, advise patient to:
  - Avoid mouth rinses with high alcohol content because of drying effects.
  - Use daily home fluoride products for anticaries effect.
  - Use sugarless gum, frequent sips of water, or saliva substitutes.

nilotinib

nye-**loe**′-ti-nib
(Tasigna)

CATEGORY AND SCHEDULE

Pregnancy Risk Category: D

Drug Class: Antineoplastic agent, tyrosine kinase inhibitor

MECHANISM OF ACTION

Selectively inhibits Bcr-Abl kinase. Binds to and stabilizes the inactive conformation of the kinase domain of Abl protein. Also exhibits activity in imatinib-resistant Bcr-Abl kinase mutations.

USES

Treatment of chronic phase and accelerated phase of Philadelphia chromosome-positive chronic myelogenous leukemia (CML) in patients resistant or intolerant to prior imatinib therapy

PHARMACOKINETICS

98% protein binding. Metabolized hepatically via oxidation and hydroxylation by CYP3A4 into inactive metabolites. Bioavailability is increased by 82% when administered 30 min after a high-fat meal. ***Half-life:*** 15–17 hr. Excreted in the feces (93%; 69% as parent drug).

INDICATIONS AND DOSAGES

Treatment of chronic phase and accelerated phase Philadelphia chromosome-positive CML in patients resistant or intolerant to prior imatinib therapy

PO

Adults. 400 mg twice daily (every 12 hr).

Dosage adjustment for concomitant use with CYP3A4 inhibitors: avoid concomitant use. If required, consider reducing nilotinib by 50% to 400 mg once daily with careful monitoring.

Dosage adjustment for concomitant use with CYP3A4 inducers: avoid concomitant use. If required, consider increasing dose of nilotinib with careful monitoring.

Dosage adjustment for hepatotoxicity: If bilirubin >3 times upper limit of normal (ULN) (= grade 3): withhold nilotinib, monitor bilirubin, resume at 400 mg once daily when bilirubin returns to = 1.5 times ULN (= grade 1). If ALT or AST >5 times ULN (= grade 3): withhold nilotinib, monitor transaminases, resume at 400 mg once daily when ALT or AST returns to = 2.5 times ULN (= grade 1).

Dosage adjustment for hematologic toxicity (neutropenia and thrombocytopenia): absolute neutrophil count (ANC) <1000/mm^3 and/or platelets <50,000/mm^3: stop

nilotinib, monitor blood counts.
ANC >1000/mm^3 and platelets >50,000/mm^3 within 2 wk: continue at 400 mg twice daily.
ANC <1000/mm^3 and/or platelets <50,000/mm^3 for >2 wk: reduce dose to 400 mg once daily.
Dosage adjustment for QT prolongation:
QTc >480 msec: stop nilotinib, monitor and correct potassium and magnesium levels. QTcF returns to <450 msec and to within 20 msec of baseline within 2 wk: continue at 400 mg twice daily.
QTcF returns to 450–480 msec within 2 wk: reduce dose to 400 mg once daily. QTcF >480 msec after dosage reduction to 400 mg once daily, discontinue therapy.

SIDE EFFECTS/ADVERSE REACTIONS

Adult

Frequent

Peripheral edema, headache, fatigue, fever, rash, pruritus, hyperglycemia, nausea, diarrhea, constipation, vomiting, increased lipase, abdominal pain, neutropenia, thrombocytopenia, anemia, arthralgia, limb pain, myalgia, weakness, muscle spasm, bone pain, back pain, cough, nasopharyngitis, dyspnea

Occasional

Flushing, hypertension, palpitation, prolonged QT interval, dizziness, dysphonia, insomnia, vertigo, alopecia, dry skin, eczema, erythema, hyperhidrosis, urticaria, hypophosphatemia (10%), hypokalemia (5%), hyperkalemia (4%), hypocalcemia (4%), hyponatremia (3%), decreased albumin (1%), abdominal discomfort, dyspepsia, pancreatitis (<1%), pleural effusion (<1%), hyperbilirubinemia (10%), increased ALT (4%), increased phosphatase (3%), increased AST (1%)

PRECAUTIONS AND CONTRAINDICATIONS

Hypokalemia
Hypomagnesemia
Long QT syndrome
Avoid comitant use with QT-prolonging agents and CYP3A4 inhibitors/inducers
Use with caution in patients with bone marrow suppression, electrolyte imbalances, pancreatitis, and hepatic impairment
Administer nilotinib on an empty stomach, at least 1 hr before and 2 hr after food

DRUG INTERACTIONS OF CONCERN TO DENTISTRY

- CYP3A4 inhibitors (e.g., erythromycin): May increase the blood levels and adverse effects of nilotinib.

SERIOUS REACTIONS

! QT prolongation, which can lead to sudden death, has been reported.
! Fetal damage can occur when used in pregnant women.

DENTAL CONSIDERATIONS

General:

- Stomatitis and mouth ulceration may complicate dental treatment and oral hygiene.
- Consider semisupine chair position for patient comfort if GI side effects occur.
- Use with caution when in combination with vasoconstrictors (epinephrine, levonordefrin) in the local anesthetic regimen due to the possible risk of QT prolongation (torsade de pointes).

Consultations:
• Medical consultation may be required to assess disease control and ability of patient to tolerate dental treatment.
Teach Patient/Family to:
• Encourage effective oral hygiene to prevent soft tissue inflammation.
• Use caution to prevent injury when using oral hygiene aids.
• Be alert for the possibility of stomatitis and mouth ulcerations and the need to see dentist immediately if signs of inflammation and ulceration occur.

nilutamide

nih-**lute**′-ah-myd
(Anandron[CAN], Nilandron)

CATEGORY AND SCHEDULE

Pregnancy Risk Category: C

Drug Class: Hormone; antineoplastic

MECHANISM OF ACTION

An antiandrogen hormone and antineoplastic agent that competitively inhibits androgen action by binding to androgen receptors in target tissue.
Therapeutic Effect: Decreases growth of abnormal prostate tissue.

USES

Treatment of cancer of the prostate gland

PHARMACOKINETICS

Rapidly and completed absorbed; excreted in urine and feces as metabolites.

INDICATIONS AND DOSAGES

▸ **Prostatic Carcinoma**
PO
Adults, Elderly. 300 mg once a day for 30 days, then 150 mg once a day. Begin on day of, or day after, surgical castration.

SIDE EFFECTS/ADVERSE REACTIONS

Frequent
Hot flashes, delay in recovering vision after bright illumination (such as sun, television, bright lights), decreased libido, diminished sexual function, mild nausea, gynecomastia, alcohol intolerance
Occasional
Constipation, hypertension, dizziness, dyspnea, UTIs

PRECAUTIONS AND CONTRAINDICATIONS

Severe hepatic impairment, severe respiratory insufficiency

DRUG INTERACTIONS OF CONCERN TO DENTISTRY

• Avoid drugs that may aggravate urinary retention when symptoms are present.
• This is an inhibitor of CYP3A4 isoenzymes; no specific studies have been done, but use caution when prescribing drugs metabolized by this enzyme.

SERIOUS REACTIONS

! Interstitial pneumonitis occurs rarely.

DENTAL CONSIDERATIONS

General:
• Monitor and record vital signs.
• If additional analgesia is required for dental pain, consider alternative analgesics (NSAIDs) in patients taking narcotics for acute or chronic pain.

• Avoid dental light in patient's eyes; offer dark glasses for patient comfort.
• This drug may be used in the hospital or on an outpatient basis. Confirm the patient's disease and treatment status.
• Short appointments and a stress-reduction protocol may be required for anxious patients.

Consultations:

• Medical consultation may be required to assess immunologic status during cancer chemotherapy and determine safety risk, if any, posed by the required dental treatment.
• Medical consultation may be required to assess disease control and patient's ability to tolerate stress.

Teach Patient/Family to:

• Encourage effective oral hygiene to prevent soft tissue inflammation.
• Prevent trauma when using oral hygiene aids.
• Report oral lesions, soreness, or bleeding to dentist.
• Update health and medication history if physician makes any changes in evaluation or drug regimens; include OTC, herbal, and nonherbal in the update.

nimodipine

nye-**mode′**-ih-peen
(Nimotop)
Do not confuse nimodipine with nifedipine.

CATEGORY AND SCHEDULE

Pregnancy Risk Category: C

Drug Class: Calcium channel blockers

MECHANISM OF ACTION

A cerebral vasospasm agent that inhibits movement of calcium ions across vascular smooth-muscle cell membranes.
Therapeutic Effect: Produces favorable effect on severity of neurologic deficits due to cerebral vasospasm. Exerts greatest effect on cerebral arteries; may prevent cerebral spasm.

USES

Relief of and control of angina pectoris (chest pain)

PHARMACOKINETICS

Rapidly absorbed from the GI tract. Protein binding: 95%. Metabolized in the liver. Excreted in urine; eliminated in feces. Not removed by hemodialysis. ***Half-life:*** terminal, 3 hr.

INDICATIONS AND DOSAGES

▸ Improvement in Neurologic Deficits after Subarachnoid Hemorrhage from Ruptured Congenital Aneurysms

PO

Adults, Elderly. 60 mg q4h for 21 days. Begin within 96 hr of subarachnoid hemorrhage.

SIDE EFFECTS/ADVERSE REACTIONS

Occasional

Hypotension, peripheral edema, diarrhea, headache

Rare

Allergic reaction (rash, hives), tachycardia, flushing of skin

PRECAUTIONS AND CONTRAINDICATIONS

Atrial fibrillation or flutter, cardiogenic shock, CHF, heart block, sinus bradycardia, ventricular tachycardia, within several hr of IV β-blocker therapy

DRUG INTERACTIONS OF CONCERN TO DENTISTRY

- Hypotension: anesthetics, other antihypertensive medications
- Antagonism of antihypertensive effect: indomethacin and possibly other NSAIDs
- Possible reduction in antihypertensive effects: sympathomimetics

SERIOUS REACTIONS

! Overdose produces nausea, weakness, dizziness, somnolence, confusion, and slurred speech.

DENTAL CONSIDERATIONS

General:

- Patients may have significant neurologic deficit; dental care may not be practical.
- Avoid vasoconstrictors or limit doses appropriately.
- Caution: potential for interactions with drugs used in dentistry.
- Determine why patient is taking the drug.
- Monitor for possible gingival enlargement.
- Monitor and record vital signs.
- After supine positioning, have patient sit upright for at least 2 min before standing to avoid orthostatic hypotension.

Consultations:

- This drug may be used in the hospital or on an outpatient basis. Confirm the patient's disease and treatment status.
- Medical consultation may be required to assess disease control and patient's ability to tolerate stress.

Teach Patient/Family to:

- Encourage effective oral hygiene to prevent soft tissue inflammation.
- Update health and medication history if physician makes any changes in evaluation or drug regimens; include OTC, herbal, and nonherbal drugs in the update.

nipradilol

ni-**pra**-dih-lole
(Hypadil [JAPAN])

CATEGORY AND SCHEDULE

Drug Class: β-adrenergic blocker (non-selective)

MECHANISM OF ACTION

Non-selective β blocker with α-1 blocking activity. Nitroglycerin-like vasodilator properties.
Therapeutic Effect: Reduces B/P, improved myocardial ischemia, reduces heart rate. Reduces intraocular pressure. Decreases peripheral vascular resistance.

USES

Essential hypertension
Angina pectoris
Open-angle glaucoma
Ocular hypertension
Cardiomyopathy
Parkinsonian tremor

PHARMACOKINETICS

Bioavailability: 29%–47%. Protein binding: less than 30%. Extensively distributed in tissues. Ophthalmic: rapidly reaches ocular tissue.
Half-life: 2 hr.

INDICATIONS AND DOSAGES

▸ Hypertension, Essential
PO
Adults. 3–9 mg twice day.

▸ Angina
PO
Adults. 3–6 mg twice a day.

▸ Cardiomyopathy
PO
Adults. 1.5–9 mg/day.

▸ Parkinsonian Tremor
PO
Adults. 3 mg twice a day.

▸ Glaucoma
Ophthalmic
Adults. Apply 0.25% twice/day.

▸ Ocular Hypertension
Ophthalmic
Adults. 0.25% twice/day.

SIDE EFFECTS/ADVERSE REACTIONS

Frequency not defined
Oral: Bradycardia, circulatory disturbances, shortness of breath, dizziness, headache, drowsiness, insomnia, GI symptoms, weakness, sweating, tinnitus, hypersensitivity, orthostatic hypotension, arrhythmias, hypoglycemia, nausea, anorexia, thrombocytosis, vertigo
Ophthalmic: Blepharitis, eyelid pruritus, punctate keratitis, corneal erosion, eyelid contact eczema, eye irritation and redness

PRECAUTIONS AND CONTRAINDICATIONS

Hypersensitivity to nipradilol or any component of the formulation
Bronchial asthma or related bronchospastic conditions
Cardiogenic shock
Pulmonary edema
Second- or third-degree AV block
Severe bradycardia
Diabetic ketoacidosis
Metabolic acidosis
Left ventricular dysfunction

Caution:
Anesthesia/surgery
Abrupt withdrawal
Bronchial asthma or related bronchospastic conditions
Cerebrovascular insufficiency
CHF
Diabetes mellitus
Hyperthyroidism/thyrotoxicosis
Myasthenic conditions
Peripheral vascular disease
Hepatic dysfunction
Renal dysfunction

DRUG INTERACTIONS OF CONCERN TO DENTISTRY

- Diuretics, other antihypertensives: May increase hypotensive effect of nipradilol.
- Sympathomimetics, xanthines: Possible increased systolic BP, bradycardia. May antagonize the effects and reduce bronchodilation.
- Oral hypoglycemics and insulin: May mask symptoms of hypoglycemia and prolong hypoglycemic effect of insulin and oral hypoglycemics.
- NSAIDs: May reduce the antihypertensive effect of nipradilol.
- Digoxin: May cause serious bradycardia.
- Calcium channel blockers (verapamil, diltiazem): May cause hypotension and bradycardia.
- Latanoprost: Additive effects.

SERIOUS REACTIONS

! Ophthalmic overdose may produce bradycardia, hypotension, bronchospasm, and acute cardiac failure.

DENTAL CONSIDERATIONS

General:
- Monitor vital signs at every appointment because of cardiovascular side effects.

• Assess salivary flow as a factor in caries, periodontal disease, and candidiasis.
• Limit use of sodium-containing products, such as saline IV fluids, for those patients with dietary salt restriction.

Consultations:

• Medical consultation may be required to assess disease control.

Teach Patient/Family to:

• Report oral lesions, soreness, or bleeding to dentist.
• When chronic dry mouth occurs, advise patient to:
  • Avoid mouth rinses with high alcohol content because of drying effects.
  • Use daily home fluoride products for anticaries effect.
  • Use sugarless gum, frequent sips of water, or saliva substitutes.

nisoldipine

nye-**soul′**-dih-peen
(Sular)
Do not confuse with nicardipine.

CATEGORY AND SCHEDULE

Pregnancy Risk Category: C

Drug Class: Calcium channel antagonist (dihydropyridine group)

MECHANISM OF ACTION

A calcium channel blocker that inhibits calcium ion movement across cell membrane, depressing contraction of cardiac and vascular smooth muscle.
Therapeutic Effect: Increases heart rate and cardiac output. Decreases systemic vascular resistance and B/P.

USES

Hypertension as a single agent or in combination with other antihypertensive medications

PHARMACOKINETICS

Poor absorption from the GI tract. Food increases bioavailability. Protein binding: more than 99%. Metabolism occurs in the gut wall. Primarily excreted in urine. Not removed by hemodialysis. ***Half-life:*** 7–12 hr.

INDICATIONS AND DOSAGES

▸ **Hypertension**

PO

Adults. Initially, 20 mg once daily, then increase by 10 mg/wk, or longer intervals until therapeutic B/P response is attained.
Initially, 10 mg once daily. Increase by 10 mg/wk to therapeutic response. Maintenance: 20–40 mg once daily. Maximum: 60 mg once daily.

SIDE EFFECTS/ADVERSE REACTIONS

Frequent

Giddiness, dizziness, light-headedness, peripheral edema, headache, flushing, weakness, nausea, oral gingival enlargement

Occasional

Transient hypotension, heartburn, muscle cramps, nasal congestion, cough, wheezing, sore throat, palpitations, nervousness, mood changes

Rare

Increase in frequency, intensity, duration of anginal attack during initial therapy

PRECAUTIONS AND CONTRAINDICATIONS

Sick-sinus syndrome or second- or third-degree AV block (except in

presence of pacemaker), hypersensitivity to nisoldipine or any component of the formulation
Caution:
Avoid high-fat meals, severe coronary artery disease, monitor B/P, CHF, severe hepatic impairment, do not break or crush tablets, lactation, geriatric patients

SERIOUS REACTIONS

May precipitate CHF and MI in patients with cardiac disease and peripheral ischemia.
Overdose produces nausea, drowsiness, confusion, and slurred speech.

DENTAL CONSIDERATIONS

General:
- Stress from dental procedures may compromise cardiovascular function; determine patient risk.
- Avoid vasoconstrictors or limit doses appropriately.
- Monitor vital signs at every appointment because of cardiovascular side effects.
- Short appointments and a stress-reduction protocol may be required for anxious patients.
- Grapefruit juice may increase plasma levels.
- Monitor for possible gingival enlargement.
- Limit use of sodium-containing products, such as saline IV fluids, for patients with a dietary salt restriction.
- After supine positioning, have patient sit upright for at least 2 min before standing to avoid orthostatic hypotension.
- Assess salivary flow as a factor in caries, periodontal disease, and candidiasis.

Consultations:
- Medical consultation may be required to assess disease control and patient's ability to tolerate stress.

Teach Patient/Family to:
- Schedule frequent oral prophylaxis if gingival enlargement occurs.
- When chronic dry mouth occurs, advise patient to:
  - Avoid mouth rinses with high alcohol content because of drying effects.
  - Use daily home fluoride products for anticaries effect.
  - Use sugarless gum, frequent sips of water, or saliva substitutes.

nitazoxanide

nigh-taz-**oks**′-ah-nide
(Alinia)

CATEGORY AND SCHEDULE

Pregnancy Risk Category: B

Drug Class: Antiprotozoals

MECHANISM OF ACTION

An antiparasitic that interferes with the body's reaction to pyruvate ferredoxin oxidoreductase, an enzyme essential for anaerobic energy metabolism.
Therapeutic Effect: Produces antiprotozoal activity, reducing or terminating diarrheal episodes.

USES

Treatment of diarrhea that is caused by certain types of protozoa (tiny, 1-celled animals)

PHARMACOKINETICS

Rapidly hydrolyzed to an active metabolite. Protein binding: 99%. Excreted in the urine, bile, and feces. ***Half-life:*** 2–4 hr.

INDICATIONS AND DOSAGES

▸ Diarrhea

PO

Children 12 yr and older. 200 mg q12h.

Children 4–11 yr. 200 mg (10 ml) q12h for 3 days.

Children 12–47 mo. 100 mg (5 ml) q12h for 3 days.

SIDE EFFECTS/ADVERSE REACTIONS

Occasional

Abdominal pain

Rare

Diarrhea, vomiting, headache

PRECAUTIONS AND CONTRAINDICATIONS

History of sensitivity to aspirin and salicylates

DRUG INTERACTIONS OF CONCERN TO DENTISTRY

- None reported

SERIOUS REACTIONS

! None known

DENTAL CONSIDERATIONS

General:

- This is an acute-use drug; patients highly unlikely to present for dental care.
- Ensure patients are well hydrated and electrolytes reestablished following recovery if they present for dental treatment.

Consultations:

- Medical consultation may be required to assess disease control.

Teach Patient/Family to:

- Maintain or reestablish oral hygiene care.

nitrofurantoin sodium

nye-troe-**fyoor′**-an-toyn **soe′**-dee-um

(Apo-Nitrofurantoin[CAN], Furadantin, Macrobid, Macrodantin, Novo-Furan[CAN], Ralodantin[AUS])

CATEGORY AND SCHEDULE

Pregnancy Risk Category: B

Drug Class: Urinary tract antiinfective

MECHANISM OF ACTION

An antibacterial UTI agent that inhibits the synthesis of bacterial DNA, RNA, proteins, and cell walls by altering or inactivating ribosomal proteins.

Therapeutic Effect: Bacteriostatic (bactericidal at high concentrations).

USES

Treatment of UTIs caused by *E. coli, Klebsiella, Pseudomonas, P. vulgaris, P. morganii, Serratia, Citrobacter, S. aureus*

PHARMACOKINETICS

Microcrystalline form rapidly and completely absorbed; macrocrystalline form more slowly absorbed. Food increases absorption. Protein binding: 40%. Primarily concentrated in urine and kidneys. Metabolized in most body tissues. Primarily excreted in urine. Removed by hemodialysis. ***Half-life:*** 20–60 min.

INDICATIONS AND DOSAGES

▸ UTIs

PO (Furadantin, Macrodantin)
Adults, Elderly. 50–100 mg q6h. Maximum: 400 mg/day.
Children. 5–7 mg/kg/day in divided doses q6h. Maximum: 400 mg/day.
PO (Macrobid)
Adults, Elderly. 100 mg twice a day. Maximum: 400 mg/day.

▸ Long-Term Prevention of UTIs

PO
Adults, Elderly. 50–100 mg at bedtime.
Children. 1–2 mg/kg/day as a single dose. Maximum: 100 mg/day.

SIDE EFFECTS/ADVERSE REACTIONS

Frequent
Anorexia, nausea, vomiting, dark urine
Occasional
Abdominal pain, diarrhea, rash, pruritus, urticaria, hypertension, headache, dizziness, drowsiness
Rare
Photosensitivity, transient alopecia, asthmatic exacerbation in those with history of asthma

PRECAUTIONS AND CONTRAINDICATIONS

Anuria, oliguria, substantial renal impairment (creatinine clearance less than 40 ml/min); infants younger than 1 mo because of the risk of hemolytic anemia
Caution:
Lactation

DRUG INTERACTIONS OF CONCERN TO DENTISTRY

• Increased effects: anticholinergic drugs

SERIOUS REACTIONS

! Superinfection, hepatotoxicity, peripheral neuropathy (may be irreversible), Stevens-Johnson syndrome, permanent pulmonary function impairment, and anaphylaxis occur rarely.

DENTAL CONSIDERATIONS

General:
• Determine why the patient is taking the drug.
Consultations:
• Medical consultation may be required to assess disease control and to select an antiinfective if a dental infection is diagnosed.

nitrofurazone

nye-troe-**fyoor′**-ah-zone
(Furacin)
Do not confuse with nitrofurantoin.

CATEGORY AND SCHEDULE

Pregnancy Risk Category: C
OTC (ointment)

Drug Class: Antibacterial, topical

MECHANISM OF ACTION

A synthetic nitrofuran that inhibits bacterial enzymes involved in carbohydrate metabolism.
Therapeutic Effect: Inhibits a variety of enzymes. Bactericidal.

USES

Surface skin infections, including *S. aureus, streptococci, E. coli, C. perfringens, E. aerogens, Proteus* spp.

PHARMACOKINETICS

Not known

INDICATIONS AND DOSAGES

▸ **Burns, Catheter-Related UTI, Skin Grafts**

Topical

Adults. Apply directly on lesion with spatula or place on a piece of gauze first. Use of a bandage is optional. Preparation should remain on lesion for at least 24 hr. Dressing may be changed several times daily or left on the lesion for a longer period.

SIDE EFFECTS/ADVERSE REACTIONS

Occasional

Itching, rash, swelling

PRECAUTIONS AND CONTRAINDICATIONS

Hypersensitivity to nitrofurazone or any of its components

DRUG INTERACTIONS OF CONCERN TO DENTISTRY

• None reported

SERIOUS REACTIONS

! Use of nitrofurazone may result in bacterial or fungal overgrowth of nonsusceptible pathogens, which may lead to secondary infection.

DENTAL CONSIDERATIONS

General:

• Dental management depends on extent and severity of burns and patient's ability to cooperate; use aseptic techniques.

• Provide palliative dental care for dental emergencies only.

• Monitor and record vital signs.

Consultations:

• Medical consultation may be required to assess disease control and patient's ability to tolerate stress.

• Consult patient's physician if an acute dental infection occurs and another antiinfective is required.

Teach Patient/Family to:

• Encourage effective oral hygiene to prevent soft tissue inflammation.

• Prevent trauma when using oral hygiene aids.

nitroglycerin

nye-troe-**gli′**-ser-in

(Anginine[AUS], Minitran, Nitradisc[AUS], Nitrek, Nitro-Bid, Nitro-Dur, Nitrogard, Nitroject[CAN], Nitrolingual, Nitrolingual Spray[AUS], Nitrong-SR, NitroQuick, Nitrostat, Nitro-Tab, Rectogesic[AUS], Transiderm Nitro[AUS], Trinipatch[CAN])

Do not confuse nitroglycerin with nitroprusside; Nitro-Bid with Nicobid; Nitro-Dur with NicoDerm; Nitrostat with Hyperstat, Nilstat, or Nystatin; or Nitrong-SR with Nizoral.

CATEGORY AND SCHEDULE

Pregnancy Risk Category: B

Drug Class: Inorganic nitrate, vasodilator

N

MECHANISM OF ACTION

A nitrate that decreases myocardial oxygen demand. Reduces left ventricular preload and afterload. ***Therapeutic Effect:*** Dilates coronary arteries and improves collateral blood flow to ischemic areas within myocardium. Produces peripheral vasodilation.

USES

Treatment of chronic stable angina pectoris, prophylaxis of angina pain, CHF associated with acute MI, controlled hypotension in surgical procedures

PHARMACOKINETICS

Route	Onset	Peak	Duration
Sublingual	1–3 min	4–8 min	30–60 min
Translingual spray	2 min	4–10 min	30–60 min
Buccal tablet	2–5 min	4–10 min	2 hr
PO (extended release)	20–45 min	45–120 min	4–8 hr
Topical	15–60 min	30–120 min	2–12 hr
Transdermal patch	40–60 min	60–180 min	18–24 hr
IV	1–2 min	Immediate	3–5 min

Well absorbed after PO, sublingual, and topical administration. Undergoes extensive first-pass metabolism. Metabolized in the liver and by enzymes in the bloodstream. Primarily excreted in urine. Not removed by hemodialysis. ***Half-life:*** 1–4 min.

INDICATIONS AND DOSAGES

▸ Acute Relief of Angina Pectoris, Acute Prophylaxis

Lingual Spray

Adults, Elderly. 1 spray onto or under tongue q3–5min until relief is noted (no more than 3 sprays in 15-min period).

Sublingual

Adults, Elderly. 0.4 mg q5min until relief is noted (no more than 3 doses in 15-min period). Use prophylactically 5–10 min before activities that may cause an acute attack.

▸ Long-Term Prophylaxis of Angina

PO (Extended-Release)

Adults, Elderly. 2.5–9 mg q8–12h.

Topical

Adults, Elderly. Initially, 1/2 inch q8h. Increase by 1/2 inch with each application. Range: 1–2 inches q8h up to 4–5 inches q4h.

Transdermal Patch

Adults, Elderly. Initially, 0.2–0.4 mg/hr. Maintenance: 0.4–0.8 mg/hr. Consider patch on for 12–14 hr, patch off for 10–12 hr (prevents tolerance).

▸ CHF Associated with Acute MI

IV

Adults, Elderly. Initially, 5 mcg/min via infusion pump. Increase in 5-mcg/min increments at 3- to 5-min intervals until B/P response is noted or until dosage reaches 20 mcg/min; then increase as needed by 10 mcg/min. Dosage may be further titrated according to clinical, therapeutic response up to 200 mcg/min.

Children. Initially, 0.25–0.5 mcg/kg/min; titrate by 0.5–1 mcg/kg/min up to 20 mcg/kg/min.

SIDE EFFECTS/ADVERSE REACTIONS

Frequent

Headache (possibly severe; occurs mostly in early therapy, diminishes rapidly in intensity, and usually disappears during continued treatment), transient flushing of face and neck, dizziness (especially if patient is standing immobile or is in a warm environment), weakness, orthostatic hypotension

Sublingual: Burning, tingling sensation at oral point of dissolution

Ointment: Erythema, pruritus

Occasional

GI upset

Transdermal: Contact dermatitis

PRECAUTIONS AND CONTRAINDICATIONS

Allergy to adhesives (transdermal), closed-angle glaucoma, constrictive pericarditis (IV), early MI (sublingual), GI hypermotility or malabsorption (extended-release), head trauma, hypotension (IV), inadequate cerebral circulation (IV), increased intracranial pressure, nitrates, orthostatic hypotension, pericardial tamponade (IV), severe anemia, uncorrected hypovolemia (IV)

Caution:

Postural hypotension, lactation

DRUG INTERACTIONS OF CONCERN TO DENTISTRY

• Increased hypotensive effects: alcohol, opioids, benzodiazepines, phenothiazines, and other drugs used in conscious sedation techniques

SERIOUS REACTIONS

! Nitroglycerin should be discontinued if blurred vision or dry mouth occurs.

! Severe orthostatic hypotension may occur, manifested by fainting, pulselessness, cold or clammy skin, and diaphoresis.

! Tolerance may occur with repeated, prolonged therapy; minor tolerance may occur with intermittent use of sublingual tablets.

! High doses of nitroglycerin tend to produce severe headache.

DENTAL CONSIDERATIONS

General:

• Take vital signs at every appointment because of cardiovascular side effects.

• After supine positioning, have patient sit upright for at least 2 min before standing to avoid orthostatic hypotension.

• Assess salivary flow as a factor in caries, periodontal disease, and candidiasis.

• Ensure that patient's drug is easily available if angina occurs.

• A benzodiazepine or nitrous oxide/oxygen may be prescribed to allay anxiety.

• Check expiration date on prescription to ensure drug activity. If bottle has been opened, the shelf life is 3 mo.

• Stress from dental procedures may compromise cardiovascular function; determine patient risk.

• Talk with patient about disease control (frequency of angina episodes).

• Use vasoconstrictors with caution, in low doses, and with careful aspiration. Avoid gingival retraction cord with epinephrine.

• Short appointments and a stress-reduction protocol may be required for anxious patients.

• Consider semisupine chair position for patients with cardiovascular disease.

Consultations:

• Medical consultation may be required to assess disease control and patient's ability to tolerate stress.

Teach Patient/Family to:

• Encourage effective oral hygiene to prevent soft tissue inflammation.

• Use caution to prevent injury when using oral hygiene aids.

• When chronic dry mouth occurs, advise patient to:

  • Avoid mouth rinses with high alcohol content because of drying effects.

  • Use daily home fluoride products for anticaries effect.

  • Use sugarless gum, frequent sips of water, or saliva substitutes.

nizatidine

ni-**za**′-ti-deen

(Apo-Nizatidine[CAN], Axid, Axid AR, Tazac[AUS])

Do not confuse Axid with Ansaid.

CATEGORY AND SCHEDULE

Pregnancy Risk Category: B

OTC (75 mg capsules)

Drug Class: Histamine H_2-receptor antagonist

MECHANISM OF ACTION

An antiulcer agent and gastric acid secretion inhibitor that inhibits histamine action at H_2 receptors of parietal cells.

Therapeutic Effect: Inhibits basal and nocturnal gastric acid secretion.

N

USES

Treatment of duodenal ulcer, Zollinger-Ellison syndrome, gastric ulcers, hypersecretory conditions, gastroesophageal reflux disease (GERD), stress ulcers; unapproved: GI symptoms associated with NSAID use in rheumatoid arthritis

PHARMACOKINETICS

Rapidly well absorbed from the GI tract. Protein binding: 35%. Metabolized in the liver. Primarily excreted in urine. Not removed by hemodialysis. ***Half-life:*** 1–2 hr (increased with impaired renal function).

INDICATIONS AND DOSAGES

▸ **Active Duodenal Ulcer**

PO

Adults, Elderly. 300 mg at bedtime or 150 mg twice a day.

▸ **Prevention of Duodenal Ulcer Recurrence**

PO

Adults, Elderly. 150 mg at bedtime.

▸ **GERD**

PO

Adults, Elderly. 150 mg twice a day.

▸ **Active Benign Gastric Ulcer**

PO

Adults, Elderly. 150 mg twice a day or 300 mg at bedtime.

PO, Oral Solution

Children 12 yr and older. 2 tsp twice a day.

▸ **Dyspepsia**

PO

Adults, Elderly. 75 mg 30–60 min before meals; no more than 2 tablets a day.

▸ **Dosage in Renal Impairment**

Dosage adjustment is based on creatinine clearance.

Creatinine Clearance	Active Ulcer	Maintenance Therapy
20–50 ml/min	150 mg every bedtime	150 mg every other day
Less than 20 ml/min	150 mg every bedtime	150 mg q3days

SIDE EFFECTS/ADVERSE REACTIONS

Occasional

Somnolence, fatigue

Rare

Diaphoresis, rash

PRECAUTIONS AND CONTRAINDICATIONS

Hypersensitivity to other H_2-antagonists

Caution:

Hepatic disease, renal disease, lactation, children younger than 16 yr

DRUG INTERACTIONS OF CONCERN TO DENTISTRY

- Increased serum salicylate when administered with high doses of aspirin
- Decreased absorption of ketoconazole (take doses 2 hr apart)

SERIOUS REACTIONS

! Asymptomatic ventricular tachycardia, hyperuricemia not associated with gout, and nephrolithiasis occur rarely.

DENTAL CONSIDERATIONS

General:

- Avoid prescribing aspirin-containing products in patients with active GI disease.

Teach Patient/Family to:

- Avoid mouth rinses with high alcohol content because of drying effects.

norethindrone

nor-**eth'**-in-drone
(Aygestin, Camila, Errin, Jolivette, Micronor, Nora-BE, Nor-QD, Norlutate[CAN])

CATEGORY AND SCHEDULE

Pregnancy Risk Category: X

Drug Class: Progesterone derivative

MECHANISM OF ACTION

A synthetic progestin that is used as a single agent or in combination with estrogens for the treatment of gynecological disorders. It inhibits secretion of pituitary gonadotropin (LH), which prevents follicular maturation and ovulation.

Therapeutic Effect: Transforms endometrium from proliferative to secretory in an estrogen-primed endometrium, promotes mammary gland development, relaxes uterine smooth muscle.

USES

Treatment of uterine bleeding (abnormal), amenorrhea, endometriosis

PHARMACOKINETICS

Rapidly absorbed from the GI tract. Widely distributed. Protein binding: 61%. Metabolized in liver. Excreted in urine and feces. ***Half-life:*** 4–13 hr.

INDICATIONS AND DOSAGES

▸ **Contraception**

PO

Adults. 1 tablet/day.

▸ **Amenorrhea and Abnormal Uterine Bleeding**

PO

Adults. 5–20 mg/day cyclically (21 days on; 7 days off or continuously) or for acetate salt formulation, 2.5–10 mg cyclically.

▸ **Endometriosis**

PO

Adults. 10 mg/day for 2 wk increase at increments of 5 mg/day every 2 wk until 30 mg/day; continue for 6–9 mo or until breakthrough bleeding demands temporary termination. For acetate salt formulation, 5 mg/day for 14 days increase at increments of 2.5 mg/day every 2 wk up to 15 mg/day; continue for 6–9 mo or until breakthrough bleeding demands temporary termination.

SIDE EFFECTS/ADVERSE REACTIONS

Occasional

Breast tenderness, dizziness, headache, breakthrough bleeding, amenorrhea, menstrual irregularity, nausea, weakness

Rare

Mental depression, fever, insomnia, rash, acne, increased breast tenderness, weight gain/loss, changes in cervical erosion and secretions, cholestatic jaundice

PRECAUTIONS AND CONTRAINDICATIONS

Acute liver disease, benign or malignant liver tumors, hypersensitivity to norethindrone and any component of the formulation, known or suspected carcinoma of the breast, known or suspected pregnancy, undiagnosed abnormal genital bleeding

Caution:

Lactation, hypertension, asthma, blood dyscrasias, gallbladder disease, CHF, diabetes mellitus, bone disease, depression, migraine headache, convulsive disorders, hepatic disease, renal disease, family history of breast or reproductive tract cancer

DRUG INTERACTIONS OF CONCERN TO DENTISTRY

- Decreased effectiveness of oral contraceptives (low risk), antibiotics, barbiturates

SERIOUS REACTIONS

! Thrombophlebitis, cerebrovascular disorders, retinal thrombosis, cholestatic jaundice, and pulmonary embolism occur rarely.

DENTAL CONSIDERATIONS

General:

- Place on frequent recall to evaluate gingival inflammation, if present.
- Increased incidence of dry socket has been reported after extraction.
- Monitor vital signs at each appointment.

Teach Patient/Family to:

- Encourage effective oral hygiene to prevent periodontal inflammation.
- Use additional method of birth control while undergoing antibiotic therapy.

N

norfloxacin

nor-**flox**′-ah-sin

(Apo-Norflox[CAN], Insensye[AUS], Norfloxacine[CAN], Noroxin, Novo-Norfloxacin[CAN], PMS-Norfloxacin[CAN], Roxin[AUS])

CATEGORY AND SCHEDULE

Pregnancy Risk Category: C

Drug Class: Fluoroquinolone antiinfective

MECHANISM OF ACTION

A quinolone that inhibits DNA gyrase in susceptible microorganisms, interfering with bacterial cell replication and repair.

Therapeutic Effect: Bactericidal.

USES

Treatment of adult UTIs (including complicated) caused by *E. coli, E. cloacae, P. mirabilis, K. pneumoniae,* group D strep, indole-positive *Proteus, C. freundii, S. aureus;* sexually transmitted disease caused by *N. gonorrhoeae;* prostatitis caused by *E. coli*

PHARMACOKINETICS

PO: Peak 1 hr, steady state 2 days. ***Half-life:*** 3–4 hr; excreted in urine as active drug, metabolites.

INDICATIONS AND DOSAGES

▸ UTIs

PO

Adults, Elderly. 400 mg twice a day for 7–21 days.

▸ Prostatitis

PO

Adults. 400 mg twice a day for 28 days.

▸ Uncomplicated Gonococcal Infections

PO

Adults. 800 mg as a single dose.

▸ Dosage in Renal Impairment

Dosage and frequency are modified on the basis of creatinine clearance.

Creatinine Clearance	Dosage
30 ml/min or higher	400 mg twice a day
Less than 30 ml/min	400 mg once a day

SIDE EFFECTS/ADVERSE REACTIONS

Frequent

Nausea, headache, dizziness

Rare

Vomiting, diarrhea, dry mouth, bitter taste, nervousness, drowsiness, insomnia, photosensitivity, tinnitus, crystalluria, rash, fever, seizures

PRECAUTIONS AND CONTRAINDICATIONS

Children younger than 18 yr because of risk of arthropathy; hypersensitivity to norfloxacin, other quinolones, or their components

Caution:

Children, renal disease, seizure disorders, tendon rupture in shoulder, hand, and Achilles tendons

DRUG INTERACTIONS OF CONCERN TO DENTISTRY

• Decreased absorption: sodium bicarbonate

SERIOUS REACTIONS

! Superinfection, anaphylaxis, Stevens-Johnson syndrome, and arthropathy occur rarely.

! Hypersensitivity reactions, including photosensitivity (as evidenced by rash, pruritus, blisters, edema, and burning skin), have occurred in patients receiving fluoroquinolones.

DENTAL CONSIDERATIONS

General:

• Assess salivary flow as a factor in caries, periodontal disease, and candidiasis.

• Determine why the patient is taking the drug.

• Because of drug interaction, do not use ingestible sodium bicarbonate products, such as the Prophy-Jet air polishing system, until 2 hr after drug use.

• Avoid dental light in patient's eyes; offer dark glasses for patient comfort.

• Ruptures of the shoulder, hand, and Achilles tendons that required surgical repair or resulted in prolonged disability have been reported.

Consultations:

• Consult with patient's physician if an acute dental infection occurs and another antiinfective is required.

Teach Patient/Family to:
• Avoid mouth rinses with high alcohol content because of drying effects.
• Discontinue treatment and inform dentist immediately if patient experiences pain or inflammation of a tendon, and to rest and refrain from exercise.

norgestrel

nor-**jes**′-trel
(Ovrette)

CATEGORY AND SCHEDULE

Pregnancy Risk Category: X

Drug Class: Progesterone derivative

MECHANISM OF ACTION

A progestin that inhibits secretion of pituitary gonadotropin (LH), which prevents follicular maturation and ovulation.
Therapeutic Effect: Transforms endometrium from proliferative to secretory in an estrogen-primed endometrium, promotes mammary gland development, relaxes uterine smooth muscle.

USES

Oral contraception

PHARMACOKINETICS

Well absorbed from the GI tract. Widely distributed. Protein binding: 97%. Metabolized in liver via reduction and conjugation. Primarily excreted in urine. ***Half-life:*** 20 hr.

INDICATIONS AND DOSAGES

▸ **Contraception, Female**

PO
Adults. 0.075 mg/day.

SIDE EFFECTS/ADVERSE REACTIONS

Frequent
Breakthrough bleeding or spotting at beginning of therapy, amenorrhea, change in menstrual flow, breast tenderness
Occasional
Edema, weight gain or loss, rash, pruritus, photosensitivity, skin pigmentation
Rare
Pain or swelling at injection site, acne, mental depression, alopecia, hirsutism

PRECAUTIONS AND CONTRAINDICATIONS

Hypersensitivity to norgestrel or any component of the formulation, hypersensitivity to tartrazine, thromboembolic disorders, severe hepatic disease; breast cancer; undiagnosed vaginal bleeding, pregnancy
Caution:
Lactation, hypertension, asthma, blood dyscrasias, gallbladder disease, CHF, diabetes mellitus, bone disease, depression, migraine headache, convulsive disorders, hepatic disease, renal disease, family history of breast or reproductive tract cancer

DRUG INTERACTIONS OF CONCERN TO DENTISTRY

• Decreased effectiveness of oral contraceptives: antibiotics, barbiturates

SERIOUS REACTIONS

! Thrombophlebitis, cerebrovascular disorders, retinal thrombosis, and pulmonary embolism occur rarely.

DENTAL CONSIDERATIONS

General:

- Place on frequent recall to evaluate gingival inflammation, if present.
- Increased incidence of dry socket has been reported after extraction.
- Monitor vital signs at each appointment.

Teach Patient/Family to:

- Encourage effective oral hygiene to prevent periodontal inflammation.
- Quit smoking because it decreases risk of serious and adverse cardiovascular side effects.
- Use an additional method of birth control while undergoing antibiotic therapy.

nortriptyline hydrochloride

nor-**trip**′-ti-leen
high-droh-**klor**′-ide
(Allegron[AUS], Apo-Nortriptyline[CAN], Aventyl, Norventyl, Novo-Nortriptyline [CAN], Pamelor)
Do not confuse nortriptyline with amitriptyline, or Aventyl with Ambenyl or Bentyl.

CATEGORY AND SCHEDULE

Pregnancy Risk Category: D

Drug Class:
Antidepressant-tricyclic

MECHANISM OF ACTION

A tricyclic antidepressant that blocks reuptake of the neurotransmitters norepinephrine and serotonin at neuronal presynaptic membranes, increasing their availability at postsynaptic receptor sites.
Therapeutic Effect: Relieves depression.

USES

Treatment of major depression

PHARMACOKINETICS

Well absorbed from the GI tract. Protein binding: 86%–95%. Metabolized in the liver. Primarily excreted in urine. ***Half-life:*** 17.6 hr.

INDICATIONS AND DOSAGES

▸ **Depression**

PO

Adults. 75–100 mg/day in 1–4 divided doses until therapeutic response is achieved. Reduce dosage gradually to effective maintenance level.
Elderly. Initially, 10–25 mg at bedtime. May increase by 25 mg every 3–7 days. Maximum: 150 mg/day.
Children 12 yr and older. 30–50 mg/day in 3–4 divided doses. Maximum: 150 mg/day.
Children 6–11 yr. 10–20 mg/day in 3–4 divided doses.

▸ **Enuresis**

PO

Children 12 yr and older. 25–35 mg/day.
Children 8–11 yr. 10–20 mg/day.
Children 6–7 yr. 10 mg/day.

SIDE EFFECTS/ADVERSE REACTIONS

Frequent
Somnolence, fatigue, dry mouth, blurred vision, constipation, delayed micturition, orthostatic hypotension, diaphoresis, impaired concentration, increased appetite, urine retention
Occasional
GI disturbances (nausea, GI distress, metallic taste), photosensitivity
Rare
Paradoxic reactions (agitation, restlessness, nightmares, insomnia), extrapyramidal symptoms (particularly fine hand tremors)

PRECAUTIONS AND CONTRAINDICATIONS

Acute recovery period after MI; use within 14 days of MAOIs

Caution:

Suicidal patients, severe depression, increased intraocular pressure, narrow-angle glaucoma, urinary retention, cardiac disease, hepatic disease, hyperthyroidism, electroshock therapy, elective surgery, MAOIs

DRUG INTERACTIONS OF CONCERN TO DENTISTRY

- Increased anticholinergic effects: muscarinic blockers, antihistamines, phenothiazines
- Increased effects of direct-acting sympathomimetics (epinephrine, levonordefrin)
- Potential risk of increased CNS depression: alcohol, barbiturates, benzodiazepines, and other CNS depressants
- Decreased antihypertensive effect: clonidine, guanadrel, guanethidine
- Avoid concurrent use with St. John's wort (herb)

N

SERIOUS REACTIONS

! Overdose may produce seizures; cardiovascular effects, such as severe orthostatic hypotension, dizziness, tachycardia, palpitations, and arrhythmias; and altered temperature regulation, such as hyperpyrexia or hypothermia.

! Abrupt discontinuation after prolonged therapy may produce headache, malaise, nausea, vomiting, and vivid dreams.

DENTAL CONSIDERATIONS

General:

- Take vital signs at every appointment because of cardiovascular side effects.
- Assess salivary flow as a factor in caries, periodontal disease, and candidiasis.
- Patients on chronic drug therapy may rarely have symptoms of blood dyscrasias, which can include infection, bleeding, and poor healing.
- After supine positioning, have patient sit upright for at least 2 min before standing to avoid orthostatic hypotension.
- Use vasoconstrictors with caution, in low doses, and with careful aspiration. Avoid use of gingival retraction cord with epinephrine.
- Place on frequent recall because of oral side effects.

Consultations:

- In patients with symptoms of blood dyscrasias, request a medical consultation for blood studies and postpone dental treatment until normal values are reestablished.
- Medical consultation may be required to assess disease control.
- Physician should be informed if significant xerostomic side effects occur (e.g., increased caries, sore tongue, problems eating or swallowing, difficulty wearing prosthesis) so that a medication change can be considered.

Teach Patient/Family to:

- Encourage effective oral hygiene to prevent soft tissue inflammation.
- Use caution to prevent injury when using oral hygiene aids.
- When chronic dry mouth occurs, advise patient to:
  - Avoid mouth rinses with high alcohol content because of drying effects.
  - Use daily home fluoride products for anticaries effect.
  - Use sugarless gum, frequent sips of water, or saliva substitutes.

nystatin

nye-**stat′**-in
(Mycostatin, Nilstat[CAN],
Nyaderm, Nystop)
Do not confuse nystatin or
Mycostatin with Nitrostat.

CATEGORY AND SCHEDULE

Pregnancy Risk Category: C

Drug Class: Antifungal

MECHANISM OF ACTION

A fungistatic antifungal that binds to sterols in the fungal cell membrane. ***Therapeutic Effect:*** Increases fungal cell-membrane permeability, allowing loss of potassium and other cellular components.

USES

Treatment of *Candida* species causing oral, vaginal, intestinal infections

PHARMACOKINETICS

PO: Poorly absorbed from the GI tract. Eliminated unchanged in feces. Topical: Not absorbed systemically from intact skin.

INDICATIONS AND DOSAGES

▸ Intestinal Infections

PO

Adults, Elderly. 500,000–1,000,000 units q8h.

▸ Oral Candidiasis

PO

Adults, Elderly, Children. 400,000–600,000 units 4 times a day.

Infants. 200,000 units 4 times a day.

▸ Vaginal Infections

Vaginal

Adults, Elderly, Adolescents. 1 tablet/day at bedtime for 14 days.

▸ Cutaneous Candidal Infections

Topical

Adults, Elderly, Children. Apply 2–4 times a day.

SIDE EFFECTS/ADVERSE REACTIONS

Occasional

PO: None known
Topical: Skin irritation
Vaginal: Vaginal irritation

PRECAUTIONS AND CONTRAINDICATIONS

Hypersensitivity

SERIOUS REACTIONS

! High dosages of oral form may produce nausea, vomiting, diarrhea, and GI distress.

DENTAL CONSIDERATIONS

General:

• Determine why the patient is taking the drug.
• Broad-spectrum antibiotic may contribute to oral *Candida* infections.

Teach Patient/Family to:

• Complete entire course of medication.
• Not use commercial mouthwashes for mouth infection unless prescribed by dentist.
• Soak full or partial dentures in a suitable antifungal solution nightly.
• Prevent reinoculation of *Candida* infection by disposing of tooth brush or other contaminated oral hygiene devices used during period of infection.

octreotide acetate

ok-**tree′**-oh-tide **ass′**-ih-tate

(Sandostatin, Sandostatin LAR)

Do not confuse octreotide with OctreoScan, or Sandostatin with Sandimmune or Sandoglobulin.

CATEGORY AND SCHEDULE

Pregnancy Risk Category: B

Drug Class: Secretory inhibitor, growth hormone suppressant

MECHANISM OF ACTION

An antidiarrheal and growth hormone suppressant that suppresses the secretion of serotonin and gastroenteropancreatic peptides and enhances fluid and electrolyte absorption from the GI tract. ***Therapeutic Effect:*** Prolongs intestinal transit time.

O

USES

Treatment of severe diarrhea and other symptoms that occur with certain intestinal tumors

PHARMACOKINETICS

Route	Onset	Peak	Duration
Subcutaneous	N/A	N/A	Up to 12 hr

Rapidly and completely absorbed from injection site. Excreted in urine. Removed by hemodialysis. ***Half-life:*** 1.5 hr.

INDICATIONS AND DOSAGES

▸ **Diarrhea**

IV (Sandostatin)

Adults, Elderly. Initially, 50–100 mcg q8h. May increase by 100 mcg/dose q48h. Maximum: 500 mcg q8h.

Subcutaneous (Sandostatin)

Adults, Elderly. 50 mcg 1–2 times a day.

IV, Subcutaneous (Sandostatin)

Children. 1–10 mcg/kg q12h.

▸ **Carcinoid Tumors**

IV, Subcutaneous (Sandostatin)

Adults, Elderly. 100–600 mcg/day in 2–4 divided doses.

IM (Sandostatin LAR)

Adults, Elderly. 20 mg q4wk.

▸ **VIPomas**

IV, Subcutaneous (Sandostatin)

Adults, Elderly. 200–300 mcg/day in 2–4 divided doses.

IM (Sandostatin LAR)

Adults, Elderly. 20 mg q4wk.

▸ **Esophageal Varices**

IV (Sandostatin)

Adults, Elderly. Bolus of 25–50 mcg followed by IV infusion of 25–50 mcg/hr.

▸ **Acromegaly**

IV, Subcutaneous (Sandostatin)

Adults, Elderly. 50 mcg 3 times a day. Increase as needed. Maximum: 500 mcg 3 times a day.

IM (Sandostatin LAR)

Adults, Elderly. 20 mg q4wk for 3 mo. Maximum: 40 mg q4wk.

SIDE EFFECTS/ADVERSE REACTIONS

Frequent

Diarrhea, nausea, abdominal discomfort, headache, injection site pain

Occasional

Vomiting, flatulence, constipation, alopecia, facial flushing, pruritus, dizziness, fatigue, arrhythmias, ecchymosis, blurred vision

Rare

Depression, diminished libido, vertigo, palpitations, dyspnea

PRECAUTIONS AND CONTRAINDICATIONS

None known

DRUG INTERACTIONS OF CONCERN TO DENTISTRY

• May cause decrease in vitamin B_{12} levels.

SERIOUS REACTIONS

! Patients using octreotide may develop cholelithiasis or, with prolonged high dosages, hypothyroidism.

! GI bleeding, hepatitis, and seizures occur rarely.

DENTAL CONSIDERATIONS

General:

• This drug is administered in several disease states; determine patient's medical and drug history and exact use to accurately plan patient management.

• Monitor and record vital signs.

• Consider semisupine chair position for patient comfort if GI side effects occur.

• Question patient about tolerance of NSAIDs or aspirin related to GI disease.

• This drug may be used in the hospital or on an outpatient basis. Confirm the patient's disease and treatment status.

• Patient may need assistance in getting into and out of dental chair. Adjust chair position for patient comfort.

• Examine for oral manifestation of opportunistic infection.

Consultations:

• Medical consultation may be required to assess disease control and patient's ability to tolerate stress.

Teach Patient/Family to:

• Encourage effective oral hygiene to prevent soft tissue inflammation.

• Prevent trauma when using oral hygiene aids.

• Use powered tooth brush if patient has difficulty holding conventional devices.

• Update health and medication history if physician makes any changes in evaluation or drug regimens; include OTC, herbal, and nonherbal drugs in the update.

ofloxacin

o-**flox**′-ah-sin

(Apo-Oflox[CAN], Floxin, Floxin Otic, Ocuflox)

Do not confuse Floxin with Flexeril or Flexon, or Ocuflox with Ocufen.

CATEGORY AND SCHEDULE

Pregnancy Risk Category: C

Drug Class: Fluoroquinolone antiinfective

MECHANISM OF ACTION

A fluoroquinolone antibiotic that inhibits DNA gyrase in susceptible microorganisms, interfering with bacterial cell replication and repair.

Therapeutic Effect: Bactericidal.

USES

Treatment of lower respiratory tract infections (pneumonia, bronchitis), genitourinary infections (prostatitis, UTIs) caused by *E. coli, K. pneumoniae, C. trachomatis, N. gonorrhoeae;* skin and skin-structure infections

PHARMACOKINETICS

Rapidly and well absorbed from the GI tract. Protein binding: 20%–25%. Widely distributed (including to CSF). Metabolized in the liver. Primarily excreted in urine. Removed by hemodialysis.

Half-life: 4.7–7 hr (increased in impaired renal function, cirrhosis, and the elderly).

INDICATIONS AND DOSAGES

▸ UTIs

PO, IV

Adults. 200 mg q12h.

▸ Pelvic Inflammatory Disease (PID)

PO

Adults. 400 mg q12h for 10–14 days.

▸ Lower Respiratory Tract, Skin and Skin-Structure Infections

PO, IV

Adults. 400 mg q12h for 10 days.

▸ Prostatitis, Sexually Transmitted Diseases (Cervicitis, Urethritis)

PO

Adults. 300 mg q12h.

▸ Prostatitis

IV

Adults. 300 mg q12h.

▸ Sexually Transmitted Diseases

IV

Adults. 400 mg as a single dose.

▸ Acute, Uncomplicated Gonorrhea

PO

Adults. 400 mg 1 time.

▸ Usual Elderly Dosage

PO

Elderly. 200–400 mg q12–24h for 7 days up to 6 wk.

▸ Bacterial Conjunctivitis

Ophthalmic

Adults, Elderly. 1–2 drops q2–4h for 2 days, then 4 times a day for 5 days.

▸ Corneal Ulcers

Ophthalmic

Adults. 1–2 drops q30min while awake for 2 days, then q60min while awake for 5–7 days, then 4 times a day.

▸ Acute Otitis Media

Otic

Children 1–12 yr. 5 drops into the affected ear 2 times a day for 10 days.

▸ Otitis Externa

Otic

Adults, Elderly, Children 12 yr and older. 10 drops into the affected ear once a day for 7 days.

Children 6 mo–11 yr. 5 drops into the affected ear once a day for 7 days.

▸ Dosage in Renal Impairment

After a normal initial dose, dosage and frequency are based on creatinine clearance.

Creatinine Clearance	Adjusted Dose	Dosage Interval
Greater than 50 ml/min	None	q12h
10–50 ml/min	None	q24h
Less than 10 ml/min	1/2	q24h

SIDE EFFECTS/ADVERSE REACTIONS

Frequent

Nausea, headache, insomnia

Occasional

Abdominal pain, diarrhea, vomiting, dry mouth, flatulence, dizziness, fatigue, drowsiness, rash, pruritus, fever

Rare

Constipation, paresthesia

PRECAUTIONS AND CONTRAINDICATIONS

Hypersensitivity to any quinolones

Caution:

Lactation, children younger than 18 yr, elderly, renal disease, seizure disorders, excessive sunlight, tendon rupture in shoulder, hand, and Achilles tendons

DRUG INTERACTIONS OF CONCERN TO DENTISTRY

- Decreased effects: antacids
- Possible increased risk of life-threatening dysrhythmias: procainamide

SERIOUS REACTIONS

! Antibiotic-associated colitis and other superinfections may occur from altered bacterial balance.

! Hypersensitivity reactions, including photosensitivity (as evidenced by rash, pruritus, blisters, edema, and burning skin), have occurred in patients receiving fluoroquinolones.

! Arthropathy (swelling, pain, and clubbing of fingers and toes, degeneration of stress-bearing portion of a joint) may occur if the drug is given to children.

DENTAL CONSIDERATIONS

General:

• Because of drug interaction, do not use ingestible sodium bicarbonate products, such as the Prophy-Jet air polishing system, until 2 hr after drug use.

• Examine for oral manifestation of opportunistic infections.

• Avoid dental light in patient's eyes; offer dark glasses for patient comfort.

• Minimize exposure to sunlight and wear sunscreen if sun exposure is planned.

• Ruptures of the shoulder, hand, and Achilles tendons that required surgical repair or resulted in prolonged disability have been reported with this drug.

Consultations:

• Consult with patient's physician if an acute dental infection occurs and another antiinfective is required.

Teach Patient/Family to:

• Encourage effective oral hygiene to prevent soft tissue inflammation.

• Avoid mouth rinses with high alcohol content because of drying effects.

• Discontinue treatment and inform dentist immediately if patient experiences pain or inflammation of a tendon, and to rest and refrain from exercise.

Ofloxacin (Optic)

General:

• Avoid dental light in patient's eyes; offer dark glasses for patient comfort and safety protection during dental treatment.

Ofloxacin Otic Solution

General:

• Determine why the patient is taking the drug.

• Severity or discomfort of infection may require postponement of elective dental treatment.

Consultations:

• Consult with patient's physician if an acute dental infection occurs and another antiinfective is required.

• Medical consultation may be required to assess disease control in the patient.

Teach Patient/Family to:

• When chronic dry mouth occurs, advise patient to:
  • Avoid mouth rinses with high alcohol content because of drying effects.
  • Use daily home fluoride products for anticaries effect.
  • Use sugarless gum, frequent sips of water, or saliva substitutes.

olanzapine

oh-**lan**′-za-peen

(Zyprexa, Zyprexa Intramuscular, Zyprexa Zydis)

Do not confuse olanzapine with olsalazine, or Zyprexa with Zyrtec.

CATEGORY AND SCHEDULE

Pregnancy Risk Category: C

Drug Class: Antipsychotic

MECHANISM OF ACTION

A dibenzepin derivative that antagonizes α_1-adrenergic, dopamine, histamine, muscarinic, and serotonin receptors. Produces anticholinergic, histaminic, and CNS depressant effects.

Therapeutic Effect: Diminishes manifestations of psychotic symptoms.

USES

Treatment of psychotic disorders, schizophrenia, bipolar disorder; acute manic episode in bipolar 1 disorder in combination with lithium or valproate

PHARMACOKINETICS

Well absorbed after PO administration. Protein binding: 93%. Extensively distributed throughout the body. Undergoes extensive first-pass metabolism in the liver. Excreted primarily in urine and, to a lesser extent, in feces. Not removed by dialysis. ***Half-life:*** 21–54 hr.

INDICATIONS AND DOSAGES

▸ Schizophrenia

PO

Adults. Initially, 5–10 mg once daily. May increase by 10 mg/day at 5–7 day intervals. If further adjustments are indicated, may increase by 5–10 mg/day at 7-day intervals. Range: 10–30 mg/day.

Elderly. Initially, 2.5 mg/day. May increase as indicated. Range: 2.5–10 mg/day.

Children. Initially, 2.5 mg/day. Titrate as needed up to 20 mg/day.

▸ Bipolar Mania

PO

Adults. Initially, 10–15 mg/day. May increase by 5 mg/day at intervals of at least 24 hr. Maximum: 20 mg/day.

Children. Initially, 2.5 mg/day. Titrate as needed up to 20 mg/day.

▸ Dosage for Elderly or Debilitated Patients and Those Predisposed to Hypotensive Reactions

The initial dosage for these patients is 5 mg/day.

▸ Control Agitation in Schizophrenic or Bipolar Patients

IM

Adults, Elderly. 2.5–10 mg. May repeat 2 hr after first dose and 4 hr after second dose. Maximum: 30 mg/day.

SIDE EFFECTS/ADVERSE REACTIONS

Frequent

Somnolence, agitation, insomnia, headache, nervousness, hostility, dizziness, rhinitis

Occasional

Anxiety, constipation, nonaggressive atypical behavior, dry mouth, weight gain, orthostatic hypotension, fever, arthralgia, restlessness, cough, pharyngitis, visual changes (dim vision)

Rare

Tachycardia; back, chest, abdominal, or extremity pain; tremors

PRECAUTIONS AND CONTRAINDICATIONS

Hypersensitivity

Caution:

Lactation, paralytic ileus, elderly; combination of age, smoking, and gender (female) may increase clearance rate; neuroleptic malignant syndrome, cardiovascular disease, cerebrovascular disease, seizures, orthostatic hypotension, Alzheimer's dementia, prostate hypertrophy, glaucoma; patients should be monitored for signs and symptoms of diabetes mellitus

DRUG INTERACTIONS OF CONCERN TO DENTISTRY

- Potentiation of orthostatic hypotension: diazepam, alcohol, other CNS depressants
- Increased anticholinergic effects: anticholinergic drugs
- Suspected reduction of plasma levels: carbamazepine

SERIOUS REACTIONS

! Rare reactions include seizures and neuroleptic malignant syndrome, a potentially fatal syndrome characterized by hyperpyrexia, muscle rigidity, irregular pulse or B/P, tachycardia, diaphoresis, and cardiac arrhythmias.

! Extrapyramidal symptoms and dysphagia may also occur.

! Overdose produces drowsiness and slurred speech.

DENTAL CONSIDERATIONS

General:

- Consider semisupine chair position for patient comfort because of GI effects of drug.
- Assess salivary flow as factor in caries, periodontal disease, and candidiasis.
- Monitor vital signs at every appointment because of cardiovascular side effects.
- After supine positioning, have patient sit upright for at least 2 min before standing to avoid orthostatic hypotension.
- Patients on chronic drug therapy may rarely have symptoms of blood dyscrasias, which can include infection, bleeding, and poor healing.
- Assess for presence of extrapyramidal motor symptoms, such as tardive dyskinesia and akathisia. Extrapyramidal motor activity may complicate dental treatment.

Consultations:

- In a patient with symptoms of blood dyscrasias, request a medical consultation for blood studies and postpone dental treatment until normal values are reestablished.
- Medical consultation may be required to assess disease control.
- Physician should be informed if significant xerostomic side effects occur (e.g., increased caries, sore tongue, problems eating or swallowing, difficulty wearing prosthesis) so that a medication change can be considered.

Teach Patient/Family to:

- Encourage effective oral hygiene to prevent soft tissue inflammation.
- Use powered tooth brush if patient has difficulty holding conventional devices.
- Use caution when driving or performing other tasks requiring alertness.
- When chronic dry mouth occurs, advise patient to:
  - Avoid mouth rinses with high alcohol content because of drying effects.
  - Use daily home fluoride products for anticaries effect.
  - Use sugarless gum, frequent sips of water, or saliva substitutes.

O

olmesartan

ol-meh-**sar′**-tan

(Benicar)

CATEGORY AND SCHEDULE

Pregnancy Risk Category: C (1st trimester) and D (2nd and 3rd trimesters).

Drug Class: Antihypertensive, angiotensin (AT) II receptor blocker.

MECHANISM OF ACTION

Blocks the vasoconstrictor effects of angiotensin II by blocking the binding of angiotensin II to the AT 1 receptor in smooth muscle. Olmesartan increases urinary flow rate.

USES

Treatment of hypertension as monotherapy or in combination with other antihypertensive agents

PHARMACOKINETICS

Rapidly, completely absorbed after PO administration. Protein binding: 99%. Olmesartan medoxomil is an inactive drug. It is hydrolyzed in the gastrointestinal tract to active olmesartan, which is absorbed. Bioavailability: 26%. Food does not affect the bioavailability of olmesartan. Dose not cross blood-brain barrier. Primarily excreted in feces and to a lesser extent in urine. ***Half-life:*** 13 hr.

INDICATIONS AND DOSAGES

▸ **Hypertension (with or without Other Antihypertensive Agents)**

PO

Adults. Initially, 20 mg once daily. May be increased to 40 mg once daily after 2 wk. Lower starting dose in patients receiving volume depleting drugs (e.g., diuretics).

Elderly. May start at 5–10 mg/day.

Dosage in Hepatic Impairment: no adjustment necessary.

Dosage in Renal Impairment: no adjustment necessary.

SIDE EFFECTS/ADVERSE REACTIONS

Adults

Frequent

Dizziness, headache, diarrhea

Occasional

Abdominal pain, chest pain, insomnia, tachycardia, cough, hyperglycemia

Children

Safety and efficacy have not been established in children

PRECAUTIONS AND CONTRAINDICATIONS

Hypertensive to olmesartan or its components

Use caution in patients with aortic/mitral stenosis, hypovolemia, renal artery stenosis, and renal impairment.

Hyperkalemia may occur.

Pregnancy: [U.S. Boxed Warning]: "Based on human data, drugs that act on the angiotensin system can cause injury and death to the developing fetus when used in the second and third trimesters. Angiotensin receptor blockers should be discontinued as soon as possible once pregnancy is detected."

DRUG INTERACTIONS OF CONCERN TO DENTISTRY

- NSAIDs: May reduce efficacy of olmesartan.

SERIOUS REACTIONS

! Allergic reactions are reported rarely with angiotensin receptor antagonists.

! Bradycardia may occur.

! Rhabdomyolysis has been reported.

DENTAL CONSIDERATIONS

General:

- Monitor vital signs at every appointment because of cardiovascular side effects.
- Avoid or limit dose of vasoconstrictor.

• After supine positioning, have patient sit upright for at least 2 min to avoid dizziness.
• Stress from dental procedure may compromise cardiovascular function; determine patient risk.

Consultations:
• Medical consultation may be required to assess disease control and to determine ability of patient to tolerate dental treatment.

Teach Patient/Family to:
• Prevent injury when using oral hygiene aids.
• Encourage effective oral hygiene to prevent soft tissue inflammation.

olmesartan medoxomil

ol-meh-**sar**′-tan mee-**dox**′-oh-mill
(Benicar)

CATEGORY AND SCHEDULE

Pregnancy Risk Category: C (D if used in second or third trimester)

Drug Class: Angiotensin II (ATI) receptor antagonist

MECHANISM OF ACTION

An angiotensin II receptor, type ATI, antagonist that blocks the vasoconstrictor and aldosterone-secreting effects of angiotensin II, inhibiting the binding of angiotensin II to the ATI receptors.
Therapeutic Effect: Causes vasodilation, decreases peripheral resistance, and decreases B/P.

USES

Treatment of hypertension, as a single drug or in combination with other antihypertensives

PHARMACOKINETICS

Rapidly and completely absorbed after PO administration. Metabolized in the liver. Recovered primarily in feces and, to a lesser extent, in urine. Not removed by hemodialysis.
Half-life: 13 hr.

INDICATIONS AND DOSAGES

▸ **Hypertension**

PO

Adults, Elderly, Patients with mildly impaired hepatic or renal function. 20 mg once a day in patients who are not volume depleted. After 2 wk of therapy, if further reduction in B/P is necessary, may increase dosage to 40 mg/day.

SIDE EFFECTS/ADVERSE REACTIONS

Occasional
Dizziness

Rare
Headache, diarrhea, upper respiratory tract infection

PRECAUTIONS AND CONTRAINDICATIONS

Bilateral renal artery stenosis

Caution:
Discontinue drug if pregnancy occurs, use in volume- or salt-depleted patients, or in nursing mothers or pediatric patients has not been established, impaired renal function, CHF, renal artery stenosis

DRUG INTERACTIONS OF CONCERN TO DENTISTRY

• No significant drug interactions have been reported, but increased hypotensive effects always are possible when used with other antihypertensives or sedatives.

SERIOUS REACTIONS

! Overdosage may manifest as hypotension and tachycardia. Bradycardia occurs less often.

DENTAL CONSIDERATIONS

General:

- Monitor vital signs at every appointment because of cardiovascular side effects.
- Avoid or limit dose of vasoconstrictor.
- Consider semisupine chair position for patient comfort if GI side effects occur.
- Limit use of sodium-containing products, such as saline IV fluids, for patients with a dietary salt restriction.
- Stress from dental procedures may compromise cardiovascular function; determine patient risk.
- Patients with hypertensive disease may be taking more than one drug to control B/P; although not specifically noted for this drug, postural hypotension is always a possibility.
- After supine positioning, have patient sit upright for at least 2 min before standing to avoid orthostatic hypotension.
- Short appointments and a stress-reduction protocol may be required for anxious patients.
- Use precaution if sedation or general anesthesia is required; risk of hypotensive episode.

Consultations:

- Medical consultation may be required to assess disease control and patient's ability to tolerate stress.

Teach Patient/Family to:

- Update health and drug history if physician makes any changes in evaluation or drug regimens; include OTC, herbal, and nonherbal drugs in the update.

O

olopatadine

(oh-loh-**pat′**-ah-deen)
(Patanase [U.S.], Pataday, Patanol, Patanol S, Opatanol [INTL.])

CATEGORY AND SCHEDULE

Pregnancy Risk Category: C

Drug Class: Ophthalmic and nasal antihistamine

MECHANISM OF ACTION

Blocks release of histamine from mast cells and blocks effect of histamine on H_1 receptors in tissues of eye.
Therapeutic Effect: Reduces effects of ophthalmic (allergic conjunctivitis) and nasal allergic reactions.

USES

Allergic conjunctivitis and rhinitis

PHARMACOKINETICS

Low systemic exposure after topical administration. ***Half-life:*** 3 hr. Excreted primarily (60%–70%) as parent drug in urine

INDICATIONS AND DOSAGES

▸ **Allergic Conjunctivitis**

Topical, Ophthalmic/Intranasal
Adult. One drop two times per day q6–8h.

SIDE EFFECTS/ADVERSE REACTIONS

Frequent

Headache

Occasional

Asthenia, blurred vision, burning or stinging, cold syndrome, dry eye, foreign body sensation, hyperemia, hypersensitivity, keratitis, lid edema, nausea, pharyngitis, rhinitis, pruritus, sinusitis, dysgeusia

PRECAUTIONS AND CONTRAINDICATIONS
Hypersensitivity
Nursing
Contraindicated by hypersensitivity to olopatadine or any of its ingredients

DRUG INTERACTIONS OF CONCERN TO DENTISTRY
- None reported

SERIOUS REACTIONS
! None reported

DENTAL CONSIDERATIONS
General:
- Consider drug as etiologic factor in dysgeusia.

Consultations:
- Consult with physician to determine disease control and ability to tolerate dental procedures.

Teach Patient/Family to:
- Report changes in taste sensation or other oral adverse effects.

olsalazine sodium
ohl-**sal′**-ah-zeen **soe′**-dee-um
(Dipentum)
Do not confuse olsalazine with olanzapine.

CATEGORY AND SCHEDULE
Pregnancy Risk Category: C

Drug Class: Antiinflammatory, salicylate derivative

MECHANISM OF ACTION
A salicylic acid derivative that is converted to mesalamine in the colon by bacterial action.
Blocks prostaglandin production in bowel mucosa.

Therapeutic Effect: Reduces colonic inflammation in inflammatory bowel disease.

USES
Maintenance of remission of ulcerative colitis in patients intolerant to sulfasalazine

PHARMACOKINETICS
PO: Partially absorbed, peak 1.5 hr. ***Half-life:*** 5–10 hr; excreted in urine as 5-aminosalicylic acid and metabolites; crosses placenta.

INDICATIONS AND DOSAGES
▸ Maintenance of Controlled Ulcerative Colitis
PO
Adults, Elderly. 1 g/day in 2 divided doses, preferably q12h.

SIDE EFFECTS/ADVERSE REACTIONS
Frequent
Headache, diarrhea, abdominal pain or cramps, nausea
Occasional
Depression, fatigue, dyspepsia, upper respiratory tract infection, decreased appetite, rash, itching, arthralgia
Rare
Dizziness, vomiting, stomatitis

PRECAUTIONS AND CONTRAINDICATIONS
History of hypersensitivity to salicylates
Caution:
Lactation, impaired hepatic function, severe allergy, bronchial asthma, renal disease

SERIOUS REACTIONS
! Sulfite sensitivity may occur in susceptible patients, manifested by cramping, headache, diarrhea, fever,

rash, hives, itching, and wheezing. Discontinue drug immediately.
! Excessive diarrhea associated with extreme fatigue is noted rarely.

DENTAL CONSIDERATIONS

General:
• Consider semisupine chair position for patient comfort because of GI effects of disease.
Consultations:
• Avoid drugs that could aggravate an inflammatory colon disease; consultation is recommended before selection of an antibiotic.
Teach Patient/Family to:
• Encourage effective oral hygiene to prevent soft tissue inflammation.
• Use caution to prevent injury when using oral hygiene aids.
• Avoid mouth rinses with high alcohol content because of drying effects.

O

omalizumab

oh-mah-**liz**′-uw-mab
(Xolair)

CATEGORY AND SCHEDULE

Pregnancy Risk Category: B

Drug Class: Anti-IgE monoclonal antibody

MECHANISM OF ACTION

A monoclonal antibody that selectively binds to human immunoglobulin E (IgE), preventing it from binding to the surface of mast cells and basophils.
Therapeutic Effect: Prevents or reduces the number of asthmatic attacks.

USES

Reduction of asthma exacerbation in patients with moderate to severe asthma who have a positive skin test or in vitro reactivity to a perennial aeroallergen not adequately controlled by inhaled glucocorticoids

PHARMACOKINETICS

Absorbed slowly after subcutaneous administration, with peak concentration in 7–8 days. Excreted in the liver, reticuloendothelial system, and endothelial cells.
Half-life: 26 days.

INDICATIONS AND DOSAGES

▸ **Moderate-to-Severe Persistent Asthma in Patients Who Are Reactive to a Perennial Allergen and Whose Asthma Symptoms Have Been Inadequately Controlled with Inhaled Corticosteroids**

Subcutaneous

Adults, Elderly, Children 12 yr and older. 150–375 mg every 2 or 4 wk; dose and dosing frequency are individualized on the basis of weight and pretreatment IgE level (as shown below).

4-wk Dosing Table

Pretreatment Serum IgE Levels (units/ml)	Weight 30–60 kg	Weight 61–70 kg	Weight 71–90 kg	Weight 91–150 kg
30–100	150 mg	150 mg	150 mg	300 mg
101–200	300 mg	300 mg	300 mg	See next table
201–300	300 mg	See next table	See next table	See next table

2-wk Dosing Table

Pretreatment Serum IgE (units/ml)	Weight 30–60 kg	Weight 61–70 kg	Weight 71–90 kg	Weight 91–150 kg
101–200	See preceding table	See preceding table	See preceding table	225 mg
201–300	See preceding table	225 mg	225 mg	300 mg
301–400	225 mg	225 mg	300 mg	Do not dose
401–500	300 mg	300 mg	375 mg	Do not dose
501–600	300 mg	375 mg	Do not dose	Do not dose
601–700	375 mg	Do not dose	Do not dose	Do not dose

SIDE EFFECTS/ADVERSE REACTIONS

Frequent

Injection site ecchymosis, redness, warmth, stinging, and urticaria; viral infections; sinusitis; headache; pharyngitis

Occasional

Arthralgia, leg pain, fatigue, dizziness

Rare

Arm pain, earache, dermatitis, pruritus

PRECAUTIONS AND CONTRAINDICATIONS

Hypersensitivity

Caution:

Possible risk of malignancy, anaphylactic reactions, not for acute asthma or status asthmaticus, do not abruptly discontinue glucocorticoid therapy, use in nursing mothers or children younger than 12 yr has not been established

DRUG INTERACTIONS OF CONCERN TO DENTISTRY

• None reported

SERIOUS REACTIONS

! Anaphylaxis occurs within 2 hr of the first dose or subsequent doses in 0.1% of patients.
! Malignant neoplasms occur in 0.5% of patients.

DENTAL CONSIDERATIONS

General:

• Determine why patient is taking the drug.
• Be aware of patient's disease, its severity, and its frequency, when known.
• Question patient about other medications used for asthma or to prevent bronchoconstriction.
• Avoid drugs that may aggravate asthma.
• Short appointments and a stress-reduction protocol may be required for anxious patients.
• Have patient bring personal short-acting bronchodilator to appointment for use in emergency.
• Acute asthmatic episodes may be precipitated in the dental office. Rapid-acting sympathomimetic inhalants should be available for emergency use. A stress-reduction protocol may be required.

Consultations:

• Consultation with physician may be necessary if sedation or general anesthesia is required.
• Medical consultation may be required to assess disease control and patient's ability to tolerate stress.

Teach Patient/Family to:

• Encourage effective oral hygiene to prevent soft tissue inflammation/infection.
• Update health and drug history and report changes in health status, drug regimen, or disease/treatment status.

omega-3 fatty acids
(Lovaza)

CATEGORY AND SCHEDULE
Pregnancy Risk Category: C

Drug Class: Antihyperlipidemic agent

MECHANISM OF ACTION
A combination of ethyl esters of omega 3 fatty acids, principally eicosapentaenoic acid (EPA) and docosahexaenoic acid (DHA) but the mechanism of action is not well understood. May inhibit acyl-CoA:1,2-diacylglycerol acyltransferase, increase mitochondrial and peroxisomal β-oxidation in the liver, decrease lipogenesis in the liver, and increase plasma lipoprotein lipase activity.
Therapeutic Effect: Lowers serum triglyceride level.

O

USES
Hypertriglyceridemia, severe (≥500 mg/dl), adjunct to diet

PHARMACOKINETICS
Absorbed when administered as ethyl esters following PO administration.

INDICATIONS AND DOSAGES
▸ **Hypertriglyceridemia, Severe (≥500 mg/dl), Adjunct to Diet**
PO
Adults. 4-g dose (4 capsules) or as two 2-g doses (2 capsules twice daily).

SIDE EFFECTS/ADVERSE REACTIONS
Frequent
Eructation, infection
Occasional
Flu syndrome, dyspepsia, back pain, pain (general), angina, rash, dysgeusia
Rare
Elevated LDL cholesterol levels

PRECAUTIONS AND CONTRAINDICATIONS
Hypersensitivity to omega-3 fatty acids or any component of the formulation
Caution:
Hepatic impairment
Fish allergy
Pregnancy
Nursing mothers
Elevated LDL cholesterol levels
Prolongation of bleeding time

DRUG INTERACTIONS OF CONCERN TO DENTISTRY
- Anticoagulants, antiplatelets: May increase the risk of bleeding.

SERIOUS REACTIONS
! ALT and AST should be monitored periodically in patients with hepatic impairment.
! Lipid profile should be monitored.

DENTAL CONSIDERATIONS
General:
- Monitor vital signs at every appointment because of cardiovascular side effects.
- After supine positioning, have patient sit upright for at least 2 min before standing to avoid orthostatic hypotension.
- Assess salivary flow as a factor in caries, periodontal disease, and candidiasis.
- Stress from dental procedures may compromise cardiovascular function; determine patient risk. Short appointments and a stress-reduction protocol may be required for anxious patients.

Consultations:
- Medical consultation may be required to assess disease control.

Teach Patient/Family to:
- Report oral lesions, soreness, or bleeding to dentist.
- When chronic dry mouth occurs, advise patient to:
  - Avoid mouth rinses with high alcohol content because of drying effects.
  - Use daily home fluoride products for anticaries effect.
  - Use sugarless gum, frequent sips of water, or saliva substitutes.

omeprazole

oh-**mep′**-rah-zole
(Losec[CAN], Maxor[AUS], Prilosec, Prilosec OTC, Probitor[AUS], Zegerid)
Do not confuse Prilosec with prilocaine, Prinivil, or Prozac.

CATEGORY AND SCHEDULE

Pregnancy Risk Category: C

Drug Class: Antisecretory, proton pump inhibitor

MECHANISM OF ACTION

A benzimidazole that is converted to active metabolites that irreversibly bind to and inhibit hydrogen-potassium adenosine triphosphatase, an enzyme on the surface of gastric parietal cells. Inhibits hydrogen ion transport into gastric lumen. ***Therapeutic Effect:*** Increases gastric pH, reduces gastric acid production.

USES

Treatment of gastroesophageal reflux disease (GERD), severe erosive esophagitis, poorly responsive systemic GERD, pathologic hypersecretory conditions (Zollinger-Ellison syndrome, systemic mastocytosis, multiple endocrine adenomas), with clarithromycin, short-term treatment of gastric ulcers; not approved for long-term ulcer maintenance therapy

PHARMACOKINETICS

Route	Onset	Peak	Duration
PO	1 hr	2 hr	72 hr

Rapidly absorbed from the GI tract. Protein binding: 99%. Primarily distributed into gastric parietal cells. Metabolized extensively in the liver. Primarily excreted in urine. Unknown if removed by hemodialysis. ***Half-life:*** 0.5–1 hr (increased in patients with hepatic impairment).

O

INDICATIONS AND DOSAGES

▸ **Erosive Esophagitis, Poorly Responsive GERD, Active Duodenal Ulcer, Prevention and Treatment of NSAID-Induced Ulcers**

PO

Adults, Elderly. 20 mg/day.

▸ **To Maintain Healing of Erosive Esophagitis**

PO

Adults, Elderly. 20 mg/day.

▸ **Pathologic Hypersecretory Conditions**

PO

Adults, Elderly. Initially, 60 mg/day up to 120 mg 3 times a day.

▸ **Duodenal Ulcer Caused by *H. pylori***

PO

Adults, Elderly. 20 mg twice a day for 10 days.

▸ **Active Benign Gastric Ulcer**
PO
Adults, Elderly. 40 mg/day for 4–8 wk.

▸ **Usual Pediatric Dosage**
Children older than 2 yr, weighing 20 kg and more. 20 mg/day.
Children older than 2 yr, weighing less than 20 kg. 10 mg/day.

SIDE EFFECTS/ADVERSE REACTIONS

Frequent
Headache
Occasional
Diarrhea, abdominal pain, nausea
Rare
Dizziness, asthenia or loss of strength, vomiting, constipation, upper respiratory tract infection, back pain, rash, cough

PRECAUTIONS AND CONTRAINDICATIONS

Hypersensitivity
Caution:
Lactation, children

DRUG INTERACTIONS OF CONCERN TO DENTISTRY

• Increased serum levels: diazepam

SERIOUS REACTIONS

! None known

DENTAL CONSIDERATIONS

General:
• Question the patient about tolerance of NSAIDs or aspirin related to GI problem.
• Consider semisupine chair position for patient comfort because of GI effects of disease.
• Assess salivary flow as a factor in caries, periodontal disease, and candidiasis.

Teach Patient/Family to:
• Use caution to prevent injury when using oral hygiene aids.
• When chronic dry mouth occurs, advise patient to:
  • Avoid mouth rinses with high alcohol content because of drying effects.
  • Use daily home fluoride products to prevent caries.
  • Use sugarless gum, frequent sips of water, or saliva substitutes.

ondansetron, oral soluble film

on-**dan′**-seh-tron
(Zuplenz)
Do not confuse with Zantac or Zosyn.

CATEGORY AND SCHEDULE

Pregnancy Risk Category: B

Drug Class: Antiemetic; selective 5-HT3 receptor antagonist

MECHANISM OF ACTION

An antiemetic that blocks serotonin, both peripherally on vagal nerve terminals and centrally in the chemoreceptor trigger zone.
Therapeutic Effect: Prevents nausea and vomiting.

USES

Prevention of nausea and vomiting associated with highly emetogenic cancer chemotherapy
Prevention of nausea and vomiting associated with initial and repeat courses of moderately emetogenic cancer chemotherapy
Prevention of nausea and vomiting associated with radiotherapy
Prevention of postoperative nausea and vomiting (PONV)

PHARMACOKINETICS
Readily absorbed from the GI tract. Protein binding: 70%–76%. Metabolized in the liver. Primarily excreted in urine. ***Half-life:*** 4 hr.

INDICATIONS AND DOSAGES
▸ Prevention of Chemotherapy-Induced Nausea and Vomiting
PO
Adults, Elderly, Children older than 11 yr. 24 mg as a single dose 30 min before starting chemotherapy, or 8 mg 30 min before chemotherapy and again 8 hr after first dose; then q12h for 1–2 days.
PO
Children 4–11 yr. 4 mg 30 min before chemotherapy and again 4 and 8 hr after chemotherapy, then q8h for 1–2 days.
▸ Prevention of Radiation-Induced Nausea and Vomiting
PO
Adults, Elderly. 8 mg 1–2 hr before radiation, followed by 8 mg 3 times a day, or if radiation is intermittent, 8-mg single dose 1–2 hr before radiation.
▸ Prevention of Postoperative Nausea and Vomiting
PO
Adults, Elderly. 16 mg given as two 8-mg tablets 1 hr before anesthesia.

SIDE EFFECTS/ADVERSE REACTIONS
Frequent
Anxiety, dizziness, somnolence, headache, fatigue, constipation, diarrhea, hypoxia, urinary retention
Occasional
Abdominal pain, xerostomia, fever, feeling of cold, rash, blurred vision

PRECAUTIONS AND CONTRAINDICATIONS
Hypersensitivity to ondansetron or any component of the formulation; concomitant use of apomorphine (profound hypotension and loss of consciousness may result). Use with caution in patients with moderate-to-severe hepatic impairment.

DRUG INTERACTIONS OF CONCERN TO DENTISTRY
• Apomorphine: can result in profound hypotension and loss of consciousness

SERIOUS REACTIONS
! Liver failure and death have been reported in patients with cancer receiving concurrent potentially hepatotoxic chemotherapy and antibiotics.

DENTAL CONSIDERATIONS
General:
• Monitor patient carefully for oral adverse effects of coexisting cancer chemotherapy, including ulcerations, stomatitis, and candidiasis.
• Consider increased risk of nausea and vomiting (e.g., during sedation, impressions).
Teach Patient/Family to:
• Avoid mouth rinses with high alcohol content because of irritating effect.
• Use home fluoride products for anticaries effect.
• Use frequent sips of water or saliva substitutes if oral irritation occurs.
• Use palliative treatments for ulcerations and oral pain (see section on "Therapeutic Management of Common Oral Lesions").

oprelvekin (interleukin-2, IL-2)

oh-**prel**′-vee-kinn
(Neumega)
Do not confuse Neumega with Neupogen.

CATEGORY AND SCHEDULE

Pregnancy Risk Category: C
Controlled substance: Schedule IV

Drug Class: Hematopoietic; platelet growth factor

MECHANISM OF ACTION

A hematopoietic that stimulates production of blood platelets, essential to the blood-clotting process.

Therapeutic Effect: Increases platelet production.

USES

Prevention of low platelet counts caused by treatment with some cancer medicines

PHARMACOKINETICS

Peak 3.2 hr following single subcutaneous dose. ***Half-life:*** 6.9 hr. Rapidly excreted by the kidneys.

INDICATIONS AND DOSAGES

▸ **Prevention of Thrombocytopenia**

Subcutaneous

Adults. 50 mcg/kg once a day.
Children. 75–100 mcg/kg once a day. Continue for 14–28 days or until platelet count reaches 50,000 cells/mcl after its nadir.

SIDE EFFECTS/ADVERSE REACTIONS

Frequent

Nausea or vomiting, fluid retention, neutropenic fever, diarrhea, rhinitis, headache, dizziness, fever, insomnia, cough, rash, pharyngitis, tachycardia, vasodilation

PRECAUTIONS AND CONTRAINDICATIONS

None known

DRUG INTERACTIONS OF CONCERN TO DENTISTRY

- No data available

SERIOUS REACTIONS

! Transient atrial fibrillation or flutter occurs in 10% of patients and may be caused by increased plasma volume; oprelvekin is not directly dysrhythmogenic. Dysrhythmias are usually brief in duration and convert spontaneously to normal sinus rhythm.
! Papilledema may occur in children.

DENTAL CONSIDERATIONS

General:

- If bleeding problem has not been diagnosed, refer for evaluation prior to any dental treatment.
- Question patient about medical and drug history in relationship to bleeding problems.
- Provide dental treatment in conjunction with hematologist.
- Patients may present with localized gingival bleeding with incomplete clotting.
- Avoid elective dental procedures if severe neutropenia (more than 500 cells/mm^3) or thrombocytopenia (fewer than 50,000 cells/mm^3) is present.
- Avoid products that affect platelet function, such as aspirin and NSAIDs.
- Monitor and record vital signs.
- Consider local hemostasis measures to prevent excessive bleeding.

• Short appointments and a stress-reduction protocol may be required for anxious patients.
• Place on frequent recall to evaluate healing response.

Consultations:

• Consultation with hematologist or physician of record required.
• Medical consultation should include routine blood counts, including platelet counts and bleeding time.
• Consultation with physician may be necessary if sedation or general anesthesia is required.
• In a patient with symptoms of blood dyscrasias, request a medical consultation for blood studies and postpone treatment until normal values are reestablished.
• Medical consultation should include PPT or INR.

Teach Patient/Family to:

• Use soft tooth brush to prevent trauma to oral tissues and risk of bleeding.
• Encourage effective oral hygiene to prevent soft tissue inflammation.
• Report oral lesions, soreness, or bleeding to dentist.
• Update health and medication history if physician makes any changes in evaluation or drug regimens; include OTC, herbal, and nonherbal drugs in the update.
• Prevent trauma when using oral hygiene aids.

orlistat

ohr′-lih-stat
(Xenical)
Do not confuse Xenical with Xeloda.

CATEGORY AND SCHEDULE

Pregnancy Risk Category: B

Drug Class: Antiobesity

MECHANISM OF ACTION

A gastric and pancreatic lipase inhibitor that inhibits absorption of dietary fats by inactivating gastric and pancreatic enzymes.
Therapeutic Effect: Resulting caloric deficit may positively affect weight control.

USES

Obesity management, including weight loss and maintenance in conjunction with a reduced-calorie diet; used in patients with a defined body mass index with other risk factors for cardiovascular disease

PHARMACOKINETICS

Minimal absorption after administration. Protein binding: 99%. Primarily eliminated unchanged in feces. Unknown if removed by hemodialysis. ***Half-life:*** 1–2 hr.

INDICATIONS AND DOSAGES

▸ **Weight Reduction**

PO

Adults, Elderly, Children 12–16 yr. 120 mg 3 times a day.

SIDE EFFECTS/ADVERSE REACTIONS

Frequent

Headache, abdominal discomfort, flatulence, fecal urgency, fatty or oily stool

Occasional

Back pain, menstrual irregularity, nausea, fatigue, diarrhea, dizziness

Rare

Anxiety, rash, myalgia, dry skin, vomiting

PRECAUTIONS AND CONTRAINDICATIONS

Cholestasis, chronic malabsorption syndrome

Caution:
Adherence to dietary guidelines, supplemental fat-soluble vitamins may be required, along with beta-carotene, nephrolithiasis, use in children not established

DRUG INTERACTIONS OF CONCERN TO DENTISTRY

• None reported

SERIOUS REACTIONS

! None known

DENTAL CONSIDERATIONS

General:
• Although no dental drug interactions are reported, observe expected outcomes of systemically administered drugs.
• Severely obese patients may have type 2 diabetes or cardiovascular diseases.
• Consider semisupine chair position for patient comfort if GI side effects occur.
• Ensure that patient is following prescribed diet and regularly takes medication.
Consultations:
• Medical consultation may be required to assess disease control.
Teach Patient/Family to:
• Update health and drug history if physician makes any changes in evaluation or drug regimens; include OTC, herbal, and nonherbal drugs in the update.

orphenadrine

or-**fen**′-ah-dreen
(Norflex, Orphenace[CAN], Rhoxal-orphenadrine[CAN])

CATEGORY AND SCHEDULE

Pregnancy Risk Category: C

Drug Class: Skeletal muscle relaxant

MECHANISM OF ACTION

A skeletal muscle relaxant that is structurally related to diphenhydramine and is thought to indirectly affect skeletal muscle by central atropine-like effects.
Therapeutic Effect: Relieves musculoskeletal pain.

USES

Treatment of pain in musculoskeletal conditions

PHARMACOKINETICS

Well absorbed after PO and IM absorption. Protein binding: low. Metabolized in liver. Primarily excreted in urine and feces.
Half-life: 14 hr.

INDICATIONS AND DOSAGES

▸ **Musculoskeletal Pain**
IM/IV
Adults, Elderly. 60 mg 2 times a day. Switch to oral form for maintenance.
PO
Adults, Elderly. 100 mg 2 times a day.

SIDE EFFECTS/ADVERSE REACTIONS

Frequent
Drowsiness, dizziness, muscular weakness, hypotension, dry mouth, nose, throat, and lips, urinary retention, thickening of bronchial secretions

Elderly. Sedation, dizziness, hypotension
Occasional
Elderly. Flushing, visual or hearing disturbances, paresthesia, diaphoresis, chill

PRECAUTIONS AND CONTRAINDICATIONS

Angle-closure glaucoma, myasthenia gravis, pyloric or duodenal obstruction, stenosing peptic ulcer, prostatic hypertrophy, obstruction of the bladder neck, achalasia, cardiospasm (megaesophagus), hypersensitivity to orphenadrine or any component of the formulation
Caution:
Children, cardiac disease, tachycardia, caution in lactation

DRUG INTERACTIONS OF CONCERN TO DENTISTRY

- Increased CNS effects: CNS depressants, alcohol
- Increased anticholinergic effect: other anticholinergics

SERIOUS REACTIONS

! Hypersensitivity reaction, such as eczema, pruritus, rash, cardiac disturbances, and photosensitivity, may occur.
! Overdosage may vary from CNS depression, including sedation, apnea, hypotension, cardiovascular collapse, or death, to severe paradoxical reaction, such as hallucinations, tremors, and seizures.

DENTAL CONSIDERATIONS

General:
- Consider semisupine chair position for patients with back pain.
- Patients on chronic drug therapy may rarely have symptoms of blood dyscrasias, which can include infection, bleeding, and poor healing.
- Assess salivary flow as a factor in caries, periodontal disease, and candidiasis.

Consultations:
- In a patient with symptoms of blood dyscrasias, request a medical consultation for blood studies and postpone dental treatment until normal values are reestablished.
- Medical consultation may be required to assess disease control.

Teach Patient/Family to:
- Encourage effective oral hygiene to prevent soft tissue inflammation.
- Use caution to prevent injury when using oral hygiene aids.
- Use caution when driving or operating equipment because of risk of dizziness.
- When chronic dry mouth occurs, advise patient to:
  - Avoid mouth rinses with high alcohol content because of drying effects.
  - Use daily home fluoride products to prevent caries.
  - Use sugarless gum, frequent sips of water, or saliva substitutes.

oseltamivir

oh-sell-**tam′**-ah-veer
(Tamiflu)

CATEGORY AND SCHEDULE

Pregnancy Risk Category: C

Drug Class: Antiviral

MECHANISM OF ACTION

A selective inhibitor of influenza virus neuraminidase, an enzyme essential for viral replication. Acts against both influenza A and B viruses.

Therapeutic Effect: Suppresses the spread of infection within the respiratory system and reduces the duration of clinical symptoms.

USES

Treatment of uncomplicated acute illness caused by influenza infection in adults who have been symptomatic for no more than 2 days; more effective against influenza type A virus; prophylaxis for adults and children older than 13 yr

PHARMACOKINETICS

Readily absorbed. Protein binding: 3%. Extensively converted to active drug in the liver. Primarily excreted in urine. ***Half-life:*** 6–10 hr.

INDICATIONS AND DOSAGES

▸ **Influenza**

PO

Adults, Elderly. 75 mg 2 times a day for 5 days.

Children weighing more than 40 kg. 75 mg twice a day.

Children weighing 24–40 kg. 60 mg twice a day.

Children weighing 15–23 kg. 45 mg twice a day.

Children weighing less than 15 kg. 30 mg twice a day.

▸ **Prevention of Influenza**

PO

Adults, Elderly. 75 mg once a day.

▸ **Dosage in Renal Impairment**

PO

Adults, Elderly. Dosage is decreased to 75 mg once a day for at least 7 days and possibly up to 6 wk.

SIDE EFFECTS/ADVERSE REACTIONS

Frequent

Nausea, vomiting, diarrhea

Occasional

Abdominal pain, bronchitis, dizziness, headache, cough, insomnia, fatigue, vertigo

PRECAUTIONS AND CONTRAINDICATIONS

Hypersensitivity

Caution:

Renal impairment, lactation

DRUG INTERACTIONS OF CONCERN TO DENTISTRY

• None reported

SERIOUS REACTIONS

! Colitis, pneumonia, and pyrexia occur rarely.

DENTAL CONSIDERATIONS

General:

• Acute influenza patients are unlikely to be seen in the dental office except for dental emergencies.

• Consider semisupine chair position for patient comfort because of respiratory effects of disease.

oxacillin

ox-ah-**sill′**-in

CATEGORY AND SCHEDULE

Pregnancy Risk Category: B

Drug Class: Broad-spectrum antiinfective; beta lactamase-resistant penicillin

MECHANISM OF ACTION

A penicillin that binds to bacterial membranes.

Therapeutic Effect: Bactericidal.

USES

Treatment of infections caused by beta lactamase-producing bacteria

PHARMACOKINETICS

PO/IM: Peak 30–60 min, duration 4–6 hr **IV:** Peak 5 min, duration 4–6 hr. ***Half-life:*** 30–60 min. Metabolized in the liver; excreted in urine, bile, breast milk, crosses placenta.

INDICATIONS AND DOSAGES

▸ Upper Respiratory Tract, Skin, and Skin-Structure Infections

IV, IM

Adults, Elderly, Children weighing 40 kg or more. 250–500 mg q4–6h.

Children weighing less than 40 kg. 50 mg/kg/day in divided doses q6h. Maximum: 12 g/day.

▸ Lower Respiratory Tract and Other Serious Infections

IV, IM

Adults, Elderly, Children weighing 40 kg or more. 1 g q4–6h. Maximum: 12 g/day.

Children weighing less than 40 kg. 100 mg/kg/day in divided doses q4–6h.

SIDE EFFECTS/ADVERSE REACTIONS

Frequent

Mild hypersensitivity reaction (fever, rash, pruritus), GI effects (nausea, vomiting, diarrhea)

Occasional

Phlebitis, thrombophlebitis (more common in elderly), hepatotoxicity (with high IV dosage)

PRECAUTIONS AND CONTRAINDICATIONS

Hypersensitivity to any penicillin

DRUG INTERACTIONS OF CONCERN TO DENTISTRY

- Increased or prolonged plasma levels: probenecid
- Aminoglycosides: injections must be separated by 1 hr
- Possible decrease in antimicrobial effectiveness: tetracyclines, erythromycins, lincomycins
- Suspected increase in methotrexate toxicity

SERIOUS REACTIONS

! Antibiotic-associated colitis and other superinfections may result from altered bacterial balance.

! A mild to severe hypersensitivity reaction may occur in those allergic to penicillins.

DENTAL CONSIDERATIONS

General:

- Determine why patient is taking the drug.
- Caution regarding allergy to medication.

Consultations:

- Consult patient's physician if an acute dental infection occurs and another antiinfective is required.
- Medical consultation may be required to assess disease control.

Teach Patient/Family to:

- Encourage effective oral hygiene to prevent soft tissue inflammation.
- Prevent trauma when using oral hygiene aids.
- When antibiotics are used for dental infection:
    - Report sore throat, oral burning sensation, fever, or fatigue, any of which could indicate presence of a superinfection.

oxaliplatin

ahks-al-eh-**plah′**-tin
(Eloxatin)

CATEGORY AND SCHEDULE

Pregnancy Risk Category: D

Drug Class: Antineoplastic; platinum coordination complex

MECHANISM OF ACTION

A platinum-containing complex that cross-links with DNA strands, preventing cell division. Cell cycle-phase nonspecific.
Therapeutic Effect: Inhibits DNA replication.

USES

Treatment of metastatic carcinoma of the colon or rectum in combination with 5-FU/leucovorin

PHARMACOKINETICS

Rapidly distributed. Protein binding: 90%. Undergoes rapid, extensive nonenzymatic biotransformation. Excreted in urine. ***Half-life:*** 70 hr.

INDICATIONS AND DOSAGES

▸ **Metastatic Colon or Rectal Cancer in Patients Whose Disease Has Recurred or Progressed During or Within 6 Mo of Completing First-Line Therapy with Bolus 5-Fluorouracil (5-FU), Leucovorin, and Irinotecan**

IV

Adults. Day 1: Oxaliplatin 85 mg/m^2 in 250–500 ml D5W and leucovorin 200 mg/m^2, both given simultaneously over more than 2 hr in separate bags using a Y-line, followed by 5-FU 400 mg/m^2 IV bolus given over 2–4 min, followed by 5-FU 600 mg/m^2 in 500 ml D5W as a 22-hr continuous IV infusion.
Day 2: Leucovorin 200 mg/m^2 IV infusion given over more than 2 hr, followed by 5-FU 400 mg/m^2 IV bolus given over 2–4 min, followed by 5-FU 600 mg/m^2 in 500 ml D5W as a 22-hr continuous IV infusion.

▸ **Ovarian Cancer**

IV

Adults. Cisplatin 100 mg/m^2 and oxaliplatin 130 mg/m^2 every 3 wk.

SIDE EFFECTS/ADVERSE REACTIONS

Frequent

Peripheral or sensory neuropathy (usually occurs in hands, feet, perioral area, and throat but may present as jaw spasm, abnormal tongue sensation, eye pain, chest pressure, or difficulty walking, swallowing, or writing), nausea, fatigue, diarrhea, vomiting, constipation, abdominal pain, fever, anorexia

Occasional

Stomatitis, earache, insomnia, cough, difficulty breathing, backache, edema

Rare

Dyspepsia, dizziness, rhinitis, flushing, alopecia

PRECAUTIONS AND CONTRAINDICATIONS

History of allergy to platinum compounds

DRUG INTERACTIONS OF CONCERN TO DENTISTRY

• None reported

SERIOUS REACTIONS

! Peripheral or sensory neuropathy can occur, sometimes precipitated or exacerbated by drinking or holding a glass of cold liquid during the IV infusion.

! Pulmonary fibrosis, characterized by a nonproductive cough, dyspnea, crackles, and radiologic pulmonary infiltrates, may require drug discontinuation.

! Hypersensitivity reaction (rash, urticaria, pruritus) occurs rarely.

DENTAL CONSIDERATIONS

General:

• If additional analgesia is required for dental pain, consider alternative analgesics (NSAIDs or acetaminophen) in patients taking opioids for acute or chronic pain.
• Examine for oral manifestation of opportunistic infection.
• Avoid products that affect platelet function, such as aspirin and NSAIDs.
• This drug may be used in the hospital or on an outpatient basis. Confirm the patient's disease and treatment status.
• Chlorhexidine mouth rinse prior to and during chemotherapy may reduce severity of mucositis.
• Patient on chronic drug therapy may rarely present with symptoms of blood dyscrasias, which can include infection, bleeding, and poor healing. If dyscrasia is present, caution patient to prevent oral tissue trauma when using oral hygiene aids.
• Palliative medication may be required for management of oral side effects.
• Short appointments and a stress-reduction protocol may be required for anxious patients.
• Provide palliative emergency dental care during drug use.
• Patients may be at risk of bleeding; check for oral signs.
• Oral infections should be eliminated and treated aggressively.
• Monitor vital signs.

Consultations:

• Medical consultation should include routine blood counts, including platelet counts and bleeding time.
• Consult physician; prophylactic or therapeutic antiinfectives may be indicated if surgery or periodontal treatment is required.
• Medical consultation may be required to assess immunologic status during cancer chemotherapy and determine safety risk, if any, posed by the required dental treatment.
• Medical consultation may be required to assess disease control and patient's ability to tolerate stress.

Teach Patient/Family to:

• See dentist immediately if secondary oral infection occurs.
• Be aware of oral side effects.
• Encourage effective oral hygiene to prevent soft tissue inflammation.
• Report oral lesions, soreness, or bleeding to dentist.
• Prevent trauma when using oral hygiene aids.
• Update health and medication history if physician makes any changes in evaluation or drug regimens; include OTC, herbal, and nonherbal drugs in the update.
• Avoid ice water rinses and exposure to cold to prevent exacerbation of neuropathy symptoms.

oxandrolone

ox-**an**′-droe-lone
(Lonavar[AUS], Oxandrin)
Do not confuse with testolactone.

CATEGORY AND SCHEDULE

Pregnancy Risk Category: X
Controlled Substance: Schedule III

Drug Class: Androgenic anabolic steroid

MECHANISM OF ACTION
A synthetic testosterone derivative that promotes growth and development of male sex organs, maintains secondary sex characteristics in androgen-deficient males.
Therapeutic Effect: Androgenic and anabolic actions.

USES
Promotion of weight gain in catabolic or tissue wasting processes, such as extensive surgery, burns, infection, or trauma; HIV wasting syndrome; Turner's syndrome

PHARMACOKINETICS
Well absorbed from the GI tract. Protein binding: 94%–97%. Metabolized in liver. Primarily excreted in urine. Unknown if removed by hemodialysis. ***Half-life:*** 5–13 hr.

INDICATIONS AND DOSAGES
▸ Weight Gain
Adults, Elderly. 2.5–20 mg in divided doses 2–4 times a day usually for 2–4 wk. Course of therapy is based on individual response. Repeat intermittently as needed.
Children. Total daily dose is 0.1 mg/kg. Repeat intermittently as needed.

SIDE EFFECTS/ADVERSE REACTIONS
Frequent
Gynecomastia, acne, amenorrhea, other menstrual irregularities
Females: Hirsutism, deepening of voice, clitoral enlargement that may not be reversible when drug is discontinued
Occasional
Edema, nausea, insomnia, oligospermia, priapism, male pattern of baldness, bladder irritability, hypercalcemia in immobilized patients or those with breast cancer, hypercholesterolemia
Rare
Polycythemia with high dosage

PRECAUTIONS AND CONTRAINDICATIONS
Nephrosis, carcinoma of breast or prostate hypercalcemia, pregnancy, hypersensitivity to oxandrolone or any component of the formulation
Caution:
Diabetes mellitus, cardiovascular disease, MI, increased risk of prostatic hypertrophy, prostatic carcinoma, virilization (women), increased PT

DRUG INTERACTIONS OF CONCERN TO DENTISTRY
- Increased risk of bleeding: aspirin
- Edema: adrenocorticotropic hormone (ACTH), adrenal steroids

SERIOUS REACTIONS
! Peliotic hepatitis of the liver, spleen replaced with blood-filled cysts, hepatic neoplasms and hepatocellular carcinoma have been associated with prolonged high-dosage, anaphylactic reactions.

DENTAL CONSIDERATIONS
General:
- Monitor vital signs at every appointment because of cardiovascular side effects.
- Determine why the patient is taking the drug.
- Consider local hemostasis measures to prevent excessive bleeding.

• Short appointments and a stress-reduction protocol may be required for anxious patients.
• Avoid prescribing aspirin-containing products.

Consultations:

• If signs of anemia are observed in oral tissues, physician consultation may be required.
• Medical consultation may be required to assess disease control and patient's ability to tolerate stress.
• Medical consultation should include INR.

Teach Patient/Family to:

• Encourage effective oral hygiene to prevent soft tissue inflammation.
• See dentist immediately if secondary oral infection occurs.

oxaprozin

ox-ah-**pro′**-zin
(Daypro)
Do not confuse oxaprozin with oxazepam.

CATEGORY AND SCHEDULE

Pregnancy Risk Category: C (D if used in third trimester or near delivery)

Drug Class: Nonsteroidal antiinflammatory

MECHANISM OF ACTION

An NSAID that produces analgesic and antiinflammatory effects by inhibiting prostaglandin synthesis. ***Therapeutic Effect:*** Reduces the inflammatory response and intensity of pain.

USES

Treatment of rheumatoid arthritis, osteoarthritis, and ankylosing spondylitis

PHARMACOKINETICS

Well absorbed from the GI tract. Protein binding: 99%. Widely distributed. Metabolized in the liver. Primarily excreted in urine; partially eliminated in feces. Not removed by hemodialysis. ***Half-life:*** 42–50 hr.

INDICATIONS AND DOSAGES

▸ **Osteoarthritis**

PO

Adults, Elderly. 1200 mg once a day (600 mg in patients with low body weight or mild disease). Maximum: 1800 mg/day.

▸ **Rheumatoid Arthritis**

PO

Adults, Elderly. 1200 mg once a day. Range: 600–1800 mg/day.

▸ **Juvenile Rheumatoid Arthritis**

Children weighing more than 54 kg. 1200 mg/day.
Children weighing 32–54 kg. 900 mg/day.
Children weighing 22–31 kg. 600 mg/day.

▸ **Dosage in Renal Impairment**

For adults and elderly patients with renal impairment, the recommended initial dose is 600 mg/day; may be increased up to 1200 mg/day.

SIDE EFFECTS/ADVERSE REACTIONS

Occasional

Nausea, diarrhea, constipation, dyspepsia, edema

Rare

Vomiting, abdominal cramps or pain, flatulence, anorexia, confusion, tinnitus, insomnia, somnolence

PRECAUTIONS AND CONTRAINDICATIONS

Active peptic ulcer disease, chronic inflammation of GI tract, GI bleeding or ulceration, history of hypersensitivity to aspirin or NSAIDs

Caution:
- Lactation, children, bleeding disorders, GI disorders, cardiac disorders, hypersensitivity to other antiinflammatory agents, diabetes

DRUG INTERACTIONS OF CONCERN TO DENTISTRY

- GI ulceration, bleeding: aspirin, alcohol, corticosteroids
- Decreased action: salicylates
- Nephrotoxicity: acetaminophen (prolonged use and high doses)
- Possible risk of decreased renal function: cyclosporine
- SSRIs: increased risk of GI side effects
- When prescribed for dental pain:
  - Risk of increased effects: oral anticoagulants, oral antidiabetics, lithium, methotrexate
  - Decreased antihypertensive effects of diuretics, β-adrenergic blockers, and ACE inhibitors

SERIOUS REACTIONS

! Hypertension, acute renal failure, respiratory depression, GI bleeding, and coma occur rarely.

DENTAL CONSIDERATIONS

General:
- Patients on chronic drug therapy may rarely have symptoms of blood dyscrasias, which can include infection, bleeding, and poor healing.
- Assess salivary flow as a factor in caries, periodontal disease, and candidiasis.
- Avoid prescribing for dental use in pregnancy.
- Consider semisupine chair position for patients with arthritic disease.
- Severe stomach bleeding may occur in patients who regularly use NSAIDs in recommended doses, when the patient is also taking another NSAID, an anticoagulant/antiplatelet drug, or steroid drug, if the patient has GI or peptic ulcer disease, if they are 60 yr or older, or when NSAIDs are taken longer than directed. Warn patients of the potential for severe stomach bleeding.

Consultations:
- Medical consultation may be required to assess disease control.
- In a patient with symptoms of blood dyscrasias, request a medical consultation for blood studies and postpone dental treatment until normal values are reestablished.

Teach Patient/Family to:
- Encourage effective oral hygiene to prevent soft tissue inflammation.
- Use caution to prevent injury when using oral hygiene aids.
- Warn patient of potential risks of NSAIDs.
- When chronic dry mouth occurs, advise patient to:
  - Avoid mouth rinses with high alcohol content because of drying effects.
  - Use daily home fluoride products to prevent caries.
  - Use sugarless gum, frequent sips of water, or saliva substitutes.

oxazepam

ox-**a**′-ze-pam
(Alepam[AUS], Apo-Oxazepam[CAN], Murelax[AUS], Serax, Serepax[AUS])
Do not confuse oxazepam with oxaprozin, or Serax with Eurax or Xerac.

CATEGORY AND SCHEDULE

Pregnancy Risk Category: D
Controlled Substance: Schedule IV

Drug Class: Benzodiazepine

MECHANISM OF ACTION

A benzodiazepine that potentiates the effects of gamma-aminobutyric acid and other inhibitory neurotransmitters by binding to specific receptors in the CNS. ***Therapeutic Effect:*** Produces anxiolytic effect and skeletal muscle relaxation.

USES

Treatment of anxiety, alcohol withdrawal

PHARMACOKINETICS

Well absorbed from the GI tract. Protein binding: 97%. Metabolized in the liver. Primarily excreted in urine. Not removed by hemodialysis. ***Half-life:*** 5–20 hr.

INDICATIONS AND DOSAGES

▸ Mild-to-Moderate Anxiety

PO

Adults. 10–15 mg 3–4 times a day.

▸ Severe Anxiety

PO

Adults. 15–30 mg 3–4 times a day.

▸ Alcohol Withdrawal

PO

Adults. 15–30 mg 3–4 times a day.
Elderly. Initially, 10–20 mg 3 times a day. May gradually increase up to 30–45 mg/day.

SIDE EFFECTS/ADVERSE REACTIONS

Frequent
Mild, transient somnolence at beginning of therapy
Occasional
Dizziness, headache
Rare
Paradoxic CNS reactions, such as hyperactivity or nervousness in children and excitement or restlessness in the elderly or debilitated (generally noted during the first 2 wk of therapy)

PRECAUTIONS AND CONTRAINDICATIONS

Angle-closure glaucoma; preexisting CNS depression; severe, uncontrolled pain
Caution:
Elderly, debilitated, hepatic disease, renal disease

DRUG INTERACTIONS OF CONCERN TO DENTISTRY

- Increased effects: CNS depressants, alcohol, and anticonvulsant medications
- Possible increase in CNS side effects of kava kava (herb)

SERIOUS REACTIONS

! Abrupt or too-rapid withdrawal may result in pronounced restlessness, irritability, insomnia, hand tremors, abdominal or muscle cramps, diaphoresis, vomiting, and seizures.
! Overdose results in somnolence, confusion, diminished reflexes, and coma.

DENTAL CONSIDERATIONS

General:
- Monitor vital signs at every appointment because of cardiovascular side effects.
- Avoid use in pregnancy.
- Psychological and physical dependence may occur with chronic administration.
- Geriatric patients are more susceptible to drug effects; use lower dose.
- Assess salivary flow as a factor in caries, periodontal disease, and candidiasis.

Consultations:
- Medical consultation may be required to assess disease control.

Teach Patient/Family to:
- Avoid mouth rinses with high alcohol content because of drying effects.

• Anxious patients may require short appointments and a stress-reduction protocol.

oxcarbazepine

oks-kar-**bays**′-uh-peen
(Trileptal)

CATEGORY AND SCHEDULE

Pregnancy Risk Category: C

Drug Class: Anticonvulsant

MECHANISM OF ACTION

An anticonvulsant that blocks sodium channels, resulting in stabilization of hyperexcited neural membranes, inhibition of repetitive neuronal firing, and diminishing synaptic impulses.
Therapeutic Effect: Prevents seizures.

USES

Monotherapy or adjunctive therapy of partial seizures in adults with epilepsy; monotherapy or adjunctive therapy for partial seizures in children (4–16 yr) with epilepsy

PHARMACOKINETICS

Completely absorbed from GI tract and extensively metabolized in the liver to active metabolite. Protein binding: 40%. Primarily excreted in urine. ***Half-life:*** 2 hr; metabolite, 6–10 hr.

INDICATIONS AND DOSAGES

▸ Adjunctive Treatment of Seizures

PO

Adults, Elderly. Initially, 600 mg/day in 2 divided doses. May increase by up to 600 mg/day at weekly intervals. Maximum: 2400 mg/day.
Children 4–16 yr. 8–10 mg/kg. Maximum: 600 mg/day.
Maintenance (based on weight): 1800 mg/day for children weighing more than 39 kg; 1200 mg/day for children weighing 29.1–39 kg; and 900 mg/day for children weighing 20–29 kg.

▸ Conversion to Monotherapy

PO

Adults, Elderly. 600 mg/day in 2 divided doses (while decreasing concomitant anticonvulsant over 3–6 wk). May increase by 600 mg/day at weekly intervals up to 2400 mg/day.
Children. Initially, 8–10 mg/kg/day in 2 divided doses with simultaneous initial reduction of dose of concomitant antiepileptic.

▸ Initiation of Monotherapy

PO

Adults, Elderly. 600 mg/day in 2 divided doses. May increase by 300 mg/day every 3 days up to 1200 mg/day.
Children. Initially, 8–10 mg/kg/day in 2 divided doses. Increase at 3 day intervals by 5 mg/kg/day to achieve maintenance dose by weight;
(70 kg): 1500–2100 mg/day;
(60–69 kg): 1200–2100 mg/day;
(50–59 kg): 1200–1800 mg/day;
(41–49 kg): 1200–1500 mg/day;
(35–40 kg): 900–1500 mg/day;
(25–34 kg): 900–1200 mg/day;
(20–24 kg): 600–900 mg/day.

▸ Dosage in Renal Impairment

For patients with creatinine clearance less than 30 ml/min, give 50% of normal starting dose, then titrate slowly to desired dose.

SIDE EFFECTS/ADVERSE REACTIONS

Frequent

Dizziness, nausea, headache

Occasional
Vomiting, diarrhea, ataxia, nervousness, heartburn, indigestion, epigastric pain, constipation
Rare
Tremors, rash, back pain, epistaxis, sinusitis, diplopia

PRECAUTIONS AND CONTRAINDICATIONS

Hypersensitivity to this drug or carbamazepine
Caution:
Development of hyponatremia, withdraw drug slowly to avoid seizures, cognitive CNS adverse effects, decreases effect of oral contraceptives, caution when used with other anticonvulsants, renal impairment, lactation

DRUG INTERACTIONS OF CONCERN TO DENTISTRY

- No dental drug interactions reported; CYP450 3A4/5 enzyme inducers may decrease plasma levels
- Possible increase in CNS depression: all CNS depressants, alcohol

SERIOUS REACTIONS

! Clinically significant hyponatremia may occur.

DENTAL CONSIDERATIONS

General:
- Monitor vital signs at every appointment because of cardiovascular side effects.
- Patients on chronic drug therapy may rarely have symptoms of blood dyscrasias, which can include infection, bleeding, and poor healing.
- Assess salivary flow as a factor in caries, periodontal disease, and candidiasis.
- Consider semisupine chair position for patient comfort if GI side effects occur.
- Short appointments and a stress-reduction protocol may be required for anxious patients.
- Determine type of epilepsy, seizure frequency, and quality of seizure control.

Consultations:
- In a patient with symptoms of blood dyscrasias, request a medical consultation for blood studies and postpone treatment until normal values are reestablished.
- Medical consultation may be required to assess disease control and patient's ability to tolerate stress.

Teach Patient/Family to:
- Encourage effective oral hygiene to prevent soft tissue inflammation.
- Prevent trauma when using oral hygiene aids.
- When chronic dry mouth occurs, advise patient to:
  - Avoid mouth rinses with high alcohol content because of drying effects.
  - Use daily home fluoride products for anticaries effect.
  - Use sugarless gum, frequent sips of water, or saliva substitutes.

oxiconazole

ox-i-**con**′-a-zole
(Oxistat, Oxizole[CAN])
Do not confuse with Nitrostat.

CATEGORY AND SCHEDULE

Pregnancy Risk Category: B

Drug Class: Antifungals, topical, dermatologics

MECHANISM OF ACTION

An antifungal agent that inhibits ergosterol synthesis.
Therapeutic Effect: Destroys cytoplasmic membrane integrity of fungi. Fungicidal.

USES

Treatment of infections caused by a fungus

PHARMACOKINETICS

Low systemic absorption. Absorbed and distributed in each layer of the dermis. Excreted in the urine.

INDICATIONS AND DOSAGES

▸ ***Tinea pedis***
Topical
Adults, Elderly, Children 12 yr and older. Apply 1–2 times a day for 1 mo or until signs and symptoms significantly improve.
▸ ***Tinea cruris, Tinea corporis***
Topical
Adults, Elderly, Children 12 yr and older. Apply 1–2 times a day for 2 wk or until signs and symptoms significantly improve.

SIDE EFFECTS/ADVERSE REACTIONS

Occasional
Itching, local irritation, stinging, dryness

PRECAUTIONS AND CONTRAINDICATIONS

Not for ophthalmic use, hypersensitivity to oxiconazole or any other azole fungals

DRUG INTERACTIONS OF CONCERN TO DENTISTRY

- None reported

SERIOUS REACTIONS

! Hypersensitivity reactions characterized by rash, swelling, pruritus, maceration, and a sensation of warmth may occur.

DENTAL CONSIDERATIONS

General:
- Determine why the patient is using this medication.

oxidized cellulose

oks′-ih-dye-zed **cell′**-you-loze
(Interceed, Surgicel)

CATEGORY AND SCHEDULE

Pregnancy Risk Category: Not reported

Drug Class: Cellulose hemostatic

MECHANISM OF ACTION

Oxidized cellulose is saturated with blood at the bleeding site and swells into a gelatinous mass that aids in clot formation. When used in small amounts, it is absorbed from the sites of implantation with minimal tissue reaction.
Therapeutic Effect: Reduces bleeding.

USES

Hemostasis in surgery, oral surgery, exodontia

PHARMACOKINETICS

Absorption occurs in 7–14 days.
Half-life: Unknown.

INDICATIONS AND DOSAGES

▸ **Surgical Procedures to Assist in the Control of Capillary, Venous, and Small Arterial Hemorrhage When Ligation or Other Conventional Methods of Control Are Impractical or Ineffective**
Topical
Adults. Minimal amounts of an appropriate size are laid on the bleeding site or held firmly against

the tissues until hemostasis is obtained.

SIDE EFFECTS/ADVERSE REACTIONS

Frequency Not Defined

Headache, nasal burning or stinging, sneezing, encapsulation of fluid

PRECAUTIONS AND CONTRAINDICATIONS

Use for packing or implantation in fractures or laminectomies, hemorrhage from large arteries, and nonhemorrhagic oozing surfaces; use as a wrap; use around the optic nerve and chiasm; applied as wadding or packing as a hemostatic agent; hypersensitivity to oxidized cellulose or any component of the formulation

Caution:

Do not autoclave; inactivation of topical thrombin

SERIOUS REACTIONS

! Pain, numbness, and paralysis have been reported.

DENTAL CONSIDERATIONS

General:

- Apply dry; use only amount needed to control bleeding.
- Place loosely and avoid packing; remove excess before closure in surgery; irrigate first, then remove using sterile technique.
- Ensure therapeutic response: decreased bleeding in surgery.
- Can be left in situ when necessary but should be removed once bleeding is controlled.
- Application of topical thrombin solution to the cellulose gauze will inactivate thrombin because of acidity.

oxybutynin

ox-ih-**byoo′**-ti-nin

(Ditropan, Ditropan XL, Oxytrol)

Do not confuse oxybutynin with OxyContin, or Ditropan with diazepam.

CATEGORY AND SCHEDULE

Pregnancy Risk Category: B

Drug Class: Antispasmodic

MECHANISM OF ACTION

An anticholinergic that exerts antispasmodic (papaverine-like) and antimuscarinic (atropine-like) action on the detrusor smooth muscle of the bladder.

Therapeutic Effect: Increases bladder capacity and delays desire to void.

USES

Antispasmodic for neurogenic bladder, overactive bladder

PHARMACOKINETICS

Route	Onset	Peak	Duration
PO	0.5–1 hr	3–6 hr	6–10 hr

Rapidly absorbed from the GI tract. Metabolized in the liver. Primarily excreted in urine. Unknown if removed by hemodialysis. ***Half-life:*** 1–2.3 hr.

INDICATIONS AND DOSAGES

▸ **Neurogenic Bladder**

PO

Adults. 5 mg 2–3 times a day up to 5 mg 4 times a day.

Elderly. 2.5–5 mg twice a day. May increase by 2.5 mg/day every 1–2 days.

Children 5 yr and older. 5 mg twice a day up to 5 mg 4 times a day.
Children 1–4 yr. 0.2 mg/kg/dose 2–4 times a day.
PO (Extended-Release)
Adults. 5–10 mg/day up to 30 mg/day.
Transdermal
Adults. 3.9 mg applied twice a week. Apply every 3–4 days.

SIDE EFFECTS/ADVERSE REACTIONS

Frequent
Constipation, dry mouth, somnolence, decreased perspiration
Occasional
Decreased lacrimation or salivation, impotence, urinary hesitancy and retention, suppressed lactation, blurred vision, mydriasis, nausea or vomiting, insomnia

PRECAUTIONS AND CONTRAINDICATIONS

GI or GU obstruction, glaucoma, myasthenia gravis, toxic megacolon, ulcerative colitis
Caution:
Lactation, suspected glaucoma, children younger than 12 yr, hiatal hernia, esophageal reflux, coronary heart disease, CHF, hypertension

DRUG INTERACTIONS OF CONCERN TO DENTISTRY

- Increased anticholinergic effect: anticholinergic drugs
- Increased depressant effect of both drugs: CNS depressants, alcohol

SERIOUS REACTIONS

! Overdose produces CNS excitation (including nervousness, restlessness, hallucinations, and irritability), hypotension or hypertension, confusion, tachycardia, facial flushing, and respiratory depression.

DENTAL CONSIDERATIONS

General:
- Assess salivary flow as a factor in caries, periodontal disease, and candidiasis.
- Monitor vital signs at every appointment because of cardiovascular side effects.
- Avoid dental light in patient's eyes; offer dark glasses for patient comfort.
- Consider semisupine chair position for patient comfort if GI side effects occur.

Consultations:
- Physician should be informed if significant xerostomic side effects occur (e.g., increased caries, sore tongue, problems eating or swallowing, difficulty wearing prosthesis) so that a medication change can be considered.

Teach Patient/Family to:
- Encourage effective oral hygiene to prevent soft tissue inflammation.
- When chronic dry mouth occurs, advise patient to:
  - Avoid mouth rinses with high alcohol content because of drying effects.
  - Use daily home fluoride products to prevent caries.
  - Use sugarless gum, frequent sips of water, or saliva substitutes.

oxycodone

ox-ee-**koe′**-done

(Endone[AUS], OxyContin, Oxydose, OxyFast, OxyIR, Oxynorm[AUS], Roxicodone, Roxicodone Intensol)

Do not confuse oxycodone with oxybutynin.

CATEGORY AND SCHEDULE

Pregnancy Risk Category: B (D if used for prolonged periods or at high dosages at term)

Controlled Substance: Schedule II

Drug Class: Synthetic opioid analgesic

MECHANISM OF ACTION

An opioid analgesic that binds with opioid receptors in the CNS. ***Therapeutic Effect:*** Alters the perception of and emotional response to pain.

USES

Treatment of moderate-to-severe pain, normally used in combination with aspirin or acetaminophen; combination products

PHARMACOKINETICS

Route	Onset	Peak	Duration
PO, immediate release	N/A	N/A	4–5 hr
PO, controlled release	N/A	N/A	12 hr

Moderately absorbed from the GI tract. Protein binding: 38%–45%. Widely distributed. Metabolized in the liver. Excreted in urine. Unknown if removed by hemodialysis. ***Half-life:*** 2–3 hr (3.2 hr controlled-release).

INDICATIONS AND DOSAGES

▸ **Analgesia**

PO (Controlled-Release)

Adults, Elderly. Initially, 10 mg q12h. May increase every 1–2 days by 25%–50%. Usual: 40 mg/day (100 mg/day for cancer pain).

PO (Immediate-Release)

Adults, Elderly. Initially, 5 mg q6h as needed. May increase up to 30 mg q4h. Usual: 10–30 mg q4h as needed.

Children. 0.05–0.15 mg/kg/dose q4–6h.

SIDE EFFECTS/ADVERSE REACTIONS

Frequent

Somnolence, dizziness, hypotension (including orthostatic hypotension), anorexia

Occasional

Confusion, diaphoresis, facial flushing, urine retention, constipation, dry mouth, nausea, vomiting, headache

Rare

Allergic reaction, depression, paradoxic CNS hyperactivity or nervousness in children, paradoxic excitement and restlessness in elderly or debilitated patients

PRECAUTIONS AND CONTRAINDICATIONS

Hypersensitivity, addiction (narcotic)

Caution:

Addictive personality, lactation, increased intracranial pressure, MI (acute), severe heart disease, respiratory depression, hepatic disease, renal disease, children younger than 18 yr, physical dependence

DRUG INTERACTIONS OF CONCERN TO DENTISTRY

• Increased effects with other CNS depressants: alcohol, other narcotics, sedative-hypnotics, skeletal muscle relaxants, phenothiazines, benzodiazepines
• Contraindication: MAOIs
• Increased effects of anticholinergics
• Partial antagonists (e.g., pentazocine) may precipitate withdrawal

SERIOUS REACTIONS

! Overdose results in respiratory depression, skeletal muscle flaccidity, cold or clammy skin, cyanosis, and extreme somnolence progressing to seizures, stupor, and coma.
! Hepatotoxicity may occur with overdose of the acetaminophen component of fixed-combination products.
! The patient who uses oxycodone repeatedly may develop a tolerance to the drug's analgesic effect and physical dependence.

DENTAL CONSIDERATIONS

General:
• Monitor vital signs at every appointment because of cardiovascular and respiratory side effects.
• Assess salivary flow as a factor in caries, periodontal disease, and candidiasis.
• Psychological and physical dependence may occur with chronic administration.
• Determine why the patient is taking the drug.

Teach Patient/Family to:
• Avoid mouth rinses with high alcohol content because of drying effects.

oxymetazoline

ox-ee-met-**az′**-oh-leen
(Afrin, Afrin 12-Hour, Afrin Children's Strength Nose Drops, OcuClear, Sinex 12 Hour Long-Acting)

CATEGORY AND SCHEDULE

Pregnancy Risk Category: C
OTC

Drug Class: Nasal decongestant, sympathomimetic amine

MECHANISM OF ACTION

A direct-acting sympathomimetic amine that acts on α-adrenergic receptors in arterioles of the nasal mucosa to produce constriction. ***Therapeutic Effect:*** Causes vasoconstriction resulting in decreased blood flow and decreased nasal congestion.

USES

Treatment of nasal congestion

PHARMACOKINETICS

Onset of action is about 10 min, and duration of action is 7 hr or more. Absorption occurs from the nasal mucosa and can produce systemic effects, primarily following overdose or excessive use. Excreted mostly in the urine, as well as the feces. ***Half-life:*** 5–8 hr.

INDICATIONS AND DOSAGES

▸ **Rhinitis**

Intranasal

Adults, Elderly, Children older than 6 yr. 2–3 drops/sprays (0.05% nasal solution) in each nostril q12h.

Children 2–5 yr. 2–4 drops or sprays (0.025% nasal solution) in each nostril q12h for up to 3 days.

▸ **Conjunctivitis**
Ophthalmic
Adults, Elderly, Children older than 6 yr: 1–2 drops (0.025% ophthalmic solution) q6h for 3–4 days.

SIDE EFFECTS/ADVERSE REACTIONS

Occasional
Burning, stinging, drying nasal mucosa, sneezing, rebound congestion, insomnia, nervousness

PRECAUTIONS AND CONTRAINDICATIONS

Narrow-angle glaucoma or hypersensitivity to oxymetazoline or other adrenergic agents
Caution:
Children younger than 6 yr, elderly, diabetes, cardiovascular disease, hypertension, hyperthyroidism, increased intracranial pressure, prostatic hypertrophy, glaucoma

DRUG INTERACTIONS OF CONCERN TO DENTISTRY

- Increased risk of hypertension: tricyclic antidepressants, but it requires adequate systemic absorption of oxymetazoline

SERIOUS REACTIONS

! Large doses may produce tachycardia, hypertension, arrhythmias, palpitations, lightheadedness, nausea, and vomiting.

DENTAL CONSIDERATIONS

General:
- Excessive use can lead to rebound congestion and cardiovascular side effects; follow recommended dosing intervals.
- Extensive nasal swelling and congestion may interfere with optimal use of nitrous oxide/oxygen sedation.

oxymetholone

ox-ee-**meth′**-oh-lone
(Anadrol, Anapolon[CAN])
Do not confuse with oxycodone.

CATEGORY AND SCHEDULE

Pregnancy Risk Category: X
Controlled Substance: Schedule III

Drug Class: Androgenic anabolic steroid

MECHANISM OF ACTION

An androgenic-anabolic steroid that is a synthetic derivative of testosterone synthesized to accentuate anabolic as opposed to androgenic effects.
Therapeutic Effect: Improves nitrogen balance in conditions of unfavorable protein metabolism with adequate caloric and protein intake, stimulates erythropoiesis, suppresses gonadotropic functions of pituitary, and may exert a direct effect upon the testes.

USES

Anemia associated with bone marrow failure and red cell production deficiencies; aplastic anemia, myelofibrosis, and anemia caused by myelotoxic drugs

PHARMACOKINETICS

Metabolized in the liver via reduction and oxidation. Unchanged oxymetholone and its metabolites are excreted in urine. ***Half-life:*** Unknown.

INDICATIONS AND DOSAGES

▸ Anemia, Chronic Renal Failure, Acquired Aplastic Anemia, Chemotherapy-Induced Myelosuppression, Fanconi's Anemia, Red Cell Aplasia

PO

Adults, Elderly, Children. 1–5 mg/kg/day. Response is not immediate, and a minimum of 3–6 mo should be given.

SIDE EFFECTS/ADVERSE REACTIONS

Frequent

Gynecomastia, acne, amenorrhea, menstrual irregularities

Females: Hirsutism, deepening of voice, clitoral enlargement that may not be reversible when drug is discontinued

Occasional

Edema, nausea, insomnia, oligospermia, priapism, male pattern of baldness, bladder irritability, hypercalcemia in immobilized patients or those with breast cancer, hypercholesterolemia, inflammation and pain at IM injection site

Transdermal: Itching, erythema, skin irritation

Rare

Liver damage, hypersensitivity

PRECAUTIONS AND CONTRAINDICATIONS

Cardiac impairment, hypercalcemia, pregnancy/lactation, prostatic or breast cancer in males, metastatic breast cancer in women with active hypercalcemia, nephrosis or nephritic phase nephritis, severe liver disease, hypersensitivity to oxymetholone or any of its components

Caution:

Diabetes mellitus, cardiovascular disease, MI, increased risk of prostatic hypertrophy, prostatic carcinoma, virilization (women), increased PT

DRUG INTERACTIONS OF CONCERN TO DENTISTRY

- Increased risk of bleeding: aspirin
- Edema: ACTH, adrenal steroids

SERIOUS REACTIONS

! Cholestatic jaundice, hepatic necrosis and death occur rarely but have been reported in association with long-term androgenic-anabolic steroid use.

DENTAL CONSIDERATIONS

General:

- Monitor vital signs at every appointment because of cardiovascular side effects.
- Determine why the patient is taking the drug.
- Consider local hemostasis measures to prevent excessive bleeding.
- Short appointments and a stress-reduction protocol may be required for anxious patients.
- Avoid prescribing aspirin-containing products.

Consultations:

- Physician consultation may be required if signs of anemia are observed in oral tissues.
- Medical consultation may be required to assess disease control and patient's ability to tolerate stress.
- Medical consultation should include INR.

Teach Patient/Family to:

- Encourage effective oral hygiene to prevent soft tissue inflammation.
- See dentist immediately if secondary oral infection occurs.

paclitaxel

pak-leh-**tax′**-ell

(Abraxane, Anzatax[AUS], Onxol, Taxol)

Do not confuse paclitaxel with Paxil, or Taxol with Taxotere.

CATEGORY AND SCHEDULE

Pregnancy Risk Category: D

Drug Class: Antineoplastic

MECHANISM OF ACTION

An antimitotic agent in the taxoids family that disrupts the microtubular cell network, which is essential for cellular function. Blocks cells in the late G_2 phase and M phase of the cell cycle.

Therapeutic Effect: Inhibits cellular mitosis and replication.

USES

Treatment of metastatic ovarian cancer, non–small-cell lung cancer; second-line treatment for AIDS-related Kaposi's sarcoma (KS); adjuvant treatment of node-positive breast cancer sequential to a course of standard doxorubicin-containing combination chemotherapy

PHARMACOKINETICS

Does not readily cross the blood-brain barrier. Protein binding: 89%–98%. Metabolized in the liver to active metabolites; eliminated by bile. Not removed by hemodialysis. ***Half-life:*** 1.3–8.6 hr.

INDICATIONS AND DOSAGES

▸ Ovarian Cancer

IV

Adults. 135–175 mg/m²/dose over 1–24 hr q3wk.

▸ Breast Carcinoma

IV (Onxol, Taxol)

Adults, Elderly. 175 mg/m² over 3 hr q3wk.

PO (Abraxane)

Adults, Elderly. 260 mg/m² over 30 min q3wk.

▸ Non–Small-Cell Lung Carcinoma

IV

Adults, Elderly. 135 mg/m² over 24 hr, followed by cisplatin 75 mg/m² q3wk.

▸ KS

IV

Adults, Elderly. 135 mg/m²/dose over 3 hr q3wk or 100 mg/m²/dose over 3 hr q2wk.

▸ Dosage in Hepatic Impairment

Total Bilirubin	Total Dose
More than 3 mg/dl	Less than 50 mg/m²
1.6–3 mg/dl	Less than 75 mg/m²
1.5 mg/dl or less	Less than 135 mg/m²

SIDE EFFECTS/ADVERSE REACTIONS

Expected

Diarrhea, alopecia, nausea, vomiting

Frequent

Myalgia or arthralgia, peripheral neuropathy

Occasional

Mucositis, hypotension during infusion, pain or redness at injection site

Rare

Bradycardia

PRECAUTIONS AND CONTRAINDICATIONS

Baseline neutropenia (neutrophil count 1500 cells/mm³), hypersensitivity to drugs developed with Cremophor EL (polyoxyethylated castor oil)

Caution:

Bone marrow depression, AV block, hepatic impairment, lactation,

P

children, recent MI, angina pectoris, CHF history, current use of drug with effect on cardiac conduction system

DRUG INTERACTIONS OF CONCERN TO DENTISTRY

- Possible (not demonstrated) increase in action by strong inhibitors of CYP2C8 and CYP3A4 isoenzymes: diazepam, ketoconazole, midazolam (monitor patient if prescribed)

SERIOUS REACTIONS

! Neutropenic nadir occurs at approximately day 11 of paclitaxel therapy.
! Anemia and leukopenia are common reactions.
! Thrombocytopenia occurs occasionally.
! A severe hypersensitivity reaction, including dyspnea, severe hypotension, angioedema, and generalized urticaria, occurs rarely.

DENTAL CONSIDERATIONS

General:

- Consider semisupine chair position for patient comfort if GI side effects occur.
- Patients receiving chemotherapy may require palliative therapy for stomatitis.
- Patients on chronic drug therapy may rarely have symptoms of blood dyscrasias, which can include infection, bleeding, and poor healing.

Consultations:

- Medical consultation may be required to assess disease control.

Teach Patient/Family to:

- Encourage effective oral hygiene to prevent soft tissue inflammation.
- Use caution to prevent trauma when using oral hygiene aids.

paliperidone

pal-ee-**per′**-i-done
(Invega, Invega Sustenna)

CATEGORY AND SCHEDULE

Pregnancy Risk Category: C

Drug Class: Antipsychotic

MECHANISM OF ACTION

The active metabolite of risperidone that may antagonize dopamine and serotonin receptors. Exhibits α-adrenergic and H_1 receptor antagonistic activity.
Therapeutic Effect: Suppresses psychotic behavior; decreases both positive and negative symptoms of schizophrenia.

USES

Schizophrenia

PHARMACOKINETICS

Paliperidone ER uses the osmotic drug-release technology that delivers the drug at a controlled rate. Oral bioavailability of paliperidone ER is 28%. Protein binding: 74%. Paliperidone dissolves slowly following IM injection. Not extensively metabolized in the liver. Extensively excreted in the kidney unchanged; minimal in feces.
Half-life: 23 hr (PO); 25–49 days (IM).

INDICATIONS AND DOSAGES

▸ **Schizophrenia**

PO (Extended-Release)
Adults. 6 mg a day, administered in the morning. Maximum: 12 mg a day. Titration should not occur more frequently than 5 days.

▸ **Renal Impairment**
PO (Extended-Release)
Creatinine clearance 50 to 80 ml/min. Initially, 3 mg/day. Maximum dose is 6 mg/day.
Creatinine clearance 10 to 50 ml/min. Initially, 1.5 mg/day. Maximum dose is 3 mg/day.

SIDE EFFECTS/ADVERSE REACTIONS

Frequent
Tachycardia, headache, somnolence, parkinsonism, insomnia, tremor
Occasional
Anxiety, extrapyramidal side effects, akathisia, dizziness, constipation, dyspepsia, nausea, weight gain, nasopharyngitis, appetite changes, sleep disturbances, back pain
Rare
Arrhythmia, fatigue, asthenia, orthostatic hypotension, abdominal pain, cough, myalgia, hyperprolactinemia, xerostomia

PRECAUTIONS AND CONTRAINDICATIONS

Hypersensitivity to paliperidone, risperidone, or its components
Caution:
Elderly with dementia-related psychosis (increased mortality)—black box warning
Renal impairment
Hepatic impairment
Neuroleptic malignant syndrome
Tardive dyskinesia
Seizures
Leukopenia, neutropenia, agranulocytosis
Patients at risk for suicide
Cognitive and motor impairment
Hyperglycemia, diabetes, patients should be monitored for signs and symptoms of hyperglycemia
QT prolongation; electrolyte disturbances; serum potassium and magnesium should be monitored as hypokalemia and hypomagnesemia may increase the risk of QT prolongation

DRUG INTERACTIONS OF CONCERN TO DENTISTRY

- CNS depressants, alcohol: Additive CNS depressant effects
- Antihypertensive agents: May enhance the hypotensive effects
- Dopamine agonists, levodopa: May block the effects of dopamine agonists and levodopa
- QT-interval prolonging drugs: May cause additive effects
- Carbamazepine: May decrease the levels of paliperidone

SERIOUS REACTIONS

! Prolongation of QT interval may produce torsades de pointes. Patients with bradycardia, hypokalemia, hypomagnesemia are at increased risk.
! Orthostatic hypotension including dizziness, tachycardia, and syncope with standing may occur.
! Agranulocytosis, leucopenia, and neutropenia may occur.

P

DENTAL CONSIDERATIONS

General:
- Monitor vital signs at every appointment because of cardiovascular side effects.
- After supine positioning, have patient sit upright for at least 2 min before standing to avoid orthostatic hypotension.
- Assess salivary flow as a factor in caries, periodontal disease, and candidiasis.
- Assess for presence of extrapyramidal motor symptoms such as tardive dyskinesia and akathisia. Extrapyramidal motor

activity may complicate dental treatment.
• Consider semisupine chair position for patient comfort if GI side effects occur.

Consultations:
• In a patient with symptoms of blood dyscrasias, request a medical consultation for blood studies and postpone treatment until normal values are reestablished.
• Medical consultation may be required to assess disease control.
• Physician should be informed if significant xerostomic side effects occur (e.g., increased caries, sore tongue, problems eating or swallowing, difficulty wearing prosthesis) so that medication change can be considered.
• Consultation with physician may be necessary if sedation or general anesthesia is required.

Teach Patient/Family to:
• Encourage effective oral hygiene to prevent soft tissue inflammation.
• Prevent trauma when using oral hygiene aids.
• When chronic dry mouth occurs, advise patient to:
  • Avoid mouth rinses with high alcohol content because of drying effects.
  • Use daily home fluoride products for anticaries effect.
  • Use sugarless gum, frequent sips of water, or saliva substitutes.

palonosetron hydrochloride

pal-oh-**noe′**-seh-tron
high-droh-**klor′**-ide
(Aloxi)

CATEGORY AND SCHEDULE

Pregnancy Risk Category: B

Drug Class: Antiemetics/antivertigo, serotonin receptor antagonists

MECHANISM OF ACTION

A 5-HT_3 receptor antagonist that acts centrally in the chemoreceptor trigger zone and peripherally at vagal nerve endings.

USES

Prevention of nausea and vomiting associated with chemotherapy

PHARMACOKINETICS

Protein binding: 52%. Eliminated in urine. ***Half-life:*** 40 hr.

INDICATIONS AND DOSAGES

▸ Chemotherapy-Induced Nausea and Vomiting

IV

Adults, Elderly. 0.25 mg as a single dose 30 min before starting chemotherapy.

SIDE EFFECTS/ADVERSE REACTIONS

Occasional

Headache, constipation

Rare

Diarrhea, dizziness, fatigue, abdominal pain, insomnia

PRECAUTIONS AND CONTRAINDICATIONS

None known

DRUG INTERACTIONS OF CONCERN TO DENTISTRY

- None reported

SERIOUS REACTIONS

! Overdose may produce a combination of CNS stimulant and depressant effects.

DENTAL CONSIDERATIONS

General:

- For acute use in hospitals or cancer treatment centers.

Teach Patient/Family to:

- Be aware of possible oral side effects from concurrent chemotherapy.

pamidronate disodium

pam-**id**′-row-nate die-**soe**′-dee-um
(Aredia, Pamisol[AUS])
Do not confuse Aredia with Adriamycin.

CATEGORY AND SCHEDULE

Pregnancy Risk Category: D

Drug Class: Bone-resorption inhibitor, electrolyte modifier

MECHANISM OF ACTION

A bisphosphate that binds to bone and inhibits osteoclast-mediated calcium resorption.

Therapeutic Effect: Lowers serum calcium concentrations.

USES

Treatment of moderate-to-severe Paget's disease, mild-to-moderate hypercalcemia associated with malignancy with or without bone metastases, osteolytic bone metastases in breast cancer, multiple myeloma patients

PHARMACOKINETICS

Route	Onset	Peak	Duration
IV	24–48 hr	5–7 days	N/A

After IV administration, rapidly absorbed by bone. Slowly excreted unchanged in urine. Unknown if removed by hemodialysis. ***Half-life:*** bone, 300 days; unmetabolized, 2.5 hr.

INDICATIONS AND DOSAGES

▸ **Hypercalcemia**

IV Infusion

Adults, Elderly. Moderate hypercalcemia (corrected serum calcium level 12–13.5 mg/dl): 60–90 mg. Severe hypercalcemia (corrected serum calcium level greater than 13.5 mg/dl): 90 mg.

▸ **Paget's Disease**

IV Infusion

Adults, Elderly. 30 mg/day for 3 days.

▸ **Osteolytic Bone Lesion**

90 mg over 4 hr once monthly.

SIDE EFFECTS/ADVERSE REACTIONS

Frequent

Temperature elevation (at least 1°C) 24–48 hr after administration; redness, swelling, induration, pain at catheter site in patients receiving 90 mg; anorexia, nausea, fatigue

Occasional

Constipation, rhinitis

PRECAUTIONS AND CONTRAINDICATIONS

Hypersensitivity to other bisphosphonates, such as etidronate, tiludronate, risedronate, and alendronate. Dental implants are contraindicated for patients taking this drug.

DRUG INTERACTIONS OF CONCERN TO DENTISTRY

• None reported

SERIOUS REACTIONS

! Hypophosphatemia, hypokalemia, hypomagnesemia, and hypocalcemia occur more frequently with higher dosages.
! Anemia, hypertension, tachycardia, atrial fibrillation, and somnolence occur more frequently with 90-mg doses.
! GI hemorrhage occurs rarely.
! Osteonecrosis of the jaw.

DENTAL CONSIDERATIONS

General:

• Evaluate patient for signs and symptoms of osteonecrosis of the jaw.
• Determine why patient is taking the drug.
• This drug may be used in the hospital or on an outpatient basis. Confirm the patient's disease and treatment status.
• Examine for oral manifestation of opportunistic infection.
• Monitor and record vital signs.
• Consider semisupine chair position for patient comfort if GI side effects occur.
• Question patient about tolerance of NSAIDs or aspirin related to GI disease.
• Be aware of the oral manifestations of Paget's disease (macrognathia, alveolar pain).
• Patients may have received other chemotherapy or radiation; confirm medical and drug history.

Consultations:

• Medical consultation may be required to assess disease control and patient's ability to tolerate stress.

Teach Patient/Family to:

• Observe regular recall schedule and practice effective oral hygiene to minimize risk of osteonecrosis of the jaw.
• Avoid drugs containing calcium, vitamin D, and antacids; possible antagonism of pamidronate.

pancreatin/ pancrelipase

pan-kree-**ah**′-tin/
pan-kree-**lie**′-pace
(pancreatin: Ku-Zyme, Pancreatin; pancrelipase: Cotazym-S[AUS], Cotazym-S Forte[AUS], Creon, Pancrease[CAN], Pancrease MT, Ultrase, Viokase)

CATEGORY AND SCHEDULE

Pregnancy Risk Category: B (Pancrease, Pancrease MT); C (Creon, Kutrase, Lipram, Pancrelipase, Panokase, Plaretase, Ultrase, Ultrase MT, Viokase)

Drug Class: Digestive enzyme, oral

MECHANISM OF ACTION

A pancreatic digestive enzyme combination (protease, lipase, amylase) that hydrolyzes fats to glycerol and fatty acids, converts proteins into peptides and amino acids, and converts starch into dextrins and maltose.

USES

Enzyme replacement therapy for pancreatic insufficiency, such as in cystic fibrosis, chronic pancreatitis, post-pancreatectomy, ductal obstructions causes by pancreatic or bile duct tumors, steatorrhea of malabsorption, and post-gastrectomy.

PHARMACOKINETICS

Locally inactivated in the GI tract by anti-enzymes, excreted by the intestinal mucosa, or by the action of protease enzymes. Digested enzyme fragments may be absorbed by blood and are excreted in urine, or excreted in feces.

INDICATIONS AND DOSAGES

▸ **Pancreatic Insufficiency**

Adult. PO 4,000 to 20,000 units as capsules or tablets with meals or snacks and with sufficient liquids.
Children 7–12 yr. PO 4,000 to 12,000 units with each meal and snacks.
Children 1–6 yr. PO 4,000 to 8,000 units with each meal and snacks.
Dosages vary from product to product and preparations are not interchangeable due to variations in bioequivalence.

SIDE EFFECTS/ADVERSE REACTIONS

Frequent
Gastrointestinal upset
Occasional
Diarrhea, abdominal pain, vomiting, intestinal obstruction or stenosis, constipation, dermatitis, flatulence, nausea, melena, weight loss, pain, bloating, cramping
Rare
Allergic reactions

PRECAUTIONS AND CONTRAINDICATIONS

Fibrotic strictures, primarily in cystic fibrosis patients. GI obstructions; hyperuricosuria and hyperuricemia (high doses)

DRUG INTERACTIONS OF CONCERN TO DENTISTRY

- None reported in dentistry

SERIOUS REACTIONS

! Hypersensitivity, hyperuricosuria, hyperuricemia, fibrotic strictures

DENTAL CONSIDERATIONS

General:
- Know why patient is taking drug.
- Plan dental care to avoid disruptions of patient's diet.

Consultations:
- Consult with physician to determine severity of systemic disease and ability to tolerate dental procedures.

Teach Patient/Family to:
- Report changes in medical status and update medical history of prescription drugs.

panitumumab

pan-ih-**tu**′-mue-mab
(Vectibix)

CATEGORY AND SCHEDULE

Pregnancy Risk Category: C

Drug Class: Antineoplastic, monoclonal antibody

MECHANISM OF ACTION

An antineoplastic agent that binds specifically to epidermal growth factor (EGFR) on normal and tumor cells, and competitively inhibits the binding of ligands for EGFR. Blocks phosphorylation and activation of intracellular tyrosine kinases, resulting in inhibition of cell survival, growth, proliferation, and transformation.
Therapeutic Effect: Inhibits growth and survival of selected human tumor cell lines expressing EGFR.

USES

Treatment of EGFR-positive metastatic colorectal cancer

PHARMACOKINETICS

Half-life: 4–11 days. Other pharmacokinetic parameters have not been clearly established.

INDICATIONS AND DOSAGES

▸ EGFR-Positive Metastatic Colorectal Cancer

IV Infusion

Adults. 6 mg/kg administered over 60 min every 14 days. Doses higher than 1000 mg should be administered over 90 min.

▸ Dosing Adjustments

Infusion Reactions

Infusion reactions, mild-to-moderate (grade 1 or 2). Reduce the infusion rate by 50% for the duration of infusion. Infusion reactions, severe (grade 3 or 4). Immediately and permanently discontinue.

▸ Dermatologic Toxicity

Dermatologic toxicity (grade 3 or 4). Withhold panitumumab if skin toxicity does not improve to grade 2 or lower within 1 mo, permanently discontinue.

Dermatologic toxicity (grade 2 or lower), and the patient is symptomatically improved after withholding no more than 2 doses of panitumumab. Treatment may be resumed at 50% of the original dose. If toxicities recur, permanently discontinue drug. If toxicities do not recur, subsequent doses may be increased in increments of 25% of the original dose until the recommended dose of 6 mg/kg is obtained.

Safety and efficacy have not been established in children.

P

SIDE EFFECTS/ADVERSE REACTIONS

Frequent

Dermatologic toxicity, erythema, acneiform rash, pruritus, hypomagnesemia, fatigue, exfoliation, abdominal pain, paronychia, nausea, rash, diarrhea, constipation, fissures, vomiting, cough, acne, peripheral edema, dry skin

Occasional

Nail disorder, stomatitis, mucositis, eyelash growth, conjunctivitis, ocular hyperemia, lacrimation increased

Rare

Infusion reactions, eye/eyelid irritation

PRECAUTIONS AND CONTRAINDICATIONS

Hypersensitivity to panitumumab or its components; sunlight may exacerbate skin reactions

DRUG INTERACTIONS OF CONCERN TO DENTISTRY

- None reported

SERIOUS REACTIONS

! Dermatologic toxicities have been reported.

! Severe infusion-related reactions have been reported.

! Pulmonary fibrosis has been reported.

DENTAL CONSIDERATIONS

General:

- Examine patient for signs of adverse drug effects, including stomatitis and mucositis.
- Be prepared to manage nausea and vomiting related to drug use.
- Avoid aspirin and NSAIDs to reduce GI irritation.

Consultations:
- Consult physician to determine degree of disease control and ability of patient to tolerate dental procedures.

Teach Patient/Family to:
- Be aware of oral side effects of drug.
- Report oral lesions, soreness or bleeding to dentist.
- Use effective, atraumatic oral hygiene to minimize soft tissue inflammation.
- Update health and medication history if physician makes any changes in evaluation or drug regimen; include OTC, herbal, and nonherbal drugs in the update.

pantoprazole

pan-**toe**′-pra-zole
(Protonix, Pantoloc, Somac[AUS])
Do not confuse Protonix with Lotronex.

CATEGORY AND SCHEDULE

Pregnancy Risk Category: B

Drug Class: Gastrointestinal, proton pump inhibitor

MECHANISM OF ACTION

A benzimidazole that is converted to active metabolites that irreversibly bind to and inhibit hydrogen-potassium adenosine triphosphate, an enzyme on the surface of gastric parietal cells. Inhibits hydrogen ion transport into gastric lumen.
Therapeutic Effect: Increases gastric pH and reduces gastric acid production.

USES

Short-term treatment of esophageal erosion and ulceration associated with gastroesophageal reflux disease (GERD)

PHARMACOKINETICS

Route	Onset	Peak	Duration
PO	N/A	N/A	24 hr

Rapidly absorbed from the GI tract. Protein binding: 98%. Primarily distributed into gastric parietal cells. Metabolized extensively in the liver. Primarily excreted in urine. Not removed by hemodialysis. ***Half-life:*** 1 hr.

INDICATIONS AND DOSAGES

▸ **Erosive Esophagitis**

PO

Adults, Elderly. 40 mg/day for up to 8 wk. If not healed after 8 wk, may continue an additional 8 wk.

IV

Adults, Elderly. 40 mg/day for 7–10 days.

▸ **Hypersecretory Conditions**

PO

Adults, Elderly. Initially, 40 mg twice a day. May increase to 240 mg/day.

IV

Adults, Elderly. 80 mg twice a day. May increase to 80 mg q8hr.

SIDE EFFECTS/ADVERSE REACTIONS

Rare

Diarrhea, headache, dizziness, pruritus, rash

PRECAUTIONS AND CONTRAINDICATIONS

Caution is warranted with a chronic or current hepatic disease. It is unknown if pantoprazole crosses the placenta or is distributed in breast milk. Safety and efficacy of pantoprazole have not been

P

established in children. No age-related precautions have been noted in the elderly. Serum chemistry laboratory values, including serum creatinine and cholesterol levels, should be obtained before therapy.

DRUG INTERACTIONS OF CONCERN TO DENTISTRY

• None reported

SERIOUS REACTIONS

! None known

DENTAL CONSIDERATIONS

General:

• Avoid aspirin and NSAIDs for pain control if GI disease requires.

• Consider semisupine chair position for patient comfort because of possible regurgitation of stomach contents.

• Patients with gastroesophageal reflux may have oral symptoms, including burning mouth, secondary candidiasis, and dental erosion

Consultations:

• Consultation is only required if GI disease is severe or associated with other systemic conditions.

Teach Patient/Family to:

• Report symptoms of oral adverse effects of GI disease.

P

papaverine hydrochloride

pa-**pav**′-er-een

(Papacon, Para-Time SR, Pavabid Plateau, Pavacot, Pavagen)

CATEGORY AND SCHEDULE

Pregnancy Risk Category: C

Drug Class: Peripheral vasodilator

MECHANISM OF ACTION

A vasodilating agent that acts directly on the heart muscle to depress conduction and prolong the refractory period.

Therapeutic Effect: Relaxes smooth muscle.

USES

Treatment of arterial spasm resulting in cerebral and peripheral ischemia; myocardial ischemia associated with vascular spasm or dysrhythmias; angina pectoris; peripheral pulmonary embolism; visceral spasm as in ureteral, biliary, and GI colic PVD; unapproved: with phentolamine or alprostadil for intracavernous injection for impotence

PHARMACOKINETICS

Protein binding: 90%. Primarily excreted in urine as inactive metabolites. ***Half-life:*** Unknown.

INDICATIONS AND DOSAGES

▸ Vascular Spasm

IV/IM

Adults, Elderly. Inject 1–4 ml slowly and repeat q3h as indicated.

PO

Adults, Elderly. One capsule q12h. In difficult cases, administration may be increased to one capsule q8h or 2 capsules q12h.

SIDE EFFECTS/ADVERSE REACTIONS

Frequency Not Defined

Capsules: Nausea, abdominal distress, anorexia, constipation, malaise, drowsiness, vertigo, perspiration, headache, diarrhea, skin rash

Injection: General discomfort, nausea, abdominal discomfort, anorexia, constipation, diarrhea, skin rash, malaise, vertigo, headache, intensive flushing of the face, perspiration, increased depth of respiration, increased heart rate, slight rise in B/P, excessive sedation

PRECAUTIONS AND CONTRAINDICATIONS

Complete atrioventricular heart block, impotence by intracorporeal injection, hypersensitivity to papaverine or any component of the formulation

Caution:

Cardiac dysrhythmias, glaucoma, pregnancy category C, lactation, drug dependency, children, hepatic hypersensitivity, Parkinson's disease

DRUG INTERACTIONS OF CONCERN TO DENTISTRY

• Increased hypotension: alcohol, other drugs that may also lower B/P

SERIOUS REACTIONS

! Hepatotoxicity has been reported.

! Priapism has been reported.

DENTAL CONSIDERATIONS

General:

• Monitor vital signs at every appointment because of cardiovascular and respiratory side effects.

• Short appointments and a stress-reduction protocol may be required for anxious patients.

Consultations:

• Stress from dental procedures may compromise cardiovascular function; determine patient risk.

• Medical consultation may be required to assess disease control.

Teach Patient/Family to:

• Avoid mouth rinses with high alcohol content.

• Encourage effective oral hygiene to prevent soft tissue inflammation.

paregoric

par-eh-**gor′**-ik

Do not confuse with opium tincture.

CATEGORY AND SCHEDULE

Pregnancy Risk Category: B (D if used for prolonged periods, high dosages at term)

Controlled Substance: Schedule III

Drug Class: Antidiarrheal

MECHANISM OF ACTION

An opioid agonist that contains many opioid alkaloids, including morphine. It inhibits gastric motility due to its morphine content.

Therapeutic Effect: Decreases digestive secretions, increases GI muscle tone, and reduces GI propulsion.

USES

Treatment of diarrhea

PHARMACOKINETICS

Variably absorbed from the GI tract. Protein binding: low. Metabolized in liver. Primarily excreted in urine primarily as morphine glucuronide conjugates and unchanged drug—morphine, codeine, papaverine, etc. Unknown if removed by hemodialysis. ***Half-life:*** 2–3 hr.

INDICATIONS AND DOSAGES

▸ **Antidiarrheal**

PO

Adults, Elderly. 5–10 ml 1–4 times a day.

Children. 0.25–0.5 ml/kg/dose 1–4 times a day.

SIDE EFFECTS/ADVERSE REACTIONS

Frequent

Constipation, drowsiness, nausea, vomiting

Occasional

Paradoxical excitement, confusion, pounding heartbeat, facial flushing, decreased urination, blurred vision, dizziness, dry mouth, headache, hypotension, decreased appetite, redness, burning, pain at injection site

Rare

Hallucinations, depression, stomach pain, insomnia

PRECAUTIONS AND CONTRAINDICATIONS

Diarrhea caused by poisoning until the toxic material is removed, hypersensitivity to morphine sulfate or any component of the formulation, pregnancy (prolonged use or high dosages near term)

Caution:

Liver disease, addiction-prone individuals, prostatic hypertrophy (severe), caution in lactation, safety and efficacy in pediatric patients not established

DRUG INTERACTIONS OF CONCERN TO DENTISTRY

- Increased action of both drugs: alcohol, all other CNS depressants
- Decreased peristalsis: anticholinergic drugs

SERIOUS REACTIONS

! Overdosage results in cold or clammy skin, confusion, convulsions, decreased B/P, restlessness, pinpoint pupils, bradycardia, respiratory depression, decreased level of consciousness, and severe weakness.

! Tolerance to analgesic effect and physical dependence may occur with repeated use.

DENTAL CONSIDERATIONS

General:

- Psychological and physical dependence may occur with chronic administration.
- Determine why the patient is taking the drug.

Teach Patient/Family to:

- Avoid mouth rinses with high alcohol content because of drying effects.

pargyline

par-gi-leen

(Eutonyl)

CATEGORY AND SCHEDULE

Pregnancy Risk Category: NA

Drug Class: Monoamine oxidase inhibitor; antihypertensive

MECHANISM OF ACTION

A monoamine oxidase inhibitor that inhibits the metabolism of catecholamines and tyramine.

Therapeutic Effect: Decreases blood pressure.

USES

Hypertension, moderate to severe

PHARMACOKINETICS

Not available

INDICATIONS AND DOSAGES

▸ **Hypertension**

PO

Adults. Initially, 25 mg daily. May be titrated by weekly intervals. Maintenance: 5–75 mg daily.

SIDE EFFECTS/ADVERSE REACTIONS

Side effects based on other monoamine oxidase inhibitors

Frequent

Orthostatic hypotension, restlessness, GI upset, insomnia, dizziness, lethargy, weakness, dry mouth, peripheral edema, fainting, palpitations

Occasional

Flushing, diaphoresis, rash, urinary frequency, increased appetite, transient impotence

Rare

Visual disturbances, impotence

PRECAUTIONS AND CONTRAINDICATIONS

Hypersensitivity to pargyline or any component of the formulation
Pheochromocytoma
Malignant hypertension
Advanced renal failure
Schizophrenia
Hyperthyroidism

Caution:

Cardiac arrhythmias
Hypertension
Suicidal tendencies
Pregnancy
Children

DRUG INTERACTIONS OF CONCERN TO DENTISTRY

• Tyramine-containing foods: May increase the risk of hypertensive crisis.

SERIOUS REACTIONS

! Manic psychosis has been reported.

DENTAL CONSIDERATIONS

General:

• Monitor vital signs at every appointment because of cardiovascular side effects.

• After supine positioning, have patient sit upright for at least 2 min before standing to avoid orthostatic hypotension.

• Assess salivary flow as a factor in caries, periodontal disease, and candidiasis.

• Stress from dental procedures may compromise cardiovascular function; determine patient risk.

Consultations:

• Medical consultation may be required to assess disease control.

Teach Patient/Family to:

• Report oral lesions, soreness, or bleeding to dentist.

• When chronic dry mouth occurs, advise patient to:

  • Avoid mouth rinses with high alcohol content because of drying effects.

  • Use daily home fluoride products for anticaries effect.

  • Use sugarless gum, frequent sips of water, or saliva substitutes.

P

paromomycin

par-oh-moe-**mye′**-sin
(Humatin)
Do not confuse with Humira.

CATEGORY AND SCHEDULE

Pregnancy Risk Category: C

Drug Class: Amoebicide antibiotic

MECHANISM OF ACTION

An antibacterial agent that acts directly on amoebas and against normal and pathogenic organisms in the GI tract. Interferes with bacterial protein synthesis by binding to 30S ribosomal subunits.

Therapeutic Effect: Produces amoebicidal effects.

USES

Treatment of intestinal amebiasis, adjunct in hepatic coma

PHARMACOKINETICS

Poorly absorbed from the GI tract and most of the dose is eliminated unchanged in feces.

INDICATIONS AND DOSAGES

▸ Intestinal Amebiasis

PO

Adults, Elderly, Children. 25–35 mg/kg/day q8h for 5–10 days.

▸ Hepatic Coma

PO

Adults, Elderly. 4 g/day q6–12h for 5–6 days.

SIDE EFFECTS/ADVERSE REACTIONS

Occasional

Diarrhea, abdominal cramps, nausea, vomiting, heartburn

Rare

Rash, pruritus, vertigo

PRECAUTIONS AND CONTRAINDICATIONS

Intestinal obstruction, renal failure, hypersensitivity to paromomycin or any of its components

DRUG INTERACTIONS OF CONCERN TO DENTISTRY

- Possible degradation by penicillins and cephalosporins

SERIOUS REACTIONS

! Overdosage may result in nausea, vomiting, and diarrhea.

DENTAL CONSIDERATIONS

General:

- Determine why patient is taking the drug.
- Consider semisupine chair position for patient comfort due to GI effects of disease.
- Question patient about tolerance of NSAIDs or aspirin related to GI disease.
- Postpone elective dental treatment until symptoms are controlled.

Consultations:

- Medical consultation may be required to assess disease control.

Teach Patient/Family to:

- Update health and medication history if physician makes any changes in evaluation or drug regimens; include OTC, herbal, and nonherbal drugs in the update.
- Report sore throat, oral burning sensation, fever, or fatigue, any of which could indicate presence of a superinfection.

paroxetine hydrochloride

par-**ox**′-eh-teen
high-droh-**klor**′-ide
(Aropax 20[AUS], Paxeva, Paxil, Paxil CR, Paxtine[AUS])
Do not confuse paroxetine with pyridoxine, or Paxil with Doxil or Taxol.

CATEGORY AND SCHEDULE

Pregnancy Risk Category: C

Drug Class: Antidepressant, SSRI

MECHANISM OF ACTION

An antidepressant, anxiolytic, and antiobsessional agent that selectively blocks uptake of the neurotransmitter serotonin at neuronal presynaptic membranes, thereby increasing its availability at postsynaptic receptor sites.
Therapeutic Effect: Relieves depression, reduces obsessive-compulsive behavior, decreases anxiety.

USES

Treatment of depression, panic disorder, obsessive-compulsive disorder, social anxiety disorder; generalized anxiety disorder, posttraumatic stress disorder; premenstrual dysphoric disorder

PHARMACOKINETICS

Well absorbed from the GI tract. Protein binding: 95%. Widely distributed. Metabolized in the liver. Excreted in urine. Not removed by hemodialysis. ***Half-life:*** 24 hr.

INDICATIONS AND DOSAGES

▸ Depression

PO

Adults. Initially, 20 mg/day. May increase by 10 mg/day at intervals of more than 1 wk. Maximum: 50 mg/day.

PO (Controlled-Release)

Adults. Initially, 25 mg/day. May increase by 12.5 mg/day at intervals of more than 1 wk. Maximum: 62.5 mg/day.

▸ Generalized Anxiety Disorder

PO

Adults. Initially, 20 mg/day. May increase by 10 mg/day at intervals of more than 1 wk. Range: 20–50 mg/day.

▸ Obsessive-Compulsive Disorder

PO

Adults. Initially, 20 mg/day. May increase by 10 mg/day at intervals of more than 1 wk. Range: 20–60 mg/day.

▸ Panic Disorder

PO

Adults. Initially, 10–20 mg/day. May increase by 10 mg/day at intervals of more than 1 wk. Range: 10–60 mg/day.

▸ Social Anxiety Disorder

PO

Adults. Initially, 20 mg/day. Range: 20–60 mg/day.

▸ Posttraumatic Stress Disorder

PO

Adults. Initially, 20 mg/day. May increase by 10 mg/day at intervals of more than 1 wk. Range: 20–50 mg/day.

▸ Premenstrual Dysphoric Disorder

PO (Paxil CR)

Adults. Initially, 12.5 mg/day. May increase by 12.5 mg at weekly intervals to a maximum of 25 mg/day.

▸ Usual Elderly Dosage

PO

Initially, 10 mg/day. May increase by 10 mg/day at intervals of more than 1 wk. Maximum: 40 mg/day.

PO (Controlled-Release)

Initially, 12.5 mg/day. May increase by 12.5 mg/day at intervals of more than 1 wk. Maximum: 50 mg/day.

SIDE EFFECTS/ADVERSE REACTIONS

Frequent

Nausea, somnolence, headache, dry mouth, asthenia, constipation, dizziness, insomnia, diarrhea, diaphoresis, tremor

Occasional

Decreased appetite, respiratory disturbance (such as increased cough), anxiety, nervousness, flatulence, paresthesia, yawning, decreased libido, sexual dysfunction, abdominal discomfort

Rare

Palpitations, vomiting, blurred vision, altered taste, confusion

PRECAUTIONS AND CONTRAINDICATIONS

Use within 14 days of MAOIs

Caution:

Lactation, elderly, oral anticoagulants, renal or hepatic impairment, children with suspected higher risk of suicide ideation, other serotonergic drugs

DRUG INTERACTIONS OF CONCERN TO DENTISTRY

- Possible increased side effects: highly protein-bound drugs (aspirin), other antidepressants, alcohol
- Possible inhibition of fluoxetine metabolism: erythromycin, clarithromycin
- Increased half-life of diazepam
- NSAIDs: increased risk of GI side effects

SERIOUS REACTIONS

! Abnormal bleeding, hyponatremia, seizures, hypomania, and suicidal thoughts have been reported.

DENTAL CONSIDERATIONS

General:

- After supine positioning, have patient sit upright for at least 2 min before standing to avoid orthostatic hypotension.
- Assess salivary flow as a factor in caries, periodontal disease, and candidiasis.
- Avoid dental light in patient's eyes; offer dark glasses for patient comfort.

Consultations:

- Medical consultation may be required to assess disease control and patient's ability to tolerate stress.
- Physician should be informed if significant xerostomic side effects occur (e.g., increased caries, sore tongue, problems eating or swallowing, difficulty wearing prosthesis) so that a medication change can be considered.

Teach Patient/Family to:

- When chronic dry mouth occurs, advise patient to:
  - Avoid mouth rinses with high alcohol content because of drying effects.
  - Use daily home fluoride products to prevent caries.
  - Use sugarless gum, frequent sips of water, or saliva substitutes.

pazopanib

pay-**zoe**′-pan-ib
(Votrient)
Do not confuse with axitinib, sunitinib, or vandetanib.

CATEGORY AND SCHEDULE

Pregnancy Risk Category: D

Drug Class: Antineoplastic agent, signal transduction inhibitor

MECHANISM OF ACTION

An oral multikinase inhibitor of angiogenesis. Pazopanib inhibits vascular endothelial growth factor receptor (VEGFR), platelet-derived growth factor receptor (PDGFR), fibroblast growth factor receptor (FGFR), cytokine receptor (Kit), interleukin-2 receptor inducible T-cell kinase (Itk), leukocyte-specific protein tyrosine kinase (Lck), and transmembrane glycoprotein receptor tyrosine kinase (c-Fms). ***Therapeutic Effect:*** Inhibits tumor growth.

USES

Treatment of advanced renal cell cancer

PHARMACOKINETICS

Well absorbed after oral administration of whole tablets. 99% plasma protein bound. Hepatic metabolism via CYP3A4 (major), CYP1A2 (minor), and CYP2C8 (minor). Eliminated via feces. ***Half-life:*** 30.9 hr.

INDICATIONS AND DOSAGES

▸ **Advanced Renal Cell Cancer**

PO

Adults, Elderly. 800 mg once daily on an empty stomach.

▸ **Dosage Adjustment for Moderate Hepatic Impairment**

200 mg orally once daily. Not recommended in patients with severe hepatic impairment.

SIDE EFFECTS/ADVERSE REACTIONS

Frequent

Diarrhea, hypertension, hair color changes (depigmentation), nausea, anorexia, fatigue, and vomiting; may decrease magnesium and phosphorus levels, cause hyperglycemia

Occasional

Alopecia, chest pain, dysgeusia (altered taste), dyspepsia, facial edema, hand-foot syndrome, proteinuria, rash, skin depigmentation, and weight loss

PRECAUTIONS AND CONTRAINDICATIONS

Hypersensitivity to pazopanib or any components of its formulation. Use with caution in patients with hepatic disease, high B/P, cardiac disease, heart failure or arrhythmia, QT prolongation, a history of stroke, GI disease with GI bleeding in the past 6 mo or a history of GI perforation or fistula, thyroid disease, had recent surgery or scheduled for surgery.

DRUG INTERACTIONS OF CONCERN TO DENTISTRY

- CYP3A4 inhibitors (e.g., macrolide antibiotics, azole antifungals): may increase blood levels and adverse effects of pazopanib
- CYP3A4 inducers (e.g., carbamazepine, barbiturates): may decrease blood levels and therapeutic effect of pazopanib
- CYP2D6 substrates (e.g., opioids): avoid use in patients taking pazopanib

SERIOUS REACTIONS

! Serious hypersensitivity reactions occur rarely and may include angioedema. May cause leukopenia, thrombocytopenia, serious bleeding, and delayed wound healing.

DENTAL CONSIDERATIONS

General:

- Avoid aspirin and NSAIDs to prevent GI irritation and excessive bleeding.
- Examine patient carefully for signs of opportunistic infections, mucositis, blood dyscrasias, stomatitis, and bleeding.
- Chlorhexidine mouth rinse prior to and during chemotherapy may reduce severity of oral inflammation.
- Patient may be taking prophylactic antiinfective drug.
- Place patient on frequent recall because of adverse oral effects of drug.

Consultations:

- Consult physician to determine disease status and ability of patient to tolerate dental procedures.
- Consult physician to determine need for prophylactic or therapeutic antiinfective drug if oral surgery or periodontal therapy is planned.
- Consult physician to determine patient's immunologic and coagulation status.

Teach Patient/Family to:

- Beware of oral adverse effects of drug.
- Use effective, atraumatic oral hygiene measures to prevent soft tissue inflammation.

• Report oral lesions, soreness, or bleeding to dentist.
• Update health and medication history regularly.

pegfilgrastim

peg-fil-**gras'**-tim
(Neulasta)
Do not confuse Neulasta with Neumega.

CATEGORY AND SCHEDULE

Pregnancy Risk Category: C

Drug Class: Hematopoietic agent

MECHANISM OF ACTION

A colony-stimulating factor that regulates production of neutrophils within bone marrow. Also a glycoprotein that primarily affects neutrophil progenitor proliferation, differentiation, and selected end-cell functional activation.
Therapeutic Effect: Increases phagocytic ability and antibody-dependent destruction; decreases incidence of infection.

USES

To decrease infection in patients receiving antineoplastics that are myelosuppressive; to increase WBC in patients with drug-induced neutropenia

PHARMACOKINETICS

Readily absorbed after subcutaneous administration. ***Half-life:*** 15–80 hr.

INDICATIONS AND DOSAGES

▸ **Myelosuppression**

Subcutaneous

Adults, Elderly. Give as a single 6-mg injection once per chemotherapy cycle.

SIDE EFFECTS/ADVERSE REACTIONS

Frequent

Bone pain, nausea, fatigue, alopecia, diarrhea, vomiting, constipation, anorexia, abdominal pain, arthralgia, generalized weakness, peripheral edema, dizziness, stomatitis, mucositis, neutropenic fever

PRECAUTIONS AND CONTRAINDICATIONS

Hypersensitivity to *Escherichia coli*–derived proteins, within 14 days before and 24 hr after cytotoxic chemotherapy

DRUG INTERACTIONS OF CONCERN TO DENTISTRY

• None reported

SERIOUS REACTIONS

! Allergic reactions, such as anaphylaxis, rash, and urticaria, occur rarely.
! Cytopenia resulting from an antibody response to growth factors occurs rarely.
! Splenomegaly occurs rarely; assess for left upper abdominal or shoulder pain.
! Adult respiratory distress syndrome (ARDS) may occur in patients with sepsis.

DENTAL CONSIDERATIONS

General:

• Patients may have a history of chemotherapy or radiation; confirm medical and drug history.
• Determine type of chemotherapeutic agents used and related oral side effects.
• Monitor and record vital signs.

• Examine for oral manifestation of opportunistic infection.

Consultations:

• Medical consultation may be required to assess disease control and patient's ability to tolerate stress.

Teach Patient/Family to:

• Encourage effective oral hygiene to prevent soft tissue inflammation.

• Prevent trauma when using oral hygiene aids.

• Report oral lesions, soreness, or bleeding to dentist.

peginterferon alfa-2a

peg-inn-ter-**fear′**-on **al′**-fah (Pegasys)

CATEGORY AND SCHEDULE

Pregnancy Risk Category: C

Drug Class: Biologic response modifier

MECHANISM OF ACTION

An immunomodulator that binds to specific membrane receptors on the cell surface, inhibiting viral replication in virus-infected cells, suppressing cell proliferation, and producing reversible decreases in leukocyte and platelet counts. ***Therapeutic Effect:*** Inhibits hepatitis C virus.

USES

Treatment of adults with chronic hepatitis C with compensated liver disease who have not been previously treated with interferon-alfa.

PHARMACOKINETICS

Subcutaneous: Peak serum levels 72–96 hr; cleared from the body at 94 ml/hr; no data in children. Readily absorbed after subcutaneous administration. Excreted by the kidneys. ***Half-life:*** 80 hr.

INDICATIONS AND DOSAGES

▸ **Hepatitis C**

Subcutaneous

Adults 18 yr and older, Elderly. 180 mcg (1 ml) injected in abdomen or thigh once weekly for 48 wk.

▸ **Dosage in Renal Impairment**

For patients who require hemodialysis, dosage is 135 mg injected in abdomen or thigh once weekly for 48 wk.

▸ **Dosage in Hepatic Impairment**

For patients with progressive ALT (SGPT) increases above baseline values, dosage is 90 mcg injected in abdomen or thigh once weekly for 48 wk.

SIDE EFFECTS/ADVERSE REACTIONS

Frequent

Headache

Occasional

Alopecia, nausea, insomnia, anorexia, dizziness, diarrhea, abdominal pain, flu-like symptoms, psychiatric reactions (depression, irritability, anxiety), injection site reaction, impaired concentration, diaphoresis, dry mouth, nausea, vomiting

PRECAUTIONS AND CONTRAINDICATIONS

Autoimmune hepatitis, decompensated hepatic disease, infants, neonates

Caution:

Preexisting cardiac disease, may aggravate hypothyroidism,

hyperthyroidism, hyperglycemia, hypoglycemia, diabetes, ophthalmologic disorders, lactation, children; closely monitor patients, severe life-threatening neuropsychiatric, autoimmune, ischemic, or infectious disorders may cause or aggravate these conditions

DRUG INTERACTIONS OF CONCERN TO DENTISTRY

• Risk of hepatotoxicity in severe liver disease: acetaminophen

SERIOUS REACTIONS

! Serious, acute hypersensitivity reactions, such as urticaria, angioedema, bronchoconstriction, and anaphylaxis, may occur. Other rare reactions include pancreatitis, colitis, endocrine disorders (e.g., diabetes mellitus), hyperthyroidism or hypothyroidism, ophthalmologic disorders, and pulmonary disorders.

DENTAL CONSIDERATIONS

General:

• Determine why patient is taking the drug.
• Assess salivary flow as a factor in caries, periodontal disease, and candidiasis.
• Consider semisupine chair position for patient comfort if GI side effects occur.
• Question patient about tolerance of NSAIDs or aspirin related to GI disease.
• Patients on chronic drug therapy may rarely have symptoms of blood dyscrasias, which can include infection, bleeding, and poor healing.
• Avoid elective dental procedures if severe neutropenia (fewer than 500 cells/mm^3) or thrombocytopenia (fewer than 50,000 cell/mm^3) is present.
• Severe side effects may require postponing elective dental procedures until drug therapy is completed.

Consultations:

• Medical consultation may be required to assess disease control in the patient.
• In a patient with symptoms of blood dyscrasias, request a medical consultation for blood studies and postpone treatment until normal values are reestablished.
• Liver function tests may be required to determine chronic liver disease.

Teach Patient/Family to:

• Encourage effective oral hygiene to prevent soft tissue inflammation/ infection.
• Evaluate efficacy of oral hygiene home care; preventive appointments may be necessary.
• Prevent trauma when using oral hygiene aids.
• When chronic dry mouth occurs, advise patient to:
  • Avoid mouth rinses with high alcohol content because of drying effects.
  • Use daily home fluoride products for anticaries effect.
  • Use sugarless gum, frequent sips of water, or saliva substitutes.

peginterferon alfa-2b

peg-inn-ter-**fear′**-on **al′**-fah
(PEG-Intron)

CATEGORY AND SCHEDULE

Pregnancy Risk Category: C

Drug Class: Biologic response modifier

MECHANISM OF ACTION

An immunomodulator that inhibits viral replication in virus-infected cells, suppresses cell proliferation, increases phagocytic action of macrophages, and augments specific cytotoxicity of lymphocytes for target cells.
Therapeutic Effect: Inhibits hepatitis C virus.

USES

Treatment of adults with chronic hepatitis C with compensated liver disease who have not been previously treated with interferon-alfa; peginterferon alfa-2b can be used with ribavirin

PHARMACOKINETICS

Subcutaneous: Peak serum levels 72–96 hr; cleared from the body at 94 ml/hr; no data in children, pharmacokinetic data are limited.

INDICATIONS AND DOSAGES

▸ Chronic Hepatitis C, Monotherapy

Subcutaneous

Adults 18 yr and older, Elderly. Administer appropriate dosage (see chart below) once weekly for 1 yr on the same day each week.

Vial Strength	Weight (kg)	mcg*	ml*
100 mcg/ml	37–45	40	0.4
	46–56	50	0.5
160 mcg/ml	57–72	64	0.4
	73–88	80	0.5
240 mcg/ml	89–106	96	0.4
	107–136	120	0.5
300 mcg/ml	137–160	150	0.5

*Of peginterferon alpha-2b to administer

▸ Chronic Hepatitis C

Subcutaneous combination therapy with ribavirin (400 mg twice a day). Initially, 1.5 mcg/kg/wk.

SIDE EFFECTS/ADVERSE REACTIONS

Frequent

Flu-like symptoms; inflammation, bruising, pruritus, and irritation at injection site

Occasional

Psychiatric reactions (depression, anxiety, emotional lability, irritability), insomnia, alopecia, diarrhea

Rare

Rash, diaphoresis, dry skin, dizziness, flushing, vomiting, dyspepsia

PRECAUTIONS AND CONTRAINDICATIONS

Autoimmune hepatitis, decompensated hepatic disease, history of psychiatric disorders

Caution:

Preexisting cardiac disease, may aggravate hypothyroidism, hyperthyroidism, hyperglycemia, hypoglycemia, diabetes, ophthalmologic disorders, lactation, children; closely monitor patients, severe life-threatening neuropsychiatric, autoimmune, ischemic, or infectious disorders may cause or aggravate these conditions

DRUG INTERACTIONS OF CONCERN TO DENTISTRY

• Risk of hepatotoxicity in severe liver disease: acetaminophen

SERIOUS REACTIONS

! Serious, acute hypersensitivity reactions (such as urticaria, angioedema, bronchoconstriction, and anaphylaxis), pulmonary disorders, endocrine disorders (e.g., diabetes mellitus), hypothyroidism, hyperthyroidism, and pancreatitis occur rarely.

! Ulcerative colitis may occur within 12 wk of starting treatment.

P

DENTAL CONSIDERATIONS

General:

• Determine why patient is taking the drug.

• Assess salivary flow as a factor in caries, periodontal disease, and candidiasis.

• Consider semisupine chair position for patient comfort if GI side effects occur.

• Question patient about tolerance of NSAIDs or aspirin related to GI disease.

• Patients on chronic drug therapy may rarely have symptoms of blood dyscrasias, which can include infection, bleeding, and poor healing.

• Avoid elective dental procedures if severe neutropenia (fewer than 500 cells/mm^3) or thrombocytopenia (fewer than 50,000 cell/mm^3) is present.

• Severe side effects may require postponing elective dental procedures until drug therapy is completed.

Consultations:

• Medical consultation may be required to assess disease control in the patient.

• In a patient with symptoms of blood dyscrasias, request a medical consultation for blood studies and postpone treatment until normal values are reestablished.

• Liver function tests may be required to determine chronic liver disease.

Teach Patient/Family to:

• Encourage effective oral hygiene to prevent soft tissue inflammation/infection.

• Evaluate efficacy of oral hygiene home care; preventive appointments may be necessary.

• Prevent trauma when using oral hygiene aids.

• When chronic dry mouth occurs, advise patient to:

  • Avoid mouth rinses with high alcohol content because of drying effects.
  • Use daily home fluoride products for anticaries effect.
  • Use sugarless gum, frequent sips of water, or saliva substitutes.

pegvisomant

peg-**vis**′-oh-mant

(Somavert)

Do not confuse Somavert with somatrem or somatropin.

CATEGORY AND SCHEDULE

Pregnancy Risk Category: B

Drug Class: Acromegaly agent

MECHANISM OF ACTION

A protein that selectively binds to growth hormone (GH) receptors on cell surfaces, blocking the binding of endogenous GHs and interfering with GH signal transduction.

Therapeutic Effect: Decreases serum concentrations of insulin-like growth factor 1 (IGF-1) and other GH-responsive serum proteins.

USES

Treatment of acromegaly in those patients who have an inadequate response to other treatment

PHARMACOKINETICS

Not distributed extensively into tissues after subcutaneous administration. Less than 1% excreted in urine. ***Half-life:*** 6 days.

INDICATIONS AND DOSAGES

▸ **Acromegaly**

Subcutaneous

Adults, Elderly. Initially, 40 mg as a loading dose, then 10 mg daily. After 4–6 wk, adjust dosage in 5-mg increments if serum IGF-1 level is still elevated, or in 5-mg decrements if IGF-1 level has decreased below the normal range. Maximum: 30 mg daily.

SIDE EFFECTS/ADVERSE REACTIONS

Frequent

Infection (cold symptoms, upper respiratory tract infection, blister, ear infection)

Occasional

Back pain, dizziness, injection site reaction, peripheral edema, sinusitis, nausea

Rare

Diarrhea, paresthesia

PRECAUTIONS AND CONTRAINDICATIONS

Latex allergy (stopper on vial contains latex)

DRUG INTERACTIONS OF CONCERN TO DENTISTRY

- Opioids: decreased serum levels

SERIOUS REACTIONS

! Pegvisomant use may markedly elevate liver function test results, including serum transaminase levels.

! Substantial weight gain occurs rarely.

DENTAL CONSIDERATIONS

General:

- Confirm history of previous medical, surgical, or radiation treatment for this disease.
- Monitor vital signs.
- Patient may complain of temporomandibular dysfunction (TMD) due to disease.
- Place on frequent recall to evaluate healing response.

Consultations:

- Physician consultation should include liver function tests.

Teach Patient/Family to:

- Encourage effective oral hygiene to prevent soft tissue inflammation.
- Prevent trauma when using oral hygiene aids.
- Update health and medication history if physician makes any changes in evaluation or drug regimens; include OTC, herbal, and nonherbal drugs in the update.

pemirolast potassium

peh-**meer′**-oh-last
poe-**tass′**-ee-um
(Alamast)

CATEGORY AND SCHEDULE

Pregnancy Risk Category: C

Drug Class: Ophthalmic

P

MECHANISM OF ACTION

An antiallergic agent that prevents activation and release of mediators of inflammation (e.g., mast cells). ***Therapeutic Effect:*** Reduces symptoms of allergic conjunctivitis.

USES

Relief of allergic conjunctivitis

PHARMACOKINETICS

Detected in plasma. Excreted in urine. ***Half-life:*** 4.5 hr.

INDICATIONS AND DOSAGES

▸ Allergic Conjunctivitis

Ophthalmic

Adults, Elderly, Children 3 yr and older. 1–2 drops in affected eye(s) 4 times a day.

SIDE EFFECTS/ADVERSE REACTIONS

Frequent

Headache, rhinitis, cold and flu symptoms

Occasional

Transient ocular stinging, burning, itching, dry eye, foreign body sensation, tearing

Rare

Sinusitis, sneezing/nasal congestion

PRECAUTIONS AND CONTRAINDICATIONS

Hypersensitivity to pemirolast potassium or any other component of the formulation

Caution:

Lactation; children; do not wear contact lens if eyes are red, may affect soft contact lens, if no red eyes wait 10 min after using to place soft contacts

DRUG INTERACTIONS OF CONCERN TO DENTISTRY

- None reported

SERIOUS REACTIONS

! None reported

DENTAL CONSIDERATIONS

General:

- Question patient about history of allergies to avoid using other potential allergens.
- Avoid dental light in patient's eyes; offer dark glasses for patient comfort.

P

pemoline

pem′-oh-leen

(Cylert, PemADD, PemADD CT)

CATEGORY AND SCHEDULE

Pregnancy Risk Category: B

Controlled Substance: Schedule IV

Drug Class: CNS stimulant

MECHANISM OF ACTION

A CNS stimulant that blocks the reuptake mechanism present in dopaminergic neurons in the cerebral cortex and subcortical structures.

Therapeutic Effect: Reduces motor restlessness and fatigue, increases alertness, elevates mood.

USES

Treatment of attention-deficit/hyperactivity disorder (ADHD)

PHARMACOKINETICS

PO: Peak 2–4 hr, duration 8 hr. ***Half-life:*** 12 hr; metabolized (50%) by liver; excreted (40%) by kidneys.

INDICATIONS AND DOSAGES

▸ ADHD

PO

Children 6 yr and older. Initially, 37.5 mg/day as a single dose in morning. May increase by 18.75 mg at weekly intervals until therapeutic response is achieved. Range: 56.25–75 mg/day. Maximum: 112.5 mg/day.

SIDE EFFECTS/ADVERSE REACTIONS

Frequent

Anorexia, insomnia

Occasional
Nausea, abdominal discomfort, diarrhea, headache, dizziness, somnolence

PRECAUTIONS AND CONTRAINDICATIONS

Family history of Tourette's syndrome, hepatic impairment, motor tics
Caution:
Renal disease, lactation, drug abuse, children younger than 6 yr; liver function monitoring recommended

DRUG INTERACTIONS OF CONCERN TO DENTISTRY

- Increased irritability, stimulation: caffeine-containing products and food

SERIOUS REACTIONS

! Visual disturbances, rash, and dyskinetic movements of the tongue, lips, face, and extremities have occurred.
! Large doses of pemoline may produce extreme nervousness and tachycardia.
! Hepatic effects, such as hepatitis and jaundice, appear to be reversible when the drug is discontinued.
! Prolonged administration to children with ADHD may temporarily delay growth.

DENTAL CONSIDERATIONS

General:
- Keep dental appointments short because of effects of disease.

Teach Patient/Family to:
- Use powered tooth brush for effective plaque control.

penbutolol

pen-**beaut′**-oh-lol
(Levatol)
Do not confuse with pindolol.

CATEGORY AND SCHEDULE

Pregnancy Risk Category: C (D if used in the second or third trimester)

Drug Class: Nonselective β-adrenergic blocker

MECHANISM OF ACTION

An antihypertensive that possesses nonselective β-blocking. Has moderate intrinsic sympathomimetic activity.
Therapeutic Effect: Reduces cardiac output, decreases B/P, increases airway resistance, and decreases myocardial ischemia severity.

USES

Treatment of hypertension alone or with other antihypertensive drugs, mild-to-moderate heart failure

PHARMACOKINETICS

Rapidly and extensively absorbed from the GI tract. Protein binding: 80%–90%. Metabolized in liver. Excreted primarily via urine.
Half-life: 17–26 hr.

INDICATIONS AND DOSAGES

▸ Hypertension

PO
Adults. Initially, 20 mg/day as a single dose. May increase to 40–80 mg/day.
Elderly. Initially, 10 mg/day.

SIDE EFFECTS/ADVERSE REACTIONS

Frequent

Decreased sexual ability, drowsiness, trouble sleeping, unusual tiredness/weakness

Occasional

Diarrhea, bradycardia, depression, cold hands/feet, constipation, anxiety, nasal congestion, nausea, vomiting

Rare

Altered taste, dry eyes, itching, numbness of fingers, toes, scalp

PRECAUTIONS AND CONTRAINDICATIONS

Bronchial asthma or related bronchospastic conditions, cardiogenic shock, pulmonary edema, second- or third-degree AV block, severe bradycardia, overt cardiac failure, hypersensitivity to penbutolol or any component of the formulation

Caution:

Diabetes mellitus, renal disease, lactation, hyperthyroidism, COPD, hepatic disease, children, myasthenia gravis, peripheral vascular disease, hypotension

DRUG INTERACTIONS OF CONCERN TO DENTISTRY

• Decreased hypotensive effect: indomethacin, NSAIDs
• Increased hypotension, myocardial depression: hydrocarbon inhalation anesthetics
• Hypertension, bradycardia: sympathomimetics (epinephrine, ephedrine)
• Slow metabolism of lidocaine

SERIOUS REACTIONS

! Abrupt withdrawal may result in sweating, palpitations, headache, and tremulousness.

! Hypoglycemia may occur in patients with previously controlled diabetes.

DENTAL CONSIDERATIONS

General:

• Monitor vital signs at every appointment because of cardiovascular side effects.
• Patients on chronic drug therapy may rarely have symptoms of blood dyscrasias, which can include infection, bleeding, and poor healing.
• Limit use of sodium-containing products, such as saline IV fluids, for patients with a dietary salt restriction.
• Assess salivary flow as a factor in caries, periodontal disease, and candidiasis.
• After supine positioning, have patient sit upright for at least 2 min before standing to avoid orthostatic hypotension.
• Stress from dental procedures may compromise cardiovascular function; determine patient risk.
• Short appointments and a stress-reduction protocol may be required for anxious patients.
• Use vasoconstrictor with caution, in low doses, and with careful aspiration.
• Avoid using gingival retraction cord containing epinephrine.

Consultations:

• In a patient with symptoms of blood dyscrasias, request a medical consultation for blood studies and postpone dental treatment until normal values are reestablished.
• Medical consultation may be required to assess disease control and patient's ability to tolerate stress.

Teach Patient/Family to:

- Use caution to prevent injury when using oral hygiene aids.
- Encourage effective oral hygiene to prevent soft tissue inflammation.
- If taste alterations occur, consider drug as potential cause.
- When chronic dry mouth occurs, advise patient to:
  - Avoid mouth rinses with high alcohol content because of drying effects.
  - Use daily home fluoride products to prevent caries.
  - Use sugarless gum, frequent sips of water, or saliva substitutes.

penciclovir

pen-**sye**′-kloe-veer

(Denavir, Vectavir[South Africa, Costa Rica, Dominican Republic, El Salvador, Germany, Guatemala, Honduras, Israel, Nicaragua, Panama])

Do not confuse with acyclovir.

CATEGORY AND SCHEDULE

Pregnancy Risk Category: B

Drug Class: Antiviral

MECHANISM OF ACTION

Penciclovir triphosphate inhibits HSV polymerase competitively with deoxyguanosine triphosphate. Consequently, herpes viral DNA synthesis and, therefore, replication are selectively inhibited.

Therapeutic Effect: An antiviral compound that has inhibitory activity against human herpes virus types 1 and 2.

USES

Treatment of recurrent herpes labialis (cold sores)

PHARMACOKINETICS

Measurable penciclovir concentrations were not detected in plasma or urine. The systemic absorption of penciclovir following topical administration has not been evaluated.

INDICATIONS AND DOSAGES

▸ Herpes Labialis (Cold Sores)

Topical

Adolescents, Adults. Penciclovir should be applied every 2 hr during waking hours for a period of 4 days. Treatment should be started as early as possible (i.e., during the prodrome or when lesions appear).

SIDE EFFECTS/ADVERSE REACTIONS

Frequent

Headache

Occasional

Dysgeusia; decreased sensitivity of skin, particularly to touch; redness of the skin; skin rash (maculopapular, erythematous), local edema, skin discoloration; pruritus; hypoesthesia; paresthesias; parosmia; urticaria; oral/pharyngeal edema

Rare

Mild pain, burning, or stinging

PRECAUTIONS AND CONTRAINDICATIONS

Hypersensitivity to penciclovir or any of its components

Caution:

Acyclovir-resistant herpes viruses, patients younger than 18 yr, use on mucous membranes not recommended, avoid applications near the eye, lactation

DRUG INTERACTIONS OF CONCERN TO DENTISTRY

- None reported

SERIOUS REACTIONS

! None reported

DENTAL CONSIDERATIONS

General:

- Use in immunocompromised patients not established.
- Postpone dental treatment when oral herpetic lesions are present.

Teach Patient/Family to:

- Dispose of tooth brush or other contaminated oral hygiene devices used during period of infection to prevent reinoculation of herpetic infection.
- Apply with a finger cot or latex glove to prevent herpes infection on fingers.

P

penicillin G benzathine

pen-ih-**sil′**-lin G **benz′**-ah-thene
(Bicillin LA, Permapen)
Do not confuse penicillin G benzathine with penicillin G potassium or penicillin G procaine.

CATEGORY AND SCHEDULE

Pregnancy Risk Category: B

Drug Class: Benzathine salt of natural penicillin G

MECHANISM OF ACTION

A penicillin that inhibits bacterial cell wall synthesis by binding to one or more of the penicillin-binding proteins of bacteria.
Therapeutic Effect: Bactericidal.

USES

Treatment of respiratory infections, scarlet fever, erysipelas, otitis media, pneumonia, skin and soft tissue infections, bejel, pinta, yaws; effective for gram-positive cocci (*Staphylococcus, S. pyogenes, S. viridans, S. faecalis, S. bovis, S. pneumoniae*), gram-negative cocci (*N. gonorrhoeae*), gram-positive bacilli (*B. anthracis, C. perfringens, C. tetani, C. diphtheriae, L. monocytogenes*), gram-negative bacilli (*E. coli, P. mirabilis, Salmonella, Shigella, Enterobacter, S. moniliformis*), spirochetes (*T. pallidum*), Actinomyces

PHARMACOKINETICS

IM: Very slow absorption, hydrolyzed to penicillin G, duration 21–28 days. ***Half-life:*** 30–60 min; excreted in urine, breast milk; crosses placenta.

INDICATIONS AND DOSAGES

▸ **Group A Streptococcal Infections**

IM

Adults, Elderly. 1.2 million units as a single dose.
Children. 25,000–50,000 units/kg as a single dose.

▸ **Prevention of Rheumatic Fever**

IM

Adults, Elderly. 1.2 million units every 3–4 wk or 600,000 units twice monthly.
Children. 25,000–50,000 units/kg every 3–4 wk.

▸ **Early Syphilis**

IM

Adults, Elderly. 2.4 million units divided and administered in 2 separate injection sites.

▸ **Congenital Syphilis**

IM

Children. 50,000 units/kg weekly for 3 wk.

▸ **Syphilis of More Than 1 Yr Duration**
IM
Adults, Elderly. 2.4 million units divided and administered in 2 separate injection sites weekly for 3 wk.
Children. 50,000 units/kg weekly for 3 wk.

SIDE EFFECTS/ADVERSE REACTIONS

Occasional
Lethargy, fever, dizziness, rash, pain at injection site
Rare
Seizures, interstitial nephritis

PRECAUTIONS AND CONTRAINDICATIONS

Hypersensitivity to any penicillin
Caution:
Hypersensitivity to cephalosporins

DRUG INTERACTIONS OF CONCERN TO DENTISTRY

- Decreased antimicrobial effect of penicillin: tetracyclines, erythromycins, lincomycins
- Increased penicillin concentrations: aspirin, probenecid
- Suspected increased risk of methotrexate toxicity

SERIOUS REACTIONS

! Hypersensitivity reactions, ranging from chills, fever, and rash to anaphylaxis, may occur.

DENTAL CONSIDERATIONS

General:
- Take precautions regarding allergy to medication.
- Determine why the patient is taking the drug.
- Place on frequent recall to evaluate healing response.

Consultations:
- Medical consultation may be required to assess disease control.

Teach Patient/Family to:
- When used for dental infection, advise patient to:
  - Report sore throat, oral burning sensation, fever, fatigue, any of which could indicate superinfection.
  - Take at prescribed intervals and complete dosage regimen.
  - Immediately notify the dentist if signs or symptoms of infection increase.

penicillin G potassium

pen-ih-**sil′**-lin G poe-**tass′**-ee-um
(Megacillin[CAN], Novepen-G[CAN], Pfizerpen)
Do not confuse penicillin G potassium with penicillin G benzathine or penicillin G procaine.

CATEGORY AND SCHEDULE

Pregnancy Risk Category: B

Drug Class: Antibiotics, penicillins

P

MECHANISM OF ACTION

A penicillin that inhibits bacterial cell wall synthesis by binding to one or more of the penicillin-binding proteins of bacteria.
Therapeutic Effect: Bactericidal.

USES

Treatment of sepsis, meningitis, pericarditis, endocarditis, pneumonia due to susceptible gram-positive organisms (not *Staphylococcus aureus*), and some gram-negative organisms

PHARMACOKINETICS

Completely absorbed from intramuscular injection sites. Peak blood levels reached rapidly after intravenous infusion. Bound primarily to albumin. Widely distributed, but has limited penetration into cerebrospinal fluid. 60% excreted within 5 hr by kidney.

INDICATIONS AND DOSAGES

▸ **Sepsis, Meningitis, Pericarditis, Endocarditis, Pneumonia Caused by Susceptible Gram-Positive Organisms (Not *Staphylococcus aureus*) and Some Gram-Negative Organisms**

IV, IM

Adults, Elderly. 2–24 million units/kg/day in divided doses q4–6h.
Children. 100,000–400,000 units/kg/day in divided doses q4–6h.

▸ **Dosage in Renal Impairment**

Dosage interval is modified on the basis of creatinine clearance.

Creatinine Clearance	Dosage Interval
10–30 ml/min	Usual dose q8–12h
Less than 10 ml/min	Usual dose q12–18h

SIDE EFFECTS/ADVERSE REACTIONS

Occasional

Lethargy, fever, dizziness, rash, electrolyte imbalance, diarrhea, thrombophlebitis

Rare

Seizures, interstitial nephritis

PRECAUTIONS AND CONTRAINDICATIONS

Hypersensitivity to any penicillin

DRUG INTERACTIONS OF CONCERN TO DENTISTRY

- Increased or prolonged plasma levels: probenecid
- Possible decrease in antimicrobial effectiveness: tetracyclines, erythromycins, lincomycins

SERIOUS REACTIONS

! Hypersensitivity reactions ranging from rash, fever, and chills to anaphylaxis occur.

DENTAL CONSIDERATIONS

General:

- Determine why patient is taking the drug.
- Caution regarding allergy to medication.
- Use with caution in patients with a history of antibiotic-associated colitis.

Consultations:

- Consult patient's physician if an acute dental infection occurs and another antiinfective is required.
- Medical consultation may be required to assess disease control.

Teach Patient/Family to:

- Encourage effective oral hygiene to prevent soft tissue inflammation.
- Prevent trauma when using oral hygiene aids.
- Report sore throat, oral burning sensation, fever, or fatigue, any of which could indicate presence of a superinfection.

penicillin V potassium

pen-ih-**sil**′-in V poe-**tass**′-ee-um
(Abbocillin VK[AUS], Apo-Pen-VK[CAN], Cilicaine VK[AUS], L.P.V.[AUS], Novo-Pen-VK[CAN], Veetids)

CATEGORY AND SCHEDULE

Pregnancy Risk Category: B

Drug Class: Semisynthetic penicillin

MECHANISM OF ACTION
A penicillin that inhibits cell wall synthesis by binding to bacterial cell membranes.
Therapeutic Effect: Bactericidal.

USES
Effective for treatment of gram-positive cocci (*S. aureus, S. viridans, S. faecalis, S. bovis, S. pneumoniae*), gram-negative cocci (*N. gonorrhoeae, N. meningitidis*), gram-positive bacilli (*B. anthracis, C. perfringens, C. tetani, C. diphtheriae*), gram-negative bacilli (*S. moniliformis*), spirochetes (*T. pallidum*), *Actinomyces, Peptococcus,* and *Peptostreptococcus* species

PHARMACOKINETICS
Moderately absorbed from the GI tract. Protein binding: 80%. Widely distributed. Metabolized in the liver. Primarily excreted in urine.
Half-life: 1 hr (increased in impaired renal function).

INDICATIONS AND DOSAGES
▸ Mild-to-Moderate Respiratory Tract or Skin or Skin-Structure Infections, Otitis Media, Necrotizing Ulcerative Gingivitis
PO
Adults, Elderly, Children 12 yr and older. 125–500 mg q6–8h.
Children younger than 12 yr. 25–50 mg/kg/day in divided doses q6–8h. Maximum: 3 g/day.
▸ Primary Prevention of Rheumatic Fever
PO
Adults, Elderly. 500 mg 2–3 times a day for 10 days.
Children. 250 mg 2–3 times a day for 10 days.

SIDE EFFECTS/ADVERSE REACTIONS
Frequent
Mild hypersensitivity reaction (chills, fever, rash), nausea, vomiting, diarrhea
Rare
Bleeding

PRECAUTIONS AND CONTRAINDICATIONS
Hypersensitivity to any penicillin
Caution:
Hypersensitivity to cephalosporins, lactation

DRUG INTERACTIONS OF CONCERN TO DENTISTRY
• Decreased antimicrobial effectiveness of penicillin: tetracyclines, erythromycins, lincomycins
• Increased penicillin concentrations: probenecid
• Food: reduced absorption and effectiveness

SERIOUS REACTIONS
! Severe hypersensitivity reactions, including anaphylaxis, may occur.
! Nephrotoxicity, antibiotic-associated colitis, and other superinfections may result from high dosages or prolonged therapy.

DENTAL CONSIDERATIONS
General:
• Take precautions regarding allergy to medication.
• Determine why the patient is taking the drug.
• If used for dental infection, place on frequent recall to evaluate healing response.
Consultations:
• Medical consultation may be required to assess disease control.

Teach Patient/Family:

- When used for dental infection, advise patient to:
  - Report sore throat, oral burning sensation, fever, fatigue, any of which could indicate superinfection.
  - Take at prescribed intervals and complete dosage regimen.
  - Immediately notify the dentist if signs or symptoms of infection or allergy occur.

pentamidine isethionate

pen-**tam′**-ih-deen ice-eth-**eyé**-oh-nate

(NebuPent, Pentacarinat[CAN], Pentam-300)

CATEGORY AND SCHEDULE

Pregnancy Risk Category: C

Drug Class: Antiprotozoal

P

MECHANISM OF ACTION

An antiinfective that interferes with nuclear metabolism and incorporation of nucleotides, inhibiting DNA, RNA, phospholipid, and protein synthesis.

Therapeutic Effect: Antibacterial and antiprotozoal.

USES

Treatment of *Pneumocystis carinii* infections in immunocompromised patients (injection); prevention in high-risk HIV-infected patients (INH)

PHARMACOKINETICS

Well absorbed after IM administration; minimally absorbed after inhalation. Widely distributed. Primarily excreted in urine. Minimally removed by hemodialysis. ***Half-life:*** 6.5 hr (increased in impaired renal function). Powder for Nebulization (NebuPent): 300 mg.

INDICATIONS AND DOSAGES

▸ *Pneumocystis carinii* Pneumonia (PCP)

IV, IM

Adults, Elderly. 4 mg/kg/day once a day for 14–21 days.

Children. 4 mg/kg/day once a day for 10–14 days.

▸ Prevention of PCP

Inhalation

Adults, Elderly. 300 mg once q4wk.

Children 5 yr and older. 300 mg q3–4wk.

Children younger than 5 yr. 8 mg/kg/dose once q3–4wk.

SIDE EFFECTS/ADVERSE REACTIONS

Frequent

Injection: Abscess, pain at injection site

Inhalation: Fatigue, metallic taste, shortness of breath, decreased appetite, dizziness, rash, cough, nausea, vomiting, chills

Occasional

Injection: Nausea, decreased appetite, hypotension, fever, rash, altered taste, confusion

Inhalation: Diarrhea, headache, anemia, muscle pain

Rare

Injection: Neuralgia, thrombocytopenia, phlebitis, dizziness

PRECAUTIONS AND CONTRAINDICATIONS

Concurrent use with didanosine

Caution:

Blood dyscrasias, hepatic disease, renal disease, diabetes mellitus, cardiac disease, hypocalcemia

DRUG INTERACTIONS OF CONCERN TO DENTISTRY

• None reported

SERIOUS REACTIONS

! Rare reactions include life-threatening or fatal hypotension, arrhythmias, hypoglycemia, leukopenia, nephrotoxicity or renal failure, anaphylactic shock, Stevens-Johnson syndrome, and toxic epidural necrolysis.

! Hyperglycemia and insulin-dependent diabetes mellitus (often permanent) may occur even months after therapy has stopped.

DENTAL CONSIDERATIONS

General:

• Monitor vital signs at every appointment because of cardiovascular side effects.

• Patients on chronic drug therapy may rarely have symptoms of blood dyscrasias, which can include infection, bleeding, and poor healing.

• Place on frequent recall to evaluate healing response.

• Assess salivary flow as a factor in caries, periodontal disease, and candidiasis.

• Consider semisupine chair position for patients with respiratory disease.

• For inhalation dosage forms, rinse mouth with water after each dose to prevent dryness.

• Place on frequent recall because of oral side effects.

Consultations:

• In a patient with symptoms of blood dyscrasias, request a medical consultation for blood studies and postpone dental treatment until normal values are reestablished.

• Medical consultation may be required to assess disease control.

Teach Patient/Family to:

• See dentist immediately if secondary oral infection occurs.

• Encourage effective oral hygiene to prevent soft tissue inflammation.

• Use caution to prevent injury when using oral hygiene aids.

• Use dietary suggestions to maintain oral and systemic health.

• When chronic dry mouth occurs, advise patient to:

  • Avoid mouth rinses with high alcohol content because of drying effects.
  • Use daily home fluoride products to prevent caries.
  • Use sugarless gum, frequent sips of water, or saliva substitutes.

pentazocine hydrochloride; naloxone hydrochloride

pen-**taz**′oh-seen high-droh-**klor**′-ide; nah-**lok**′-sohn high-droh-**klor**′-ide
(Talwin Nx)

CATEGORY AND SCHEDULE

Pregnancy Risk Category: C
Controlled Substance: Schedule IV

Drug Class: Synthetic opioid/mixed agonist/antagonist

MECHANISM OF ACTION

Pentazocine is both an opioid agonist and antagonist that induces analgesia by stimulating the kappa and sigma opioid receptors. Naloxone is an opioid antagonist that displaces opiates at opiate-occupied receptor sites in the CNS.

Therapeutic Effect: Pentazocine: induces analgesia. Naloxone: blocks opioid effects if injected; reverses opiate-induced sleep or sedation; increases respiratory rate, returns B/P to normal.

USES

Treatment of moderate-to-severe pain alone or in combination with aspirin or acetaminophen

PHARMACOKINETICS

Well absorbed. Metabolized in liver. Primarily excreted in urine. Minimal excretion in bile and feces.
Half-life: 2–3 hr.

INDICATIONS AND DOSAGES

▸ **Pain, Moderate-to-Severe**

PO

Adults, Elderly, Children 12 yr and older. 1 tablet every 3–4 hr. May be increased to 2 tablets when needed. Maximum: 12 tablets/day.

SIDE EFFECTS/ADVERSE REACTIONS

Occasional

Confusion, dizziness, fatigue, light-headedness, drowsiness, mood changes, headache, GI upset, vomiting, constipation, stomach pain, rash, difficulty urinating

PRECAUTIONS AND CONTRAINDICATIONS

Hypersensitivity to pentazocine or naloxone or any component on the formulation

Caution:

Addictive personality, lactation, increased intracranial pressure, head injury, MI (acute), severe heart disease, respiratory depression, hepatic disease, renal disease, children 12 yr, acute abdominal conditions, Addison's disease, prostatic hypertrophy, patients taking other narcotics

DRUG INTERACTIONS OF CONCERN TO DENTISTRY

- Increased effects: all CNS depressants, alcohol
- Contraindication: MAOIs
- Do not mix in solutions or syringe with barbiturates
- Additive side effects of opioid agonists
- Increased effects of anticholinergics
- Decreased effects of opioid agonists, precipitation of withdrawal

SERIOUS REACTIONS

! Respiratory depression and serious skin reactions, such as Stevens-Johnson syndrome, have been reported but occur rarely.

DENTAL CONSIDERATIONS

General:

- Monitor vital signs at every appointment because of cardiovascular and respiratory side effects.
- Assess salivary flow as a factor in caries, periodontal disease, and candidiasis.
- Consider semisupine chair position for patient comfort if GI side effects occur.
- Psychological and physical dependence may occur with chronic administration.

Teach Patient/Family:

- When chronic dry mouth occurs, advise patient to:
  - Avoid mouth rinses with high alcohol content because of drying effects.
  - Use daily home fluoride products to prevent caries.
  - Use sugarless gum, frequent sips of water, or saliva substitutes.

P

pentazocine

pen-**tah**′-zoe-seen
(Talwin)

COMBINATION PRODUCTS

With naloxone, an opioid antagonist (oral) (Talwin NX); with aspirin (oral) (Talwin Compound); w/acetaminophen (oral) (Talacen)

CATEGORY AND SCHEDULE

Pregnancy Risk Category: C
Controlled Substance: Schedule IV

Drug Class: Opioid analgesics

MECHANISM OF ACTION

An opioid antagonist that binds with opioid receptors within CNS. ***Therapeutic Effect:*** Alters processes affecting pain perception, emotional response to pain.

USES

Relief of moderate-to-severe pain associated with surgical procedures

PHARMACOKINETICS

Well absorbed after administration. Widely distributed including in CSF. Metabolized in liver via oxidative and glucuronide conjugation pathways, extensive first-pass effect. Excreted in small amounts as unchanged drug. ***Half-life:*** 2–3 hr, prolonged with hepatic impairment.

INDICATIONS AND DOSAGES

▸ **Analgesia**

PO (with Naloxone)
Adults. 50 mg q3–4h. May increase to 100 mg q3–4h, if needed. Maximum: 600 mg/day.
Elderly. 50 mg q4h.

▸ **Subcutaneous/IM/IV (without Naloxone)**

Adults. 30 mg q3–4h. Do not exceed 30 mg IV or 60 mg subcutaneous/IM per dose. Maximum: 360 mg/day.
IM
Elderly. 25 mg q4h.

▸ **Obstetric Labor (without Naloxone)**

IM
Adults. 30 mg as a single dose.
IV
Adults. 20 mg when contractions are regular. May repeat 2–3 times q2–3h.

SIDE EFFECTS/ADVERSE REACTIONS

Frequent
Drowsiness, euphoria, nausea, vomiting
Occasional
Allergic reaction, histamine reaction (decreased B/P, increased sweating, flushing, wheezing), decreased urination, altered vision, constipation, dizziness, dry mouth, headache, hypotension, pain/burning at injection site

PRECAUTIONS AND CONTRAINDICATIONS

Hypersensitivity to pentazocine or any component of the formulation

DRUG INTERACTIONS OF CONCERN TO DENTISTRY

- Increased effects: all CNS depressants, alcohol
- Contraindication: MAOIs
- Do not mix with barbiturates in solutions or syringe
- Additive side effects of opioid agonists
- Increased effects of anticholinergics
- Decreased effects of opioid agonists, precipitation of withdrawal

SERIOUS REACTIONS

! Overdosage results in severe respiratory depression, skeletal muscle flaccidity, cyanosis, extreme somnolence progressing to convulsions, stupor, and coma.
! Abrupt withdrawal after prolonged use may produce symptoms of narcotic withdrawal (abdominal cramps, rhinorrhea, lacrimation, nausea, vomiting, restlessness, anxiety, increased temperature, piloerection).

DENTAL CONSIDERATIONS

General:

- Monitor vital signs at every appointment because of cardiovascular and respiratory side effects.
- Assess salivary flow as a factor in caries, periodontal disease, and candidiasis.
- Consider semisupine chair position for patient comfort if GI side effects occur.
- Psychological and physical dependence may occur with chronic administration.

Teach Patient/Family:

- When chronic dry mouth occurs, advise patient to:
  - Avoid mouth rinses with high alcohol content because of drying effects.
  - Use daily home fluoride products to prevent caries.
  - Use sugarless gum, frequent sips of water, or saliva substitutes.

P

pentobarbital

pen-toe-**bar′**-bi-tal
(Nembutal, Phenobarbitone[AUS])
Do not confuse with phenobarbital.

CATEGORY AND SCHEDULE

Pregnancy Risk Category: D
Controlled Substance: Schedule II (capsules, injection), Schedule III (suppositories)

Drug Class: Sedative-hypnotic barbiturate

MECHANISM OF ACTION

A barbiturate that binds at the gamma-aminobutyric acid (GABA) receptor complex, enhancing GABA activity.
Therapeutic Effect: Depresses CNS activity and reticular activating system.

USES

Treatment of insomnia, sedation, preoperative medication, increased intracranial pressure (ICP), dental anesthetic

PHARMACOKINETICS

Well absorbed after PO, parenteral administration. Protein binding: 35%–55%. Rapidly, widely distributed. Metabolized in liver. Primarily excreted in urine. Removed by hemodialysis. ***Half-life:*** 15–48 hr.

INDICATIONS AND DOSAGES

▸ **Preanesthetic**

PO
Adults, Elderly. 100 mg.
Children. 2–6 mg/kg. Maximum: 100 mg/dose.
IM

Adults, Elderly. 150–200 mg.
Children. 2–6 mg/kg. Maximum: 100 mg/dose.
Rectal
Children 12–14 yr. 60 or 120 mg.
Children 5–12 yr. 60 mg.
Children 1–4 yr. 30–60 mg.
Children 2 mo–1 yr. 30 mg.

▸ **Hypnotic**
PO
Adults, Elderly. 100 mg at bedtime.
IM
Adults, Elderly. 150–200 mg at bedtime.
Children. 2–6 mg/kg. Maximum: 100 mg/dose at bedtime.
IV
Adults, Elderly. 100 mg initially then, after 1 min, may give additional small doses at 1-min intervals, up to 500 mg total.
Children. 50 mg initially then, after 1 min, may give additional small doses at 1-min intervals, up to desired effect.
Rectal
Adults, Elderly. 120–200 mg at bedtime.
Children 12–14 yr. 60 or 120 mg at bedtime.
Children 5–12 yr. 60 mg at bedtime.
Children 1–4 yr. 30–60 mg at bedtime.
Children 2 mo–1 yr. 30 mg at bedtime.

▸ **Anticonvulsant**
IV
Adults, Elderly. 2–15 mg/kg loading dose given slowly over 1–2 hr. Maintenance infusion: 0.5–5 mg/kg/hr.
Children. 5–15 mg/kg loading dose given slowly over 1–2 hr. Maintenance infusion: 0.5–3 mg/kg/hr.

SIDE EFFECTS/ADVERSE REACTIONS

Occasional
Agitation, confusion, dizziness, somnolence

Rare
Confusion, paradoxic CNS hyperactivity or nervousness in children, excitement or restlessness in elderly

PRECAUTIONS AND CONTRAINDICATIONS

Porphyria, hypersensitivity to barbiturates

Caution:
Anemia, lactation, hepatic disease, renal disease, hypertension, elderly, acute/chronic pain

DRUG INTERACTIONS OF CONCERN TO DENTISTRY

- Hepatotoxicity: halogenated-hydrocarbon anesthetics
- Increased CNS depression: alcohol, all other CNS depressants
- Increased metabolism of carbamazepine, tricyclic antidepressants, corticosteroids
- Decreased half-life of doxycycline

SERIOUS REACTIONS

! Agranulocytosis, megaloblastic anemia, apnea, hypoventilation, bradycardia, hypotension, syncope, hepatic damage, and Stevens-Johnson syndrome occur rarely.
! Abrupt withdrawal after prolonged therapy may produce effects ranging from markedly increased dreaming, nightmares or insomnia, tremor, sweating and vomiting, to hallucinations, delirium, seizures, and status epilepticus.
! Skin eruptions appear as hypersensitivity reactions.
! Overdosage produces cold or clammy skin, hypothermia, severe

CNS depression, cyanosis, and rapid pulse.

DENTAL CONSIDERATIONS

General:

- Determine why the patient is taking the drug.
- Monitor vital signs at every appointment because of cardiovascular side effects. Evaluate respiration characteristics and rate.
- Patients on chronic drug therapy may rarely have symptoms of blood dyscrasias, which can include infection, bleeding, and poor healing.
- When used for sedation in dentistry:
  - Assess vital signs before use and q30min after use as sedative.
  - Observe respiratory dysfunction: respiratory depression, character, rate, rhythm; hold drug if respirations are fewer than 10/min or if pupils are dilated.
  - After supine positioning, have patient sit upright for at least 2 min before standing to avoid orthostatic hypotension.
  - Have someone escort patient to and from dental office when drug is used for conscious sedation.
  - Barbiturates induce liver microsomal enzymes, which alter the metabolism of other drugs.
  - Geriatric patients are more susceptible to drug effects; use lower dose.

Consultations:

- In a patient with symptoms of blood dyscrasias, request a medical consultation for blood studies and postpone dental treatment until normal values are reestablished.

Teach Patient/Family to:

- Avoid driving or other activities requiring alertness.
- Avoid alcohol ingestion or CNS depressants; serious CNS depression may result.
- Avoid OTC preparations (antihistamines, cold remedies) that contain CNS depressants.

pentosan polysulfate

pen′-toe-san poll-ee-**sull′**-fate
(Elmiron)
Do not confuse with pentostatin.

CATEGORY AND SCHEDULE

Pregnancy Risk Category: B

Drug Class: Anticoagulant

MECHANISM OF ACTION

A negatively charged synthetic sulfated polysaccharide with heparin-like properties that appear to adhere to bladder wall mucosal membrane, may act as a buffering agent to control cell permeability, preventing irritating solutes in the urine. Has anticoagulant/fibrinolytic effects.
Therapeutic Effect: Relieves bladder pain.

USES

Relief of interstitial cystitis symptoms

PHARMACOKINETICS

Poorly and erratically absorbed from the gastrointestinal tract. Distributed in uroepithelium of GU tract with lesser amount found in the liver, spleen, lung, skin, periosteum, and bone marrow. Metabolized in liver and kidney (secondary). Eliminated in the urine. ***Half-life:*** 4.8 hr.

INDICATIONS AND DOSAGES

▸ **Interstitial Cystitis**

PO

Adults, Elderly. 100 mg 3 times a day.

SIDE EFFECTS/ADVERSE REACTIONS

Frequent

Alopecia areata (a single area on the scalp), diarrhea, nausea, headache, rash, abdominal pain, dyspepsia

Occasional

Dizziness, depression, increased liver function tests

PRECAUTIONS AND CONTRAINDICATIONS

Hypersensitivity to pentosan polysulfate sodium or structurally related compounds

DRUG INTERACTIONS OF CONCERN TO DENTISTRY

• Potential risk of bleeding: high-dose aspirin

SERIOUS REACTIONS

! Ecchymosis, epistaxis, gum hemorrhage have been reported (drug produces weak anticoagulant effect).

! Overdose may produce liver function abnormalities.

DENTAL CONSIDERATIONS

General:

• Possesses weak anticoagulant activity; question patient about bleeding or bruising.

• Consider semisupine chair position for patient comfort if GI side effects occur.

• Question patient about tolerance of NSAIDs or aspirin related to GI disease.

• Do not discontinue pentosan therapy for routine dental procedures.

• Avoid products that affect platelet function, such as aspirin and NSAIDs.

• Consider local hemostasis measures to prevent excessive bleeding.

Consultations:

• Confer with physician if bleeding is a problem; epistaxis, spontaneous gingival bleeding.

• Medical consultation should include routine blood counts, including platelet counts and bleeding time.

Teach Patient/Family to:

• Encourage effective oral hygiene to prevent soft tissue inflammation.

• Prevent trauma when using oral hygiene aids.

• Report oral lesions, soreness, or bleeding to dentist.

• Importance of updating health and medication history if physician makes any changes in evaluation or drug regimens; include OTC, herbal, and nonherbal drugs in the update.

pentostatin

pen-toe-**stat′**-in

(Nipent)

Do not confuse with pravastatin.

CATEGORY AND SCHEDULE

Pregnancy Risk Category: D

Drug Class: Antineoplastic, enzyme inhibitor

MECHANISM OF ACTION

An antimetabolite that inhibits the enzyme adenosine deaminase (ADA) (increases intracellular levels of adenine deoxynucleotide). Greatest activity in T cells of lymphoid system. Inhibits ADA and RNA synthesis. Produces DNA damage.

Therapeutic Effect: Leads to death of tumor cells.

USES

Treatment of α-interferon–refractory hairy cell leukemia

PHARMACOKINETICS

After IV administration, rapidly distributed to body tissues (poorly distributed to cerebrospinal fluid). Protein binding: 4%. Excreted primarily in urine unchanged or as active metabolite. ***Half-life:*** 5.7 hr (2.6–10 hr).

INDICATIONS AND DOSAGES

▸ Hairy Cell Leukemia

IV

Adults, Elderly. 4 mg/m^2 q2wk until complete response attained (without any major toxicity). Discontinue if no response in 6 mo; partial response in 12 mo.

▸ Dosage in Renal Impairment

Only when benefits justify risks, give 2–3 mg/m^2 in patients with creatinine clearance 50–60 ml/min.

SIDE EFFECTS/ADVERSE REACTIONS

Frequent

Nausea, vomiting, fever, fatigue, rash, pain, cough, upper respiratory tract infection, anorexia, diarrhea

Occasional

Headache, pharyngitis, sinusitis, myalgia, chills, arthralgia, peripheral edema, anorexia, blurred vision, conjunctivitis, skin discoloration, sweating, anxiety, depression, dizziness, confusion

PRECAUTIONS AND CONTRAINDICATIONS

Hypersensitivity to pentostatin

SERIOUS REACTIONS

! Bone marrow depression is manifested as hematologic toxicity (principally leukopenia, anemia, thrombocytopenia).

! Doses higher than recommended (20–50 mg/m^2 in divided doses for more than 5 days) may produce severe renal, hepatic, pulmonary, or CNS toxicity.

DENTAL CONSIDERATIONS

- Increased susceptibility to infections.
- Increased bleeding.
- Anemia.
- Oral ulcerations, mucositis (use palliative measures for relief).
- Increased nausea, vomiting.
- Consult physician to determine disease control and ability of patient to tolerate dental procedures.

pentoxifylline

pen-tox-**if**′-ih-lin

(Albert[CAN], Apo-Pentoxifylline SR[CAN], Pentoxifylline[CAN], Pentoxyl, Trental)

Do not confuse Trental with Tegretol or Trandate.

CATEGORY AND SCHEDULE

Pregnancy Risk Category: C

Drug Class: Hemorheologic agent

MECHANISM OF ACTION

A blood viscosity-reducing agent that alters the flexibility of RBCs; inhibits production of tumor necrosis factor, neutrophil activation, and platelet aggregation.

Therapeutic Effect: Reduces blood viscosity and improves blood flow.

USES
Treatment of intermittent claudication related to chronic occlusive arterial disease of the limbs

PHARMACOKINETICS
Well absorbed after oral administration. Undergoes first-pass metabolism in the liver. Primarily excreted in urine. Unknown if removed by hemodialysis.
Half-life: 24–48 min; metabolite, 60–90 min.

INDICATIONS AND DOSAGES
▸ **Intermittent Claudication**
PO
Adults, Elderly. 400 mg 3 times a day. Decrease to 400 mg twice a day if GI or CNS adverse effects occur. Continue for at least 8 wk.

SIDE EFFECTS/ADVERSE REACTIONS
Occasional
Dizziness, nausea, altered taste, dyspepsia, marked by heartburn, epigastric pain, and indigestion
Rare
Rash, pruritus, anorexia, constipation, dry mouth, blurred vision, edema, nasal congestion, anxiety

PRECAUTIONS AND CONTRAINDICATIONS
History of intolerance to xanthine derivatives, such as caffeine, theophylline, or theobromine; recent cerebral or retinal hemorrhage
Caution:
Angina pectoris, cardiac disease, lactation, children, impaired renal function

DRUG INTERACTIONS OF CONCERN TO DENTISTRY
- Increased bleeding: ASA, NSAIDs

SERIOUS REACTIONS
! Angina and chest pain occur rarely and may be accompanied by palpitations, tachycardia, and arrhythmias.
! Signs and symptoms of overdose, such as flushing, hypotension, nervousness, agitation, hand tremor, fever, and somnolence, appear 4–5 hr after ingestion and last for 12 hr.

DENTAL CONSIDERATIONS
General:
- Monitor vital signs at every appointment because of cardiovascular side effects.
- Assess salivary flow as a factor in caries, periodontal disease, and candidiasis.
- Stress from dental procedures may compromise cardiovascular function; determine patient risk.
- Short appointments and a stress-reduction protocol may be required for anxious patients.
- Talk with patient about potential systemic diseases (e.g., diabetes, cardiovascular disease) that may be associated with claudication.

Consultations:
- Medical consultation may be required to assess disease control and patient's ability to tolerate stress.

Teach Patient/Family to:
- Encourage effective oral hygiene to prevent soft tissue inflammation.
- Prevent injury when using oral hygiene aids.
- When chronic dry mouth occurs, advise patient to:
  - Avoid mouth rinses with high alcohol content because of drying effects.
  - Use home fluoride products to prevent caries.

• Use sugarless gum, frequent sips of water, or saliva substitutes.

perindopril

per-**in**′-doh-pril
(Aceon)

CATEGORY AND SCHEDULE

Pregnancy Risk Category: C (D if used in second or third trimester)

Drug Class: Angiotensin-converting enzyme (ACE) inhibitor

MECHANISM OF ACTION

An ACE inhibitor that suppresses the renin-angiotensin-aldosterone system and prevents conversion of angiotensin I to angiotensin II, a potent vasoconstrictor; may also inhibit angiotensin II at local vascular and renal sites.
Therapeutic Effect: Reduces peripheral arterial resistance and B/P.

USES

Treatment of essential hypertension as monotherapy or in combination with other antihypertensive medication

PHARMACOKINETICS

PO: Absolute bioavailability 20%–30%, metabolized to active metabolite, perindoprilat, peak plasma levels 1 hr, active metabolite 3–4 hr; protein binding 10%–20%, hepatic metabolism, excreted mostly in urine (75%)

INDICATIONS AND DOSAGES

▸ **Hypertension**

PO

Adults, Elderly. 2–8 mg/day as single dose or in 2 divided doses. Maximum: 16 mg/day.

SIDE EFFECTS/ADVERSE REACTIONS

Occasional

Cough, back pain, sinusitis, upper extremity pain, dyspepsia, fever, palpitations, hypotension, dizziness, fatigue, syncope

PRECAUTIONS AND CONTRAINDICATIONS

History of angioedema from previous treatment with ACE inhibitors

Caution:

Renal insufficiency, hypertension with CHF, severe CHF, renal artery stenosis, autoimmune disease, collagen vascular disease, pregnancy category C (first trimester); pregnancy category D (second and third trimesters), lactation

DRUG INTERACTIONS OF CONCERN TO DENTISTRY

• Decreased hypotensive effects: NSAIDs, aspirin
• Increased hypotension: caution in use of other drugs that have hypotensive effects
• Suspected reduction in the antihypertensive and vasodilator effects by salicylates; monitor B/P if used concurrently

SERIOUS REACTIONS

! Excessive hypotension ("first-dose syncope") may occur in patients with CHF and in those who are severely salt or volume depleted.
! Angioedema (swelling of face and lips) and hyperkalemia occur rarely.

! Agranulocytosis and neutropenia may be noted in those with collagen vascular disease, including scleroderma and systemic lupus erythematosus, and impaired renal function.

! Nephrotic syndrome may be noted in those with history of renal disease.

DENTAL CONSIDERATIONS

General:

• Monitor vital signs at every appointment because of cardiovascular side effects.

• Limit use of sodium-containing products, such as saline IV fluids, for patients with a dietary salt restriction.

• Stress from dental procedures may compromise cardiovascular function; determine patient risk.

• Short appointments and a stress-reduction protocol may be required for anxious patients.

• After supine positioning, have patient sit upright for at least 2 min before standing to avoid orthostatic hypotension.

• Use precaution if sedation or general anesthesia is required; risk of hypotensive episode.

• Assess salivary flow as a factor in caries, periodontal disease, and candidiasis.

• Consider semisupine chair position for patient comfort if GI or respiratory side effects occur.

• Patients on chronic drug therapy may rarely have symptoms of blood dyscrasias, which can include infection, bleeding, and poor healing.

Consultations:

• In a patient with symptoms of blood dyscrasias, request a medical consultation for blood studies and postpone treatment until normal values are reestablished.

• Medical consultation may be required to assess disease control and patient's ability to tolerate stress.

Teach Patient/Family to:

• Update health and drug history if physician makes any changes in evaluation or drug regimens; include OTC, herbal, and nonherbal drugs in the update.

• Encourage effective oral hygiene to prevent soft tissue inflammation.

• Prevent trauma when using oral hygiene aids.

• When chronic dry mouth occurs, advise patient to:

  • Avoid mouth rinses with high alcohol content because of drying effects.

  • Use daily home fluoride products for anticaries effect.

  • Use sugarless gum, frequent sips of water, or saliva substitutes.

perphenazine

per-**fen**′-ah-zeen

(Trilafon)

Do not confuse perphenazine with promazine.

CATEGORY AND SCHEDULE

Pregnancy Risk Category: C

Drug Class: Phenothiazine antipsychotic

MECHANISM OF ACTION

An antipsychotic agent and antiemetic that blocks postsynaptic dopamine receptor sites in the brain.

Therapeutic Effect: Suppresses behavioral response in psychosis, and relieves nausea and vomiting.

USES

Treatment of psychotic disorders, schizophrenia, alcoholism, nausea, vomiting

PHARMACOKINETICS

PO: Onset erratic, peak 2–4 hr IM: Onset 10 min, peak 1–2 hr, duration 6 hr, occasionally 12–24 hr Metabolized by liver, excreted in urine, crosses placenta, excreted in breast milk.

INDICATIONS AND DOSAGES

▸ Severe Schizophrenia

PO

Adults. 4–16 mg 2–4 times a day. Maximum: 64 mg/day.

Elderly. Initially, 2–4 mg/day. May increase at 4–7 day intervals by 2–4 mg/day up to 32 mg/day.

▸ Severe Nausea and Vomiting

PO

Adults. 8–16 mg/day in divided doses up to 24 mg/day.

SIDE EFFECTS/ADVERSE REACTIONS

Occasional

Marked photosensitivity, somnolence, dry mouth, blurred vision, lethargy, constipation or diarrhea, nasal congestion, peripheral edema, urine retention

Rare

Ocular changes, altered skin pigmentation, hypotension, dizziness, syncope

PRECAUTIONS AND CONTRAINDICATIONS

Coma, myelosuppression, severe cardiovascular disease, severe CNS depression, subcortical brain damage

Caution:

Lactation, seizure disorders, hypertension, hepatic disease, cardiac disease

DRUG INTERACTIONS OF CONCERN TO DENTISTRY

- Increased sedation: other CNS depressants, alcohol, barbiturate anesthetics, opioid analgesics
- Hypotension, tachycardia: epinephrine
- Increased extrapyramidal effects: phenothiazines and related drugs (haloperidol, droperidol), metoclopramide
- Additive photosensitization: tetracyclines, fluoroquinolones
- Increased anticholinergic effects: anticholinergics

SERIOUS REACTIONS

! Extrapyramidal symptoms appear to be dose-related and are divided into three categories: akathisia (characterized by inability to sit still, tapping of feet), parkinsonian symptoms (including mask-like face, tremors, shuffling gait, hypersalivation), and acute dystonias (such as torticollis, opisthotonos, and oculogyric crisis).

! Tardive dyskinesia occurs rarely.

! Abrupt withdrawal after long-term therapy may precipitate nausea, vomiting, gastritis, dizziness, and tremors.

DENTAL CONSIDERATIONS

General:

- Monitor vital signs at every appointment because of cardiovascular side effects.
- Patients on chronic drug therapy may rarely have symptoms of blood dyscrasias, which can include infection, bleeding, and poor healing.
- After supine positioning, have patient sit upright for at least 2 min before standing to avoid orthostatic hypotension.

- Assess salivary flow as a factor in caries, periodontal disease, and candidiasis.
- Avoid dental light in patient's eyes; offer dark glasses for patient comfort.
- Assess for presence of extrapyramidal motor symptoms, such as tardive dyskinesia and akathisia. Extrapyramidal motor activity may complicate dental treatment.
- Geriatric patients are more susceptible to drug effects; use lower dose.
- Use vasoconstrictors with caution, in low doses, and with careful aspiration. Avoid use of gingival retraction cord with epinephrine.

Consultations:

- In a patient with symptoms of blood dyscrasias, request a medical consultation for blood studies and postpone dental treatment until normal values are reestablished.
- Take precautions if dental surgery is anticipated and anesthesia is required.
- If signs of tardive dyskinesia or akathisia are present, refer to physician.
- Physician should be informed if significant xerostomic side effects occur (e.g., increased caries, sore tongue, problems eating or swallowing, difficulty wearing prosthesis) so that a medication change can be considered.

Teach Patient/Family to:

- Encourage effective oral hygiene to prevent soft tissue inflammation.
- Use caution to prevent injury when using oral hygiene aids.
- Use powered tooth brush if patient has difficulty holding conventional devices.
- When chronic dry mouth occurs, advise patient to:
  - Avoid mouth rinses with high alcohol content because of drying effects.
  - Use daily home fluoride products to prevent caries.
  - Use sugarless gum, frequent sips of water, or saliva substitutes.

phenazopyridine hydrochloride

fen-az-oh-**peer′**-ih-deen high-droh-**klor′**-ide
(Azo-Gesic, Azo-Standard, Phenazo[CAN], Prodium, Pyridium, Uristat)
Do not confuse phenazopyridine with pyridoxine, or Prodium with Perdiem.

CATEGORY AND SCHEDULE

Pregnancy Risk Category: B

Drug Class: Urinary tract analgesic

MECHANISM OF ACTION

An interstitial cystitis agent that exerts topical analgesic effect on urinary tract mucosa.
Therapeutic Effect: Relieves urinary pain, burning, urgency, and frequency.

USES

Treatment of urinary tract irritation/infection

PHARMACOKINETICS

Well absorbed from the GI tract. Partially metabolized in the liver. Primarily excreted in urine.

INDICATIONS AND DOSAGES

▸ Urinary Analgesic

PO

Adults. 100–200 mg 3–4 times a day.

Children 6 yr and older. 12 mg/kg/day in 3 divided doses for 2 days.

▸ Dosage in Renal Impairment

Dosage interval is modified on the basis of creatinine clearance.

Creatinine Clearance	Interval
50–80 ml/min	Usual dose q8–16h
Less than 50 ml/min	Avoid use

SIDE EFFECTS/ADVERSE REACTIONS

Occasional

Headache, GI disturbance, rash, pruritus

PRECAUTIONS AND CONTRAINDICATIONS

Hepatic or renal insufficiency

Caution:

Renal disease

P

DRUG INTERACTIONS OF CONCERN TO DENTISTRY

- None reported

SERIOUS REACTIONS

! Overdose may lead to hemolytic anemia, nephrotoxicity, or hepatotoxicity. Patients with renal impairment or severe hypersensitivity to the drug may also develop these reactions.

! A massive and acute overdose may result in methemoglobinemia.

DENTAL CONSIDERATIONS

General:

- Consider semisupine chair position for patient comfort if GI side effects occur.
- Patients on chronic drug therapy may rarely have symptoms of blood dyscrasias, which can include infection, bleeding, and poor healing.
- Be aware that patient might have UTI; question if antiinfectives are also being used.

phendimetrazine

fen-dye-**me**′-tra-zeen

(Adipost, Bontril PDM, Bontril Slow-Release, Melfiat, Obezine, Phendiet, Phendiet-105, Plegine, Prelu-2)

CATEGORY AND SCHEDULE

Pregnancy Risk Category: C

Controlled Substance: Schedule III

Drug Class: Anorexiant, amphetamine-like

MECHANISM OF ACTION

A phenylalkylamine sympathomimetic with activity similar to amphetamines that stimulates the CNS and elevates B/P most likely mediated via norepinephrine and dopamine metabolism. Causes stimulation of the hypothalamus.

Therapeutic Effect: Decreases appetite.

USES

Treatment of exogenous obesity

PHARMACOKINETICS

The pharmacokinetics of phendimetrazine tartrate have not been well established. Metabolized to active metabolite, phendimetrazine. Excreted in urine. ***Half-life:*** 2–4 hr.

INDICATIONS AND DOSAGES

▸ **Obesity**

PO

Adults, Elderly. 105 mg/day in the morning or before the morning meal (sustained release); 35 mg 2–3 times a day (immediate release). Maximum: 70 mg 3 times a day.

SIDE EFFECTS/ADVERSE REACTIONS

Occasional

Constipation, nausea, diarrhea, dry mouth, dysuria, libido changes, flushing, hypertension, insomnia, nervousness, headache, dizziness, irritability, agitation, restlessness, palpitations, increased heart rate, sweating, tremor, urticaria

PRECAUTIONS AND CONTRAINDICATIONS

Advanced arteriosclerosis, agitated states, glaucoma, history of drug abuse, history of hypersensitivity to sympathomimetic amines, hyperthyroidism, moderate-to-severe hypertension, symptomatic cardiovascular disease, use within 14 days of discontinuation MAOI, hypersensitivity to phendimetrazine or sympathomimetics

Caution:

Drug abuse, anxiety, lactation

DRUG INTERACTIONS OF CONCERN TO DENTISTRY

- Hypertensive crisis: MAOIs or within 14 days of MAOIs
- Increased risk of dysrhythmia: hydrocarbon inhalation, general anesthetics, epinephrine
- Decreased effect: tricyclic antidepressants, ascorbic acid, phenothiazines
- Caffeine or caffeine-containing products: may increase risk of insomnia and dry mouth

SERIOUS REACTIONS

! Multivalvular heart disease, primary pulmonary hypertension, and arrhythmias occur rarely.

! Overdose may produce flushing, arrhythmias, and psychosis.

! Abrupt withdrawal following prolonged administration of high doses may produce extreme fatigue and depression.

DENTAL CONSIDERATIONS

General:

- Monitor vital signs at every appointment because of cardiovascular side effects.
- Avoid or limit dose of vasoconstrictor.
- Assess salivary flow as a factor in caries, periodontal disease, and candidiasis.
- Determine why the patient is taking the drug.
- Psychological and physical dependence may occur with chronic administration.
- Patients on chronic drug therapy may rarely have symptoms of blood dyscrasias, which can include infection, bleeding, and poor healing.

Consultations:

- In a patient with symptoms of blood dyscrasias, request a medical consultation for blood studies and postpone dental treatment until normal values are reestablished.

Teach Patient/Family to:

- Encourage effective oral hygiene to prevent soft tissue inflammation.
- Report oral lesions, soreness, or bleeding to dentist.
- Use caution to prevent injury when using oral hygiene aids.
- When chronic dry mouth occurs, advise patient to:
  - Avoid mouth rinses with high alcohol content because of drying effects.

• Use daily home fluoride products to prevent caries.
• Use sugarless gum, frequent sips of water, or saliva substitutes.

phenelzine sulfate

fen′-el-zeen **sull′**-fate
(Nardil)

CATEGORY AND SCHEDULE

Pregnancy Risk Category: C

Drug Class: Antidepressant, monoamine oxidase inhibitor (MAOI)

MECHANISM OF ACTION

An MAOI that inhibits the activity of the enzyme monoamine oxidase at CNS storage sites, leading to increased levels of the neurotransmitters epinephrine, norepinephrine, serotonin, and dopamine at neuronal receptor sites.
Therapeutic Effect: Relieves depression.

USES

Treatment of depression when uncontrolled by other means

PHARMACOKINETICS

Well absorbed from GI tract. Metabolized in the liver. Primarily excreted in urine. ***Half-life:*** 1.2 hr.

INDICATIONS AND DOSAGES

▸ Depression Refractory to Other Antidepressants or Electroconvulsive Therapy

PO
Adults. 5 mg 3 times a day. May increase to 60–90 mg/day.
Elderly. Initially, 7.5 mg/day. May increase by 7.5–15 mg/day q3–4wk up to 60 mg/day in divided doses.

SIDE EFFECTS/ADVERSE REACTIONS

Frequent
Orthostatic hypotension, restlessness, GI upset, insomnia, dizziness, headache, lethargy, asthenia, dry mouth, peripheral edema
Occasional
Flushing, diaphoresis, rash, urinary frequency, increased appetite, transient impotence
Rare
Visual disturbances

PRECAUTIONS AND CONTRAINDICATIONS

Cardiovascular or cerebrovascular disease, hepatic or renal impairment, pheochromocytoma
Caution:
Suicidal patients, convulsive disorders, severe depression, schizophrenia, hyperactivity, diabetes mellitus

DRUG INTERACTIONS OF CONCERN TO DENTISTRY

• Increased anticholinergic effect: anticholinergics, haloperidol, phenothiazines, antihistamines
• Hyperpyretic crisis, convulsions, hypertensive episode: meperidine, carbamazepine, cyclobenzaprine
• Cardiac dysrhythmia: caffeine-containing medications
• Increased risk of serotonin syndrome: tricyclic antidepressants, other serotonin reuptake inhibitors
• Increased sedative effects of alcohol, barbiturates, benzodiazepines, CNS depressants
• Increased pressor effects: indirect-acting sympathomimetics, such as ephedrine, amphetamine

SERIOUS REACTIONS

! Hypertensive crisis occurs rarely and is marked by severe

P

hypertension, occipital headache radiating frontally, neck stiffness or soreness, nausea, vomiting, diaphoresis, fever or chilliness, clammy skin, dilated pupils, palpitations, tachycardia or bradycardia, and constricting chest pain.

! Intracranial bleeding has been reported in association with severe hypertension.

DENTAL CONSIDERATIONS

General:

- Monitor vital signs at every appointment because of cardiovascular side effects.
- Assess salivary flow as a factor in caries, periodontal disease, and candidiasis.
- After supine positioning, have patient sit upright for at least 2 min before standing to avoid orthostatic hypotension.
- Hypertensive episodes are possible even though there are no specific contraindications to vasoconstrictor use in local anesthetics.
- Avoid prescribing caffeine-containing products.
- Take precautions if dental surgery is anticipated and general anesthesia is required.

Consultations:

- Medical consultation may be required to assess disease control and patient's ability to tolerate stress.

Teach Patient/Family to:

- Use powered tooth brush if patient has difficulty holding conventional devices.
- When chronic dry mouth occurs, advise patient to:
  - Avoid mouth rinses with high alcohol content because of drying effects.
  - Use daily home fluoride products to prevent caries.
  - Use sugarless gum, frequent sips of water, or saliva substitutes.

phenobarbital

fee-noe-**bar′**-bi-tal

(Luminal, Phenobarbitone[AUS])

Do not confuse phenobarbital with pentobarbital, or Luminal with Tuinal.

CATEGORY AND SCHEDULE

Pregnancy Risk Category: D

Controlled Substance: Schedule IV

Drug Class: Barbiturate anticonvulsant

MECHANISM OF ACTION

A barbiturate that enhances the activity of gamma-aminobutyric acid (GABA) by binding to the GABA receptor complex.

Therapeutic Effect: Depresses CNS activity.

USES

Treatment of all forms of epilepsy, status epilepticus, febrile seizures in children, sedation, insomnia; unapproved: hyperbilirubinemia, chronic cholestasis

PHARMACOKINETICS

Route	Onset	Peak	Duration
PO	20–60 min	N/A	6–10 hr
IV	5 min	30 min	4–10 hr

Well absorbed after PO or parenteral administration. Protein binding: 35%–50%. Rapidly and widely distributed. Metabolized in the liver.

P

Primarily excreted in urine. Removed by hemodialysis. ***Half-life:*** 53–118 hr.

INDICATIONS AND DOSAGES

▸ **Status Epilepticus**

IV

Adults, Elderly, Children, Neonates. Loading dose of 15–20 mg/kg as a single dose or in divided doses.

▸ **Seizure Control**

PO, IV

Adults, Elderly, Children older than 12 yr. 1–3 mg/kg/day.
Children 6–12 yr. 4–6 mg/kg/day.
Children 1–5 yr. 6–8 mg/kg/day.
Children younger than 1 yr. 5–6 mg/kg/day.
Neonates. 3–4 mg/kg/day.

▸ **Sedation**

PO, IM

Adults, Elderly. 30–120 mg/day in 2–3 divided doses.
Children. 2 mg/kg 3 times a day.

▸ **Hypnotic**

PO, IV, IM, Subcutaneous

Adults, Elderly. 100–320 mg at bedtime.
Children. 3–5 mg/kg at bedtime.

P

SIDE EFFECTS/ADVERSE REACTIONS

Occasional

Somnolence

Rare

Confusion; paradoxic CNS reactions, such as hyperactivity or nervousness in children and excitement or restlessness in the elderly (generally noted during first 2 wk of therapy, particularly in presence of uncontrolled pain)

PRECAUTIONS AND CONTRAINDICATIONS

Porphyria, preexisting CNS depression, severe pain, severe respiratory disease

Caution:

Anemia

DRUG INTERACTIONS OF CONCERN TO DENTISTRY

- Increased effects: alcohol, all CNS depressants, saquinavir, protease inhibitors
- Decreased effects of corticosteroids, doxycycline, carbamazepine

SERIOUS REACTIONS

! Abrupt withdrawal after prolonged therapy may produce increased dreaming, nightmares, insomnia, tremor, diaphoresis, vomiting, hallucinations, delirium, seizures, and status epilepticus.
! Skin eruptions may be a sign of a hypersensitivity reaction.
! Blood dyscrasias, hepatic disease, and hypocalcemia occur rarely.
! Overdose produces cold or clammy skin, hypothermia, severe CNS depression, cyanosis, tachycardia, and Cheyne-Stokes respirations.
! Toxicity may result in severe renal impairment.

DENTAL CONSIDERATIONS

General:

- Determine why the patient is taking the drug.
- Monitor vital signs at every appointment because of cardiovascular side effects. Evaluate respiration characteristics and rate.
- Patients on chronic drug therapy may rarely have symptoms of blood dyscrasias, which can include infection, bleeding, and poor healing.
- When used for sedation in dentistry:
  - Assess vital signs before and during use and after use as sedative.

- Observe respiratory dysfunction: respiratory depression, character, rate, rhythm; hold drug if respirations are less frequent than 10/min or if pupils are dilated.
- After supine positioning, have patient sit upright for at least 2 min before standing to avoid orthostatic hypotension.
- Have someone escort patient to and from dental office when drug used for conscious sedation.
- Barbiturates induce liver microsomal enzymes, which alters the metabolism of other drugs.
- Geriatric patients are more susceptible to drug effects; use lower dose.

Consultations:

- In a patient with symptoms of blood dyscrasias, request a medical consultation for blood studies and postpone dental treatment until normal values are reestablished.

Teach Patient/Family to:

- Avoid driving or other activities requiring alertness.
- Avoid alcohol ingestion or CNS depressants; serious CNS depression may result.
- Use OTC preparations with caution because they may contain other CNS depressants (e.g., antihistamines, cold remedies).

phenoxybenzamine

fen-ox-ee-**ben′**-za-meen
(Dibenzyline)

CATEGORY AND SCHEDULE

Pregnancy Risk Category: C

Drug Class: Antihypertensive, pheochromocytoma

MECHANISM OF ACTION

An antihypertensive that produces long-lasting, noncompetitive α-adrenergic blockade of postganglionic synapses in exocrine glands and smooth muscles. Relaxes urethra and increases opening of the bladder.

Therapeutic Effect: Controls hypertension.

USES

Treatment of hypertension caused by pheochromocytoma

PHARMACOKINETICS

Well absorbed from the GI tract. Distributed into fatty tissue. Metabolized in liver. Eliminated in urine and feces. Not removed by hemodialysis. ***Half-life:*** 24 hr.

INDICATIONS AND DOSAGES

▸ **Pheochromocytoma**

PO

Adults. Initially, 10 mg twice daily. May increase dose every other day to 20–40 mg 2–3 times/day.

Children. 1–2 mg/kg/day in divided doses.

SIDE EFFECTS/ADVERSE REACTIONS

Frequent

Headache, lethargy, confusion, fatigue

Occasional

Nausea, postural hypotension, syncope, dry mouth

Rare

Palpitations, diarrhea, constipation, inhibition of ejaculation, weakness, altered vision, dizziness

PRECAUTIONS AND CONTRAINDICATIONS

Any condition compromised by hypotension, hypersensitivity to phenoxybenzamine or any component of the formulation

DRUG INTERACTIONS OF CONCERN TO DENTISTRY

• Exaggerated hypotension, tachycardia: epinephrine, other α-adrenergic agonists

SERIOUS REACTIONS

! Overdosage produces severe hypotension, irritability, lethargy, tachycardia, dizziness, and shock.

DENTAL CONSIDERATIONS

General:

• Medication may be used in anticipation of surgery to remove the adrenal tumor.
• Hypertension may preclude all dental care except for palliative emergency treatment.
• Question patient about compliance with drug therapy.
• Risk of increased CNS depression when other CNS depressants are used.
• Determine why patient is taking the drug.
• Monitor and record vital signs.
• Use vasoconstrictor with caution, in low doses, and with careful aspiration. Avoid using gingival retraction cord containing epinephrine.
• After supine positioning, have patient sit upright for at least 2 min before standing to avoid orthostatic hypotension.

Consultations:

• Medical consultation may be required to assess disease control and patient's ability to tolerate stress.

Teach Patient/Family to:

• Encourage effective oral hygiene to prevent soft tissue inflammation.
• Not drive or perform other tasks requiring mental alertness.

P

phentermine

fen′-ter-meen
(Adipex-P, Fastin, Ionamin, Oby-Cap, Phentercot, Pro-Fast HS, Pro-Fast SA, Pro-Fast SR, T-Diet, Teramine, Zantryl)

CATEGORY AND SCHEDULE

Pregnancy Risk Category: B
Controlled Substance: Schedule IV

Drug Class: Sympathomimetic, anorexiant

MECHANISM OF ACTION

A sympathomimetic amine structurally similar to dextroamphetamine and is most likely mediated via norepinephrine and dopamine metabolism. Causes stimulation of the hypothalamus.
Therapeutic Effect: Decreased appetite.

USES

Treatment of exogenous obesity

PHARMACOKINETICS

Well absorbed from the GI tract; resin absorbed slower. Excreted unchanged in urine. ***Half-life:*** 20 hr.

INDICATIONS AND DOSAGES

▸ **Obesity**

PO

Adults, Children older than 16 yr.
Adipex-P: 37.5 mg as a single daily dose or in divided doses.
Ionamin: 15–37.5 mg/day before breakfast or 1–2 hr after breakfast.
Fastin: 30 mg/day taken in the morning.

SIDE EFFECTS/ADVERSE REACTIONS

Occasional

Restlessness, insomnia, tremor, palpitations, tachycardia, elevation in B/P, headache, dizziness, dry mouth, unpleasant taste, diarrhea or constipation, changes in libido

PRECAUTIONS AND CONTRAINDICATIONS

Advanced arteriosclerosis, agitated states, cardiovascular disease, concurrent use or within 14 days of discontinuation of MAOI therapy, glaucoma, history of drug abuse, hypertension (moderate to severe), hyperthyroidism, hypersensitivity to phentermine or sympathomimetic amines

Caution:

Lactation, drug abuse, anxiety, tolerance

DRUG INTERACTIONS OF CONCERN TO DENTISTRY

- Hypertensive crisis: MAOIs or within 14 days of MAOIs
- Increased risk of dysrhythmia: hydrocarbon inhalation general anesthetics
- Decreased effect: tricyclic antidepressants, ascorbic acid, phenothiazines
- Caffeine or caffeine-containing products may increase risk of insomnia

SERIOUS REACTIONS

! Primary pulmonary hypertension (PPH), psychotic episodes, and valvular heart disease rarely occur.

! Anorectic agents have been associated with regurgitant multivalvular heart disease involving mitral, aortic, and/or tricuspid valves.

! Prolonged use may cause physical or psychological dependence.

DENTAL CONSIDERATIONS

General:

- Monitor vital signs at every appointment because of cardiovascular side effects.
- Assess salivary flow as a factor in caries, periodontal disease, and candidiasis.
- Determine why the patient is taking the drug.
- Psychological and physical dependence may occur with chronic administration.
- Patients on chronic drug therapy may rarely have symptoms of blood dyscrasias, which can include infection, bleeding, and poor healing.

Consultations:

- In a patient with symptoms of blood dyscrasias, request a medical consultation for blood studies and postpone dental treatment until normal values are reestablished.
- Determine need for possible antibiotic prophylaxis.

Teach Patient/Family to:

- Encourage effective oral hygiene to prevent soft tissue inflammation.
- Prevent injury when using oral hygiene aids.
- Report oral lesions, soreness, or bleeding to dentist.
- When chronic dry mouth occurs, advise patient to:
  - Avoid mouth rinses with high alcohol content because of drying effects.
  - Use daily home fluoride products to prevent caries.
  - Use sugarless gum, frequent sips of water, or saliva substitutes.

phentolamine

fen-**tole**′-ah-meen
(Regitine, Oraverse)

CATEGORY AND SCHEDULE
Pregnancy Risk Category: C

Drug Class: Antihypertensive

MECHANISM OF ACTION

Blocks α-adrenergic receptors. ***Therapeutic Effect:*** Produces relaxation of vascular smooth muscle, vasodilation and increased blood flow, systemically reducing B/P and locally increasing the rate of vascular uptake of dental local anesthetics containing a vasoconstrictor.

USES

Treatment of hypertension, diagnosis of pheochromocytoma, control of acute hypertension, prevention and treatment of dermal necrosis following extravasation of norepinephrine or dopamine (unapproved with papaverine for intracavernous injection for impotence) (Regitine); reversal of dental local anesthetic-related soft-tissue anesthesia and associated functional deficits (Oraverse)

PHARMACOKINETICS

Poorly absorbed from the GI tract; rapidly absorbed after parenteral administration. Protein binding 72%. Metabolized primarily in the liver; metabolites excreted in urine and feces. ***Half-life***: 2–3 hr.

INDICATIONS AND DOSAGES

▸ Extravasation of Norepinephrine
Subcutaneous
Adults, Elderly. Infiltrate area with a small amount (1 ml) of solution made by diluting 5–10 mg in 10 ml of normal saline within 12 hr of extravasation. Do not exceed 0.1–0.2 mg/kg or 5 mg total. If dose is effective, normal skin color should return to the blanched area within 1 hr.
Children. Infiltrate area with small amount (1 ml) of solution made by diluting 5–10 mg in 10 ml of normal saline within 12 hr of extravasation. Do not exceed 0.1–0.2 mg/kg or 5 mg total.

▸ Diagnosis of Pheochromocytoma
IM/IV
Adults, Elderly. 5 mg as a single dose.
Children. 0.05–0.1 mg/kg/dose, maximum single dose 5 mg.

▸ Surgery for Pheochromocytoma Hypertension
IM/IV
Adults, Elderly. 5 mg given 1–2 hr before procedure and repeated as needed every 2–4 hr.
Children. 0.05–0.1 mg/kg/dose given 1–2 hr before procedure. Repeat as needed every 2–4 hr until hypertension is controlled.
Maximum single dose: 5 mg

▸ Hypertensive Crisis
IV
Adults, Elderly. 5–20 mg as a single dose.

▸ Reversal of Soft-Tissue Anesthesia Related to Dental Local Anesthetics
0.2 to 0.8 mg (0.25–2 1.7-ml dental cartridges), using the same location(s) and technique(s) employed for the administration of the vasoconstrictor-containing local anesthetic (infiltration or block technique).

SIDE EFFECTS/ADVERSE REACTIONS

Occasional
Hypotension, tachycardia, bradycardia, flushing, orthostatic

hypotension, weakness, dizziness, nausea, vomiting, diarrhea, nasal congestion, pulmonary hypertension, injection site pain

Rare

Acute, prolonged hypotension, cardiac dysrhythmias

Contraindications

Hypersensitivity

PRECAUTIONS AND CONTRAINDICATIONS

Myocardial infarction, cerebrovascular spasm and cerebrovascular occlusion have been reported following parenteral administration of phentolamine, in association with hypotension producing shock-like states. Contraindicated in patients with hypersensitivity to phentolamine.

DRUG INTERACTIONS OF CONCERN TO DENTISTRY

- None reported

SERIOUS REACTIONS

! Symptoms of overdosage include tachycardia, shock, vomiting, and dizziness.

! Mixed-acting (e.g., epinephrine) agents may result in greater hypotension.

DENTAL CONSIDERATIONS

General:

- When used for reversal of soft-tissue anesthesia associated with dental local anesthetic, use to reverse soft-tissue effects of vasoconstrictor-containing local anesthetics and explain use and effects of drug to patient.
- This is an acute-use drug for hypertension and pheochromocytoma, which are the principal immediate, systemic concerns.
- Assess vital signs at each appointment because of nature of disease.
- Patients with untreated pheochromocytoma or with extreme, uncontrolled hypertension are not candidates for elective dental treatment.
- Stress from dental procedures may compromise cardiovascular function; determine patient risk.
- Short appointments and stress-reduction protocol may be required for anxious patients.
- Use vasoconstrictors with caution, in low doses and with careful aspiration.

Consultations:

- Consult with physician to determine disease control and ability to tolerate dental procedures.

Teach Patient/Family to:

- Update medical history based on most recent medical evaluation.

phenylephrine hydrochloride

fen-ill-**eh′**-frin high-droh-**klor′**-ide (AD-Nephrin, AK-Dilate, Isopto Frin[AUS], Mydfrin, Neo-Synephrine, Neo-Synephrine Ophthalmic Viscous 10%[AUS], Prefrin)

CATEGORY AND SCHEDULE

Pregnancy Risk Category: C
OTC (nasal solution, nasal spray, ophthalmic solution)

Drug Class: Nasal decongestant, sympathomimetic

MECHANISM OF ACTION

A sympathomimetic, α receptor stimulant that acts on the α-adrenergic receptors of vascular smooth muscle. Causes vasoconstriction of arterioles of nasal mucosa or conjunctiva, activates dilator muscle of the pupil to cause contraction, produces systemic arterial vasoconstriction. ***Therapeutic Effect:*** Decreases mucosal blood flow and relieves congestion and increases systolic B/P.

USES

Treatment of nasal congestion (temporary relief)

PHARMACOKINETICS

Route	Onset	Peak	Duration
IV	Immediate	N/A	15–20 min
IM	10–15 min	N/A	0.5–2 hr
Subcutaneous	10–15 min	N/A	1 hr

Minimal absorption after intranasal and ophthalmic administration. Metabolized in the liver and GI tract. Primarily excreted in urine. ***Half-life:*** 2.5 hr.

INDICATIONS AND DOSAGES

▸ Nasal Decongestant

Nasal Spray, Nasal Solution

Adults, Elderly, Children 12 yr and older. 2–3 drops or 1–2 sprays of 0.25%–0.5% solution into each nostril.

Children 6–11 yr. 2–3 drops or 1–2 sprays of 0.25% solution into each nostril.

Children younger than 6 yr. 2–3 drops of 0.125% solution (dilute 0.5% solution with 0.9% NaCl to achieve 0.125%) in each nostril. Repeat q4h as needed. Do not use for more than 3 days.

▸ Conjunctival Congestion, Itching, and Minor Irritation; Whitening of Sclera

Ophthalmic

Adults, Elderly, Children 12 yr and older. 1–2 drops of 0.12% solution q3–4h.

▸ Hypotension, Shock

IM, Subcutaneous

Adults, Elderly. 2–5 mg/dose q1–2h.

Children. 0.1 mg/kg/dose q1–2h.

IV Bolus

Adults, Elderly. 0.1–0.5 mg/dose q10–15min as needed.

Children. 5–20 mcg/kg/dose q10–15min.

IV Infusion

Adults, Elderly. 100–180 mcg/min.

Children. 0.1–0.5 mcg/kg/min.

Titrate to desired effect.

SIDE EFFECTS/ADVERSE REACTIONS

Frequent

Nasal: Rebound nasal congestion caused by overuse, especially when used longer than 3 days

Occasional

Mild CNS stimulation (restlessness, nervousness, tremors, headache, insomnia, particularly in those hypersensitive to sympathomimetics, such as elderly patients)

Nasal: Stinging, burning, drying of nasal mucosa

Ophthalmic: Transient burning or stinging, brow ache, blurred vision

PRECAUTIONS AND CONTRAINDICATIONS

Acute pancreatitis, heart disease, hepatitis, narrow-angle glaucoma, pheochromocytoma, severe hypertension, thrombosis, ventricular tachycardia

Caution:

Children younger than 6 yr, elderly, diabetes, cardiovascular disease, hypertension, hyperthyroidism, increased intraocular pressure, prostatic hypertrophy, glaucoma, ischemic heart disease, excessive use

DRUG INTERACTIONS OF CONCERN TO DENTISTRY

• None reported with normal topical use

SERIOUS REACTIONS

! Large doses may produce tachycardia and palpitations (particularly in those with cardiac disease), light-headedness, nausea, and vomiting.
! Overdose in those older than 60 yr may result in hallucinations, CNS depression, and seizures.
! Prolonged nasal use may produce chronic swelling of nasal mucosa and rhinitis.

DENTAL CONSIDERATIONS

General:

• Consider semisupine chair position for patient comfort because of respiratory effects of disease.
• Assess salivary flow as a factor in caries, periodontal disease, and candidiasis.
• Patients with significant nasal congestion may complicate nasal administration of nitrous oxide/oxygen sedation.

Teach Patient/Family:

• That this product is not indicated for prolonged use because of congestion rebound.

phenylephrine hydrochloride; sulfacetamide sodium

fen-ill-**eh′**-frin high-droh-**klor′**-ide; sul-fa-**see′**-ta-mide **soe′**-dee-um
(Vasosulf)

CATEGORY AND SCHEDULE

Pregnancy Risk Category: C

Drug Class: Antibacterial, sympathomimetic, ophthalmic

MECHANISM OF ACTION

Phenylephrine is a sympathomimetic that acts on α-adrenergic receptors of vascular smooth muscle. Sulfacetamide is a sulfonamide that interferes with synthesis of folic acid that bacteria require for growth.
Therapeutic Effect: Increases systolic/diastolic B/P, produces constriction of blood vessels, conjunctival arterioles, nasal arterioles. Prevents bacterial growth.

USES

Treatment of generalized tonic-clonic (grand mal) seizures, status epilepticus, nonepileptic seizures, trigeminal neuralgia, cardiac dysrhythmias (class Ib) caused by digitalis-type drugs

PHARMACOKINETICS

Minimal absorption following ophthalmic administration.

INDICATIONS AND DOSAGES

▸ **Topical Application to Conjunctiva That Relieves Congestion, Itching, Minor Irritation; Whitens Sclera of Eye**

Ophthalmic

Adults, Elderly, Children 12 yr and older. Instill 1–2 drops q3–4h.

SIDE EFFECTS/ADVERSE REACTIONS

Occasional

Transient burning/stinging, brow ache, blurred vision

PRECAUTIONS AND CONTRAINDICATIONS

Angle-closure glaucoma, those with soft contact lenses, hypersensitivity to phenylephrine, sulfacetamide, or any component of the formulation

DRUG INTERACTIONS OF CONCERN TO DENTISTRY

- None reported with normal topical use

SERIOUS REACTIONS

! None reported

DENTAL CONSIDERATIONS

General:

- Consider semisupine chair position for patient comfort because of respiratory effects of disease.
- Assess salivary flow as a factor in caries, periodontal disease, and candidiasis.
- Patients with significant nasal congestion may complicate nasal administration of nitrous oxide/oxygen sedation.

Teach Patient/Family:

- That this product is not indicated for prolonged use because of congestion rebound.

phenytoin

fen′-ih-toyn

(Dilantin)

CATEGORY AND SCHEDULE

Pregnancy Risk Category: D

Drug Class: Anticonvulsant, hydantoin; antiarrhythmic agent, class Ib

MECHANISM OF ACTION

Phenytoin is an anticonvulsant drug that can stabilize neuronal membranes and decreases seizure activity by increasing efflux or decreasing influx of sodium ions across cell membranes from neurons of the motor cortex.

Acts as an antiarrhythmic by suppressing abnormal ventricular automaticity of cardiac tissue and shortening refractory period and QT interval.

USES

Status epilepticus, other seizure disorders

Prevention and treatment of seizures following head trauma/neurosurgery

Cardiac dysrhythmias

PHARMACOKINETICS

Slowly absorbed after oral administration. Highly protein bound: neonates greater or equal to 80%, infants greater or equal to 85%, and adults between 90% and 95%. ***Half-life:*** 7–42 hr. Renal excretion (<5% as unchanged drug) and its metabolites occur partly with glomerular filtration but more importantly by tubular secretion.

INDICATIONS AND DOSAGES

IV

Adults, Elderly. Status epilepticus: Loading dose: 10–15 mg/kg; Maintenance dose: 300 mg/day or 4–6 mg/kg/day in 2–3 divided doses. Cardiac dysrhythmia: 1.25 mg/kg every 5 min as needed. May repeat to a max dose of 15 mg/kg.

IM

Seizure, during and following neurosurgery; treatment and prophylaxis: 100–200 mg IM every 4 hr during surgery and continued during the postoperative period.

PO

Adults, Elderly. Seizure control: Loading dose: 15–20 mg/kg in 3 divided doses 2–4 hr apart. Maintenance dose: 300 mg/day or 4–6 mg/kg/day in 2–3 divided doses.

▸ Status Epilepticus

IV

Children 10–16 yr. 6–7 mg/kg/day.
Children 7–9 yr. 7–8 mg/kg/day.
Children 4–6 yr. 7.5–9 mg/kg/day.
Children 6 mo–3 yr. 8–10 mg/kg/day.
Neonates. Loading dose: 15–20 mg/kg; Maintenance dose: 5–8 mg/kg/day.

PO

Seizure control: Loading dose: 15–20 mg/kg in 3 divided doses 2–4 hr apart. Maintenance dose: 300 mg/day or 4–6 mg/kg/day in 2–3 divided doses.

Dosage adjustments

Dosage adjustments may be required in the elderly: Initially, 3 mg/kg/day, in divided doses, the dosage being adjusted according to serum hydantoin concentrations and patient response.

Obese patients: the IV loading dose should be calculated on the basis of ideal body weight plus 1.33 times the excess weight over ideal weight, because phenytoin preferentially distributes into fat.

Pregnancy: phenytoin requirements are greater during pregnancy, requiring increases in doses in some patients. After delivery, the dose should be decreased to avoid toxicity.

Liver disease: there may be an increase in unbound phenytoin concentrations in patients with hepatic insufficiency, recommended to measuring unbound phenytoin concentrations level.

Renal impairment: there may be an increase in unbound phenytoin concentrations in patients with renal impairment, recommended to measuring unbound phenytoin concentrations level.

SIDE EFFECTS/ADVERSE REACTIONS

▸ Dose-Related

Frequent

Headache, blurred vision, sleepy, nausea and vomiting, constipation

Occasional

Confusion, rash, feeling nervous, hypokalemia

Frequent

Headache, blurred vision, sleepy, nausea and vomiting, constipation

Occasional

Confusion, rash, feeling nervous, hypokalemia

PRECAUTIONS AND CONTRAINDICATIONS

Contraindications

Hypersensitivity to phenytoin, fosphenytoin, or hydantoins

Sinus bradycardia, SA block, second and third-degree AV block and Adams-Stokes syndrome (intravenous phenytoin only)

Seizures Caused by Hypoglycemia
Use caution in patients with respiratory depression, CHF, MI, or damaged myocardium (IV route only).
Use with caution in patients with preexisting diseases such as liver impairment, diabetes mellitus (hyperglycemia has occurred in diabetics), history of renal disease, and alcohol use (acute use: increases levels; chronic use: decrease levels); hypotension.
Do not abruptly withdraw this medicine because of precipitate status epilepticus.
It is important to discontinue if skin rash occurs (do not resume if rash is exfoliative, purpuric, or bullous, or if lupus erythematosus or Stevens-Johnson syndrome is suspected).

DRUG INTERACTIONS OF CONCERN TO DENTISTRY

- Alcohol, other CNS depressants: May increase CNS depression.
- Fluconazole, ketoconazole, miconazole: May increase phenytoin blood concentration.
- Glucocorticoids: Phenytoin may decrease the effects of glucocorticoids.
- Lidocaine, propranolol: Phenytoin may increase cardiac depressant effects.

SERIOUS REACTIONS

! Increased risk of suicidal behavior has been observed.
! Phenytoin should be discontinued if a skin rash appears.
! Hyperglycemia, resulting from the drug's inhibitory effects on insulin release, has been reported.
! Osteomalacia has been associated with phenytoin therapy and is considered to be due to phenytoin's interference with vitamin D metabolism.

DENTAL CONSIDERATIONS

General:

- Gingival enlargement is a common problem observed primarily during the first 6 months of phenytoin therapy, appearing with gingivitis.
- To minimize severity and growth rate of gingival tissue, begin a program of professional cleaning and patient plaque control within 10 days of starting anticonvulsant therapy.
- Consider semisupine chair position for patient comfort because of GI side effects.
- Monitor vital signs every appointment because of cardiovascular side effects.
- Avoid or limit dose of vasoconstrictor in patients with dysrhythmias.
- Avoid any agents that contain alcohol (propylene glycol and ethanol) due to increased risk of hypotension, bradycardia, and arrhythmias.

Consultations:

- Medical consultation may be required to assess disease control and patient's ability to tolerate stress.

Teach Patient/Family to:

- Update health and drug history, reporting changes in health status, drug regimen changes.
- Avoid mouth rinses with high alcohol content because of drying effects.
- When chronic dry mouth occurs advise patient to:
  - Suggest xylitol gum/products to stimulate saliva and for anticaries effect.

physostigmine

fih-zoe-**stig**′-meen
(Antilirium)
Do not confuse physostigmine with Prostigmin or pyridostigmine.

CATEGORY AND SCHEDULE

Pregnancy Risk Category: C

Drug Class:
Parasympathomimetic (cholinergic)

MECHANISM OF ACTION

A cholinergic that inhibits destruction of acetylcholine by enzyme acetylcholinesterase, thus enhancing impulse transmission across the myoneural junction.
Therapeutic Effect: Improves skeletal muscle tone, stimulates salivary and sweat gland secretions.

USES

Antidote for reversal of toxic CNS effects due to anticholinergic drugs, tricyclic antidepressants

INDICATIONS AND DOSAGES

▸ To Reverse CNS Effects of Anticholinergic Drugs and Tricyclic Antidepressants

IV, IM
Adults, Elderly. Initially, 0.5–2 mg. If no response, repeat q20min until response or adverse cholinergic effects occur. If initial response occurs, may give additional doses of 1–4 mg q30–60 min as life-threatening signs, such as arrhythmias, seizures, and deep coma, recur.
Children. 0.01–0.03 mg/kg. May give additional doses q5–10 min until response or adverse cholinergic effects occur or total dose of 2 mg given.

SIDE EFFECTS/ADVERSE REACTIONS

Expected
Miosis, increased GI and skeletal muscle tone, bradycardia, sweating, excessive salivation
Occasional
Marked drop in B/P (hypertensive patients)
Rare
Allergic reaction

PRECAUTIONS AND CONTRAINDICATIONS

Active uveal inflammation, angle-closure glaucoma before iridectomy, asthma, cardiovascular disease, concurrent use of ganglionic-blocking agents, diabetes, gangrene, glaucoma associated with iridocyclitis, hypersensitivity to cholinesterase inhibitors or their components, mechanical obstruction of intestinal or urogenital tract, vagotonic state

DRUG INTERACTIONS OF CONCERN TO DENTISTRY

- Contraindicated: succinylcholine

SERIOUS REACTIONS

! Parenteral overdose produces a cholinergic crisis manifested as abdominal discomfort or cramps, nausea, vomiting, diarrhea, flushing, facial warmth, excessive salivation, diaphoresis, urinary urgency, and blurred vision. If overdose occurs, stop all anticholinergic drugs and immediately administer 0.6–1.2 mg atropine sulfate IM or IV for adults, or 0.01 mg/kg for infants and children younger than 12 yr.

DENTAL CONSIDERATIONS

General:

• For acute use in hospitals and emergency rooms.

Teach Patient/Family to:

• Avoid driving at night or participating in activities requiring visual acuity in the presence of dim lighting.

phytonadione

(vitamin K_1)
fye-toe-na-**dye′**-own
(Aqua Mephyton, Mephyton)

CATEGORY AND SCHEDULE

Pregnancy Risk Category: C

Drug Class: Vitamin K_1, fat-soluble vitamin

MECHANISM OF ACTION

Needed for adequate blood clotting (factors II, VII, IX, X)

P

USES

Treatment of vitamin K malabsorption, hypoprothrombinemia, prevention of hypoprothrombinemia caused by oral anticoagulants

PHARMACOKINETICS

PO/Injection: Readily absorbed from duodenum and requires bile salts, rapid hepatic metabolism, onset of action 6–12 hr, normal PT in 12–24 hr, crosses placenta, renal and biliary excretion; because of severe side effects, restrict IV route when other administration routes are not available.

INDICATIONS AND DOSAGES

▸ **Hypoprothrombinemia Caused by Vitamin K Malabsorption**

PO/IM

Adult. 2–25 mg; may repeat or increase to 50 mg.

Child. 5–10 mg.

Infants. 2 mg.

▸ **Prevention of Hemorrhagic Disease of the Newborn**

Subcutaneous/IM

Neonate. 0.5–1 mg after birth; repeat in 6–8 hr if required.

▸ **Hypoprothrombinemia Caused by Oral Anticoagulants**

PO/Subcutaneous/IM

Adult. 2.5–10 mg; may repeat 12–48 hr after PO dose or 6–8 hr after subcutaneous/IM dose, based on PT.

SIDE EFFECTS/ADVERSE REACTIONS

Occasional

Dysgeusia, headache, cardiac irregularities (tachycardia), nausea, vomiting, hemoglobinuria, rash, urticaria, flushing, erythema, sweating, bronchospasms, dyspnea, cramplike pain

Rare

Hyperbilirubinemia

PRECAUTIONS AND CONTRAINDICATIONS

Hypersensitivity, severe hepatic disease, last few weeks of pregnancy

DRUG INTERACTIONS OF CONCERN TO DENTISTRY

• Decreased action: broad-spectrum antibiotics, salicylates (high doses)
• Antagonist to oral anticoagulants

SERIOUS REACTIONS

! Severe hypersensitivity reactions

DENTAL CONSIDERATIONS

General:

• Determine why the patient is taking this drug. Medical consultation should be made before dental treatment.

• Patients on chronic drug therapy may rarely have symptoms of blood dyscrasias, which can include infection, bleeding, and poor healing.

Consultations:

• Medical consultation to determine coagulation stability.

pilocarpine hydrochloride

pye-loe-**kar′**-peen high-droh-**klor′**-ide
(Isopto Carpin[AUS], Ocusert Pilo-20[AUS], Ocusert Pilo-40[AUS], Pilopt Eye Drops[AUS], P.V. Carpine Liquifilm Ophthalmic Solution[AUS], Salagen)

CATEGORY AND SCHEDULE

Pregnancy Risk Category: C

Drug Class: Miotic, cholinergic agonist

MECHANISM OF ACTION

A cholinergic that increases exocrine gland secretions by stimulating cholinergic receptors.
Therapeutic Effect: Improves symptoms of dry mouth in patients with salivary gland hypofunction.

USES

Treatment of primary glaucoma, early stages of wide-angle glaucoma (less useful in advanced stages), chronic open-angle glaucoma, acute narrow-angle glaucoma before emergency surgery; also used to neutralize mydriatics used during eye exam; may be used alternately with mydriatics to break adhesions between iris and lens

PHARMACOKINETICS

Route	Onset	Peak	Duration
PO	20 min	1 hr	3–5 hr

Absorption decreased if taken with a high-fat meal. Inactivation of pilocarpine thought to occur at neuronal synapses and probably in plasma. Excreted in urine. ***Half-life:*** 4–12 hr.

INDICATIONS AND DOSAGES

▸ Dry Mouth Associated with Radiation Treatment for Head and Neck Cancer

PO

Adults, Elderly. 5 mg 3 times a day. Range: 15–30 mg/day. Maximum: 2 tablets/dose.

▸ Dry Mouth Associated with Sjögren's Syndrome

PO

Adults, Elderly. 5 mg 4 times a day. Range: 20–40 mg/day.

▸ Dosage in Hepatic Impairment

Dosage decreased to 5 mg twice a day for adults and elderly with hepatic impairment.

SIDE EFFECTS/ADVERSE REACTIONS

Frequent

Diaphoresis, excessive salivation

Occasional

Headache, dizziness, urinary frequency, flushing, dyspepsia, nausea, asthenia, lacrimation, visual disturbances

Rare

Diarrhea, abdominal pain, peripheral edema, chills

PRECAUTIONS AND CONTRAINDICATIONS

Conditions in which miosis is undesirable, such as acute iritis and angle-closure glaucoma; uncontrolled asthma

Caution:

Bronchial asthma, hypertension

DRUG INTERACTIONS OF CONCERN TO DENTISTRY

• Anticholinergic drugs, which reduce salivation antagonize therapeutic action

SERIOUS REACTIONS

! Patients with diaphoresis who don't drink enough fluids may develop dehydration.

DENTAL CONSIDERATIONS

General:

• Avoid drugs with anticholinergic activity, such as antihistamines, opioids, benzodiazepines, propantheline, atropine, and scopolamine.

• Avoid dental light in patient's eyes; offer dark glasses for patient comfort.

• Monitor vital signs at every appointment because of cardiovascular and respiratory side effects.

Consultations:

• Medical consultation may be required to assess disease control.

▸ Pilocarpine HCl (Oral)

General:

• Patients receiving chemotherapy may require palliative treatment for stomatitis.

• Assess salivary flow as a factor in caries, periodontal disease, and candidiasis.

• Monitor vital signs at every appointment because of cardiovascular side effects.

• Place on frequent recall because of oral effects of head and neck radiation.

Consultations:

• Medical consultation may be required to assess disease control.

• Medical consultation may be necessary before prescribing for patients with cardiovascular, retinal, or respiratory disease.

Teach Patient/Family to:

• Use caution when driving at night or performing hazardous activities in reduced lighting (visual blurring).

• Take plenty of fluids, observe for dehydration, or discontinue drug.

pimecrolimus

pim-eh-crow-**lee**′-mus
(Elidel)

CATEGORY AND SCHEDULE

Pregnancy Risk Category: C

Drug Class: Topical antiinflammatory

MECHANISM OF ACTION

An immunomodulator that inhibits release of cytokine, an enzyme that produces an inflammatory reaction. ***Therapeutic Effect:*** Produces antiinflammatory activity.

USES

Short-term and intermittent long-term treatment of mild to moderate atopic dermatitis in non-immunocompromised patients age 2 yr and older in whom conventional therapies cannot be used because of potential risks; in patients with an inadequate response; or in patients who are not responsive to conventional therapies

PHARMACOKINETICS
Minimal systemic absorption with topical application. Metabolized in liver. Excreted in feces.

INDICATIONS AND DOSAGES
▸ **Atopic Dermatitis (Eczema)**
Topical
Adults, Elderly, Children 2–17 yr. Apply to affected area twice daily for up to 3 wk (up to 6 wk in adolescents, children 2–17 yr). Rub in gently and completely.

SIDE EFFECTS/ADVERSE REACTIONS
Rare
Transient application-site sensation of burning or feeling of heat

PRECAUTIONS AND CONTRAINDICATIONS
Hypersensitivity to pimecrolimus or any component of the formulation, Netherton's syndrome (potential for increased systemic absorption), application to active cutaneous viral infections
Caution:
Do not use for active cutaneous viral infections, infected dermatitis, natural or artificial sunlight exposure, no data on excretion in human milk, children younger than 2 yr

DRUG INTERACTIONS OF CONCERN TO DENTISTRY
• Drug interactions have not been evaluated. Low blood levels were measured in some patients. Use drugs that inhibit CYP3A4 isoenzymes with caution in patients with widespread and erythrodermic disease.

SERIOUS REACTIONS
! Lymphadenopathy and phototoxicity occur rarely.

DENTAL CONSIDERATIONS
General:
• Determine why the patient is taking this drug.

pimozide
pim′-oh-zide
(Orap)

CATEGORY AND SCHEDULE
Pregnancy Risk Category: C

Drug Class: Antipsychotic, antidyskinetic

MECHANISM OF ACTION
A diphenylbutylpiperidine that blocks dopamine at postsynaptic receptor sites in the brain.
Therapeutic Effect: Suppresses behavioral response in psychosis.

USES
Treatment of motor and phonic tics in Gilles de la Tourette's syndrome; unapproved: psychotic disorders

PHARMACOKINETICS
PO: Onset erratic, peak 6–8 hr.
Half-life: 50–55 hr; metabolized by liver; excreted in urine, feces.

INDICATIONS AND DOSAGES
▸ **Tourette's Disorder**
PO
Adults, Elderly. 1–2 mg/day in divided doses 3 times a day. Maximum: 10 mg/day.
Children older than 12 yr. Initially, 0.5 mg/kg/day. Maximum: 10 mg/day.

SIDE EFFECTS/ADVERSE REACTIONS
Occasional
Akathisia, dystonic extrapyramidal effects, parkinsonian extrapyramidal

effects, tardive dyskinesia, blurred vision, ocular changes, constipation, decreased sweating, dry mouth, nasal congestion, dizziness, drowsiness, orthostatic hypotension, urinary retention, somnolence

Rare

Rash, cholestatic jaundice, priapism

PRECAUTIONS AND CONTRAINDICATIONS

Aggressive schizophrenics when sedation is required; concurrent administration of pemoline; methylphenidate or amphetamines; concurrent administration with dofetilide, sotalol, quinidine, other Class IA and III anti-arrhythmics, mesoridazine, thioridazine, chlorpromazine, droperidol, sparfloxacin, gatifloxacin, moxifloxacin, halofantrine, mefloquine, pentamidine, arsenic trioxide, levomethadyl acetate, dolasetron mesylate, probucol, tacrolimus, ziprasidone, sertraline, macrolide antibiotics, drugs that cause QT prolongation, and less potent inhibitors of CYP3A4; congenital or drug-induced long QT syndrome; doses greater than 10 mg daily; history of cardiac arrhythmias, Parkinson's disease; patients with known hypokalemia or hypomagnesemia; severe central nervous system depression; simple tics or tics not associated with Tourette's syndrome; hypersensitivity to pimozide or any of its components

Caution:

Children younger than 12 yr, lactation, hypertension, hepatic disease, cardiac disease, renal disease, breast cancer, hypokalemia

DRUG INTERACTIONS OF CONCERN TO DENTISTRY

- Increased CNS depression: alcohol, CNS depressants
- Increased effects of both drugs: phenothiazines
- Increased effects of anticholinergic drugs
- Prolonged QT interval, fatal cardiac arrhythmia; contraindicated: clarithromycin, erythromycin, azithromycin, dirithromycin, itraconazole

SERIOUS REACTIONS

! Serious reactions such as blood dyscrasias, agranulocytosis, leukocytopenia, thrombocytopenia, cholestatic jaundice, neuroleptic malignant syndrome (NMS), constipation or paralytic ileus, priapism, QT prolongation and torsades de pointes, seizure, systemic lupus erythematosus-like syndrome, and temperature regulation dysfunction (heatstroke or hypothermia) occur rarely.

! Abrupt withdrawal following long-term therapy may precipitate nausea, vomiting, gastritis, dizziness, and tremors.

DENTAL CONSIDERATIONS

General:

- Assess salivary flow as a factor in caries, periodontal disease, and candidiasis.
- Monitor vital signs at every appointment because of cardiovascular side effects.
- Assess for presence of extrapyramidal motor symptoms, such as tardive dyskinesia and akathisia. Extrapyramidal motor activity may complicate dental treatment.
- After supine positioning, have patient sit upright for at least 2 min

before standing to avoid orthostatic hypotension.

- Consider action of drug in assessment of dysgeusia.

Consultations:

- Medical consultation may be required to assess disease control.
- If signs of tardive dyskinesia or akathisia are present, refer to physician.

Teach Patient/Family to:

- Encourage effective oral hygiene to prevent soft tissue inflammation.
- Use caution to prevent injury when using oral hygiene aids.
- When chronic dry mouth occurs, advise patient to:
  - Avoid mouth rinses with high alcohol content because of drying effects.
  - Use daily home fluoride products to prevent caries.
  - Use sugarless gum, frequent sips of water, or saliva substitutes.

pindolol

pin′-doe-loll

(Apo-Pindol[CAN], Visken)

CATEGORY AND SCHEDULE

Pregnancy Risk Category: B (D if used in second or third trimester)

Drug Class: Nonselective β-adrenergic blocker

MECHANISM OF ACTION

A nonselective beta blocker that blocks β_1- and β_2-adrenergic receptors.

Therapeutic Effect: Slows heart rate, decreases cardiac output, decreases B/P, and exhibits antiarrhythmic activity. Decreases myocardial ischemia severity by decreasing oxygen requirements.

USES

Treatment of mild-to-moderate hypertension, mild-to-moderate heart failure

PHARMACOKINETICS

Completely absorbed from GI tract. Metabolized in liver. Primarily excreted in urine. ***Half-life:*** 3–4 hr (half-life increased with impaired renal function, elderly).

INDICATIONS AND DOSAGES

▸ Mild-to-Moderate Hypertension

PO

Adults. Initially, 5 mg 2 times a day. Gradually increase dose by 10 mg/day at 2- to 4-wk intervals. Maintenance: 10–30 mg/day in 2–3 divided doses. Maximum: 60 mg/day.

▸ Usual Elderly Dosage

PO

Initially, 5 mg/day. May increase by 5 mg q3–4wk.

P

SIDE EFFECTS/ADVERSE REACTIONS

Frequent

Decreased sexual ability, drowsiness, trouble sleeping, unusual tiredness or weakness

Occasional

Bradycardia, depression, cold hands/feet, diarrhea, constipation, anxiety, nasal congestion, nausea, vomiting

Rare

Altered taste, dry eyes, itching, numbness of fingers, toes, and scalp

PRECAUTIONS AND CONTRAINDICATIONS

Bronchial asthma, COPD, uncontrolled cardiac failure, sinus

bradycardia, heart block greater than first degree, cardiogenic shock, CHF, unless secondary to tachyarrhythmias

Caution:

Major surgery, diabetes mellitus, renal disease, thyroid disease, COPD, well-compensated heart failure, CAD, nonallergic bronchospasm, impaired hepatic function, children

DRUG INTERACTIONS OF CONCERN TO DENTISTRY

- Increased hypotension, bradycardia: anticholinergics, hydrocarbon inhalation anesthetics, fentanyl derivatives
- Decreased antihypertensive effects: indomethacin, sympathomimetics
- Increased effect of both drugs: phenothiazines, xanthines
- Decreased bronchodilation: theophyllines
- Hypertension, bradycardia: epinephrine, ephedrine
- Slow metabolism of drug: lidocaine

SERIOUS REACTIONS

! Overdosage may produce profound bradycardia and hypotension.

! Abrupt withdrawal may result in sweating, palpitations, headache, and tremulousness.

! May precipitate CHF or MI in patients with heart disease; thyroid storm in those with thyrotoxicosis; or peripheral ischemia in those with existing peripheral vascular disease.

! Hypoglycemia may occur in previously controlled diabetics.

! Signs of thrombocytopenia, such as unusual bleeding or bruising, occur rarely.

DENTAL CONSIDERATIONS

General:

- Monitor vital signs at every appointment because of cardiovascular side effects.
- Patients on chronic drug therapy may rarely have symptoms of blood dyscrasias, which can include infection, bleeding, and poor healing.
- Stress from dental procedures may compromise cardiovascular function; determine patient risk; use stress-reduction protocol.
- Use vasoconstrictors with caution, in low doses, and with careful aspiration. Avoid use of gingival retraction cord with epinephrine.
- Consider semisupine chair position for patient comfort if GI side effects occur.
- Assess salivary flow as a factor in caries, periodontal disease, and candidiasis.
- Consider drug effects if taste alteration occurs.

Consultations:

- In a patient with symptoms of blood dyscrasias, request a medical consultation for blood studies and postpone dental treatment until normal values are reestablished.
- Medical consultation may be required to assess disease control and patient's ability to tolerate stress.

Teach Patient/Family to:

- Encourage effective oral hygiene to prevent soft tissue inflammation.
- Use caution to prevent injury when using oral hygiene aids.
- When chronic dry mouth occurs, advise patient to:
    - Avoid mouth rinses with high alcohol content because of drying effects.
    - Use daily home fluoride products to prevent caries.

• Use sugarless gum, frequent sips of water, or saliva substitutes.

pioglitazone

pye-oh-**gli′**-ta-zone
(Actos)

CATEGORY AND SCHEDULE

Pregnancy Risk Category: C

Drug Class: Antidiabetic, oral

MECHANISM OF ACTION

An antidiabetic that improves target-cell response to insulin without increasing pancreatic insulin secretion. Decreases hepatic glucose output and increases insulin-dependent glucose utilization in skeletal muscle.
Therapeutic Effect: Lowers blood glucose concentration.

USES

Monotherapy, as an adjunct to diet and exercise in patients with type 2 diabetes mellitus; may also be used with metformin when metformin, diet, and exercise are not adequate for control

PHARMACOKINETICS

Rapidly absorbed. Highly protein bound (99%), primarily to albumin. Metabolized in the liver. Excreted in urine. Unknown if removed by hemodialysis. ***Half-life:*** 16–24 hr.

INDICATIONS AND DOSAGES

▸ Diabetes Mellitus, Combination Therapy

PO

Adult, Elderly. With insulin: Initially, 15–30 mg once a day. Initially continue current insulin dosage; then decrease insulin dosage by 10%–25% if hypoglycemia occurs or plasma glucose level decreases to less than 100 mg/dl. Maximum: 45 mg/day. With sulfonylureas: Initially, 15–30 mg/day. Decrease sulfonylurea dosage if hypoglycemia occurs. With metformin: Initially, 15–30 mg/day. As monotherapy: Monotherapy is not to be used if patient is well controlled with diet and exercise alone. Initially, 15–30 mg/day. May increase dosage in increments until 45 mg/day is reached.

SIDE EFFECTS/ADVERSE REACTIONS

Frequent

Headache, upper respiratory tract infection

Occasional

Sinusitis, myalgia, pharyngitis, aggravated diabetes mellitus

PRECAUTIONS AND CONTRAINDICATIONS

Active hepatic disease; diabetic ketoacidosis; increased serum transaminase levels, including ALT (SGPT) greater than 2.5 times normal serum level

Caution:

Hepatic dysfunction (reduce dose), renal impairment, lactation, children younger than 18 yr

DRUG INTERACTIONS OF CONCERN TO DENTISTRY

• None reported

SERIOUS REACTIONS

! None known

DENTAL CONSIDERATIONS

General:

• Ensure that patient is following prescribed diet and regularly takes medication.

• Place on frequent recall to evaluate healing response.
• Short appointments and a stress-reduction protocol may be required for anxious patients.
• Diabetics may be more susceptible to infection and have delayed wound healing.
• Question patient about self-monitoring of drug's antidiabetic effect, including blood glucose values or finger-stick records.
• Consider semisupine chair position for patient comfort if GI side effects occur.

Consultations:

• Medical consultation may be required to assess disease control and patient's ability to tolerate stress.
• Medical consultation may include data from patient's blood glucose monitoring, including glycosylated hemoglobin or HbA_{1c} testing.

Teach Patient/Family to:

• Prevent trauma when using oral hygiene aids.
• Update health and drug history if physician makes any changes in evaluation or drug regimens; include OTC, herbal, and nonherbal drugs in the update.
• Encourage effective oral hygiene to prevent soft tissue inflammation.

P

pirbuterol

peer-**beut′**-er-all
(Maxair, Maxair Autohaler)

CATEGORY AND SCHEDULE

Pregnancy Risk Category: C

Drug Class: Bronchodilator

MECHANISM OF ACTION

A sympathomimetic, adrenergic agonist, that stimulates β_2-adrenergic receptors in the lungs, resulting in relaxation of bronchial smooth muscle.

Therapeutic Effect: Relieves bronchospasm, reduces airway resistance.

USES

Treatment of reversible bronchospasm (prevention, treatment), including asthma; may be given with theophylline or steroids

PHARMACOKINETICS

Absorbed from bronchi following inhalation. Metabolized in liver. Primarily excreted in urine. Unknown if removed by hemodialysis. ***Half-life:*** 2–3 hr.

INDICATIONS AND DOSAGES

▸ **Prevention of Bronchospasm**

Inhalation

Adults, Elderly, Children 12 yr and older. 2 inhalations q4–6h. Maximum: 12 inhalations daily.

▸ **Treatment of Bronchospasm**

Inhalation

Adults, Elderly, Children 12 yr and older. 2 inhalations separated by at least 1–3 min, followed by a third inhalation. Maximum: 12 inhalations daily.

SIDE EFFECTS/ADVERSE REACTIONS

Occasional

Nervousness, tremor, headache, palpitations, nausea, dizziness, tachycardia, cough

PRECAUTIONS AND CONTRAINDICATIONS

History of hypersensitivity to pirbuterol, albuterol, or any of its components

Caution:
Lactation, cardiac disorders, hyperthyroidism, diabetes mellitus, prostatic hypertrophy

DRUG INTERACTIONS OF CONCERN TO DENTISTRY

- None reported

SERIOUS REACTIONS

! Excessive sympathomimetic stimulation may produce palpitations, extrasystoles, tachycardia, chest pain, slight increases in B/P followed by a substantial decrease, chills, sweating and blanching of skin.
! Too-frequent or excessive use may lead to loss of bronchodilating effectiveness and severe, paradoxical bronchoconstriction.

DENTAL CONSIDERATIONS

General:

- Acute asthmatic episodes may be precipitated in the dental office. Sympathomimetic inhalants should be available for emergency use.
- Be aware that aspirin or sulfite preservatives in vasoconstrictor-containing products can exacerbate asthma.
- Monitor vital signs at every appointment because of cardiovascular and respiratory side effects.
- Assess salivary flow as a factor in caries, periodontal disease, and candidiasis.
- Consider semisupine chair position for patients with respiratory disease.
- Short appointments and a stress-reduction protocol may be required for anxious patients.

Consultations:

- Medical consultation may be required to assess disease control and patient's ability to tolerate stress.

Teach Patient/Family to:

- Rinse mouth with water after each dose to prevent dryness (for inhalation dosage forms).
- When chronic dry mouth occurs, advise patient to:
  - Avoid mouth rinses with high alcohol content because of drying effects.
  - Use daily home fluoride products to prevent caries.
  - Use sugarless gum, frequent sips of water, or saliva substitutes.

piroxicam

peer-**ox**′-ih-kam
(Apo-Piroxicam[CAN], Candyl-D[AUS], Feldene, Fexicam[CAN], Mobilis[AUS], Novo-Pirocam[CAN], Pyrahexyl-D [AUS], Rosig[AUS], Rosig-D[AUS])
Do not confuse Feldene with Seldane.

CATEGORY AND SCHEDULE

Pregnancy Risk Category: C (D if used in third trimester or near delivery)

Drug Class: Nonsteroidal antiinflammatory

MECHANISM OF ACTION

An NSAID that produces analgesic and antiinflammatory effects by inhibiting prostaglandin synthesis.
Therapeutic Effect: Reduces inflammatory response and intensity of pain.

USES

Treatment of osteoarthritis, rheumatoid arthritis; unapproved: gouty arthritis

PHARMACOKINETICS

PO: Peak 2 hr. ***Half-life:*** 3–3.5 hr; 99% protein binding; metabolized in liver; excreted in urine (metabolites), breast milk.

INDICATIONS AND DOSAGES

▸ Acute or Chronic Rheumatoid Arthritis and Osteoarthritis

PO

Adults, Elderly. Initially, 10–20 mg/day as a single dose or in divided doses. Some patients may require up to 30–40 mg/day.

Children. 0.2–0.3 mg/kg/day. Maximum: 15 mg/day.

SIDE EFFECTS/ADVERSE REACTIONS

Frequent

Dyspepsia, nausea, dizziness

Occasional

Diarrhea, constipation, abdominal cramps or pain, flatulence, stomatitis

Rare

Hypertension, urticaria, dysuria, ecchymosis, blurred vision, insomnia, phototoxicity

P

PRECAUTIONS AND CONTRAINDICATIONS

Active peptic ulcer disease, chronic inflammation of the GI tract, GI bleeding or ulceration, history of hypersensitivity to aspirin or NSAIDs

Caution:

Lactation, children, bleeding disorders, GI disorders, cardiac disorders, hypersensitivity to other antiinflammatory agents, hypertension

DRUG INTERACTIONS OF CONCERN TO DENTISTRY

- GI ulceration, bleeding: aspirin, alcohol, corticosteroids
- Nephrotoxicity: acetaminophen (prolonged use and high doses)
- Possible risk of decreased renal function: cyclosporine
- Decreased action: salicylates
- SSRIs: increased risk of GI side effects
- When prescribed for dental pain:
  - Risk of increased effects of oral anticoagulants, oral antidiabetics, lithium, methotrexate
  - Decreased antihypertensive effects of diuretics, α-adrenergic blockers, ACE inhibitors

SERIOUS REACTIONS

! Rare reactions with long-term use include peptic ulcer disease, GI bleeding, gastritis, severe hepatic reaction (cholestasis, jaundice), nephrotoxicity (dysuria, hematuria, proteinuria, nephrotic syndrome), hematologic sensitivity (anemia, leukopenia, eosinophilia, thrombocytopenia), and a severe hypersensitivity reaction (fever, chills, bronchospasm).

DENTAL CONSIDERATIONS

General:

- Patients on chronic drug therapy may rarely have symptoms of blood dyscrasias, which can include infection, bleeding, and poor healing.
- Assess salivary flow as a factor in caries, periodontal disease, and candidiasis.
- Avoid prescribing during pregnancy.
- Minimize use of aspirin-containing products.
- Consider semisupine chair position for patients with arthritic disease or if GI side effects occur.

Consultations:

- In a patient with symptoms of blood dyscrasias, request a medical consultation for blood studies and

postpone dental treatment until normal values are reestablished.

• Medical consultation may be required to assess disease control.

Teach Patient/Family to:

• Encourage effective oral hygiene to prevent soft tissue inflammation.

• Use caution to prevent injury when using oral hygiene aids.

• Report oral lesions, soreness, or bleeding to dentist.

• When chronic dry mouth occurs, advise patient to:

  • Avoid mouth rinses with high alcohol content because of drying effects.
  • Use daily home fluoride products to prevent caries.
  • Use sugarless gum, frequent sips of water, or saliva substitutes.

pitavastatin

pit′-a-**vah′**-stah-tin
(Livalo)
Do not confuse with Levatol.

CATEGORY AND SCHEDULE

Pregnancy Risk Category: X

Drug Class: Antihyperlipidemics, HMG-CoA reductase inhibitors

MECHANISM OF ACTION

An antihyperlipidemic that inhibits HMG-CoA reductase, the enzyme that catalyzes the early step in cholesterol synthesis.

Therapeutic Effect: Increases the amount of LDL receptors on hepatocyte membranes thereby decreasing LDL and VLDL cholesterol as well as plasma triglyceride levels; also increases HDL cholesterol.

USES

Hypercholesterolemia
Mixed dyslipidemia

PHARMACOKINETICS

Rapidly and well absorbed after PO administration. Bioavailability: 51%. Protein binding: >99%. Distributed primarily to the liver. Major metabolite is a lactone, formed by glucuronidation. Metabolized in the liver, via UGT1A3 and UGT2B7; mildly by CYP2C9 and 2C8. Primarily excreted in feces; minimally in urine. ***Half-life:*** 9–12 hr.

INDICATIONS AND DOSAGES

▸ Hypercholesterolemia, Mixed Dyslipidemia

PO

Adults. Initially, 2 mg a day. May increase after 4 wk. Range: 1–4 mg/day. Maximum: 4 mg/day.
Concomitant use with erythromycin: Maximum: 1 mg/day.
Concomitant use with rifampin: Maximum: 2 mg/day.

▸ Dosage in Renal Impairment

Mild to moderate impairment (CrCl 30 to less than 60 ml/min or ESRD on hemodialysis). 1 mg a day (Maximum: 2 mg/day).
Moderate to severe impairment (CrCl less than 30 ml/min and not on hemodialysis). Not recommended.

SIDE EFFECTS/ADVERSE REACTIONS

Pitavastatin is generally well tolerated. Side effects are usually mild and transient.

Occasional

Constipation, diarrhea, back pain, myalgia, arthralgia, pain in extremities, headache, rash or pruritus, allergy, influenza, nasopharyngitis, headache, increased

CPK, increased alkaline phosphatase and bilirubin
Rare
Rhabdomyolysis

PRECAUTIONS AND CONTRAINDICATIONS

Hypersensitivity to pitavastatin or its components
Active liver disease
Lactation
Pregnancy
Unexplained elevated hepatic function test results
Concomitant use with cyclosporine or lopinavir/ritonavir
Severe renal impairment (CrCl <30 ml/min without dialysis)
Cholestasis or jaundice
Hepatitis
Hepatic encephalopathy
Caution:
Mild to moderate renal impairment
Alcohol consumption
Seizure disorder
Major surgery or trauma

DRUG INTERACTIONS OF CONCERN TO DENTISTRY

- Cyclosporine, lopinavir/ritonavir: May potentiate the effects of pitavastatin
- CYP450 inducers: May decrease pitavastatin levels
- CYP450 inhibitors: May increase pitavastatin levels (e.g., macrolide antibiotics)
- Fibric acids, niacin: May cause additive effects; increase risk of myopathy

SERIOUS REACTIONS

! Cases of rhabdomyolysis have been reported with pitavastatin.
! Discontinue pitavastatin if myopathy or elevated CK levels occur.
! Elevated liver transaminases have been reported. Liver function should be assessed before therapy, at 4 wk after starting or when increasing dose, then periodically. Reduce dose if serum transaminases are 3 times ULN.

DENTAL CONSIDERATIONS

General:
- Consider semisupine chair position for patient comfort if GI side effects occur.

Consultations:
- Medical consultation may be required to assess disease control.

Teach Patient/Family to:
- Encourage effective oral hygiene to prevent soft tissue inflammation.
- Prevent trauma when using oral hygiene aids.
- Be alert for the possibility of secondary oral infection and the need to see dentist immediately if signs of infection occur.

podofilox

poe-**dof′**-il-lox
(Condyline[CAN], Condyline Paint[AUS], Condylox)

CATEGORY AND SCHEDULE

Pregnancy Risk Category: C

Drug Class: Antimitotic agent

MECHANISM OF ACTION

An active component of podophyllin resin that binds to tubulin to prevent formation of microtubules resulting in mitotic arrest. Exercises many biological effects, such as damages endothelium of small blood vessels, attenuates nucleoside transport, suppresses immune responses, inhibits macrophage metabolism, induces interleukin-1 and interleukin-2, decreases lymphocytes' response to mitogens, and enhances macrophage growth. ***Therapeutic Effect:*** Removes genital warts.

USES

Removal of certain types of warts on the outside skin of the genital areas (penis or vulva)

PHARMACOKINETICS

Time to peak occurs in 1–2 hr. Some degree of absorption. ***Half-life:*** 1–4.5 hr.

INDICATIONS AND DOSAGES

▸ **Anogenital Warts**

Topical

Adults. Apply 0.5% gel for 3 days, then withhold for 4 days. Repeat cycle up to 4 times.

▸ **Genital Warts (Condylomata Acuminate)**

Topical

Adults. Apply 0.5% solution or gel q12h in the morning and evening for 3 days, then withhold for 4 days. Repeat cycle up to 4 times.

SIDE EFFECTS/ADVERSE REACTIONS

Occasional

Erosion, inflammation, itching, pain, burning

Rare

Nausea, vomiting

PRECAUTIONS AND CONTRAINDICATIONS

Bleeding warts, moles, birthmarks or unusual warts with hair, diabetes, poor blood circulation, pregnancy, steroid use, hypersensitivity to podofilox or any component of its formulation

DRUG INTERACTIONS OF CONCERN TO DENTISTRY

- None reported

SERIOUS REACTIONS

! Nausea and vomiting occur rarely and usually after cumulative doses.

DENTAL CONSIDERATIONS

General:

- Determine why patient is taking the drug.
- Examine oral mucous membranes for lesions; overuse may be associated with oral ulcers.
- Tactful questions related to STD may be appropriate.
- Explore medical and drug history.
- Not for use on mucous membranes.

Consultations:

- Medical consultation may be required to assess disease control.

Teach Patient/Family to:

- Encourage effective oral hygiene to prevent soft tissue inflammation.
- Prevent trauma when using oral hygiene aids.
- Update health and medication history if physician makes any changes in evaluation or drug regimens; include OTC, herbal, and nonherbal drugs in the update.

P

podophyllum resin

po-**dof**′-fil-um rez-in

(Podocon-25, Pododerm)

CATEGORY AND SCHEDULE

Pregnancy Risk Category: X

Drug Class: Cytotoxic, topical

MECHANISM OF ACTION

A cytotoxic agent that directly affects epithelial cell metabolism by arresting mitosis through binding to a protein subunit of spindle microtubules.

Therapeutic Effect: Removes soft genital warts.

USES
Removal of benign growths

PHARMACOKINETICS
Topical podophyllum is systemically absorbed. Absorption may be increased if applied to bleeding, friable, or recently biopsied warts.

INDICATIONS AND DOSAGES
▸ **Genital Warts (Condylomata Acuminate)**

Topical

Adults, Elderly, Children. Apply 10%–25% solution in compound benzoin tincture to dry surface. Use 1 drop at a time allowing drying between drops until area is covered. Total volume should be limited to less than 0.5 ml per treatment session.

SIDE EFFECTS/ADVERSE REACTIONS
Occasional

Pruritus, nausea, vomiting, abdominal pain, diarrhea

PRECAUTIONS AND CONTRAINDICATIONS
Diabetes mellitus, concomitant steroid therapy, circulation disorders, bleeding warts, moles, birthmarks or unusual warts with hair growing from them, pregnancy, hypersensitivity to podophyllum resin preparations

DRUG INTERACTIONS OF CONCERN TO DENTISTRY
- None reported

SERIOUS REACTIONS
! Paresthesia, polyneuritis, paralytic ileus, pyrexia, leukopenia, thrombocytopenia, coma, and death have been reported with podophyllum resin use.

DENTAL CONSIDERATIONS
General:
- Determine why patient is taking the drug.
- This medication is applied in physician's office.
- Questions related to sexually transmitted diseases may be appropriate.

Consultations:
- Medical consultation may be required to assess disease control.

Teach Patient/Family to:
- Encourage effective oral hygiene to prevent soft tissue inflammation.
- Prevent trauma when using oral hygiene aids.
- Update health and medication history if physician makes any changes in evaluation or drug regimens; include OTC, herbal, and nonherbal drugs in the update.

polymyxin B
polly-**mix′**-in

(Aerosporin)

CATEGORY AND SCHEDULE
Pregnancy Risk Category: B

Drug Class: Antibiotics, polymyxins

MECHANISM OF ACTION
An antibiotic that alters cell membrane permeability in susceptible microorganisms.

Therapeutic Effect: Bactericidal.

USES
Treatment of superficial external infections

PHARMACOKINETICS
Negligible absorption. Protein binding: low. Excreted in urine. Poor

removal in hemodialysis. ***Half-life:*** 6 hr.

INDICATIONS AND DOSAGES

▸ Mild-to-Moderate Infections

IV

Adults, Elderly, Children 2 yr and older. 15,000–25,000 units/kg/day in divided doses q12h.

Infants. Up to 40,000 units/kg/day.

IM

Adults, Elderly, Children 2 yr and older. 25,000–30,000 units/kg/day in divided doses q4–6h.

Infants. Up to 40,000 units/kg/day.

▸ Usual Irrigation Dosage

Continuous Bladder Irrigation

Adults, Elderly. 1 ml urogenital concentrate (contains 200,000 units polymyxin B, 57 mg neomycin) added to 1000 ml 0.9% NaCl. Give each 1000 ml >24 hr for up to 10 days (may increase to 2000 ml/day when urine output is greater than 2 L/day).

▸ Usual Ophthalmic Dosage

Ophthalmic

Adults, Elderly, Children. 1 drop q3–4h.

SIDE EFFECTS/ADVERSE REACTIONS

Frequent

Severe pain, irritation at IM injection sites, phlebitis, thrombophlebitis with IV administration

Occasional

Fever, urticaria

PRECAUTIONS AND CONTRAINDICATIONS

Hypersensitivity to polymyxin B or any component of the formulation

Caution:

Hypokalemia, renal disease, hepatic disease, gout, COPD, lupus erythematosus, diabetes mellitus

SERIOUS REACTIONS

! Nephrotoxicity, especially with concurrent/sequential use of other nephrotoxic drugs, renal impairment, concurrent/sequential use of muscle relaxants.

! Superinfection, especially with fungi, may occur.

DENTAL CONSIDERATIONS

General:

- Avoid dental light in patient's eyes; offer dark glasses for patient comfort and safety during dental treatment.

polymyxin B sulfate; trimethoprim sulfate

pol-ee-**mix′**-in bee **sul′**-fate; trye-**meth′**-oh-prim **sul′**-fate

(Polytrim)

CATEGORY AND SCHEDULE

Pregnancy Risk Category: C

Drug Class: Antiinfective, ophthalmic

MECHANISM OF ACTION

Polymyxin B damages bacterial cytoplasmic membrane that causes leakage of intracellular components. Trimethoprim is a folate antagonist that blocks bacterial biosynthesis of nucleic acids and proteins by interfering with metabolism of folinic acid.

Therapeutic Effect: Prevents inflammatory process. Interferes with bacterial protein synthesis. Produces antibacterial activity.

USES

Treatment of superficial external ocular infections

PHARMACOKINETICS

Absorption through intact skin and mucous membranes is insignificant.

INDICATIONS AND DOSAGES

▸ Treatment of Surface Ocular Bacterial Conjunctivitis and Blepharoconjunctivitis

Ophthalmic

Adults, Elderly, Children. Instill 1–2 drops in eye(s) every 3 hr for 7–10 days. Maximum: 6 doses/day.

SIDE EFFECTS/ADVERSE REACTIONS

Occasional

Local irritation, redness, burning, stinging, itching

PRECAUTIONS AND CONTRAINDICATIONS

Hypersensitivity to polymyxin B, trimethoprim sulfate, or any component of the formulation

DRUG INTERACTIONS OF CONCERN TO DENTISTRY

P

• None reported

SERIOUS REACTIONS

! Prolonged use may result in overgrowth of nonsusceptible organisms, including superinfection.

! Hypersensitivity reactions consisting of lid edema, itching, increased redness, tearing, and/or circumocular rash have been reported.

! Photosensitivity has been reported in patients taking oral trimethoprim.

DENTAL CONSIDERATIONS

General:

• Avoid dental light in patient's eyes; offer dark glasses for patient comfort and safety during dental treatment.

posaconazole

poe-sah-**kone′**-ah-zole

(Noxafil)

CATEGORY AND SCHEDULE

Pregnancy Risk Category: C

Drug Class: Antifungal

MECHANISM OF ACTION

A triazole antifungal that blocks the synthesis of ergosterol, a key component of fungal cell membrane, through the inhibition of the enzyme lanosterol 14a-α-demethylase and accumulation of methylated sterol precursors.

Therapeutic Effect: Inhibits fungal cell membrane formation.

USES

Prophylaxis of invasive *Aspergillus* and *Candida* infections in patients who are severely immunocompromised

PHARMACOKINETICS

Food increases absorption. Protein binding: greater than 98%. Not significantly metabolized; undergoes glucuronidation into metabolites. Primarily eliminated in feces (71%, 66% unchanged); partial excretion in urine (13%, less than 0.2% unchanged). ***Half-life:*** 35 hr.

INDICATIONS AND DOSAGES

▸ Prophylaxis of Invasive Fungal Infections

PO

Adults, Children 13 yr and older. 200 mg (5 ml) three times a day.

▸ Oropharyngeal Candidiasis

PO

Adults, Children 13 yr and older. Initially, 100 mg (2.5 ml) twice a day on the first day. Maintenance:

100 mg (2.5 ml) once a day for 13 days.

▸ **Oropharyngeal Candidiasis, Refractory to Itraconazole and/or Fluconazole**

PO

Adults, Children 13 yr and older: 400 mg (10 ml) twice a day.

SIDE EFFECTS/ADVERSE REACTIONS

Adult

Frequent

Diarrhea

Occasional

Nausea, neutropenia, headache, vomiting, abdominal pain, flatulence, QTc prolongation, rash, hypokalemia, anemia, fever, bilirubin increased, ALT increased, AST increased, GGT increased, dizziness, weakness, anorexia, fatigue, insomnia, mucositis, thrombocytopenia, alkaline phosphatase increased, serum creatinine increased, myalgia, pruritus, dyspepsia, xerostomia

Rare

Hypertension, blurred vision, tremor, hepatocellular damage, taste perversion, constipation, somnolence

PRECAUTIONS AND CONTRAINDICATIONS

Hypersensitivity to azole antifungals, posaconazole or its components; avoid coadministration with ergot alkaloids

Caution:

Do not breast-feed, hepatic impairment, patients with an increased risk of arrhythmia, electrolyte abnormalities

DRUG INTERACTIONS OF CONCERN TO DENTISTRY

- Calcium channel blockers: may increase the levels and effects of calcium channel blockers
- Cimetidine: may decrease the levels and effects of posaconazole; avoid concurrent use
- Cyclosporine: may increase the levels and effects of cyclosporine
- CYP3A4 substrates: may increase the levels and effects of CYP3A4 substrates (e.g., midazolam, triazolam)
- Ergot alkaloids: may increase the levels and effects of ergot alkaloids
- HMG-CoA reductase inhibitors: may increase the levels and effects of HMG-CoA reductase inhibitors
- Phenytoin: may increase the levels and effects of phenytoin; avoid concurrent use
- QT-prolonging agents: increased risk of arrhythmia (torsades de pointes)
- Rifabutin: may increase the levels and effects of rifabutin; avoid concurrent use
- Sirolimus: may increase the levels and effects of sirolimus
- Tacrolimus: may increase the levels and effects of tacrolimus
- Vinca alkaloids: may increase the levels and effects of vinca alkaloids

SERIOUS REACTIONS

! Hepatic dysfunction may occur.

! Arrhythmia (torsades de pointes) has been reported.

DENTAL CONSIDERATIONS

General:

- Monitor vital signs at every appointment due to possible adverse cardiovascular effects.
- Determine why patient is taking the drug.
- Consider semisupine chair position for patient comfort due to adverse GI effects of drug.
- To prevent reinoculation of candidal infection, dispose of tooth brush and other contaminated oral

hygiene devices used during period of infection.

• Assess salivary flow as a factor in caries, periodontal disease, and candidiasis.

• Disinfect or remake removable prostheses that may harbor residual candidal organisms.

• Consider drug effect in evaluating taste changes versus restorative materials.

Consultations:

• Medical consult may be necessary to determine patient's ability to tolerate dental procedures.

Teach Patient/Family to:

• Avoid mouth rinses with high alcohol content because of drying effects.

potassium chloride

poe-**tass**′-ee-um **klor**′-ide

(Apo-K[CAN], Cena K; Ed K10, KCare; K-10, K-8, Kaochlor, Kaochlor S-F, Kaon-CI, Kaon-CL 10, Kaon-CL 20%, Kato, Kay Ciel, KCl-20, KCl-40, K-Dur 10, K-Dur 20, K-Lor; Klor-Con, Klor-Con/25, Klor-Con 10, Klor-Con 8, Klor-Con M10, Klor-Con M15, Klor-Con M20, Klotrix, K-Lyte CI, K-Norm, K-Sol, K-Tab, Micro-K, Micro-K 10, Rum-K)

Do not confuse with Cardura or Slow-FE.

CATEGORY AND SCHEDULE

Pregnancy Risk Category: C

Drug Class: Potassium electrolyte

MECHANISM OF ACTION

An electrolyte that is necessary for multiple cellular metabolic processes. Primary action is intracellular.

Therapeutic Effect: Necessary for nerve impulse conduction, contraction of cardiac, skeletal, and smooth muscle; maintains normal renal function and acid-base balance.

USES

Prevention and treatment of hypokalemia

PHARMACOKINETICS

Well absorbed from the GI tract. Enters cells via active transport from extracellular fluid. Primarily excreted in urine.

INDICATIONS AND DOSAGES

▸ **Prevention of Hypokalemia (on Diuretic Therapy)**

PO

Adults, Elderly. 20–40 mEq/day in 1–2 divided doses.

Children. 1–2 mEq/kg in 1–2 divided doses.

▸ **Treatment of Hypokalemia**

IV

Adults, Elderly. 5–10 mEq/hr. Maximum: 400 mEq/day.

Children. 1 mEq/kg over 1–2 hr.

PO

Adults, Elderly. 40–80 mEq/day, further doses based on laboratory values.

Children. 1–2 mEq/day, further doses based on laboratory values.

SIDE EFFECTS/ADVERSE REACTIONS

Occasional

Nausea, vomiting, diarrhea, flatulence, abdominal discomfort with distention, phlebitis with IV administration (particularly when potassium concentration of greater than 40 mEq/L is infused)

Rare
Rash

PRECAUTIONS AND CONTRAINDICATIONS

Digitalis toxicity, heat cramps, hyperkalemia, patients receiving potassium-sparing diuretics, postoperative oliguria, severe burns, severe renal impairment, shock with dehydration or hemolytic reaction, untreated Addison's disease, hypersensitivity to any component of the formulation

Caution:
Cardiac disease, potassium-sparing diuretic therapy, systemic acidosis, pregnancy category A, renal impairment

DRUG INTERACTIONS OF CONCERN TO DENTISTRY

- Decreased potassium requirement: corticosteroids
- Increased GI side effects: anticholinergic drugs, NSAIDs
- Increased serum potassium: NSAIDs, cyclosporine

SERIOUS REACTIONS

! Hyperkalemia (observed particularly in elderly or in patients with impaired renal function) manifested as paresthesia of extremities, heaviness of legs, cold skin, grayish pallor, hypotension, mental confusion, irritability, flaccid paralysis, and cardiac arrhythmias.

DENTAL CONSIDERATIONS

General:

- Patients taking potassium supplements will normally be taking a diuretic. Compliance with potassium supplements can be a problem. Verify serum potassium levels as required.
- Consider semisupine chair position for patient comfort if GI side effects occur.

potassium acetate/ potassium bicarbonate-citrate/ potassium chloride/ potassium gluconate

poe-**tah′**-see-um **ass′**-eh-tayte
(potassium bicarbonate-citrate: K-Lyte, Klor-Con EF, Effer K, K-Lyte DS; potassium chloride: Apo-K[CAN], Kaochlor, K-Dur, K-Lor, K-Lor-Con M 15, Kaon-Cl, KSR[AUS], KSR-600[AUS], Micro-K, Slow-K[AUS], Span-K[AUS]; potassium gluconate: Kaon)
Do not confuse K-dur with Cardura.

CATEGORY AND SCHEDULE

Pregnancy Risk Category: C (A for potassium chloride)

Drug Class: Potassium electrolyte

MECHANISM OF ACTION

An electrolyte that is necessary for multiple cellular metabolic processes. Primary action is intracellular.
Therapeutic Effect: Is necessary for nerve impulse conduction and contraction of cardiac, skeletal, and smooth muscle; maintains normal renal function and acid-base balance.

USES

Prevention and treatment of hypokalemia

PHARMACOKINETICS

Well absorbed from the GI tract. Enters cells by active transport from extracellular fluid. Primarily excreted in urine.

INDICATIONS AND DOSAGES

▸ Prevention of Hypokalemia (in Patients on Diuretic Therapy)

PO

Adults, Elderly. 20–40 mEq/day in 1–2 divided doses.
Children. 1–2 mEq/kg/day in 1–2 divided doses.

▸ Treatment of Hypokalemia

PO

Adults, Elderly. 40–80 mEq/day; further doses based on laboratory values.
Children. 2–5 mEq/day; further doses based on laboratory values.

IV

Adults, Elderly. 5–10 mEq/hr. Maximum: 400 mEq/day.
Children. 1 mEq/kg over 1–2 hr.

P

SIDE EFFECTS/ADVERSE REACTIONS

Occasional

Nausea, vomiting, diarrhea, flatulence, abdominal discomfort with distention, phlebitis with IV administration (particularly when higher concentrations are infused IV)

Rare

Rash

PRECAUTIONS AND CONTRAINDICATIONS

Concurrent use of potassium-sparing diuretics, digitalis toxicity, heat cramps, hyperkalemia, postoperative oliguria, severe burns, severe renal impairment, shock with dehydration or hemolytic reaction, untreated Addison's disease

Caution:

Cardiac disease, potassium-sparing diuretic therapy, systemic acidosis, renal impairment

DRUG INTERACTIONS OF CONCERN TO DENTISTRY

- Decreased potassium requirement: corticosteroids
- Increased GI side effects: anticholinergic drugs, NSAIDs
- Increased serum potassium: NSAIDs, cyclosporine

SERIOUS REACTIONS

! Hyperkalemia (more common in elderly patients and those with impaired renal function) may be manifested as paresthesia, feeling of heaviness in the lower extremities, cold skin, grayish pallor, hypotension, confusion, irritability, flaccid paralysis, and cardiac arrhythmias.

DENTAL CONSIDERATIONS

General:

- Patients taking potassium supplements will normally be taking a diuretic. Compliance with potassium supplements can be a problem. Verify serum potassium levels as required.
- Consider semisupine chair position for patient comfort if GI side effects occur.

povidone iodine

poe′-vi-done
(ACU-dyne, Aerodine, Betadine, Betagen, Biodyne, Efodine, Iodex-P, Mallisol, Minidyne, Operand, Polydine Proviodine)

CATEGORY AND SCHEDULE

Pregnancy Risk Category: D (vaginal antiseptic)

Drug Class: Iodophor disinfectant

MECHANISM OF ACTION

Destroys a wide variety of microorganisms by germicidal action.

USES

Cleansing wounds, disinfection, preoperative skin preparation removal

INDICATIONS AND DOSAGES

Topical
Adults, Children. Use as needed on infected body surface.

SIDE EFFECTS/ADVERSE REACTIONS

Frequent
Skin irritation

PRECAUTIONS AND CONTRAINDICATIONS

Hypersensitivity to iodine
Caution:
Extensive burns

DRUG INTERACTIONS OF CONCERN TO DENTISTRY

• Do not use with alcohol or hydrogen peroxide

SERIOUS REACTIONS

! Severe allergic reactions

DENTAL CONSIDERATIONS

General:
• Assess for allergies to seafood; if present, drug should not be used.
• Store in tight, light-resistant container.
• Evaluate area of the body involved for irritation, rash, breaks, dryness, and scales.
Teach Patient/Family to:
• Discontinue use if rash, irritation, or redness occurs.

pramipexole

pram-eh-**pex**′-ol
(Mirapex)
Do not confuse Mirapex with Mifeprex or MiraLAX.

CATEGORY AND SCHEDULE

Pregnancy Risk Category: C

Drug Class: Antiparkinson agent

MECHANISM OF ACTION

An antiparkinson agent that stimulates dopamine receptors in the striatum.
Therapeutic Effect: Relieves signs and symptoms of Parkinson’s disease.

USES

Treatment of idiopathic Parkinson’s disease

PHARMACOKINETICS

Rapidly and extensively absorbed after PO administration. Protein binding: 15%. Widely distributed. Steady-state concentrations achieved within 2 days. Primarily eliminated in urine. Not removed by hemodialysis. ***Half-life:*** 8 hr (12 hr in patients older than 65 yr).

INDICATIONS AND DOSAGES

▸ Parkinson's Disease

PO

Adults, Elderly. Initially, 0.375 mg/day in 3 divided doses. Do not increase dosage more frequently than every 5–7 days. Maintenance: 1.5–4.5 mg/day in 3 equally divided doses.

▸ Dosage in Renal Impairment

Dosage and frequency are modified on the basis of creatinine clearance.

Creatinine Clearance	Initial Dose	Maximum Dose
Greater than 60 ml/min	0.125 mg 3 times a day	1.5 mg 3 times a day
35–59 ml/min	0.125 mg twice a day	1.5 mg twice a day
15–34 ml/min	0.125 mg once a day	1.5 mg once a day

SIDE EFFECTS/ADVERSE REACTIONS

Frequent

Early Parkinson's disease: Nausea, asthenia, dizziness, somnolence, insomnia, constipation

Advanced Parkinson's disease: Orthostatic hypotension, extrapyramidal reactions, insomnia, dizziness, hallucinations

Occasional

Early Parkinson's disease: Edema, malaise, confusion, amnesia, akathisia, anorexia, dysphagia, peripheral edema, vision changes, impotence

Advanced Parkinson's disease: Asthenia, somnolence, confusion, constipation, abnormal gait, dry mouth

Rare

Advanced Parkinson's disease: General edema, malaise, chest pain, amnesia, tremor, urinary frequency or incontinence, dyspnea, rhinitis, vision changes

PRECAUTIONS AND CONTRAINDICATIONS

History of hypersensitivity to pramipexole

Caution:

Orthostatic hypotension, hallucination risk higher than 65 yr, renal insufficiency, caution in driving a car (somnolence), risk of falling asleep while performing daily activities, lactation, use not established in children

DRUG INTERACTIONS OF CONCERN TO DENTISTRY

- Increased CNS depression: all CNS depressants
- Possible decreased effects: dopamine antagonists (phenothiazines, butyrophenones, or thioxanthenes) and metoclopramide

SERIOUS REACTIONS

! None known

DENTAL CONSIDERATIONS

General:

- Monitor vital signs at every appointment because of cardiovascular side effects.
- Assess salivary flow as factor in caries, periodontal disease, and candidiasis.
- Consider semisupine chair position for patient comfort if GI side effects occur.
- After supine positioning, have patient sit upright for at least 2 min before standing to avoid orthostatic hypotension.

Consultations:

- Medical consultation may be required to assess disease control and patient's ability to tolerate stress.

Teach Patient/Family to:

- Encourage effective oral hygiene to prevent soft tissue inflammation.
- Use caution to prevent trauma when using oral hygiene aids.
- Use powered tooth brush if patient has difficulty holding conventional devices.
- Update health and drug history if physician makes any changes in evaluation or drug regimens; include OTC, herbal, and nonherbal drugs in the update.
- When chronic dry mouth occurs, advise patient to:
  - Avoid mouth rinses with high alcohol content because of drying effects.
  - Use daily home fluoride products for anticaries effect.
  - Use sugarless gum, frequent sips of water, or saliva substitutes.

prasugrel

pra-soo-grel

(Effient)

Do not confuse with prazosin.

CATEGORY AND SCHEDULE

Pregnancy Risk Category: C

Drug Class: Platelet aggregation inhibitor

MECHANISN OF ACTION

Binds selectively and irreversibly to platelet P2Y12 receptors and inhibits ADP-induced platelet activation and aggregation.

USES

Reduction of adverse thrombotic cardiovascular events, including stent thrombosis, in patients with acute coronary syndrome, with unstable angina or non-ST-elevation myocardial infarction and those with ST-elevation myocardial infarction managed with primary or delayed percutaneous coronary intervention (PCI)

PHARMACOKINETICS

Rapidly hydrolyzed in the intestine to a thiolactone metabolite, which is then absorbed. Metabolized in the liver primarily by CYP3A4 and 2B6, with numerous metabolites. ***Half-life:*** 7 hr. 70% excreted by the kidneys, 25% in the feces. Metabolism and excretion not significantly affected by mild-to-moderate hepatic or renal impairment.

INDICATIONS AND DOSAGES

▸ Antiplatelet Therapy

PO

Adult, Elderly (under the age of 75). 60-mg loading dose, then 10 mg once daily, in combination with low-dose aspirin (75–325 mg).

SIDE EFFECTS/ADVERSE REACTIONS

Frequent

Bleeding, hypertension, hypercholesterolemia, hyperlipidemia, headache, back pain, dyspnea, nausea, dizziness, cough, hypotension, fatigue, non-cardiac chest pain

Occasional

Anemia

Rare

Thrombocytopenia, abnormal hepatic function, allergic reactions, angioedema

PRECAUTIONS AND CONTRAINDICATIONS

Severe bleeding, especially elderly over the age of 75 and less than 60 kg body weight

DRUG INTERACTIONS OF CONCERN TO DENTISTRY

- Increased risk of serious bleeding: NSAIDs
- Epinephrine: coexisting cardiovascular disease
- CYP Inhibitors: increased bleeding (erythromycin, clarithromycin, azole antifungal drugs, benzodiazepines)

SERIOUS REACTIONS

! Excessive bleeding, hypersensitivity

DENTAL CONSIDERATIONS

General:

- Avoid discontinuation for dental procedures because of increased risk of thromboembolism.
- Use careful surgical technique and local hemostatic measures to prevent excessive bleeding.
- Question patient about concurrent use of aspirin, other NSAIDs.
- Avoid or limit doses of epinephrine in local anesthetic due to cardiovascular disease status.
- Monitor vital signs at every appointment due to cardiovascular disease status.

Consultations:

- Medical consultation may be required to assess disease control and patient's ability to tolerate stress.
- Consultation should include data on bleeding time.
- In a patient with signs or symptoms of blood dyscrasias, request a medical consultation for blood studies and postpone treatment until normal values are reestablished.

Teach Patient/Family to:

- Update health and drug history if physician makes any changes in evaluation or drug regimens.
- Use caution to prevent trauma when using oral hygiene aids.
- Report any unusual or prolonged bleeding episodes after dental treatment.

pravastatin

prav-ih-**sta′**-tin

(Pravachol)

Do not confuse pravastatin with Prevacid, or Pravachol with propranolol.

CATEGORY AND SCHEDULE

Pregnancy Risk Category: X

Drug Class: Antihyperlipidemic

MECHANISM OF ACTION

An HMG-CoA reductase inhibitor that interferes with cholesterol biosynthesis by preventing the conversion of HMG-CoA reductase to mevalonate, a precursor to cholesterol.

Therapeutic Effect: Lowers serum low-density lipoproteins (LDLs) and very low-density lipoproteins (VLDLs), cholesterol, and plasma triglyceride levels; increases serum high-density lipoprotein (HDL) concentration.

USES

As an adjunct in homozygous or heterozygous familial hypercholesterolemia, mixed hyperlipidemia, elevated serum triglyceride levels, and type IV hyperproteinemia; also reduces total cholesterol LDL-C, apo B, and triglyceride levels; patient should first be placed on cholesterol-lowering diet; primary prevention of coronary events, secondary prevention of cardiovascular events

PHARMACOKINETICS

Poorly absorbed from the GI tract. Protein binding: 50%. Metabolized in the liver (minimal active metabolites). Primarily excreted in feces via the biliary system. Not removed by hemodialysis. ***Half-life:*** 2.7 hr.

INDICATIONS AND DOSAGES

▸ **Hyperlipidemia, Primary and Secondary Prevention of Cardiovascular Events in Patients with Elevated Cholesterol Levels**

PO

Adults, Elderly. Initially, 40 mg/day. Titrate to desired response. Range: 10–80 mg/day.
Children 14–18 yr. 40 mg/day.
Children 8–13 yr. 20 mg/day.

▸ **Dosage in Hepatic and Renal Impairment**

For adults, give 10 mg/day initially. Titrate to desired response.

SIDE EFFECTS/ADVERSE REACTIONS

Pravastatin is generally well tolerated. Side effects are usually mild and transient.

Occasional

Nausea, vomiting, diarrhea, constipation, abdominal pain, headache, rhinitis, rash, pruritus

Rare

Heartburn, myalgia, dizziness, cough, fatigue, flu-like symptoms

PRECAUTIONS AND CONTRAINDICATIONS

Active hepatic disease or unexplained, persistent elevations of liver function test results

Caution:

Past liver disease, alcoholics, severe acute infections, trauma, hypotension, uncontrolled seizure disorders, severe metabolic disorders, electrolyte imbalances

DRUG INTERACTIONS OF CONCERN TO DENTISTRY

- Increased risk of myopathy or rhabdomyolysis: erythromycin, itraconazole

SERIOUS REACTIONS

! Malignancy and cataracts may occur.
! Hypersensitivity occurs rarely.

DENTAL CONSIDERATIONS

General:

- Monitor vital signs at every appointment because of possible cardiovascular disease.
- Consider semisupine chair position for patient comfort if GI side effects occur.

prazosin hydrochloride

pra′-zoe-sin high-droh-**klor′**-ide
(Minipress, Prasig[AUS], Pratisol[AUS], Pressin[AUS])

P

CATEGORY AND SCHEDULE

Pregnancy Risk Category: C

Drug Class: Antihypertensive, α-adrenergic antagonist

MECHANISM OF ACTION

An antidote, antihypertensive, and vasodilator that selectively blocks α_1-adrenergic receptors, decreasing peripheral vascular resistance. ***Therapeutic Effect:*** Produces vasodilation of veins and arterioles, decreases total peripheral resistance, and relaxes smooth muscle in bladder neck and prostate.

USES

Treatment of hypertension; unapproved: CHF, urinary retention in prostatic hypertrophy, pheochromocytoma

PHARMACOKINETICS

PO: Onset 2 hr, peak 1–3 hr, duration 6–12 hr. ***Half-life:*** 2–4 hr; metabolized in liver; excreted via bile, feces (greater than 90%), in urine (less than 10%).

INDICATIONS AND DOSAGES

▸ Mild-to-Moderate Hypertension

PO

Adults, Elderly. Initially, 1 mg 2–3 times a day. Maintenance: 3–15 mg/day in divided doses. Maximum: 20 mg/day.

Children. 5 mcg/kg/dose q6h. Gradually increase up to 25 mcg/kg/dose.

SIDE EFFECTS/ADVERSE REACTIONS

Frequent

Dizziness, somnolence, headache, asthenia (loss of strength, energy)

Occasional

Palpitations, nausea, dry mouth, nervousness

Rare

Angina, urinary urgency

P

PRECAUTIONS AND CONTRAINDICATIONS

Hypersensitivity, severe CHF

Caution:

Children

DRUG INTERACTIONS OF CONCERN TO DENTISTRY

- Increased effects: epinephrine
- Decreased effect: indomethacin, NSAIDs

SERIOUS REACTIONS

! First-dose syncope (hypotension with sudden loss of consciousness) may occur 30–90 min following initial dose of more than 2 mg, a too-rapid increase in dosage, or addition of another antihypertensive agent to therapy. First-dose syncope may be preceded by tachycardia (pulse rate of 120–160 beats/min).

DENTAL CONSIDERATIONS

General:

- Monitor vital signs at every appointment because of cardiovascular side effects.
- Avoid or limit dose of vasoconstrictor.
- After supine positioning, have patient sit upright for at least 2 min before standing to avoid orthostatic hypotension.
- Assess salivary flow as a factor in caries, periodontal disease, and candidiasis.
- Limit use of sodium-containing products, such as saline IV fluids, for patients with a dietary salt restriction.
- Stress from dental procedures may compromise cardiovascular function; determine patient risk.
- Short appointments and a stress-reduction protocol may be required.

Consultations:

- Medical consultation may be required to assess disease control.

Teach Patient/Family to:

- When chronic dry mouth occurs, advise patient to:
  - Avoid mouth rinses with high alcohol content because of drying effects.
  - Use daily home fluoride products to prevent caries.
  - Use sugarless gum, frequent sips of water, or saliva substitutes.

prednisolone

pred-**niss**′-oh-lone
(AK-Pred, AK-Tate[CAN], Inflamase Forte, Inflamase Mild, Minims-Prednisolone[CAN], Novo-Prednisolone[CAN], Orapred, Pediapred, Pred Forte, Pred Mild, Prelone, Solone[AUS])
Do not confuse prednisolone with prednisone or primidone.

CATEGORY AND SCHEDULE

Pregnancy Risk Category: C (D if used in first trimester)

Drug Class: Glucocorticoid, immediate acting

MECHANISM OF ACTION

An adrenocortical steroid that inhibits accumulation of inflammatory cells at inflammation sites, phagocytosis, lysosomal enzyme release and synthesis, and release of mediators of inflammation.
Therapeutic Effect: Prevents or suppresses cell-mediated immune reactions. Decreases or prevents tissue response to inflammatory process.

USES

Treatment of severe inflammation, immunosuppression, neoplasms, adrenal insufficiency, acute exacerbation of multiple sclerosis

PHARMACOKINETICS

PO: Peak 1–2 hr, duration 2 days.
IM: Peak 3–45 hr.

INDICATIONS AND DOSAGES

▸ **Substitution Therapy for Deficiency States: Acute or Chronic Adrenal Insufficiency, Congenital Adrenal Hyperplasia, and Adrenal Insufficiency Secondary to Pituitary Insufficiency; Nonendocrine Disorders: Arthritis; Rheumatic Carditis; Allergic, Collagen, Intestinal Tract, Liver, Ocular, Renal, Skin Diseases; Bronchial Asthma; Cerebral Edema; Malignancies**

PO

Adults, Elderly. 5–60 mg/day in divided doses.
Children. 0.1–2 mg/kg/day in 1–4 divided doses.

▸ **Treatment of Conjunctivitis and Corneal Injury**

Ophthalmic

Adults, Elderly. 1–2 drops every hr during day and q2h during night. After response, decrease dosage to 1 drop q4h, then 1 drop 3–4 times a day.

SIDE EFFECTS/ADVERSE REACTIONS

Frequent

Insomnia, heartburn, nervousness, abdominal distention, increased sweating, acne, mood swings, increased appetite, facial flushing, delayed wound healing, increased susceptibility to infection, diarrhea or constipation

Occasional

Headache, edema, change in skin color, frequent urination

Rare

Tachycardia, allergic reaction (such as rash and hives), psychological changes, hallucinations, depression
Ophthalmic: stinging or burning, posterior subcapsular cataracts

PRECAUTIONS AND CONTRAINDICATIONS

Acute superficial herpes simplex keratitis, systemic fungal infections, varicella

Caution:

Diabetes mellitus, glaucoma, osteoporosis, seizure disorders, ulcerative colitis, CHF, myasthenia gravis, ulcerative GI disease, rifampin

DRUG INTERACTIONS OF CONCERN TO DENTISTRY

- Decreased action: barbiturates, rifampin, rifabutin
- Increased side effects: alcohol, salicylates, NSAIDs
- Increased action: ketoconazole, macrolide antibiotics (erythromycin, clarithromycin, azithromycin)
- Hepatotoxicity: acetaminophen (chronic use, high doses)

SERIOUS REACTIONS

! Long-term therapy may cause hypocalcemia, hypokalemia, muscle wasting (especially in the arms and legs), osteoporosis, spontaneous fractures, amenorrhea, cataracts, glaucoma, peptic ulcer disease, and CHF.

! Abruptly withdrawing the drug after long-term therapy may cause anorexia, nausea, fever, headache, severe or sudden joint pain, rebound inflammation, fatigue, weakness, lethargy, dizziness, and orthostatic hypotension.

! Suddenly discontinuing prednisolone may be fatal.

P

DENTAL CONSIDERATIONS

General:

- Monitor vital signs at every appointment because of cardiovascular side effects.
- Patients on chronic drug therapy may rarely have symptoms of blood dyscrasias, which can include infection, bleeding, and poor healing.
- Assess salivary flow as a factor in caries, periodontal disease, and candidiasis.
- Avoid prescribing aspirin-containing products.
- Place on frequent recall to evaluate healing response.
- Prophylactic antibiotics may be indicated to prevent infection if surgery or deep scaling is planned.
- Symptoms of oral infections may be masked.
- Determine dose and duration of steroid therapy for each patient to assess risk for stress tolerance and immunosuppression.
- Patients who have been or are currently on chronic steroid therapy longer than 2 wk may require supplemental steroids for some dental procedures.
- Determine why the patient is taking the drug.

Consultations:

- In a patient with symptoms of blood dyscrasias, request a medical consultation for blood studies and postpone dental treatment until normal values are reestablished.
- Medical consultation may be required to assess disease control.
- Consultation may be required to confirm steroid dose and duration of use.

Teach Patient/Family to:

- Encourage effective oral hygiene to prevent soft tissue inflammation.
- Use caution to prevent injury when using oral hygiene aids.
- When chronic dry mouth occurs, advise patient to:
    - Avoid mouth rinses with high alcohol content because of drying effects.

• Use daily home fluoride products to prevent caries.
• Use sugarless gum, frequent sips of water, or saliva substitutes.

prednisolone acetate

pred-**niss**′-oh-lone **as**′-ih-tate
(AK-Pred, Econopred Plus, Inflamase Forte, Inflamase Mild, Ocu-Pred, Ocu-Pred-A, Ocu-Pred Forte, Pred Forte, Pred Mild, Prednisol)

CATEGORY AND SCHEDULE

Pregnancy Risk Category: C

Drug Class: Glucocorticoid, immediate acting

MECHANISM OF ACTION

An adrenal corticosteroid that inhibits accumulation of inflammatory cells at inflammation sites, phagocytosis, lysosomal enzyme release and synthesis, and release of mediators of inflammation.

Therapeutic Effect: Prevents or suppresses cell-mediated immune reactions. Decreases or prevents tissue response to inflammatory process.

USES

Treatment of severe inflammation, immunosuppression, neoplasms, adrenal insufficiency, acute exacerbation of multiple sclerosis

PHARMACOKINETICS

Absorbed into aqueous humor, cornea, iris, choroids, ciliary body, and retina. Systemic absorption may occur, but significant only at high dosages.

INDICATIONS AND DOSAGES

▸ **Conjunctivitis**

Ophthalmic

Adults, Elderly, Children. 1–2 drops 2–4 times a day.

SIDE EFFECTS/ADVERSE REACTIONS

Occasional

Stinging or burning

PRECAUTIONS AND CONTRAINDICATIONS

Fungal, mycobacterial, or viral infections of the eye, hypersensitivity to prednisolone acetate or any component of the formulation

Caution:

Diabetes mellitus, glaucoma, osteoporosis, seizure disorders, ulcerative colitis, CHF, myasthenia gravis, ulcerative GI disease, rifampin

DRUG INTERACTIONS OF CONCERN TO DENTISTRY

• Decreased action: barbiturates, rifampin, rifabutin
• Increased side effects: alcohol, salicylates, NSAIDs
• Increased action: ketoconazole, macrolide antibiotics (erythromycin, clarithromycin, azithromycin)
• Hepatotoxicity: acetaminophen (chronic use, high doses)

SERIOUS REACTIONS

! Prolonged use of corticosteroids may result in glaucoma with damage to the optic nerve, defects in visual acuity and fields of vision, posterior subcapsular cataract formation, and delayed wound healing.

! Long-term use may cause corneal and scleral thinning.

! Systemic effects are uncommon, but systemic hypercorticoidism has been reported.

! Acute anterior uveitis and perforation of the globe, keratitis, conjunctivitis, corneal ulcers, mydriasis, conjunctival hyperemia, loss of accommodation, and ptosis have occasionally been reported.
! The development of secondary ocular infection has occurred. Fungal and viral infections of the cornea may develop with long-term applications of steroid.

DENTAL CONSIDERATIONS

General:

- Monitor vital signs at every appointment because of cardiovascular side effects.
- Patients on chronic drug therapy may rarely have symptoms of blood dyscrasias, which can include infection, bleeding, and poor healing.
- Assess salivary flow as a factor in caries, periodontal disease, and candidiasis.
- Avoid prescribing aspirin-containing products.
- Place on frequent recall to evaluate healing response.
- Prophylactic antibiotics may be indicated to prevent infection if surgery or deep scaling is planned.
- Symptoms of oral infections may be masked.
- Determine dose and duration of steroid therapy for each patient to assess risk for stress tolerance and immunosuppression.
- Patients who have been or are currently on chronic steroid therapy longer than 2 wk may require supplemental steroids for some dental procedures.
- Determine why the patient is taking the drug.

Consultations:

- In a patient with symptoms of blood dyscrasias, request a medical consultation for blood studies and postpone dental treatment until normal values are reestablished.
- Medical consultation may be required to assess disease control.
- Consultation may be required to confirm steroid dose and duration of use.

Teach Patient/Family to:

- Encourage effective oral hygiene to prevent soft tissue inflammation.
- Use caution to prevent injury when using oral hygiene aids.
- When chronic dry mouth occurs, advise patient to:
  - Avoid mouth rinses with high alcohol content because of drying effects.
  - Use daily home fluoride products to prevent caries.
  - Use sugarless gum, frequent sips of water, or saliva substitutes.

prednisolone acetate; sulfacetamide sodium

pred-**niss′**-oh-lone **ass′**-eh-tate; sul-fa-**see′**-ta-mide **soe′**-dee-um
(AK-Cide; Blephamide; Blephamide S.O.P.; Medasulf; Metimyd; Ocu-Lone C; Vasocidin)

CATEGORY AND SCHEDULE

Pregnancy Risk Category: C

Drug Class: Glucocorticoid, immediate acting

MECHANISM OF ACTION

Prednisolone is an adrenal corticosteroid that inhibits accumulation of inflammatory cells at inflammation sites, phagocytosis, lysosomal enzyme release and

synthesis, and release of mediators of inflammation. Sulfacetamide is a sulfonamide that interferes with synthesis of folic acid that bacteria require for growth.
Therapeutic Effect: Prevents or suppresses cell-mediated immune reactions. Decreases or prevents tissue response to inflammatory process. Prevents further bacterial growth; bacteriostatic.

USES

Treatment of severe inflammation, immunosuppression, neoplasms, adrenal insufficiency, acute exacerbation of multiple sclerosis

PHARMACOKINETICS

None reported

INDICATIONS AND DOSAGES

▸ Steroid-Responsive Inflammatory Ocular Conditions for Which a Corticosteroid is Indicated and Where Superficial Bacterial Ocular Infection or a Risk of Bacterial Ocular Infection Exists

Ophthalmic Ointment
Adults, Elderly, Children. Apply 3 or 4 times a day and once at bedtime.
Ophthalmic Suspension
Adults, Elderly, Children. Instill 2–3 drops every 1–2 hr while awake.

SIDE EFFECTS/ADVERSE REACTIONS

Occasional
Local irritation
Rare
Elevation of intraocular pressure

PRECAUTIONS AND CONTRAINDICATIONS

Epithelial herpes simplex keratitis (dendritic keratitis), vaccinia, varicella, and other viral diseases of the cornea or conjunctiva, mycobacterial infection of the eye, and fungal diseases of ocular structure, known or suspected hypersensitivity to other sulfonamides or other corticosteroids or any component of the formulation

DRUG INTERACTIONS OF CONCERN TO DENTISTRY

- Decreased action: barbiturates, rifampin, rifabutin
- Increased side effects: alcohol, salicylates, NSAIDs
- Increased action: ketoconazole, macrolide antibiotics (erythromycin, clarithromycin, azithromycin)
- Hepatotoxicity: acetaminophen (chronic use, high doses)

SERIOUS REACTIONS

! Prolonged use of corticosteroids may result in glaucoma with damage to the optic nerve, defects in visual acuity and fields of vision, posterior subcapsular cataract formation, and delayed wound healing.
! Long-term use may cause corneal and scleral thinning.
! Systemic effects are uncommon, but systemic hypercorticoidism has been reported.
! Acute anterior uveitis and perforation of the globe, keratitis, conjunctivitis, corneal ulcers, mydriasis, conjunctival hyperemia, loss of accommodation, and ptosis have occasionally been reported.
! The development of secondary ocular infection has occurred. Fungal and viral infections of the cornea may develop with long-term applications of steroid.
! Fatalities caused by reactions to sulfonamides including Stevens-Johnson syndrome, toxic epidermal necrolysis, fulminant hepatic necrosis, agranulocytosis, aplastic anemia, and other blood dyscrasias have occurred.

DENTAL CONSIDERATIONS

General:
- Monitor vital signs at every appointment because of cardiovascular side effects.
- Patients on chronic drug therapy may rarely have symptoms of blood dyscrasias, which can include infection, bleeding, and poor healing.
- Assess salivary flow as a factor in caries, periodontal disease, and candidiasis.
- Avoid prescribing aspirin-containing products.
- Place on frequent recall to evaluate healing response.
- Prophylactic antibiotics may be indicated to prevent infection if surgery or deep scaling is planned.
- Symptoms of oral infections may be masked.
- Determine dose and duration of steroid therapy for each patient to assess risk for stress tolerance and immunosuppression.
- Patients who have been or are currently on chronic steroid therapy longer than 2 wk may require supplemental steroids for stressful dental treatment.
- Determine why the patient is taking the drug.

Consultations:
- In a patient with symptoms of blood dyscrasias, request a medical consultation for blood studies and postpone dental treatment until normal values are reestablished.
- Medical consultation may be required to assess disease control.
- Consultation may be required to confirm steroid dose and duration of use.

Teach Patient/Family to:
- Encourage effective oral hygiene to prevent soft tissue inflammation.
- Use caution to prevent injury when using oral hygiene aids.
- When chronic dry mouth occurs, advise patient to:
  - Avoid mouth rinses with high alcohol content because of drying effects.
  - Use daily home fluoride products to prevent caries.
  - Use sugarless gum, frequent sips of water, or saliva substitutes.

prednisolone sodium phosphate

pred-**nis**′-oh-lone **soe**′-dee-um **foss**′-fate
(AK-Pred, Inflamase Forte, Inflamase Mild, Orapred, Pediapred)

CATEGORY AND SCHEDULE

Pregnancy Risk Category: C

Drug Class: Glucocorticoid, antiinflammatory

MECHANISM OF ACTION

An adrenal corticosteroid that inhibits accumulation of inflammatory cells at inflammation sites, phagocytosis, lysosomal enzyme release and synthesis, and release of mediators of inflammation.

Therapeutic Effect: Prevents or suppresses cell-mediated immune reactions. Decreases or prevents tissue response to inflammatory process.

USES

Primary or secondary adrenocortical insufficiency; adjunctive therapy of rheumatoid arthritis; collagen diseases; skin inflammatory disorders; allergy; respiratory diseases; hematologic disorders;

neoplastic diseases; multiple sclerosis

PHARMACOKINETICS

Rapidly and well absorbed from the GI tract following oral administration. Protein binding: 90%–95%. Widely distributed. Metabolized in the liver. Excreted in the urine as sulfate and glucuronide conjugates. ***Half-life:*** 2–4 hr. Absorbed into aqueous humor, cornea, iris, choroid, ciliary body, and retina following ocular administration. Systemic absorption occurs but may be significant only at higher dosages or in extended pediatric therapy.

INDICATIONS AND DOSAGES

▸ **Asthma**

PO

Children. 1–2 mg/kg/day in single or divided doses for 3–10 days.

▸ **Endocrine Disorders, Hematologic and Neoplastic Disorders, Inflammatory Conditions**

PO

Adults, Elderly. 5–60 mg/day.
Children. 0.14–2 mg/kg/day divided into 3 or 4 doses.

▸ **Multiple Sclerosis Exacerbations**

PO

Adults, Elderly. 200 mg/day for 1 wk, followed by 80 mg every other day for 1 mo.

▸ **Nephrotic Syndrome**

PO

Children. 60 mg/m^2 daily. Maximum: 80 mg/day divided 3 times a day for 4 wk, then 40 mg/m^2 every other day for 4 wk.

▸ **Ophthalmic Disorders**

Ophthalmic Suspension

Adults, Elderly, Children. Instill 1 or 2 drops up to 6 times a day.

SIDE EFFECTS/ADVERSE REACTIONS

Frequent

Insomnia, heartburn, nervousness, abdominal distention, increased sweating, acne, mood swings, increased appetite, facial flushing, delayed wound healing, increased susceptibility to infection, diarrhea or constipation

Occasional

Headache, edema, change in skin color, frequent urination

Rare

Tachycardia, allergic reaction, such as rash and hives, psychic changes, hallucinations, depression
Ophthalmic: stinging or burning, posterior subcapsular cataracts

PRECAUTIONS AND CONTRAINDICATIONS

Systemic fungal infections, live or live attenuated vaccines, hypersensitivity to prednisolone sodium phosphate or any component of the formulation

DRUG INTERACTIONS OF CONCERN TO DENTISTRY

- Decreased action: barbiturates, rifampin, rifabutin
- Increased side effects: alcohol, salicylates, NSAIDs
- Increased action: ketoconazole, macrolide antibiotics (erythromycin, clarithromycin, azithromycin)
- Hepatotoxicity: acetaminophen (chronic use, high doses)

SERIOUS REACTIONS

! Prolonged use of corticosteroids may result in glaucoma with damage to the optic nerve, defects in visual acuity and fields of vision, posterior subcapsular cataract formation, and delayed wound healing.

! Long-term use may cause corneal and scleral thinning.
! Systemic effects are uncommon, but systemic hypercorticoidism has been reported.
! Acute anterior uveitis and perforation of the globe, keratitis, conjunctivitis, corneal ulcers, mydriasis, conjunctival hyperemia, loss of accommodation and ptosis have occasionally been reported.
! The development of secondary ocular infection has occurred. Fungal and viral infections of the cornea may develop with long-term applications of steroid.

DENTAL CONSIDERATIONS

General:
- Monitor vital signs at every appointment because of cardiovascular side effects.
- Patients on chronic drug therapy may rarely have symptoms of blood dyscrasias, which can include infection, bleeding, and poor healing.
- Assess salivary flow as a factor in caries, periodontal disease, and candidiasis.
- Avoid prescribing aspirin-containing products.
- Place on frequent recall to evaluate healing response.
- Prophylactic antibiotics may be indicated to prevent infection if surgery or deep scaling is planned.
- Symptoms of oral infections may be masked.
- Determine dose and duration of steroid therapy for each patient to assess risk for stress tolerance and immunosuppression.
- Patients who have been or are currently on chronic steroid therapy longer than 2 wk may require supplemental steroids for some dental procedures.
- Determine why the patient is taking the drug.

Consultations:
- In a patient with symptoms of blood dyscrasias, request a medical consultation for blood studies and postpone dental treatment until normal values are reestablished.
- Medical consultation may be required to assess disease control.
- Consultation may be required to confirm steroid dose and duration of use.

Teach Patient/Family to:
- Encourage effective oral hygiene to prevent soft tissue inflammation.
- Use caution to prevent injury when using oral hygiene aids.
- When chronic dry mouth occurs, advise patient to:
  - Avoid mouth rinses with high alcohol content because of drying effects.
  - Use daily home fluoride products to prevent caries.
  - Use sugarless gum, frequent sips of water, or saliva substitutes.

prednisone

pred′-ni-sone
(Apo-Prednisone[CAN], Deltasone, Panafcort[AUS], Prednisone Intensol, Sone[AUS], Sterapred, Sterapred DS, Winpred[CAN])
Do not confuse prednisone with prednisolone or primidone.

CATEGORY AND SCHEDULE

Pregnancy Risk Category: C (D if used in first trimester)

Drug Class: Glucocorticoid, intermediate acting

MECHANISM OF ACTION

An adrenocortical steroid that inhibits accumulation of inflammatory cells at inflammation sites, phagocytosis, lysosomal enzyme release and synthesis, and release of mediators of inflammation.
Therapeutic Effect: Prevents or suppresses cell-mediated immune reactions. Decreases or prevents tissue response to inflammatory process.

USES

Treatment of severe inflammation, immunosuppression, neoplasms, multiple sclerosis, collagen disorders, dermatologic disorders, acute exacerbation of multiple sclerosis

PHARMACOKINETICS

Well absorbed from the GI tract. Protein binding: 70%–90%. Widely distributed. Metabolized in the liver and converted to prednisolone. Primarily excreted in urine. Not removed by hemodialysis. ***Half-life:*** 3.4–3.8 hr.

INDICATIONS AND DOSAGES

▸ **Substitution Therapy in Deficiency States: Acute or Chronic Adrenal Insufficiency, Congenital Adrenal Hyperplasia, and Adrenal Insufficiency Secondary to Pituitary Insufficiency; Nonendocrine Disorders: Arthritis; Rheumatic Carditis; Allergic, Collagen, Intestinal Tract, Liver, Ocular, Renal, Skin Diseases; Bronchial Asthma; Cerebral Edema; Malignancies**
PO
Adults, Elderly. 5–60 mg/day in divided doses.
Children. 0.05–2 mg/kg/day in 1–4 divided doses.

SIDE EFFECTS/ADVERSE REACTIONS

Frequent
Insomnia, heartburn, nervousness, abdominal distention, increased sweating, acne, mood swings, increased appetite, facial flushing, delayed wound healing, increased susceptibility to infection, diarrhea or constipation
Occasional
Headache, edema, change in skin color, frequent urination
Rare
Tachycardia, allergic reaction (including rash and hives), psychological changes, hallucinations, depression

PRECAUTIONS AND CONTRAINDICATIONS

Acute superficial herpes simplex keratitis, systemic fungal infections, varicella
Caution:
Diabetes mellitus, glaucoma, osteoporosis, seizure disorders, ulcerative colitis, CHF, myasthenia gravis, renal disease, esophagitis, peptic ulcer, rifampin

DRUG INTERACTIONS OF CONCERN TO DENTISTRY

- Decreased action: barbiturates, rifampin, rifabutin
- Increased side effects: alcohol, salicylates, NSAIDs
- Increased action: ketoconazole, macrolide antibiotics
- Hepatotoxicity: acetaminophen (chronic, high doses)

SERIOUS REACTIONS

! Long-term therapy may cause muscle wasting in the arms and legs, osteoporosis, spontaneous fractures, amenorrhea, cataracts, glaucoma, peptic ulcer disease, and CHF.

! Abruptly withdrawing the drug following long-term therapy may cause anorexia, nausea, fever, headache, sudden or severe joint pain, rebound inflammation, fatigue, weakness, lethargy, dizziness, and orthostatic hypotension.
! Suddenly discontinuing prednisone may be fatal.

DENTAL CONSIDERATIONS

General:
- Monitor vital signs at every appointment because of cardiovascular side effects.
- Patients on chronic drug therapy may rarely have symptoms of blood dyscrasias, which can include infection, bleeding, and poor healing.
- Avoid aspirin-containing products.
- Assess salivary flow as a factor in caries, periodontal disease, and candidiasis.
- Symptoms of oral infections may be masked.
- Place on frequent recall to evaluate healing response.
- Prophylactic antibiotics may be indicated to prevent infection if surgery or deep scaling is planned.
- Determine dose and duration of steroid therapy for each patient to assess risk for stress tolerance and immunosuppression.
- Patients who have been or are currently on chronic steroid therapy longer than 2 wk may require supplemental steroids for some dental procedures.
- Determine why the patient is taking the drug.

Consultations:
- In a patient with symptoms of blood dyscrasias, request a medical consultation for blood studies and postpone dental treatment until normal values are reestablished.
- Medical consultation may be required to assess disease control.
- Consultation may be required to confirm steroid dose and duration of use.

Teach Patient/Family to:
- Encourage effective oral hygiene to prevent soft tissue inflammation.
- Use caution to prevent injury when using oral hygiene aids.
- When chronic dry mouth occurs, advise patient to:
  - Avoid mouth rinses with high alcohol content because of drying effects.
  - Use daily home fluoride products to prevent caries.
  - Use sugarless gum, frequent sips of water, or saliva substitutes.

pregabalin

pre-**gab**-a-lin
(Lyrica)
Do not confuse with Premarin.

CATEGORY AND SCHEDULE

Pregnancy Risk Category: C

Drug Class: Anticonvulsant, analgesic

MECHANISM OF ACTION

An anticonvulsant and antineuralgic agent whose exact mechanism is unknown but may be related to binding to and modulation of calcium channels with a resulting decrease in the calcium-dependent release of neurotransmitters.

USES

Partial-onset seizures, post-herpetic neuralgia, neuropathic pain associated with diabetic neuropathy

PHARMACOKINETICS

Well absorbed following oral administration (90%), can be taken with food. Peak plasma concentrations reached in 0.7–1.5 hr, widely distributed, not protein-bound. Does not undergo hepatic metabolism. ***Half-life:*** 4.6–6.8 hr. 98% excreted unchanged by the kidneys.

INDICATIONS AND DOSAGES

▸ **Partial-Onset Seizures**

PO

Adults. 150–600 mg per day, beginning at 150 mg/day (75 mg bid or 50 mg tid). May be increased to a maximum dose of 600 mg/day based on efficacy and tolerability.

▸ **Neuropathic Pain Associated with Diabetic Neuropathy**

PO

Adults. 50 mg tid initially; increased to 300 mg per day within 1 wk based on efficacy and tolerability.

▸ **Post-Herpetic Neuralgia**

PO

Adults. 75–100 mg bid or 50–100 mg tid, beginning at 75 mg bid or 50 mg tid. May be increased to 300 mg/day within 1 wk based on efficacy and tolerability.

SIDE EFFECTS/ADVERSE REACTIONS

Frequent

Dizziness, somnolence, peripheral edema, dry mouth, constipation, accidental injury, asthenia, weight gain, blurred vision, abnormal thought

Occasional

Amnesia, speech impairment, abnormal gait, twitching, confusion, myoclonus, constipation, diplopia, ecchymosis, arthralgia, leg cramps, myalgia, myasthenia

PRECAUTIONS AND CONTRAINDICATIONS

Hypersensitivity to pregabalin or any of its ingredients, weight gain, peripheral edema, creatine kinase elevations (associated with myopathy), thrombocytopenia, mild PR prolongation, may cause dizziness, somnolence and mental impairment. Can cause blurring or other changes in vision. Abrupt discontinuation can result in recurrence of seizures and insomnia, nausea, headache, and diarrhea. Safety in children not established.

DRUG INTERACTIONS OF CONCERN TO DENTISTRY

Increased risk of CNS depression: all CNS depressants, alcohol. May potentiate mental impairment and somnolence.

SERIOUS REACTIONS

! Increased risk of congestive circulatory failure in patients at-risk for peripheral edema

DENTAL CONSIDERATIONS

General:

• Assess salivary flow as a factor in caries, periodontal disease, and candidiasis.

• Early-morning appointments and stress-reduction protocol may be needed for anxious patients.

• Be prepared to manage seizures.

• After supine positioning, allow patient to sit upright for 2 min to avoid occurrence of dizziness.

Consultations:

• Consult with physician to determine seizure control and ability to tolerate dental procedures.

Teach Patient/Family to:

• Avoid mouth rinses with high alcohol content because of drying effect.

• Use home fluoride products for anticaries effect.
• Use sugarless/xylitol gum, frequent sips of water, or saliva substitutes if dry mouth occurs.

prilocaine hydrochloride (local)

pry′-lo-kane high-droh-**klor′**-ide
(Citanest)
With vasoconstrictor:
(Citanest Forte with epinephrine)

CATEGORY AND SCHEDULE

Pregnancy Risk Category: B

Drug Class: Amide local anesthetic

MECHANISM OF ACTION

Inhibits ion fluxes across membranes; decreases rise of depolarization phase of action potential; blocks nerve action potential.

USES

Local dental anesthesia

PHARMACOKINETICS

Injection: Onset 2–10 min, duration 2–4 hr; metabolized in liver; excreted in urine.

INDICATIONS AND DOSAGES

▸ Dental Injection: Infiltration or Conduction Block

Prilocaine 4% without vasoconstrictor: Maximum aggregate dose of 600 mg/kg per dental appointment for healthy adult patient; doses must be adjusted for medically compromised, debilitated, or elderly and for each individual patient. Doses in excess of 400 mg have caused methemoglobinemia. Always use the lowest effective dose, a slow injection rate, and a careful aspiration technique. In considering the dose of local anesthesia with vasoconstrictor, the dose of epinephrine must also be considered. The recommended dose of epinephrine in a local anesthetic solution is 3 mcg/kg, not to exceed a total dose of 0.2 mg per appointment for a healthy adult. For adult patients with clinically significant cardiovascular disease, the dose limit of epinephrine is 0.04 mg per appointment. The dose limits of epinephrine will affect the amount of local anesthetic allowable in a given appointment.

▸ Example Calculations Illustrating Amount of Drug Administered per Dental Cartridge(s):

No. of Dental Cartridges (1.8 ml)*	mg of Prilocaine (4%)
1	72
2	144
3	216
4	288

*Also available in 1.7-ml cartridges.

▸ Example Calculations Illustrating Amount of Drug Administered per Dental Cartridge(s):

No. of Dental Cartridges (1.8 ml)	mg of Prilocaine (4%)	mg (mcg) Vasoconstrictor (1:200,000)
1	72	0.009 (9)
2	144	0.018 (18)
4	288	0.036 (36)

Available forms include: 4% solution, 4% solution with epinephrine 1:200,000.

SIDE EFFECTS/ADVERSE REACTIONS

Occasional

Numbness, tingling, trismus, convulsions, loss of consciousness, drowsiness, disorientation, tremors, shivering, anxiety, restlessness, myocardial depression, cardiac arrest, dysrhythmias, bradycardia, hypotension, hypertension, nausea, vomiting, methemoglobinemia, rash, urticaria, allergic reactions

Rare

Status asthmaticus, respiratory arrest, anaphylaxis

PRECAUTIONS AND CONTRAINDICATIONS

Hypersensitivity, cross-sensitivity among amides (rare), severe liver disease

Caution:

Elderly, large doses of local anesthetic in myasthenia gravis, risk of methemoglobinemia

DRUG INTERACTIONS OF CONCERN TO DENTISTRY

- CNS depressants: increased risk of CNS depression with all CNS depressants, especially in children and when larger doses are used
- Avoid placing dental cartridges in disinfection solutions
- Avoid excessive exposure of dental cartridges to light or heat; hastens deterioration of vasoconstrictor; observe for color change in local anesthetic solution
- Risk of cardiovascular side effects; rapid intravascular administration of local anesthetic containing vasoconstrictor, either alone or in patients taking tricyclic antidepressants, MAOIs, digitalis drugs, cocaine, phenothiazines, β-blockers, and in the presence of halogenated-hydrocarbon general anesthetics; use smallest effective vasoconstrictor dose and careful aspiration technique
- Avoid use of vasoconstrictors in patients with uncontrolled hyperthyroidism, diabetes, angina, or hypertension; refer these patients for medical treatment before elective dental treatment

SERIOUS REACTIONS

! Methemoglobinemia (at higher doses)

P

DENTAL CONSIDERATIONS

General:

- Monitor vital signs at every appointment because of cardiovascular side effects.
- Often used with vasoconstrictor for increased duration of action.
- Lubricate dry lips before injection or dental treatment as required.

Teach Patient/Family to:

- Use care to prevent injury while numbness exists and to refrain from chewing gum and eating following dental anesthesia.
- Report any signs of infection, muscle pain, or fever to dentist when feeling returns.
- Report any unusual soft tissue reactions (e.g., paresthesia).

primaquine

prim′-ah-kween

(Primacin[AUS])

Do not confuse with primidone.

CATEGORY AND SCHEDULE

Pregnancy Risk Category: C

Drug Class: Antiprotozoal

MECHANISM OF ACTION

An antimalarial and antirheumatic that eliminates tissue exoerythrocytic forms of *Plasmodium falciparum.* Disrupts mitochondria and binds to DNA.

Therapeutic Effect: Inhibits parasite growth.

USES

Treatment of malaria caused by *P. vivax;* unapproved: with clindamycin in the treatment of *P. carinii* in AIDS

P

PHARMACOKINETICS

Well absorbed. Metabolized in the liver to the active metabolite, carboxyprimaquine. Excreted in the urine in small amounts as unchanged drug. ***Half-life:*** 4–6 hr.

INDICATIONS AND DOSAGES

▸ **Treatment of Malaria**

PO

Adults, Elderly. 15-mg base daily for 14 days.

Children. 0.3-mg base/kg/wk once daily for 14 days.

▸ **Malaria Prophylaxis**

PO

Adults, Elderly. 30 mg base daily. Begin 1 day before departure and continue for 7 days after leaving malarious area.

SIDE EFFECTS/ADVERSE REACTIONS

Frequent

Abdominal pain, nausea, vomiting

Rare

Leukopenia, hemolytic anemia, methemoglobinemia

PRECAUTIONS AND CONTRAINDICATIONS

Concomitant medications that cause bone marrow suppression, rheumatoid arthritis, lupus erythematosus, glucose-6-phosphate dehydrogenase deficiency, pregnancy, hypersensitivity to primaquine or any of its components

DRUG INTERACTIONS OF CONCERN TO DENTISTRY

- None reported

SERIOUS REACTIONS

! Leukopenia, hemolytic anemia, methemoglobinemia occur rarely.

! Overdosage include symptoms of abdominal cramps, vomiting, burning epigastric distress, central nervous system and cardiovascular disturbances, cyanosis, methemoglobinemia, moderate leukocytosis or leukopenia, and anemia.

! Acute hemolysis occurs, but patients recover completely if the dosage is discontinued.

DENTAL CONSIDERATIONS

General:

- Patients on chronic drug therapy may rarely have symptoms of blood dyscrasias, which can include infection, bleeding, and poor healing.
- Avoid dental light in patient's eyes; offer dark glasses for patient comfort.

Consultations:

• In a patient with symptoms of blood dyscrasias, request a medical consultation for blood studies and postpone dental treatment until normal values are reestablished.

Teach Patient/Family to:

• Encourage effective oral hygiene to prevent soft tissue inflammation.
• Use caution to prevent injury when using oral hygiene aids.

primidone

prih′-mih-done

(Apo-Primidone[CAN], Mysoline)

Do not confuse primidone with prednisone.

CATEGORY AND SCHEDULE

Pregnancy Risk Category: D

Controlled Substance: Schedule IV

Drug Class: Anticonvulsant, barbiturate derivative

MECHANISM OF ACTION

A barbiturate that decreases motor activity from electrical and chemical stimulation and stabilizes the seizure threshold against hyperexcitability.

Therapeutic Effect: Reduces seizure activity.

USES

Treatment of generalized tonic-clonic (grand mal), complex-partial psychomotor seizures

PHARMACOKINETICS

PO: Peak 4 hr. ***Half-life:*** 3–24 hr; excreted by kidneys, in breast milk.

INDICATIONS AND DOSAGES

▸ **Seizure Control**

PO

Adults, Elderly, Children 8 yr and older. 125–150 mg/day at bedtime. May increase by 125–250 mg/day every 3–7 days. Maximum: 2 g/day.

Children younger than 8 yr. Initially, 50–125 mg/day at bedtime. May increase by 50–125 mg/day every 3–7 days. Usual dose: 10–25 mg/kg/day in divided doses.

Neonates. 12–20 mg/kg/day in divided doses.

SIDE EFFECTS/ADVERSE REACTIONS

Frequent

Ataxia, dizziness

Occasional

Anorexia, drowsiness, mental changes, nausea, vomiting, paradoxical excitement

Rare

Rash

PRECAUTIONS AND CONTRAINDICATIONS

History of bronchopneumonia, porphyria

Caution:

COPD, hepatic disease, renal disease, abrupt withdrawal, lactation, hyperactive children

DRUG INTERACTIONS OF CONCERN TO DENTISTRY

• Increased CNS depression: alcohol, other CNS depressants
• Increased metabolism/hepatotoxicity: halothane, halogenated-hydrocarbon inhalation anesthetics
• Increased seizure threshold: haloperidol, phenothiazines
• Decreased effects of acetaminophen, corticosteroids, doxycycline, fenoprofen

• Lower blood concentrations: carbamazepine

SERIOUS REACTIONS

! Abrupt withdrawal after prolonged therapy may produce effects ranging from increased dreaming, nightmares, insomnia, tremor, diaphoresis, and vomiting to hallucinations, delirium, seizures, and status epilepticus.
! Skin eruptions may be a sign of a hypersensitivity reaction.
! Blood dyscrasias, hepatic disease, and hypocalcemia occur rarely.
! Overdose produces cold or clammy skin, hypothermia, and severe CNS depression, followed by high fever and coma.

DENTAL CONSIDERATIONS

General:
• Ask about type of epilepsy, seizure frequency, and quality of seizure control.
• After supine positioning, have patient sit upright for at least 2 min before standing to avoid orthostatic hypotension.
• Patients on chronic drug therapy may rarely have symptoms of blood dyscrasias, which can include infection, bleeding, and poor healing.
• Short appointments and a stress-reduction protocol may be required for anxious patients.
Consultations:
• Medical consultation may be required to assess disease control and patient's ability to tolerate stress.
• In a patient with symptoms of blood dyscrasias, request a medical consultation for blood studies and postpone dental treatment until normal values are reestablished.
Teach Patient/Family to:
• Encourage effective oral hygiene to prevent soft tissue inflammation.
• Use caution to prevent injury when using oral hygiene aids.
• Avoid mouth rinses with high alcohol content because of drying effects.

probenecid

proe-**ben**′-eh-sid
(Benuryl[CAN], Pro-Cid[AUS])
Do not confuse probenecid with procainamide.

CATEGORY AND SCHEDULE

Pregnancy Risk Category: C

Drug Class: Uricosuric

MECHANISM OF ACTION

A uricosuric that competitively inhibits reabsorption of uric acid at the proximal convoluted tubule. Also, inhibits renal tubular secretion of weak organic acids, such as penicillins.
Therapeutic Effect: Promotes uric acid excretion, reduces serum uric acid level, and increases plasma levels of penicillins and cephalosporins.

USES

Treatment of hyperuricemia in gout, gouty arthritis, adjunct to cephalosporin or penicillin treatment by reducing excretion and maintaining high blood levels

PHARMACOKINETICS

Hyperuricemia in gout, gouty arthritis, adjunct to cephalosporin or penicillin treatment by reducing excretion and maintaining high blood levels.

INDICATIONS AND DOSAGES

▸ **Gout**

PO

Adults, Elderly. Initially, 250 mg twice a day for 1 wk; then 500 mg twice a day. May increase by 500 mg q4wk. Maximum: 2–3 g/day. Maintenance: Dosage that maintains normal uric acid level.

▸ **As Adjunct to Penicillin or Cephalosporin Therapy to Prolong Antibiotic Plasma Levels**

PO

Adults, Elderly. 2 g/day in divided doses.

Children weighing more than 50 kg. Receive adult dosage.

Children 2–14 yr. Initially, 25 mg/kg. Maintenance: 40 mg/kg/day in 4 divided doses.

▸ **Gonorrhea**

PO

Adults, Elderly. 1 g 30 min before penicillin, ampicillin, or amoxicillin.

SIDE EFFECTS/ADVERSE REACTIONS

Frequent

Headache, anorexia, nausea, vomiting

Occasional

Lower back or side pain, rash, hives, itching, dizziness, flushed face, frequent urge to urinate, gingivitis

PRECAUTIONS AND CONTRAINDICATIONS

Blood dyscrasias, children younger than 2 yr, concurrent high-dose aspirin therapy, severe renal impairment, uric acid calculi

Caution:

Severe respiratory disease, lactation, cardiac edema

DRUG INTERACTIONS OF CONCERN TO DENTISTRY

- Increased toxicity: dapsone, indomethacin, other NSAIDs, acyclovir
- Increased sedation: benzodiazepines
- Decreased action: alcohol, salicylates
- Increased duration of action: penicillins, cephalosporins

SERIOUS REACTIONS

! Severe hypersensitivity reactions, including anaphylaxis, occur rarely and usually within a few hr after administration following previous use. If severe hypersensitivity reactions develop, discontinue the drug immediately and contact the physician.

! Pruritic maculopapular rash, possibly accompanied by malaise, fever, chills, arthralgia, nausea, vomiting, leukopenia, and aplastic anemias should be considered a toxic reaction.

DENTAL CONSIDERATIONS

General:

- Avoid prescribing aspirin-containing products.

Teach Patient/Family to:

- Encourage effective oral hygiene to prevent soft tissue inflammation.
- Use caution to prevent injury when using oral hygiene aids.
- Avoid mouth rinses with high alcohol content because of drying effects.

procaine

proe'-kane
(Novocain, Mericaine)

CATEGORY AND SCHEDULE
Pregnancy Risk Category: C

Drug Class: Anesthetics, local

MECHANISM OF ACTION

Procaine causes a reversible blockade of nerve conduction by decreasing nerve membrane permeability to sodium.
Therapeutic Effect: Local anesthesia.

USES

Treatment of pain by local infiltration, nerve block, spinal

PHARMACOKINETICS

Highly plasma protein-bound and distributed to all body tissues. Excreted in the urine (80%).
Half-life: 40 ± 9 sec in adults, 84 ± 30 sec in neonates.

INDICATIONS AND DOSAGES

▸ Spinal Anesthesia
Intrathecal
Adults. 0.5–1 ml of a 10% solution (50–100 mg) mixed with an equal volume of diluent injected into the third or fourth lumbar interspace (perineum and lower extremities).
2 ml of a 10% solution (200 mg) mixed with 1 ml of diluent injected into the second, third, or fourth interspace.

▸ Infiltration Anesthesia, Dental Anesthesia, Control of Severe Pain (Postherpetic Neuralgia, Cancer Pain, or Burns)
Topical
Adults. A single dose of 350–600 mg using a 0.25 or 0.5% solution. Use 0.9% sodium chloride for dilution.
Children. 15 mg/kg of a 0.5% solution is the maximum recommended dose.

▸ Peripheral or Sympathetic Nerve Block (Regional Anesthesia)
Topical
Adults. Up to 200 ml of a 0.5% solution (1 g), 100 ml of a 1% solution (1 g), or 50 ml of a 2% solution (1 g). The 2% solution should only be used when a small volume of anesthetic is required.

SIDE EFFECTS/ADVERSE REACTIONS

Frequent
Numbness or tingling of the face or mouth, pain at the injection site, dizziness, drowsiness, lightheadedness, nausea, vomiting, back pain, headache
Rare
Anxiety, restlessness, difficulty breathing, shortness of breath, seizures (convulsions), skin rash, itching (hives), slow, irregular heartbeat (palpitations), swelling of the face or mouth, tremors, QT prolongation, PR prolongation, atrial fibrillation, sinus bradycardia, hypotension, angina, cardiovascular collapse, fecal or urinary incontinence, loss of perineal sensation and sexual function, persistent motor, sensory, and/or autonomic (sphincter control) deficit

PRECAUTIONS AND CONTRAINDICATIONS

Hypersensitivity to ester local anesthetics, sulfites, PABA, patients on anticoagulant therapy, and in patients with coagulopathy, infection, thrombocytopenia. Should not be given by the intraarterial, intrathecal, or intravenous routes.

DRUG INTERACTIONS OF CONCERN TO DENTISTRY

• Possible prolonged effects of succinylcholine
• Increased CNS depression with all CNS depressants, especially in children and when larger doses are used
• Risk of cardiovascular side effects: rapid intravascular injection
• Suspected interference with antimicrobial activity of sulfonamides

SERIOUS REACTIONS

! Procaine-induced CNS toxicity usually presents with symptoms of stimulation, such as anxiety, apprehension, restlessness, nervousness, disorientation, confusion, dizziness, blurred vision, tremor, nausea/vomiting, shivering, or seizures. Subsequently, depressive symptoms can occur including drowsiness, unconsciousness, and respiratory arrest.
! If higher concentrations are introduced into the bloodstream, depression of cardiac excitability and contractility may cause AV block, ventricular arrhythmias, or cardiac arrest. CNS toxicity including dizziness, tongue numbness, visual impairment and disturbances, and muscular twitching appear to occur before cardiotoxic effects.
Alert
! Procaine should be used with caution in patients that have asthma because there is the increased risk of anaphylactoid reactions including bronchospasm and status asthmaticus.
Alert
! Local anesthetics can cause varying degrees of maternal, fetal, and neonatal toxicities during labor and obstetric delivery. Fetal heart rate should be monitored, as well as the presence of symptoms indicating fetal bradycardia, fetal acidosis, and maternal hypotension. Epidural procaine may cause decreased uterine contractility or maternal expulsion efforts and alter the forces of parturition.
Alert
! Unintentional fetal intracranial injection of procaine occurring during pudendal or paracervical block has been shown to lead to neonatal depression at birth and can lead to seizures within 6 hr as a result of high serum concentrations.

DENTAL CONSIDERATIONS

General:
• Not available for use in dental local anesthetic cartridges.

procarbazine hydrochloride

pro-**car′**-bah-zeen
high-droh-**klor′**-ide
(Matulane, Natulan[CAN])
Do not confuse procarbazine with dacarbazine.

CATEGORY AND SCHEDULE

Pregnancy Risk Category: D

Drug Class: Antineoplastic, miscellaneous

MECHANISM OF ACTION

A methylhydrazine derivative that inhibits DNA, RNA, and protein synthesis. May also directly damage DNA. Cell cycle-phase specific for S phase of cell division.
Therapeutic Effect: Causes cell death.

USES

Treatment of lymphoma, Hodgkin's disease, cancers resistant to other therapy

PHARMACOKINETICS

PO: Peak levels 1 hr; concentrates in liver, kidney, skin; metabolized in liver, excreted in urine.

INDICATIONS AND DOSAGES

▸ Advanced Hodgkin's Disease

PO

Adults, Elderly. Initially, 2–4 mg/kg/day as a single dose or in divided doses for 1 wk, then 4–6 mg/kg/day. Maintenance: 1–2 mg/kg/day.
Children. 50–100 mg/m^2/day for 10–14 days of a 28-day cycle. Continue until maximum response occurs, leukocyte count falls below $4000/mm^3$, or platelet count falls below $100,000/mm^3$. Maintenance: 50 mg/m^2/day.

SIDE EFFECTS/ADVERSE REACTIONS

Frequent
Severe nausea, vomiting, respiratory disorders (cough, effusion), myalgia, arthralgia, drowsiness, nervousness, insomnia, nightmares, diaphoresis, hallucinations, seizures
Occasional
Hoarseness, tachycardia, nystagmus, retinal hemorrhage, photophobia, photosensitivity, urinary frequency, nocturia, hypotension, diarrhea, stomatitis, paresthesia, unsteadiness, confusion, decreased reflexes, footdrop
Rare
Hypersensitivity reaction (dermatitis, pruritus, rash, urticaria), hyperpigmentation, alopecia

PRECAUTIONS AND CONTRAINDICATIONS

Myelosuppression, hypersensitivity, thrombocytopenia, bone marrow depression
Caution:
Renal disease, hepatic disease, radiation therapy

DRUG INTERACTIONS OF CONCERN TO DENTISTRY

- Increased CNS depression: barbiturates, antihistamines, narcotics
- Disulfiram-like reaction: ethyl alcohol
- Hypertension: indirect-acting sympathomimetics
- Increased anticholinergic effect: anticholinergic drugs, antihistamines
- Increased risk of severe toxic reactions: tricyclic antidepressants, meperidine and other opioids, tyramine-containing foods and other MAOIs; may include cyclobenzaprine and carbamazepine

SERIOUS REACTIONS

! Major toxic effects are myelosuppression manifested as hematologic toxicity (mainly leukopenia, thrombocytopenia, and anemia) and hepatotoxicity manifested as jaundice and ascites.
! UTIs may occur secondary to leukopenia.

DENTAL CONSIDERATIONS

General:
- Patients on chronic drug therapy may rarely have symptoms of blood dyscrasias, which can include infection, bleeding, and poor healing.
- Monitor vital signs at every appointment because of cardiovascular side effects.

• Consider semisupine chair position for patient comfort if GI side effects occur.
• Assess salivary flow as a factor in caries, periodontal disease, and candidiasis.
• After supine positioning, have patient sit upright for at least 2 min before standing to avoid orthostatic hypotension.
• Avoid dental light in patient's eyes; offer dark glasses for patient comfort.
• Avoid aspirin-containing products because of bleeding risk.
• Avoid use of gingival retraction cord with epinephrine.
• Patients receiving chemotherapy may require palliative treatment for stomatitis.

Consultations:
• In a patient with symptoms of blood dyscrasias, request a medical consultation for blood studies and postpone dental treatment until normal values are reestablished.
• Take precautions if dental surgery is anticipated and sedation or general anesthesia is required (risk of hypotension).

Teach Patient/Family to:
• Encourage effective oral hygiene to prevent soft tissue inflammation.
• Use caution to prevent injury when using oral hygiene aids.
• Report oral lesions, soreness, or bleeding to dentist.
• When chronic dry mouth occurs, advise patient to:
  • Avoid mouth rinses with high alcohol content because of drying effects.
  • Use daily home fluoride products to prevent caries.
  • Use sugarless gum, frequent sips of water, or saliva substitutes.

prochlorperazine

proe-klor-**per**′-ah-zeen
(Compazine, Stemetil[CAN], Stemzine[AUS])
Do not confuse prochlorperazine with chlorpromazine, or Compazine with Copaxone.

CATEGORY AND SCHEDULE

Pregnancy Risk Category: C

Drug Class: Antipsychotic

MECHANISM OF ACTION

A phenothiazine that acts centrally to inhibit or block dopamine receptors in the chemoreceptor trigger zone and peripherally to block the vagus nerve in the GI tract.
Therapeutic Effect: Relieves nausea and vomiting and improves psychotic conditions.

PHARMACOKINETICS

Route	Onset*	Peak	Duration
Tablets, oral solution	30–40 min	N/A	3–4 hr
Capsules (extended release)	30–40 min	N/A	10–12 hr
Rectal	60 min	N/A	3–4 hr

*As an antiemetic.

Variably absorbed after PO administration. Widely distributed. Metabolized in the liver and GI mucosa. Primarily excreted in urine. Unknown if removed by hemodialysis. ***Half-life:*** 23 hr.

INDICATIONS AND DOSAGES

▸ **Nausea and Vomiting**

PO

Adults, Elderly. 5–10 mg 3–4 times a day.

P

Children. 0.4 mg/kg/day in 3–4 divided doses.
PO (Extended-Release)
Adults, Elderly. 10 mg twice a day or 15 mg once a day.
IV
Adults, Elderly. 2.5–10 mg. May repeat q3–4h.
Children. 0.1–0.15 mg/kg/dose q8–12h. Maximum: 40 mg/day.
IM
Adults, Elderly. 5–10 mg q3–4h.
Children. 0.1–0.15 mg/kg/dose q8–12h. Maximum: 40 mg/day.
Rectal
Adults, Elderly. 25 mg twice a day.
Children. 0.4 mg/kg/day in 3–4 divided doses.

▸ **Psychosis**
PO
Adults, Elderly. 5–10 mg 3–4 times a day. Maximum: 150 mg/day.
Children. 2.5 mg 2–3 times a day. Maximum: 25 mg for children 6–12 yr; 20 mg for children 2–5 yr.
IM
Adults, Elderly. 10–20 mg q4h.
Children. 0.13 mg/kg/dose.

SIDE EFFECTS/ADVERSE REACTIONS

Frequent
Somnolence, hypotension, dizziness, fainting (commonly occurring after first dose, occasionally after subsequent doses, and rarely with oral form)
Occasional
Dry mouth, blurred vision, lethargy, constipation, diarrhea, myalgia, nasal congestion, peripheral edema, urine retention

PRECAUTIONS AND CONTRAINDICATIONS

Angle-closure glaucoma, CNS depression, coma, myelosuppression, severe cardiac or hepatic impairment, severe hypotension or hypertension
Caution:
Children younger than 2 yr, elderly

DRUG INTERACTIONS OF CONCERN TO DENTISTRY

- Increased sedation: other CNS depressants, alcohol, barbiturate anesthetics, opioid analgesics
- Hypotension, tachycardia: epinephrine
- Increased extrapyramidal effects: phenothiazines and related drugs (haloperidol, droperidol), metoclopramide
- Additive photosensitization: tetracyclines
- Increased anticholinergic effects: anticholinergics

SERIOUS REACTIONS

! Extrapyramidal symptoms appear to be dose-related and are divided into three categories: akathisia (marked by inability to sit still, tapping of feet), parkinsonian symptoms (including mask-like face, tremors, shuffling gait, hypersalivation), and acute dystonias (such as torticollis, opisthotonos, and oculogyric crisis). A dystonic reaction may also produce diaphoresis or pallor.
! Tardive dyskinesia, manifested as tongue protrusion, puffing of the cheeks, and puckering of the mouth, is a rare reaction that may be irreversible.
! Abrupt withdrawal after long-term therapy may precipitate nausea, vomiting, gastritis, dizziness, and tremors.
! Blood dyscrasias, particularly agranulocytosis and mild leukopenia, may occur.
! Prochlorperazine use may lower the seizure threshold.

DENTAL CONSIDERATIONS

General:

- Monitor vital signs at every appointment because of cardiovascular side effects.
- Patients on chronic drug therapy may rarely have symptoms of blood dyscrasias, which can include infection, bleeding, and poor healing.
- After supine positioning, have patient sit upright for at least 2 min before standing to avoid orthostatic hypotension.
- Assess salivary flow as a factor in caries, periodontal disease, and candidiasis.
- Avoid dental light in patient's eyes; offer dark glasses for patient comfort.
- Assess for presence of extrapyramidal motor symptoms, such as tardive dyskinesia and akathisia. Extrapyramidal motor activity may complicate dental treatment.
- Geriatric patients are more susceptible to drug effects; use lower dose.
- Use vasoconstrictors with caution, in low doses, and with careful aspiration.

Consultations:

- In a patient with symptoms of blood dyscrasias, request a medical consultation for blood studies and postpone dental treatment until normal values are reestablished.
- Take precautions if dental surgery is anticipated and anesthesia is required.
- If signs of tardive dyskinesia or akathisia are present, refer to physician.

Teach Patient/Family to:

- Encourage effective oral hygiene to prevent soft tissue inflammation.
- Use caution to prevent injury when using oral hygiene aids.
- Use powered tooth brush if patient has difficulty holding conventional devices.
- When chronic dry mouth occurs, advise patient to:
    - Avoid mouth rinses with high alcohol content because of drying effects.
    - Use daily home fluoride products to prevent caries.
    - Use sugarless gum, frequent sips of water, or saliva substitutes.

procyclidine

proe-**sye**′-kli-deen

(Kemadrin)

CATEGORY AND SCHEDULE

Pregnancy Risk Category: C

Drug Class: Anticholinergic, antidyskinetic

P

MECHANISM OF ACTION

An anticholinergic agent that exerts an atropine-like action and produces an antispasmodic effect on smooth muscle, is a potent mydriatic, and inhibits salivation.

Therapeutic Effect: Relieves symptoms of Parkinson's disease and drug-induced extrapyramidal symptoms.

USES

Treatment of Parkinson symptoms, extrapyramidal symptoms associated with neuroleptic drugs

PHARMACOKINETICS

Well absorbed from the GI tract. Protein binding: extensive. Metabolized in liver, undergoes extensive first-pass effect. Primarily excreted in urine. Unknown if removed by hemodialysis. ***Half-life:*** 7.7–16.1 hr.

INDICATIONS AND DOSAGES

▸ Drug-Induced Extrapyramidal Reactions

PO

Adults, Elderly. Initially, 2.5 mg 3 times a day. May increase by 2.5 mg/day as needed. Maintenance: 10–20 mg/day in divided doses 3 times a day.

▸ Parkinson's Disease

PO

Adults, Elderly. Initially, 2.5 mg 3 times a day after meals. Maintenance: 2.5–5 mg mg/day in divided doses 3 times a day after meals.

▸ Hepatic Function Impairment

PO

Adults, Elderly. 2.5–5 mg mg/day in divided doses twice a day after meals.

P

SIDE EFFECTS/ADVERSE REACTIONS

Frequent

Blurred vision, mydriasis, disorientation, light-headedness, nausea, vomiting, dry mouth, nose, throat, and lips

PRECAUTIONS AND CONTRAINDICATIONS

Angle-closure glaucoma

Elderly, lactation, tachycardia, prostatic hypertrophy, children, kidney or liver disease, drug abuse, hypotension, hypertension, psychiatric patients

DRUG INTERACTIONS OF CONCERN TO DENTISTRY

- Increased anticholinergic effect: antihistamines, anticholinergics, meperidine
- Increased CNS depression: alcohol, CNS depressants

SERIOUS REACTIONS

! Overdosage may vary from severe anticholinergic effects, such as unsteadiness, severe drowsiness, severe dryness of mouth, nose, or throat, tachycardia, shortness of breath, and skin flushing.

! Also produces severe paradoxical reaction, marked by hallucinations, tremor, seizures, and toxic psychosis.

DENTAL CONSIDERATIONS

General:

- Monitor vital signs at every appointment because of cardiovascular side effects.
- Assess salivary flow as a factor in caries, periodontal disease, and candidiasis.
- After supine positioning, have patient sit upright for at least 2 min before standing to avoid orthostatic hypotension.
- Avoid dental light in patient's eyes; offer dark glasses for patient comfort.
- Do not ingest sodium bicarbonate products, such as the Prophy-Jet air polishing system, until 1 hr after drug use.
- Place on frequent recall because of oral side effects.

Consultations:

- Medical consultation may be required to assess disease control.
- Medical consultation may be required to assess patient's ability to tolerate stress.

Teach Patient/Family to:

- Use powered tooth brush if patient has difficulty holding conventional devices.
- Encourage effective oral hygiene to prevent soft tissue inflammation.

- Use caution to prevent injury when using oral hygiene aids.
- When chronic dry mouth occurs, advise patient to:
  - Avoid mouth rinses with high alcohol content because of drying effects.
  - Use daily home fluoride products for anticaries effect.
  - Use sugarless gum, frequent sips of water, or saliva substitutes.

progesterone

proe-**jess**′-ter-one
(Crinone, Prochieve, Prometrium)

CATEGORY AND SCHEDULE

Pregnancy Risk Category: D

Drug Class: Contraceptives, hormones/hormone modifiers, progestins

MECHANISM OF ACTION

A natural steroid hormone that promotes mammary gland development and relaxes uterine smooth muscle.

Therapeutic Effect: Decreases abnormal uterine bleeding; transforms endometrium from proliferative to secretory in an estrogen-primed endometrium.

USES

Prevention of endometrial hyperplasia, secondary amenorrhea, abnormal uterine bleeding, treatment of infertility

PHARMACOKINETICS

IM, Rectal, Vaginal: Duration 24 hr, excreted in urine, feces; metabolized in liver.

INDICATIONS AND DOSAGES

▸ **Amenorrhea**

PO

Adults. 400 mg daily in evening for 10 days.

IM

Adults. 5–10 mg for 6–8 days. Withdrawal bleeding expected in 48–72 hr if ovarian activity produced proliferative endometrium.

Vaginal

Adults. Apply 45 mg (4% gel) every other day for 6 or fewer doses.

▸ **Abnormal Uterine Bleeding**

IM

Adults. 5–10 mg for 6 days. When estrogen given concomitantly, begin progesterone after 2 wk of estrogen therapy; discontinue when menstrual flow begins.

▸ **Prevention of Endometrial Hyperplasia**

PO

Adults. 200 mg in evening for 12 days per 28-day cycle in combination with daily conjugated estrogen.

▸ **Infertility**

Vaginal

Adults. 90 mg (8% gel) once a day (twice a day in women with partial or complete ovarian failure).

SIDE EFFECTS/ADVERSE REACTIONS

Frequent

Breakthrough bleeding or spotting at beginning of therapy, amenorrhea, change in menstrual flow, breast tenderness

Gel: drowsiness

Occasional

Edema, weight gain or loss, rash, pruritus, photosensitivity, skin pigmentation

Rare

Pain or swelling at injection site, acne, depression, alopecia, hirsutism

PRECAUTIONS AND CONTRAINDICATIONS

Breast cancer; history of active cerebral apoplexy; thromboembolic disorders or thrombophlebitis; missed abortion; severe hepatic dysfunction; undiagnosed vaginal bleeding; use as a pregnancy test

DRUG INTERACTIONS OF CONCERN TO DENTISTRY

- None reported

SERIOUS REACTIONS

! Thrombophlebitis, cerebrovascular disorders, retinal thrombosis, and pulmonary embolism occur rarely.

DENTAL CONSIDERATIONS

General:

- Determine why patient is taking the drug.
- Advise patient if dental drugs prescribed have a potential for photosensitivity.
- Monitor vital signs.
- Some patients may experience drowsiness; inquire before using CNS depressants.

Teach Patient/Family to:

- Not drive or perform other tasks requiring mental alertness.
- Encourage effective oral hygiene to prevent soft tissue inflammation.
- Prevent trauma when using oral hygiene aids.
- Update health and medication history if physician makes any changes in evaluation or drug regimens; include OTC, herbal, and nonherbal drugs in the update.

P

promethazine hydrochloride

proe-**meth′**-ah-zeen high-droh-**klor′**-ide
(Insomn-Eze[AUS], Phenadoz, Phenergan)
Do not confuse promethazine with promazine.

CATEGORY AND SCHEDULE

Pregnancy Risk Category: C

Drug Class: Antihistamine, H_1 receptor antagonist

MECHANISM OF ACTION

A phenothiazine that acts as an antihistamine, antiemetic, and sedative-hypnotic. As an antihistamine, inhibits histamine at histamine receptor sites. As an antiemetic, diminishes vestibular stimulation, depresses labyrinthine function, and acts on the chemoreceptor trigger zone. As a sedative-hypnotic, produces CNS depression by decreasing stimulation of the brainstem reticular formation.
Therapeutic Effect: Prevents allergic responses mediated by histamine, such as rhinitis, urticaria, and pruritus. Prevents and relieves nausea and vomiting.

USES

Motion sickness, rhinitis, allergy symptoms, sedation, nausea, preoperative or postoperative sedation

PHARMACOKINETICS

Route	Onset	Peak	Duration
PO	20 min	N/A	2–8 hr
IV	3–5 min	N/A	2–8 hr
IM	20 min	N/A	2–8 hr
Rectal	20 min	N/A	2–8 hr

Well absorbed from the GI tract after IM administration. Widely distributed. Metabolized in the liver. Primarily excreted in urine. Not removed by hemodialysis. ***Half-life:*** 16–19 hr.

INDICATIONS AND DOSAGES

▸ Allergic Symptoms

PO

Adults, Elderly. 6.25–12.5 mg 3 times a day plus 25 mg at bedtime.

Children. 0.1 mg/kg/dose (maximum: 12.5 mg) 3 times a day plus 0.5 mg/kg/dose (maximum: 25 mg) at bedtime.

IV, IM

Adults, Elderly. 25 mg. May repeat in 2 hr.

▸ Motion Sickness

PO

Adults, Elderly. 25 mg 30–60 min before departure; may repeat in 8–12 hr, then every morning on rising and before evening meal.

Children. 0.5 mg/kg 30–60 min before departure; may repeat in 8–12 hr, then every morning on rising and before evening meal.

▸ Prevention of Nausea and Vomiting

PO, IV, IM, Rectal

Adults, Elderly. 12.5–25 mg q4–6h as needed.

Children. 0.25–1 mg/kg q4–6h as needed.

▸ Preoperative and Postoperative Sedation; Adjunct to Analgesics

IV, IM

Adults, Elderly. 25–50 mg.

Children. 12.5–25 mg.

▸ Sedative

PO, IV, IM, Rectal

Adults, Elderly. 25–50 mg/dose. May repeat q4–6h as needed.

Children. 0.5–1 mg/kg/dose q6h as needed. Maximum: 50 mg/dose.

SIDE EFFECTS/ADVERSE REACTIONS

Expected

Somnolence, disorientation; in elderly, hypotension, confusion, syncope

Frequent

Dry mouth, nose, or throat; urine retention; thickening of bronchial secretions

Occasional

Epigastric distress, flushing, visual disturbances, hearing disturbances, wheezing, paresthesia, diaphoresis, chills

Rare

Dizziness, urticaria, photosensitivity, nightmares

PRECAUTIONS AND CONTRAINDICATIONS

Angle-closure glaucoma, GI or GU obstruction, severe CNS depression or coma

Caution:

Increased intraocular pressure, renal disease, cardiac disease, hypertension, bronchial asthma, seizure disorder, stenosed peptic ulcers, hyperthyroidism, prostatic hypertrophy, bladder neck obstruction

DRUG INTERACTIONS OF CONCERN TO DENTISTRY

- Increased CNS depression: alcohol, all CNS depressants
- Hypotension: general anesthetics
- Increased effect of anticholinergic drugs

SERIOUS REACTIONS

! Children may experience paradoxical reactions, such as excitation, nervousness, tremor, hyperactive reflexes, and seizures.

! Infants and young children have experienced CNS depression

P

manifested as respiratory depression, sleep apnea, and sudden infant death syndrome.
! Long-term therapy may produce extrapyramidal symptoms, such as dystonia (abnormal movements), pronounced motor restlessness (most frequently in children), and parkinsonian symptoms (most frequently in elderly patients).
! Blood dyscrasias, particularly agranulocytosis, occur rarely.

DENTAL CONSIDERATIONS

General:

- Determine why the patient is taking the drug.
- Patients on chronic drug therapy may rarely have symptoms of blood dyscrasias, which can include infection, bleeding, and poor healing.
- Monitor vital signs at every appointment because of cardiovascular side effects.
- Assess salivary flow as a factor in caries, periodontal disease, and candidiasis.
- Assess vital signs q30min after use as sedative.

Teach Patient/Family to:

- When chronic dry mouth occurs, advise patient to:
  - Avoid mouth rinses with high alcohol content because of drying effects.
  - Use daily home fluoride products to prevent caries.
  - Use sugarless gum, frequent sips of water, or saliva substitutes.

propafenone hydrochloride

proe-**pah′**-eh-none
high-droh-**klor′**-ide
(Rythmol, Rythmol SR)

CATEGORY AND SCHEDULE

Pregnancy Risk Category: C

Drug Class: Antidysrhythmic (class Ic)

MECHANISM OF ACTION

An antidysrhythmic that decreases the fast sodium current in Purkinje or myocardial cells. Decreases excitability and automaticity; prolongs conduction velocity and the refractory period.
Therapeutic Effect: Suppresses dysrhythmias.

USES

Treatment of documented life-threatening dysrhythmias; unapproved: sustained ventricular tachycardia

PHARMACOKINETICS

Peak 3–5 hr. ***Half-life:*** 2–10 hr; metabolized in liver; excreted in urine (metabolite).

INDICATIONS AND DOSAGES

▸ Documented, Life-Threatening Ventricular Arrhythmias, such as Sustained Ventricular Tachycardia

PO (Prompt-Release)
Adults, Elderly. Initially, 150 mg q8h; may increase at 3- to 4-day intervals to 225 mg q8h, then to 300 mg q8h. Maximum: 900 mg/day.
PO (Extended-Release)
Adults, Elderly. Initially, 225 mg q12h. May increase at 5-day intervals. Maximum: 425 mg q12h.

P

SIDE EFFECTS/ADVERSE REACTIONS

Frequent

Dizziness, nausea, vomiting, altered taste, constipation

Occasional

Headache, dyspnea, blurred vision, dyspepsia (heartburn, indigestion, epigastric pain)

Rare

Rash, weakness, dry mouth, diarrhea, edema, hot flashes

PRECAUTIONS AND CONTRAINDICATIONS

Bradycardia; bronchospastic disorders; cardiogenic shock; electrolyte imbalance; sinoatrial, AV, and intraventricular impulse generation or conduction disorders, such as sick sinus syndrome or AV block, without the presence of a pacemaker; uncontrolled CHF

Caution:

CHF, hypokalemia, hyperkalemia, recent MI, nonallergic bronchospasm, lactation, children, hepatic or renal disease

DRUG INTERACTIONS OF CONCERN TO DENTISTRY

• No specific interactions are reported; however, any drug that could affect the cardiac action of propafenone (other local anesthetics, vasoconstrictors, anticholinergics) should be used in the lowest effective dose.

SERIOUS REACTIONS

! Propafenone may produce or worsen existing arrhythmias.

! Overdose may produce hypotension, somnolence, bradycardia, and atrioventricular conduction disturbances.

DENTAL CONSIDERATIONS

General:

• Monitor vital signs at every appointment because of cardiovascular side effects.

• Avoid or limit dose of vasoconstrictor.

• Patients on chronic drug therapy may rarely have symptoms of blood dyscrasias, which can include infection, bleeding, and poor healing.

• Assess salivary flow as a factor in caries, periodontal disease, and candidiasis.

• Stress from dental procedures may compromise cardiovascular function; determine patient risk and consider a stress-reduction protocol.

• Consider semisupine chair position for patients with respiratory distress.

Consultations:

• In a patient with symptoms of blood dyscrasias, request a medical consultation for blood studies and postpone dental treatment until normal values are reestablished.

• Medical consultation may be required to assess disease control and patient's ability to tolerate stress.

Teach Patient/Family to:

• Encourage effective oral hygiene to prevent soft tissue inflammation.

• Use caution to prevent injury when using oral hygiene aids.

• When chronic dry mouth occurs, advise patient to:

  • Avoid mouth rinses with high alcohol content because of drying effects.

  • Use daily home fluoride products to prevent caries.

  • Use sugarless gum, frequent sips of water, or saliva substitutes.

propantheline

proe-**pan**′-the-leen
(Pro-Banthine, Propanthl[CAN])

CATEGORY AND SCHEDULE

Pregnancy Risk Category: C

Drug Class: Anticholinergic

MECHANISM OF ACTION

A quaternary ammonium compound that has anticholinergic properties and that inhibits action of acetylcholine at postganglionic parasympathetic sites.
Therapeutic Effect: Reduces gastric secretions and urinary frequency, urgency and urge incontinence.

USES

Treatment of peptic ulcer disease, irritable bowel syndrome, duodenography, urinary incontinence; unapproved: reduction in salivary flow

P

PHARMACOKINETICS

Onset occurs within 90 min. but less than 50% is absorbed from GI tract. Extensive hepatic metabolism. Excreted in the urine and feces. ***Half-life:*** 2.9 hr.

INDICATIONS AND DOSAGES

▸ **Peptic Ulcer**

PO

Adults, Elderly. 15 mg 3 times a day 30 min. before meals and 30 mg at bedtime.
Children. 1–2 mg/kg/day, divided q4–6h and at bedtime.

SIDE EFFECTS/ADVERSE REACTIONS

Frequent
Dry mouth, decreased sweating, constipation, hyperthermia
Occasional
Blurred vision, intolerance to light, urinary hesitancy, drowsiness, agitation, excitement
Rare
Confusion, increased intraocular pressure, orthostatic hypotension, tachycardia

PRECAUTIONS AND CONTRAINDICATIONS

GI or GU obstruction, myasthenia gravis, narrow-angle glaucoma, toxic megacolon, severe ulcerative colitis, unstable cardiovascular adjustment in acute hemorrhage, hypersensitivity to propantheline or other anticholinergics
Caution:
Hyperthyroidism, CAD, dysrhythmias, CHF, ulcerative colitis, hypertension, hiatal hernia, hepatic disease, renal disease, pregnancy category C, urinary retention, prostatic hypertrophy

DRUG INTERACTIONS OF CONCERN TO DENTISTRY

- Increased anticholinergic effect: other anticholinergic drugs
- Constipation, urinary retention: opioid analgesics
- Decreased absorption of ketoconazole; take doses 2 hr apart

SERIOUS REACTIONS

! Overdosage may produce temporary paralysis of ciliary muscle, pupillary dilation, tachycardia, palpitations, hot, dry, or flushed skin, absence of bowel sounds, hyperthermia, increased respiratory rate, ECG abnormalities, nausea, vomiting, rash over face or upper trunk, CNS stimulation, and psychosis, marked by agitation, restlessness, rambling speech, visual hallucinations, paranoid behavior, and delusions, followed by depression.

DENTAL CONSIDERATIONS

General:

- Assess salivary flow as a factor in caries, periodontal disease, and candidiasis.
- Avoid dental light in patient's eyes; offer dark glasses for patient comfort.
- Place on frequent recall because of oral side effects.
- Avoid prescribing aspirin-containing products.
- Consider semisupine chair position for patient comfort because of GI effects of disease.
- Caution against exercise or exposure to heat or bright light while taking.

Consultations:

- Physician should be informed if significant xerostomic side effects occur (e.g., increased caries, sore tongue, problems eating or swallowing, difficulty wearing prosthesis) so that a medication change can be considered.

Teach Patient/Family to:

- When chronic dry mouth occurs, advise patient to:
    - Avoid mouth rinses with high alcohol content because of drying effects.
    - Use daily home fluoride products to prevent caries.
    - Use sugarless gum, frequent sips of water, or saliva substitutes.

propofol

pro-poe-**fall′**
(Diprivan, Recofol[AUS])

CATEGORY AND SCHEDULE

Pregnancy Risk Category: B

Drug Class: General anesthetic

MECHANISM OF ACTION

A rapidly acting general anesthetic that inhibits sympathetic vasoconstrictor nerve activity and decreases vascular resistance.
Therapeutic Effect: Produces hypnosis rapidly.

USES

Induction or maintenance of anesthesia as part of balanced anesthetic technique, in-patient sedation

PHARMACOKINETICS

Route	Onset	Peak	Duration
IV	40 sec	N/A	3–10 min

Rapidly and extensively distributed. Protein binding: 97%–99%. Metabolized in the liver. Primarily excreted in urine. Unknown if removed by hemodialysis. ***Half-life:*** 3–12 hr.

INDICATIONS AND DOSAGES

▸ **Intensive Care Unit Sedation**

IV

Adults, Elderly. Initially, 0.3 mg/kg/hr. May increase by 0.3–0.6 mg/kg/hr q5–10 min until desired effect is obtained. Maintenance: 0.3–3 mg/kg/h.

▸ **Anesthesia**

IV

Adults, American Society of Anesthesiologists (ASA) I and II patients. 2–2.5 mg/kg (about 40 mg q10sec until onset of anesthesia). Maintenance: 0.1–0.2 mg/kg/min.
Elderly, Debilitated, Hypovolemic, ASA III or IV patients. 1–1.5 mg/kg (about 20 mg q10sec until onset of anesthesia). Maintenance: 0.05–0.1 mg/kg/min.
Children 3 yr and older, ASA I or II patients. 2.5–3.5 mg/kg (lower dosage for ASA III or IV patients).

P

Children 2 mo–16 yr. Maintenance dose: 0.125–0.15 mg/kg/min.

SIDE EFFECTS/ADVERSE REACTIONS

Frequent

Involuntary muscle movements, apnea (common during induction; lasts longer than 60 sec), hypotension, nausea, vomiting, IV site burning or stinging

Occasional

Twitching, bucking, jerking, thrashing, headache, dizziness, bradycardia, hypertension, fever, abdominal cramps, paresthesia, coldness, cough, hiccups, facial flushing, greenish-colored urine

Rare

Rash, dry mouth, agitation, confusion, myalgia, thrombophlebitis

PRECAUTIONS AND CONTRAINDICATIONS

Impaired cerebral circulation, increased intracranial pressure

Caution:

Elderly, debilitated, respiratory depression, severe respiratory disorders, cardiac dysrhythmias, pregnancy category B, labor and delivery, lactation, children younger than 3 yr, epilepsy

DRUG INTERACTIONS OF CONCERN TO DENTISTRY

• Increased CNS depression: alcohol, narcotics, sedative-hypnotics, antipsychotics, skeletal muscle relaxants, inhalational anesthetics

SERIOUS REACTIONS

! A continuous infusion or repeated intermittent infusions of propofol may result in extreme somnolence, respiratory depression, and circulatory depression.

! Too-rapid IV administration may produce severe hypotension, respiratory depression, and involuntary muscle movements.

! The patient may experience an acute allergic reaction, characterized by abdominal pain, anxiety, restlessness, dyspnea, erythema, hypotension, pruritus, rhinitis, and urticaria.

DENTAL CONSIDERATIONS

General:

- Monitor vital signs at regular intervals during recovery after use as anesthetic.
- Have someone escort patient to and from dental office if used for general anesthesia.
- Geriatric patients are more susceptible to drug effects; use lower dose.
- Use only with resuscitative equipment available and only by qualified persons trained in general anesthesia.
- Monitor:
  - Injection site: phlebitis, burning/stinging.
  - ECG for changes: PVC, PAC, ST-segment changes.
  - Allergic reactions: hives.
- Administer:
  - After diluting with D5W, use only glass containers when mixing; not stable in plastic.
  - By IV injection only.
  - Alone; do not mix with other agents before using.
- Perform/provide:
  - Storage in light-resistant area at room temperature.
  - Coughing, turning, deep breathing for postoperative patients.
  - Safety measures: side rails, night light, call bell within reach.

P

- Evaluate:
  - CNS changes: movement, jerking, tremors, dizziness, LOC, pupil reaction.
  - Respiratory dysfunction: respiratory depression, character, rate, rhythm; notify physician if respirations are <10/min.
  - Treatment of overdose: discontinue drug, artificial ventilation, administer vasopressor agents or anticholinergics.

propranolol hydrochloride

proe-**pran′**-oh-lole high-droh-**klor′**-ide
(Apo-Propranolol[CAN], Deralin[AUS], Inderal, Inderal LA, InnoPran XL, Nu-Propranolol[CAN], Propranolol Intensol)
Do not confuse Inderal with Adderall or Isordil, or propranolol with Pravachol.

CATEGORY AND SCHEDULE

Pregnancy Risk Category: C (D if used in second or third trimester)

Drug Class: Nonselective β-adrenergic blocker

MECHANISM OF ACTION

An antihypertensive, antianginal, antiarrhythmic, and antimigraine agent that blocks β_1- and β_2-adrenergic receptors. Decreases oxygen requirements. Slows AV conduction and increases refractory period in AV node. Large doses increase airway resistance. ***Therapeutic Effect:*** Slows sinus heart rate; decreases cardiac output, B/P, and myocardial ischemia severity. Exhibits antiarrhythmic activity.

USES

Treatment of chronic stable angina pectoris, hypertension, supraventricular dysrhythmias (class II), migraine, MI prophylaxis, pheochromocytoma, essential tremor, hypertrophic cardiomyopathy, anxiety

PHARMACOKINETICS

Route	Onset	Peak	Duration
PO	1–2 hr	N/A	6 hr

Well absorbed from the GI tract. Protein binding: 93%. Widely distributed. Metabolized in the liver. Primarily excreted in urine. Not removed by hemodialysis. ***Half-life:*** 3–5 hr.

INDICATIONS AND DOSAGES

▸ **Hypertension**

PO

Adults, Elderly. Initially, 40 mg twice a day. May increase dose q3–7 days. Range: Up to 320 mg/day in divided doses. Maximum: 640 mg/day.

Children. Initially, 0.5–1 mg/kg/day in divided doses q6–12h. May increase at 3- to 5-day intervals. Usual dose: 1–5 mg/kg/day. Maximum: 16 mg/kg/day.

▸ **Angina**

PO

Adults, Elderly. 80–320 mg/day in divided doses. Long acting: Initially, 80 mg/day. Maximum: 320 mg/day.

▸ **Arrhythmias**

IV

Adults, Elderly. 1 mg/dose. May repeat q5min. Maximum: 5 mg total dose.

Children. 0.01–0.1 mg/kg.
Maximum: infants, 1 mg; children, 3 mg.
PO
Adults, Elderly. Initially, 10–20 mg q6–8h. May gradually increase dose. Range: 40–320 mg/day.
Children. Initially, 0.5–1 mg/kg/day in divided doses q6–8h. May increase q3–5 days. Usual dosage: 2–4 mg/kg/day. Maximum: 16 mg/kg/day or 60 mg/day.

▸ **Life-Threatening Arrhythmias**
IV
Adults, Elderly. 0.5–3 mg. Repeat once in 2 min. Give additional doses at intervals of at least 4 hr.
Children. 0.01–0.1 mg/kg.

▸ **Hypertrophic Subaortic Stenosis**
PO
Adults, Elderly. 20–40 mg in 3–4 divided doses. Or 80–160 mg/day as extended-release capsule.

▸ **Adjunct to α-Blocking Agents to Treat Pheochromocytoma**
PO
Adults, Elderly. 60 mg/day in divided doses with α-blocker for 3 days before surgery. Maintenance (inoperable tumor): 30 mg/day with α-blocker.

▸ **Migraine Headache**
PO
Adults, Elderly. 80 mg/day in divided doses. Or 80 mg once daily as extended-release capsule. Increase up to 160–240 mg/day in divided doses.
Children. 0.6–1.5 mg/kg/day in divided doses q8h. Maximum: 4 mg/kg/day.

▸ **Reduction of Cardiovascular Mortality and Reinfarction in Patients with Previous MI**
PO
Adults, Elderly. 180–240 mg/day in divided doses.

▸ **Essential Tremor**
PO
Adults, Elderly. Initially, 40 mg twice a day increased up to 120–320 mg/day in 3 divided doses.

SIDE EFFECTS/ADVERSE REACTIONS

Frequent
Diminished sexual ability, drowsiness, difficulty sleeping, unusual fatigue or weakness
Occasional
Bradycardia, depression, sensation of coldness in extremities, diarrhea, constipation, anxiety, nasal congestion, nausea, vomiting
Rare
Altered taste, dry eyes, pruritus, paresthesia

PRECAUTIONS AND CONTRAINDICATIONS

Asthma, bradycardia, cardiogenic shock, COPD, heart block, Raynaud's syndrome, uncompensated CHF
Caution:
Diabetes mellitus, renal disease, lactation, hyperthyroidism, COPD, hepatic disease, children, myasthenia gravis, peripheral vascular disease, hypotension

DRUG INTERACTIONS OF CONCERN TO DENTISTRY

- Decreased hypotensive effect: indomethacin, NSAIDs
- Increased hypotension, myocardial depression: hydrocarbon inhalation anesthetics
- Hypertension, bradycardia: sympathomimetics (epinephrine, ephedrine)
- Suspected increase in plasma levels: diphenhydramine
- Slow metabolism of lidocaine
- Decreased effects: didanosine (take 2 hr before didanosine tabs)

SERIOUS REACTIONS

! Overdose may produce profound bradycardia and hypotension.
! Abrupt withdrawal may result in sweating, palpitations, headache, and tremors.
! Propranolol administration may precipitate CHF and MI in patients with cardiac disease, thyroid storm in those with thyrotoxicosis, and peripheral ischemia in those with existing peripheral vascular disease.
! Hypoglycemia may occur in patients with previously controlled diabetes.

DENTAL CONSIDERATIONS

General:

- Monitor vital signs at every appointment because of cardiovascular side effects.
- Patients on chronic drug therapy may rarely have symptoms of blood dyscrasias, which can include infection, bleeding, and poor healing.
- Limit use of sodium-containing products, such as saline IV fluids, for patients with a dietary salt restriction.
- Assess salivary flow as a factor in caries, periodontal disease, and candidiasis.
- After supine positioning, have patient sit upright for at least 2 min before standing to avoid orthostatic hypotension.
- Stress from dental procedures may compromise cardiovascular function; determine patient risk.
- Short appointments and a stress-reduction protocol may be required for anxious patients.
- Consider semisupine chair position for patients with respiratory distress.
- Use vasoconstrictors with caution, in low doses, and with careful aspiration. Avoid use of gingival retraction cord with epinephrine.

Consultations:

- In a patient with symptoms of blood dyscrasias, request a medical consultation for blood studies and postpone dental treatment until normal values are reestablished.
- Medical consultation may be required to assess disease control and patient's ability to tolerate stress.

Teach Patient/Family to:

- Use caution to prevent injury when using oral hygiene aids.
- Encourage effective oral hygiene to prevent soft tissue inflammation.
- When chronic dry mouth occurs, advise patient to:
  - Avoid mouth rinses with high alcohol content because of drying effects.
  - Use daily home fluoride products to prevent caries.
  - Use sugarless gum, frequent sips of water, or saliva substitutes.

P

propylthiouracil

proe-pill-thye-oh-**yoor′**-ah-sill
(Propylthiouracil, Propyl-Thyracil[CAN])

CATEGORY AND SCHEDULE

Pregnancy Risk Category: D

Drug Class: Thyroid hormone antagonist

MECHANISM OF ACTION

A thiourea derivative that blocks oxidation of iodine in the thyroid gland and blocks synthesis of thyroxine and triiodothyronine.

Therapeutic Effect: Inhibits synthesis of thyroid hormone.

USES

Preparation for thyroidectomy, thyrotoxic crisis, hyperthyroidism, thyroid storm

PHARMACOKINETICS

PO: Onset 30–40 min, duration 2–4 hr. ***Half-life:*** 1–2 hr; excreted in urine, bile, breast milk; crosses placenta.

INDICATIONS AND DOSAGES

▸ Hyperthyroidism

PO

Adults, Elderly. Initially: 300–450 mg/day in divided doses q8h. Maintenance: 100–150 mg/day in divided doses q8–12h.

Children. Initially: 5–7 mg/kg/day in divided doses q8h. Maintenance: 33%–66% of initial dose in divided doses q8–12h.

Neonates. 5–10 mg/kg/day in divided doses q8h.

P

SIDE EFFECTS/ADVERSE REACTIONS

Frequent

Urticaria, rash, pruritus, nausea, skin pigmentation, hair loss, headache, paresthesia

Occasional

Somnolence, lymphadenopathy, vertigo

Rare

Drug fever, lupus-like syndrome

PRECAUTIONS AND CONTRAINDICATIONS

Infection, bone marrow depression, hepatic disease

Caution:

Infection, bone marrow depression, hepatic disease

DRUG INTERACTIONS OF CONCERN TO DENTISTRY

- Increased cardiovascular side effects in uncontrolled patients: anticholinergics and sympathomimetics
- Patients with uncontrolled hyperthyroidism are at risk when vasoconstrictors are used
- Patients with uncontrolled hypothyroidism may be more responsive to CNS depressants

SERIOUS REACTIONS

! Agranulocytosis as long as 4 mo after therapy, pancytopenia, and fatal hepatitis have occurred.

DENTAL CONSIDERATIONS

General:

- Patients on chronic drug therapy may rarely have symptoms of blood dyscrasias, which can include infection, bleeding, and poor healing.
- Patients with uncontrolled hyperthyroidism should not be treated in the dental office until thyroid values are normalized.
- Uncontrolled patients should be referred for medical evaluation and treatment.
- Monitor vital signs at every appointment because of cardiovascular side effects.
- Consider semisupine chair position for patient comfort if GI side effects occur, and stress-reduction protocol.

Consultations:

- Medical consultation may be required to assess disease control and patient's ability to tolerate stress.

protein C, human
(Ceprotin)

CATEGORY AND SCHEDULE
Pregnancy Risk Category: C

Drug Class: Vitamin K antagonist, anticoagulant

MECHANISM OF ACTION
Protein C is a precursor of a vitamin K-dependent anticoagulant glycoprotein. Once activated, protein C inactivates factors V and VIII resulting in decreased thrombin formation. Protein C also has profibrinolytic effects.
Therapeutic Effect: Decrease in thrombin formation.

USES
Severe congenital Protein C deficiency for the prevention and treatment of venous thrombosis and purpura fulminans, replacement therapy for pediatric and adult patients

PHARMACOKINETICS
Half-life: 4.9–14.7 hr, median of 9.8 hr.

INDICATIONS AND DOSAGES
▸ **Severe Congenital Protein C Deficiency for the Prevention and Treatment of Venous Thrombosis and Purpura Fulminans, Replacement Therapy for Pediatric and Adult Patients**
Injection, Powder for Reconstitution
Adults. Ceprotin dosing schedule for acute episodes, short-term prophylaxis, and long-term prophylaxis:

	Initial Dose	Subsequent Dose	Maintenance Dose
Acute episode/ short-term prophylaxis	100–120 IU/kg	60–80 IU/kg q6 hr	45–60 IU/kg q6 or 12 hr
Long-term prophylaxis	NA	NA	45–60 IU/kg q12 hr

SIDE EFFECTS/ADVERSE REACTIONS
Occasional
Bleeding, rash, itching, and light-headedness

PRECAUTIONS AND CONTRAINDICATIONS
Hypersensitivity to protein C or any component of the formulation including mouse proteins and/or heparin
Caution:
Made from pooled human plasma; possibility of transmitting infectious agents may occur
Concurrent use with tPA and/or other anticoagulants
Renal impairment (contains sodium)
Elderly
Immunocompromised patients
Sodium-restricted patients (e.g., heart failure patients)

DRUG INTERACTIONS OF CONCERN TO DENTISTRY
• tPA and/or anticoagulants: may increase risk of bleeding

SERIOUS REACTIONS
! Hemothorax has been reported.
! Hypotension may occur.
! Contains heparin; if heparin-induced thrombocytopenia is suspected, check platelets.

DENTAL CONSIDERATIONS

General:

• Do not discontinue drug for routine dental procedures.

• Monitor vital signs at every appointment because of cardiovascular side effects.

• Assess salivary flow as a factor in caries, periodontal disease, and candidiasis.

• Stress from dental procedures may compromise cardiovascular function; determine patient risk.

Consultations:

• Medical consultation may be required to assess disease control.

Teach Patient/Family to:

• Report oral lesions, soreness, or bleeding to dentist.

• When chronic dry mouth occurs, advise patient to:

  • Avoid mouth rinses with high alcohol content because of drying effects.

  • Use daily home fluoride products for anticaries effect.

  • Use sugarless gum, frequent sips of water, or saliva substitutes.

P

protriptyline

proe-**trip**′-ti-leen

(Vivactil, Triptil[CAN])

CATEGORY AND SCHEDULE

Pregnancy Risk Category: C

Drug Class: Tricyclic antidepressant

MECHANISM OF ACTION

A tricyclic antidepressant that increases synaptic concentration of norepinephrine and/or serotonin by inhibiting their reuptake by presynaptic membranes.

Therapeutic Effect: Produces antidepressant effect.

USES

Depression; unapproved use: adjunctive use in narcolepsy and attention-deficit disorders

PHARMACOKINETICS

Well absorbed from the GI tract. Protein binding: 92%. Widely distributed. Extensively metabolized in liver. Excreted in urine. Not removed by hemodialysis. ***Half-life:*** 54–92 hr.

INDICATIONS AND DOSAGES

▸ Depression

PO

Adults. 15–40 mg/day divided into 3–4 doses/day. Maximum: 600 mg/day.

Elderly. 5 mg 3 times a day. May increase gradually.

SIDE EFFECTS/ADVERSE REACTIONS

Frequent

Drowsiness, weight gain, fatigue, dry mouth, blurred vision, constipation, delayed micturition, postural hypotension, diaphoresis, disturbed concentration, increased appetite, urinary retention

Occasional

GI disturbances, such as nausea, diarrhea, GI distress, metallic taste sensation

Rare

Paradoxical reaction, marked by agitation, restlessness, nightmares, insomnia, extrapyramidal symptoms, particularly fine hand tremor

PRECAUTIONS AND CONTRAINDICATIONS

Acute recovery period after myocardial infarction, coadministration with cisapride, use

of MAOIs within 14 days, hypersensitivity to protriptyline or any component of the formulation
Caution:
Suicidal patients, severe depression, increased intraocular pressure, narrow-angle glaucoma, urinary retention, cardiac disease, hepatic disease, hyperthyroidism, electroshock therapy, elective surgery, MAOIs

DRUG INTERACTIONS OF CONCERN TO DENTISTRY

• Increased anticholinergic effects: muscarinic blockers, antihistamines, phenothiazines
• Increased effects of direct-acting sympathomimetics (epinephrine, levonordefrin)
• Possible risk of increased CNS depression: alcohol, barbiturates, benzodiazepines, and other CNS depressants
• Decreased antihypertensive effects of: clonidine, guanadrel, guanethidine
• Avoid concurrent use with St. John's wort (herb)

SERIOUS REACTIONS

! High dosage may produce confusion, seizures, severe drowsiness, arrhythmias, fever, hallucinations, agitation, shortness of breath, vomiting, and unusual tiredness or weakness.
! Abrupt withdrawal from prolonged therapy may produce severe headache, malaise, nausea, vomiting, and vivid dreams.

DENTAL CONSIDERATIONS

General:
• Monitor vital signs at every appointment because of cardiovascular side effects.
• Consider stress-reduction protocol for anxious patients.
• Assess salivary flow as a factor in caries, periodontal disease, and candidiasis.
• Patients on chronic drug therapy may rarely have symptoms of blood dyscrasias, which can include infection, bleeding, and poor healing.
• After supine positioning, have patient sit upright for at least 2 min before standing to avoid orthostatic hypotension.
• Use vasoconstrictors with caution, in low doses, and with careful aspiration. Avoid use of gingival retraction cord with epinephrine.
• Place on frequent recall because of oral side effects.
Consultations:
• In a patient with symptoms of blood dyscrasias, request a medical consultation for blood studies and postpone dental treatment until normal values are reestablished.
• Medical consultation may be required to assess disease control.
• Physician should be informed if significant xerostomic side effects occur (e.g., increased caries, sore tongue, problems eating or swallowing, difficulty wearing prosthesis) so that a medication change can be considered.
Teach Patient/Family to:
• Encourage effective oral hygiene to prevent soft tissue inflammation.
• Use caution to prevent injury when using oral hygiene aids.
• When chronic dry mouth occurs, advise patient to:
  • Avoid mouth rinses with high alcohol content because of drying effects.
  • Use daily home fluoride products to prevent caries.
  • Use sugarless gum, frequent sips of water, or saliva substitutes.

pseudoephedrine

soo-doe-eh-**fed'**-rin

(Balminil Decongestant[CAN], Bio Contac Cold 12 Hour Relief Non Drowsy[CAN], Decofed, Dimetapp 12 Hour Non Drowsy Extentabs, Dimetapp Decongestant, Dimetapp Sinus Liquid Caps[AUS], Genaphed, PMS-Pseudoephedrine[CAN], Robidrine[CAN], Sudafed, Sudafed 12h[AUS], Sudafed 12 Hour, Sudafed 24 Hour)

CATEGORY AND SCHEDULE

Pregnancy Risk Category: C
OTC

Drug Class: α-adrenergic agonist

MECHANISM OF ACTION

A sympathomimetic that directly stimulates α-adrenergic and β-adrenergic receptors.
Therapeutic Effect: Produces vasoconstriction of respiratory tract mucosa; shrinks nasal mucous membranes; reduces edema and nasal congestion.

USES

Decongestant, treatment of nasal congestion

PHARMACOKINETICS

Route	Onset	Peak	Duration
PO	15–30 min	N/A	4–6 hr
PO	N/A	N/A	8–12 hr

Well absorbed from the GI tract. Partially metabolized in the liver. Primarily excreted in urine. Not removed by hemodialysis. ***Half-life:*** 9–16 hr (children, 3.1 hr).

INDICATIONS AND DOSAGES

▸ **Decongestant**

PO

Adults, Children 12 yr and older. 60 mg q4–6h. Maximum: 240 mg/day.

Children 6–11 yr. 30 mg q6h. Maximum: 120 mg/day.

Children 2–5 yr. 15 mg q6h. Maximum: 60 mg/day.

Children younger than 2 yr. 4 mg/kg/day in divided doses q6h.

Elderly. 30–60 mg q6h as needed.

PO (Extended Release)

Adults, Children 12 yr and older. 120 mg q12h.

SIDE EFFECTS/ADVERSE REACTIONS

Occasional

Nervousness, restlessness, insomnia, tremor, headache

Rare

Diaphoresis, weakness

PRECAUTIONS AND CONTRAINDICATIONS

Breast-feeding women, coronary artery disease, severe hypertension, use within 14 days of MAOIs

Caution:

Cardiac disorders, hyperthyroidism, diabetes mellitus, prostatic hypertrophy

DRUG INTERACTIONS OF CONCERN TO DENTISTRY

- Dysrhythmia: hydrocarbon inhalation anesthetics
- Increased CNS, cardiovascular effects: sympathomimetics

SERIOUS REACTIONS

! Large doses may produce tachycardia, palpitations (particularly in patients with cardiac disease), light-headedness, nausea, and vomiting.

! Overdose in patients older than 60 yr may result in hallucinations, CNS depression, and seizures.

DENTAL CONSIDERATIONS

General:

- Assess salivary flow as a factor in caries, periodontal disease, and candidiasis.
- Monitor vital signs at every appointment because of cardiovascular side effects.
- Consider semisupine chair position for patient comfort if GI side effects occur.

Teach Patient/Family to:

- Use powered tooth brush if patient has difficulty holding conventional devices.
- When chronic dry mouth occurs, advise patient to:
  - Avoid mouth rinses with high alcohol content because of drying effects.
  - Use daily home fluoride products to prevent caries.
  - Use sugarless gum, frequent sips of water, or saliva substitutes.

pyrazinamide

pye-ra-**zin′**-ah-mide
(Pyrazinamide, Tebrazid[CAN], Zinamide[AUS])

CATEGORY AND SCHEDULE

Pregnancy Risk Category: C

Drug Class: Antitubercular

MECHANISM OF ACTION

An antitubercular whose exact mechanism of action is unknown.
Therapeutic Effect: Either bacteriostatic or bactericidal, depending on the drug's concentration at the infection site and the susceptibility of infecting bacteria.

USES

Treatment of tuberculosis (TB), as an adjunct with other drugs

PHARMACOKINETICS

PO: Peak 2 hr. ***Half-life:*** 9–10 hr; metabolized in liver, excreted in urine (metabolites/unchanged drug).

INDICATIONS AND DOSAGES

▸ TB (in Combination with Other Antituberculars)

PO

Adults. 15–30 mg/kg/day in 1–4 doses. Maximum: 3 g/day.
Children. 20–40 mg/kg/day in 1 or 2 doses. Maximum: 2 g/day.

SIDE EFFECTS/ADVERSE REACTIONS

Frequent

Arthralgia, myalgia (usually mild and self-limiting)

Rare

Hypersensitivity reaction (rash, pruritus, urticaria), photosensitivity, gouty arthritis

PRECAUTIONS AND CONTRAINDICATIONS

Severe hepatic dysfunction

Caution:

Children younger than 13 yr

DRUG INTERACTIONS OF CONCERN TO DENTISTRY

- None reported

SERIOUS REACTIONS

! Hepatotoxicity, gouty arthritis, thrombocytopenia, and anemia occur rarely.

DENTAL CONSIDERATIONS

General:

- Determine why the patient is taking the drug (for prophylaxis or active therapy).
- Determine that noninfectious status exists by ensuring that (1) anti-TB drugs have been taken for longer than 3 wk, (2) culture has confirmed TB susceptibility to antiinfectives, (3) patient has had three consecutive negative sputum smears, and (4) patient is not in the coughing stage.
- Do not treat patients with active tuberculosis.

Consultations:

- Medical consultation may be required to assess disease control.

Teach Patient/Family to:

- Take medications for full length of regimen to ensure effectiveness of treatment and to prevent the emergence of resistant strains.

P

pyridostigmine bromide

peer-id-oh-**stig′**-meen **broe′**-mide
(Mestinon, Mestinon SR[CAN], Mestinon Timespan)
Do not confuse pyridostigmine with physostigmine or Mesitonin with Mesantoin or Metatensin.

CATEGORY AND SCHEDULE

Pregnancy Risk Category: C

Drug Class: Cholinergic

MECHANISM OF ACTION

A cholinergic that prevents destruction of acetylcholine by inhibiting the enzyme acetylcholinesterase, thus enhancing impulse transmission across the myoneural junction.

Therapeutic Effect: Produces miosis; increases tone of intestinal, skeletal muscle; stimulates salivary and sweat gland secretions.

USES

Nondepolarizing muscle relaxant antagonist, myasthenia gravis

PHARMACOKINETICS

PO: Onset 20–30 min, duration 3–6 hr
IM/IV/Subcutaneous: Onset 2–15 min, duration 2.5–4 hr; metabolized in liver, excreted in urine

INDICATIONS AND DOSAGES

▸ Myasthenia Gravis

PO
Adults, Elderly. Initially, 60 mg 3 times a day. Dosage increased at 48-hr intervals. Maintenance: 60 mg–1.5 g a day.
PO (Extended-Release)
Adults, Elderly. 180–540 mg once or twice a day with at least a 6 hr interval between doses.
IV, IM
Adults, Elderly. 2 mg q2–3h.
Children, Neonates. 0.05–0.15 mg/kg/dose. Maximum single dose: 10 mg.

▸ Reversal of Nondepolarizing Neuromuscular Blockade

IV
Adults, Elderly. 10–20 mg with, or shortly after, 0.6–1.2 mg atropine sulfate or 0.3–0.6 mg glycopyrrolate.
Children. 0.1–0.25 mg/kg/dose preceded by atropine or glycopyrrolate.

SIDE EFFECTS/ADVERSE REACTIONS

Frequent

Miosis, increased GI and skeletal muscle tone, bradycardia,

constriction of bronchi and ureters, diaphoresis, increased salivation

Occasional

Headache, rash, temporary decrease in diastolic B/P with mild reflex tachycardia, short periods of atrial fibrillation (in hyperthyroid patients), marked drop in B/P (in hypertensive patients)

PRECAUTIONS AND CONTRAINDICATIONS

Mechanical GI or urinary tract obstruction

Caution:

Seizure disorders, bronchial asthma, coronary occlusion, hyperthyroidism, dysrhythmias, peptic ulcer, megacolon, poor GI motility, elderly, lactation

DRUG INTERACTIONS OF CONCERN TO DENTISTRY

• Decreased effects: atropine, scopolamine, and other anticholinergic drugs; methocarbamol

• Reduced rate of metabolism of ester local anesthetics

• Avoid anticholinergic drugs to control excessive salivation

SERIOUS REACTIONS

! Overdose may produce a cholinergic crisis, manifested as increasingly severe muscle weakness that appears first in muscles involving chewing and swallowing and is followed by muscle weakness of the shoulder girdle and upper extremities, respiratory muscle paralysis, and pelvis girdle and leg muscle paralysis. If overdose occurs, stop all cholinergic drugs and immediately administer 1–4 mg atropine sulfate IV for adults or 0.01 mg/kg for infants and children younger than 12 yr.

DENTAL CONSIDERATIONS

General:

• Monitor vital signs at every appointment because of cardiovascular and respiratory side effects.

• After supine positioning, have patient sit upright for at least 2 min before standing to avoid orthostatic hypotension.

• Schedule short appointments because of effects of disease on oral musculature.

• Avoid dental light in patient's eyes; offer dark glasses for patient comfort.

• Place on frequent recall because of oral side effects.

• Consider semisupine chair position for patient comfort if GI side effects occur.

Consultations:

• Medical consultation may be required to assess disease control.

• Consult with physician about adjusting dose if excessive salivation becomes a problem.

Teach Patient/Family to:

• Use powered tooth brush or other oral hygiene aids if patient has difficulty in maintaining oral hygiene.

• Encourage effective oral hygiene to prevent soft tissue inflammation.

• Prevent injury when using oral hygiene aids.

pyridoxine hydrochloride (vitamin B_6)

peer-ih-**dox**′-een
high-droh-**klor**′-ide
(Aminoxin, Beesix, Doxine, Nestrex, Pryi, Pyroxin[AUS], Rodex, Vitabee 6)
Do not confuse pyridoxine with paroxetine, pralidoxime, or Pyridium.

CATEGORY AND SCHEDULE

Pregnancy Risk Category: A
OTC

Drug Class: Vitamin B_6, water-soluble vitamin

MECHANISM OF ACTION

Acts as a coenzyme for various metabolic functions, including metabolism of proteins, carbohydrates, and fats. Aids in the breakdown of glycogen and in the synthesis of gamma-aminobutyric acid in the CNS.

Therapeutic Effect: Prevents pyridoxine deficiency. Increases the excretion of certain drugs, such as isoniazid, that are pyridoxine antagonists.

USES

Treatment of vitamin B_6 deficiency associated with inborn errors of metabolism, inadequate diet; unapproved: drug-induced deficiencies

PHARMACOKINETICS

Readily absorbed primarily in jejunum. Stored in the liver, muscle, and brain. Metabolized in the liver. Primarily excreted in urine. Removed by hemodialysis. ***Half-life:*** 15–20 days.

INDICATIONS AND DOSAGES

▸ Pyridoxine Deficiency

PO
Adults, Elderly. Initially, 2.5–10 mg/day; then 2.5 mg/day when clinical signs are corrected.
Children. Initially, 5–25 mg/day for 3 wk, then 1.5–2.5 mg/day.

▸ Pyridoxine Dependent Seizures

PO, IV, IM
Infants. Initially, 10–100 mg/day. Maintenance: PO: 50–100 mg/day.

▸ Drug-Induced Neuritis

PO (Treatment)
Adults, Elderly. 100–300 mg/day in divided doses.
Children. 10–50 mg/day.
PO (Prophylaxis)
Adults, Elderly. 25–100 mg/day.
Children. 1–2 mg/kg/day.

SIDE EFFECTS/ADVERSE REACTIONS

Occasional
Stinging at IM injection site
Rare
Headache, nausea, somnolence; sensory neuropathy (paresthesia, unstable gait, clumsiness of hands) with high doses

PRECAUTIONS AND CONTRAINDICATIONS

Hypersensitivity, Parkinson's disease

DRUG INTERACTIONS OF CONCERN TO DENTISTRY

- Decreased serum levels of phenytoin, phenobarbital

SERIOUS REACTIONS

! Long-term megadoses (2–6 g over more than 2 mo) may produce sensory neuropathy (reduced deep tendon reflexes, profound impairment of sense of position in distal limbs, gradual sensory ataxia). Toxic symptoms subside when drug is discontinued.

! Seizures have occurred after IV megadoses.

DENTAL CONSIDERATIONS

General:

- Vitamin B deficiency and peripheral neuropathy may manifest with oral symptoms of glossitis and cheilosis.

pyrimethamine

pye-ri-**meth′**-ah-meen

(Daraprim, Malocide[FRANCE])

Do not confuse with Dantrium, Daranide.

CATEGORY AND SCHEDULE

Pregnancy Risk Category: C

Drug Class: Antimalarial

MECHANISM OF ACTION

An antiprotozoal with blood and some tissue schizonticidal activity against malaria parasites of humans. Highly selective activity against plasmodia and *Toxoplasma gondii*. ***Therapeutic Effect:*** Inhibition of tetrahydrofolic acid synthesis.

USES

Malaria prophylaxis

PHARMACOKINETICS

Well absorbed, peak levels occurring between 2 and 6 hr following administration. Protein binding: 87%. Eliminated slowly. ***Half-life:*** approximately 96 hr.

INDICATIONS AND DOSAGES

▸ Toxoplasmosis

PO

Adults. Initially, 50–75 mg daily, with 1–4 g daily of a sulfonamide of the sulfapyrimidine type (e.g., sulfadoxine). Continue for 1–3 wk, depending on response of patient and tolerance to therapy, then reduce dose to one-half that previously given for each drug and continue for additional 4–5 wk.

Children. 1 mg/kg/day divided into 2 equal daily doses; after 2–4 days reduce to one-half and continue for approximately 1 month. The usual pediatric sulfonamide dosage is used in conjunction with pyrimethamine.

▸ Acute Malaria

PO

Adults (in combination with sulfonamide). 25 mg daily for 2 days with a sulfonamide.

Adults (without concomitant sulfonamide). 50 mg for 2 days.

Children 4–10 yr. 25 mg daily for 2 days.

▸ Chemoprophylaxis of Malaria

PO

Adults and pediatric patients over 10 yr. 25 mg once a wk.

Children 4–10 yr. 12.5 mg once a wk.

Infants and children under 4 yr. 6.25 mg once a wk.

SIDE EFFECTS/ADVERSE REACTIONS

Frequent

Anorexia, vomiting

Occasional

Hypersensitivity reactions, Stevens-Johnson syndrome, toxic epidermal necrolysis, erythema multiforme, anaphylaxis, hyperphenylalaninemia, megaloblastic anemia, leukopenia, thrombocytopenia, pancytopenia, atrophic glossitis, hematuria, and disorders of cardiac rhythm

Rare

Pulmonary eosinophilia

PRECAUTIONS AND CONTRAINDICATIONS

Hypersensitivity to pyrimethamine, megaloblastic anemia due to folate deficiency, monotherapy for treatment of acute malaria

DRUG INTERACTIONS OF CONCERN TO DENTISTRY

• Possible mild hepatotoxicity: lorazepam

SERIOUS REACTIONS

! None known

DENTAL CONSIDERATIONS

General:

• Determine why patient is taking the drug.

• Consider semisupine chair position for patient comfort if GI side effects occur.

• Question patient about tolerance of NSAIDs or aspirin related to GI disease.

• Patient on chronic drug therapy may rarely present with symptoms of blood dyscrasias, which can include infection, bleeding, and poor healing. If dyscrasia is present, advise patient to prevent oral tissue trauma when using oral hygiene aids.

• Determine why patient is taking drug (prophylaxis or active therapy).

Consultations:

• Medical consultation may be required to assess disease control and patient's ability to tolerate stress.

Teach Patient/Family to:

• Report sore throat, pallor, purpura, or glossitis, which may be symptoms of serious effects.

• Encourage effective oral hygiene to prevent soft tissue inflammation.

• Prevent trauma when using oral hygiene aids.

• Update health and medication history if physician makes any changes in evaluation or drug regimens; include OTC, herbal, and nonherbal drug in the update.

quazepam

kwaz′-eh-pam
(Doral)

CATEGORY AND SCHEDULE

Pregnancy Risk Category: X
Controlled Substance: Schedule IV

Drug Class: Benzodiazepine, sedative-hypnotic

MECHANISM OF ACTION

A BZ-1 receptor selective benzodiazepine with sedative properties.
Therapeutic Effect: Produces sedative effect from its CNS depressant action.

USES

Treatment of insomnia

PHARMACOKINETICS

Rapidly absorbed from GI tract. Food increases absorption. Protein binding: 95%. Extensively metabolized in liver. Excreted in urine and feces. Unknown if removed by hemodialysis. ***Half-life:*** 25–41 hr.

INDICATIONS AND DOSAGES

▸ Insomnia

PO

Adults (older than 18 yr). Initially, 15 mg at bedtime. Adjust dose up or down from 7.5 mg to 30 mg at bedtime, depending on initial response.
Elderly, debilitated, liver disease. Initially, 7.5–15 mg at bedtime. Adjust dose depending on initial response.

SIDE EFFECTS/ADVERSE REACTIONS

Frequent

Muscular incoordination (ataxia), light-headedness, transient mild drowsiness, slurred speech (particularly in elderly or debilitated patients)

Occasional

Confusion, depression, blurred vision, constipation, diarrhea, dry mouth, headache, nausea

Rare

Behavioral problems such as anger, impaired memory; paradoxic reactions, such as insomnia, nervousness, or irritability

PRECAUTIONS AND CONTRAINDICATIONS

Pregnancy, sleep apnea, hypersensitivity to quazepam or any component of the formulation

Caution:

Hepatic disease, renal disease, suicidal individuals, drug abuse, elderly, psychosis, children younger than 18 yr, lactation, depression, pulmonary insufficiency

DRUG INTERACTIONS OF CONCERN TO DENTISTRY

- Increased effects: CNS depressants, alcohol
- Delayed elimination: erythromycin
- Contraindicated with saquinavir, ritonavir
- Increased serum levels and prolonged effect of benzodiazepines: erythromycin, ketoconazole, itraconazole, fluconazole, miconazole (systemic)

SERIOUS REACTIONS

! Abrupt or too-rapid withdrawal may result in pronounced restlessness, irritability, insomnia, hand tremors, abdominal and muscle cramps, sweating, vomiting, and seizures.

! Overdosage results in somnolence, confusion, diminished reflexes, and coma.

! Blood dyscrasias have been reported rarely.

DENTAL CONSIDERATIONS

General:

- Assess salivary flow as a factor in caries, periodontal disease, and candidiasis.
- Psychological and physical dependence may occur with chronic administration.
- Geriatric patients are more susceptible to drug effects; use a lower dose.
- Avoid using this drug in a patient with a history of drug abuse or alcoholism.

Consultations:

- Medical consultation may be required to assess disease control.

Teach Patient/Family to:

- When chronic dry mouth occurs, advise patient to:
  - Avoid mouth rinses with high alcohol content because of drying effects.
  - Use daily home fluoride products to prevent caries.
  - Use sugarless gum, frequent sips of water, or saliva substitutes.

Q

quetiapine

kwe-**tye**′-ah-peen

(Seroquel)

CATEGORY AND SCHEDULE

Pregnancy Risk Category: C

Drug Class: Antipsychotic, atypical

MECHANISM OF ACTION

A dibenzothiazepine derivative that antagonizes dopamine, serotonin, histamine, and α_1-adrenergic receptors.

Therapeutic Effect: Diminishes manifestations of psychotic disorders. Produces moderate sedation, few extrapyramidal effects, and no anticholinergic effects.

USES

Treatment of schizophrenia

PHARMACOKINETICS

Well absorbed after PO administration. Protein binding: 83%. Widely distributed in tissues; CNS concentration exceeds plasma concentration. Undergoes extensive first-pass metabolism in the liver. Primarily excreted in urine. ***Half-life:*** 6 hr.

INDICATIONS AND DOSAGES

▸ To Manage Manifestations of Psychotic Disorders, Bipolar Disorder

PO

Adults, Elderly. Initially, 25 mg twice a day, then 25–50 mg 2–3 times a day on the second and third days, up to 300–400 mg/day in divided doses 2–3 times a day by the fourth day. Further adjustments of 25–50 mg twice a day may be made at intervals of 2 days or longer. Maintenance: 300–800 mg/day (adults); 50–200 mg/day (elderly).

▸ Dosage in Hepatic Impairment, Elderly or Debilitated Patients, and Those Predisposed to Hypotensive Reactions

These patients should receive a lower initial dose and lower dosage increases.

SIDE EFFECTS/ADVERSE REACTIONS

Frequent
Headache, somnolence, dizziness
Occasional
Constipation, orthostatic hypotension, tachycardia, dry mouth, dyspepsia, rash, asthenia, abdominal pain, rhinitis
Rare
Back pain, fever, weight gain

PRECAUTIONS AND CONTRAINDICATIONS

Renal impairment, hepatic impairment, cardiovascular disease, thyroid disease, hyperprolactinemia, neuromalignant syndrome, tardive dyskinesia, seizure disorders, cataracts, dementia, suicide tendency, lactation; patients should be monitored for signs and symptoms of diabetes mellitus, severe CNS depression

DRUG INTERACTIONS OF CONCERN TO DENTISTRY

- Risk of increased CNS depression: CNS depressants

SERIOUS REACTIONS

! Overdose may produce heart block, hypotension, hypokalemia, and tachycardia.

DENTAL CONSIDERATIONS

General:

- Monitor vital signs at every appointment because of cardiovascular and respiratory side effects.
- Assess salivary flow as factor in caries, periodontal disease, and candidiasis.
- Assess for presence of extrapyramidal motor symptoms, such as tardive dyskinesia and akathisia.
- Extrapyramidal motor activity may complicate dental treatment.
- After supine positioning, have patient sit upright for at least 2 min before standing to avoid orthostatic hypotension.
- Consider semisupine chair position for patient comfort if GI side effects occur.
- Patients on chronic drug therapy may rarely have symptoms of blood dyscrasias, which can include infection, bleeding, and poor healing.
- Place on frequent recall because of oral side effects.

Consultations:

- In a patient with symptoms of blood dyscrasias, request a medical consultation for blood studies and postpone treatment until normal values are reestablished.
- Medical consultation may be required to assess disease control and patient's ability to tolerate stress.
- If signs of tardive dyskinesia or akathisia are present, refer to physician.
- Consultation with physician may be necessary if sedation or general anesthesia is required.
- Physician should be informed if significant xerostomic side effects occur (e.g., increased caries, sore tongue, problems eating or swallowing, difficulty wearing prosthesis) so that a medication change can be considered.

Teach Patient/Family to:

- Use caution to prevent trauma when using oral hygiene aids.
- Use powered tooth brush if patient has difficulty holding conventional devices.
- Encourage effective oral hygiene to prevent soft tissue inflammation.
- Update health and drug history if physician makes any changes in

evaluation or drug regimens; include OTC, herbal, and nonherbal drugs in the update.

• Be aware of oral side effects and potential sequelae.
• When chronic dry mouth occurs, advise patient to:
  • Avoid mouth rinses with high alcohol content because of drying effects.
  • Use daily home fluoride products for anticaries effect.
  • Use sugarless gum, frequent sips of water, or saliva substitutes.

quinapril

kwin′-ah-pril

(Accupril, Asig[AUS])

Do not confuse Accupril with Accolate or Accutane.

CATEGORY AND SCHEDULE

Pregnancy Risk Category: C (D if used in second or third trimester)

Drug Class: Angiotensin-converting enzyme (ACE) inhibitor

MECHANISM OF ACTION

An ACE inhibitor that suppresses the renin-angiotensin-aldosterone system and prevents the conversion of angiotensin I to angiotensin II, a potent vasoconstrictor; may also inhibit angiotensin II at local vascular and renal sites. ***Therapeutic Effect:*** Reduces peripheral arterial resistance, B/P, and pulmonary capillary wedge pressure; improves cardiac output.

USES

Treatment of hypertension, alone or in combination with thiazide diuretics, heart failure

PHARMACOKINETICS

Route	Onset	Peak	Duration
PO	1 hr	N/A	24 hr

Readily absorbed from the GI tract. Protein binding: 97%. Metabolized in the liver, GI tract, and extravascular tissue to active metabolite. Primarily excreted in urine. Minimal removal by hemodialysis. ***Half-life:*** 1–2 hr; metabolite, 3 hr (increased in those with impaired renal function).

INDICATIONS AND DOSAGES

▸ **Hypertension (Monotherapy)**

PO

Adults. Initially, 10–20 mg/day. May adjust dosage at intervals of at least 2 wk or longer. Maintenance: 20–80 mg/day as single dose or 2 divided doses. Maximum: 80 mg/day.

Elderly. Initially, 2.5–5 mg/day. May increase by 2.5–5 mg q1–2wk.

▸ **Hypertension (Combination Therapy)**

PO

Adults. Initially, 5 mg/day titrated to patient's needs.

Elderly. Initially, 2.5–5 mg/day. May increase by 2.5–5 mg q1–2wk.

▸ **Adjunct to Manage Heart Failure**

PO

Adults, Elderly. Initially, 5 mg twice a day. Range: 20–40 mg/day.

▸ **Dosage in Renal Impairment**

Dosage is titrated to the patient's needs after the following initial doses:

Creatinine Clearance	Initial Dose
More than 60 ml/min	10 mg
30–60 ml/min	5 mg
10–29 ml/min	2.5 mg

SIDE EFFECTS/ADVERSE REACTIONS

Frequent
Headache, dizziness
Occasional
Fatigue, vomiting, nausea, hypotension, chest pain, cough, syncope
Rare
Diarrhea, cough, dyspnea, rash, palpitations, impotence, insomnia, drowsiness, malaise

PRECAUTIONS AND CONTRAINDICATIONS

Bilateral renal artery stenosis
Caution:
Pregnancy category D, impaired renal/liver function, dialysis patients, hypovolemia, blood dyscrasias, CHF, COPD, asthma, elderly, lactation

DRUG INTERACTIONS OF CONCERN TO DENTISTRY

• Increased hypotension: alcohol, phenothiazines
• Decreased hypotensive effects: indomethacin and possibly other NSAIDs, sympathomimetics
• Suspected reduction in the antihypertensive and vasodilator effects by salicylates; monitor B/P if used concurrently

SERIOUS REACTIONS

! Excessive hypotension ("first-dose syncope") may occur in patients with CHF and in those who are severely salt or volume depleted.
! Angioedema and hyperkalemia occur rarely.
! Agranulocytosis and neutropenia may be noted in those with collagen vascular disease, including scleroderma and systemic lupus erythematosus, and impaired renal function.
! Nephrotic syndrome may be noted in those with history of renal disease.

DENTAL CONSIDERATIONS

General:
• Monitor vital signs at every appointment because of cardiovascular side effects.
• After supine positioning, have patient sit upright for at least 2 min before standing to avoid orthostatic hypotension.
• Patients on chronic drug therapy may rarely have symptoms of blood dyscrasias, which can include infection, bleeding, and poor healing.
• Assess salivary flow as a factor in caries, periodontal disease, and candidiasis.
• Limit use of sodium-containing products, such as saline IV fluids, for patients with a dietary salt restriction.
• Use vasoconstrictors with caution, in low doses, and with careful aspiration.
• Stress from dental procedures may compromise cardiovascular function; determine patient risk.
• Short appointments and a stress-reduction protocol may be required for anxious patients.
Consultations:
• Medical consultation may be required to assess disease control and patient's ability to tolerate stress.
• In a patient with symptoms of blood dyscrasias, request a medical consultation for blood studies and postpone dental treatment until normal values are reestablished.
• Take precautions if dental surgery is anticipated and sedation or general anesthesia is required; risk of hypotensive episode.

Teach Patient/Family to:

- Encourage effective oral hygiene to prevent soft tissue inflammation.
- Use caution to prevent injury when using oral hygiene aids.
- When chronic dry mouth occurs, advise patient to:
  - Avoid mouth rinses with high alcohol content because of drying effects.
  - Use daily home fluoride products to prevent caries.
  - Use sugarless gum, frequent sips of water, or saliva substitutes.

quinidine

kwin′-ih-deen

(Apo-Quin-G[CAN], Apo-Quinidine[CAN], BioQuin Durules[CAN], Kinidin Durules[AUS], Quinaglute Dura-Tabs, Quinate[CAN], Quinidex Extentabs)

Do not confuse quinidine with clonidine or quinine.

CATEGORY AND SCHEDULE

Pregnancy Risk Category: C

Drug Class: Antidysrhythmic (class Ia)

Q

MECHANISM OF ACTION

An antidysrhythmic that decreases sodium influx during depolarization, potassium efflux during repolarization, and reduces calcium transport across the myocardial cell membrane. Decreases myocardial excitability, conduction velocity, and contractility.

Therapeutic Effect: Suppresses cardiac dysrhythmias.

USES

Treatment of premature ventricular contractions (PVCs), atrial flutter and fibrillation, PAT, ventricular tachycardia

PHARMACOKINETICS

PO: Peak 0.5–6 hr (depending on form given), duration 6–8 hr, ***Half-life:*** 6–7 hr; metabolized in liver; excreted unchanged by kidneys.

INDICATIONS AND DOSAGES

▸ **Maintenance of Normal Sinus Rhythm after Conversion of Atrial Fibrillation or Flutter; Prevention of Premature Atrial, AV, and Ventricular Contractions; Paroxysmal Atrial Tachycardia; Paroxysmal AV Junctional Rhythm; Atrial Fibrillation; Atrial Flutter; Paroxysmal Ventricular Tachycardia Not Associated with Complete Heart Block**

PO

Adults, Elderly. 100–600 mg q4–6h. Long-acting: 324–972 mg q8–12h.

Children. 30 mg/kg/day in divided doses q4–6h.

IV

Adults, Elderly. 200–400 mg.

Children. 2–10 mg/kg.

SIDE EFFECTS/ADVERSE REACTIONS

Frequent

Abdominal pain and cramps, nausea, diarrhea, vomiting (can be immediate, intense)

Occasional

Mild cinchonism (ringing in ears, blurred vision, hearing loss) or severe cinchonism (headache, vertigo, diaphoresis, light-headedness, photophobia, confusion, delirium)

Rare
Hypotension (particularly with IV administration), hypersensitivity reaction (fever, anaphylaxis, photosensitivity reaction)

PRECAUTIONS AND CONTRAINDICATIONS

Complete AV block, intraventricular conduction defects (widening of QRS complex)

Caution:
Lactation, children, renal disease, potassium imbalance, liver disease, CHF, respiratory depression

DRUG INTERACTIONS OF CONCERN TO DENTISTRY

- May decrease effects of quinidine: barbiturates
- Increased anticholinergic effect: anticholinergic drugs
- Increased effects of neuromuscular blockers, tricyclic antidepressants
- Contraindicated with itraconazole
- Prevention of action: cholinergics

SERIOUS REACTIONS

! Cardiotoxic effects occur most commonly with IV administration, particularly at high concentrations, and are observed as conduction changes (50% widening of QRS complex, prolonged QT interval, flattened T waves, and disappearance of P wave), ventricular tachycardia or flutter, frequent PVCs, or complete AV block.
! Quinidine-induced syncope may occur with the usual dosage.
! Severe hypotension may result from high dosages.
! Patients with atrial flutter and fibrillation may experience a paradoxical, extremely rapid ventricular rate that may be prevented by prior digitalization.
! Hepatotoxicity with jaundice caused by drug hypersensitivity may occur.

DENTAL CONSIDERATIONS

General:

- Monitor vital signs at every appointment because of cardiovascular and respiratory side effects.
- Minimize; use stress-reduction protocol.
- Patients on chronic drug therapy may rarely have symptoms of blood dyscrasias, which can include infection, bleeding, and poor healing.
- After supine positioning, have patient sit upright for at least 2 min before standing to avoid orthostatic hypotension.
- Use vasoconstrictors with caution, in low doses, and with careful aspiration. Avoid use of gingival retraction cord with epinephrine.
- Consider semisupine chair position for patient comfort if GI side effects occur.

Consultations:

- In a patient with symptoms of blood dyscrasias, request a medical consultation for blood studies and postpone dental treatment until normal values are reestablished.
- Medical consultation may be required to assess patient's ability to tolerate stress.

Teach Patient/Family to:

- Encourage effective oral hygiene to prevent soft tissue inflammation.

quinine

kwye′-nine
(Quinine)
Do not confuse with quinidine.

CATEGORY AND SCHEDULE

Pregnancy Risk Category: X

Drug Class: Antimalarial

MECHANISM OF ACTION

A cinchona alkaloid that relaxes skeletal muscle by increasing the refractory period, decreasing excitability of motor end plates (curare-like), and affecting distribution of calcium with muscle fiber. Antimalarial: Depresses oxygen uptake, carbohydrate metabolism, elevates pH in intracellular organelles of parasites. ***Therapeutic Effect:*** Relaxes skeletal muscle; produces parasite death.

USES

Treatment of *P. falciparum* malaria, nocturnal leg cramps

Q

PHARMACOKINETICS

Rapidly absorbed mainly from upper small intestine. Protein binding: 70%–95%. Metabolized in liver. Excreted in feces, saliva, and urine. ***Half-life:*** 8–14 hr (adults), 6–12 hr (children).

INDICATIONS AND DOSAGES

▸ Nocturnal Leg Cramps

PO

Adults, Elderly. 260–300 mg at bedtime as needed.

▸ Treatment of Malaria

PO

Adults, Elderly. 260–650 mg 3 times a day for 6–12 days.

Children. 10 mg/kg q8h for 5–7 days.

▸ Dosage in Renal Impairment

Creatinine Clearance	Dosage Interval
10–50 ml/min	75% of normal dose or q12h
Less than 10 ml/min	30%–50% of normal dose or q24h

SIDE EFFECTS/ADVERSE REACTIONS

Frequent

Nausea, headache, tinnitus, slight visual disturbances (mild cinchonism)

Occasional

Extreme flushing of skin with intense generalized pruritus is most typical hypersensitivity reaction; also rash, wheezing, dyspnea, angioedema

Prolonged therapy: cardiac conduction disturbances, decreased hearing

PRECAUTIONS AND CONTRAINDICATIONS

Hypersensitivity to quinine (possible cross-sensitivity to quinidine), G-6-PD deficiency, tinnitus, optic neuritis, history of thrombocytopenia during previous quinine therapy, blackwater fever

Caution:

Blood dyscrasias, severe GI disease, neurologic disease, severe hepatic disease, psoriasis, cardiac dysrhythmias, tinnitus

DRUG INTERACTIONS OF CONCERN TO DENTISTRY

- Decreased absorption: magnesium or aluminum salts
- Prolonged duration of neuromuscular blocking drugs

SERIOUS REACTIONS

! Overdosage (severe cinchonism) may result in cardiovascular effects, severe headache, intestinal cramps with vomiting and diarrhea, apprehension, confusion, seizures, blindness, and respiratory depression.

! Hypoprothrombinemia, thrombocytopenic purpura, hemoglobinuria, asthma, agranulocytosis, hypoglycemia, deafness, and optic atrophy occur rarely.

DENTAL CONSIDERATIONS

General:

• Patients on chronic drug therapy rarely may have symptoms of blood dyscrasias, which can include infection, bleeding, and poor healing.

• Avoid dental light in patient's eyes; offer dark glasses for patient comfort.

• Monitor vital signs at every appointment because of cardiovascular side effects.

• Consider semisupine chair position for patient comfort if GI side effects occur.

Consultations:

• Medical consultation may be required to assess disease control.

• In a patient with symptoms of blood dyscrasias, request a medical consultation for blood studies and postpone dental treatment until normal values are reestablished.

Teach Patient/Family to:

• Encourage effective oral hygiene to prevent soft tissue inflammation.

rabeprazole sodium

rah-**bep'**-rah-zole **soe'**-dee-um
(AcipHex, Pariet[CAN])
Do not confuse AcipHex with Accupril or Aricept.

CATEGORY AND SCHEDULE

Pregnancy Risk Category: B

Drug Class: Antisecretory, proton pump inhibitor

MECHANISM OF ACTION

A proton pump inhibitor that converts to active metabolites that irreversibly bind to and inhibit hydrogen-potassium adenosine triphosphate, an enzyme on the surface of gastric parietal cells. Actively secretes hydrogen ions for potassium ions, resulting in an accumulation of hydrogen ions in gastric lumen.
Therapeutic Effect: Increases gastric pH, reducing gastric acid production.

USES

Treatment of gastroesophageal reflux disease (GERD), duodenal ulcers, and hypersecretory conditions (Zollinger-Ellison disease); eradication of *Helicobacter pylori* infection (with amoxicillin and clarithromycin), *H. pylori* eradication to reduce risk of duodenal ulcer

PHARMACOKINETICS

Rapidly absorbed from the GI tract after passing through the stomach relatively intact. Protein binding: 96%. Metabolized extensively in the liver. Primarily excreted in urine. Unknown if removed by hemodialysis. ***Half-life:*** 1–2 hr (increased with hepatic impairment).

R

INDICATIONS AND DOSAGES

▸ **GERD**
PO
Adults, Elderly. 20 mg/day for 4–8 wk. Maintenance: 20 mg/day.

▸ **Duodenal Ulcer**
PO
Adults, Elderly. 20 mg/day after morning meal for 4 wk.

▸ **NSAID-Induced Ulcer**
PO
Adults, Elderly. 20 mg/day.

▸ **Pathologic Hypersecretory Conditions**
PO
Adults, Elderly. Initially, 60 mg/day. May increase to 60 mg twice a day.

▸ ***Helicobacter pylori*** **Infection**
PO
Adults, Elderly. 20 mg twice a day for 7 days (given with amoxicillin 1000 mg and clarithromycin 500 mg).

SIDE EFFECTS/ADVERSE REACTIONS

Rare
Headache, nausea, dizziness, rash, diarrhea, malaise

PRECAUTIONS AND CONTRAINDICATIONS

Hypersensitivity
Caution:
Do not break, crush, or chew tablets; avoid nursing; pediatric use not studied

DRUG INTERACTIONS OF CONCERN TO DENTISTRY

- None reported

SERIOUS REACTIONS

! Hyperglycemia, hypokalemia, hyponatremia, and hyperlipemia occur rarely.

DENTAL CONSIDERATIONS

General:

• Assess salivary flow as a factor in caries, periodontal disease, and candidiasis.
• Consider semisupine chair position for patient comfort because of GI side effects of disease.
• Patients with gastroesophageal reflux may have oral symptoms, including burning mouth, secondary candidiasis, and signs of tooth erosion.
• Question the patient about tolerance of NSAIDs or aspirin related to GI problems.

Teach Patient/Family to:

• Prevent trauma when using oral hygiene aids.
• When chronic dry mouth occurs, advise patient to:
  • Avoid mouth rinses with high alcohol content because of drying effects.
  • Use daily home fluoride products for anticaries effect.
  • Use sugarless gum, frequent sips of water, or saliva substitutes.

raloxifene

ra-**lox**′-ih-feen
(Evista)

CATEGORY AND SCHEDULE

Pregnancy Risk Category: X

Drug Class: Synthetic estrogen

MECHANISM OF ACTION

A selective estrogen receptor modulator that affects some receptors like estrogen.

Therapeutic Effect: Like estrogen, prevents bone loss and improves lipid profiles.

USES

Prevention and treatment of osteoporosis in postmenopausal women, supplemented with calcium as based on need

PHARMACOKINETICS

Rapidly absorbed after PO administration. Highly bound to plasma proteins (>95%) and albumin. Undergoes extensive first-pass metabolism in liver. Excreted mainly in feces and, to a lesser extent, in urine. Unknown if removed by hemodialysis. ***Half-life:*** 27.7 hr.

INDICATIONS AND DOSAGES

▸ **Prevention or Treatment of Osteoporosis**

PO

Adults, Elderly. 60 mg/day.

SIDE EFFECTS/ADVERSE REACTIONS

Frequent

Hot flashes, flu-like symptoms, arthralgia, sinusitis

Occasional

Weight gain, nausea, myalgia, pharyngitis, cough, dyspepsia, leg cramps, rash, depression

Rare

Vaginitis, UTI, peripheral edema, flatulence, vomiting, fever, migraine, diaphoresis

PRECAUTIONS AND CONTRAINDICATIONS

Active or history of venous thromboembolic events, such as deep vein thrombosis, pulmonary embolism, and retinal vein thrombosis; women who are or may become pregnant.

Caution:
Hepatic impairment, risk of thromboembolic events, pregnancy category X, lactation

DRUG INTERACTIONS OF CONCERN TO DENTISTRY

- Reduced absorption: ampicillin
- Risk of potential drug interactions with other highly plasma protein–bound drugs, such as NSAIDs, aspirin, and diazepam, is unknown

SERIOUS REACTIONS

! Pneumonia, gastroenteritis, chest pain, vaginal bleeding, and breast pain occur rarely.

DENTAL CONSIDERATIONS

General:

- Drug should be discontinued 72 hr before prolonged immobilization, such as hospitalization, postsurgical recovery, and bed rest.
- Consider short appointments and dental chair position if needed for patient comfort.

Consultations:

- Medical consultation may be required to assess disease control and patient's ability to tolerate stress.

R

raltegravir

ral-**teg**′-ra-veer
(Isentress)

CATEGORY AND SCHEDULE

Pregnancy Risk Category: C

Drug Class: Antiretroviral agent, integrase inhibitor

MECHANISM OF ACTION

Inhibits the catalytic activity of HIV-1 integrase, an HIV-1–encoded enzyme required for viral replication.

USES

HIV-1 infection, multidrug resistance, in combination with other antiretroviral agents

PHARMACOKINETICS

Absorption: 19% increase in AUC after a high-fat meal. Protein binding: 83%. Primarily metabolized by glucuronidation mediated by UGT1A1. ***Half-life:*** 9 hr. Excreted in the feces (51%) and urine (32%).

INDICATIONS AND DOSAGES

▸ HIV Infection

PO
Adults. 400 mg twice a day.
Adolescents (16 yr). 400 mg twice a day.

SIDE EFFECTS/ADVERSE REACTIONS

▸ Adult

Frequent
Increased total cholesterol
Occasional
Hypertension, fatigue, dizziness, insomnia, rash, pruritus, folliculitis, increased glucose (<250 mg/dl: 9%), increased LDL-cholesterol, hypertriglyceridemia, hyperbilirubinemia, increased AST, increased ALT, increased alkaline phosphatase, arthralgia, extremity pain, increased creatine kinase, increased creatinine, nasopharyngitis, cough, influenza, sinusitis, herpes zoster, lymphadenopathy, anogenital warts

PRECAUTIONS AND CONTRAINDICATIONS

Use with caution in patients taking medications that cause rhabdomyolysis or other risk factors for creatine kinase elevations and/or skeletal muscle abnormalities due to the risk of myopathy (e.g., statins). Immune reconstitution syndrome (occurrence of an inflammatory response to an indolent or residual opportunistic infection) may occur. Use with caution when combining with UGT1A1 glucuronidation inducers, such as rifampin and inhibitors such as atazanavir.

DRUG INTERACTIONS OF CONCERN TO DENTISTRY

• None reported

SERIOUS REACTIONS

! Myopathy and rhabdomyolysis have been reported.
! Immune reconstitution syndrome has been reported.

DENTAL CONSIDERATIONS

General:

• Examine for oral manifestations of opportunistic infections.
• Patients on chronic drug therapy may rarely have symptoms of blood dyscrasias, which can include infection, bleeding, and poor healing.
• Palliative medication may be required for management of oral side effects.

Consultations:

• Medical consultation may be required to assess disease control and ability of patient to tolerate dental treatment.
• In a patient with symptoms of blood dyscrasias, request a medical consultation for blood studies and postpone dental treatment until normal values are reestablished.

Teach Patient/Family to:

• Encourage effective oral hygiene to prevent soft tissue inflammation.
• Use caution to prevent trauma when using oral hygiene aids.
• See dentist immediately if secondary oral infection occurs.

ramipril

ram′-ih-pril
(Altace, Ramace[AUS], Tritace[AUS])
Do not confuse Altace with Alteplase or Artane.

CATEGORY AND SCHEDULE

Pregnancy Risk Category: C (D if used in second or third trimester)

Drug Class: Angiotensin-converting enzyme (ACE) inhibitor

MECHANISM OF ACTION

An ACE inhibitor that suppresses the renin-angiotensin-aldosterone system. Decreases plasma angiotensin II, increases plasma renin activity, and decreases aldosterone secretion.
Therapeutic Effect: Reduces peripheral arterial resistance and B/P.

USES

Treatment of hypertension; alone or in combination with thiazide diuretics; CHF immediately after MI; reduce risk of MI, stroke, and death from cardiovascular causes

PHARMACOKINETICS

Route	Onset	Peak	Duration
PO	1–2 hr	3–6 hr	24 hr

Well absorbed from the GI tract. Protein binding: 73%. Metabolized in the liver to active metabolite. Primarily excreted in urine. Not removed by hemodialysis. ***Half-life:*** 5.1 hr.

INDICATIONS AND DOSAGES

▸ Hypertension (Monotherapy)

PO

Adults, Elderly. Initially, 2.5 mg/day. Maintenance: 2.5–20 mg/day as single dose or in 2 divided doses.

▸ Hypertension (in Combination with Other Antihypertensives)

PO

Adults, Elderly. Initially, 1.25 mg/day titrated to patient's needs.

▸ CHF

PO

Adults, Elderly. Initially, 1.25–2.5 mg twice a day. Maximum: 5 mg twice a day.

▸ Risk Reduction for MI Stroke

PO

Adults, Elderly. Initially, 2.5 mg/day for 7 days, then 5 mg/day for 21 days, then 10 mg/day as a single dose or in divided doses.

▸ Dosage in Renal Impairment

Creatinine clearance 40 ml/min or less. 25% of normal dose.

Hypertension. Initially, 1.25 mg/day titrated upward.

CHF. Initially, 1.25 mg/day, titrated up to 2.5 mg twice a day.

SIDE EFFECTS/ADVERSE REACTIONS

Frequent

Cough, headache

Occasional

Dizziness, fatigue, nausea, asthenia (loss of strength)

Rare

Palpitations, insomnia, nervousness, malaise, abdominal pain, myalgia

PRECAUTIONS AND CONTRAINDICATIONS

Bilateral renal artery stenosis

Caution:

Impaired renal/liver function, dialysis patients, hypovolemia, blood dyscrasias, CHF, COPD, asthma, elderly

DRUG INTERACTIONS OF CONCERN TO DENTISTRY

- Increased hypotension: alcohol, phenothiazines
- Decreased hypotensive effects: indomethacin and possibly other NSAIDs, sympathomimetics
- Suspected reduction in the antihypertensive and vasodilator effects by salicylates; monitor B/P if used concurrently

SERIOUS REACTIONS

! Excessive hypotension ("first-dose syncope") may occur in patients with CHF and in those who are severely salt or volume depleted.

! Angioedema and hyperkalemia occur rarely.

! Agranulocytosis and neutropenia may be noted in those with collagen vascular disease, including scleroderma and systemic lupus erythematosus, and impaired renal function.

! Nephrotic syndrome may be noted in those with history of renal disease.

DENTAL CONSIDERATIONS

General:

- Monitor vital signs at every appointment because of cardiovascular and respiratory side effects.
- After supine positioning, have patient sit upright for at least 2 min before standing to avoid orthostatic hypotension.
- Patients on chronic drug therapy may rarely have symptoms of blood dyscrasias, which can include

infection, bleeding, and poor healing.
• Assess salivary flow as a factor in caries, periodontal disease, and candidiasis.
• Limit use of sodium-containing products, such as saline IV fluids, for patients with a dietary salt restriction.
• Use vasoconstrictors with caution, in low doses, and with careful aspiration.
• Stress from dental procedures may compromise cardiovascular function; determine patient risk.
• Short appointments and a stress-reduction protocol may be required for anxious patients.

Consultations:
• Medical consultation may be required to assess patient's ability to tolerate stress.
• In a patient with symptoms of blood dyscrasias, request a medical consultation for blood studies and postpone dental treatment until normal values are reestablished.
• Take precautions if dental surgery is anticipated and sedation or general anesthesia is required; risk of hypotensive episode.

Teach Patient/Family to:
• Encourage effective oral hygiene to prevent soft tissue inflammation.
• Use caution to prevent injury when using oral hygiene aids.
• When chronic dry mouth occurs, advise patient to:
  • Avoid mouth rinses with high alcohol content because of drying effects.
  • Use daily home fluoride products to prevent caries.
  • Use sugarless gum, frequent sips of water, or saliva substitutes.

ranitidine hydrochloride/ ranitidine bismuth citrate

ra-**ni**′-ti-deen high-droh-**klor**′-ide/ ra-**ni**′-ti-deen **biss**′-mooth **sih**′-trate
(ranitidine hydrochloride: Apo-Ranitidine[CAN], Ausran[AUS], Novo-Ranitidine[CAN], Rani-2[AUS], Ranihexal[AUS], Zantac, Zantac-75, Zantac-150, Zantac-300, Zantac EFFERdose, Zantac-25 EFFERdose, Zantac-150 EFFERdose, Zantac-150 Maximum Strength; ranitidine bismuth citrate: Pylorid[AUS], Tritec)
Do not confuse Zantac with Xanax, Ziac, or Zyrtec.

CATEGORY AND SCHEDULE

Pregnancy Risk Category: B
OTC (75 mg tablets)

Drug Class: H_2 histamine receptor antagonist

MECHANISM OF ACTION

An antiulcer agent that inhibits histamine action at H_2 receptors of gastric parietal cells.
Therapeutic Effect: Inhibits gastric acid secretion when fasting, at night, or when stimulated by food, caffeine, or insulin. Reduces volume and hydrogen ion concentration of gastric juice.

USES

Treatment of duodenal ulcer, Zollinger-Ellison syndrome, benign gastric ulcers, hypersecretory conditions, gastroesophageal reflux disease, erosive esophagitis, stress ulcers; unapproved: treatment of GI symptoms associated with NSAID use in rheumatoid arthritis

PHARMACOKINETICS

Rapidly absorbed from the GI tract. Protein binding: 15%. Widely distributed. Metabolized in the liver. Primarily excreted in urine. Not removed by hemodialysis. ***Half-life:*** PO, 2.5 hr; IV, 2–2.5 hr (increased with impaired renal function).

INDICATIONS AND DOSAGES

▸ **Duodenal Ulcers, Gastric Ulcers, Gastroesophageal Reflux Disease**

PO

Adults, Elderly. 150 mg twice a day or 300 mg at bedtime. Maintenance: 150 mg at bedtime.

Children. 2–4 mg/kg/day in divided doses twice a day. Maximum: 300 mg/day.

▸ **Duodenal Ulcers Associated with *H. pylori* Infection**

PO

Adults, Elderly. 400 mg twice a day for 4 wk in combination with clarithromycin 500 mg 2–3 times a day for the first 2 wk.

▸ **Erosive Esophagitis**

PO

Adults, Elderly. 150 mg 4 times a day. Maintenance: 150 mg twice a day or 300 mg at bedtime.

Children. 4–10 mg/kg/day in 2 divided doses. Maximum: 600 mg/day.

▸ **Hypersecretory Conditions**

PO

Adults, Elderly. 150 mg twice a day. May increase up to 6 g/day.

▸ **OTC Use**

PO

Adults, Elderly. 75 mg 30–60 min before eating food or drinking beverages that cause heartburn. Maximum: 150 mg per 24-hr period and/or longer than 14 days.

▸ **Usual Parenteral Dosage**

IV, IM

Adults, Elderly. 50 mg/dose q6–8h. Maximum: 400 mg/day.

Children. 2–4 mg/kg/day in divided doses q6–8h. Maximum: 200 mg/day.

▸ **Usual Neonatal Dosage**

PO

Neonates. 2 mg/kg/day in divided doses q12h.

IV

Neonates. Initially, 1.5 mg/kg/dose; then 1.5–2 mg/kg/day in divided doses q12h.

▸ **Dosage in Renal Impairment**

For patients with creatinine clearance less than 50 ml/min, give 150 mg PO q24h or 50 mg IV or IM q18–24h.

SIDE EFFECTS/ADVERSE REACTIONS

Occasional

Diarrhea

Rare

Constipation, headache (may be severe)

PRECAUTIONS AND CONTRAINDICATIONS

History of acute porphyria

Caution:

Pregnancy category B, lactation, children younger than 12 yr, hepatic disease, renal disease

DRUG INTERACTIONS OF CONCERN TO DENTISTRY

- Decreased absorption of diazepam, anticholinergics, ketoconazole (take doses 2 hr apart)

SERIOUS REACTIONS

! Reversible hepatitis and blood dyscrasias occur rarely.

DENTAL CONSIDERATIONS

General:

• Avoid prescribing aspirin-containing products in patients with active GI disease.

• Consider semisupine chair position for patient comfort because of GI effects of disease.

rasagiline

rah-**sa**′-ji-leen
(Azilect)

CATEGORY AND SCHEDULE

Pregnancy Risk Category: C

Drug Class: Monoamine oxidase inhibitor

MECHANISM OF ACTION

An antiparkinson agent that irreversibly inhibits monoamine oxidase type B (more selective for MOA type B than type A).
Therapeutic Effect: Relieves signs and symptoms of Parkinson's disease.

USES

Parkinson's disease, monotherapy or adjunct therapy

PHARMACOKINETICS

Rapidly absorbed after PO administration. Protein binding: 88%–94%. Extensively metabolized in liver, primarily by CYP1A2. Less than 1% is excreted unchanged in the urine. ***Half-life:*** 1.34 hr.

INDICATIONS AND DOSAGES

▸ **Parkinson's Disease, Monotherapy**

PO

Adults. 1 mg a day.

▸ **Parkinson's Disease, Adjunct**

PO

Adults. 0.5 mg a day. May increase to 1 mg a day if clinical response is not achieved.

▸ **Hepatic Impairment**

Mild to moderate. 0.5 mg a day.
Severe hepatic impairment. Not recommended.

SIDE EFFECTS/ADVERSE REACTIONS

Frequent

Headache, orthostatic hypotension, rash, weight loss, GI upset, arthralgia, dyspepsia, depression, fall, flu syndrome, vertigo

Occasional

Conjunctivitis, fever, gastroenteritis, rhinitis, arthritis, ecchymosis, malaise, neck pain, paresthesia

PRECAUTIONS AND CONTRAINDICATIONS

Hypersensitivity to rasagiline or its components
Concurrent use with meperidine, tramadol, propoxyphene, dextromethorphan, St. John's wort, cyclobenzaprine, or other MAO inhibitors

Caution:

Hepatic impairment
Concurrent use with sympathomimetics, tyramine-containing foods, CYP1A2 inhibitors
Melanoma

DRUG INTERACTIONS OF CONCERN TO DENTISTRY

• Opioids (particularly meperidine): potentially fatal interaction; serotonin syndrome

• St. John's wort, cyclobenzaprine: contraindicated

• Dextromethorphan: concurrent use may cause psychosis or bizarre behavior; contraindicated

• MOA inhibitors: may increase the risk of hypertensive crisis
• Potent CYP1A2 inhibitors (cimetidine, ciprofloxacin, fluvoxamine): may increase levels of rasagiline
• CYP inducers: may reduce rasagiline levels
• Sympathomimetics, tyramine-containing foods: may increase the risk of hypertensive crisis
• Antidepressants (SSRIs, SNRIs, TCAs): increased risk of serotonin syndrome

SERIOUS REACTIONS

! Rasagiline may cause low blood pressure; increased risk of postural hypotension.
! May cause or exacerbate hallucinations and psychotic behavior.
! Symptoms of overdose may vary from CNS depression, characterized by sedation, apnea, cardiovascular collapse, and death, to severe paradoxical reactions, such as hallucinations, tremor, and seizures.
! Other serious effects may include involuntary movements, impaired motor coordination, loss of balance, blepharospasm, facial grimaces, feeling of heaviness in the lower extremities, depression, nightmares, delusions, overstimulation, sleep disturbance, and anger.

DENTAL CONSIDERATIONS

General:
• Monitor vital signs at every appointment because of cardiovascular side effects.
• After supine positioning, have patient sit upright for at least 2 min before standing to avoid orthostatic hypotension.
• Assess for presence of extrapyramidal motor symptoms, such as tardive dyskinesia and akathisia. Extrapyramidal motor activity may complicate dental treatment.
• Assess salivary flow as a factor in caries, periodontal disease, and candidiasis.
• Consider semisupine chair position for patient comfort if GI side effects occur.

Consultations:
• Medical consultation may be required to assess disease control and patient's ability to tolerate stress.
• If signs of tardive dyskinesia or akathisia present, refer to physician.

Teach Patient/Family to:
• When chronic dry mouth occurs, advise patient to:
  • Avoid mouth rinses with high alcohol content because of drying effects.
  • Use daily home fluoride products for anticaries effect.
  • Use sugarless gum, frequent sips of water, or saliva substitutes.

repaglinide

re-**pag'**-lih-nide
(GlucoNorm[CAN], Novo Norm[AUS], Prandin)

CATEGORY AND SCHEDULE

Pregnancy Risk Category: C

Drug Class: Oral antidiabetic, meglitinide class

MECHANISM OF ACTION

An antihyperglycemic that stimulates release of insulin from

beta cells of the pancreas by depolarizing beta cells, leading to an opening of calcium channels. Resulting calcium influx induces insulin secretion.
Therapeutic Effect: Lowers blood glucose concentration.

USES

Treatment of type 2 diabetes mellitus when hyperglycemia cannot be controlled by diet and exercise; may also be used in combination with metformin, rosiglitazone maleate, or pioglitazone HCl

PHARMACOKINETICS

Rapidly, completely absorbed from the GI tract. Protein binding: 98%. Metabolized in the liver to inactive metabolites. Excreted primarily in feces with a lesser amount in urine. Unknown if removed by hemodialysis. ***Half-life:*** 1 hr.

INDICATIONS AND DOSAGES

▸ Diabetes Mellitus

PO

Adults, Elderly. 0.5–4 mg 2–4 times a day. Maximum: 16 mg/day.

SIDE EFFECTS/ADVERSE REACTIONS

Frequent

Upper respiratory tract infection, headache, rhinitis, bronchitis, back pain

Occasional

Diarrhea, dyspepsia, sinusitis, nausea, arthralgia, UTI

Rare

Constipation, vomiting, paresthesia, allergy

PRECAUTIONS AND CONTRAINDICATIONS

Diabetic ketoacidosis, type 1 diabetes mellitus

Caution:

Increased cardiac mortality risk, hypoglycemia, hypoglycemia in patients taking adrenergic blockers, monitor laboratory values, lactation, pediatric patients

DRUG INTERACTIONS OF CONCERN TO DENTISTRY

- Clinical studies have not been completed; metabolism may be inhibited by ketoconazole, miconazole, erythromycin
- Risk of increased hypoglycemia: NSAIDs, salicylates
- Suspected increase in plasma levels: clarithromycin, erythromycin

SERIOUS REACTIONS

! Hypoglycemia occurs in 16% of patients.

! Chest pain occurs rarely.

DENTAL CONSIDERATIONS

General:

- If dentist prescribes any of the drugs listed in the drug interactions section, monitor patient blood sugar levels.
- Be prepared to manage hypoglycemia.
- Consider semisupine chair position for patient comfort because of GI side effects of drug.
- Ensure that patient is following prescribed diet and regularly takes medication.
- Place on frequent recall to evaluate healing response.
- Short appointments and a stress-reduction protocol may be required.
- Diabetics may be more susceptible to infection and have delayed wound healing.

Consultations:

- Medical consultation may include data from patient's blood glucose monitoring, including glycosylated hemoglobin or HbA_{1c} testing.

• Medical consultation may be required to assess disease control and patient's ability to tolerate stress.

Teach Patient/Family to:

• Prevent trauma when using oral hygiene aids.

• Update health and drug history if physician makes any changes in evaluation or drug regimens; include OTC, herbal, and nonherbal drugs in the update.

reserpine

reh-**zer**′-peen

(Serpalan, Maviserpin[MEX], Novoreserpine[CAN], Rauserpine[TAIWAN], Rauverid[PHILIPPINES], Reserfia[CAN], Serpasil[CAN, INDONESIA], Serpasol[SPAIN])

Do not confuse with Risperdal, risperidone

CATEGORY AND SCHEDULE

Pregnancy Risk Category: C

Drug Class: Antiadrenergic agent, antihypertensive

MECHANISM OF ACTION

An antihypertensive that depletes stores of catecholamines and 5-hydroxytryptamine in many organs, including the brain and adrenal medulla. Depression of sympathetic nerve function results in a decreased heart rate and a lowering of arterial B/P. Depletion of catecholamines and 5-hydroxytryptamine from the brain is thought to be the mechanism of the sedative and tranquilizing properties.

Therapeutic Effects: Decrease B/P and heart rate; sedation.

USES

Treatment of refractory hypertension

PHARMACOKINETICS

Characterized by slow onset of action and sustained effects. Both cardiovascular and CNS effects may persist for a period of time following withdrawal of the drug. Mean maximum plasma levels were attained after a median of 3.5 hr. Bioavailability was approximately 50% of that of a corresponding intravenous dose. Protein binding: 96%. ***Half-life:*** 33 hr.

INDICATIONS AND DOSAGES

▸ Hypertension

PO

Adults. Usual initial dosage 0.5 mg/day for 1 or 2 wk. For maintenance, reduce to 0.1–0.25 mg/day.

Children. Reserpine is not recommended for use in children. If it is to be used in treating a child, the usual recommended starting dose is 20 mcg/kg daily. The maximum recommended dose is 0.25 mg (total) daily.

▸ Psychiatric Disorders

PO

Adults. Initial dosage 0.5 mg/day, may range from 0.1 to 1.0 mg. Adjust dosage upward or downward according to response.

SIDE EFFECTS/ADVERSE REACTIONS

Occasional

Burning in the stomach, nausea, vomiting, diarrhea, dry mouth, nosebleed, stuffy nose, dizziness, headache, nervousness, nightmares, drowsiness, muscle aches, weight gain, redness of the eyes

Rare

Irregular heart beat, difficulty breathing, heart problems, feeling faint, swelling, gynecomastia, decreased libido

PRECAUTIONS AND CONTRAINDICATIONS

Hypersensitivity, mental depression or history of mental depression (especially with suicidal tendencies), active peptic ulcer, ulcerative colitis, patients receiving electroconvulsive therapy

Caution:

Lactation, seizure disorders, renal disease

DRUG INTERACTIONS OF CONCERN TO DENTISTRY

- Increased CNS depression: barbiturates, alcohol, opioids
- Increased pressor effects: epinephrine
- Decreased pressor effects: ephedrine, tricyclic antidepressants
- Decreased hypotensive effect: NSAIDs

SERIOUS REACTIONS

! None known

DENTAL CONSIDERATIONS

General:

- After supine positioning, have patient sit upright for at least 2 min before standing to avoid orthostatic hypotension.
- Use vasoconstrictors with caution, in low doses, and with careful aspiration.
- Avoid stress; consider a stress-reduction protocol.

Consultations:

- Medical consultation may be required to assess disease control.

Teach Patient/Family to:

- Encourage effective oral hygiene to prevent soft tissue inflammation.
- When chronic dry mouth occurs, advise patient to:
  - Avoid mouth rinses with high alcohol content because of drying effects.
  - Use daily home fluoride products to prevent caries.
  - Use sugarless gum, frequent sips of water, or saliva substitutes.

retapamulin

ee-te-**pam′**-ue-lin

(Altabax)

CATEGORY AND SCHEDULE

Pregnancy Risk Category: B

Drug Class: Antibiotic

MECHANISM OF ACTION

Bacteriostatic binds to protein L2 on the ribosomal 50S subunit, inhibits peptidyl transfer and blocks P-site interaction to prevent formation of this subunit; therefore, inhibits bacterial protein biosynthesis.

USES

Impetigo caused by *Staphylococcus aureus* or *Streptococcus pyogenes*

PHARMACOKINETICS

When applied topically, low systemic absorption. Absorption increased when applied to abraded skin. Protein binding is 94%. Extensively metabolized in the liver via CYP3A4.

INDICATIONS AND DOSAGES

▸ **Impetigo Caused by *Staphylococcus aureus* or *Streptococcus pyogenes***

Topical

Adults. Apply to the affected area (up to 100 cm^2 in total area) twice a day for 5 days.

Children (9 mo or older). Apply to the affected area (2% total body surface area) twice a day for 5 days.

SIDE EFFECTS/ADVERSE REACTIONS

Occasional

▸ **Adults**

Headache, application site irritation, diarrhea, nausea, nasopharyngitis, increased creatinine phosphokinase.

▸ **Children**

Application site pruritus, diarrhea, nasopharyngitis, pruritus, eczema, headache, pyrexia.

PRECAUTIONS AND CONTRAINDICATIONS

Contraindicated in patients with hypersensitivity to retapamulin or components of the formulation. Sensitization or severe local irritation may occur.

Retapamulin is for external use only and has not been proven for intranasal, intravaginal, ophthalmic, oral, or mucosal application.

DRUG INTERACTIONS OF CONCERN TO DENTISTRY

- None reported

R

SERIOUS REACTIONS

! Superinfections may result from altered bacterial balance.

DENTAL CONSIDERATIONS

General:

- Consider semisupine chair position for patient comfort if GI side effects occur.

Consultations:

- Medical consultation may be required to assess disease control.

Teach Patient/Family to:

- Encourage effective oral hygiene to prevent soft tissue inflammation.
- Use caution to prevent injury when using oral hygiene aids.

reteplase, recombinant

reh′-te-place

(Rapilysin[AUS], Retavase)

Do not confuse reteplase or Retavase with Restasis.

CATEGORY AND SCHEDULE

Pregnancy Risk Category: C

Drug Class: Thrombolytic

MECHANISM OF ACTION

A tissue plasminogen activator that activates the fibrinolytic system by directly cleaving plasminogen to generate plasmin, an enzyme that degrades the fibrin of the thrombus.

Therapeutic Effect: Exerts thrombolytic action.

USES

Dissolving of blood clots that have formed in certain blood vessels

PHARMACOKINETICS

Rapidly cleared from plasma. Eliminated primarily by the liver and kidney. ***Half-life:*** 13–16 min.

INDICATIONS AND DOSAGES

▸ **Acute MI, CHF**

IV Bolus

Adults, Elderly. 10 units over 2 min; repeat in 30 min.

SIDE EFFECTS/ADVERSE REACTIONS

Frequent

Bleeding at superficial sites, such as venous injection sites, catheter insertion sites, venous cutdowns, arterial punctures, and sites of recent surgical procedures, gingival bleeding

PRECAUTIONS AND CONTRAINDICATIONS

Active internal bleeding, AV malformation or aneurysm, bleeding diathesis, history of cerebrovascular accident, intracranial neoplasm, recent intracranial or intraspinal surgery or trauma, severe uncontrolled hypertension

DRUG INTERACTIONS OF CONCERN TO DENTISTRY

• Increased risk of bleeding: drugs that interfere with coagulation or platelet function, such as NSAIDs or aspirin

SERIOUS REACTIONS

! Bleeding at internal sites may occur, including intracranial, retroperitoneal, GI, GU, and respiratory sites.

! Lysis or coronary thrombi may produce atrial or ventricular arrhythmias and stroke.

DENTAL CONSIDERATIONS

General:

• Acute-use drug for use in hospitals or emergency rooms.

• Patients are at risk for bleeding, check for oral signs.

• Monitor and record vital signs.

• Avoid products that affect platelet function, such as aspirin and NSAIDs.

• Patients who have been treated with this drug may present with cardiovascular disease or stroke, review medical and drug history.

Consultations:

• Medical consultation should include routine blood counts including platelet counts and bleeding time.

• In a patient with symptoms of blood dyscrasias, request a medical consultation for blood studies and postpone treatment until normal values are reestablished.

• Medical consultation may be required to assess disease control and patient's ability to tolerate stress.

Teach Patient/Family to:

• Use soft tooth brush to reduce risk of bleeding.

• Encourage effective oral hygiene to prevent soft tissue inflammation.

• Report oral lesions, soreness, or bleeding to dentist.

• Prevent trauma when using oral hygiene aids.

• Update health and medication history if physician makes any changes in evaluation or drug regimens; include OTC, herbal, and nonherbal remedies in the update.

ribavirin

rye-ba-**vye**′-rin

(Copegus, Rebetol, Rebetron, Virazole)

Do not confuse ribavirin with riboflavin.

CATEGORY AND SCHEDULE

Pregnancy Risk Category: X

Drug Class: Antiviral

MECHANISM OF ACTION

A synthetic nucleoside that inhibits influenza virus RNA polymerase activity and interferes with expression of messenger RNA.

Therapeutic Effect: Inhibits viral protein synthesis and replication of viral RNA and DNA.

USES

Treatment of adults and children with chronic hepatitis C but only in combination with interferon alfa-2b or peginterferon alfa-2a; patients must have compensated liver disease and not previously been treated with interferons; respiratory syncytial virus (RSV) in hospitalized infants and young children, unapproved use in influenza A or B or in lower respiratory tract pneumonia associated with an adenovirus

PHARMACOKINETICS

Rapidly absorbed from the GI tract following oral administration. A small amount is systemically absorbed following inhalation. Primarily excreted in urine. ***Half-life:*** 298 hr (oral); 9.5 hr (inhalation).

INDICATIONS AND DOSAGES

▸ Chronic Hepatitis C

PO (Capsule or Oral Solution in Combination with Interferon Alfa-2b)

Adults, Elderly. 1000–1200 mg/day in 2 divided doses.

Children weighing 60 kg or more. Use adult dosage. (51–60 kg): 400 mg twice a day. (37–50 kg): 200 mg in morning, 400 mg in evening. (24–36 kg): 200 mg twice a day.

PO (Capsules in Combination with Peginterferon Alfa-2b)

Adults, Elderly. 800 mg/day in 2 divided doses.

PO (Tablets in Combination with Peginterferon Alfa-2b)

Adults, Elderly. 800–1200 mg/day in 2 divided doses.

▸ Severe Lower Respiratory Tract Infection Caused by RSV

Inhalation

Children, Infants. Use with Vivatek small-particle aerosol generator at a concentration of 20 mg/ml (6 g reconstituted with 300 ml sterile water) over 12–18 hr/day for 3–7 days.

SIDE EFFECTS/ADVERSE REACTIONS

Frequent

Dizziness, headache, fatigue, fever, insomnia, irritability, depression, emotional lability, impaired concentration, alopecia, rash, pruritus, nausea, anorexia, dyspepsia, vomiting, decreased hemoglobin, hemolysis, arthralgia, musculoskeletal pain, dyspnea, sinusitis, flu-like symptoms

Occasional

Nervousness, altered taste, weakness

PRECAUTIONS AND CONTRAINDICATIONS

Autoimmune hepatitis, creatinine clearance less than 50 ml/min, hemoglobinopathies, hepatic decompensation, hypersensitivity to ribavirin products, pregnancy, significant or unstable cardiac disease, women of childbearing age who will not use contraception reliably

Caution:

Must not be used alone for hepatitis C, severe side effects occur, pregnancy category X, aggravation of sarcoidosis, stop therapy if pancreatitis occurs, use aerosol only for RSV, extra contraception required to prevent pregnancy during use and for up to 6 mo after discontinuing use

DRUG INTERACTIONS OF CONCERN TO DENTISTRY

- None reported

SERIOUS REACTIONS

! Cardiac arrest, apnea, and ventilator dependence, bacterial pneumonia, pneumonia, and pneumothorax occur rarely.

! Anemia may occur if ribavirin therapy exceeds 7 days.

DENTAL CONSIDERATIONS

General:

- Patients taking this drug will also be taking an interferon drug; be sure to conduct a thorough drug history.
- Assess salivary flow as a factor in caries, periodontal disease, and candidiasis.
- Patients on chronic drug therapy may rarely have symptoms of blood dyscrasias, which can include infection, bleeding, and poor healing.
- Consider semisupine chair position for patient comfort if GI side effects occur.
- Examine for oral manifestation of opportunistic infection.
- Take precautions if dental surgery is anticipated and general anesthesia is required.
- Monitor vital signs at every appointment because of cardiovascular side effects.

Consultations:

- In a patient with symptoms of blood dyscrasias, request a medical consultation for blood studies and postpone treatment until normal values are reestablished.
- Medical consultation may be required to assess disease control and patient's ability to tolerate stress.
- Consultation with physician may be necessary if sedation or general anesthesia is required.

Teach Patient/Family to:

- Update health and drug history if physician makes any changes in evaluation or drug regimens; include OTC, herbal, and nonherbal drugs in the update.
- Encourage effective oral hygiene to prevent soft tissue inflammation.
- Prevent trauma when using oral hygiene aids.
- When chronic dry mouth occurs, advise patient to:
  - Avoid mouth rinses with high alcohol content because of drying effects.
  - Use daily home fluoride products for anticaries effect.
  - Use sugarless gum, frequent sips of water, or saliva substitutes.

rifabutin

rif′-ah-**byoo′**-ten

(Mycobutin)

Do not confuse rifabutin with rifampin.

CATEGORY AND SCHEDULE

Pregnancy Risk Category: B

Drug Class: Antimycobacterial

MECHANISM OF ACTION

An antitubercular that inhibits DNA-dependent RNA polymerase, an enzyme in susceptible strains of *Escherichia coli* and *Bacillus subtilis.* Rifabutin has a broad spectrum of antimicrobial activity, including against mycobacteria such as *Mycobacterium avium* complex (MAC).

Therapeutic Effect: Prevents MAC disease.

USES

Prevention of disseminated MAC disease with advanced HIV infection

PHARMACOKINETICS

Readily absorbed from the GI tract (high-fat meals delay absorption). Protein binding: 85%. Widely distributed. Crosses the blood-brain barrier. Extensive intracellular tissue uptake. Metabolized in the liver to active metabolite. Excreted in urine; eliminated in feces. Unknown if removed by hemodialysis. ***Half-life:*** 16–69 hr.

INDICATIONS AND DOSAGES

▸ Prevention of MAC Disease (First Episode)

PO

Adults, Elderly. 300 mg as a single dose or in 2 divided doses if GI upset occurs.

▸ Prevention of Recurrent MAC Disease

PO

Adults, Elderly. 300 mg/day (in combination).

▸ Dosage in Renal Impairment

Dosage is modified on the basis of creatinine clearance. If creatinine clearance is less than 30 ml/min, reduce dosage by 50%.

SIDE EFFECTS/ADVERSE REACTIONS

Frequent

Red-orange or red-brown discoloration of urine, feces, saliva, skin, sputum, sweat, or tears

Occasional

Rash, nausea, abdominal pain, diarrhea, dyspepsia, belching, headache, altered taste, uveitis, corneal deposits

Rare

Anorexia, flatulence, fever, myalgia, vomiting, insomnia

PRECAUTIONS AND CONTRAINDICATIONS

Active tuberculosis; hypersensitivity to other rifamycins, including rifampin

Caution:

Pregnancy category B, lactation, concurrent corticosteroid therapy

DRUG INTERACTIONS OF CONCERN TO DENTISTRY

- Decreases plasma concentrations of corticosteroids; may be significant
- May induce CYP3A4 isoenzymes, possible reduction in action of ketoconazole, itraconazole, benzodiazepines, doxycycline, erythromycin, clarithromycin

SERIOUS REACTIONS

! Hepatitis and thrombocytopenia occur rarely. Anemia and neutropenia may also occur.

DENTAL CONSIDERATIONS

General:

- Examine for evidence of oral signs of opportunistic disease.
- Determine why the patient is taking the drug.
- Patients on chronic drug therapy may rarely have symptoms of blood dyscrasias, which can include infection, bleeding, and poor healing.

Consultations:

- Medical consultation may be required to assess patient's ability to tolerate stress.
- In a patient with symptoms of blood dyscrasias, request a medical consultation for blood studies and postpone dental treatment until normal values are reestablished.

Teach Patient/Family to:

- Avoid mouth rinses with high alcohol content because of drying effects.
- Encourage effective oral hygiene to prevent soft tissue inflammation.

rifampin

rye′-fam-pin
(Rifadin, Rimactane, Rimycin[AUS], Rofact[CAN])
Do not confuse rifampin with rifabutin, Rifamate, rifapentine, or Ritalin.

CATEGORY AND SCHEDULE

Pregnancy Risk Category: C

Drug Class: Antitubercular antiinfective

MECHANISM OF ACTION

An antitubercular that interferes with bacterial RNA synthesis by binding to DNA-dependent RNA polymerase, thus preventing its attachment to DNA and blocking RNA transcription.
Therapeutic Effect: Bactericidal in susceptible microorganisms.

USES

Pulmonary tuberculosis (TB), meningococcal carriers (prevention); unapproved: leprosy and atypical mycobacterial infections

PHARMACOKINETICS

Well absorbed from the GI tract (food delays absorption). Protein binding: 80%. Widely distributed. Metabolized in the liver to active metabolite. Primarily eliminated by the biliary system. Not removed by hemodialysis. ***Half-life:*** 3–5 hr (increased in hepatic impairment).

INDICATIONS AND DOSAGES

▸ **Tuberculosis**
PO, IV
Adults, Elderly. 10 mg/kg/day. Maximum: 600 mg/day.
Children. 10–20 mg/kg/day in divided doses q12–24h.

▸ **Prevention of Meningococcal Infections**
PO, IV
Adults, Elderly. 600 mg q12h for 2 days.
Children 1 mo and older. 20 mg/kg/day in divided doses q12–24h. Maximum: 600 mg/dose.
Infants younger than 1 mo. 10 mg/kg/day in divided doses q12h for 2 days.

▸ **Staphylococcal Infections**
PO, IV
Adults, Elderly. 600 mg/day.
Children. 15 mg/kg/day in divided doses q12h.

▸ ***Staphylococcus aureus*** **Infections (in Combination with Other Antiinfectives)**
PO
Adults, Elderly. 300–600 mg twice a day.
Neonates. 5–20 mg/kg/day in divided doses q12h.

▸ **Prevention of *Haemophilus influenzae* Infection**
PO
Adults, Elderly. 600 mg/day for 4 days.
Children 1 mo and older. 20 mg/kg/day in divided doses q12h for 5–10 days.
Children younger than 1 mo. 10 mg/kg/day in divided doses q12h for 2 days.

SIDE EFFECTS/ADVERSE REACTIONS

Expected
Red-orange or red-brown discoloration of urine, feces, saliva, skin, sputum, sweat, or tears
Occasional
Hypersensitivity reaction (such as flushing, pruritus, or rash)
Rare
Diarrhea, dyspepsia, nausea, candida as evidenced by sore mouth or tongue

PRECAUTIONS AND CONTRAINDICATIONS

Concomitant therapy with amprenavir, hypersensitivity to rifampin or any other rifamycins

Caution:

Lactation, hepatic disease, blood dyscrasias, concurrent therapy with corticosteroids

Reduced effectiveness of oral contraceptives

DRUG INTERACTIONS OF CONCERN TO DENTISTRY

- Increased risk of hepatotoxicity: acetaminophen (chronic use and high doses), alcohol, hydrocarbon inhalation anesthetics (except isoflurane)
- Decreased effects of corticosteroids, dapsone, ketoconazole, fluconazole, itraconazole, oral contraceptives, benzodiazepines, doxycycline, erythromycin, clarithromycin, opioid analgesics (induces CYP450 isoenzymes)
- Suspected decrease in fexofenadine effects

SERIOUS REACTIONS

! Rare reactions include hepatotoxicity (risk is increased when rifampin is taken with isoniazid), hepatitis, blood dyscrasias, Stevens-Johnson syndrome, and antibiotic-associated colitis.

DENTAL CONSIDERATIONS

General:

- Examine for oral manifestation of opportunistic infections.
- Do not treat patients with active tuberculosis.
- Patients on chronic drug therapy may rarely have symptoms of blood dyscrasias, which can include infection, bleeding, and poor healing.
- Determine why the patient is taking the drug (prophylaxis or active therapy).
- Determine that noninfectious status exists by ensuring that (1) anti-TB drugs have been taken for longer than 3 wk, (2) culture has confirmed TB susceptibility to antiinfectives, (3) patient has had three consecutive negative sputum smears, and (4) patient is not in the coughing stage.

Consultations:

- Medical consultation may be required to assess patient's ability to tolerate stress.
- In a patient with symptoms of blood dyscrasias, request a medical consultation for blood studies and postpone dental treatment until normal values are reestablished.

Teach Patient/Family to:

- Avoid mouth rinses with high alcohol content because of drying effects.
- Encourage effective oral hygiene to prevent soft tissue inflammation.
- Take medications for full length of regimen to ensure effectiveness of treatment and to prevent the emergence of resistant strains.

rifapentine

rif-ah-**pen′**-teen

(Priftin)

Do not confuse rifapentine with rifampin.

CATEGORY AND SCHEDULE

Pregnancy Risk Category: C

Drug Class: Antimycobacterial

R

MECHANISM OF ACTION

An antitubercular that inhibits bacterial RNA synthesis by binding to DNA-dependent RNA polymerase in *Mycobacterium tuberculosis*. This action prevents the enzyme from attaching to DNA, thereby blocking RNA transcription.
Therapeutic Effect: Bactericidal.

USES

Treatment of pulmonary tuberculosis (TB) in combination with other anti-TB drugs; unlabeled use includes prophylaxis of *Mycobacterium avium* complex (MAC) in patients with AIDS

PHARMACOKINETICS

PO: Slow absorption, peak levels 5–6 hr, highly plasma protein bound (97%–93%), hepatic metabolism, 25-desacetylrifapentine is active metabolite, hepatic metabolism, excreted in feces (70%) and urine (17%).

INDICATIONS AND DOSAGES

▸ TB

PO

Adults, Elderly. Intensive phase: 600 mg twice a wk for 2 mo (interval between doses no less than 3 days). Continuation phase: 600 mg/wk for 4 mo.

SIDE EFFECTS/ADVERSE REACTIONS

Rare

Red-orange or red-brown discoloration of urine, feces, saliva, skin, sputum, sweat, or tears; arthralgia, pain, nausea, vomiting, headache, dyspepsia, hypertension, dizziness, diarrhea

PRECAUTIONS AND CONTRAINDICATIONS

Hypersensitivity to rifampin, rifabutin

Caution:

Significant hepatic dysfunction, induces hepatic microsomal enzymes, pregnancy category C, lactation, children younger than 12 yr

DRUG INTERACTIONS OF CONCERN TO DENTISTRY

- May accelerate metabolism of clarithromycin, doxycycline, ciprofloxacin, fluconazole, ketoconazole, itraconazole, diazepam, barbiturates, corticosteroids, opioids, zolpidem, sildenafil, tricyclic antidepressants
- Inducer of CYP3A4 and CYP2C8/9 isoenzymes may cause drug interactions

SERIOUS REACTIONS

! Hyperuricemia, neutropenia, proteinuria, hematuria, and hepatitis occur rarely.

DENTAL CONSIDERATIONS

General:

- Determine why patient is taking the drug (prophylaxis or active therapy).
- Examine for oral manifestation of opportunistic infections.
- Do not treat patients with active tuberculosis.
- Patients on chronic drug therapy may rarely have symptoms of blood dyscrasias, which can include infection, bleeding, and poor healing.
- Determine that noninfectious status exists by ensuring that (1) anti-TB drugs have been taken for longer than 3 wk, (2) culture has confirmed TB susceptibility to

antiinfectives, (3) patient has had three consecutive negative sputum smears, and (4) patient is not in the coughing stage.
• Consider semisupine chair position for patient comfort because of GI side effects of drug.

Consultations:
• Medical consultation may be required to assess disease control and patient's ability to tolerate stress.
• In a patient with symptoms of blood dyscrasias, request a medical consultation for blood studies and postpone treatment until normal values are reestablished.

Teach Patient/Family to:
• Avoid mouth rinses with high alcohol content because of drying effects.
• Prevent trauma when using oral hygiene aids.
• Encourage effective oral hygiene to prevent soft tissue inflammation.
• Take medication for full length of regimen to ensure effectiveness of treatment and prevent emergence of resistant strains.
• Be aware of potential for extrinsic oral staining side effect.

R

rifaximin

rye-fax′-ih-min
(Xifaxan)
Do not confuse with rifampin.

CATEGORY AND SCHEDULE

Pregnancy Risk Category: C

Drug Class: Antibiotic

MECHANISM OF ACTION

An anti-infective that inhibits bacterial RNA synthesis by binding to the beta subunit of bacterial DNA-dependent RNA polymerase. Resulting in inhibition of bacterial RNA synthesis.
Therapeutic Effect: Bactericidal.

USES

Traveler's diarrhea
Hepatic encephalopathy

PHARMACOKINETICS

Less than 0.4% absorbed after PO administration. Protein binding: 62%–67.5%. Primarily eliminated in feces; minimal excretion in urine. ***Half-life:*** 1.8–4.8 hr.

INDICATIONS AND DOSAGES

▸ Traveler's Diarrhea

PO
Adults, Elderly, Children 12 yr and older. 200 mg 3 times a day for 3 days.

▸ Hepatic Encephalopathy

PO
Adults, Elderly. One 550 mg tablet 2 times/day.

SIDE EFFECTS/ADVERSE REACTIONS

Frequent
Diarrhea, peripheral edema, nausea, dizziness, fatigue, ascites (HE), headache, flatulence, muscle spasms, pruritus, abdominal pain, abdominal distention, anemia

Occasional
Rectal tenesmus, defecation urgency, cough, depression, insomnia, nasopharyngitis, arthralgia, back pain, constipation, dyspnea

Rare
Rash, fever, vomiting, immunohypersensitivity reaction

PRECAUTIONS AND CONTRAINDICATIONS

Hypersensitivity to rifaximin, other rifamycin antibiotics, or any component of the formulation

Caution:
Hepatic impairment, severe
Clostridium difficile-associated diarrhea
Pseudomembranous colitis
Use only if *E. coli* is the causative pathogen

DRUG INTERACTIONS OF CONCERN TO DENTISTRY

- None reported

SERIOUS REACTIONS

! Hypersensitivity reactions, including dermatitis, angioneurotic edema, pruritus, rash, and urticaria may occur.
! Superinfection occurs rarely.

DENTAL CONSIDERATIONS

General:
- Assess salivary flow as a factor in caries, periodontal disease, and candidiasis.
- Determine why the patient is taking the drug.
- Examine for evidence oral signs of opportunistic infection.

Consultations:
- Medical consultation may be required to assess disease control.

Teach Patient/Family to:
- Report oral lesions, soreness, or bleeding to dentist.
- When chronic dry mouth occurs, advise patient to:
  - Avoid mouth rinses with high alcohol content because of drying effects.
  - Use daily home fluoride products for anticaries effect.
  - Use sugarless gum, frequent sips of water, or saliva substitutes.

rilpivirine

ril′-pi-**vir′**-een
(Edurant)

CATEGORY AND SCHEDULE

Pregnancy Risk Category: B

Drug Class: Antiretroviral agent, reverse transcriptase inhibitor (nonnucleoside)

MECHANISM OF ACTION

As a nonnucleoside reverse transcriptase inhibitor, rilpivirine has activity against HIV-1 by binding to reverse transcriptase. It consequently blocks the RNA-dependent and DNA-dependent DNA polymerase activities, including HIV-1 replication.
Therapeutic Effect: Slows HIV replication and reduces viral load.

USES

Treatment of HIV-1 infections in combination with at least two other antiretroviral agents

PHARMACOKINETICS

99.7% plasma protein bound. Hepatic metabolism via CYP3A4. Excreted primarily in feces as unchanged drug. ***Half-life:*** 50 hr.

INDICATIONS AND DOSAGES

▸ Treatment of HIV-1 Infection

PO
Adults. 25 mg once daily.

SIDE EFFECTS/ADVERSE REACTIONS

Frequent
Rash, increased cholesterol and triglycerides
Occasional
Abdominal discomfort/pain, abnormal dreams, anxiety, decreased

appetite, cholecystitis, cholelithiasis, diarrhea, dizziness, fatigue, glomerulonephritis (membranous and mesangioproliferative), nausea, somnolence, sleep disorders, vomiting

PRECAUTIONS AND CONTRAINDICATIONS

Concomitant use of carbamazepine, oxcarbazepine, phenobarbital, phenytoin, proton pump inhibitors (PPIs), rifabutin, rifampin, rifapentine, or St. John's wort

DRUG INTERACTIONS OF CONCERN TO DENTISTRY

• CYP3A4 inhibitors (e.g., macrolide antibiotics, azole antifungals): increased blood levels and toxicity of rilpivirine
• CYP3A4 inducers (e.g., carbamazepine, barbiturates): decreased blood levels and efficacy of rilpivirine
• Highly bioavailable benzodiazepines (e.g., triazolam): increased blood levels and sedation if coadministered with rilpivirine

SERIOUS REACTIONS

! May cause depression, depressed mood, dysphoria, mood changes, negative thoughts, suicide attempts, or suicidal ideation

DENTAL CONSIDERATIONS

General:
• Examine for oral manifestation of opportunistic infections.
Consultations:
• Consult physician to determine disease status and ability of patient to tolerate dental procedures.
Teach Patient/Family to:
• Report changes in disease status and drug regimen.

R

riluzole

rye′-loo-zole
(Rilutek)

CATEGORY AND SCHEDULE

Pregnancy Risk Category: C

Drug Class: Glutamate antagonist

MECHANISM OF ACTION

An amyotrophic lateral sclerosis (ALS) agent that inhibits presynaptic glutamate release in the CNS and interferes postsynaptically with the effects of excitatory amino acids.
Therapeutic Effect: Extends survival of ALS patients.

USES

Treatment of ALS (Lou Gehrig's disease)

PHARMACOKINETICS

PO: Well absorbed, extensively metabolized by liver (CYP1A2), excreted in urine/feces.

INDICATIONS AND DOSAGES

▸ **ALS**

PO

Adults, Elderly. 50 mg q12h.

SIDE EFFECTS/ADVERSE REACTIONS

Frequent
Nausea, asthenia, reduced respiratory function
Occasional
Edema, tachycardia, headache, dizziness, somnolence, depression, vertigo, tremor, pruritus, alopecia, abdominal pain, diarrhea, anorexia, dyspepsia, vomiting, stomatitis, increased cough

PRECAUTIONS AND CONTRAINDICATIONS

Hypersensitivity, hepatic impairment, renal impairment, hypertension, other CNS disorders, pregnancy category C, lactation, children

DRUG INTERACTIONS OF CONCERN TO DENTISTRY

• No data reported with dental drugs, but use with caution when given with inducers or inhibitors of CYP1A2

SERIOUS REACTIONS

! None known

DENTAL CONSIDERATIONS

General:

• Short appointments may be required because of nature of disease process.

• Monitor vital signs at every appointment because of cardiovascular and respiratory side effects.

• Consider semisupine chair position for patient comfort.

• Assess salivary flow as factor in caries, periodontal disease, and candidiasis.

• Examine for oral manifestation of opportunistic infection.

• Patients on chronic drug therapy may rarely have symptoms of blood dyscrasias, which can include infection, bleeding, and poor healing.

• After supine positioning, have patient sit upright for at least 2 min before standing to avoid orthostatic hypotension.

Consultations:

• Medical consultation may be required to assess disease control.

• In a patient with symptoms of blood dyscrasias, request a medical consultation for blood studies and postpone treatment until normal values are reestablished.

Teach Patient/Family to:

• Encourage effective oral hygiene, including use of powered tooth brush if patient has difficulty holding conventional devices or directions for caregiver.

• Use caution to prevent trauma when using oral hygiene aids.

• When chronic dry mouth occurs, advise patient to:

  • Avoid mouth rinses with high alcohol content because of drying effects.

  • Use daily home fluoride products for anticaries effect.

  • Use sugarless gum, frequent sips of water, or saliva substitutes.

rimantadine hydrochloride

ri-**man**′-ta-deen
high-droh-**klor**′-ide
(Flumadine)

Do not confuse rimantadine with ranitidine or Flumadine with flunisolide or flutamide.

CATEGORY AND SCHEDULE

Pregnancy Risk Category: C

Drug Class: Antiviral

MECHANISM OF ACTION

An antiviral that appears to exert an inhibitory effect early in the viral replication cycle. May inhibit uncoating of the virus.

Therapeutic Effect: Prevents replication of influenza A virus.

USES
Adult: prophylaxis and treatment of illnesses caused by strains of influenza A virus; children: prophylaxis against influenza A virus

PHARMACOKINETICS
PO: Peak plasma levels 6 hr; 40% plasma protein binding; hepatic metabolism; renal excretion.

INDICATIONS AND DOSAGES
▸ **Influenza A Virus**
PO
Adults, Elderly. 100 mg twice a day for 7 days.
Elderly nursing home patients, Patients with severe hepatic or renal impairment. 100 mg/day for 7 days.
▸ **Prevention of Influenza A Virus**
PO
Adults, Elderly, Children 10 yr and older. 100 mg twice a day for at least 10 days after known exposure (usually for 6–8 wk).
Children younger than 10 yr. 5 mg/kg/day. Maximum: 150 mg.
Elderly nursing home patients, Patients with severe hepatic or renal impairment. 100 mg/day.

R

SIDE EFFECTS/ADVERSE REACTIONS
Occasional
Insomnia, nausea, nervousness, impaired concentration, dizziness
Rare
Vomiting, anorexia, dry mouth, abdominal pain, asthenia, fatigue

PRECAUTIONS AND CONTRAINDICATIONS
Hypersensitivity to amantadine or rimantadine
Caution:
Pregnancy category C, elderly, epilepsy, hepatic or renal impairment, emergence of resistant viral strains

DRUG INTERACTIONS OF CONCERN TO DENTISTRY
• Tramadol: increased risk of seizures

SERIOUS REACTIONS
! None known

DENTAL CONSIDERATIONS
General:
• Monitor vital signs at every appointment because of cardiovascular side effects.
• Determine why the patient is taking the drug (probably will be used only during peak seasons for influenza).
• Assess salivary flow as a factor in caries, periodontal disease, and candidiasis.
Teach Patient/Family to:
• Encourage effective oral hygiene to prevent soft tissue inflammation.
• When chronic dry mouth occurs, advise patient to:
  • Avoid mouth rinses with high alcohol content because of drying effects.
  • Use daily home fluoride products to prevent caries.
  • Use sugarless gum, frequent sips of water, or saliva substitutes.

rimexolone
rye-**mex′**-oh-lone
(Vexol)
Do not confuse with riluzole.

CATEGORY AND SCHEDULE
Pregnancy Risk Category: C

Drug Class: Corticosteroid

MECHANISM OF ACTION

An ophthalmic agent that suppresses migration of polymorphonuclear leukocytes and reverses increased capillary permeability.
Therapeutic Effect: Decreases inflammation.

USES

Treatment of inflammation of the eye associated with ocular surgery and uveitis

PHARMACOKINETICS

Absorbed through aqueous humor. Metabolized in liver. Excreted in urine and feces.

INDICATIONS AND DOSAGES

▸ **Inflammation after Ocular Surgery, Treatment of Anterior Uveitis**
Ophthalmic
Adults, Elderly. Instill 1 drop 2–4 times a day up to q4h. May use q1–2h during the first 1–2 days.

SIDE EFFECTS/ADVERSE REACTIONS

Occasional
Temporary mild blurred vision

PRECAUTIONS AND CONTRAINDICATIONS

Fungal, viral, or untreated pus-forming bacterial ocular infections, hypersensitivity to rimexolone or any component of the formulation
Caution:
Increased intraocular pressure, lactation, children, secondary ocular infections

DRUG INTERACTIONS OF CONCERN TO DENTISTRY

- None reported

SERIOUS REACTIONS

! Prolonged use has been associated with the development of corneal or scleral perforation and posterior subcapsular cataracts.
! Cataracts, corneal thinning, glaucoma, increased intraocular pressure, optic nerve damage, secondary ocular infection, and visual acuity defects occur rarely.

DENTAL CONSIDERATIONS

General:
- Determine why the patient is taking the drug.
- Avoid dental light in patient's eyes; offer dark glasses for patient comfort.

risedronate sodium

rih-**sed′**-roe-nate **soe′**-dee-um
(Actonel)

CATEGORY AND SCHEDULE

Pregnancy Risk Category: C

Drug Class: Bisphosphonate

R

MECHANISM OF ACTION

A bisphosphonate that binds to bone hydroxyapatite and inhibits osteoclasts.
Therapeutic Effect: Reduces bone turnover (the number of sites at which bone is remodeled) and bone resorption.

USES

Treatment of Paget's disease of bone; treatment and prevention of osteoporosis in postmenopausal women and glucocorticoid-induced osteoporosis

INDICATIONS AND DOSAGES

▸ Paget's Disease

PO

Adults, Elderly. 30 mg/day for 2 mo. Retreatment may occur after 2-mo posttreatment observation period.

▸ Prevention and Treatment of Postmenopausal Osteoporosis

PO

Adults, Elderly. 5 mg/day or 35 mg once a wk.

▸ Glucocorticoid-Induced Osteoporosis

PO

Adults, Elderly. 5 mg/day.

SIDE EFFECTS/ADVERSE REACTIONS

Frequent

Arthralgia

Occasional

Rash, flu-like symptoms, peripheral edema

Rare

Bone pain, sinusitis, asthenia, dry eye, tinnitus

PRECAUTIONS AND CONTRAINDICATIONS

Hypersensitivity to other bisphosphonates, including etidronate, tiludronate, risedronate, and alendronate; hypocalcemia; inability to stand or sit upright for at least 20 min; renal impairment when serum creatinine clearance is greater than 5 mg/dl

Caution:

Upper GI disease, avoid use in significant renal impairment, pregnancy category C, lactation, pediatric patients

DRUG INTERACTIONS OF CONCERN TO DENTISTRY

- Retarded absorption: calcium, antacids, medications with divalent cations
- Increased GI side effects: NSAIDs, aspirin

SERIOUS REACTIONS

! Overdose causes hypocalcemia, hypophosphatemia, and significant GI disturbances.

DENTAL CONSIDERATIONS

General:

- Bisphosphonates may increase the risk of osteonecrosis of the jaw.
- Be aware of the oral manifestations of Paget's disease (macrognathia, alveolar pain).
- Consider semisupine chair position for patient comfort because of GI side effects of drug.
- Short appointments may be required for patient comfort.

Consultations:

- Medical consultation may be required to assess disease control.

Teach Patient/Family to:

- Observe regular recall schedule and practice effective oral hygiene to minimize risk of osteonecrosis of the jaw.
- Use powered tooth brush if patient has difficulty holding conventional devices.

risperidone

ris-**per′**-ih-done

(Risperdal, Risperdal Consta, Risperdal M-Tabs)

Do not confuse risperidone with reserpine.

CATEGORY AND SCHEDULE

Pregnancy Risk Category: C

Drug Class: Antipsychotic (benzisoxazole derivative)

MECHANISM OF ACTION

A benzisoxazole derivative that may antagonize dopamine and serotonin receptors.

Therapeutic Effect: Suppresses psychotic behavior.

USES

Treatment of schizophrenia

PHARMACOKINETICS

Well absorbed from the GI tract; unaffected by food. Protein binding: 90%. Extensively metabolized in the liver to active metabolite. Primarily excreted in urine. ***Half-life:*** 3–20 hr; metabolite: 21–30 hr (increased in elderly).

INDICATIONS AND DOSAGES

▸ Psychotic Disorder

PO

Adults. 0.5–1 mg twice a day. May increase dosage slowly. Range: 2–6 mg/day.

Elderly. Initially, 0.25–2 mg/day in 2 divided doses. May increase dosage slowly. Range: 2–6 mg/day.

IM

Adults, Elderly. 25 mg q2wk. Maximum: 50 mg q2wk.

▸ Mania

PO

Adults, Elderly. Initially, 2–3 mg as a single daily dose. May increase at 24-hr intervals of 1 mg/day. Range: 2–6 mg/day.

▸ Dosage in Renal Impairment

Initial dosage for adults and elderly patients is 0.25–0.5 mg twice a day. Dosage is titrated slowly to desired effect.

SIDE EFFECTS/ADVERSE REACTIONS

Frequent

Agitation, anxiety, insomnia, headache, constipation

Occasional

Dyspepsia, rhinitis, somnolence, dizziness, nausea, vomiting, rash, abdominal pain, dry skin, tachycardia

Rare

Visual disturbances, fever, back pain, pharyngitis, cough, arthralgia, angina, aggressive behavior, orthostatic hypotension, breast swelling

PRECAUTIONS AND CONTRAINDICATIONS

Hypersensitivity, pregnancy category C, lactation, seizures, suicidal patients, cardiac diseases, renal or hepatic impairment, elderly; patients should be monitored for signs and symptoms of diabetes mellitus

DRUG INTERACTIONS OF CONCERN TO DENTISTRY

- Increased excretion: chronic use of carbamazepine
- Increased sedation: other CNS depressants, alcohol, barbiturate anesthesia, opioid analgesics
- Increased extrapyramidal effects: phenothiazines and related drugs (haloperidol, droperidol), metoclopramide
- Additive photosensitization: tetracyclines
- Increased anticholinergic effects: anticholinergics, such as atropine and scopolamine

SERIOUS REACTIONS

! Rare reactions include tardive dyskinesia (characterized by tongue protrusion, puffing of the cheeks, and chewing or puckering of the mouth) and neuroleptic malignant syndrome (marked by hyperpyrexia, muscle rigidity, change in mental status, irregular pulse or B/P, tachycardia, diaphoresis, cardiac arrhythmias, rhabdomyolysis, and acute renal failure).

DENTAL CONSIDERATIONS

General:

- Monitor vital signs at every appointment because of cardiovascular side effects.
- Patients on chronic drug therapy may rarely have symptoms of blood dyscrasias, which can include infection, bleeding, and poor healing.
- After supine positioning, have patient sit upright for at least 2 min before standing to avoid orthostatic hypotension.
- Assess salivary flow as a factor in caries, periodontal disease, and candidiasis.
- Consider semisupine chair position for patient comfort because of GI effects of drug.
- Assess for presence of extrapyramidal motor symptoms, such as tardive dyskinesia and akathisia. Extrapyramidal motor activity may complicate dental treatment.
- Use vasoconstrictors with caution, in low doses, and with careful aspiration; avoid use of gingival retraction cord with epinephrine.

Consultations:

- In a patient with symptoms of blood dyscrasias, request a medical consultation for blood studies and postpone dental treatment until normal values are reestablished.
- Take precautions if dental surgery is anticipated and anesthesia is required.
- If signs of tardive dyskinesia or other extrapyramidal symptoms are present, refer to physician.
- Physician should be informed if significant xerostomic side effects occur (e.g., increased caries, sore tongue, problems eating or swallowing, difficulty wearing prosthesis) so that a medication change can be considered.

Teach Patient/Family to:

- Encourage effective oral hygiene to prevent soft tissue inflammation.
- Use caution to prevent injury when using oral hygiene aids.
- Use powered tooth brush if patient has difficulty holding conventional devices.
- When chronic dry mouth occurs, advise patient to:
  - Avoid mouth rinses with high alcohol content because of drying effects.
  - Use daily home fluoride products for anticaries effect.
  - Use sugarless gum, frequent sips of water, or saliva substitutes.

ritonavir

ri-**tone**′-ah-veer
(Norvir, Norvisec[CAN])
Do not confuse ritonavir with Retrovir.

CATEGORY AND SCHEDULE

Pregnancy Risk Category: B

Drug Class: Antiviral, protease inhibitor

MECHANISM OF ACTION

Inhibits HIV-1 and HIV-2 proteases, rendering these enzymes incapable of processing the polypeptide precursors; this results in the production of noninfectious, immature HIV particles.
Therapeutic Effect: Impedes HIV replication, slowing the progression of HIV infection.

USES

Treatment of HIV infection in adults and children as single-drug therapy or in combination with nucleoside analogues

R

PHARMACOKINETICS

Well absorbed after PO administration (absorption increased with food). Protein binding: 98%–99%. Extensively metabolized in the liver to active metabolite. Primarily eliminated in feces. Unknown if removed by hemodialysis. ***Half-life:*** 2.7–5 hr.

INDICATIONS AND DOSAGES

▸ HIV Infection

PO

Adults, Children 12 yr and older. 600 mg twice a day. If nausea occurs at this dosage, give 300 mg twice a day for 1 day, 400 mg twice a day for 2 days, 500 mg twice a day for 1 day, then 600 mg twice a day thereafter.

Children younger than 12 yr. Initially, 250 mg/m^2/dose twice a day. Increase by 50 mg/m^2/dose up to 400 mg/m^2/dose. Maximum: 600 mg/dose twice a day.

SIDE EFFECTS/ADVERSE REACTIONS

Frequent

GI disturbances (abdominal pain, anorexia, diarrhea, nausea, vomiting), circumoral and peripheral paresthesias, altered taste, headache, dizziness, fatigue, asthenia

Occasional

Allergic reaction, flu-like symptoms, hypotension

Rare

Diabetes mellitus, hyperglycemia

PRECAUTIONS AND CONTRAINDICATIONS

Concurrent use of amiodarone, astemizole, bepridil, bupropion, cisapride, clozapine, encainide, flecainide, meperidine, piroxicam, propafenone, propoxyphene, quinidine, rifabutin, or terfenadine (increased risk of serious or life-threatening drug interactions, such as arrhythmias, hematologic abnormalities, and seizures); concurrent use of alprazolam, clorazepate, diazepam, estazolam, flurazepam, midazolam, triazolam, or zolpidem (may produce extreme sedation and respiratory depression)

Caution:

Hepatic impairment, lactation, children younger than 12 yr, alters lab chemistry values (triglycerides, ALT, AST, GGT, CPK, uric acid)

DRUG INTERACTIONS OF CONCERN TO DENTISTRY

- Alprazolam, clorazepate, diazepam, bupropion, estazolam, flurazepam, midazolam, triazolam, zolpidem, meperidine, piroxicam, propoxyphene, chlordiazepoxide, halazepam, quazepam (increased CNS depression)
- Increased plasma level drugs metabolized by CYP3A4 (clarithromycin, fluconazole), macrolide antibiotics, azole antifungals
- Possible alcohol–disulfiram reaction: metronidazole, disulfiram
- Decreased plasma levels with carbamazepine, dexamethasone, phenobarbital, St. John's wort (herb)
- Increased plasma levels of fentanyl

SERIOUS REACTIONS

! None known

DENTAL CONSIDERATIONS

General:

- Monitor vital signs at every appointment because of cardiovascular side effects.
- Examine for oral manifestation of opportunistic infection.
- Place on frequent recall to evaluate healing response.

• Assess salivary flow as a factor in caries, periodontal disease, and candidiasis.
• Consider semisupine chair position for patient comfort because of GI effects of drug.

Consultations:

• Medical consultation may be required to assess disease control.

Teach Patient/Family to:

• Encourage effective oral hygiene to prevent soft tissue inflammation.
• See dentist immediately if secondary oral infection occurs.
• When chronic dry mouth occurs, advise patient to:
  • Avoid mouth rinses with high alcohol content because of drying effects.
  • Use daily home fluoride products for anticaries effect.
  • Use sugarless gum, frequent sips of water, or saliva substitutes.

rituximab

rye-**tucks′**-ih-mab
(Mabthera[AUS], Rituxan)

CATEGORY AND SCHEDULE

Pregnancy Risk Category: C

Drug Class: Antineoplastics, monoclonal antibodies

MECHANISM OF ACTION

Binds to CD20, the antigen found on the surface of B lymphocytes and B-cell non-Hodgkin's lymphomas. ***Therapeutic Effect:*** Produces cytotoxicity, reducing tumor size.

USES

Treatment of a type of cancer called non-Hodgkin's lymphoma. It can be used alone or with other cancer medicines or chemotherapy.

PHARMACOKINETICS

Rapidly depletes B cells. ***Half-life:*** 59.8 hr after first infusion and 174 hr after fourth infusion.

INDICATIONS AND DOSAGES

▸ **Non-Hodgkin's Lymphoma**

IV

Adults. 375 mg/m^2 once a wk for 4–8 wk. May administer a second 4-wk course.

SIDE EFFECTS/ADVERSE REACTIONS

Frequent

Fever, chills, nausea, asthenia, headache, angioedema, hypotension, rash or pruritus

Occasional

Myalgia, dizziness, abdominal pain, throat irritation, vomiting, neutropenia, rhinitis, bronchospasm, urticaria

PRECAUTIONS AND CONTRAINDICATIONS

Hypersensitivity to murine proteins

DRUG INTERACTIONS OF CONCERN TO DENTISTRY

• None reported

SERIOUS REACTIONS

! A hypersensitivity reaction marked by hypotension, bronchospasm, and angioedema may occur.

! Arrhythmias may occur, particularly in those with a history of preexisting cardiac conditions.

DENTAL CONSIDERATIONS

General:

• Monitor and record vital signs.
• If additional analgesia is required for dental pain, consider alternative analgesics (NSAIDs) in patients taking narcotics for acute or chronic pain.

• After supine positioning, have patient sit upright for at least 2 min before standing to avoid orthostatic hypotension.
• Patient on chronic drug therapy may rarely present with symptoms of blood dyscrasias, which can include infection, bleeding, and poor healing. If dyscrasia is present, caution patient to prevent oral tissue trauma when using oral hygiene aids.
• Provide emergency dental care only during drug use.
• Hypersensitivity reactions may occur.
• Oral infections should be eliminated and treated aggressively.

Consultations:

• Medical consultation should include routine blood counts including platelet counts and bleeding time.
• Consult physician; prophylactic or therapeutic antiinfectives may be indicated if surgery or periodontal treatment is required.
• Medical consultation may be required to assess immunologic status during cancer chemotherapy and determine safety risk, if any, posed by the required dental treatment.
• Medical consultation may be required to assess disease control and patient's ability to tolerate stress.

Teach Patient/Family to:

• Encourage effective oral hygiene to prevent soft tissue inflammation.
• Report oral lesions, soreness, or bleeding to dentist.
• Prevent trauma when using oral hygiene aids.
• Update health and medication history if physician makes any changes in evaluation or drug regimens; include OTC, herbal, and nonherbal remedies in the update.

rivaroxaban

riv-a-**rox′**-a-ban
(Xarelto)

CATEGORY AND SCHEDULE

Pregnancy Risk Category: C

Drug Class: Factor Xa inhibitor

MECHANISM OF ACTION

Inhibits platelet activation and fibrin clot formation via direct, selective, and reversible inhibition of factor Xa (FXa) in both the intrinsic and extrinsic coagulation pathways.
Therapeutic Effect: Produces anticoagulation.

USES

Postoperative thromboprophylaxis in patients who have undergone hip or knee replacement surgery; prevention of stroke and systemic embolism in patients with nonvalvular atrial fibrillation

PHARMACOKINETICS

Rapid absorption after oral administration. 92%–95% plasma protein bound. Hepatic metabolism via CYP3A4/5 and CYP2J2. Excreted via urine (66%) and feces (28%). ***Half-life:*** 5–9 hr.

INDICATIONS AND DOSAGES

▸ **Nonvalvular Atrial Fibrillation (to Prevent Stroke and Systemic Embolism)**

Adults. 20 mg once daily.

▸ **Postoperative Thromboprophylaxis**

Knee replacement:
PO
Adults. 10 mg once daily; recommended total duration of therapy: 12–14 days.
Hip replacement:

R

PO

Adults. 10 mg once daily; total duration of therapy: 35 days.

SIDE EFFECTS/ADVERSE REACTIONS

Frequent

Dyspepsia, abdominal discomfort and pain, bleeding

Occasional

GERD, esophagitis, anemia, hematuria, hematoma, epistaxis, wound secretion, anaphylaxis

PRECAUTIONS AND CONTRAINDICATIONS

Hypersensitivity to rivaroxaban or any component of the formulation; active pathological bleeding. Avoid use in patients with moderate-to-severe hepatic and renal impairment. Avoid concomitant use with other anticoagulant and antiplatelet agents, CYP3A4 inhibitors (ketoconazole, itraconazole, ritonavir, conivaptan) and inducers (carbamazepine, phenytoin, rifampin, St. John's wort)

DRUG INTERACTIONS OF CONCERN TO DENTISTRY

- Increased risk of bleeding: NSAIDs, aspirin, aspiring-containing products
- CYP3A4 inducers (e.g., carbamazepine, St. John's wort): reduced blood levels and efficacy of dabigatran, rivaroxaban
- CYP3A4 inhibitors (e.g., macrolide antibiotics, azole antifungals): increased blood levels and adverse effects of dabigatran, rivaroxaban

SERIOUS REACTIONS

! Spinal or epidural hematomas, including subsequent paralysis, may occur with neuraxial anesthesia (epidural or spinal anesthesia) or spinal puncture in patients who are anticoagulated. Discontinuing rivaroxaban for elective and/or invasive procedures increases the risk of stroke, which is sometimes fatal.

DENTAL CONSIDERATIONS

General:

- Expect increased intraoperative and postoperative bleeding; additional hemostatic measures are indicated.
- Monitor vital signs at every visit due to existing cardiovascular disease.
- Avoid discontinuation of drug therapy for routine dental procedures without consulting patient's prescribing physician.

Consultations:

- Consult physician to determine patient's coagulation status and risk for complications.

Teach Patient/Family to:

- Report changes in drug regimen.
- Report signs and symptoms of excessive postoperative bleeding.

rivastigmine tartrate

riv-ah-**stig′**-meen **tar′**-trate

(Exelon)

CATEGORY AND SCHEDULE

Pregnancy Risk Category: B

Drug Class: Reversible cholinesterase inhibitor

MECHANISM OF ACTION

A cholinesterase inhibitor that inhibits the enzyme acetylcholinesterase, thus increasing the concentration of acetylcholine at cholinergic synapses and enhancing cholinergic function in the CNS.

Therapeutic Effect: Slows the progression of symptoms of Alzheimer's disease.

PHARMACOKINETICS

Rapidly and completely absorbed. Protein binding: 60%. Widely distributed throughout the body. Rapidly and extensively metabolized. Primarily excreted in urine. ***Half-life:*** 1.5 hr.

INDICATIONS AND DOSAGES

▸ Alzheimer's Disease

PO

Adults, Elderly. Initially, 1.5 mg twice a day. May increase at intervals of least 2 wk to 3 mg twice a day, then 4.5 mg twice a day, and finally 6 mg twice a day. Maximum: 6 mg twice a day.

SIDE EFFECTS/ADVERSE REACTIONS

Frequent

Nausea, vomiting, dizziness, diarrhea, headache, anorexia

Occasional

Abdominal pain, insomnia, dyspepsia (heartburn, indigestion, epigastric pain), confusion, UTI, depression

Rare

Anxiety, somnolence, constipation, malaise, hallucinations, tremor, flatulence, rhinitis, hypertension, flu-like symptoms, weight loss, syncope

PRECAUTIONS AND CONTRAINDICATIONS

Hypersensitivity to this drug or other carbamate derivatives

Caution:

Significant GI reactions, nausea, vomiting, and weight-loss occur; history of GI ulcers or GI bleeding, patients taking NSAIDs, seizures, asthma, COPD, lactation, pediatric patients (no studies); smoking increases renal clearance

DRUG INTERACTIONS OF CONCERN TO DENTISTRY

- Caution in use of NSAIDs if GI side effects are significant
- Decreased response to neuromuscular blocking agents used in general anesthesia
- Increased cholinergic response: other cholinergic drugs
- Decreased cholinergic response: anticholinergics or other drugs with anticholinergic actions

SERIOUS REACTIONS

! Overdose may result in cholinergic crisis, characterized by severe nausea and vomiting, increased salivation, diaphoresis, bradycardia, hypotension, respiratory depression, and seizures.

DENTAL CONSIDERATIONS

General:

- Determine why patient is taking the drug.
- Monitor vital signs at every appointment because of cardiovascular side effects.
- Drug is used early in the disease; ensure that patient or caregiver understands informed consent.
- Place on frequent recall because early attention to dental health is important for Alzheimer's patients.
- Assess salivary flow as a factor in caries, periodontal disease, and candidiasis.
- Use precaution if sedation or general anesthesia is required; risk of hypotensive episode.
- Consider semisupine chair position for patient comfort if GI side effects occur.
- Patients on chronic drug therapy may rarely have symptoms of blood dyscrasias, which can include infection, bleeding, and poor healing.

Consultations:

• Consultation with physician may be necessary if sedation or general anesthesia is required.

• In a patient with symptoms of blood dyscrasias, request a medical consultation for blood studies and postpone treatment until normal values are reestablished.

• Medical consultation may be required to assess disease control and patient's ability to tolerate stress.

Teach Patient/Family to:

• Use powered tooth brush if patient has difficulty holding conventional devices.

• Prevent trauma when using oral hygiene aids.

• Encourage effective oral hygiene to prevent soft tissue inflammation.

rizatriptan benzoate

rize-ah-**trip**′-tan **ben**′-zoe-ate
(Maxalt, Maxalt-MLT)

CATEGORY AND SCHEDULE

Pregnancy Risk Category: C

Drug Class: Serotonin agonist

R

MECHANISM OF ACTION

A serotonin receptor agonist that binds selectively to vascular receptors, producing a vasoconstrictive effect on cranial blood vessels.

Therapeutic Effect: Relieves migraine headache.

USES

Acute treatment of migraine attacks with or without aura

PHARMACOKINETICS

Well absorbed after PO administration. Protein binding: 14%. Crosses the blood-brain barrier. Metabolized by the liver to inactive metabolite. Eliminated primarily in urine and, to a lesser extent, in feces. ***Half-life:*** 2–3 hr.

INDICATIONS AND DOSAGES

▸ **Acute Migraine Attack**

PO

Adults older than 18 yr, Elderly. 5–10 mg. If headache improves, but then returns, dose may be repeated after 2 hr. Maximum: 30 mg/24 hr.

SIDE EFFECTS/ADVERSE REACTIONS

Frequent

Dizziness, somnolence, paresthesia, fatigue

Occasional

Nausea, chest pressure, dry mouth

Rare

Headache; neck, throat, or jaw pressure; photosensitivity

PRECAUTIONS AND CONTRAINDICATIONS

Basilar or hemiplegic migraine, coronary artery disease, ischemic heart disease (including angina pectoris, history of MI, silent ischemia, and Prinzmetal's angina), uncontrolled hypertension, use within 24 hr of ergotamine-containing preparations or another serotonin receptor agonist, use within 14 days of MAOIs

Caution:

Risk of serious cardiovascular events, renal/hepatic impairment, SSRI antidepressants, lactation, use in children not established, orally disintegrating tabs contain aspartame

DRUG INTERACTIONS OF CONCERN TO DENTISTRY

• No specific interactions with dental drugs reported
• Increased plasma levels: propranolol
• Should not be used within 24 hr of another 5-HT agonist

SERIOUS REACTIONS

! Cardiac reactions (such as ischemia, coronary artery vasospasm, and MI) and noncardiac vasospasm-related reactions (including hemorrhage and CVA) occur rarely, particularly in patients with hypertension, diabetes, or a strong family history of coronary artery disease; obese patients; smokers; males older than 40 yr; and postmenopausal women.

DENTAL CONSIDERATIONS

General:
• This is an acute-use drug; it is doubtful that patients will be treated in the office if acute migraine is present.
• Be aware of patient's disease, its severity, and its frequency, when known.
• Avoid dental light in patient's eyes; offer dark glasses for patient comfort.
• Short appointments and a stress-reduction protocol may be required for anxious patients.
• After supine positioning, have patient sit upright for at least 2 min before standing to avoid orthostatic hypotension.
Consultations:
• If treating chronic orofacial pain, consult with physician of record.
• Medical consultation may be required to assess disease control and patient's ability to tolerate stress.
Teach Patient/Family to:
• Update health and drug history if physician makes any changes in evaluation or drug regimens; include OTC, herbal, and nonherbal drugs in the update.

roflumilast

roe-**flue**′-mi-last
(Daliresp)

CATEGORY AND SCHEDULE

Pregnancy Risk Category: C

Drug Class: Phosphodiesterase -4 enzyme inhibitor

MECHANISM OF ACTION

Roflumilast selectively inhibits phosphodiesterase-4 (PDE4), leading to an accumulation of cyclic AMP (cAMP) within inflammatory and structural cells important in the pathogenesis of COPD.
Therapeutic Effect: Reduces frequency of COPD. flare-ups

USES

Adjunct to bronchodilator therapy in the maintenance treatment of severe chronic obstructive pulmonary disease (COPD) associated with chronic bronchitis

PHARMACOKINETICS

99% plasma protein bound. Hepatic metabolism via CYP3A4 and CYP1A2 to active metabolite. Excreted primarily via urine. ***Half-life:*** 17 hr.

INDICATIONS AND DOSAGES

▸ **COPD**
PO
Adults. 500 mcg once daily.

SIDE EFFECTS/ADVERSE REACTIONS

Frequent
Diarrhea, weight loss
Occasional
Headache, dizziness, insomnia, back pain

PRECAUTIONS AND CONTRAINDICATIONS

May cause neuropsychiatric effects, including anxiety and depression

DRUG INTERACTIONS OF CONCERN TO DENTISTRY

- CYP3A4 inhibitors (e.g., macrolide antibiotics, azole antifungals): increased blood levels of roflumilast and increased adverse effects
- CYP3A4 inducers (e.g., carbamazepine, barbiturates): reduced blood levels and decreased efficacy of roflumilast

SERIOUS REACTIONS

! None known

DENTAL CONSIDERATIONS

General:

- Roflumilast is not a rescue inhaler and should not be used to treat acute respiratory distress.
- Consider semisupine position for patient comfort due to respiratory disease.
- Monitor patients for signs of psychiatric changes, including insomnia, increased anxiety, and mood changes.
- Take precautions when seating and dismissing patient due to possible dizziness.
- Possible increased nausea and vomiting (e.g., during sedation, impressions).

Teach Patient/Family to:

- Rinse mouth with water and expectorate following use of inhaler.
- Use home fluoride products for anticaries effect.

R

ropinirole hydrochloride

roe-**pin′**-ih-role
high-droh-**klor′**-ide
(Requip)

CATEGORY AND SCHEDULE

Pregnancy Risk Category: C

Drug Class: Antiparkinson agent

MECHANISM OF ACTION

An antiparkinson agent that stimulates dopamine receptors in the striatum.
Therapeutic Effect: Relieves signs and symptoms of Parkinson's disease.

USES

Treatment of Parkinson's disease

PHARMACOKINETICS

Rapidly absorbed after PO administration. Protein binding: 40%. Extensively distributed throughout the body. Extensively metabolized. Steady-state concentrations achieved within 2 days. Eliminated in urine. Unknown if removed by hemodialysis.
Half-life: 6 hr.

INDICATIONS AND DOSAGES

▸ **Parkinson's Disease**

PO
Adults, Elderly. Initially, 0.25 mg 3 times a day. May increase dosage every 7 days.

SIDE EFFECTS/ADVERSE REACTIONS

Frequent
Nausea, dizziness, somnolence

Occasional
Syncope, vomiting, fatigue, viral infection, dyspepsia, diaphoresis, asthenia, orthostatic hypotension, abdominal discomfort, pharyngitis, abnormal vision, dry mouth, hypertension, hallucinations, confusion
Rare
Anorexia, peripheral edema, memory loss, rhinitis, sinusitis, palpitations, impotence

PRECAUTIONS AND CONTRAINDICATIONS: HYPERSENSITIVITY

Cardiovascular disease, severely impaired renal or hepatic function, lactation, pregnancy category C, syncope, hypotension

DRUG INTERACTIONS OF CONCERN TO DENTISTRY

• Possible increase in sedation with all CNS depressants
• Possible diminished effects: dopamine antagonists, phenothiazines, haloperidol, droperidol, and metoclopramide

SERIOUS REACTIONS

! None known

DENTAL CONSIDERATIONS

General:
• Monitor vital signs at every appointment because of cardiovascular side effects.
• Assess salivary flow as factor in caries, periodontal disease, and candidiasis.
• After supine positioning, have patient sit upright for at least 2 min before standing to avoid orthostatic hypotension.
• Patients on chronic drug therapy may rarely have symptoms of blood dyscrasias, which can include infection, bleeding, and poor healing.
• Consider semisupine chair position for patient comfort if GI side effects occur.
Consultations:
• In a patient with symptoms of blood dyscrasias, request a medical consultation for blood studies and postpone treatment until normal values are reestablished.
• Medical consultation may be required to assess disease control and patient's ability to tolerate stress.
Teach Patient/Family to:
• Use caution to prevent trauma when using oral hygiene aids.
• Use powered tooth brush if patient has difficulty holding conventional devices.
• Encourage effective oral hygiene to prevent soft tissue inflammation.
• Update health and drug history if physician makes any changes in evaluation or drug regimens; include OTC, herbal, and nonherbal drugs in the update.
• When chronic dry mouth occurs, advise patient to:
  • Avoid mouth rinses with high alcohol content because of drying effects.
  • Use daily home fluoride products for anticaries effect.
  • Use sugarless gum, frequent sips of water, or saliva substitutes.

rosiglitazone maleate

roz-ih-**gli′**-tah-zone **mal′**-ee-ate
(Avandia)
Do not confuse Avandia with Avalide, Avinza, or Prandin.

CATEGORY AND SCHEDULE

Pregnancy Risk Category: C

Drug Class: Oral antidiabetic

MECHANISM OF ACTION

An antidiabetic that improves target-cell response to insulin without increasing pancreatic insulin secretion. Decreases hepatic glucose output and increases insulin-dependent glucose utilization in skeletal muscle.

Therapeutic Effect: Lowers blood glucose concentration.

USES

Monotherapy, as an adjunct to diet and exercise in patients with type 2 diabetes mellitus; may also be used with metformin when metformin, diet, and exercise are not adequate for control

PHARMACOKINETICS

Rapidly absorbed. Protein binding: 99%. Metabolized in the liver. Excreted primarily in urine, with a lesser amount in feces. Not removed by hemodialysis. ***Half-life:*** 3–4 hr.

INDICATIONS AND DOSAGES

▸ Diabetes Mellitus, Combination Therapy

PO

Adults, Elderly. Initially, 4 mg as a single daily dose or in divided doses twice a day. May increase to 8 mg/day after 12 wk of therapy if fasting glucose level is not adequately controlled.

▸ Diabetes Mellitus, Monotherapy

Adults, Elderly. Initially, 4 mg as single daily dose or in divided doses twice a day. May increase to 8 mg/day after 12 wk of therapy.

SIDE EFFECTS/ADVERSE REACTIONS

Frequent

Upper respiratory tract infection

Occasional

Headache, edema, back pain, fatigue, sinusitis, diarrhea

PRECAUTIONS AND CONTRAINDICATIONS

Active hepatic disease, diabetic ketoacidosis, increased serum transaminase levels, including ALT (SGPT) greater than 2.5 times the normal serum level, type 1 diabetes mellitus

Caution:

May cause resumption of ovulation in premenopausal anovulatory women (risk of pregnancy), patients with edema, advanced heart failure, hepatic impairment, monitor liver enzymes, lactation

DRUG INTERACTIONS OF CONCERN TO DENTISTRY

• None reported

SERIOUS REACTIONS

! None known

DENTAL CONSIDERATIONS

General:

• Ensure that patient is following prescribed diet and regularly takes medication.

• Be prepared to manage hypoglycemia.

• Place on frequent recall to evaluate healing response.

• Short appointments and a stress-reduction protocol may be required for anxious patients.

• Diabetics may be more susceptible to infection and have delayed wound healing.

• Question patient about self-monitoring of drug's antidiabetic effect, including blood glucose values or finger-stick records.

Consultations:

• Medical consultation may include data from patient's blood glucose monitoring, including glycosylated hemoglobin or HbA_{1c} testing.

• Medical consultation may be required to assess disease control and patient's ability to tolerate stress.
Teach Patient/Family to:
• Prevent trauma when using oral hygiene aids.
• Update health and drug history if physician makes any changes in evaluation or drug regimens; include OTC, herbal, and nonherbal drugs in the update.

rosuvastatin calcium

ross-uh-vah-**stah**′-tin **kal**′-see-um
(Crestor)

CATEGORY AND SCHEDULE

Pregnancy Risk Category: X

Drug Class: Antihyperlipidemic

MECHANISM OF ACTION

An antihyperlipidemic that interferes with cholesterol biosynthesis by inhibiting the conversion of the enzyme HMG-CoA to mevalonate, a precursor to cholesterol.
Therapeutic Effect: Decreases low-density lipoprotein (LDL) cholesterol, very low-density lipoprotein (VLDL), and plasma triglyceride levels; increases high-density lipoprotein (HDL) concentration.

USES

An adjunct to diet in primary hypercholesterolemia, mixed lipidemia (Fredricksen types IIa and IIb), and homozygous familial hypercholesterolemia and to lower triglycerides in Fredrickson type IV hyperlipidemia

PHARMACOKINETICS

Protein binding: 88%. Minimal hepatic metabolism. Primarily eliminated in the feces. ***Half-life:*** 19 hr (increased in patients with severe renal dysfunction).

INDICATIONS AND DOSAGES

▸ **Hyperlipidemia, Dyslipidemia**
PO
Adults, Elderly. 5 to 40 mg/day. Usual starting dosage is 10 mg/day, with adjustments based on lipid levels; monitor q2–4wk until desired level is achieved.
▸ **Renal Impairment (Creatinine Clearance <30 ml/min)**
PO
Adults, Elderly. 5 mg/day; do not exceed 10 mg/day.
▸ **Concurrent Cyclosporine Use**
PO
Adults, Elderly. 5 mg/day.
▸ **Concurrent Lipid-Lowering Therapy**
PO
Adults, Elderly. 10 mg/day.

SIDE EFFECTS/ADVERSE REACTIONS

Rosuvastatin is generally well tolerated. Side effects are usually mild and transient.
Occasional
Pharyngitis, headache, diarrhea, dyspepsia, including heartburn and epigastric distress, nausea
Rare
Myalgia, asthenia or unusual fatigue and weakness, back pain

PRECAUTIONS AND CONTRAINDICATIONS

Active hepatic disease, breast-feeding, pregnancy, unexplained, persistent elevations of serum transaminase levels

Caution:
Severe renal impairment, hepatic impairment, pregnancy category X, liver function test recommended, alcoholics, efficacy and safety in pediatric patients unknown

DRUG INTERACTIONS OF CONCERN TO DENTISTRY

• No dental drug interactions reported; however, interactions with cyclosporine, warfarin, and gemfibrozil are noted
• Does not inhibit CYP3A4

SERIOUS REACTIONS

! Lens opacities may occur.
! Hypersensitivity reaction and hepatitis occur rarely.

DENTAL CONSIDERATIONS

General:
• Monitor vital signs because patients with high cholesterol levels are predisposed to cardiovascular disease.
• Consider semisupine chair position for patient comfort if GI side effects occur.

R

rotigotine

roe-**tig**′-oh-teen
(Neupro)
Do not confuse Neupro with Neupogen.

CATEGORY AND SCHEDULE

Pregnancy Risk Category: C

Drug Class: Antiparkinson agent, dopamine agonist

MECHANISM OF ACTION

Rotigotine is a nonergot dopamine agonist within the substantia nigra in the brain that improves dopaminergic transmission in the motor areas of the basal ganglia.
Therapeutic Effect: Reduces symptoms of Parkinson's disease and RLS.

USES

Treatment of the signs and symptoms of idiopathic Parkinson's disease (early-stage to advanced-stage disease); treatment of moderate-to-severe primary restless legs syndrome (RLS)

PHARMACOKINETICS

90% plasma protein bound. Extensive hepatic metabolism. Excreted via urine (71%) and feces (23%). ***Half-life:*** 5–7 hr after removal of patch.

INDICATIONS AND DOSAGES

▸ Parkinson's Disease

Transdermal
Adults. Early-stage: Initially, apply 2 mg/24 hr patch once daily; may increase by 2 mg/24 hr weekly, based on clinical response and tolerability; lowest effective dose: 4 mg/24 hr (maximum dose: 6 mg/24 hr).
Advanced-stage: Initially, apply 4 mg/24 hr patch once daily; may increase by 2 mg/24 hr weekly, based on clinical response and tolerability (maximum dose: 8 mg/24 hr).
Discontinuation of treatment in Parkinson's disease: Decrease by ≤2 mg/24 hr preferably every other day until withdrawal complete.

▸ Restless Legs Syndrome

Transdermal
Adults. Initially, apply 1 mg/24 hr patch once daily; may increase by 1 mg/24 hr weekly, based on clinical response and tolerability; lowest effective dose: 1 mg/24 hr (maximum dose: 3 mg/24 hr)

Discontinuation of treatment for RLS: Decrease by 1 mg/24 hr preferably every other day until withdrawal complete.

SIDE EFFECTS/ADVERSE REACTIONS

Frequent

Peripheral edema, somnolence, dizziness, orthostatic hypotension, headache, fatigue, sleep disorder, application site reactions, nausea, dyskinesia

Occasional

Erectile dysfunction, vision changes, nasopharyngitis, hiccups

PRECAUTIONS AND CONTRAINDICATIONS

Hypersensitivity to rotigotine or any component of the formulation.

DRUG INTERACTIONS OF CONCERN TO DENTISTRY

• Increased risk of CNS and respiratory depression: all CNS depressants, alcohol. May potentiate mental impairment and somnolence, postural hypotension.

SERIOUS REACTIONS

! May cause hallucinations, psychotic-like behavior, compulsive disorders

DENTAL CONSIDERATIONS

General:

• Avoid postural hypotension. Allow patient to sit upright for 2 min prior to dismissing.

• Use precaution when seating and dismissing patient due to dizziness and dyskinesia.

• Increased risk of nausea and vomiting (e.g., during impressions).

• Possible hallucinations and psychotic behavioral manifestations.

Consultations:

• Consult physician to determine disease status and ability of patient to tolerate dental procedures.

Teach Patient/Family to:

• Report changes in disease status and drug regimen.

• Use special oral hygiene aids if patient has difficulty managing regular tooth brushes and floss due to underlying Parkinson's disease.

salmeterol

sal-**me**′-teh-rol
(Serevent Diskus, Serevent Inhaler and Disks[AUS])
Do not confuse Serevent with Serentil.

CATEGORY AND SCHEDULE

Pregnancy Risk Category: C

Drug Class: Long-acting selective β_2-adrenergic receptor agonist

MECHANISM OF ACTION

An adrenergic agonist that stimulates β_2-adrenergic receptors in the lungs, resulting in relaxation of bronchial smooth muscle.
Therapeutic Effect: Relieves bronchospasm and reduces airway resistance.

USES

Treatment of bronchospasm associated with COPD, maintenance treatment of bronchospasm associated with COPD, asthma, and exercise-induced bronchospasm

PHARMACOKINETICS

S

Route	Onset	Peak	Duration
Inhalation	10–20 min	3 hr	12 hr

Low systemic absorption; acts primarily in the lungs. Protein binding: 95%. Metabolized by hydroxylation. Primarily eliminated in feces. ***Half-life:*** 3–4 hr.

INDICATIONS AND DOSAGES

▸ **Prevention and Maintenance Treatment of Asthma**
Inhalation (Diskus)
Adults, Elderly, Children 4 yr and older. 1 inhalation (50 mcg) q12h.

▸ **Prevention of Exercise-Induced Bronchospasm**
Inhalation
Adults, Elderly, Children 4 yr and older. 1 inhalation at least 30 min before exercise.

▸ **COPD**
Inhalation
Adults, Elderly. 1 inhalation q12h.

SIDE EFFECTS/ADVERSE REACTIONS

Frequent
Headache
Occasional
Cough, tremor, dizziness, vertigo, throat dryness or irritation, pharyngitis
Rare
Palpitations, tachycardia, nausea, heartburn, GI distress, diarrhea

PRECAUTIONS AND CONTRAINDICATIONS

History of hypersensitivity to sympathomimetics
Caution:
Lactation, children younger than 12 yr, hepatic impairment, coronary insufficiency, dysrhythmias, hypertension, convulsive disorders; not for acute symptoms, not to exceed recommended dose, paradoxic bronchospasm may occur with use; not recommended for use with a spacer or other aerosol device

DRUG INTERACTIONS OF CONCERN TO DENTISTRY

- Increased cardiovascular effects: tricyclic antidepressants

SERIOUS REACTIONS

! Salmeterol may prolong the QT interval, which may precipitate ventricular arrhythmias.
! Hypokalemia and hyperglycemia may occur.

DENTAL CONSIDERATIONS

General:

• Monitor vital signs at every appointment because of cardiovascular and respiratory side effects.
• Be aware that aspirin or sulfite preservatives in vasoconstrictor-containing products can exacerbate asthma.
• Acute asthmatic episodes may be precipitated in the dental office. Rapid-acting sympathomimetic inhalants should be available for emergency use. Salmeterol is not a rapid-acting drug and is not intended for use in acute asthmatic attacks.
• Consider semisupine chair position for patients with respiratory disease.
• Midmorning appointments and a stress-reduction protocol may be required for anxious patients.

Consultations:

• Medical consultation may be required to assess disease control and patient's ability to tolerate stress.

Teach Patient/Family to:

• Encourage effective oral hygiene to prevent soft tissue inflammation.

salsalate

sal′-sa-late
(Amigesic, Disalcid, Mono-Gesic, Salflex)

CATEGORY AND SCHEDULE

Pregnancy Risk Category: C

Drug Class: Salicylate, non-opioid analgesic

MECHANISM OF ACTION

An NSAID that inhibits prostaglandin synthesis, reducing the inflammatory response and the intensity of pain stimuli reaching the sensory nerve endings.
Therapeutic Effect: Produces analgesic and antiinflammatory effects.

USES

Treatment of mild-to-moderate pain or fever, including arthritis, juvenile rheumatoid arthritis

PHARMACOKINETICS

Half-life: 7–8 hr.

INDICATIONS AND DOSAGES

▸ **Rheumatoid Arthritis, Osteoarthritis Pain**
PO
Adults, Elderly. Initially, 3 g/day in 2–3 divided doses. Maintenance: 2–4 g/day.

SIDE EFFECTS/ADVERSE REACTIONS

Occasional

Nausea, dyspepsia (including heartburn, indigestion, and epigastric pain)

PRECAUTIONS AND CONTRAINDICATIONS

Bleeding disorders, hypersensitivity to salicylates or NSAIDs

Caution:

Anemia, hepatic disease, renal disease, Hodgkin's disease, lactation

DRUG INTERACTIONS OF CONCERN TO DENTISTRY

• Increased risk of GI complaints and occult blood loss: alcohol, NSAIDs, corticosteroids
• Increased risk of bleeding: oral anticoagulants, valproic acid, dipyridamole
• Avoid prolonged or concurrent use with NSAIDs, corticosteroids, acetaminophen

• Increased risk of hypoglycemia: oral antidiabetics
• Increased risk of toxicity: methotrexate, lithium, zidovudine
• Decreased effects of probenecid, sulfinpyrazone
• Suspected reduction in the antihypertensive and vasodilator effects of ACE inhibitors; monitor B/P if used concurrently

SERIOUS REACTIONS

! Tinnitus may be the first indication that the serum salicylic acid concentration is reaching or exceeding the upper therapeutic range.
! Salsalate use may also produce vertigo, headache, confusion, drowsiness, diaphoresis, hyperventilation, vomiting, and diarrhea.
! Reye's syndrome may occur in children with chickenpox or the flu.
! Severe overdose may result in electrolyte imbalance, hyperthermia, dehydration, and blood pH imbalance.
! GI bleeding, peptic ulcer, and Reye's syndrome rarely occur.

DENTAL CONSIDERATIONS

S

General:
• Patients on chronic drug therapy rarely have symptoms of blood dyscrasias, which can include infection, bleeding, and poor healing.
• Potential cross-allergies with other salicylates such as aspirin.
• Consider semisupine chair position for patients with inflammatory joint diseases.
• Avoid prescribing aspirin-containing products because this drug is a salicylate.
• If used for dental patients, take with food or milk to decrease GI complaints; give 30 min before meals or 2 hr after meals; take with a full glass of water.
• Severe stomach bleeding may occur in patients who regularly use NSAIDs in recommended doses, when the patient is also taking another NSAID, a blood thinning, or steroid drug, if the patient has GI or peptic ulcer disease, if they are 60 yr or older, or when NSAIDs are taken longer than directed. Warn patients of the potential for severe stomach bleeding.

Consultations:
• In a patient with symptoms of blood dyscrasias, request a medical consultation for blood studies and postpone dental treatment until normal values are reestablished.
• Medical consultation may be required to assess disease control.

Teach Patient/Family to:
• Not place directly on a tooth or oral mucosa because of risk of chemical burns.
• Not exceed recommended dosage; acute toxicity may result.
• Read label on other OTC drugs; many contain aspirin.
• Avoid alcohol ingestion; GI bleeding may occur.
• Encourage effective oral hygiene to prevent soft tissue inflammation.
• Use caution to prevent injury when using oral hygiene aids.
• Warn patient of potential risks of increased GI adverse effects of NSAIDs.

sapropterin

sa-**prop**′-ter-in
(Kuvan)

CATEGORY AND SCHEDULE

Pregnancy Risk Category: C

Drug Class: Synthetic enzyme cofactor

MECHANISM OF ACTION

Promotes action of phenylalanine-4-hydroxylase as a cofactor for the enzyme.
Therapeutic Effect: Replaces tetrahydrobiopterin in phenylketonuria (PKU) to reduce blood phenylalanine levels.

USES

Treatment of hyperphenylalanemia (PKU), in conjunction with a phenylalanine-restricted diet

PHARMACOKINETICS

Absorbed after oral administration. Metabolized primarily in the liver (CYP3A4); metabolites excreted in urine

INDICATIONS AND DOSAGES

▸ **Management of Phenylketonuria**
Adult. PO 10 mg/kg/day for a period of up to 1 month (may be increased up to 20 mg/kg/day if phenylalanine levels do not decrease from baseline).

SIDE EFFECTS/ADVERSE REACTIONS

Frequent
Headache, peripheral edema, arthralgia, polyuria, agitation, dizziness, upper respiratory tract infection, diarrhea, abdominal pain, upper respiratory tract infection, pharyngolaryngeal pain, nausea, vomiting

Occasional
Confusion, rash, nasal congestion

PRECAUTIONS AND CONTRAINDICATIONS

Hypersensitivity
Blood phenylalanine levels need to be monitored carefully during therapy
Nonresponders to therapy need to be identified
Monitor carefully in the presence of hepatic impairment
Use with caution with inhibitors of folate metabolism (e.g., methotrexate)
Possible hypotension if used with PDE-5 inhibitors (e.g., sildenafil, vardenafil)
Use with caution in patients taking levodopa (seizures, overstimulation)

DRUG INTERACTIONS OF CONCERN TO DENTISTRY

• None reported

SERIOUS REACTIONS

! Gastritis, spinal cord injury, streptococcal infection
! Testicular carcinoma, urinary tract infection, neutropenia
! Convulsions
! Dizziness
! GI bleeding, postprocedural bleeding, headache, irritability, MI, overstimulation and respiratory tract infection
! Safety during nursing is not known

DENTAL CONSIDERATIONS

General:
• Monitor patient carefully for adverse reactions/side effects of drug.
• Phenylketonuric patients frequently exhibit manifestations of neurologic injury, including mental retardation

and must be managed accordingly, including knowledge of the patient's dietary restrictions.
• Early-morning appointments and stress-reduction protocol may be needed for anxious patients.
• Position patient for comfort if GI adverse effects occur.
Consultations:
• Consult with physician to determine disease control, dietary restrictions and ability to tolerate dental procedures.
Teach Patient/Family to:
• Avoid recommending artificially sweetened products that may otherwise be recommended in routine oral hygiene programs.
• Use home fluoride products for anticaries effect.
• Encourage effective oral hygiene measures to prevent soft tissue inflammation.

saquinavir

sa-**kwin′**-ah-veer
(Fortovase, Invirase)
Do not confuse saquinavir with Sinequan.

CATEGORY AND SCHEDULE

Pregnancy Risk Category: B

Drug Class: Antiviral

S

MECHANISM OF ACTION

Inhibits HIV protease, rendering the enzyme incapable of processing the polyprotein precursors needed to generate functional proteins in HIV-infected cells.
Therapeutic Effect: Interferes with HIV replication, slowing the progression of HIV infection.

USES

Treatment of AIDS in combination with nucleoside analogues, zidovudine, or zalcitabine

PHARMACOKINETICS

Poorly absorbed after PO administration (absorption increased with high-calorie and high-fat meals). Protein binding: 99%. Metabolized in the liver to inactive metabolite. Primarily eliminated in feces. Unknown if removed by hemodialysis. ***Half-life:*** 13 hr.

INDICATIONS AND DOSAGES

▸ **HIV Infection in Combination with Other Antiretrovirals**
PO
Adults, Elderly. 1200 mg Fortovase 3 times a day or 600 mg Invirase 3 times a day within 2 hr after a full meal.
▸ **Dosage Adjustments When Given in Combination Therapy**
Delavirdine: Fortovase 800 mg 3 times a day.
Lopinavir/ritonavir: Fortovase 800 mg 2 times a day.
Nelfinavir: Fortovase 800 mg 3 times/day or 1200 mg 2 times a day.
Ritonavir: Fortovase or Invirase 1000 mg 2 times a day.

SIDE EFFECTS/ADVERSE REACTIONS

Occasional
Diarrhea, abdominal discomfort and pain, nausea, photosensitivity, stomatitis
Rare
Confusion, ataxia, asthenia, headache, rash

PRECAUTIONS AND CONTRAINDICATIONS

Clinically significant hypersensitivity to saquinavir; concurrent use with ergot medications, lovastatin, midazolam, simvastatin, or triazolam

Caution:

Hepatic impairment, children younger than 16 yr, pregnancy category B, lactation (unknown), bone marrow suppression, renal impairment

DRUG INTERACTIONS OF CONCERN TO DENTISTRY

- Increased plasma levels of clindamycin, troleandomycin, ketoconazole, itraconazole, fentanyl, clarithromycin, midazolam, triazolam (inhibits CYP3A4 isoenzymes)
- Increased metabolism of carbamazepine, dexamethasone, phenobarbital

SERIOUS REACTIONS

! Ketoacidosis occurs rarely.

DENTAL CONSIDERATIONS

General:

- Examine for oral manifestations of opportunistic infections.
- Patients on chronic drug therapy may rarely have symptoms of blood dyscrasias, which can include infection, bleeding, and poor healing.
- Palliative medication may be required for management of oral side effects.

Consultations:

- Medical consultation may be required to assess disease control.
- In a patient with symptoms of blood dyscrasias, request a medical consultation for blood studies and postpone dental treatment until normal values are reestablished.

Teach Patient/Family to:

- Encourage effective oral hygiene to prevent soft tissue inflammation.
- Use caution to prevent trauma when using oral hygiene aids.
- See dentist immediately if secondary oral infection occurs.
- Update medical/drug history if physician makes any changes in evaluation or drug regimen; include OTC, herbal, and nonherbal drugs in the update.

sargramostim (granulocyte macrophage colony-stimulating factor, GM-CSF)

sar-gra-**moh′**-stim

(Leukine)

Do not confuse Leukine with Leukeran.

CATEGORY AND SCHEDULE

Pregnancy Risk Category: C

Drug Class: Chemotherapeutic

MECHANISM OF ACTION

A colony-stimulating factor that stimulates proliferation and differentiation of hematopoietic cells to activate mature granulocytes and macrophages.

Therapeutic Effect: Assists bone marrow in making new WBCs and increases their chemotactic, antifungal, and antiparasitic activity. Increases cytoneoplastic cells and activates neutrophils to inhibit tumor cell growth.

USES

Acute myelogenous leukemia; myeloid reconstitution after bone marrow transplantation

PHARMACOKINETICS

Effect	Onset	Peak	Duration
Increase WBCs	7–14 days	N/A	1 wk

Detected in serum within 5 min after subcutaneous administration. ***Half-life:*** IV, 1 hr; subcutaneous, 3 hr.

INDICATIONS AND DOSAGES

▸ Myeloid Recovery Following Bone Marrow Transplant (BMT)

IV Infusion

Adults, Elderly. Usual parenteral dosage: 250 mcg/m^2/day for 21 days (as 2-hr infusion). Begin 2–4 hr after autologous bone marrow infusion and not less than 24 hr after last dose of chemotherapy or not less than 12 hr after last radiation treatment. Discontinue if blast cells appear or underlying disease progresses.

▸ BMT Failure, Engraftment Delay

IV Infusion

Adults, Elderly. 250 mcg/m^2/day for 14 days. Infuse over 2 hr. May repeat after 7 days off therapy if engraftment has not occurred with 500 mcg/m^2/day for 14 days.

▸ Stem Cell Transplant

IV, Subcutaneous

Adults. 250 mcg/m^2/day.

SIDE EFFECTS/ADVERSE REACTIONS

Frequent

GI disturbances, including nausea, diarrhea, vomiting, stomatitis, anorexia, and abdominal pain; arthralgia or myalgia; headache; malaise; rash; pruritus

Occasional

Peripheral edema, weight gain, dyspnea, asthenia, fever, leukocytosis, capillary leak syndrome (such as fluid retention, irritation at local injection site, and peripheral edema)

Rare

Rapid or irregular heartbeat, thrombophlebitis

PRECAUTIONS AND CONTRAINDICATIONS

Use 12 hr before or after radiation therapy; 24 hr before or after chemotherapy; excessive leukemic myeloid blasts in bone marrow or peripheral blood (10%); known hypersensitivity to GM-CSF, yeast-derived products, or components of drug

DRUG INTERACTIONS OF CONCERN TO DENTISTRY

- Potentiation of myeloproliferative effects: corticosteroids

SERIOUS REACTIONS

! Pleural or pericardial effusion occurs rarely after infusion.

DENTAL CONSIDERATIONS

General:

- Caution: graft patients or myelosuppressed patients may be at high risk for infection.
- Provide palliative care for dental emergencies only.
- Oral infections should be eliminated and/or treated aggressively.
- If additional analgesia is required for dental pain, consider alternative analgesics (NSAIDs) in patients taking narcotics for acute or chronic pain.
- Monitor and record vital signs.
- Avoid products that affect platelet function, such as aspirin and NSAIDs.
- Patient on chronic drug therapy may rarely present with symptoms of blood dyscrasias, which can include

infection, bleeding, and poor healing. If dyscrasia is present, caution patient to prevent oral tissue trauma when using oral hygiene aids.

• Examine for oral manifestation of opportunistic infection.

• Palliative medication may be required for management of oral side effects.

Consultations:

• Medical consultation should include routine blood counts, including platelet counts and bleeding time.

• Consult physician; prophylactic or therapeutic antiinfectives may be indicated if surgery or periodontal treatment is required.

• In a patient with symptoms of blood dyscrasias, request a medical consultation for blood studies and postpone treatment until normal values are reestablished.

• Medical consultation may be required to assess disease control and patient's ability to tolerate stress.

Teach Patient/Family to:

• Use soft tooth brush to reduce risk of bleeding.

• Encourage effective oral hygiene to prevent soft tissue inflammation.

• Prevent trauma when using oral hygiene aids.

• Report oral lesions, soreness, or bleeding to dentist.

saxagliptin

sax′-a-**glip**′-tin

(Onglyza)

Do not confused with sitagliptin or sumatriptan.

CATEGORY AND SCHEDULE

Pregnancy Risk Category: B

Drug Class: Antidiabetic agent, Dipeptidyl peptidase 4 inhibitors

MECHANISM OF ACTION

A competitive inhibitor of dipeptidyl peptidase (DPP4) that delays the inactivation of incretin hormones. ***Therapeutic Effect:*** Reduces fasting and postprandial glucose concentrations.

USES

Type 2 diabetes mellitus

PHARMACOKINETICS

Rapidly and well absorbed following PO administration. Protein binding: negligible. Metabolized in by CYP3A4/5. Partial excretion in feces, partial excretion in urine. ***Half-life:*** 2.5 hr; 3.1 hr (active metabolite).

INDICATIONS AND DOSAGES

▸ **Type 2 Diabetes Mellitus**

PO

Adults. 2.5–5 mg a day.

Concurrent use with strong CYP3A4/5 inhibitors. 2.5 mg a day.

▸ **Dosage in Renal Impairment**

Mild impairment (CrCl greater than 50 ml/min). No adjustment needed.

Moderate to severe impairment (CrCl 50 ml/min or less). 2.5 mg a day.

ESRD requiring dialysis. 2.5 mg a day after dialysis.

SIDE EFFECTS/ADVERSE REACTIONS

Frequent

Headache, urinary tract infection, hypoglycemia, peripheral edema, upper respiratory tract infection, nasopharyngitis

Occasional

Sinusitis, abdominal pain, gastroenteritis, vomiting, decrease lymphocyte count, hypersensitivity reaction

Rare

Lymphopenia

PRECAUTIONS AND CONTRAINDICATIONS

Hypersensitivity to saxigliptin or its components

Caution:

Renal impairment

Concurrent use with insulin secretagogues; increase risk of hypoglycemia

DRUG INTERACTIONS OF CONCERN TO DENTISTRY

- Antacids: May decrease the levels and effects of saxagliptin
- CYP3A4 inducers: May decrease the levels and effects of saxagliptin
- CYP3A4 inhibitors: May increase the levels and effects of saxagliptin
- Insulin secretagogues; increase risk of hypoglycemia

SERIOUS REACTIONS

! A hypersensitivity reaction may be life threatening. Signs and symptoms include fever, rash, fatigue, intractable nausea and vomiting, severe diarrhea, abdominal pain, cough, pharyngitis, and dyspnea.

! Overdose or insufficient food intake may produce hypoglycemia, especially with increased glucose demands.

! Bone fracture has been reported.

DENTAL CONSIDERATIONS

General:

- Short appointments and a stress-reduction protocol may be required for anxious patients.
- Be prepared to manage hypoglycemia.
- Diabetics may be more susceptible to infection and have delayed wound healing.
- Question the patient about self-monitoring of drug's antidiabetic effect including blood glucose values or finger-stick records.
- Avoid prescribing aspiring-containing products.
- Consider semisupine chair position for patient comfort if GI side effects occur.

Consultations:

- Medical consultation may include data from patient's blood glucose monitoring, including glycosylated hemoglobin or HbA_{1c} testing.
- Medical consultation may be required to assess disease control.

Teach Patient/Family to:

- Encourage effective oral hygiene to prevent soft tissue inflammation.
- Prevent trauma when using oral hygiene aids.
- Avoid mouth rinses with high alcohol content because of drying effects.

scopolamine

skoe-**pol′**-ah-meen
(Trans-Derm Scop, Transderm-V)

CATEGORY AND SCHEDULE

Pregnancy Risk Category: C

Drug Class: Antiemetic, anticholinergic

MECHANISM OF ACTION

An anticholinergic that reduces excitability of labyrinthine receptors, depressing conduction in the vestibular cerebellar pathway.

Therapeutic Effect: Prevents motion-induced nausea and vomiting.

USES

Prevention of motion sickness; prevention of nausea, vomiting associated with anesthesia or opiate analgesia

PHARMACOKINETICS
Patch: Onset 4–5 hr, duration 72 hr.

INDICATIONS AND DOSAGES
▸ **Prevention of Motion Sickness**
Transdermal
Adults. 1 system q72h.
▸ **Postoperative Nausea or Vomiting**
Transdermal
Adults, Elderly. 1 system no sooner than 1 hr before surgery and removed 24 hr after surgery.

SIDE EFFECTS/ADVERSE REACTIONS
Frequent
Dry mouth, somnolence, blurred vision
Rare
Dizziness, restlessness, hallucinations, confusion, difficulty urinating, rash

PRECAUTIONS AND CONTRAINDICATIONS
Angle-closure glaucoma, GI or GU obstruction, myasthenia gravis, paralytic ileus, tachycardia, thyrotoxicosis
Caution:
Children, elderly, pyloric, urinary, bladder neck, intestinal obstruction; liver, kidney disease

DRUG INTERACTIONS OF CONCERN TO DENTISTRY
- Increased anticholinergic effects: propantheline and other anticholinergic drugs
- Increased risk of CNS depression: alcohol, all CNS depressants

SERIOUS REACTIONS
! None known

DENTAL CONSIDERATIONS
General:
- Avoid dental light in patient's eyes; offer dark glasses for patient comfort.
- Caution patients about driving or performing other tasks requiring mental alertness.

Teach Patient/Family to:
- Avoid mouth rinses with high alcohol content because of drying effects.
- Avoid exposure to heat or exercise while taking.

secobarbital
see-koe-**bar′**-bih-tal
Schedule II
(Seconal)

CATEGORY AND SCHEDULE
Pregnancy Risk Category: D
Controlled Substance: Schedule II

Drug Class: Sedative-hypnotic barbiturate

MECHANISM OF ACTION
A barbiturate that depresses the CNS activity by binding to barbiturate site at the gamma-aminobutyric acid (GABA)-receptor complex, enhancing GABA activity and depressing the reticular activity system.
Therapeutic Effect: Produces hypnotic effect due to CNS depression.

USES
Treatment of insomnia, sedation, preoperative medication, status epilepticus, acute tetanus convulsions

PHARMACOKINETICS
Well absorbed from the GI tract. Protein binding: 52%–57%. Crosses blood-brain barrier. Widely distributed. Metabolized in liver by microsomal enzyme system to inactive and active metabolites.

Primarily excreted in urine. Not removed by hemodialysis. ***Half-life:*** 15–40 hr.

INDICATIONS AND DOSAGES

▸ Insomnia

PO

Adults. 100 mg at bedtime.

▸ Preoperative Sedation

PO

Adults. 100–300 mg 1–2 hr. before procedure.

Children. 2–6 mg/kg 1–2 hr. before procedure. Maximum: 100 mg/dose.

▸ Sedation, Daytime

PO

Adults. 30–50 mg 3–4 times a day.

Children. 2 mg/kg 3 times a day.

SIDE EFFECTS/ADVERSE REACTIONS

Frequent

Somnolence

Occasional

Agitation, confusion, hyperkinesia, ataxia, CNS depression, nightmares, nervousness, psychiatric disturbance, hallucinations, insomnia, anxiety, dizziness, abnormality in thinking, hypoventilation, apnea, bradycardia, hypotension, syncope, nausea, vomiting, constipation, headache

Rare

Hypersensitivity reactions, fever, liver damage, megaloblastic anemia

S

PRECAUTIONS AND CONTRAINDICATIONS

History of manifest or latent porphyria, marked liver dysfunction, marked respiratory disease in which dyspnea or obstruction is evident, and hypersensitivity to secobarbital or barbiturates

Caution:

Anemia, lactation, hepatic disease, renal disease, hypertension, elderly, acute/chronic pain

DRUG INTERACTIONS OF CONCERN TO DENTISTRY

- Hepatotoxicity: halogenated hydrocarbon anesthetics
- Increased CNS depression: alcohol, all CNS depressants
- Increased metabolism of carbamazepine, tricyclic antidepressants, corticosteroids
- Decreased half-life of doxycycline

SERIOUS REACTIONS

! Agranulocytosis, megaloblastic anemia, apnea, hypoventilation, bradycardia, hypotension, syncope, hepatic damage, and Stevens-Johnson syndrome rarely occur.

! Tolerance and physical dependence may occur with repeated use.

DENTAL CONSIDERATIONS

General:

- Determine why the patient is taking the drug.
- Monitor vital signs at every appointment because of cardiovascular side effects. Evaluate respiration characteristics and rate.
- Patients on chronic drug therapy may rarely have symptoms of blood dyscrasias, which can include infection, bleeding, and poor healing.
- When used for sedation in dentistry:
    - Assess vital signs before and after use as sedative.
    - Observe respiratory dysfunction: respiratory depression, character, rate, rhythm; hold drug if respirations are less than 10/min or if pupils are dilated.
    - After supine positioning, have patient sit upright for at least 2 min before standing to avoid orthostatic hypotension.

• Have someone drive patient to and from dental office when drug used for conscious sedation.

• Barbiturates induce liver microsomal enzymes, which alter the metabolism of other drugs.

• Geriatric patients are more susceptible to drug effects; use a lower dose.

Consultations:

• In a patient with symptoms of blood dyscrasias, request a medical consultation for blood studies and postpone dental treatment until normal values are reestablished.

Teach Patient/Family to:

• Avoid driving or other activities requiring mental alertness.

• Avoid alcohol ingestion and CNS depressants; serious CNS depression may result.

• Use caution when using OTC preparations (antihistamines, cold remedies) that contain CNS depressants.

selegiline hydrochloride

seh-**ledge**′-ill-ene high-droh-**klor**′-ide

(Apo-Selegiline[CAN], Eldepryl, Novo-Selegiline[CAN], Selgene[AUS])

Do not confuse selegiline with Stelazine, or Eldepryl with enalapril.

CATEGORY AND SCHEDULE

Pregnancy Risk Category: C

Drug Class: Antiparkinson agent

MECHANISM OF ACTION

An antiparkinson agent that irreversibly inhibits the activity of monoamine oxidase type B, the enzyme that breaks down dopamine, thereby increasing dopaminergic action.

Therapeutic Effect: Relieves signs and symptoms of Parkinson's disease.

USES

Adjunct management of Parkinson's disease in patients being treated with levodopa or carbidopa

PHARMACOKINETICS

Rapidly absorbed from the GI tract. Crosses the blood-brain barrier. Metabolized in the liver to the active metabolites. Primarily excreted in urine. ***Half-life:*** 17 hr (amphetamine), 20 hr (methamphetamine).

INDICATIONS AND DOSAGES

▸ Adjunctive Treatment for Parkinsonism

PO

Adults. 10 mg/day in divided doses, such as 5 mg at breakfast and lunch, given concomitantly with each dose of carbidopa and levodopa.

Elderly. Initially, 5 mg in the morning. May increase up to 10 mg/day.

SIDE EFFECTS/ADVERSE REACTIONS

Frequent

Nausea, dizziness, light-headedness, syncope, abdominal discomfort

Occasional

Confusion, hallucinations, dry mouth, vivid dreams, dyskinesia

Rare

Headache, myalgia, anxiety, diarrhea, insomnia

PRECAUTIONS AND CONTRAINDICATIONS

Hypersensitivity: fluoxetine, meperidine

Caution:
Lactation, children

DRUG INTERACTIONS OF CONCERN TO DENTISTRY

• Fatal interaction: opioids (especially meperidine); do not administer together
• Risk of serotonin syndrome: serotonin uptake inhibitors (fluoxetine, sertraline, paroxetine)

SERIOUS REACTIONS

! Symptoms of overdose may vary from CNS depression, characterized by sedation, apnea, cardiovascular collapse, and death, to severe paradoxic reactions, such as hallucinations, tremor, and seizures.
! Other serious effects may include involuntary movements, impaired motor coordination, loss of balance, blepharospasm, facial grimaces, feeling of heaviness in the lower extremities, depression, nightmares, delusions, overstimulation, sleep disturbance, and anger.

DENTAL CONSIDERATIONS

General:
• Monitor vital signs at every appointment because of cardiovascular side effects.
• After supine positioning, have patient sit upright for at least 2 min before standing to avoid orthostatic hypotension.
• Assess for presence of extrapyramidal motor symptoms, such as tardive dyskinesia and akathisia. Extrapyramidal motor activity may complicate dental treatment.
• Assess salivary flow as a factor in caries, periodontal disease, and candidiasis.

Consultations:
• Medical consultation may be required to assess disease control and patient's ability to tolerate stress.
• If signs of tardive dyskinesia or akathisia are present, refer to physician.

Teach Patient/Family to:
• Use powered tooth brush if patient has difficulty holding conventional devices.
• When chronic dry mouth occurs, advise patient to:
  • Avoid mouth rinses with high alcohol content because of drying effects.
  • Use daily home fluoride products to prevent caries.
  • Use sugarless gum, frequent sips of water, or saliva substitutes.

sertaconazole

sir-tah-**con′**-ah-zole
(Ertaczo)

CATEGORY AND SCHEDULE

Pregnancy Risk Category: C

Drug Class: Antifungal

MECHANISM OF ACTION

An imidazole derivative that inhibits synthesis of ergosterol, a vital component of fungal cell formation.
Therapeutic Effect: Damages the fungal cell membrane, altering its function.

USES

Fungal infections

PHARMACOKINETICS

Half-life: 60 hr.

S

INDICATIONS AND DOSAGES

▸ **Tinea Pedis**

Topical

Adults, Elderly, Children 12 yr and older. Apply to affected area twice a day for 4 wk.

SIDE EFFECTS/ADVERSE REACTIONS

Rare

Burning, tenderness, erythema, dryness, pruritus, hyperpigmentation, and contact dermatitis at application site

PRECAUTIONS AND CONTRAINDICATIONS

None known

DRUG INTERACTIONS OF CONCERN TO DENTISTRY

• None reported

SERIOUS REACTIONS

! None known

DENTAL CONSIDERATIONS

General:

• Determine why patient is taking this drug.

sertraline

sir′-trall-een

(Apo-Sertraline[CAN], Novo-Sertraline[CAN], PMS-Sertraline[CAN], Zoloft)

Do not confuse sertraline with Serentil.

CATEGORY AND SCHEDULE

Pregnancy Risk Category: B

Drug Class: Antidepressant

MECHANISM OF ACTION

An antidepressant, anxiolytic, and obsessive-compulsive disorder adjunct that blocks the reuptake of the neurotransmitter serotonin at CNS neuronal presynaptic membranes, increasing its availability at postsynaptic receptor sites.

Therapeutic Effect: Relieves depression, reduces obsessive-compulsive behavior, decreases anxiety.

USES

Treatment of major depression, obsessive-compulsive disorder (OCD), panic disorder, posttraumatic stress disorder, premenstrual dysphoric mood disorder, social anxiety disorder

PHARMACOKINETICS

Incompletely and slowly absorbed from the GI tract; food increases absorption. Protein binding: 98%. Widely distributed. Undergoes extensive first-pass metabolism in the liver to active compound. Excreted in urine and feces. Not removed by hemodialysis. ***Half-life:*** 26 hr.

INDICATIONS AND DOSAGES

▸ **Depression**

PO

Adults. Initially, 50 mg/day. May increase by 50 mg/day at 7-day intervals up to 200 mg/day.

Elderly. Initially, 25 mg/day. May increase by 25–50 mg/day at 7-day intervals up to 200 mg/day.

▸ **OCD**

PO

Adults, Children 13–17 yr. Initially, 50 mg/day with morning or evening meal. May increase by 50 mg/day at 7-day intervals.

Elderly, Children 6–12 yr. Initially, 25 mg/day. May increase by 25–50 mg/day at 7-day intervals. Maximum: 200 mg/day.

▸ **Panic Disorder, Posttraumatic Stress Disorder, Social Anxiety Disorder**

PO

Adults, Elderly. Initially, 25 mg/day. May increase by 50 mg/day at 7-day intervals. Range: 50–200 mg/day. Maximum: 200 mg/day.

▸ **Premenstrual Dysphoric Disorder**

PO

Adults. Initially, 50 mg/day. May increase up to 150 mg/day in 50-mg increments.

SIDE EFFECTS/ADVERSE REACTIONS

Frequent

Headache, nausea, diarrhea, insomnia, somnolence, dizziness, fatigue, rash, dry mouth

Occasional

Anxiety, nervousness, agitation, tremor, dyspepsia, diaphoresis, vomiting, constipation, abnormal ejaculation, visual disturbances, altered taste

Rare

Flatulence, urinary frequency, paresthesia, hot flashes, chills

S

PRECAUTIONS AND CONTRAINDICATIONS

Use within 14 days of MAOIs

Caution:

Lactation, elderly, hepatic/renal disease, epilepsy

DRUG INTERACTIONS OF CONCERN TO DENTISTRY

• Increased CNS depression: alcohol, CNS depressants, St. John's wort (herb)
• Increased side effects: highly protein-bound drugs (aspirin), tricyclic antidepressants
• Increased half-life of diazepam
• Possible inhibition of sertraline metabolism: erythromycin, clarithromycin
• Potent inhibitor of CYP2D6; use drugs metabolized by the enzyme only with caution
• Possible risk of serotonin syndrome with tramadol, oxycodone
• Decreased effects: carbamazepine
• NSAIDs: increased risk of GI side effects

SERIOUS REACTIONS

! None known

DENTAL CONSIDERATIONS

General:

• Monitor vital signs at every appointment because of cardiovascular side effects.
• After supine positioning, have patient sit upright for at least 2 min before standing to avoid orthostatic hypotension.
• Assess salivary flow as a factor in caries, periodontal disease, and candidiasis.
• Avoid dental light in patient's eyes; offer dark glasses for patient comfort.
• Consider semisupine chair position for patient comfort if GI side effects occur.

Consultations:

• Medical consultation may be required to assess patient's ability to tolerate stress.
• Physician should be informed if significant xerostomic side effects occur (e.g., increased caries, sore tongue, problems eating or swallowing, difficulty wearing prosthesis) so that a medication change can be considered.

Teach Patient/Family to:

- Use powered tooth brush if patient has difficulty holding conventional devices.
- When chronic dry mouth occurs, advise patient to:
  - Avoid mouth rinses with high alcohol content because of drying effects.
  - Use daily home fluoride products to prevent caries.
  - Use sugarless gum, frequent sips of water, or saliva substitutes.

sevelamer hydrochloride

seh-**vel**′-ah-mer
high-droh-**klor**′-ide
(Renagel)
Do not confuse Renagel with Reglan or Regonol.

CATEGORY AND SCHEDULE

Pregnancy Risk Category: C

Drug Class: Chelating agent

MECHANISM OF ACTION

An antihyperphosphatemic agent that binds with dietary phosphorus in the GI tract, thus allowing phosphorus to be eliminated through the normal digestive process and decreasing the serum phosphorus level.

Therapeutic Effect: Decreases incidence of hypercalcemic episodes in patients receiving calcium acetate treatment.

USES

Adjunct to peritoneal dialysis

PHARMACOKINETICS

Not absorbed systemically. Unknown if removed by hemodialysis.

INDICATIONS AND DOSAGES

▸ **Hyperphosphatemia**

PO

Adults, Elderly. 800–1600 mg with each meal, depending on severity of hyperphosphatemia.

SIDE EFFECTS/ADVERSE REACTIONS

Frequent

Infection, pain, hypotension, diarrhea, dyspepsia, nausea, vomiting

Occasional

Headache, constipation, hypertension, thrombosis, increased cough

PRECAUTIONS AND CONTRAINDICATIONS

Bowel obstruction, hypophosphatemia

DRUG INTERACTIONS OF CONCERN TO DENTISTRY

- Possible decrease in bioavailability: orally administered, rapidly absorbed drugs; give at least 1 hr before or 3 hr after sevelamer doses.

SERIOUS REACTIONS

! None known

DENTAL CONSIDERATIONS

General:

- Patients taking this drug may be undergoing renal dialysis; confirm the medical and drug history to plan appropriate management.
- If you prescribe medications for dental needs, have patient take medication 1 hr before or 3 hr after sevelamer doses.

• Monitor and record vital signs.
• Consider semisupine chair position for patient comfort if GI side effects occur.
• Patient may need assistance getting into and out of dental chair. Adjust chair position for patient comfort.
• Consultation with physician may be necessary if sedation or general anesthesia is required.

Consultations:

• Medical consultation may be required to assess disease control and patient's ability to tolerate stress.

Teach Patient/Family to:

• Report oral lesions, soreness, or bleeding to dentist.
• Encourage effective oral hygiene to prevent soft tissue inflammation.
• Prevent trauma when using oral hygiene aids.
• Update health and medication history if physician makes any changes in evaluation or drug regimens; include OTC, herbal, and nonherbal remedies in the update.

sibutramine

sih-**byoo′**-tra-meen
(Meridia)

CATEGORY AND SCHEDULE

Pregnancy Risk Category: C
Controlled Substance: Schedule IV

Drug Class: Amphetamine analogue anorexiant

MECHANISM OF ACTION

A CNS stimulant that inhibits reuptake of serotonin (enhancing satiety) and norepinephrine (raises metabolic rate) centrally.

Therapeutic Effect: Induces and maintains weight loss.

USES

Treatment of obesity

PHARMACOKINETICS

Rapidly absorbed from the GI tract. Protein binding: 95%–97%. Metabolized in liver, undergoes first-pass metabolism. Primarily excreted in urine, minimal elimination in feces. ***Half-life:*** 1.1 hr.

INDICATIONS AND DOSAGES

▸ **Weight Loss**

PO

Adults 16 yr and older. Initially, 10 mg/day. May increase up to 15 mg/day. Maximum: 20 mg/day.

SIDE EFFECTS/ADVERSE REACTIONS

Frequent

Headache, dry mouth, anorexia, constipation, insomnia, rhinitis, pharyngitis

Occasional

Back pain, flu syndrome, dizziness, nausea, asthenia (loss of strength, energy), arthralgia, nervousness, dyspepsia, sinusitis, abdominal pain, anxiety, dysmenorrhea

Rare

Depression, rash, cough, sweating, tachycardia, migraine, increased B/P, paresthesia, altered taste

PRECAUTIONS AND CONTRAINDICATIONS

Anorexia nervosa, concomitant MAOI use, concomitant use of centrally acting appetite suppressants, hypersensitivity to sibutramine or any component of the formulation

Caution:
Requires monitoring of B/P, risk of serotonin syndrome with other serotonin reuptake inhibitors, glaucoma, lactation, children younger than 16 yr, elderly, seizures

DRUG INTERACTIONS OF CONCERN TO DENTISTRY

• Avoid use of meperidine: risk of serotonin syndrome

SERIOUS REACTIONS

! Seizures, thrombocytopenia, and deaths have been reported.
! Serotonin syndrome can occur with concomitant use of drugs that increase serotonin.
! Large doses may produce extreme nervousness and tachycardia.

DENTAL CONSIDERATIONS

General:
• Monitor vital signs at every appointment because of cardiovascular side effects.
• Avoid or limit dose of vasoconstrictor.
• Assess salivary flow as factor in caries, periodontal disease, and candidiasis.
• Information on any abuse liability is unknown.
• Determine why patient is taking the drug.

Teach Patient/Family:
• When chronic dry mouth occurs, advise patient to:
  • Avoid mouth rinses with high alcohol content because of drying effects.
  • Use daily home fluoride products to prevent caries.
  • Use sugarless gum, frequent sips of water, or saliva substitutes.

sildenafil citrate

sill-**den′**-ah-fill **sih′**-trate
(Viagra)
Do not confuse Viagra with Vaniqa.

CATEGORY AND SCHEDULE

Pregnancy Risk Category: B

Drug Class: Impotence therapy

MECHANISM OF ACTION

An erectile dysfunction agent that inhibits phosphodiesterase type 5, the enzyme responsible for degrading cyclic guanosine monophosphate in the corpus cavernosum of the penis, resulting in smooth muscle relaxation and increased blood flow.
Therapeutic Effect: Facilitates an erection.

USES

Treatment of male erectile dysfunction

PHARMACOKINETICS

PO: Rapid oral absorption, bioavailability 40%, peak plasma levels 30 min–2 hr, hepatic metabolism by CYP3A4 (major) and CYP2C9 (minor) isoenzymes, active metabolite, highly plasma protein bound (96%), major excretion route in feces, lesser route in urine.

INDICATIONS AND DOSAGES

▸ **Erectile Dysfunction**
PO
Adults. 50 mg (30 min–4 hr before sexual activity). Range: 25–100 mg. Maximum dosing frequency is once daily.
Elderly older than 65 yr. Consider starting dose of 25 mg.

SIDE EFFECTS/ADVERSE REACTIONS

Frequent
Headache, flushing
Occasional
Dyspepsia, nasal congestion, UTI, abnormal vision, diarrhea
Rare
Dizziness, rash

PRECAUTIONS AND CONTRAINDICATIONS

Concurrent use of sodium nitroprusside or nitrates in any form
Caution:
Complete medical and physical exam to determine cause of erectile dysfunction; because of cardiac risk associated with sexual activity, cardiovascular status should be evaluated; anatomic deformation of penis, conditions predisposing to priapism (sickle cell anemia, anemia, multiple myeloma, leukemia), retinitis pigmentosa, not indicated for women, children, or newborns, pregnancy category B; hepatic or renal impairment, men 65 yr or older

DRUG INTERACTIONS OF CONCERN TO DENTISTRY

- Avoid use of nitroglycerin within 24 hr
- Increased plasma levels caused by interference with metabolism: cimetidine, erythromycin, ketoconazole, itraconazole
- Inhibitors of CYP3A4 or CYP2C9 isoenzymes: should be used with caution

SERIOUS REACTIONS

! Prolonged erections (lasting over 4 hr) and priapism (painful erections lasting over 6 hr) occur rarely.

DENTAL CONSIDERATIONS

General:
- This is an acute-use drug intended to be taken just before sexual activity, and the reported incidence of oral side effects does not differ from a placebo. However, the potential interacting drugs should be avoided.

silodosin

si-**lo**′-doe-sin
(Rapaflo)
Do not confuse silodosin with sildenafil, or Rapaflo with Rapamune.

CATEGORY AND SCHEDULE

Pregnancy Risk Category: B

Drug Class: α_1-blocker

MECHANISM OF ACTION

Silodosin is a selective α_1 antagonist. Smooth muscle tone in the prostate is mediated by α_{1A} receptors; blocking them leads to relaxation of smooth muscle in the bladder neck and prostate, causing an improvement of urine flow and a decrease in symptoms of BPH.
Therapeutic Effect: Reduces size of prostate gland and symptoms of BPH.

USES

Treatment of signs and symptoms of benign prostatic hyperplasia (BPH)

PHARMACOKINETICS

Well absorbed and widely distributed. 97% plasma protein bound. Extensive hepatic metabolism via CYP3A4 enzymes. Excreted via urine (34%) and feces (55%). ***Half-life:*** 5–21 hr.

INDICATIONS AND DOSAGES

▸ **Benign Prostatic Hyperplasia**

PO

Adults. 8 mg once daily with a meal.

▸ **Renal Impairment**

Cl_{cr} 30–50 ml/min: 4 mg once daily.
Cl_{cr} <30 ml/min: Use is contraindicated.

SIDE EFFECTS/ADVERSE REACTIONS

Frequent

Retrograde ejaculation

Occasional

Dizziness, headache, diarrhea, nasal congestion

PRECAUTIONS AND CONTRAINDICATIONS

Hypersensitivity to silodosin or any component of the formulation. Potential syncope risk caused by hypotension, vertigo, dizziness, carcinoma of prostate. Avoid use with other adrenoreceptor antagonists. Not for use in women or children or during lactation. Avoid in patients with previous severe allergic reaction to sulfonamides.

DRUG INTERACTIONS OF CONCERN TO DENTISTRY

- α-blockers (e.g., phentolamine mesylate, phenothiazine sedatives): increased risk of hypotension
- CYP3A4 inhibitors and P-glycoprotein inhibitors (e.g., macrolide antibiotics, azole antifungals): potential increase in silodosin blood level and toxicity
- Opioids, alcohol, sedatives: increased risk of hypotension

SERIOUS REACTIONS

! First-dose syncope (hypotension with sudden loss of consciousness) may occur within 30–90 min after administration of initial dose and may be preceded by tachycardia (pulse rate of 120–160 beats/min).

DENTAL CONSIDERATIONS

General:

- Avoid orthostatic hypotension. Allow patient to sit upright for 2 min before standing.
- Take precaution when seating and dismissing patient due to dizziness and possibility of syncope.
- Consider nasal congestion associated with silodosin when performing diagnosis of orofacial conditions.
- Avoid or reduce dose of opioids, phentolamine mesylate, or sedatives due to excessive hypotension.

Teach Patient/Family to:

- Report changes in disease status and drug regimen.

silver sulfadiazine

sul-fah-**dye′**-ah-zeen
(Flamazine[CAN], SSD, SSD AF, Silvadene)

CATEGORY AND SCHEDULE

Pregnancy Risk Category: B

Drug Class: Antimicrobial

S

MECHANISM OF ACTION

An antiinfective that acts upon the cell wall and cell membrane. Releases silver slowly in concentrations selectively toxic to bacteria.

Therapeutic Effect: Bactericidal.

USES

Treatment of urinary tract infections

PHARMACOKINETICS

Variably absorbed. Significant systemic absorption may occur if applied to extensive burns. Absorbed medication excreted unchanged in urine. ***Half-life:*** 10 hr (half-life increased with impaired renal function).

INDICATIONS AND DOSAGES

▸ **Burns**

Topical

Adults, Elderly, Children. Apply 1–2 times daily.

SIDE EFFECTS/ADVERSE REACTIONS

Side effects characteristic of all sulfonamides may occur when systemically absorbed, such as extensive burn areas, anorexia, nausea, vomiting, headache, diarrhea, dizziness, photosensitivity, joint pain

Frequent

Burning feeling at treatment site

Occasional

Brown-gray skin discoloration, rash, itching

Rare

Increased sensitivity of skin to sunlight

PRECAUTIONS AND CONTRAINDICATIONS

Hypersensitivity to silver sulfadiazine or any component of the formulation

DRUG INTERACTIONS OF CONCERN TO DENTISTRY

• None reported

SERIOUS REACTIONS

! If significant systemic absorption occurs, less often but serious are hemolytic anemia, hypoglycemia, diuresis, peripheral neuropathy, Stevens-Johnson syndrome, agranulocytosis, disseminated lupus erythematosus, anaphylaxis, hepatitis, and toxic nephrosis.

! Fungal superinfections may occur.

! Interstitial nephritis occurs rarely.

DENTAL CONSIDERATIONS

General:

• Dental management depends on extent and severity of burns and patient's ability to cooperate; above all use aseptic techniques.

• Provide palliative dental care for dental emergencies only.

Consultations:

• Medical consultation may be required to assess disease control and patient's ability to tolerate stress.

• Consult patient's physician if an acute dental infection occurs and another antiinfective is required.

Teach Patient/Family to:

• Encourage effective oral hygiene to prevent soft tissue inflammation.

• Prevent trauma when using oral hygiene aids.

simethicone

sih-**meth**′-ih-kone

(Alka-Seltzer Gas Relief, Gas-X, Genasyme, Infant Mylicon, Mylanta Gas, Ovol[CAN], Phazyme)

CATEGORY AND SCHEDULE

Pregnancy Risk Category: C

OTC

Drug Class: Antiflatulent

MECHANISM OF ACTION

An antiflatulent that changes surface tension of gas bubbles, allowing easier elimination of gas.

Therapeutic Effect: Prevents formation of gas pockets in the GI tract.

USES

Relief of bloating, discomfort, and pain caused by excessive gas in the stomach

PHARMACOKINETICS

Does not appear to be absorbed from GI tract. Excreted unchanged in feces.

INDICATIONS AND DOSAGES

▸ Antiflatulent

PO

Adults, Elderly, Children 12 yr and older. 40–250 mg after meals and at bedtime. Maximum: 500 mg/day.
Children 2–11 yr. 40 mg 4 times a day.
Children younger than 2 yr. 20 mg 4 times a day.

SIDE EFFECTS/ADVERSE REACTIONS

None known

PRECAUTIONS AND CONTRAINDICATIONS

None known

DRUG INTERACTIONS OF CONCERN TO DENTISTRY

• None reported

SERIOUS REACTIONS

! None known

DENTAL CONSIDERATIONS

General:

• Determine why patient is taking the drug.
• Consider semisupine chair position for patient comfort because of GI effects of disease.
• Question patient about tolerance of NSAIDs or aspirin related to GI disease.
• Patients with gastroesophageal reflux may present with oral symptoms, including burning mouth, secondary candidiasis, and signs of tooth erosion.
• Patients using this drug may have GI disease; review medical and drug history.

Teach Patient/Family to:

• Update health and medication history if physician makes any changes in evaluation or drug regimens; include OTC, herbal, and nonherbal remedies in the update.
• Encourage effective oral hygiene to prevent soft tissue inflammation.

simvastatin

sim′-vah-sta-tin
(Apo-Simvastatin[CAN], Lipex[AUS], Zocor)
Do not confuse Zocor with Cozaar.

CATEGORY AND SCHEDULE

Pregnancy Risk Category: X

Drug Class: Antihyperlipidemic

MECHANISM OF ACTION

A HMG-CoA reductase inhibitor that interferes with cholesterol biosynthesis by inhibiting the conversion of the enzyme HMG-CoA to mevalonate.
Therapeutic Effect: Decreases serum low-density lipoproteins (LDLs), cholesterol, very low-density lipoproteins (VLDLs), and plasma triglyceride levels; slightly increases serum high-density lipoprotein (HDL) concentration.

USES

An adjunct in homozygous familial hypercholesterolemia, mixed hyperlipidemia, elevated serum triglyceride levels, and type IV hyperproteinemia; also reduces total cholesterol LDL-C, apo B, and triglyceride levels; patient should first be placed on cholesterol-lowering diet; effective in reducing risk of heart attacks and strokes

PHARMACOKINETICS

Route	Onset	Peak	Duration
PO to reduce cholesterol	3 days	14 days	N/A

Well absorbed from the GI tract. Protein binding: 95%. Undergoes extensive first-pass metabolism. Hydrolyzed to active metabolite. Primarily eliminated in feces. Unknown if removed by hemodialysis.

INDICATIONS AND DOSAGES

▸ Adjunct to Diet to Decrease Heterozygous Familial Hypercholesterolemia in Adolescents 10–17 Yr of Age (Girls at Least 1-Yr Post-menarche) Heterozygous Familial Hypercholesterolemia

PO

Pediatric. 10 mg once daily in evening. Range: 10–40 mg/day. Maximum: 40 mg/day.

▸ To Decrease Elevated Total and LDL Cholesterol in Hypercholesterolemia (Types IIA and IIIB), Lower Triglyceride Levels, and Increase HDL Levels; to Reduce Risk of Death and Prevent MI in Patients with Heart Disease and Elevated Cholesterol Level; to Reduce Risk of Revascularization Procedures; to Decrease Risk of Stroke or Transient Ischemic Attack; to Prevent Cardiovascular Events

PO

Adults. Initially, 10–40 mg/day in evening. Dosage adjusted at 4-wk intervals.

Elderly. Initially, 10 mg/day. May increase by 5–10 mg/day q4wk. Range: 5–80 mg/day. Maximum: 80 mg/day.

SIDE EFFECTS/ADVERSE REACTIONS

Simvastatin is generally well tolerated; side effects are usually mild and transient

Occasional

Headache, abdominal pain or cramps, constipation, upper respiratory tract infection

Rare

Diarrhea, flatulence, asthenia (loss of strength and energy), nausea or vomiting

PRECAUTIONS AND CONTRAINDICATIONS

Active hepatic disease or unexplained, persistent elevations of liver function test results, age younger than 18 yr, pregnancy

Caution:

Past liver disease, alcoholics (first-pass metabolism with CYP3A4 isoenzymes); severe acute infections, trauma, hypotension, uncontrolled seizure disorders, severe metabolic disorders, electrolyte imbalances

DRUG INTERACTIONS OF CONCERN TO DENTISTRY

- Increased myalgia, myositis: erythromycin, cyclosporine, itraconazole, ketoconazole
- Caution with use of drugs that are strong inhibitors of CYP3A4 isoenzymes

SERIOUS REACTIONS

! Lens opacities may occur.

! Hypersensitivity reaction and hepatitis occur rarely.

DENTAL CONSIDERATIONS

General:

• Consider semisupine chair position for patient comfort because of GI side effects.

• Assess patient for possible cardiovascular disease.

sirolimus

sir-oh-**leem′**-us

(Rapamune)

CATEGORY AND SCHEDULE

Pregnancy Risk Category: C

Drug Class: Immunosuppressant

MECHANISM OF ACTION

An immunosuppressant that inhibits T-lymphocyte proliferation induced by stimulation of cell surface receptors, mitogens, alloantigens, and lymphokines. Prevents activation of the enzyme target of rapamycin, a key regulatory kinase in cell cycle progression.

Therapeutic Effect: Inhibits proliferation of T and B cells, essential components of the immune response; prevents organ transplant rejection.

USES

Adjunct to organ transplantation

PHARMACOKINETICS

Rapidly absorbed from the GI tract. Peak levels 1 hr (inhibited by food). Protein binding: 92%. Extensively metabolized by the CYP3A4 isoenzyme in the intestinal wall and liver. Primarily excreted in feces.

INDICATIONS AND DOSAGES

▸ Prevention of Organ Transplant Rejection

PO

Adults. Loading dose: 6 mg. Maintenance: 2 mg/day.

Children 13 yr and older weighing less than 40 kg. Loading dose: 3 mg/m^2. Maintenance: 1 mg/m^2/day.

SIDE EFFECTS/ADVERSE REACTIONS

Occasional

Hypercholesterolemia, hyperlipidemia, hypertension, rash; with high doses (5 mg/day): anemia, arthralgia, diarrhea, hypokalemia, and thrombocytopenia

PRECAUTIONS AND CONTRAINDICATIONS

Hypersensitivity to sirolimus, malignancy

DRUG INTERACTIONS OF CONCERN TO DENTISTRY

• Increased blood levels: potent inhibitors of CYP3A4 isoenzymes (clarithromycin, clotrimazole, erythromycin, fluconazole, itraconazole, ritonavir, indinavir, grapefruit juice)

• Decreased blood levels: potent inducers of CYP3A4 isoenzymes (phenobarbital, carbamazepine, St. John's wort [herb])

SERIOUS REACTIONS

! None known

DENTAL CONSIDERATIONS

General:

• Caution: patients on immunosuppressive therapy may be at high risk for infection.

• Provide palliative dental care for dental emergencies only.

• Oral infections should be eliminated and/or treated aggressively.
• Patients may be at risk for bleeding; check oral signs.
• Examine for evidence of oral candidiasis. Topically acting antifungals may be preferred: note potential drug interactions.
• Monitor and record vital signs.
• Avoid products that affect platelet function, such as aspirin and NSAIDs.
• Patient on chronic drug therapy may rarely present with symptoms of blood dyscrasias, which can include infection, bleeding, and poor healing. If dyscrasia is present, caution patient to prevent oral tissue trauma when using oral hygiene aids.
• Consider local hemostasis measures to prevent excessive bleeding.

Consultations:

• Medical consultation should include routine blood counts, including platelet counts and bleeding time.
• Consult physician; prophylactic or therapeutic antiinfectives may be indicated if surgery or periodontal treatment is required.
• In a patient with symptoms of blood dyscrasias, request a medical consultation for blood studies and postpone treatment until normal values are reestablished.
• Medical consultation may be required to assess disease control and patient's ability to tolerate stress.

Teach Patient/Family to:

• Use soft tooth brush to reduce risk of bleeding.
• Encourage effective oral hygiene to prevent soft tissue inflammation.
• Prevent trauma when using oral hygiene aids.
• Report oral lesions, soreness, or bleeding to dentist.
• Use powered tooth brush if patient has difficulty holding conventional devices.

sitagliptin

sit-ah-**glip**′-tin
(Januvia)

CATEGORY AND SCHEDULE

Pregnancy Risk Category: B

Drug Class: Antihyperglycemic (type 2 diabetes mellitus)

MECHANISM OF ACTION

Therapeutic Effect: Increases and prolongs active incretin levels, thereby increasing insulin release and decreasing glucagon levels in the circulation in a glucose-dependent manner

USES

Improves glycemic control in type 2 diabetes mellitus in combination with metformin or a PPAR-gamma agonist (e.g., thiazolidinediones) when the single agent alone, with diet and exercise, does not provide adequate glycemic control

PHARMACOKINETICS

Rapidly absorbed after oral administration. Protein binding: 38%. Primarily excreted unchanged in the urine (79%) by active tubular secretion, minor fraction metabolized in the liver (CYP3A4, 2C8)

INDICATIONS AND DOSAGES

▸ **Monotherapy of Type 2 Diabetes Mellitus (or Combination Therapy**

with Metformin or a PPAR-gamma Agonist)
PO
Adult. 100 mg once daily.

SIDE EFFECTS/ADVERSE REACTIONS

Frequent
Hypoglycemia, nasopharyngitis, upper respiratory tract infection, headache
Occasional
Abdominal pain, nausea, diarrhea
Rare
Anaphylaxis, angioedema, rash, urticaria, exfoliative skin reactions

PRECAUTIONS AND CONTRAINDICATIONS

Hypersensitivity
Renal insufficiency (requires dosage adjustment)
Safety in nursing not established
Increased possibility of hypoglycemia when used with other antidiabetic agents

DRUG INTERACTIONS OF CONCERN TO DENTISTRY

• None reported

SERIOUS REACTIONS

! Anaphylaxis, angioedema, Stevens-Johnson syndrome

DENTAL CONSIDERATIONS

General:
• Short appointments and a stress-reduction protocol may be required for anxious patients.
• Be prepared to manage hypoglycemia.
• Question patient about self-monitoring of blood glucose values.
• Ensure that patient is following prescribed diet and medication regimen.
• Consider semisupine chair position for patient comfort if GI side/adverse effects occur.
• Diabetics may be more susceptible to infection and have delayed wound healing.
• Place on frequent recall to evaluate oral hygiene and healing response.
Consultations:
• Consult with physician to determine disease control and ability to tolerate dental procedures.
• Notify physician immediately if symptoms of lactic acidosis are observed (myalgia, respiratory distress, weakness, diarrhea, malaise, muscle cramps, somnolence).
• Medical consultation may include data from patient's blood glucose monitoring, including glycosylated hemoglobin or HbA_{1c} testing.
• Oral and maxillofacial surgical procedures associated with significantly restricted food intake require a medical consultation and may require physician adjusting medication regimen.
Teach Patient/Family to:
• Encourage effective oral hygiene to prevent soft tissue inflammation.
• Update medical history when disease status/glycemic control or medication regimen change.

sitagliptin + simvastatin

sit a glip tin & sim va stat in
(Juvisync)

CATEGORY AND SCHEDULE

Pregnancy Risk Category: X

Drug Class: Antidiabetic agent, dipeptidyl peptidase IV (DPP-IV) inhibitor; antilipemic agent, HMG-CoA reductase inhibitor

MECHANISM OF ACTION

Simvastatin: A derivative of lovastatin that inhibits HMG-CoA reductase, the enzyme that catalyzes the rate-limiting step in cholesterol biosynthesis. Sitagliptin: Inhibits dipeptidyl peptidase IV (DPP-IV) enzyme, resulting in prolonged activity of incretin hormones, which regulate glucose homeostasis by increasing insulin synthesis and release from pancreatic beta cells and decreasing glucagon secretion from pancreatic alpha cells. ***Therapeutic Effect:*** Reduces serum glucose and serum cholesterol.

USES

Management of type 2 diabetes mellitus (noninsulin dependent, NIDDM) as an adjunct to diet and exercise as monotherapy or in combination therapy with other antidiabetic agents. Secondary prevention of cardiovascular morbidity and mortality in hypercholesterolemic patients with established coronary heart disease (CHD) or at high risk for CHD

PHARMACOKINETICS

Sitagliptin: Rapidly absorbed after oral administration. Protein binding: 38%. Primarily excreted unchanged in the urine (79%). Simvastatin: Well absorbed from the GI tract. Protein binding: 95%. Undergoes extensive first-pass metabolism. Hydrolyzed to active metabolite. Primarily eliminated in feces. ***Half-life:*** Sitagliptin: 12.4 hr. Simvastatin: 3 hr.

INDICATIONS AND DOSAGES

▸ Hyperlipidemia and Type 2 Diabetes

PO

Adults. Initial dose: Sitagliptin 100 mg and simvastatin 40 mg once daily.

SIDE EFFECTS/ADVERSE REACTIONS

Frequent

Hypoglycemia, nasopharyngitis, upper respiratory tract infection, headache

Occasional

Abdominal pain, nausea, diarrhea

PRECAUTIONS AND CONTRAINDICATIONS

Hypersensitivity to simvastatin, sitagliptin, or any component of the formulation; active liver disease; unexplained persistent elevations of serum transaminases

DRUG INTERACTIONS OF CONCERN TO DENTISTRY

- CYP3A4 inhibitors (e.g., macrolide antibiotics, azole antifungals): increased risk of simvastatin-induced rhabdomyolysis

SERIOUS REACTIONS

! Rare hypersensitivity reactions, including anaphylaxis, angioedema, and/or severe dermatologic reactions such as Stevens-Johnson syndrome, have been reported with sitagliptin. Patients receiving HMG-CoA reductase inhibitors like simvastatin have developed rhabdomyolysis with acute renal failure and/or myopathy.

DENTAL CONSIDERATIONS

General:

- Short appointments and a stress-reduction protocol may be required for anxious patients.
- Be prepared to manage hypoglycemia.
- Question patient about self-monitoring of blood glucose values and glycemic control.
- Ensure that patient is following prescribed diet and medication regimen.
- Consider semisupine chair position for patient comfort if adverse GI effects occur.

• Diabetics may be more susceptible to infection and have delayed wound healing.
• Place on frequent recall to evaluate oral hygiene and healing response.
Consultations:
• Consult physician to determine disease control and ability of patient to tolerate dental procedures.
• Notify physician immediately if symptoms of lactic acidosis are observed (myalgia, respiratory distress, weakness, diarrhea, malaise, muscle cramps, somnolence).
• Medical consultation may include data from patient's blood glucose monitoring, including glycosylated hemoglobin or HbA1c testing.
• Oral and maxillofacial procedures associated with significantly restricted food intake require a medical consultation and may require physician adjustment of medication regimen.
Teach Patient/Family to:
• Encourage effective oral hygiene to prevent soft tissue inflammation.
• Update medical history when disease status/glycemic control or medication regimen changes.

sodium fluoride

soe′-dee-um **flor**′-ide
(Fluoritab, Flura-Drops, Fluor-A-Day, Fluotic, Fluoridex Karidium, Luride Lozi-Tabs, Pediaflor, PediDent, Solu-Flur; also found in pediatric vitamin formulas)

CATEGORY AND SCHEDULE

Pregnancy Risk Category: Not established

Drug Class: Fluoride ion

MECHANISM OF ACTION

Interacts with tooth structure to increase resistance to acid dissolution; promotes enamel remineralization and inhibits dental plaque microorganisms.

USES

Prevention of dental caries

PHARMACOKINETICS

PO: Efficient oral absorption (75%–90%); distributed to calcified tissues (bones and teeth); excreted in urine, feces; crosses placenta, excreted in breast milk.

INDICATIONS AND DOSAGES

▸ **Prevention of Dental Caries**

Topical

Adult, Children older than 12 yr. 10 ml 0.2% solution daily after brushing teeth; rinse mouth for at least 1 min with solution. Do not swallow.

PO

Children 6–12 yr. 5 ml 0.2% solution. Must ascertain fluoride concentration in patient's drinking water before prescribing, as shown in the following tables:

▸ **USA—Fluoride Supplementation Schedule***

Drinking Water [F^-]

Child's Age	Less than 0.3 ppm	0.3–0.6 ppm	More than 0.6 ppm
Birth–6 mo	0	0	0
6 mo–3 yr	0.25 mg/day	0	0
3–6 yr	0.50 mg/day	0.25 mg/day	0
6–16 yr	1.0 mg/day	0.50 mg/day	0

*Must consider ALL dietary sources of F^-.

S

Canada-Fluoride Supplementation Schedule

Age	Canadian Paediatric Society (Applies to all Children)	Canadian Dental Association (Applies to Children with High Risk of Caries)
6 mo–2 yr	0.25 mg/day	0
3–5 yr	0.50 mg/day	0.25 mg/day (0.5 mg/day if fluoridated toothpaste is not used regularly)
6–12 yr	Not applicable	1.00 mg/day
6–16 yr	1.0 mg/day	Not applicable

SIDE EFFECTS/ADVERSE REACTIONS

Occasional

Mottled, stained enamel (chronic use), stomatitis

Acute overdose: Black tarry stools, bloody vomit, diarrhea, decreased respiration, increased salivation, watery eyes

Chronic overdose: Hypocalcemia, tetany, respiratory arrest, constipation, loss of appetite, nausea, vomiting, weight loss

S

PRECAUTIONS AND CONTRAINDICATIONS

Hypersensitivity, renal insufficiency, GI ulcerations

Caution:

Children younger than 6 yr (must evaluate total fluoride ingestion)

DRUG INTERACTIONS OF CONCERN TO DENTISTRY

- Avoid use with dairy products and gastric alkalinizers

SERIOUS REACTIONS

! Cardiac arrhythmias, renal failure

DENTAL CONSIDERATIONS

General:

- Determine fluoride concentration in water supply, and then calculate dosage.
- Recommended dose should not be exceeded or dental fluorosis and osseous changes may occur.
- To reduce risk of accidental ingestion and overdosage, ADA recommends that a limit of 264 mg sodium fluoride be dispensed in prepackaged containers.
- Give drops after meals with fluids or undiluted tablets; may be chewed; do not swallow whole; may be given with water or juice; avoid milk.
- Systemic fluoride use during pregnancy has not been shown to prevent tooth decay in children.
- Treatment of acute overdose:
  - Gastric lavage with calcium chloride or calcium hydroxide solution to precipitate fluoride.
  - Maintenance of high urine output.
  - Refer to hospital emergency facility.

Teach Patient/Family to:

- Monitor children using gel or rinse; not to be swallowed.
- Not drink, eat, or rinse mouth for at least 0.5 hr after topical use.
- Apply after brushing and flossing at bedtime.
- Store out of children's reach.

sodium fluoride (topical)

soe′-dee-um **flor**′-ide
(nonabrasive: Karigel, NeutraCare, PreviDent; with abrasive: PreviDent 5000 Plus)

CATEGORY AND SCHEDULE

Pregnancy Risk Category: Not established

Drug Class: Fluoride ion

MECHANISM OF ACTION

Interacts with enamel surface to increase resistance to acid dissolution; promotes enamel remineralization and inhibits dental plaque microorganisms

USES

Prevention of dental caries, hypersensitive root surfaces

PHARMACOKINETICS

PO: Efficient oral absorption (75%–90%); distributed to calcified tissues (bones and teeth); excreted in urine, feces; crosses placenta, excreted in breast milk.

INDICATIONS AND DOSAGES

▸ Prevention of Dental Caries

Topical

Adults, Children older than 6 yr. Nonabrasive gels—use daily; apply thin ribbon to tooth brush for at least 1 min after regular brushing, preferably at bedtime; expectorate and refrain from eating, drinking, and rinsing; children should use under parental supervision.
Available forms include: Gel or cream 2 oz (56 g) squeeze tube 0.5% (as 1.1% sodium fluoride) with and without mild abrasive.

Other fluoride topical products include the following daily-use gels. 1.1% APF (Thera-Flur); 0.4% Sn F2 (Control, Easy-Gel, Flocare, Flo-Gel, Florentine, Gel-Kam, Gel-Pro, Gel-Tin, Perfect Choice, Quick-Gel, Stan-Gard, Stop Gel). Rinses: 0.05% APF daily use (NaFrinse, Phos-Flur) and 0.2% NaF weekly use (NaFrinse, Point-Two, Preventive, PreviDent).

Product Strength	F-Ion (%)	ppm F Equivalence
1.1% NaF	0.5	4950
0.4% SnF2	0.10	970
0.2 % NaF	0.10	910
0.05% NaF	0.02	230

SIDE EFFECTS

Occasional

Mottled, stained enamel (chronic use), stomatitis
Acute overdose: Black tarry stools, bloody vomit, diarrhea, decreased respiration, increased salivation, watery eyes
Chronic overdose*:* Hypocalcemia, tetany, respiratory arrest, constipation, loss of appetite, nausea, vomiting, weight loss

PRECAUTIONS AND CONTRAINDICATIONS

Hypersensitivity; may be used in areas of fluoridated drinking water
Caution:
Children younger than 6 yr (repeated swallowing of agent could cause dental fluorosis); do not use in pediatric patients younger than 6 yr, infants. Supervise children younger than 6 yr. A 2-oz tube of 1.1% NaF contains 250 mg fluoride, more than twice the amount that the ADA recommends to be dispensed in 1 container. Ingestion of as little as 0.29 oz could cause acute toxicity in

a 1-yr-old child. Repeated swallowing could cause fluorosis.

DRUG INTERACTIONS OF CONCERN TO DENTISTRY

• None reported

SERIOUS REACTIONS

! Cardiac arrhythmias, renal failure

DENTAL CONSIDERATIONS

General:

• Neutral sodium fluoride preparations are recommended for patients with exposed root surfaces, which may be hypersensitive.

Teach Patient/Family to:

• Apply daily a thin ribbon of dental cream or gel to tooth brush and brush thoroughly for 2 min, preferably at bedtime.

• Expectorate after use and not to eat, drink, or rinse for 30 min.

• Have children use under parental supervision.

somatropin

soe-mah-**troe**′-pin

(Accretropin; Genotropin, Genotropin MiniQuick, Humatrope, Norditropin, Norditropin Cartridge, Nutropin, Nutropin AQ, Nutropin Depot, Saizen, Serostim, Zorbtive)

CATEGORY AND SCHEDULE

Pregnancy Risk Category: C

Drug Class: Growth hormone

MECHANISM OF ACTION

Somatotropin, a purified polypeptide hormone of recombinant DNA origin, contains the identical sequence of amino acids found in human growth hormone that stimulates growth of linear bone, skeletal muscle, and organs. Human growth hormone also stimulates erythropoietin, which increases red blood cell mass, exerts both insulin-like and diabetogenic effects, and enhances the transmucosal transport of water, electrolytes, and nutrients across the gut.

USES

Growth hormone deficiency
Turner syndrome
AIDS-related wasting
Short bowel syndrome

PHARMACOKINETICS

Bioavailability: 70% when administered subcutaneously. Metabolized in the liver and kidneys. ***Half life***: IV, 20–30 min; subcutaneous, IM, 3–5 hr.

INDICATIONS AND DOSAGES

▸ **Growth Hormone Deficiency**

SC (Accretropin)
Children. 0.18–0.3 mg/kg body weight divided 6 or 7 times per week.
SC (Humatrope)
Adults. 0.006 mg/kg once daily.
Children. 0.18–0.3 mg/kg weekly divided into alternate-day doses or 6 doses/wk.
SC (Nutropin)
Adults. 0.006 mg/kg once daily.
Children. 0.3–0.7 mg/kg weekly divided into daily doses.
SC (Nutropin AQ)
Adults. 0.006 mg/kg once daily.
SC (Genotropin)
Adults. 0.04–0.08 mg/kg weekly divided into 6–7 equal doses/wk.
Children. 0.16–0.24 mg/kg weekly divided into daily doses.
SC (Protopine)
Children. 0.3 mg/kg weekly divided into daily doses.
SC (Norditropin)

Children. 0.024–0.036 mg/kg/dose 6–7 times a week.
SC (Saizen)
Children. 0.06 mg/kg 3 times a week.
SC only (Nutropin Depot)
Children. 0.75 mg/kg twice monthly or 1.5 mg/kg once monthly.

▸ **Turner Syndrome**
SC (Accretropin)
Children. 0.36 mg/kg divided in doses of 6 or 7 times a week.
SC (Humatrope, Nutropin, Nutropin AQ)
Children. 0.375 mg/kg weekly divided into equal doses 3–7 times a week.

▸ **AIDS-Related Wasting**
SC
Adults weighing more than 55 kg. 6 mg once a day at bedtime.
Adults weighing 45–55 kg. 5 mg once a day at bedtime.
Adults weighing 35–44 kg. 4 mg once a day at bedtime.
Adults weighing less than 35 kg. 0.1 mg/kg once a day at bedtime.

▸ **Short Bowel Syndrome**
SC (Zorbtive)
Adults. 0.1 mg/kg/day. Maximum: 8 mg/day.

SIDE EFFECTS/ADVERSE REACTIONS

Frequent
Bruising, erythema, hemorrhage, edema, pain, pruritus, rash, swelling, injection site reaction

Occasional
Nausea, headache, fatigue, scoliosis

PRECAUTIONS AND CONTRAINDICATIONS

Hypersensitivity to growth hormone, *E. coli*, or any component of the formulation
Closed epiphyses (Accretropin)
Local or systemic allergic reaction may occur.
Use with caution in patients with intracranial hypertension.
Progression of scoliosis may occur.
Use with caution in patients with risk factors for diabetes since somatropin may decrease insulin sensitivity.
Use with caution in patients with hypopituitarism, hypothyroidism, and preexisting tumors or growth hormone deficiency secondary to an intracranial lesion.

DRUG INTERACTIONS OF CONCERN TO DENTISTRY

• Corticosteroids: May inhibit growth response.

SERIOUS REACTIONS

! Intracranial hypertension with papilledema, visual changes, headache, nausea, and/ or vomiting may occur.
! Glucose intolerance can occur with overdosage. Long-term overdosage with growth hormone could result in signs and symptoms of acromegaly.

DENTAL CONSIDERATIONS

General:
• Consider semisupine chair position for patient comfort if GI side effects occur.
• Avoid dental light in patient's eyes; offer dark glasses for patient comfort.

Consultations:
• Medical consultation may be required to assess disease control.

Teach Patient/Family to:
• Encourage effective oral hygiene to prevent soft tissue inflammation.
• Use caution to prevent injury when using oral hygiene aids.

sotalol hydrochloride

soe′-tah-lole high-droh-**klor**′-ide
(Apo-Sotalol[CAN], Betapace, Betapace AF, Cardol[AUS], Novo-Sotalol[CAN], PMS-Sotalol[CAN], Solavert[AUS], Sorine, Sotab[AUS], Sotacor[AUS], Sotahexal[AUS])

Do not confuse sotalol with Stadol.

CATEGORY AND SCHEDULE

Pregnancy Risk Category: B (D if used in second or third trimester)

Drug Class: Nonselective β-adrenergic blocker

MECHANISM OF ACTION

A β-adrenergic blocking agent that prolongs action potential, effective refractory period, and QT interval. Decreases heart rate and AV node conduction; increases AV node refractoriness.

Therapeutic Effect: Produces antiarrhythmic activity.

USES

Treatment of life-threatening ventricular dysrhythmias (class II), atrial fibrillation (Betapace AF only), mild-to-moderate heart failure

PHARMACOKINETICS

Well absorbed from the GI tract. Protein binding: None. Widely distributed. Primarily excreted unchanged in urine. Removed by hemodialysis. ***Half-life:*** 12 hr (increased in the elderly and patients with impaired renal function).

INDICATIONS AND DOSAGES

▸ Documented, Life-Threatening Arrhythmias

PO

Adults, Elderly. Initially, 80 mg twice a day. May increase gradually at 2- to 3-day intervals. Range: 240–320 mg/day.

▸ Dosage in Renal Impairment

Dosage interval is modified on the basis of creatinine clearance.

Creatinine Clearance	Dosage Interval
31–60 ml/min	24 hr
10–30 ml/min	36–48 hr
Less than 10 ml/min	Individualized

SIDE EFFECTS/ADVERSE REACTIONS

Frequent

Diminished sexual function, drowsiness, insomnia, unusual fatigue or weakness

Occasional

Depression, cold hands or feet, diarrhea, constipation, anxiety, nasal congestion, nausea, vomiting

Rare

Altered taste, dry eyes, itching, numbness of fingers, toes, or scalp

PRECAUTIONS AND CONTRAINDICATIONS

Bronchial asthma, cardiogenic shock, prolonged QT syndrome (unless functioning pacemaker is present), second- and third-degree heart block, sinus bradycardia, uncontrolled cardiac failure

Caution:

Lactation, diabetes mellitus, renal disease. Before initiating doses, place patient in cardiac care facility to monitor for drug-induced arrhythmia

DRUG INTERACTIONS OF CONCERN TO DENTISTRY

- Decreased hypotensive effect: NSAIDs, indomethacin
- Increased hypotension, myocardial depression: hydrocarbon inhalation anesthetics
- Hypertension, bradycardia: sympathomimetics
- Slow metabolism of lidocaine

SERIOUS REACTIONS

! Bradycardia, CHF, hypotension, bronchospasm, hypoglycemia, prolonged QT interval, torsades de pointes, ventricular tachycardia, and premature ventricular complexes may occur.

DENTAL CONSIDERATIONS

General:

- Monitor vital signs at every appointment because of cardiovascular side effects.
- After supine positioning, have patient sit upright for at least 2 min before standing to avoid orthostatic hypotension.
- Stress from dental procedures may compromise cardiovascular function; determine patient risk.
- Use vasoconstrictors with caution, in low doses, and with careful aspiration. Avoid use of gingival retraction cord with epinephrine.
- Short appointments and a stress-reduction protocol may be required for anxious patients.

Consultations:

- Medical consultation should be made to assess disease control and patient's ability to tolerate stress.

spironolactone

speer-on-oh-**lak′**-tone
(Aldactone, Novo-Spiroton[CAN], Spiractin[AUS])
Do not confuse Aldactone with Aldactazide.

CATEGORY AND SCHEDULE

Pregnancy Risk Category: C (D if used in pregnancy-induced hypertension)

Drug Class: Potassium-sparing diuretic

MECHANISM OF ACTION

A potassium-sparing diuretic that interferes with sodium reabsorption by competitively inhibiting the action of aldosterone in the distal tubule, thus promoting sodium and water excretion and increasing potassium retention.
Therapeutic Effect: Produces diuresis; lowers B/P; diagnostic aid for primary aldosteronism.

USES

Edema, hypertension, diuretic-induced hypokalemia, primary hyperaldosteronism (diagnosis, short-term treatment, long-term treatment), nephrotic syndrome, cirrhosis of the liver with ascites

PHARMACOKINETICS

Route	Onset	Peak	Duration
PO	24–48 hr	48–72 hr	48–72 hr

Well absorbed from the GI tract (absorption increased with food). Protein binding: 91%–98%. Metabolized in the liver to active metabolite. Primarily excreted in urine. Unknown if removed by hemodialysis. ***Half-life:*** 0–24 hr (metabolite, 13–24 hr).

INDICATIONS AND DOSAGES

▸ **Edema**

PO

Adults, Elderly. 25–200 mg/day as a single dose or in 2 divided doses.

Children. 1.5–3.3 mg/kg/day in divided doses.

Neonates. 1–3 mg/kg/day in 1–2 divided doses.

▸ **Hypertension**

PO

Adults, Elderly. 25–50 mg/day in 1–2 doses/day.

Children. 1.5–3.3 mg/kg/day in divided doses.

▸ **Hypokalemia**

PO

Adults, Elderly. 25–200 mg/day as a single dose or in 2 divided doses.

▸ **Male Hirsutism**

PO

Adults, Elderly. 50–200 mg/day as a single dose or in 2 divided doses.

▸ **Primary Aldosteronism**

PO

Adults, Elderly. 100–400 mg/day as a single dose or in 2 divided doses.

Children. 100–400 mg/m^2/day as a single dose or in 2 divided doses.

▸ **Dosage in Renal Impairment**

Dosage interval is modified on the basis of creatinine clearance.

Creatinine Clearance	Interval
10–50 ml/min	Usual dose q12h–24h
Less than 10 ml/min	Avoid use

S

SIDE EFFECTS/ADVERSE REACTIONS

Frequent

Hyperkalemia (in patients with renal insufficiency and those taking potassium supplements), dehydration, hyponatremia, lethargy

Occasional

Nausea, vomiting, anorexia, abdominal cramps, diarrhea, headache, ataxia, somnolence, confusion, fever

Male: Gynecomastia, impotence, decreased libido

Female: Menstrual irregularities (including amenorrhea and postmenopausal bleeding), breast tenderness

Rare

Rash, urticaria, hirsutism

PRECAUTIONS AND CONTRAINDICATIONS

Acute renal insufficiency, anuria, BUN and serum creatinine levels more than twice normal values, hyperkalemia

Caution:

Dehydration, hepatic disease, lactation, hyponatremia

DRUG INTERACTIONS OF CONCERN TO DENTISTRY

- Nephrotoxicity: indomethacin and possibly other NSAIDs
- Decreased antihypertensive effect: indomethacin and possibly other NSAIDs

SERIOUS REACTIONS

! Severe hyperkalemia may produce arrhythmias, bradycardia, and ECG changes (tented T waves, widening QRS complex and ST segment depression). These may proceed to cardiac standstill or ventricular fibrillation.

! Cirrhosis patients are at risk for hepatic decompensation if dehydration or hyponatremia occurs.

! Patients with primary aldosteronism may experience rapid weight loss and severe fatigue during high-dose therapy.

DENTAL CONSIDERATIONS

General:

- Monitor vital signs at every appointment because of cardiovascular side effects.
- Assess salivary flow as a factor in caries, periodontal disease, and candidiasis.
- If dry mouth occurs, follow usual preventive and palliative measures, but consider hyponatremia as a contributing factor.
- Consider semisupine chair position for patient comfort if GI side effects occur.

Consultations:

- Medical consultation may be required to assess disease control and patient's ability to tolerate stress.

Teach Patient/Family:

- When chronic dry mouth occurs, advise patient to:
  - Avoid mouth rinses with high alcohol content because of drying effects.
  - Use daily home fluoride products to prevent caries.
  - Use sugarless gum, frequent sips of water, or saliva substitutes.

streptomycin

strep-toe-**mye′**-sin

CATEGORY AND SCHEDULE

Pregnancy Risk Category: D

Drug Class: Antibiotics, aminoglycosides, antitubercular agent

MECHANISM OF ACTION

An aminoglycoside that binds directly to the 30S ribosomal subunits causing a faulty peptide sequence to form in the protein chain.

Therapeutic Effect: Inhibits bacterial protein synthesis.

USES

Tuberculosis, brucellosis, endocarditis, mycobacterium avium complex (adjunct), plague, tularemia, gram-negative bacteremia (adjunct)

PHARMACOKINETICS

Protein binding: 34%–35%. Excreted in urine by glomerular filtration. ***Half-life:*** 2.5 hr.

INDICATIONS AND DOSAGES

▸ Tuberculosis

IM

Adults. 15 mg/kg/day. Maximum: 1 g/day.

Elderly. 10 mg/kg/day. Maximum: 750 mg/day.

Children. 20–40 mg/kg/day. Maximum: 1 g/day.

▸ Bacterial Endocarditis

IM

▸ Streptococcal

Adults. 1 g twice daily for the first week, and 500 mg twice daily for the second week.

Elderly (over 60 yr of age). 500 mg twice daily for the entire 2-wk period.

▸ Enterococcal

Adults. 1 g twice daily for 2 wk and 500 mg twice daily for an additional 4 wk concomitantly with penicillin. Ototoxicity may require early termination.

▸ Plague

IM

Adults. 2 g in two divided doses for a minimum of 10 days.

▸ **Tularemia**
IM
Adults. 1 to 2 g daily in divided doses for 7–10 days or until patient is afebrile for 5–7 days.

Dosage in Renal Impairment

GFR (mL/min)	Dosage Interval
Greater than 50	24 hr
10–50	24–72 hr
Less than 10	72–96 hr

SIDE EFFECTS/ADVERSE REACTIONS

Frequent
Vestibular ototoxicity (nausea, vomiting, and vertigo), paresthesia of face, rash, fever, urticaria, angioneurotic edema, and eosinophilia

Less Frequent
Deafness, exfoliative dermatitis, anaphylaxis, azotemia, leucopenia, thrombocytopenia, pancytopenia, hemolytic anemia, muscular weakness, and amblyopia

PRECAUTIONS AND CONTRAINDICATIONS

Hypersensitivity to streptomycin, other aminoglycosides, or sulfites

Caution:
Antibiotic hypersensitivity
Preexisting kidney or auditory impairment
Concomitant nephrotoxic, ototoxic, or neurotoxic drugs
Concomitant anesthesia or certain muscle relaxing drugs because of the risk of neuromuscular blockade

DRUG INTERACTIONS OF CONCERN TO DENTISTRY

• Increased risk of nephrotoxicity: amphotericin, loop diuretics
• May increase the effects of streptomycin: neuromuscular blockers

SERIOUS REACTIONS

! Nephrotoxicity (as evidenced by increased BUN and serum creatinine levels and decreased creatinine clearance) may be reversible if the drug is stopped at the first sign of nephrotoxic symptoms.
! Irreversible ototoxicity (manifested as tinnitus, dizziness, ringing or roaring in the ears, and impaired hearing) and neurotoxicity (as evidenced by headache, dizziness, lethargy, tremor, and visual disturbances) occur occasionally. Symptoms of ototoxicity, nephrotoxicity, and neuromuscular toxicity may occur.
! Superinfections, particularly with fungal infections, may result from bacterial imbalance.

DENTAL CONSIDERATIONS

General:
• Caution patient regarding allergy to medication.
• Do not treat patients with active tuberculosis.
• Determine why the patient is using this medication.
• Determine if the patient is pregnant.

Consultation:
• Laboratory tests may be required to assess hearing, kidney function, and streptomycin blood levels.

Teach Patient/Family to:
• Advise the patient to report any ringing in the ears, hearing loss, balance problems, or changes in vision.

sucralfate

soo-**kral**′-fate
(Apo-Sucralate[CAN], Carafate, Novo-Sucralate[CAN], Ulcyte[AUS])
Do not confuse Carafate with Cafergot.

CATEGORY AND SCHEDULE

Pregnancy Risk Category: B

Drug Class: Protectant, aluminum salt of a sulfated sucrose

MECHANISM OF ACTION

An antiulcer agent that forms an ulcer-adherent complex with proteinaceous exudate, such as albumin, at ulcer site. Also forms a viscous adhesive barrier on the surface of intact mucosa of the stomach or duodenum.
Therapeutic Effect: Protects damaged mucosa from further destruction by absorbing gastric acid, pepsin, and bile salts.

USES

Treatment of duodenal ulcer

PHARMACOKINETICS

Minimally absorbed from the GI tract. Eliminated in feces, with small amount excreted in urine. Not removed by hemodialysis.

INDICATIONS AND DOSAGES

▸ Active Duodenal Ulcers
PO
Adults, Elderly. 1 g 4 times a day (before meals and at bedtime) for up to 8 wk.
▸ Maintenance Therapy after Healing of Acute Duodenal Ulcers
PO
Adults, Elderly. 1 g twice a day.

SIDE EFFECTS/ADVERSE REACTIONS

Frequent
Constipation
Occasional
Dry mouth, backache, diarrhea, dizziness, somnolence, nausea, indigestion, rash, hives, itching, abdominal discomfort

PRECAUTIONS AND CONTRAINDICATIONS

Caution:
Lactation, children

DRUG INTERACTIONS OF CONCERN TO DENTISTRY

• Gastric irritation: chloral hydrate
• Decreased absorption of tetracyclines, fluoroquinolones
• Decreased effects of diclofenac, ketoconazole

SERIOUS REACTIONS

! None known

DENTAL CONSIDERATIONS

General:
• Prescribe acetaminophen for analgesia if needed. ASA and NSAIDs are contraindicated in active upper GI disease.
• Consider semisupine chair position for patient comfort because of GI effects of disease.
• Tetracycline doses should be given 2 hr before or after the sucralfate dose.
Teach Patient/Family to:
• Avoid mouth rinses with high alcohol content because of drying effects.

sulconazole nitrate

sul-**kon**′-ah-zole **nye**′-trate
(Exelderm)

CATEGORY AND SCHEDULE

Pregnancy Risk Category: C

Drug Class: Topical antifungal

MECHANISM OF ACTION

An imidazole derivative that inhibits synthesis of ergosterol (a vital component of fungal cell formation), the damaging cell membrane.
Therapeutic Effect: Fungistatic.

USES

Treatment of tinea pedis, tinea corporis, tinea cruris, tinea versicolor; unapproved: cutaneous candidiasis

PHARMACOKINETICS

Minimal systemic absorption following topical administration. Excreted in urine. ***Half-life:*** Unknown.

INDICATIONS AND DOSAGES

▸ **Tinea Pedis**

Topical

Adults, Elderly, Children 12 yr and older. Apply 2 times a day until signs and symptoms significantly improve.

▸ **Tinea Corporis, Tinea Cruris, Tinea Versicolor**

Topical

Adults, Elderly, Children 12 yr and older. Apply 1–2 times a day until signs and symptoms significantly improve.

SIDE EFFECTS/ADVERSE REACTIONS

Occasional
Headache, nausea

Rare
Burning or stinging, pruritus, redness

PRECAUTIONS AND CONTRAINDICATIONS

Hypersensitivity to sulconazole nitrate or any component of the formulation

Caution:
Pregnancy Category: C

DRUG INTERACTIONS OF CONCERN TO DENTISTRY

• None reported

SERIOUS REACTIONS

! None known

DENTAL CONSIDERATIONS

General:

• There are no significant dental considerations. One possible concern is the few patients with topical candidiasis, in whom broad-spectrum antiinfectives could potentially contribute to a suprainfection.

sulfacetamide

sul-fa-**see**′-ta-mide
(AK-Sulf, Bleph-10, Isopto Cetamide, Diosulf[CAN], Ophthacet, Sodium Sulamyd, Sulfair)

CATEGORY AND SCHEDULE

Pregnancy Risk Category: C

Drug Class: Antibacterial sulfonamide

MECHANISM OF ACTION

Interferes with synthesis of folic acid that bacteria require for growth.

Therapeutic Effect: Prevents further bacterial growth. Bacteriostatic.

USES

Treatment of conjunctivitis, superficial eye infections, corneal ulcers, trachoma

PHARMACOKINETICS

Small amounts may be absorbed into the cornea. Excreted rapidly in urine. ***Half-life:*** 7–13 hr.

INDICATIONS AND DOSAGES

▸ Treatment of Corneal Ulcers, Conjunctivitis, and Other Superficial Infections of the Eye, Prophylaxis after Injuries to the Eye/Removal of Foreign Bodies, Adjunctive Therapy for Trachoma and Inclusion Conjunctivitis

Ophthalmic

Adults, Elderly. Ointment: Apply small amount in lower conjunctival sac 1–4 times a day and at bedtime. Solution: 1–3 drops to lower conjunctival sac q2–3h. Seborrheic dermatitis, seborrheic sicca (dandruff), secondary bacterial skin infections.

Topical

Adults, Elderly. Apply 1–4 times a day.

SIDE EFFECTS/ADVERSE REACTIONS

Frequent

Transient ophthalmic burning, stinging

Occasional

Headache

Rare

Hypersensitivity (erythema, rash, itching, swelling, photosensitivity)

PRECAUTIONS AND CONTRAINDICATIONS

Hypersensitivity to sulfonamides or any component of preparation (some products contain sulfite), use in combination with silver-containing products

Caution:

Cross-sensitivity with other sulfas; pregnancy category C

DRUG INTERACTIONS OF CONCERN TO DENTISTRY

- None reported

SERIOUS REACTIONS

! Superinfection, drug-induced lupus erythematosus, Stevens-Johnson syndrome occur rarely; nephrotoxicity with high dermatologic concentrations.

DENTAL CONSIDERATIONS

General:

- Avoid dental light in patient's eyes; offer dark glasses for patient comfort.

sulfasalazine

sul-fa-**sal′**-ah-zeen

(Alti-Sulfasalazine[CAN], Azulfidine, Azulfidine EN-tabs, Pyralin EN[AUS], Salazopyrin[CAN], Salazopyrin EN[AUS], Salazopyrin EN-Tabs[CAN])

Do not confuse Azulfidine with azathioprine, or sulfasalazine with sulfadiazine or sulfisoxazole.

CATEGORY AND SCHEDULE

Pregnancy Risk Category: B (D if given near term)

Drug Class: Sulfonamide derivative with antiinflammatory action

S

MECHANISM OF ACTION

A sulfonamide that inhibits prostaglandin synthesis, acting locally in the colon.
Therapeutic Effect: Decreases inflammatory response, interferes with GI secretion.

USES

Treatment of ulcerative colitis, Crohn's disease, rheumatoid arthritis, juvenile rheumatoid arthritis; unapproved: ankylosing spondylitis

PHARMACOKINETICS

Poorly absorbed from the GI tract. Cleaved in colon by intestinal bacteria, forming sulfapyridine and mesalamine (5-ASA). Absorbed in colon. Widely distributed. Metabolized in the liver. Primarily excreted in urine. ***Half-life:*** sulfapyridine, 6–14 hr; 5-ASA, 0.6–1.4 hr.

INDICATIONS AND DOSAGES

▸ Ulcerative Colitis

PO

Adults, Elderly. 1 g 3–4 times a day in divided doses q4–6h. Maintenance: 2 g/day in divided doses q6–12h. Maximum: 6 g/day.
Children. 40–75 mg/kg/day in divided doses q4–6h. Maintenance: 30–50 mg/kg/day in divided doses q4–8h. Maximum: 2 g/day. Maximum: 6 g/day.

▸ Rheumatoid Arthritis

PO

Adults, Elderly. Initially, 0.5–1 g/day for 1 wk. Increase by 0.5 g/wk, up to 3 g/day.

▸ Juvenile Rheumatoid Arthritis

PO

Children. Initially, 10 mg/kg/day. May increase by 10 mg/kg/day at weekly intervals. Range: 30–50 mg/kg/day. Maximum: 2 g/day.

SIDE EFFECTS/ADVERSE REACTIONS

Frequent

Anorexia, nausea, vomiting, headache, oligospermia (generally reversed by withdrawal of drug)

Occasional

Hypersensitivity reaction (rash, urticaria, pruritus, fever, anemia)

Rare

Tinnitus, hypoglycemia, diuresis, photosensitivity

PRECAUTIONS AND CONTRAINDICATIONS

Children younger than 2 yr; hypersensitivity to carbonic anhydrase inhibitors, local anesthetics, salicylates, sulfonamides, sulfonylureas, sunscreens containing PABA, or thiazide or loop diuretics; intestinal or urinary tract obstruction; porphyria; pregnancy at term; severe hepatic or renal dysfunction

Caution:

Lactation, impaired hepatic function, severe allergy, bronchial asthma, impaired renal function, intolerance to aspirin

DRUG INTERACTIONS OF CONCERN TO DENTISTRY

- Increased photosensitizing effects: tetracycline
- Decreased absorption: folic acid

SERIOUS REACTIONS

! Anaphylaxis, Stevens-Johnson syndrome, hematologic toxicity (leukopenia, agranulocytosis), hepatotoxicity, and nephrotoxicity occur rarely.

DENTAL CONSIDERATIONS

General:

- Patients on chronic drug therapy may rarely have symptoms of blood

dyscrasias, which can include infection, bleeding, and poor healing.

- Question patient about response to antibiotics to avoid responses that might provoke pseudomembranous colitis.
- Palliative medication may be required for management of oral side effects.
- Consider semisupine chair position for patient comfort because of GI effects of disease.

Consultations:

- Medical consultation may be required to assess disease control and patient's ability to tolerate stress.
- In a patient with symptoms of blood dyscrasias, request a medical consultation for blood studies and postpone dental treatment until normal values are reestablished.

Teach Patient/Family to:

- Use caution to prevent injury when using oral hygiene aids.

sulfinpyrazone

sul-fin-**pyr**′-ah-zone
(Anturane, Apo-Sulfinpyrazone[CAN], Nu-Sulfinpyrazone[CAN])
Do not confuse Anturane with Accutane.

CATEGORY AND SCHEDULE

Pregnancy Risk Category: C/D (near term)

Drug Class: Uricosuric

MECHANISM OF ACTION

A uricosuric that increases urinary excretion of uric acid, thereby decreasing blood urate levels.

Therapeutic Effect: Promotes uric acid excretion and reduces serum uric acid levels.

USES

Treatment of chronic gouty arthritis

PHARMACOKINETICS

Rapidly and completely absorbed from GI tract. Widely distributed. Metabolized in liver to 2 active metabolites, *p*-hydroxy-sulfinpyrazone and a sulfide analogue. Excreted primarily in urine. Not removed by hemodialysis. ***Half-life:*** 2.7–6 hr.

INDICATIONS AND DOSAGES

▸ **Gout**

PO

Adults, Elderly. 100–200 mg 2 times a day. Maximum: 800 mg/day.

SIDE EFFECTS/ADVERSE REACTIONS

Frequent

Nausea, vomiting, stomach pain

Occasional

Flushed face, headache, dizziness, frequent urge to urinate, rash

Rare

Increased bleeding time, hepatic necrosis, nephrotic syndrome, uric acid stones

PRECAUTIONS AND CONTRAINDICATIONS

Active peptic ulcer, blood dyscrasias, GI inflammation, pregnancy (near term), hypersensitivity to sulfinpyrazone or any of its components, phenylbutazone, or other pyrazoles

DRUG INTERACTIONS OF CONCERN TO DENTISTRY

- Increased bleeding: NSAIDs, aspirin
- Decreased effects of salicylates

SERIOUS REACTIONS

! Hematological toxicity including anemia, leucopenia, agranulocytosis, thrombocytopenia, and aplastic anemia occur rarely.
! Overdose causes drowsiness, dizziness, anorexia, abdominal pain, hemolytic anemia, acidosis, jaundice, fever, and agranulocytosis.

DENTAL CONSIDERATIONS

General:
- Consider local hemostasis measures to prevent excessive bleeding.
- Avoid prescribing aspirin-containing products.
- Patients on chronic drug therapy may rarely have symptoms of blood dyscrasias, which can include infection, bleeding, and poor healing.
- Consider semisupine chair position for patient comfort if GI side effects occur.
- Evaluate respiration characteristics and rate.

Consultations:
- In a patient with symptoms of blood dyscrasias, request a medical consultation for blood studies and postpone dental treatment until normal values are reestablished.

Teach Patient/Family to:
- Use caution to prevent injury when using oral hygiene aids.

S

sulfisoxazole

sul-fi-**sox**′-ah-zole
(Gantrisin, Novo-Soxazole[CAN], Sulfizole[CAN], Truxazole)
Do not confuse with sulfadiazine, sulfamethoxazole, sulfasalazine, Gastrosed

CATEGORY AND SCHEDULE

Pregnancy risk category: B/D (near term)

Drug Class: Sulfonamide, antiinfective

MECHANISM OF ACTION

An antibacterial sulfonamide that inhibits bacterial synthesis of dihydrofolic acid by preventing condensation of pteridine with aminobenzoic acid through competitive inhibition of the enzyme dihydropteroate synthetase.
Therapeutic Effect: Bacteriostatic.

USES

Treatment of urinary tract, systemic infections; chancroid; trachoma; toxoplasmosis; acute otitis media; lymphogranuloma venereum; eye infections

PHARMACOKINETICS

Rapidly and completely absorbed. Small intestine is major site of absorption, but some absorption occurs in the stomach. Exists in the blood as unbound, protein-bound, and conjugated forms. Sulfisoxazole is metabolized primarily by acetylation and oxidation in the liver. The free form is considered to be the therapeutically active form. Protein binding: 85%. ***Half-life:*** 5–8 hr.

INDICATIONS AND DOSAGES

▸ **Acute, Recurrent or Chronic UTI, Meningococcal Meningitis, Acute Otitis Media Caused by *Haemophilus influenzae***

PO

Infants older than 2 mo, Children. One-half of the 24-hr dose initially then 150 mg/kg daily or 4 g/m^2 daily for maintenance divided q4–6h. Maximum dose: 6 g daily.

Adults. 2–4 g initially, then 4–8 g daily divided q4–6h.

SIDE EFFECTS/ADVERSE REACTIONS

Anaphylaxis, erythema multiforme (Stevens-Johnson syndrome), toxic epidermal necrolysis, exfoliative dermatitis, angioedema, arteritis and vasculitis, allergic myocarditis, serum sickness, rash, urticaria, pruritus, photosensitivity, conjunctival and scleral injection, generalized allergic reactions, generalized skin eruptions, tachycardia, palpitations, syncope, cyanosis, goiter, diuresis, hypoglycemia, arthralgia, myalgia, headache, dizziness, peripheral neuritis, paresthesia, convulsions, tinnitus, vertigo, ataxia, intracranial hypertension, cough, shortness of breath, pulmonary infiltrates

PRECAUTIONS AND CONTRAINDICATIONS

Patients with a known hypersensitivity to sulfonamides, children younger than 2 mo (except in the treatment of congenital toxoplasmosis as adjunctive therapy with pyrimethamine), pregnant women at term, and mothers nursing infants younger than 2 mo of age

Caution:

Lactation, impaired hepatic function, severe allergy, bronchial asthma

DRUG INTERACTIONS OF CONCERN TO DENTISTRY

- Decreased effect: ester-type local anesthetics (procaine, tetracaine)
- Increased photosensitizing effect: tetracycline
- Decreased effect of penicillins, cephalosporins

SERIOUS REACTIONS

! Fatalities associated with the administration of sulfonamides, including Stevens-Johnson syndrome toxic epidermal necrolysis; fulminant hepatic necrosis, agranulocytosis, aplastic anemia, and other blood dyscrasias occur rarely.

! Clinical signs, such as rash, sore throat, fever, arthralgia, pallor, purpura, or jaundice, may be early indications of serious reactions.

DENTAL CONSIDERATIONS

General:

- Patients on chronic drug therapy may rarely have symptoms of blood dyscrasias, which can include infection, bleeding, and poor healing.
- Determine why the patient is taking the drug.
- Palliative medication may be required for management of oral side effects.
- Consider semisupine chair position for patient comfort if GI side effects occur.

Consultations:

- Medical consultation may be required to assess disease control.
- In a patient with symptoms of blood dyscrasias, request a medical consultation for blood studies and postpone dental treatment until normal values are reestablished.

Teach Patient/Family to:

- Encourage effective oral hygiene to prevent soft tissue inflammation.

sulindac

sul-**in**′-dak
(Aclin[AUS], Apo-Sulin[CAN], Clinoril, Novo Sundac[CAN])
Do not confuse Clinoril with Clozaril.

CATEGORY AND SCHEDULE

Pregnancy Risk Category: B (D if used in third trimester or near delivery)

Drug Class: Nonsteroidal antiinflammatory

MECHANISM OF ACTION

An NSAID that produces analgesic and antiinflammatory effects by inhibiting prostaglandin synthesis. ***Therapeutic Effect:*** Reduces inflammatory response and intensity of pain.

USES

Treatment of osteoarthritis, rheumatoid arthritis, acute gouty arthritis, tendinitis, bursitis, ankylosing spondylitis

PHARMACOKINETICS

Route	Onset	Peak	Duration
PO (Anti-rheumatic)	7 days	2–3 wk	N/A

Well absorbed from the GI tract. Metabolized in liver to active metabolite. Primarily excreted in urine. Not removed by hemodialysis. ***Half-life:*** 7.8 hr; metabolite: 16.4 hr.

INDICATIONS AND DOSAGES

▸ **Rheumatoid Arthritis, Osteoarthritis, Ankylosing Spondylitis**

PO

Adults, Elderly. Initially, 150 mg twice a day; may increase up to 400 mg/day.

▸ **Acute Shoulder Pain, Gouty Arthritis, Bursitis, Tendinitis**

PO

Adults, Elderly 200 mg twice a day.

SIDE EFFECTS/ADVERSE REACTIONS

Frequent

Diarrhea or constipation, indigestion, nausea, maculopapular rash, dermatitis, dizziness, headache

Occasional

Anorexia, abdominal cramps, flatulence

PRECAUTIONS AND CONTRAINDICATIONS

Active peptic ulcer disease, chronic inflammation of GI tract, GI bleeding or ulceration, history of hypersensitivity to aspirin or NSAIDs

Caution:

Lactation, children, bleeding disorders, GI disorders, cardiac disorders, hypersensitivity to other NSAIDs, geriatric patients

DRUG INTERACTIONS OF CONCERN TO DENTISTRY

- Increased bleeding, GI effects: alcohol, aspirin, steroids, other NSAIDs
- Renal toxicity: acetaminophen (prolonged use)
- Possible risk of decreased renal function: cyclosporine
- Increased photosensitizing effect: tetracycline
- Increased toxicity of methotrexate, cyclosporine

- Decreased plasma levels: diflunisal
- SSRIs: increased risk of GI side effects

SERIOUS REACTIONS

! Rare reactions with long-term use include peptic ulcer disease

! GI bleeding, gastritis, nephrotoxicity (glomerular nephritis, interstitial nephritis, nephrotic syndrome), severe hepatic reactions (cholestasis, jaundice), and severe hypersensitivity reactions (fever, chills, and joint pain)

DENTAL CONSIDERATIONS

General:

- Patients on chronic drug therapy may rarely have symptoms of blood dyscrasias, which can include infection, bleeding, and poor healing.
- Potential for increased adverse events in patients at risk of thromboembolism.
- Assess salivary flow as a factor in caries, periodontal disease, and candidiasis.
- Avoid prescribing in last trimester of pregnancy.
- Should oral inflammation or lesions occur, refer to physician and consider palliative treatment for the lesions.
- Consider semisupine chair position for patient comfort because of GI side effects.

Consultations:

- Medical consultation may be required to assess disease control.
- In a patient with symptoms of blood dyscrasias, request a medical consultation for blood studies and postpone dental treatment until normal values are reestablished.

Teach Patient/Family to:

- Report oral lesions, soreness, or bleeding to dentist.
- Use caution to prevent injury in use of oral hygiene aids.
- Encourage effective oral hygiene to prevent soft tissue inflammation.
- When chronic dry mouth occurs, advise patient to:
  - Avoid mouth rinses with high alcohol content because of drying effects.
  - Use daily home fluoride products to prevent caries.
  - Use sugarless gum, frequent sips of water, or saliva substitutes.

sumatriptan

soo-ma-**trip**′-tan

(Imigran[AUS], Imitrex, Suvalan[AUS])

Do not confuse sumatriptan with somatropin.

CATEGORY AND SCHEDULE

Pregnancy Risk Category: C

Drug Class: Serotonin agonist

MECHANISM OF ACTION

A serotonin receptor agonist that binds selectively to vascular receptors, producing a vasoconstrictive effect on cranial blood vessels.

Therapeutic Effect: Relieves migraine headache.

USES

Treatment of migraine headaches; cluster headaches

PHARMACOKINETICS

Route	Onset	Peak	Duration
Nasal	15 min	N/A	24–48 hr
PO	30 min	2 hr	24–48 hr
Subcutaneous	10 min	1 hr	24–48 hr

S

Rapidly absorbed after subcutaneous administration. Absorption after PO administration is incomplete, with significant amounts undergoing hepatic metabolism, resulting in low bioavailability (about 14%). Protein binding: 10%–21%. Widely distributed. Undergoes first-pass metabolism in the liver. Excreted in urine. ***Half-life:*** 2 hr.

INDICATIONS AND DOSAGES

▸ Acute Migraine Attack

PO

Adults, Elderly. 25–50 mg. Dose may be repeated after at least 2 hr. Maximum: 100 mg/single dose; 200 mg/24 hr.

Subcutaneous

Adults, Elderly. 6 mg. Maximum: Two 6-mg injections/24 hr (separated by at least 1 hr).

Intranasal

Adults, Elderly. 5–20 mg; may repeat in 2 hr. Maximum: 40 mg/24 hr.

SIDE EFFECTS/ADVERSE REACTIONS

Frequent

Oral: Tingling, nasal discomfort

Subcutaneous: Injection site reactions, tingling, warm or hot sensation, dizziness, vertigo

Nasal: Bad or unusual taste, nausea, vomiting

Occasional

Oral: Flushing, asthenia, visual disturbances

Subcutaneous: Burning sensation, numbness, chest discomfort, drowsiness, asthenia

Nasal: Nasopharyngeal discomfort, dizziness

Rare

Oral: Agitation, eye irritation, dysuria

Subcutaneous: Anxiety, fatigue, diaphoresis, muscle cramps, myalgia

Nasal: Burning sensation

PRECAUTIONS AND CONTRAINDICATIONS

CVA, ischemic heart disease (including angina pectoris, history of MI, silent ischemia, and Prinzmetal's angina), severe hepatic impairment, transient ischemic attack, uncontrolled hypertension, use within 14 days of MAOIs, use within 24 hr of ergotamine preparations

Caution:

Hepatic and renal impairment, elderly, lactation, children

DRUG INTERACTIONS OF CONCERN TO DENTISTRY

• None reported; avoid ergot-containing medications.

SERIOUS REACTIONS

! Excessive dosage may produce tremor, red extremities, reduced respirations, cyanosis, seizures, and paralysis.

! Serious arrhythmias occur rarely, especially in patients with hypertension, diabetes, or a strong family history of coronary artery disease; obese patients; and smokers.

DENTAL CONSIDERATIONS

General

• Be aware of the patient's disease, its severity, and its frequency, when known.

• Monitor vital signs at every appointment because of cardiovascular side effects.

• Avoid dental light in patient's eyes; offer dark glasses for patient comfort.

Consultations:
• If treating chronic orofacial pain, consult with physician of record.
Teach Patient/Family:
• That oral symptoms rarely occur and will disappear when drug is discontinued.

sunitinib
soo-**nih**′-tih-nib
(Sutent)

CATEGORY AND SCHEDULE
Pregnancy Risk Category: D

Drug Class: Antineoplastic (tyrosine kinase inhibitor)

MECHANISM OF ACTION
An antineoplastic agent that inhibits multiple receptor tyrosine kinases (RTK) inducing platelet-derived growth factor (PDGF), vascular endothelial growth factor receptors (VEGFR1, VEGFR2, and VEGFR3), stem cell factor receptor (KIT), FMS-like tyrosine kinase-3 (FLT3), colony stimulation factor receptor Type 1 (CSF-1R), and glial cell-line derived neurotrophic factor receptor (RET).
Therapeutic Effect: Decreases tumor cell growth.

USES
Treatment of GI stromal tumor after disease progression on or intolerance to imatinib; also used for treatment of advanced renal cell carcinoma

PHARMACOKINETICS
Protein binding: 90%–95% (primary metabolite). Primarily metabolized in liver by CYP450 3A4. Primarily eliminated in feces (61%); partial excretion in urine (16%). ***Half-life:*** 40–60 hr; 80–110 hr (primary metabolite).

INDICATIONS AND DOSAGES
▸ GI Stromal Tumor after Disease Progression on or Intolerance to Imatinib
PO
Adults. 50 mg once a day, on a schedule of 4 wk on treatment followed by 2 wk off.
▸ Renal Cell Carcinoma, Advanced
PO
Adults. 50 mg once a day, on a schedule of 4 wk on treatment followed by 2 wk off.
▸ Dosage Adjustment
Concurrent CYP3A4 inhibitor (such as ketoconazole). Reduce sunitinib to a minimum of 37.5 mg daily.
Concurrent CYP3A4 inducer (such as rifampin). Increase sunitinib to a maximum of 87.5 mg daily.

SIDE EFFECTS/ADVERSE REACTIONS
Frequent
Fatigue, diarrhea, nausea, mucositis/stomatitis, neutropenia, dyspepsia, taste perversion, AST/ALT increased, lymphopenia, rash, thrombocytopenia, vomiting, constipation, anorexia, hyperpigmentation, abdominal pain, hypertension, arthralgia, dyspnea, bleeding, anemia, hyperlipasemia, headache, alkaline phosphatase increased, weakness, limb pain, fever, edema, dry skin, myalgia, back pain, cough, hair color changes, amylase increased, dizziness, hyperbilirubinemia, glossodynia, hyperuricemia, flatulence, hand-foot syndrome, hypokalemia, creatinine increased, alopecia, dehydration, hypernatremia, neuropathy, hypophosphatemia, LVEF decreased

Occasional
Appetite disturbance, skin blistering, periorbital edema, hypothyroidism, lacrimation increased, oral pain, hyperkalemia, hyponatremia, DVT
Rare
Myocardial ischemia, pulmonary embolism

PRECAUTIONS AND CONTRAINDICATIONS

Hypersensitivity to sunitinib or its components
Caution:
Do not breast-feed, left ventricular dysfunction, hypertension

DRUG INTERACTIONS OF CONCERN TO DENTISTRY

- CYP3A4 inducers: may decrease the levels and effects of sunitinib.
- CYP3A4 inhibitors (e.g., macrolide antibiotics, azole antifungal agents): may increase the blood levels and effects of sunitinib.

SERIOUS REACTIONS

! Severe GI complications have been reported.
! Hemorrhagic events have been reported.
! Hypertension may occur.
! Left ventricular dysfunction has been reported.
! Adrenal toxicities have been noted.

S

DENTAL CONSIDERATIONS

General:
- Avoid aspirin and NSAIDs to prevent GI irritation and excessive bleeding.
- Examine patient carefully for signs of opportunistic infections, mucositis, blood dyscrasias, stomatitis and bleeding.
- Confirm patient's disease status and treatment regimen.
- Chlorhexidine mouth rinse prior to and during chemotherapy may reduce severity of oral inflammation.
- Palliative medication may be required for management of oral adverse effects of drug.
- Patient may be taking prophylactic antiinfective drug.
- Place patient on frequent recall because of adverse oral effects of drug.

Consultations:
- Consult physician to determine control of disease and ability of patient to tolerate dental procedures.
- Consult physician to determine need for prophylactic or therapeutic antiinfective medications if oral surgery or periodontal treatment is planned.
- Consult physician to determine patient's immunologic and coagulation status and determine safety risk, if any, posed by the required dental treatment.

Teach Patient/Family to:
- Be aware of oral adverse effects of drugs.
- Use effective, atraumatic oral hygiene measures to prevent soft tissue inflammation.
- Report oral lesions, soreness, or bleeding to dentist.
- Update health and medication history if physician makes any changes in evaluation or drug regimen; include OTC, herbal, and nonherbal drugs in update.

tacrine hydrochloride

tack′-rin high-droh-**klor′**-ide
(Cognex)

CATEGORY AND SCHEDULE
Pregnancy Risk Category: C

Drug Class: Cholinesterase Inhibitor

MECHANISM OF ACTION
A cholinesterase inhibitor that inhibits the enzyme acetylcholinesterase, thus increasing the concentration of acetylcholine at cholinergic synapses and enhancing cholinergic function in the CNS.
Therapeutic Effect: Slows the progression of Alzheimer's disease.

USES
Treatment of mild-to-moderate cognitive defects associated with Alzheimer's disease

PHARMACOKINETICS
PO: Peak plasma levels 1–2 hr; plasma levels are higher in females; hepatic metabolism (CYP1A2 isoenzymes); renal excretion.

INDICATIONS AND DOSAGES
▸ **Alzheimer's Disease**
PO
Adults, Elderly. Initially, 10 mg 4 times a day for 6 wk, followed by 20 mg 4 times a day for 6 wk, 30 mg 4 times a day for 12 wk, then 40 mg 4 times a day if needed.
▸ **Dosage in Hepatic Impairment**
For patients with ALT (SGPT) greater than 3–5 times normal, decrease the dose by 40 mg/day and resume the normal dose when ALT (SGPT) returns to normal. For patients with ALT (SGPT) greater than 5 times normal, stop treatment and resume it when ALT (SGPT) returns to normal.

SIDE EFFECTS/ADVERSE REACTIONS
Frequent
Headache, nausea, vomiting, diarrhea, dizziness
Occasional
Fatigue, chest pain, dyspepsia, anorexia, abdominal pain, flatulence, constipation, confusion, agitation, rash, depression, ataxia, insomnia, rhinitis, myalgia
Rare
Weight loss, anxiety, cough, facial flushing, urinary frequency, back pain, tremor

PRECAUTIONS AND CONTRAINDICATIONS
Known hypersensitivity to tacrine, patients previously treated with tacrine who developed jaundice
Caution:
Cardiovascular disease, GI ulcers, general anesthesia, smokers, liver disease, seizures, asthma, lactation, children, decrease in absolute neutrophil count; liver enzyme monitoring required

DRUG INTERACTIONS OF CONCERN TO DENTISTRY
- Potential increase in GI complaints: NSAIDs
- Action inhibited by anticholinergic drugs
- Increased effects with succinylcholine and other cholinergic agonists

SERIOUS REACTIONS
! Overdose can cause cholinergic crisis, marked by increased salivation, lacrimation, bradycardia, respiratory depression, hypotension, and increased muscle weakness.

Treatment usually consists of supportive measures and an anticholinergic, such as atropine.

DENTAL CONSIDERATIONS

General:

- Patients on chronic drug therapy may rarely have symptoms of blood dyscrasias, which can include infection, bleeding, and poor healing.
- Monitor vital signs at every appointment because of cardiovascular and respiratory side effects.
- After supine positioning, have patient sit upright for at least 2 min before standing to avoid orthostatic hypotension.
- Assess salivary flow as a factor in caries, periodontal disease, and candidiasis.
- Take precautions if dental surgery is anticipated and anesthesia is required.
- Consider semisupine chair position for patient comfort because of GI effects of drug.
- Place on frequent recall because early attention to dental health is important for Alzheimer's patients.

Consultations:

- Medical consultation may be required to assess disease control.
- In a patient with symptoms of blood dyscrasias, request a medical consultation for blood studies and postpone dental treatment until normal values are reestablished.

Teach Patient/Family to:

- Encourage effective oral hygiene to prevent soft tissue inflammation.
- Prevent injury when using oral hygiene aids.
- Use powered tooth brush if patient has difficulty holding conventional devices.

tacrolimus

tak-roe-**leem′**-us

(Prograf, Protopic)

Do not confuse Protopic with Protonix, Protopam, Protropin.

CATEGORY AND SCHEDULE

Pregnancy Risk Category: C

Drug Class: Immunosuppressant

MECHANISM OF ACTION

An immunologic agent that inhibits T-lymphocyte activation by binding to intracellular proteins, forming a complex and inhibiting phosphatase activity.

Therapeutic Effect: Suppresses the immunologically mediated inflammatory response; prevents organ transplant rejection.

USES

Treatment of short-term and intermittent long-term treatment of moderate-to-severe atopic dermatitis in patients not able to use or who do not respond to alternative, conventional therapies.

PHARMACOKINETICS

Variably absorbed after PO administration (food reduces absorption). Protein binding: 75%–97%. Extensively metabolized in the liver. Excreted in urine. Not removed by hemodialysis. ***Half-life:*** 11.7 hr.

T

INDICATIONS AND DOSAGES

▸ Prevention of Liver Transplant Rejection

PO

Adults, Elderly. 0.1–0.15 mg/kg/day in 2 divided doses 12 hr apart.

Children. 0.15–0.2 mg/kg/day in 2 divided doses 12 hr apart.

IV

Adults, Elderly, Children. 0.03–0.15 mg/kg/day as a continuous infusion.

▸ Prevention of Kidney Transplant Rejection

PO

Adults, Elderly. 0.2 mg/kg/day in 2 divided doses 12 hr apart.

IV

Adults, Elderly. 0.03–0.15 mg/kg/day as continuous infusion.

▸ Atopic Dermatitis

Topical

Adults, Elderly, Children 2 yr and older. Apply 0.03% ointment to affected area twice a day. 0.1% ointment may be used in adults and the elderly. Continue until 1 wk after symptoms have cleared.

SIDE EFFECTS/ADVERSE REACTIONS

Frequent

Headache, tremor, insomnia, paresthesia, diarrhea, nausea, constipation, vomiting, abdominal pain, hypertension

Occasional

Rash, pruritus, anorexia, asthenia, peripheral edema, photosensitivity

PRECAUTIONS AND CONTRAINDICATIONS

Concurrent use with cyclosporine (increases the risk of nephrotoxicity), hypersensitivity to HCO-60 polyoxyl 60 hydrogenated castor oil (used in solution for injection), hypersensitivity to tacrolimus

Caution:

Infections at treatment site; lymphadenopathy, acute infections, mononucleosis, reduce exposure to sunlight or artificial sunlight, lactation, use has not been established in children younger than 2 yr

DRUG INTERACTIONS OF CONCERN TO DENTISTRY

Topical

- No drug interactions are documented, but use with caution in patients taking CYP3A4 inhibitors: erythromycin, itraconazole, ketoconazole, fluconazole
- Avoid drugs with potential for renal impairment
- Risk of decreased blood levels with carbamazepine, phenobarbital, St. John's wort (herb)

SERIOUS REACTIONS

! Nephrotoxicity (characterized by increased serum creatinine level and decreased urine output), neurotoxicity (including tremor, headache, and mental status changes), and pleural effusion are common adverse reactions. Thrombocytopenia, leukocytosis, anemia, atelectasis, sepsis, and infection occur occasionally.

DENTAL CONSIDERATIONS

T

Topical

General:

- Advise patient if dental drugs prescribed have a potential for photosensitivity.

FK506

General:

- Patients on immunosuppressant therapy have increased susceptibility to infection.
- Patients on chronic drug therapy may rarely have symptoms of blood

dyscrasias, which can include infection, bleeding, and poor healing.

- Monitor vital signs at every appointment because of cardiovascular side effects.
- Prophylactic antibiotics may be indicated to prevent infection if surgery or deep scaling is planned.
- Examine for evidence of oral candidiasis. Topically acting antifungals may be preferred.

Consultations:

- Medical consultation may be required to assess disease control.
- In a patient with symptoms of blood dyscrasias, request a medical consultation for blood studies and postpone dental treatment until normal values are reestablished.
- Consult with patient's physician for recommendations on possible antibiotic prophylaxis before dental treatment or when considering use of systemic antifungals.

Teach Patient/Family to:

- Encourage effective oral hygiene to prevent soft tissue inflammation.
- Use caution to prevent injury when using oral hygiene aids.
- Use powered tooth brush if patient has difficulty holding conventional devices.
- See dentist immediately if secondary oral infection occurs.
- Report oral lesions, soreness, or bleeding to dentist.

T

tadalafil

tah-**da**′-la-fil

(Adcirca)

Do not confuse with tadalafil with sildenafil or vardenafil, or Adcirca with Advair or Advicor.

CATEGORY AND SCHEDULE

Pregnancy Risk Category: B

Drug Class: Phosphodiesterase-5 enzyme inhibitor

MECHANISM OF ACTION

Inhibits phosphodiesterase type 5 (PDE-5) in smooth muscle of pulmonary vasculature where PDE-5 is responsible for the degradation of cyclic guanosine monophosphate (cGMP). Increased cGMP concentration results in pulmonary vasculature relaxation; vasodilation in the pulmonary bed and the systemic circulation (to a lesser degree) may occur.

Therapeutic Effect: Facilitates vasodilation in pulmonary vasculature.

USES

Treatment of pulmonary arterial hypertension (PAH) to improve exercise ability

PHARMACOKINETICS

Rapidly absorbed after oral administration. 94% plasma protein bound. Hepatic metabolism via CYP3A4 to inactive metabolites. Excreted via feces (61%) and urine (36%). ***Half-life:*** 15–17.5 hr.

INDICATIONS AND DOSAGES

▸ Pulmonary Arterial Hypertension

PO

Adults. 40 mg once daily.

▸ **Renal Impairment**
Cl_{cr} >80 ml/min: No dosage adjustment necessary.
Cl_{cr} 31–80 ml/min: Initially, 20 mg once daily; increase to 40 mg once daily based on individual tolerability.
Cl_{cr} ≤30 ml/min: Avoid use due to increased tadalafil exposure, limited clinical experience, and lack of ability to influence clearance by dialysis.

▸ **Hepatic Impairment**
Mild-to-moderate hepatic impairment (Child-Pugh class A or B): Use with caution; consider initial dose of 20 mg once daily.
Severe hepatic impairment (Child-Pugh class C): Avoid use; has not been studied in patients with severe hepatic cirrhosis.

SIDE EFFECTS/ADVERSE REACTIONS

Frequent
Headache, dizziness, flushing, nausea

Occasional
Back pain, nasal congestion, nasopharyngitis, color vision change

PRECAUTIONS AND CONTRAINDICATIONS

Hypersensitivity to tadalafil or any component of the formulation. Concurrent use of nitrates in any form. May cause auditory and visual disturbances, including hearing and vision loss. Not recommended for use in patients with severe cardiovascular disease (hypotension, uncontrolled hypertension, angina, arrhythmias, stroke) and bleeding disorders.

DRUG INTERACTIONS OF CONCERN TO DENTISTRY

- CYP3A4 inhibitors (e.g., macrolide antibiotics, azole antifungals, midazolam, triazolam): increased hypotension.
- Opioids, alcohol: hypotension.
- Nitrates (e.g., nitroglycerin) can potentiate hypotension associated with tadalafil, with potential loss of consciousness and cardiovascular depression.

SERIOUS REACTIONS

! Prolonged erections (lasting longer than 4 hr) and priapism (painful erections lasting longer than 6 hr) occur rarely. Instruct patients to seek immediate medical attention if erection persists for more than 4 hr.

DENTAL CONSIDERATIONS

General:
- Monitor vital signs due to coexisting cardiovascular disease.
- Short appointments and a stress-reduction protocol may be required for anxious patients.
- Allow patient to sit upright for 2 min prior to dismissing due to possible orthostatic hypotension.

Consultations:
- Consult physician to determine disease status and ability of patient to tolerate dental procedures.

Teach Patient/Family to:
- Report changes in disease or drug regimen.

tafluprost

ta′-floo-prost
(Zioptan)

CATEGORY AND SCHEDULE

Pregnancy Risk Category: C

Drug Class: Ophthalmic agent, antiglaucoma; prostaglandin

MECHANISM OF ACTION
Tafluprost acid is a fluorinated prostaglandin F2-alpha analogue believed to reduce intraocular pressure by increasing outflow of aqueous humor via the uveoscleral pathway.
Therapeutic Effect: Reduces intraocular pressure.

USES
Reduction of intraocular pressure (IOP) in patients with open-angle glaucoma or ocular hypertension

PHARMACOKINETICS
Minimal systemic absorption.
Half-life: None reported.

INDICATIONS AND DOSAGES
▸ **Treatment of Glaucoma**
Ophthalmic
Adults. 1 drop in the affected eye(s) once daily in the evening; do not exceed the once-daily dosage because it has been shown that more frequent administration may decrease the IOP-lowering effect.

SIDE EFFECTS/ADVERSE REACTIONS
Frequent
Conjunctival hyperemia, headache, cough
Occasional
Ocular: Stinging/irritation, conjunctivitis, cataract, dry eye, ocular pain, eyelash darkening, eyelash growth, blurred vision

PRECAUTIONS AND CONTRAINDICATIONS
Use with caution in patients with intraocular inflammation, aphakic patients, pseudophakic patients with a torn posterior lens capsule, or patients with risk factors for macular edema.

DRUG INTERACTIONS OF CONCERN TO DENTISTRY
• None reported

SERIOUS REACTIONS
! May permanently change/increase brown pigmentation of the iris, the eyelid skin, and eyelashes; in addition, may increase the length and/or number of eyelashes

DENTAL CONSIDERATIONS
General:
• Use protective eyewear for patient; avoid splatter in patient's eyes.

tamoxifen citrate
ta-**mox**′-ih-fen **sih**′-trate
(Apo-Tamox[CAN], Genox[AUS], Istubol, Nolvadex, Nolvadex-D[CAN], Novo-Tamoxifen[CAN], Tamofen[CAN], Tamosin[AUS])

CATEGORY AND SCHEDULE
Pregnancy Risk Category: D

Drug Class: Antineoplastic, antiestrogen hormone

MECHANISM OF ACTION
A nonsteroidal antiestrogen that competes with estradiol for estrogen-receptor binding sites in the breasts, uterus, and vagina.
Therapeutic Effect: Inhibits DNA synthesis and estrogen response.

USES
Advanced breast carcinoma that has not responded to other therapy in estrogen receptor-positive patients (usually postmenopausal), to reduce the incidence of breast cancer in healthy women with high risk of developing the disease; ductal carcinoma in situ

PHARMACOKINETICS

Well absorbed from the GI tract. Metabolized in the liver. Primarily eliminated in feces by biliary system. ***Half-life:*** 7 days.

INDICATIONS AND DOSAGES

▸ Adjunctive Treatment of Breast Cancer

PO

Adults, Elderly. 20–40 mg/day. Give doses greater than 20 mg/day in divided doses.

▸ Prevention of Breast Cancer in High-Risk Women

PO

Adults, Elderly. 20 mg/day.

SIDE EFFECTS/ADVERSE REACTIONS

Frequent

Women: Hot flashes, nausea, vomiting

Occasional

Women: Changes in menstruation, genital itching, vaginal discharge, endometrial hyperplasia or polyps

Men: Impotence, decreased libido

Men and women: Headache, nausea, vomiting, rash, bone pain, confusion, weakness, somnolence

PRECAUTIONS AND CONTRAINDICATIONS

Concomitant coumarin-type therapy when used in the treatment of breast cancer in high-risk women, history of deep vein thrombosis or pulmonary embolism in high-risk women, pregnancy

Caution:

Leukopenia, thrombocytopenia, lactation, cataracts, risk of stroke, pulmonary emboli, and uterine malignancy

DRUG INTERACTIONS OF CONCERN TO DENTISTRY

• None reported

SERIOUS REACTIONS

! Retinopathy, corneal opacity, and decreased visual acuity have been noted in patients receiving extremely high dosages (240–320 mg/day) for longer than 17 mo.

! There has been an increased number of incidences of endometrial changes, thromboembolic events, and uterine malignancies while using tamoxifen.

DENTAL CONSIDERATIONS

General:

• Patients on chronic drug therapy may rarely have symptoms of blood dyscrasias, which can include infection, bleeding, and poor healing.

• Consider semisupine chair position for patient comfort if GI side effects occur.

Consultations:

• Medical consultation may be required to assess disease control.

• In a patient with symptoms of blood dyscrasias, request a medical consultation for blood studies and postpone dental treatment until normal values are reestablished.

Teach Patient/Family:

• Importance of good oral hygiene to prevent soft tissue inflammation.

tamsulosin hydrochloride

tam-**sool′**-oh-sin

high-droh-**klor′**-ide

(Flomax)

Do not confuse Flomax with Fosamax or Volmax.

CATEGORY AND SCHEDULE

Pregnancy Risk Category: B (not indicated for use in women)

Drug Class: Adrenoreceptor antagonist

T

MECHANISM OF ACTION

An α_1 antagonist that targets receptors around bladder neck and prostate capsule.

Therapeutic Effect: Relaxes smooth muscle and improves urinary flow and symptoms of prostatic hypertrophy.

USES

Treatment of benign prostatic hyperplasia (BPH)

PHARMACOKINETICS

Well absorbed and widely distributed. Protein binding: 94%–99%. Metabolized in the liver. Primarily excreted in urine. Unknown if removed by hemodialysis. ***Half-life:*** 9–13 hr.

INDICATIONS AND DOSAGES

▸ BPH

PO

Adults. 0.4 mg once a day, approximately 30 min after same meal each day. May increase dosage to 0.8 mg if inadequate response in 2–4 wk.

SIDE EFFECTS/ADVERSE REACTIONS

Frequent

Dizziness, somnolence

Occasional

Headache, anxiety, insomnia, orthostatic hypotension

Rare

Nasal congestion, pharyngitis, rhinitis, nausea, vertigo, impotence

PRECAUTIONS AND CONTRAINDICATIONS

History of sensitivity to tamsulosin

Caution:

Potential syncope risk caused by hypotension, vertigo, dizziness, carcinoma of prostate; avoid use with other-adrenoreceptor antagonists; not for use in women, children; lactation

DRUG INTERACTIONS OF CONCERN TO DENTISTRY

- Potential risk of orthostatic hypotension with conscious sedation techniques.
- Opioids and anticholinergic drugs may enhance urinary retention.
- Caution in use or avoid concurrent use with other adrenergic antagonists.

SERIOUS REACTIONS

! First-dose syncope (hypotension with sudden loss of consciousness) may occur within 30–90 min after administration of initial dose and may be preceded by tachycardia (pulse rate of 120–160 beats/min).

DENTAL CONSIDERATIONS

General:

- Monitor vital signs at every appointment because of cardiovascular and respiratory side effects.
- Consider semisupine chair position for patient comfort when GI side effects occur.
- After supine positioning, have patient sit upright for at least 2 min before standing to avoid orthostatic hypotension.

tapentadol hydrochloride

tay-**pen**-tah-dole hi-dro-**klor**-ide
(Nucynta)
Do not confuse with tramadol.

CATEGORY AND SCHEDULE

Pregnancy Risk Category: C
Controlled Substance: Schedule II

Drug Class: Analgesic

MECHANISM OF ACTION

Centrally-acting analgesic, mu opioid receptor agonist and inhibitor of norepinephrine reuptake. ***Therapeutic Effect:*** reduces perception of pain in CNS.

USES

Moderate to severe acute pain

PHARMACOKINETICS

Limited oral bioavailability (32%) due to extensive hepatic first-pass metabolism. Peak concentration reached at 1.25 hr, widely distributed. Protein binding: 20%. Metabolized in the liver, primarily by glucuronide conjugation. ***Half-life:*** 4 hr. 99% excreted by the kidneys. No active metabolites.

INDICATIONS AND DOSAGES

▸ Analgesia

PO

Adults, Elderly. 50–100 mg every 4 to 6 hr, 700 mg total dose on first day of therapy, 600 mg/day subsequently.

SIDE EFFECTS/ADVERSE REACTIONS

Frequent

Dizziness, nausea, vomiting, somnolence, constipation

Occasional

Fatigue, insomnia, pruritus, hyperhidrosis, dry mouth, dyspepsia, decreased appetite

RARE

Hypotension, bradycardia, tachycardia, agitation, ataxia, euphoria, depressed consciousness, restlessness, syncope, seizures, delayed gastric emptying, urinary retention, involuntary muscle contractions, cough, dyspnea, drug withdrawal, hypersensitivity

PRECAUTIONS AND CONTRAINDICATIONS

Hypersensitivity to tapentadol hydrochloride or its ingredients, children under the age of 18

Caution:

Respiratory depression, CNS depression, head injury/increased intracranial pressure, seizures, serotonin syndrome risk, pancreatic/biliary tract disease, renal function impairment, moderate to severe hepatic impairment, drug abuse/dependence, hazardous tasks, pregnancy/lactation

DRUG INTERACTIONS OF CONCERN TO DENTISTRY

- Increased risk of CNS depression: all CNS depressants, alcohol. May potentiate mental impairment and somnolence, respiratory depression, hypotension (avoid alcohol)
- MAOIs: increased toxicity of tapentadol
- SSRIs (e.g., fluoxetine): potentially life-threatening serotonin syndrome

SERIOUS REACTIONS

! CNS depression with or without respiratory depression

! Serotonin syndrome (agitation, coma, autonomic instability including tachycardia,

neuromuscular abnormalities, diarrhea, nausea, vomiting)
! Drug abuse, withdrawal syndrome with abrupt discontinuation of prolonged use

DENTAL CONSIDERATIONS

General:
- Assess salivary flow as a factor in caries, periodontal disease, and candidiasis.
- Geriatric patients may be more susceptible to adverse effects.
- Avoid or reduce doses of co adminsistered sedatives.
- Avoid in patients taking MAOIs or selective serotonin reuptake inhibitors (SSRIs).

Teach Patient/Family to:
- Avoid mouth rinses with high alcohol content because of drying effect.
- Use home fluoride products for anticaries effect.
- Use sugarless/xylitol gum, frequent sips of water, or saliva substitutes if dry mouth occurs.

tegaserod

teh-**gas**′-er-od
(Zelnorm)

CATEGORY AND SCHEDULE

Pregnancy Risk Category: B

Drug Class: Serotonin agonist, a prokinetic drug

MECHANISM OF ACTION

An anti-irritable bowel syndrome agent that binds to 5-HT4 receptors in the GI tract.
Therapeutic Effect: Triggers a peristaltic reflex in the gut, increasing bowel motility.

USES

Short-term treatment of irritable bowel syndrome in women whose primary bowel symptom is constipation

PHARMACOKINETICS

Rapidly absorbed. Widely distributed. Protein binding: 98%. Metabolized by hydrolysis in the stomach and by oxidation and conjugation of the primary metabolite. Primarily excreted in feces. ***Half-life:*** 11 hr.

INDICATIONS AND DOSAGES

▸ Irritable Bowel Syndrome
PO
Adults, Elderly women. 6 mg twice a day for 4–6 wk.

▸ Chronic Constipation
PO
Adults. 6 mg twice a day.

SIDE EFFECTS/ADVERSE REACTIONS

Frequent
Headache, abdominal pain, diarrhea, nausea, flatulence
Occasional
Dizziness, migraine, back pain, extremity pain

PRECAUTIONS AND CONTRAINDICATIONS

Abdominal adhesions, diarrhea, history of bowel obstruction, moderate to severe hepatic impairment, severe renal impairment, suspected sphincter of Oddi dysfunction, symptomatic gallbladder disease
Caution:
Avoid use in patients with diarrhea, pregnancy category B, lactation (discontinue drug or discontinue nursing), safety and usefulness in children younger than 18 yr not established

DRUG INTERACTIONS OF CONCERN TO DENTISTRY

• No dental drug interactions reported; does not induce CYP450 isoenzymes.
• Avoid use of drugs (opioids, anticholinergics) that could lead to risk of constipation.
• Use NSAIDs or acetaminophen for mild or moderate pain.

SERIOUS REACTIONS

! None known

DENTAL CONSIDERATIONS

General:

• Monitor vital signs at every appointment because of cardiovascular side effects.
• Consider semisupine chair position for patient comfort if GI side effects occur.
• Short appointments and a stress-reduction protocol may be required for anxious patients.
• Avoid drugs with anticholinergic activity, such as antihistamines, opioids, benzodiazepines, propantheline, atropine, and scopolamine.
• Question patient about tolerance of NSAIDs or aspirin related to GI disease.

Consultations:

• Consult with physician before prescribing drugs that can cause constipation (opioids).
• Consultation with physician may be necessary if sedation or general anesthesia is required.
• Medical consultation may be required to assess disease control and patient's ability to tolerate stress.

Teach Patient/Family to:

• Update health and drug history if physician makes any changes in evaluation or drug regimens; include OTC, herbal, and nonherbal drugs in the update.

telaprevir

tel-**a**′-pre-vir
(Incivek)

CATEGORY AND SCHEDULE

Pregnancy Risk Category: B (X when combined with ribavirin)

Drug Class: Antiviral agent, protease inhibitor

MECHANISM OF ACTION

Binds reversibly to nonstructural protein 3 (NS 3) serine protease and inhibits replication of the hepatitis C virus.
Therapeutic Effect: Inhibits replication of hepatitis C virus, slowing progression of, or improving the clinical status of, hepatitis C infection.

USES

Treatment of chronic hepatitis C (in combination with peginterferon alfa and ribavirin) in adult patients with compensated liver disease (including cirrhosis) who are treatment naive or who have received previous interferon-based treatment

PHARMACOKINETICS

59%–76% plasma protein bound. Hepatic metabolism to inactive metabolites. Excreted primarily in feces (82%). ***Half-life:*** 4–5 hr.

INDICATIONS AND DOSAGES

▸ Treatment of Chronic Hepatitis C (CHC)

PO

Adults. 750 mg 3 times/day (in combination with peginterferon alfa and ribavirin) with a meal.

T

SIDE EFFECTS/ADVERSE REACTIONS

Frequent

Fatigue, rash, hyperuricemia, anemia, nausea, vomiting, diarrhea

Occasional

Abnormal taste, thrombocytopenia

PRECAUTIONS AND CONTRAINDICATIONS

Concomitant administration with CYP3A4 substrates (alfuzosin, cisapride, lovastatin, midazolam, sildenafil, simvastatin, triazolam) or CYP3A4 inducers (rifampin, St. John's wort)

DRUG INTERACTIONS OF CONCERN TO DENTISTRY

- CYP3A4 inhibitors (e.g., macrolide antibiotics, azole antifungals): increased blood levels and adverse effects of telaprevir
- CYP3A4 inducers (e.g., carbamazepine, barbiturates): decreased blood levels and efficacy of telaprevir
- Midazolam, triazolam: increased risk of excessive sedation

SERIOUS REACTIONS

! Mild-to-severe skin reactions, including DRESS (drug rash with eosinophilia with systemic symptoms [fever, facial edema, hepatitis, or nephritis with or without eosinophilia]) and Stevens-Johnson syndrome (SJS), have been reported.

T

DENTAL CONSIDERATIONS

General:

- Dysgeusia may alter patient response to restorative materials and oral hygiene regimen.
- Monitor vital signs for possible adverse cardiovascular effects.
- Increased risk of nausea and vomiting (e.g., during sedation); consider semisupine patient positioning.
- Examine for oral manifestation of opportunistic infections.

Consultations:

- Consult physician to determine disease status and patient's ability to tolerate dental procedures.

Teach Patient/Family to:

- Use effective oral hygiene to prevent soft tissue inflammation.
- Report oral lesions or soreness to dentist.
- Update health history and medication record regularly.

telmisartan

tel-meh-**sar′**-tan

(Micardis, Pritor[AUS])

CATEGORY AND SCHEDULE

Pregnancy Risk Category: C (D if used in second or third trimester)

Drug Class: Angiotensin II (AT1) receptor antagonist

MECHANISM OF ACTION

An angiotensin II receptor, type AT1, antagonist that blocks vasoconstrictor and aldosterone-secreting effects of angiotensin II, inhibiting the binding of angiotensin II to the AT1 receptors.

Therapeutic Effect: Causes vasodilation, decreases peripheral resistance, and decreases B/P.

USES

Treatment of hypertension as a single drug or in combination with other antihypertensives

PHARMACOKINETICS

Rapidly and completely absorbed after PO administration. Protein binding: greater than 99%. Undergoes metabolism in the liver to inactive metabolite. Excreted in feces. Unknown if removed by hemodialysis. ***Half-life:*** 24 hr.

INDICATIONS AND DOSAGES

▸ Hypertension

PO

Adults, Elderly. 40 mg once a day. Range: 20–80 mg/day.

SIDE EFFECTS/ADVERSE REACTIONS

Occasional

Upper respiratory tract infection, sinusitis, back or leg pain, diarrhea

Rare

Dizziness, headache, fatigue, nausea, heartburn, myalgia, cough, peripheral edema

PRECAUTIONS AND CONTRAINDICATIONS

Hypersensitivity, discontinue if pregnancy occurs, risk of fetal and neonatal injury, correct volume depletion if present, hepatic impairment, impaired renal function

Caution:

Discontinue if pregnancy occurs, risk of fetal and neonatal injury, correct volume depletion if present, hepatic impairment, impaired renal function; lactation

DRUG INTERACTIONS OF CONCERN TO DENTISTRY

- None reported; CYP450 isoenzymes are not involved with metabolism of this drug.

SERIOUS REACTIONS

! Overdosage may manifest as hypotension and tachycardia. Bradycardia occurs less often.

DENTAL CONSIDERATIONS

General:

- Monitor vital signs at every appointment because of cardiovascular side effects.
- Stress from dental procedures may compromise cardiovascular function; determine patient risk.
- Use precaution if sedation or general anesthesia is required; risk of hypotensive episode.
- Short appointments and a stress-reduction protocol may be required for anxious patients.
- Limit use of sodium-containing products, such as saline IV fluids, for patients with a dietary salt restriction.

Consultations:

- Medical consultation may be required to assess disease control and patient's ability to tolerate stress.

temazepam

te-**maz**′-eh-pam

(Apo-Temazepam[CAN], Novo-Temazepam[CAN], PMS-Temazepam[CAN], Restoril)

Do not confuse Restoril with Vistaril or Zestril.

CATEGORY AND SCHEDULE

Pregnancy Risk Category: X

Controlled Substance: Schedule IV

Drug Class: Benzodiazepine, sedative-hypnotic

MECHANISM OF ACTION

A benzodiazepine that enhances the action of the inhibitory neurotransmitter gamma-aminobutyric acid (GABA), resulting in CNS depression. ***Therapeutic Effect:*** Induces sleep.

USES

A sedative and hypnotic for treatment of insomnia

PHARMACOKINETICS

Well absorbed from the GI tract. Protein binding: 96%. Widely distributed. Crosses the blood-brain barrier. Metabolized in the liver. Primarily excreted in urine. Not removed by hemodialysis. ***Half-life:*** 4–18 hr.

INDICATIONS AND DOSAGES

▸ Insomnia

PO

Adults, Children 18 yr and older. 15–30 mg at bedtime.

Elderly, Debilitated. 7.5–15 mg at bedtime.

SIDE EFFECTS/ADVERSE REACTIONS

Frequent

Somnolence, sedation, rebound insomnia (may occur for 1–2 nights after drug is discontinued), dizziness, confusion, euphoria

Occasional

Asthenia, anorexia, diarrhea

Rare

Paradoxic CNS excitement or restlessness (particularly in elderly or debilitated patients)

T

PRECAUTIONS AND CONTRAINDICATIONS

Angle-closure glaucoma; CNS depression; pregnancy or breast-feeding; severe, uncontrolled pain; sleep apnea

Caution:

Anemia, hepatic disease, renal disease, suicidal individuals, drug abuse, elderly, psychosis, children younger than 18 yr, acute narrow-angle glaucoma

DRUG INTERACTIONS OF CONCERN TO DENTISTRY

- Increased action: alcohol, all CNS depressants
- Increased bioavailability: macrolide antibiotics

SERIOUS REACTIONS

! Abrupt or too-rapid withdrawal may result in pronounced restlessness, irritability, insomnia, hand tremor, abdominal or muscle cramps, vomiting, diaphoresis, and seizures. Overdose results in somnolence, confusion, diminished reflexes, respiratory depression, and coma.

DENTAL CONSIDERATIONS

General:

- Psychological and physical dependence may occur with chronic administration.
- Geriatric patients are more susceptible to drug effects; use lower dose.

Teach Patient/Family to:

- Encourage effective oral hygiene to prevent soft tissue inflammation.

temozolomide

teh-moe-**zoll′**-oh-mide

(Temodal[AUS], Temodar)

CATEGORY AND SCHEDULE

Pregnancy Risk Category: D

Drug Class: Antineoplastic

MECHANISM OF ACTION

An imidazotetrazine derivative that acts as a prodrug and is converted to a highly active cytotoxic metabolite. Its cytotoxic effect is associated with methylation of DNA.

Therapeutic Effect: Inhibits DNA replication, causing cell death.

USES

Treatment of specific types of cancer of the brain

PHARMACOKINETICS

Rapidly and completely absorbed after PO administration. Protein binding: 15%. Peak plasma concentration occurs in 1 hr. Penetrates the blood-brain barrier. Eliminated primarily in urine and, to a much lesser extent, in feces. *Half-life:* 1.6–1.8 hr.

INDICATIONS AND DOSAGES

▸ Anaplastic Astrocytoma

PO

Adults, Elderly. Initially, 150 mg/m^2/day for 5 consecutive days of a 28-day treatment cycle. Subsequent doses based on platelet count and ANC during previous cycle. ANC greater than 1500 per microliter and platelet: more than 100,000 per microliter. Maintenance: 200 mg/m^2/day for 5 days q4wk. Minimum: 100 mg/m^2/day for 5 days q4wk.

SIDE EFFECTS/ADVERSE REACTIONS

Frequent

Nausea, vomiting, headache, fatigue, constipation

Occasional

Diarrhea, asthenia, fever, dizziness, peripheral edema, incoordination, insomnia

Rare

Paresthesia, drowsiness, anorexia, urinary incontinence, anxiety, pharyngitis, cough

PRECAUTIONS AND CONTRAINDICATIONS

Hypersensitivity to dacarbazine, pregnancy

DRUG INTERACTIONS OF CONCERN TO DENTISTRY

- None reported

SERIOUS REACTIONS

! Elderly patients and women are at increased risk for developing severe myelosuppression, characterized by neutropenia and thrombocytopenia and usually occurring within the first few cycles. Neutrophil and platelet counts reach their nadirs approximately 26–28 days after administration and recover within 14 days of the nadir.

DENTAL CONSIDERATIONS

General:

- Caution: patients may be at high risk for infection.
- Provide palliative dental care for dental emergencies only.
- Oral infections should be eliminated and/or treated aggressively.
- Patients may be at risk for bleeding; check oral signs.
- Caution: potential drug interactions with drugs used in dentistry.
- Monitor and record vital signs.
- If additional analgesia is required for dental pain, consider alternative analgesics (NSAIDs) in patients taking opioids for acute or chronic pain.
- Avoid products that affect platelet function, such as aspirin and NSAIDs.
- Patient on chronic drug therapy may rarely present with symptoms of blood dyscrasias, which can include infection, bleeding, and poor healing. If dyscrasia is present, caution patient to prevent oral tissue trauma when using oral hygiene aids.
- Consider local hemostasis measures to prevent excessive bleeding.

• Consider semisupine chair position for patient comfort if GI side effects occur.

Consultations:

• Medical consultation should include routine blood counts including platelet counts and bleeding time.

• Consult physician; prophylactic or therapeutic antiinfectives may be indicated if surgery or periodontal treatment is required.

• In a patient with symptoms of blood dyscrasias, request a medical consultation for blood studies and postpone treatment until normal values are reestablished.

• Medical consultation may be required to assess disease control and patient's ability to tolerate stress.

Teach Patient/Family to:

• Use soft tooth brush to reduce risk of bleeding.

• Encourage effective oral hygiene to prevent soft tissue inflammation.

• Prevent trauma when using oral hygiene aids.

• Report oral lesions, soreness, or bleeding to dentist.

• Use powered tooth brush if patient has difficulty holding conventional devices.

temsirolimus

tem-sir-**oh**′-lee-mus

(Torisel)

CATEGORY AND SCHEDULE

Pregnancy Risk Category: D

Drug Class: Antineoplastic agent, mTOR kinase inhibitor

MECHANISM OF ACTION

Temsirolimus and sirolimus, its active metabolite, bind to FKBP-12, an intracellular protein, to form a complex that blocks the effects of mTOR (an enzyme that regulates the synthesis of proteins that control cell division). Inhibition of mTOR results in stopping the cell cycle at the G1 phase in tumor cells. When mTOR is inhibited, the process of p70S6k and S6 ribosomal protein phosphorylation, induced by mTOR, is in turn blocked.

USES

Renal cell cancer (RCC), advanced

PHARMACOKINETICS

Metabolized in the liver via CYP3A4 to sirolimus and other minor metabolites. ***Half-life***: 17 hr for temsirolimus and 55 hr for sirolimus. Excreted in the feces (78%) and urine (5%).

INDICATIONS AND DOSAGES

▸ Advanced Renal Cell Cancer

IV

Adults. 25 mg infused over a 20–60 min period once a week. Note: Patients should be given prophylactic IV diphenhydramine 25–50 mg (or similar antihistamine) about 30 min before the start of each dose.

Avoid concomitant use of CYP3A4 inhibitors. If these drugs are necessary, a dose adjustment of 12.5 mg/week of temsirolimus may be considered. If the CYP3A4 inhibitor is discontinued, allow for a washout period of 1 wk before administering temsirolimus.

Avoid concomitant use of CYP3A4 inducers. If these drugs are necessary, a dose adjustment from 25 mg/week up to 50 mg/week may be considered. If the CYP3A4 inducer is discontinued, the temsirolimus dose should be returned to the dose used prior to initiation of CYP3A4 inducer.

Dose adjustment for toxicity: ANC <1000/mm^3, platelet count <75,000/mm^3, or NCI CTCAE grade 3 or greater, stop temsirolimus. Consider restart with the dose reduced by 5 mg/week to a dose no lower than 15 mg/week only if toxicities come back to grade 2 or less.

SIDE EFFECTS/ADVERSE REACTIONS

Adult

Frequent

Edema, peripheral edema, chest pain, pain, fever, headache, insomnia, rash, pruritus, nail disorder/thinning, dry skin, hypoglycemia, hypercholesterolemia, hyperlipidemia, hypophosphatemia, hypokalemia, mucositis, nausea, anorexia, diarrhea, abdominal pain, constipation, stomatitis, taste disturbance, vomiting, weight loss, urinary tract infection, anemia, lymphopenia, thrombocytopenia, leukopenia, neutropenia, increased alkaline phosphatase, increased AST, weakness, back pain, arthralgia, increased creatinine, dyspnea, cough, epistaxis, pharyngitis, infection

Occasional

Hypertension, venous thromboembolism, thrombophlebitis, chills, depression, acne, impaired wound healing, bowel perforation, hyperbilirubinemia, myalgia, conjunctivitis, rhinitis, pneumonia, upper respiratory tract infection, interstitial lung disease, allergic/hypersensitivity reaction

PRECAUTIONS AND CONTRAINDICATIONS

Handle and dispose with caution since temsirolimus is a hazardous agent.

Hypersensitivity to temsirolimus, sirolimus, or any other components of the formulation. Hypersensitivity reactions may occur. Symptoms include anaphylaxis, dyspnea, flushing, and chest pain.

Fatal cases of renal failure, bowel perforation, and interstitial lung disease have occurred.

Avoid live vaccines.

Infection may occur as a result of immunosuppression.

DRUG INTERACTIONS OF CONCERN TO DENTISTRY

- CYP3A4 inhibitors (e.g., macrolide antibiotics and azole antifungals): May increase the effects of sirolimus (active metabolite).

SERIOUS REACTIONS

! Renal failure, sometimes fatal, has occurred. Monitor renal function at baseline and while on temsirolimus.

! Angioedema, asthenia, anemia, dyspnea, immunosuppression, interstitial lung disease, hyperglycemia, hyperlipidemia, bowel perforation (fatal), wound healing complications, and intracerebral hemorrhage have been reported.

DENTAL CONSIDERATIONS

General:

- Mucositis, stomatitis, and taste disturbances may complicate oral hygiene and dental treatment.
- Examine for oral manifestation of infections.
- Consider semisupine chair position for patient comfort if gastrointestinal (GI) side effects occur.

Consultations:

- Medical consultation may be required to assess disease control and ability of patient to tolerate dental treatment.

Teach Patient/Family to:

- Be alert for the possibility of mucositis, stomatitis, and taste disturbances and the need to be consulted by a dentist if any signs and symptoms occur.
- Encourage effective oral hygiene to prevent soft tissue inflammation.
- Prevent trauma when using oral hygiene aids.

tenecteplase

ten-**eck**′-teh-place

(Metalyse[AUS], TNKase)

CATEGORY AND SCHEDULE

Pregnancy Risk Category: C

Drug Class: Thrombolytic

MECHANISM OF ACTION

A tissue plasminogen activator produced by recombinant DNA that binds to fibrin and converts plasminogen to plasmin. Initiates fibrinolysis by degrading fibrin clots, fibrinogen, other plasma proteins. ***Therapeutic Effect:*** Exerts thrombolytic action.

USES

Dissolving blood clots

PHARMACOKINETICS

Extensively distributed to tissues. Completely eliminated by hepatic metabolism. ***Half-life:*** 11–20 min.

INDICATIONS AND DOSAGES

▸ **Acute MI**

IV

Adults. Dosage is based on patient's weight. Treatment should be initiated as soon as possible after onset of symptoms.

Weight (kg)	(mg)	(ml)
90 or more	50	10
80 to less than 90	45	9
70 to less than 80	40	8
60 to less than 70	35	7
Less than 60	30	6

SIDE EFFECTS/ADVERSE REACTIONS

Frequent

Bleeding (major, 4.7%; minor, 21.8%)

PRECAUTIONS AND CONTRAINDICATIONS

Active internal bleeding, aneurysm, AV malformation, bleeding diathesis, history of cerebrovascular accident, intracranial or intraspinal surgery or trauma within past 2 mo, intracranial neoplasm, severe uncontrolled hypertension

DRUG INTERACTIONS OF CONCERN TO DENTISTRY

- Increased risk of bleeding: drugs that interfere with coagulation or platelet function, such as NSAIDs and aspirin, ginkgo biloba (herb)

SERIOUS REACTIONS

! Bleeding at internal sites may occur, including intracranial, retroperitoneal, GI, GU, and respiratory sites. Lysis or coronary thrombi may produce atrial or ventricular arrhythmias and stroke.

DENTAL CONSIDERATIONS

General:

- An acute use drug for use in hospitals or emergency departments.
- Patients are at risk for bleeding; check for oral signs.

• Avoid products that affect platelet function, such as aspirin and NSAIDs.
• Monitor and record vital signs.
• Review medical and drug history.

Consultations:

• Medical consultation should include routine blood counts, including platelet counts and bleeding time.
• In a patient with symptoms of blood dyscrasias, request a medical consultation for blood studies and postpone treatment until normal values are reestablished.
• Medical consultation may be required to assess disease control and patient's ability to tolerate stress.

Teach Patient/Family to:

• Use soft tooth brush to reduce risk of bleeding.
• Encourage effective oral hygiene to prevent soft tissue inflammation.
• Report oral lesions, soreness, or bleeding to dentist.
• Prevent trauma when using oral hygiene aids.
• Update health and medication history if physician makes any changes in evaluation or drug regimens; include OTC, herbal, and nonherbal remedies in the update.

teniposide

ten-**ih**′-poe-side
(Vumon)

CATEGORY AND SCHEDULE

Pregnancy Risk Category: D

Drug Class: Antineoplastics, epipodophyllotoxins

MECHANISM OF ACTION

An epipodophyllotoxin that induces single- and double-strand breaks in DNA, inhibiting or altering DNA synthesis. Acts in the late S and early G2 phases of cell cycle.
Therapeutic Effect: Prevents cells from entering mitosis.

USES

Treatment of childhood acute lymphocytic leukemia

PHARMACOKINETICS

Plasma levels decline biexponentially over 1–2.5 hr, with a mean terminal half-life of 5 hr. Protein binding: >99%, excreted in the urine, primarily as metabolites.

INDICATIONS AND DOSAGES

▸ Induction Therapy in Patients with Refractory Childhood Acute Lymphoblastic Leukemia (in Combination with Other Antineoplastic Agents)

Children. Dosage is individualized on the basis of the patient's clinical response and tolerance of the drug's adverse effects. When used in combination therapy, consult specific protocols for optimum dosage or sequence of drug administration.

SIDE EFFECTS/ADVERSE REACTIONS

Frequent

Mucositis, nausea, vomiting, diarrhea, anemia

Occasional

Alopecia, rash

Rare

Hepatic dysfunction, fever, renal dysfunction, peripheral neurotoxicity

PRECAUTIONS AND CONTRAINDICATIONS

Absolute neutrophil count less than 500/mm^3; hypersensitivity to

Cremophor EL (polyoxyethylated castor oil), etoposide, or teniposide; platelet count less than 50,000/mm^3

DRUG INTERACTIONS OF CONCERN TO DENTISTRY

- None reported

SERIOUS REACTIONS

! Myelosuppression manifested as hematologic toxicity (principally leukopenia, neutropenia, and thrombocytopenia) may be severe and may increase the risk of infection or bleeding.
Hypersensitivity reaction may include anaphylaxis (marked by chills, fever, tachycardia, bronchospasm, dyspnea, and facial flushing).

DENTAL CONSIDERATIONS

General:

- If additional analgesia is required for dental pain, consider alternative analgesics (NSAIDs) in patients taking opioids for acute or chronic pain.
- Examine for oral manifestation of opportunistic infection.
- Avoid products that affect platelet function, such as aspirin and NSAIDs.
- This drug may be used in the hospital or on an outpatient basis. Confirm the patient's disease and treatment status.
- Chlorhexidine mouth rinse prior to and during chemotherapy may reduce severity of mucositis.
- Patient on chronic drug therapy may rarely present with symptoms of blood dyscrasias, which can include infection, bleeding, and poor healing. If dyscrasia is present, caution patient to prevent oral tissue trauma when using oral hygiene aids.
- Palliative medication may be required for management of oral side effects.
- Short appointments and a stress-reduction protocol may be required for anxious patients.
- Consider semisupine chair position for patient comfort if GI side effects occur.
- Caution: patients may be at high risk for infection.
- Patients may be at risk for bleeding; check oral signs.
- Oral infections should be eliminated and/or treated aggressively.

Consultations:

- Medical consultation should include routine blood counts, including platelet counts and bleeding time.
- Consult physician; prophylactic or therapeutic antiinfectives may be indicated if surgery or periodontal treatment is required.
- Medical consultation may be required to assess immunologic status during cancer chemotherapy and determine safety risk, if any, posed by the required dental treatment.
- Medical consultation may be required to assess disease control and patient's ability to tolerate stress.
- In a patient with symptoms of blood dyscrasias, request a medical consultation for blood studies and postpone treatment until normal values are reestablished.

Teach Patient/Family to:

- See dentist immediately if secondary oral infection occurs.
- Be aware of oral side effects.
- Encourage effective oral hygiene to prevent soft tissue inflammation.
- Report oral lesions, soreness, or bleeding to dentist.

• Prevent trauma when using oral hygiene aids.
• Update health and medication history if physician makes any changes in evaluation or drug regimens; include OTC, herbal, and nonherbal remedies in the update.

tenofovir

ten-**oh**′-foh-veer
(Viread)

CATEGORY AND SCHEDULE

Pregnancy Risk Category: B

Drug Class: Antiviral

MECHANISM OF ACTION

A nucleotide analogue that inhibits HIV reverse transcriptase by being incorporated into viral DNA, resulting in DNA chain termination.
Therapeutic Effect: Slows HIV replication and reduces HIV RNA levels (viral load).

USES

Treatment of HIV-1 infection in combination with other antiretroviral drugs

PHARMACOKINETICS

PO: Bioavailability 5% (improves with meal); maximum serum levels 0.6–1.4 hr; low plasma protein binding less than 7%; minimal systemic metabolism; excreted by glomerular filtration and active tubular secretion; use in children not evaluated.

INDICATIONS AND DOSAGES

▸ **HIV Infection (in combination with other antiretrovirals)**
PO
Adults, Elderly, Children 18 yr and older. 300 mg once a day.

SIDE EFFECTS/ADVERSE REACTIONS

Occasional
GI disturbances (diarrhea, flatulence, nausea, vomiting)

PRECAUTIONS AND CONTRAINDICATIONS

Hypersensitivity; avoid breast-feeding; obesity and prolonged nucleoside use; risk of lactic acidosis/severe hepatomegaly with steatosis; no data on hepatic impairment; redistribution of body fat
Caution:
Obesity and prolonged nucleoside use; risk of lactic acidosis/severe hepatomegaly with steatosis; no data on hepatic impairment; redistribution of body fat

DRUG INTERACTIONS OF CONCERN TO DENTISTRY

• Potential for competition for renal clearance: acyclovir, valacyclovir

SERIOUS REACTIONS

! Lactic acidosis and hepatomegaly with steatosis occur rarely but may be severe.

DENTAL CONSIDERATIONS

General:
• Examine for oral manifestation of opportunistic infection.
Consultations:
• Medical consultation may be required to assess disease control and patient's ability to tolerate stress.

Teach Patient/Family to:
• Encourage effective oral hygiene to prevent soft tissue inflammation/infection.

terazosin hydrochloride

ter-**ah**′-zoe-sin high-droh-**klor**′-ide
(Apo-Terazosin[CAN], Hytrin, Novo-Terazosin[CAN])

CATEGORY AND SCHEDULE

Pregnancy Risk Category: C

Drug Class: Antihypertensive, antiadrenergic

MECHANISM OF ACTION

An antihypertensive and benign prostatic hypertrophy agent that blocks α-adrenergic receptors. Produces vasodilation, decreases peripheral resistance, and targets receptors around bladder neck and prostate.
Therapeutic Effect: In hypertension, decreases B/P. In benign prostatic hyperplasia, relaxes smooth muscle and improves urine flow.

USES

Treatment of hypertension as a single agent or in combination with diuretics or β-blockers; benign prostatic hypertrophy

PHARMACOKINETICS

Rapidly, completely absorbed from the GI tract. Protein binding: 90%–94%. Metabolized in the liver to active metabolite. Primarily eliminated in feces via biliary system; excreted in urine. Not removed by hemodialysis. ***Half-life:*** 12 hr.

Route	Onset	Peak	Duration
PO	15 min	1–2 hr	12–24 hr

INDICATIONS AND DOSAGES

▸ Mild-to-Moderate Hypertension
PO
Adults, Elderly. Initially, 1 mg at bedtime. Slowly increase dosage to desired levels. Range: 1–5 mg/day as single or 2 divided doses. Maximum: 20 mg.

▸ Benign Prostatic Hyperplasia
PO
Adults, Elderly. Initially, 1 mg at bedtime. May increase up to 10 mg/day. Maximum: 20 mg/day.

SIDE EFFECTS/ADVERSE REACTIONS

Frequent
Dizziness, headache, unusual tiredness
Rare
Peripheral edema, orthostatic hypotension, myalgia, arthralgia, blurred vision, nausea, vomiting, nasal congestion, somnolence

PRECAUTIONS AND CONTRAINDICATIONS

Hypersensitivity, children, lactation

DRUG INTERACTIONS OF CONCERN TO DENTISTRY

• Decreased antihypertensive effects: NSAIDs, indomethacin

SERIOUS REACTIONS

! First-dose syncope (hypotension with sudden loss of consciousness) may occur 30–90 min after initial dose of 2 mg or more, a too-rapid increase in dosage, or addition of another antihypertensive agent to therapy. First-dose syncope may be preceded by tachycardia (pulse rate of 120–160 beats/min).

DENTAL CONSIDERATIONS

General:

- Monitor vital signs at every appointment because of cardiovascular side effects.
- After supine positioning, have patient sit upright for at least 2 min before standing to avoid orthostatic hypotension.
- Assess salivary flow as a factor in caries, periodontal disease, and candidiasis.
- Limit use of sodium-containing products, such as saline IV fluids, for patients with a dietary salt restriction.
- Consider semisupine chair position for patient comfort if GI side effects occur.

Teach Patient/Family:

- When chronic dry mouth occurs, advise patient to:
  - Avoid mouth rinses with high alcohol content because of drying effects.
  - Use daily home fluoride to prevent caries.
  - Use sugarless gum, frequent sips of water, or saliva substitutes.

terbinafine hydrochloride

ter-**been′**-ah-feen
high-droh-**klor′**-ide
(Apo-Terbinafine[CAN], Lamisil, Lamisil AT, Novo-Terbinafine [CAN])
Do not confuse terbinafine with terbutaline or Lamisil with Lamictal.

CATEGORY AND SCHEDULE

Pregnancy Risk Category: B

Drug Class: Antifungal

MECHANISM OF ACTION

A fungicidal antifungal that inhibits the enzyme squalene epoxidase, thereby interfering with fungal biosynthesis.
Therapeutic Effect: Fungicidal.

USES

Treatment of tinea pedis, tinea cruris, tinea corporis; unapproved uses: treatment of cutaneous candidiasis, tinea versicolor; treatment of onychomycosis of the toenail or fingernail caused by dermatophytes (tinea unguium)

PHARMACOKINETICS

PO: Bioavailability 40%, peak plasma levels approximately 2 hr; highly plasma protein bound (99%), extensive metabolism, excreted in urine (70%).

INDICATIONS AND DOSAGES

▸ **Tinea Pedis**

Topical

Adults, Elderly, Children 12 yr and older. Apply twice a day until signs and symptoms significantly improve.

▸ **Tinea Cruris, Tinea Corporis**

Topical

Adults, Elderly, Children 12 yr and older. Apply 1–2 times a day until signs and symptoms significantly improve.

▸ **Onychomycosis**

PO

Adults, Elderly, Children 12 yr and older. 250 mg/day for 6 wk (fingernails) or 12 wk (toenails).

▸ **Tinea Versicolor**

Topical Solution

Adults, Elderly. Apply to the affected area twice a day for 7 days.

▸ **Systemic Mycosis**

PO

Adults, Elderly. 250–500 mg/day for up to 16 mo.

SIDE EFFECTS/ADVERSE REACTIONS

Frequent
Oral: Headache
Occasional
Oral: Diarrhea, rash, dyspepsia, pruritus, taste disturbance, nausea, abdominal pain, flatulence, urticaria, visual disturbance
Topical: Irritation, burning, pruritus, dryness

PRECAUTIONS AND CONTRAINDICATIONS

Oral: Children younger than 12 yr, preexisting hepatic or renal impairment (creatinine clearance of less than 50 ml/min)
Caution:
Preexisting liver or renal disease, use not recommended during nursing, pediatric patients

DRUG INTERACTIONS OF CONCERN TO DENTISTRY

- None reported

SERIOUS REACTIONS

! Hepatobiliary dysfunction (including cholestatic hepatitis), serious skin reactions, and severe neutropenia occur rarely. Ocular lens and retinal changes have been noted.

DENTAL CONSIDERATIONS

T

General:
- Determine why patient is taking the drug.
- Consider semisupine chair position for patient comfort if GI side effects occur.
- Patients on chronic drug therapy may rarely have symptoms of blood dyscrasias, which can include infection, bleeding, and poor healing.

Consultations:
- In a patient with symptoms of blood dyscrasias, request a medical consultation for blood studies and postpone treatment until normal values are reestablished.

Teach Patient/Family to:
- Encourage effective oral hygiene to prevent soft tissue inflammation.
- Prevent trauma when using oral hygiene aids.

terconazole

ter-**kon**′-ah-zole
(Terazol[CAN], Terazol 3, Terazol 7)

CATEGORY AND SCHEDULE

Pregnancy Risk Category: C

Drug Class: Local antifungal

MECHANISM OF ACTION

An antifungal that disrupts fungal cell membrane permeability.
Therapeutic Effect: Fungicidal.

USES

Treatment of vaginal, vulval, vulvovaginal candidiasis (moniliasis)

PHARMACOKINETICS

Extent of systemic absorption after vaginal administration may be dependent on presence of a uterus, 5%–8% in women who had a hysterectomy versus 12%–16% in nonhysterectomy women.

INDICATIONS AND DOSAGES

▸ **Vulvovaginal Candidiasis**
Intravaginal
Adults, Elderly. 1 suppository vaginally at bedtime for 3 days.
Adults, Elderly. 1 applicatorful at bedtime for 7 days (0.4% cream) or for 3 days (0.8% cream).

SIDE EFFECTS/ADVERSE REACTIONS

Frequent
Headache, vulvovaginal burning
Occasional
Dysmenorrhea, pain in female genitalia, abdominal pain, fever, itching
Rare
Chills

PRECAUTIONS AND CONTRAINDICATIONS

Hypersensitivity to terconazole or any component of the formulation
Caution:
Children younger than 2 yr, pregnancy, lactation

DRUG INTERACTIONS OF CONCERN TO DENTISTRY

- None reported

SERIOUS REACTIONS

! Flu-like syndrome has been reported.

DENTAL CONSIDERATIONS

General:
- Broad-spectrum antibiotics can exacerbate vaginal candidiasis.

teriparatide

ter-ih-**par′**-ah-tide
(Forteo)

CATEGORY AND SCHEDULE

Pregnancy Risk Category: C

Drug Class: Bone resorption inhibitor (a synthetic polypeptide of rDNA origin, contains recombinant human parathyroid hormone [rhPTH(1–34)])

MECHANISM OF ACTION

A synthetic polypeptide hormone that acts on bone to mobilize calcium; also acts on kidney to reduce calcium clearance, increase phosphate excretion.
Therapeutic Effect: Promotes an increased rate of release of calcium from bone into blood, stimulates new bone formation.

USES

Treatment of postmenopausal women with osteoporosis at high risk for fracture; to increase bone mass in men with primary or hypogonadal osteoporosis at high risk for fracture

PHARMACOKINETICS

Subcutaneous: Absolute bioavailability 95%, peak serum levels 30 min. ***Half-life:*** 1 hr, no excretion or metabolism studies have been done, may be the same as PTH with hepatic metabolism and renal excretion.

INDICATIONS AND DOSAGES

▸ **Osteoporosis**
Subcutaneous
Adults, Elderly. 20 mcg once daily into the thigh or abdominal wall.

SIDE EFFECTS/ADVERSE REACTIONS

Occasional
Leg cramps, nausea, dizziness, headache, orthostatic hypotension, increased heart rate

PRECAUTIONS AND CONTRAINDICATIONS

Serum calcium above normal level, those at increased risk for osteosarcoma (Paget's disease, unexplained elevations of alkaline phosphatase, open epiphyses, prior radiation therapy that includes the skeleton), hypercalcemic disorder (e.g., hyperparathyroidism), hypersensitivity to teriparatide or any of the components of the formulation

Caution:

Active or recent urolithiasis, use longer than 2 yr, postinjection orthostatic hypotension, symptoms of hypercalcemia, pregnancy category C, avoid in nursing mothers, not for use in children

DRUG INTERACTIONS OF CONCERN TO DENTISTRY

• None reported

SERIOUS REACTIONS

! None known

DENTAL CONSIDERATIONS

General:

• Patients with osteoporosis and risk of fracture should be asked if they use this drug; otherwise, some patients may not report its use.

• Patients may need special assistance in the dental office to avoid risk of falling.

Teach Patient/Family to:

• Update health and drug history, reporting changes in health status, drug regimen, or disease/treatment status.

• Contact physician if symptoms of hypercalcemia appear (nausea, vomiting, constipation, lethargy, muscle weakness).

testosterone

tess-**toss**′-ter-one

(Andriol[CAN], Androderm, AndroGel, Andropository[CAN], Delatestryl, Depotest[CAN], Depo-Testosterone, Everone[CAN], Striant, Testim, Testoderm, Testopel, Virilon IM[CAN])

Do not confuse testosterone with testolactone.

CATEGORY AND SCHEDULE

Pregnancy Risk Category: X

Controlled Substance: Schedule III

Drug Class: Androgen, anabolic steroid

MECHANISM OF ACTION

A primary endogenous androgen that promotes growth and development of male sex organs and maintains secondary sex characteristics in androgen-deficient males.

Therapeutic Effect: Helps relieve androgen deficiency.

USES

Treatment of androgen deficiency, delayed puberty, female breast cancer, certain anemias, gender changes, hypogonadism, cryptorchidism

PHARMACOKINETICS

Well absorbed after IM administration. Protein binding: 98%. Undergoes first-pass metabolism in the liver. Primarily excreted in urine. Unknown if removed by hemodialysis. ***Half-life:*** 10–20 min.

INDICATIONS AND DOSAGES

▸ Male Hypogonadism

IM
Adults. 50–400 mg q2–4wk.
Adolescents. Initially, 40–50 mg/m^2/dose monthly until growth rate falls to prepubertal levels. 100 mg/m^2/dose until growth ceases.
Maintenance virilizing dose: 100 mg/m^2/dose twice a mo.
Subcutaneous (Pellets)
Adults, Adolescents. 150–450 mg q3–6mo.
Transdermal (Patch [Testoderm])
Adults, Elderly. Start therapy with 6 mg/day patch. Apply patch to scrotal skin.
Transdermal (Patch [Testoderm TTS])
Adults, Elderly. Apply TTS patch to arm, back, or upper buttocks.
Transdermal (Patch [Androderm])
Adults, Elderly. Start therapy with 5 mg/day patch applied at night. Apply patch to abdomen, back, thighs, or upper arms.
Transdermal (Gel [AndroGel])
Adults, Elderly. Initial dose of 5 mg delivers 50 mg testosterone and is applied once daily to the abdomen, shoulders, or upper arms. May increase to 7.5 g, then to 10 g, if necessary.
Transdermal (Gel [Testim])
Adults, Elderly. Initial dose of 5 g delivers 50 mg testosterone and is applied once a day to the shoulders or upper arms. May increase to 10 g.
Buccal System (Striant)
Adults, Elderly. 30 mg q12h.

▸ Delayed Puberty

IM
Adults. 50–200 mg q2–4wk.
Adolescents. 40–50 mg/m^2/dose every mo for 6 mo.
Subcutaneous (Pellets)
Adults, Adolescents. 150–450 mg q3–6mo.

▸ Breast Carcinoma

IM (Testosterone Aqueous)
Adults. 50–100 mg 3 times a wk.
IM (Testosterone Cypionate or Testosterone Ethanate)
Adults. 200–400 mg q2–4wk.
IM (Testosterone Propionate)
Adults. 50–100 mg 3 times a wk.

SIDE EFFECTS/ADVERSE REACTIONS

Frequent
Gynecomastia, acne
Females: Hirsutism, amenorrhea or other menstrual irregularities, deepening of voice, clitoral enlargement that may not be reversible when drug is discontinued
Occasional
Edema, nausea, insomnia, oligospermia, priapism, male-pattern baldness, bladder irritability, hypercalcemia (in immobilized patients or those with breast cancer), hypercholesterolemia, inflammation and pain at IM injection site
Transdermal: Pruritus, erythema, skin irritation
Rare
Polycythemia (with high dosage), hypersensitivity

PRECAUTIONS AND CONTRAINDICATIONS

Cardiac impairment, hypercalcemia, pregnancy, prostate or breast cancer in males, severe hepatic or renal disease
Caution:
Diabetes mellitus, cardiovascular disease, MI, increased risk of prostatic hypertrophy, prostatic carcinoma, virilization (women), increased PT

DRUG INTERACTIONS OF CONCERN TO DENTISTRY

- Edema: ACTH, adrenal steroids

T

SERIOUS REACTIONS

! Peliosis hepatitis (presence of blood-filled cysts in parenchyma of liver), hepatic neoplasms, and hepatocellular carcinoma have been associated with prolonged high-dose therapy. Anaphylactic reactions occur rarely.

DENTAL CONSIDERATIONS

General:

- Determine why the patient is taking the drug.
- Consider local hemostasis measures to prevent excessive bleeding.
- Short appointments and a stress-reduction protocol may be required for anxious patients.
- Prophylactic antibiotics may be indicated to prevent infection if surgery or deep scaling is planned.

Consultations:

- Physician consultation may be required if signs of anemia are observed in oral tissues.
- Medical consultation may be required to assess disease control and patient's ability to tolerate stress.
- Medical consultation should include PPT or PT.

Teach Patient/Family to:

- Encourage effective oral hygiene to prevent soft tissue inflammation.
- Be aware of the possibility of secondary oral infection and the need to see dentist immediately if infection occurs.

tetrabenazine

tet′-ra-**ben**′-a-zeen
(Xenazine)

CATEGORY AND SCHEDULE

Pregnancy Risk Category: C

Drug Class: CNS agent, monoamine depleter

MECHANISM OF ACTION

A monoamine depleter that inhibits the human vesicular monoamine transporter type 2 (VMAT2), resulting in decreased uptake of monoamines into synaptic vesicles and depletion of monoamine stores; depletes stores of dopamine, serotonin, and noradrenalin.
Therapeutic Effect: Reduces uncontrolled muscle movements.

USES

Chorea associated with Huntington's disease

PHARMACOKINETICS

Well absorbed following PO administration. Protein binding: 82%–85%. Metabolized in liver, primarily by CYP2D6. Primarily excreted in urine; minimal elimination in feces. ***Half-life:*** 2–8 hr.

INDICATIONS AND DOSAGES

▸ Chorea Associated with Huntington's Disease

PO

Adults. 12.5 mg a day given once in the morning. After 1 wk, the dose should be increased to 25 mg a day given as 12.5 mg twice a day. Titrate slowly at weekly intervals by 12.5 mg. If a dose of 37.5 to 50 mg per day is needed, give in a three times a day regimen. Maximum single dose: 25 mg.

SIDE EFFECTS/ADVERSE REACTIONS

Frequent

Extrapyramidal events, sedation, fatigue, insomnia, akathisia, depression, anxiety, difficulty balancing, bradykinesia, nausea, dysphagia, upper respiratory tract infection, falling, parkinsonism

Occasional

Irritability, decreased appetite, dizziness, dysarthria, headache, obsessive reaction, unsteady gait, vomiting, dysuria, ecchymosis, bronchitis, shortness of breath, head laceration, hyperprolactinemia, orthostatic hypotension

Rare

Neuroleptic malignant syndrome, QT prolongation

PRECAUTIONS AND CONTRAINDICATIONS

Hypersensitivity to tetrabenazine or its components

Hepatic impairment

Concurrent use with monoamine oxidase inhibitors or reserpine; initiation of tetrabenazine less than 20 days after discontinuation of reserpine

Use in suicidal or depressed patients (not treated or inadequately treated)

Caution:

Concurrent use with CYP2D6 inhibitors and inducers

History of depression or suicidal behavior

History of cardiac arrhythmias

Congenital ong QTc syndrome

Hypokalemia and/or hypomagnesemia

DRUG INTERACTIONS OF CONCERN TO DENTISTRY

- CYP2D6 inhibitors (fluoxetine, paroxetine, quinidine): May increase tetrabenazine levels; reduce dose by half
- Alcohol, CNS depressants: Additive CNS depressant effects
- Drugs that prolong QT interval: Increased risk of arrhythmias
- Neuroleptic agents: May increase the risk of tetrabenazine adverse effects
- Monoamine oxidase inhibitors, reserpine: Contraindicated

SERIOUS REACTIONS

! Black box warning: May increase the risk of depression and suicidal thoughts or behavior.

! Neuroleptic malignant syndrome (NMS), akathisia, agitation, parkinsonism, dysphagia, and QT prolongation–related arrhythmias have been reported.

DENTAL CONSIDERATIONS

General:

- Examine for oral manifestation of opportunistic infection.
- Patient on chronic drug therapy may rarely have symptoms of blood dyscrasias, which include infection, bleeding, and poor healing.
- Avoid dental light in patient's eyes; offer dark glasses for patient comfort.
- Place on frequent recall because of oral side effects.
- Consider semisupine chair position for patient comfort if GI side effects occur.

Consultations:

- In a patient with symptoms of blood dyscrasias, request a medical consultation for blood studies and postpone treatment until normal values are reestablished.

• Medical consultation may be required to assess disease control.

Teach Patient/Family to:

• Encourage effective oral hygiene to prevent soft tissue inflammation.
• Prevent trauma when using oral hygiene aids.
• Be alert for the possibility of secondary oral infection and the need to see dentist immediately if signs of infection occur.

tetracaine

tet′-ra-cane
(AK-T Caine, Cepacol, Opticaine, Pontocaine, Viractin)
Do not confuse with procaine, lidocaine, tetracycline

CATEGORY AND SCHEDULE

Pregnancy Risk Category: C

Drug Class: Topical anesthetic (ester group)

MECHANISM OF ACTION

Tetracaine causes a reversible blockade of nerve conduction by decreasing nerve membrane permeability to sodium.
Therapeutic Effect: Local anesthetic.

USES

Local anesthesia of mucous membranes, pruritus, sunburn, sore throat, cold sores, oral pain, rectal pain and irritation, control of gagging

PHARMACOKINETICS

Systemic absorption of tetracaine is variable. Metabolized by plasma pseudocholinesterases. Excreted in the urine.

INDICATIONS AND DOSAGES

▸ **Anesthetize Lower Abdomen**
Spinal
Adults. 3–4 ml (9–12 mg) of a 0.3% solution.

▸ **Anesthetize Perineum**
Spinal
Adults. 1–2 ml (3–6 mg) of a 0.3% solution.

▸ **Anesthetize Upper Abdomen**
Spinal
Adults. 5 ml (15 mg) of a 0.3% solution.

▸ **Obstetric Anesthesia, Low Spinal (Saddle Block) Anesthesia**
Spinal
Adults. 1–2 ml (2–14 mg) of a 0.2% solution.

▸ **Anesthesia of the Perineum**
Intrathecal
Adults. 0.5 ml (5 mg) as a 1% solution, diluted with equal amount of CSF or 10% dextrose injection.

▸ **Anesthesia of the Perineum and Lower Extremities**
Intrathecal
Adults. 1 ml (10 mg) as a 1% solution, diluted with equal amount of CSF or 10% dextrose injection.

▸ **Anesthesia up to the Costal Margin**
Intrathecal
Adults. 1.5–2 ml (15–20 mg) as a 1% solution, diluted with equal amount of CSF.

▸ **Topical Anesthesia**
Topical
Adults. Apply to the affected areas as needed. Maximum dosage is 28 g/24 hr.
Children. Apply to the affected areas as needed. Maximum dosage is 7 g in a 24-hr period.

T

▸ **Topical Anesthesia of Nose and Throat, Abolish Laryngeal and Esophageal Reflexes Prior to Diagnostic Procedure**
Topical
Adults. Direct application of a 0.25% or 0.5% topical solution or by oral inhalation of a nebulized 0.5% solution. Total dose should not exceed 20 mg.
▸ **Mild Pain, Burning, and/or Pruritus Associated with Herpes Labialis (Cold Sores or Fever Blisters)**
Topical
Adults, Children 2 yr and older. Apply to the affected area no more than 3–4 times a day.
▸ **Ophthalmic Anesthesia**
Topical
Adults. 1–2 drops of a 0.5% solution.

SIDE EFFECTS/ADVERSE REACTIONS

Frequent
Burning, stinging, or tenderness; skin rash; itching, redness, or inflammation; numbness or tingling of the face or mouth; pain at the injection site; sensitivity to light; swelling of the eye or eyelid; watering of the eyes; acute ocular pain and ocular irritation (burning, stinging, or redness)
Occasional
Paresthesias, weakness and paralysis of lower extremity, hypotension, high or total spinal block, urinary retention or incontinence, fecal incontinence, headache, back pain, septic meningitis, meningismus, arachnoiditis, shivering, cranial nerve palsies due to traction on nerves from loss of CSF, and loss of perineal sensation and sexual function
Rare
Anxiety; restlessness; difficulty breathing; shortness of breath; dizziness; drowsiness; light-headedness; nausea; vomiting; seizures (convulsions); slow, irregular heartbeat (palpitations); swelling of the face or mouth; skin rash; itching (hives); tremors; visual impairment

PRECAUTIONS AND CONTRAINDICATIONS

Hypersensitivity to ester local anesthetics, sulfites, PABA; infection or inflammation at the injection site, bacteremia, platelet abnormalities, thrombocytopenia, increased bleeding time, uncontrolled coagulopathy, anticoagulant therapy, sulfonamide therapy
Caution:
Children younger than 12 yr, sepsis, lactation, local infection, geriatric, debilitated patient

DRUG INTERACTIONS OF CONCERN TO DENTISTRY

• Caution in patients taking tocainide, mexiletine; significant systemic absorption could lead to synergistic and potentially toxic effects.

SERIOUS REACTIONS

! Tetracaine-induced CNS toxicity usually presents with symptoms of CNS stimulation, such as anxiety, apprehension, restlessness, nervousness, disorientation, confusion, dizziness, tinnitus, blurred vision, tremor, and/or seizures. Subsequently, depressive symptoms may occur, including drowsiness, respiratory arrest, or coma.
! Depression or cardiac excitability and contractility may cause AV block, ventricular arrhythmias, or cardiac arrest. Symptoms of local anesthetic CNS toxicity, such as dizziness, tongue numbness, visual

impairment or disturbances, and muscular twitching appear to occur before cardiotoxic effects. Cardiotoxic effects include angina, QT prolongation, PR prolongation, atrial fibrillation, sinus bradycardia, hypotension, palpitations, and cardiovascular collapse. Maternal seizures and cardiovascular collapse may occur following paracervical block in early pregnancy due to rapid systemic absorption.

Alert

! Tetracaine is more likely than any other topical anesthetic to cause contact reactions, including skin rash (unspecified), mucous membrane irritation, erythema, pruritus, urticaria, burning, stinging, edema, or tenderness.

Alert

! During labor and obstetric delivery, local anesthetics can cause varying degrees of maternal, fetal, and neonatal toxicities. Fetal heart rate should be monitored continuously because fetal bradycardia may occur in patients receiving tetracaine anesthesia and may be associated with fetal acidosis. Maternal hypotension can result from regional anesthesia; patient position can alleviate this problem. Spinal tetracaine may cause decreased uterine contractility or maternal expulsion efforts and alter the forces of parturition.

T

DENTAL CONSIDERATIONS

General:

- Apply smallest effective dose; apply to small area because significant absorption can occur, especially from denuded areas.
- Absorption of excessive amounts of drug may lead to signs of local anesthetic toxicity; with correct use, toxicity is a rare event.
- Use for topical anesthesia or temporary relief of symptoms; reevaluate if symptoms persist.
- Toxic amounts can be absorbed from denuded mucosa or skin.
- Apply with cotton-tipped applicator by pressing, not rubbing, paste on lesion.

Teach Patient/Family to:

- Apply correctly.
- Not chew gum or eat while numbness is present after dental treatment.
- Recognize the symptoms of systemic toxicity, which can include nervousness, nausea, excitement followed by drowsiness, convulsions, and cardiac and respiratory depression.
- Be aware that symptoms may vary because they depend on the amount of drug actually absorbed.

tetracycline hydrochloride

tet-ra-**sye′**-kleen
high-droh-**klor′**-ide
(Apo-Tetra[CAN], Latycin[AUS], Mysteclin[AUS], Novotetra[CAN], Nu-Tetra[CAN], Sumycin, Tetrex[AUS])

CATEGORY AND SCHEDULE

Pregnancy Risk Category: D (B with topical form)

Drug Class: Tetracycline, broad-spectrum antibiotic

MECHANISM OF ACTION

A tetracycline antibiotic that inhibits bacterial protein synthesis by binding to ribosomes.

Therapeutic Effect: Bacteriostatic.

USES

Treatment of syphilis, *C. trachomatis,* gonorrhea, lymphogranuloma venereum, *M. pneumoniae,* rickettsial infections, acne, actinomycosis, anthrax, bronchitis, GU infections, sinusitis, and many other infections produced by susceptible organisms; *H. pylori*–associated duodenal ulcer

PHARMACOKINETICS

Readily absorbed from the GI tract. Protein binding: 30%–60%. Widely distributed. Excreted in urine; eliminated in feces through biliary system. Not removed by hemodialysis. ***Half-life:*** 6–11 hr (increased in impaired renal function).

INDICATIONS AND DOSAGES

▸ **Inflammatory Acne Vulgaris, Lyme Disease, Mycoplasmal Disease, Legionella Infections, Rocky Mountain Spotted Fever, Chlamydial Infections in Patients with Gonorrhea**

PO

Adults, Elderly. 250–500 mg q6–12h.

Children 8 yr and older. 25–50 mg/kg/day in 4 divided doses. Maximum: 3 g/day.

▸ ***H. pylori*** **Infections**

PO

Adults, Elderly. 500 mg 2–4 times a day (in combination).

Topical

Adults, Elderly. Apply twice a day (once in the morning, once in the evening).

▸ **Dosage in Renal Impairment**

Dosage interval is modified on the basis of creatinine clearance.

Creatinine Clearance	Dosage Interval
50–80 ml/min	Usual dose q8–12h
10–50 ml/min	Usual dose q12–24h
Less than 10 ml/min	Usual dose q24h

SIDE EFFECTS/ADVERSE REACTIONS

Frequent

Dizziness, light-headedness, diarrhea, nausea, vomiting, abdominal cramps, possibly severe photosensitivity

Topical: Dry, scaly skin; stinging or burning sensation

Occasional

Pigmentation of skin or mucous membranes, rectal or genital pruritus, stomatitis

Topical: Pain, redness, swelling, or other skin irritation.

PRECAUTIONS AND CONTRAINDICATIONS

Children 8 yr and younger, hypersensitivity to tetracyclines or sulfites.

The use of tetracycline drugs during tooth development (last half of pregnancy, infancy, and childhood up to the age of 8 may cause permanent discoloration of the teeth (yellow-gray-brown). Enamel hypoplasia has also been reported. May also cause retardation of skeletal development and deformations.

Caution:

Renal disease, hepatic disease

DRUG INTERACTIONS OF CONCERN TO DENTISTRY

- Decreased absorption: $NaHCO_3$, other antacids
- Decreased effect of penicillins, cephalosporins
- Possible increase in serum levels of methotrexate

• Suspected increase in effects of warfarin, theophylline

SERIOUS REACTIONS

! Superinfection (especially fungal), anaphylaxis, and benign intracranial hypertension may occur. Bulging fontanelles occur rarely in infants.

DENTAL CONSIDERATIONS

General:

• Determine why the patient is taking tetracycline.

• Broad-spectrum antibiotics may be a factor in oral or vaginal *Candida* infections.

• Advise patient if dental drugs prescribed have a potential for photosensitivity.

• Dental staining or enamel hypoplasia may be associated with exposure to this drug before birth or up to the age of 8. Tetracycline stains may be extremely resistant to ordinary tooth-whitening procedures.

Consultations:

• Medical consultation may be required to assess disease control.

Teach Patient/Family to:

• Encourage effective oral hygiene to prevent soft tissue inflammation.

• Prevent injury when using oral hygiene aids.

• Avoid milk products; take with a full glass of water.

• Take tetracycline doses 1 hr before or 2 hr after air polishing device (Prophy-Jet), if used.

• When used for dental infection, advise patient to:

  • Use additional method of contraception for duration of cycle if taking birth control pill.

  • Report sore throat, oral burning sensation, fever, fatigue, any of which could indicate superinfection.

  • Take at prescribed intervals and complete dosage regimen.

  • Immediately notify the dentist if signs or symptoms of infection increase.

tetracycline periodontal fiber

tet-ra-**sye**′-kleen pare-ee-oh-**don**′-tal **fye**′-ber
(Actisite)

CATEGORY AND SCHEDULE

Pregnancy Risk Category: C

Drug Class: Tetracycline, broad-spectrum antiinfective

MECHANISM OF ACTION

Antimicrobial effect related to inhibition of protein synthesis; decreases incidence of postsurgical inflammation and edema; suppresses bacteria and acts as a barrier to bacterial entry; acts on cementum or fibroblasts to enhance periodontal ligament regeneration.

USES

Adjunctive treatment in adult periodontitis.

PHARMACOKINETICS

Topical: In vitro release rate 2 mcg/cm/hr; gingival concentration maintained over 10 days; plasma levels below detectable limits

INDICATIONS AND DOSAGES

Fiber: Adjust length to fit pocket depth and contour of teeth treated; fiber should contact base of pocket; apply cyanoacrylate adhesive to secure fiber for 10 days; replace if lost before 7 days; up to 11 teeth can be treated.

T

SIDE EFFECTS/ADVERSE REACTIONS

Oral: Gingival inflammation and pain, glossitis, local erythema, candidiasis, staining of tongue
EENT: Minor throat irritation
INTEG: Photosensitivity

PRECAUTIONS AND CONTRAINDICATIONS

Hypersensitivity, children younger than 8 yr, acutely abscessed periodontal pocket
Caution:
Lactation, children, superinfection, patients with predisposition to candidiasis; must remove fibers after 10 days

DRUG INTERACTIONS OF CONCERN TO DENTISTRY

• It is not known if the tetracycline fiber will decrease the effectiveness of oral contraceptives; however, manufacturer recommends suggesting the use of an alternative form of contraception during the remaining cycle to female patients taking oral contraceptives.

SERIOUS REACTIONS

! Serious systemic toxicity unlikely by this route of administration.

DENTAL CONSIDERATIONS

General:
• Take precautions regarding allergy to tetracyclines.
• Examine oral mucosa for candidiasis before placing fiber.
Teach Patient/Family to:
• Not chew hard, crusty, or sticky foods.
• Not brush or floss near treated area but clean other teeth.
• Avoid other oral hygienic practices that could dislodge fibers, such as the use of toothpicks.
• Do not irritate the treated area.
• Notify dentist if fiber dislodges or falls out.
• Notify dentist if pain, swelling, or other symptoms occur.

thalidomide

thah-**lid**′-owe-mide
(Thalomid)

CATEGORY AND SCHEDULE

Pregnancy Risk Category: X

Drug Class: Immunomodulators, tumor necrosis factor modulators

MECHANISM OF ACTION

An immunomodulator whose exact mechanism is unknown. Has sedative, antiinflammatory, and immunosuppressive activity, which may be caused by selective inhibition of the production of tumor necrosis factor-α.
Therapeutic Effect: Improves muscle wasting in HIV patients; reduces local and systemic effects of leprosy.

USES

Treatment of and prevention of erythema nodosum leprosum (ENL)

PHARMACOKINETICS

Slowly absorbed from GI tract; peak blood level in 2.9–5.7 hr. Protein binding 55%–66%; metabolized in plasma. ***Half-life:*** 5–7 hr; elimination in urine and by other routes.

INDICATIONS AND DOSAGES

▸ **AIDS-Related Muscle Wasting**
PO
Adults. 100–300 mg a day.

▸ **Leprosy**
PO
Adults, Elderly. Initially, 100–300 mg/day as single bedtime dose, at least 1 hr after the evening meal. Continue until active reaction subsides, then reduce dose q2–4 wk in 50 mg increments.

SIDE EFFECTS/ADVERSE REACTIONS

Frequent
Somnolence, dizziness, mood changes, constipation, dry mouth, peripheral neuropathy
Occasional
Increased appetite, weight gain, headache, loss of libido, edema of face and limbs, nausea, alopecia, dry skin, rash, hypothyroidism

PRECAUTIONS AND CONTRAINDICATIONS

Neutropenia, peripheral neuropathy; pregnancy, sensitivity to thalidomide

DRUG INTERACTIONS OF CONCERN TO DENTISTRY

- Increased sedative effects of: alcohol, barbiturates, phenothiazines
- Increased risk of peripheral neuropathy: metronidazole
- May interfere with hormonal contraceptives: patient must use two alternative methods of contraception

T

SERIOUS REACTIONS

! Neutropenia, peripheral neuropathy, and thromboembolism occur rarely.

DENTAL CONSIDERATIONS

General:
- Determine why patient is taking the drug.
- Consider semisupine chair position for patient comfort if GI side effects occur.
- Assess salivary flow as a factor in caries, periodontal disease, and candidiasis.
- Examine for oral manifestation of opportunistic infection.
- Patient on chronic drug therapy may rarely present with symptoms of blood dyscrasias, which can include infection, bleeding, and poor healing. If dyscrasia is present, caution patient to prevent oral tissue trauma when using oral hygiene aids.
- After supine positioning, have patient sit upright for at least 2 min before standing to avoid orthostatic hypotension.
- Can be prescribed only by S.T.E.P.S. (System for Thalidomide Education and Prescribing Safety) registered prescribers.
- Absolutely contraindicated in pregnancy.

Consultations:
- Refer patients to attending physician if symptoms of peripheral neuropathy are present (numbness, tingling or pain in hands or feet).
- Consultation with physician may be necessary if sedation or general anesthesia is required.
- Medical consultation may be required to assess disease control and patient's ability to tolerate stress.
- In a patient with symptoms of blood dyscrasias, request a medical consultation for blood studies and postpone treatment until normal values are reestablished.
- Precaution if dental surgery is anticipated or general anesthesia required.

Teach Patient/Family to:
- Not drive or perform other tasks requiring mental alertness.
- When chronic dry mouth occurs, advise patient to:

• Avoid mouth rinses with high alcohol content due to drying effects.
• Use daily home fluoride products for anticaries effect.
• Use sugarless gum, frequent sips of water, or saliva substitutes.
• Encourage effective oral hygiene to prevent soft tissue inflammation.
• Prevent trauma when using oral hygiene aids.
• Report oral lesions, soreness, or bleeding to dentist.
• Update health and medication history if physician makes any changes in evaluation or drug regimens; include OTC, herbal, and nonherbal remedies in the update.

theophylline

thee-**off′**-ih-lin
(Accurbron, Aquaphyllin, Asmalix, Bronkodyl, Elixomin, Elixophyllin, Lanophyllin, Quibron-T, Respbid, Slo-Bid, Slo-Phyllin, Sustaire, T-Phyl, Theobid, Theoclear LA, Theolair, Theo-Dur, Theo-24, Theolair-24, Theochron, Theo-Sav, Theovent, Theo-X, Uni-Dur, Uniphyl)

CATEGORY AND SCHEDULE

Pregnancy Risk Category: C

Drug Class: Xanthine

MECHANISM OF ACTION

An antiasthmatic medication with two distinct actions in the airways of patients with reversible obstruction; smooth muscle relaxation and suppression of the response of airways to stimuli. Mechanisms of action are not known with certainty. It is known that theophylline increases force of contraction of diaphragmatic muscles by enhancing calcium uptake through adenosine-mediated channels.
Therapeutic Effect: Bronchodilation and decreased airway reactivity.

USES

Treatment of bronchial asthma, bronchospasm of COPD, chronic bronchitis; unapproved use: apnea in the neonate

PHARMACOKINETICS

The pharmacokinetics of theophylline vary widely among similar patients and cannot be predicted by age, sex, body weight or other characteristics. Rapidly and completely absorbed after oral administration in solution or immediate-release solid oral dosage form. Distributed freely into fat-free tissues. Extensively metabolized in liver. ***Half-life:*** 4–8 hr.

INDICATIONS AND DOSAGES

▸ **Chronic Asthma/Lung Diseases**
PO
Adults. Acute symptoms: 5 mg/kg as a loading dose, maintenance 3 mg/kg every 8 hr (nonsmokers), 3 mg/kg every 6 hr (smokers), 2 mg/kg every 8 hr (older patients), 1–2 mg/kg every 12 hr (CHF); IV 5 mg/kg load over 20 min, maintenance 0.2 mg/kg/hr (CHF, elderly), 0.43 mg/kg/hr (nonsmokers), 0.7 mg/kg/hr (young adult smokers). Slow titration. Initial dose 16 mg/kg/day or 400 mg daily, whichever is less, doses divided every 6–8 hr.

SIDE EFFECTS/ADVERSE REACTIONS

Anxiety, dizziness, headache, insomnia, light-headedness, muscle twitching, restlessness, seizures, dysrhythmias, fluid retention with tachycardia, hypotension, palpitations, pounding heartbeat, sinus tachycardia, anorexia, bitter taste, diarrhea, dyspepsia, gastroesophageal reflux, nausea, vomiting, urinary frequency, increased respiratory rate, flushing, urticaria

PRECAUTIONS AND CONTRAINDICATIONS

Hypersensitivity to theophylline or any component of the formulation, active peptic ulcer disease, underlying seizure disorders unless receiving appropriate anticonvulsant medication

Caution:

Elderly, CHF, cor pulmonale, hepatic disease, active peptic ulcer disease, diabetes mellitus, hyperthyroidism, hypertension, children

DRUG INTERACTIONS OF CONCERN TO DENTISTRY

• Increased action: erythromycin, ciprofloxacin, glucocorticoids
• Increased risk of cardiac dysrhythmia: halothane inhalation anesthesia, CNS stimulants
• Decreased effect: barbiturates, carbamazepine, ketoconazole
• May decrease effects of benzodiazepines and other sedative agents

T

SERIOUS REACTIONS

! Severe toxicity from theophylline overdose is a relatively rare event.

DENTAL CONSIDERATIONS

General:

• Consider semisupine chair position for patients with respiratory disease.
• Monitor vital signs at every appointment because of cardiovascular side effects.
• Assess salivary flow as a factor in caries, periodontal disease, and candidiasis.
• Be aware that aspirin or sulfite preservatives in vasoconstrictor-containing products can exacerbate asthma.
• Acute asthmatic episodes may be precipitated in the dental office. Sympathomimetic inhalants should be available for emergency use.
• Midday appointments and a stress-reduction protocol may be required for anxious patients.

Consultations:

• Medical consultation may be required to assess disease control.

Teach Patient/Family:

• When chronic dry mouth occurs, advise patient to:
  • Avoid mouth rinses with high alcohol content because of drying effects.
  • Use daily home fluoride products to prevent caries.
  • Use sugarless gum, frequent sips of water, or saliva substitutes.

thiabendazole

thye-ah-**ben′**-da-zole
(Mintezol)

CATEGORY AND SCHEDULE

Pregnancy Risk Category: C

Drug Class: Anthelmintic, systemic

MECHANISM OF ACTION

An anthelmintic agent that inhibits helminth-specific mitochondrial fumarate reductase.

Therapeutic Effect: Suppresses parasite production.

USES
Treatment of worm infections

PHARMACOKINETICS
Rapidly and well absorbed from the GI tract. Rapidly metabolized in liver. Primarily excreted in urine; partially eliminated in feces.
Half-life: 1.2 hr.

INDICATIONS AND DOSAGES
Dose is based on patient's body weight.

▸ **Cutaneous Lava Migrans (Creeping Eruption)**
PO
Adults, Elderly, Children. 50 mg/kg/day q12h for 2 days. Maximum: 3 g/day.

▸ **Intestinal Roundworms**
PO
Adults, Elderly, Children. 50 mg/kg/day q12h for 2 days. Maximum: 3 g/day.

▸ **Strongyloidiasis (Thread Worms)**
PO
Adults, Elderly, Children. 50 mg/kg/day q12h for 2 days. Maximum: 3 g/day.

▸ **Trichinosis**
PO
Adults, Elderly, Children. 50 mg/kg/day q12h for 2–4 days. Maximum: 3 g/day.

▸ **Visceral Larva Migrans**
PO
Adults, Elderly, Children. 50 mg/kg/day q12h for 7 days. Maximum: 3 g/day.

SIDE EFFECTS/ADVERSE REACTIONS
Occasional
Dizziness, drowsiness, nausea, vomiting, diarrhea
Rare
Erythema multiforme, liver damage

PRECAUTIONS AND CONTRAINDICATIONS
Prophylactic treatment of pinworm infestation, hypersensitivity to thiabendazole or its components

DRUG INTERACTIONS OF CONCERN TO DENTISTRY
• Suspected interference with xanthine metabolism

SERIOUS REACTIONS
! Overdose includes symptoms of altered mental status and visual problems. Erythema multiforme, liver damage, and Stevens-Johnson syndrome occur rarely.

DENTAL CONSIDERATIONS
General:
• Determine why patient is taking the drug.
• Patient on chronic drug therapy may rarely present with symptoms of blood dyscrasias, which can include infection, bleeding, and poor healing. If dyscrasia is present, caution patient to prevent oral tissue trauma when using oral hygiene aids.
• Assess salivary flow as a factor in caries, periodontal disease, and candidiasis.
• Pinworm infections are easily spread to persons in close contact.
• Question patients about other drugs they may be using.
Consultations:
• In a patient with symptoms of blood dyscrasias, request a medical consultation for blood studies and postpone treatment until normal values are reestablished.
• Medical consultation may be required to assess disease control in the patient.

Teach Patient/Family:

- When chronic dry mouth occurs, advise patient to:
  - Avoid mouth rinses with high alcohol content because of drying effects.
  - Use daily home fluoride products for anticaries effect.
  - Use sugarless gum, frequent sips of water, or saliva substitutes.

thiamine hydrochloride (vitamin B_1)

thy′-ah-min high-droh-**klor**′-ide (Beta-Sol[AUS], Betaxin[CAN], Thiamilate)

CATEGORY AND SCHEDULE

Pregnancy Risk Category: A (C if used in doses above recommended daily allowance)
OTC (tablets)

Drug Class: Vitamin B_1, water soluble

MECHANISM OF ACTION

A water-soluble vitamin that combines with adenosine triphosphate in the liver, kidneys, and leukocytes to form thiamine diphosphate, a coenzyme that is necessary for carbohydrate metabolism.

Therapeutic Effect: Prevents and reverses thiamine deficiency.

USES

Treatment of vitamin B_1 deficiency or prophylaxis, beriberi, Wernicke-Korsakoff syndrome

PHARMACOKINETICS

Readily absorbed from the GI tract, primarily in duodenum, after IM administration. Widely distributed. Metabolized in the liver. Primarily excreted in urine.

INDICATIONS AND DOSAGES

▸ **Dietary Supplement**

PO

Adults, Elderly. 1–2 mg/day.
Children. 0.5–1 mg/day.
Infants. 0.3–0.5 mg/day.

▸ **Thiamine Deficiency**

PO

Adults, Elderly. 5–30 mg/day, as a single dose or in 3 divided doses, for 1 mo.
Children. 10–50 mg/day in 3 divided doses.

▸ **Thiamine Deficiency on Patients Who Are Critically Ill or Have Malabsorption Syndrome**

IV, IM

Adults, Elderly. 5–100 mg, 3 times a day.
Children. 10–25 mg/day.

▸ **Metabolic Disorders**

PO

Adults, Elderly, Children. 10–20 mg/day; increased up to 4 g/day in divided doses.

SIDE EFFECTS/ADVERSE REACTIONS

Frequent

Pain, induration, and tenderness at IM injection site

PRECAUTIONS AND CONTRAINDICATIONS

Sensitivity to thiamin, Wernicke's encephalopathy

DRUG INTERACTIONS OF CONCERN TO DENTISTRY

- None reported

SERIOUS REACTIONS

! IV administration may result in a rare, severe hypersensitivity reaction marked by a feeling of warmth, pruritus, urticaria, weakness, diaphoresis, nausea, restlessness, tightness in throat, angioedema, cyanosis, pulmonary edema, GI tract bleeding, and cardiovascular collapse.

DENTAL CONSIDERATIONS

General:

• Determine why the patient is taking this vitamin.

Teach Patient/Family:

• Food sources to be included in diet: yeast, whole grain, beef, liver, legumes.

thiethylperazine

thye-eth-il-**per′**-ah-zeen

(Torecan)

Do not confuse with thioridazine.

CATEGORY AND SCHEDULE

Pregnancy Risk Category: X

Drug Class: Phenothiazine-type antiemetic

MECHANISM OF ACTION

A piperazine phenothiazine that acts centrally to block dopamine receptors in chemoreceptor trigger zone (CTZ) in CNS.

Therapeutic Effect: Relieves nausea and vomiting.

USES

Treatment of nausea, vomiting

PHARMACOKINETICS

PO: Onset 45–60 min. Rectal: Onset 45–60 min. Metabolized by liver; excreted by kidneys; crosses placenta; excreted in breast milk.

INDICATIONS AND DOSAGES

▸ **Nausea or Vomiting**

PO/Rectal/IM

Adults, Elderly. 10 mg 1–3 times a day.

SIDE EFFECTS/ADVERSE REACTIONS

Frequent

Drowsiness, dizziness

Occasional

Blurred vision, decreased color/night vision, fever, headache, orthostatic hypotension, rash, ringing in ears, constipation, dry mouth, decreased sweating

PRECAUTIONS AND CONTRAINDICATIONS

Comatose states, severe CNS depression, pregnancy, hypersensitivity to phenothiazines

Caution:

Children younger than 12 yr, elderly

DRUG INTERACTIONS OF CONCERN TO DENTISTRY

• Increased anticholinergic action: anticholinergics

• Increased CNS depression, hypotension: alcohol, CNS depressants

SERIOUS REACTIONS

! Extrapyramidal symptoms manifested as torticollis (neck muscle spasm), oculogyric crisis (rolling back of eyes), and akathisia (motor restlessness, anxiety) occur rarely.

DENTAL CONSIDERATIONS

General:

• Postpone elective dental treatment when symptoms are present.

Consultations:

- Medical consultation may be required to assess disease control.

thioridazine

thye-oh-**rid′**-ah-zeen

(Aldazine[AUS], Apo-Thioridazine [CAN], Mellaril, Mellaril [AUS], Thioridazine Intensol)

Do not confuse thioridazine with thiothixene or Thorazine, or Mellaril with Mebaral.

CATEGORY AND SCHEDULE

Pregnancy Risk Category: C

Drug Class: Phenothiazine antipsychotic

MECHANISM OF ACTION

A phenothiazine that blocks dopamine at postsynaptic receptor sites. Possesses strong anticholinergic and sedative effects. ***Therapeutic Effect:*** Suppresses behavioral response in psychosis; reduces locomotor activity and aggressiveness.

USES

Treatment of psychotic disorders, schizophrenia, behavioral problems in children, alcohol withdrawal as adjunct, anxiety, major depressive disorders, organic brain syndrome

PHARMACOKINETICS

PO: Onset erratic, peak 2–4 hr. ***Half-life:*** 26–36 hr; metabolized by liver; excreted in urine; crosses placenta; excreted in breast milk.

INDICATIONS AND DOSAGES

▸ **Psychosis**

PO

Adults, Elderly, Children 12 yr and older. Initially, 25–100 mg 3 times a day; dosage increased gradually. Maximum: 800 mg/day.

Children 2–11 yr. Initially, 0.5 mg/kg/day in 2–3 divided doses. Maximum: 3 mg/kg/day.

SIDE EFFECTS/ADVERSE REACTIONS

Occasional

Drowsiness during early therapy, dry mouth, blurred vision, lethargy, constipation or diarrhea, nasal congestion, peripheral edema, urine retention

Rare

Ocular changes, altered skin pigmentation (in those taking high doses for prolonged periods), photosensitivity, darkening of urine

PRECAUTIONS AND CONTRAINDICATIONS

Angle-closure glaucoma, blood dyscrasias, cardiac arrhythmias, cardiac or hepatic impairment, concurrent use of drugs that prolong QT interval, severe CNS depression

Caution:

Lactation, seizure disorders, hypertension, hepatic disease, cardiac disease

DRUG INTERACTIONS OF CONCERN TO DENTISTRY

- Increased sedation: other CNS depressants, alcohol, barbiturate anesthetics, opioid analgesics
- Hypotension, tachycardia: epinephrine (systemic)
- Increased extrapyramidal effects: phenothiazines and related drugs (haloperidol, droperidol), metoclopramide
- Additive photosensitization: tetracyclines
- Increased anticholinergic effects: anticholinergics

SERIOUS REACTIONS

! Prolonged QT interval may produce torsades de pointes, a form of ventricular tachycardia, and sudden death.

DENTAL CONSIDERATIONS

General:

• Monitor vital signs at every appointment because of cardiovascular side effects.
• Patients on chronic drug therapy may rarely have symptoms of blood dyscrasias, which can include infection, bleeding, and poor healing.
• After supine positioning, have patient sit upright for at least 2 min before standing to avoid orthostatic hypotension.
• Assess salivary flow as a factor in caries, periodontal disease, and candidiasis.
• Avoid dental light in patient's eyes; offer dark glasses for patient comfort.
• Assess for presence of extrapyramidal motor symptoms, such as tardive dyskinesia and akathisia. Extrapyramidal motor activity may complicate dental treatment.
• Geriatric patients are more susceptible to drug effects; use lower dose.
• Use vasoconstrictors with caution, in low doses, and with careful aspiration.

Consultations:

• In a patient with symptoms of blood dyscrasias, request a medical consultation for blood studies and postpone dental treatment until normal values are reestablished.
• Take precautions if dental surgery is anticipated and anesthesia is required.
• Refer to physician if signs of tardive dyskinesia or akathisia are present.
• Physician should be informed if significant xerostomic side effects occur (e.g., increased caries, sore tongue, problems eating or swallowing, difficulty wearing prosthesis) so that a medication change can be considered.

Teach Patient/Family to:

• Encourage effective oral hygiene to prevent soft tissue inflammation.
• Use caution to prevent injury when using oral hygiene aids.
• Use powered tooth brush if patient has difficulty holding conventional devices.
• When chronic dry mouth occurs, advise patient to:
  • Avoid mouth rinses with high alcohol content because of drying effects.
  • Use daily home fluoride products to prevent caries.
  • Use sugarless gum, frequent sips of water, or saliva substitutes.

thiotepa

thigh-oh-**teh′**-pah
(Thioplex)

CATEGORY AND SCHEDULE

Pregnancy Risk Category: D

Drug Class: Antineoplastic

T

MECHANISM OF ACTION

An alkylating agent that inhibits DNA and RNA protein synthesis by cross-linking with DNA and RNA strands, preventing cell growth. Cell cycle–phase nonspecific.
Therapeutic Effect: Interferes with DNA and RNA function.

USES

Treatment of some kinds of cancer

PHARMACOKINETICS

Peak serum levels reached rapidly; elimination half-life of 2.4 hr. Excreted in urine primarily as TEPA metabolite and parent drug.

INDICATIONS AND DOSAGES

▸ Adenocarcinoma of Breast and Ovary, Hodgkin's Disease, Lymphosarcoma, Superficial Papillary Carcinoma of Urinary Bladder

IV

Adults, Elderly. Initially, 0.3–0.4 mg/kg every 1–4 wk. Maintenance dose adjusted weekly on the basis of blood counts.

Children. 25–65 mg/m^2 as a single dose every 3–4 wk.

▸ Control of Pericardial, Peritoneal, or Pleural Effusions Caused by Metastatic Tumors

Intracavitary Injection

Adults, Elderly. 0.6–0.8 mg/kg every 1–4 wk.

SIDE EFFECTS/ADVERSE REACTIONS

Occasional

Pain at injection site, headache, dizziness, urticaria, rash, nausea, vomiting, anorexia, stomatitis

Rare

Alopecia, cystitis, hematuria (after intravesical dose)

PRECAUTIONS AND CONTRAINDICATIONS

Pregnancy, severe myelosuppression (leukocyte count less than 3000/mm^3 or platelet count less than 150,000/mm^3)

DRUG INTERACTIONS OF CONCERN TO DENTISTRY

• Suspected decrease in effects: probenecid
• Prolonged neuromuscular blockade: pancuronium

SERIOUS REACTIONS

! Hematologic toxicity, manifested as leukopenia, anemia, thrombocytopenia, and pancytopenia, may occur from bone marrow depression. Although the WBC count falls to its lowest point 10–14 days after initial therapy, the initial effects on bone marrow may not be evident for 30 days. Stomatitis and ulceration of intestinal mucosa may occur.

DENTAL CONSIDERATIONS

General:

• If additional analgesia is required for dental pain, consider alternative analgesics (NSAIDs) in patients taking opioids for acute or chronic pain.
• Examine for oral manifestation of opportunistic infection.
• Avoid products that affect platelet function, such as aspirin and NSAIDs.
• This drug may be used in the hospital or on an outpatient basis. Confirm the patient's disease and treatment status.
• Patient on chronic drug therapy may rarely present with symptoms of blood dyscrasias, which can include infection, bleeding, and poor healing. If dyscrasia is present, caution patient to prevent oral tissue trauma when using oral hygiene aids.
• Palliative medication may be required for management of oral side effects.
• Patient may need assistance in getting into and out of dental chair. Adjust chair position for patient comfort.
• Consider semisupine chair position for patient comfort if GI side effects occur.
• Caution: patients may be at high risk for infection.

• Patients may be at risk for bleeding; check oral signs.
• Oral infections should be eliminated and/or treated aggressively.

Consultations:

• Medical consultation should include routine blood counts including platelet counts and bleeding time.
• In a patient with symptoms of blood dyscrasias, request a medical consultation for blood studies and postpone treatment until normal values are reestablished.
• Consult physician; prophylactic or therapeutic antiinfectives may be indicated if surgery or periodontal treatment is required.
• Medical consultation may be required to assess immunologic status during cancer chemotherapy and determine safety risk, if any, posed by the required dental treatment.
• Medical consultation may be required to assess disease control and patient's ability to tolerate stress.

Teach Patient/Family to:

• Encourage effective oral hygiene to prevent soft tissue inflammation.
• Report oral lesions, soreness, or bleeding to dentist.
• Prevent trauma when using oral hygiene aids.
• Update health and medication history if physician makes any changes in evaluation or drug regimens; include OTC, herbal, and nonherbal remedies in the update.

thiothixene

thye-oh-**thix′**-een
(Navane)
Do not confuse thiothixene with thioridazine.

CATEGORY AND SCHEDULE

Pregnancy Risk Category: C

Drug Class: Thioxanthene/antipsychotic

MECHANISM OF ACTION

An antipsychotic that blocks postsynaptic dopamine receptor sites in brain. Has α-adrenergic blocking effects, and depresses the release of hypothalamic and hypophyseal hormones.
Therapeutic Effect: Suppresses psychotic behavior.

USES

Treatment of psychotic disorders, schizophrenia, acute agitation

PHARMACOKINETICS

Well absorbed from the GI tract after IM administration. Widely distributed. Metabolized in the liver. Primarily excreted in urine. Unknown if removed by hemodialysis. ***Half-life:*** 34 hr.

INDICATIONS AND DOSAGES

▸ **Psychosis**

PO

Adults, Elderly, Children older than 12 yr: Initially, 2 mg 3 times a day. Maximum: 60 mg/day.

IM

Adults, Elderly, Children older than 12 yr: Initially, 4 mg 2–4 times a day. Maximum: 30 mg/day.

SIDE EFFECTS/ADVERSE REACTIONS

Expected

Hypotension, dizziness, syncope (occur frequently after first injection, occasionally after subsequent injections, and rarely with oral form)

Frequent

Transient drowsiness, dry mouth, constipation, blurred vision, nasal congestion

Occasional

Diarrhea, peripheral edema, urine retention, nausea

Rare

Ocular changes, altered skin pigmentation (in those taking high doses for prolonged periods), photosensitivity

PRECAUTIONS AND CONTRAINDICATIONS

Blood dyscrasias, circulatory collapse, CNS depression, coma, history of seizures

Caution:

Lactation, seizure disorders, hypertension, hepatic disease

DRUG INTERACTIONS OF CONCERN TO DENTISTRY

- Increased sedation: other CNS depressants, alcohol, barbiturate anesthetics, opioid analgesics
- Hypotension, tachycardia: epinephrine (systemic)
- Increased extrapyramidal effects: phenothiazines and related drugs (haloperidol, droperidol), metoclopramide
- Additive photosensitization: tetracyclines
- Increased anticholinergic effects: anticholinergics

SERIOUS REACTIONS

! The most common extrapyramidal reaction is akathisia, characterized by motor restlessness and anxiety. Akinesia, marked by rigidity, tremor, increased salivation, mask-like facial expression, and reduced voluntary movements, occurs less frequently. Dystonias, including torticollis, opisthotonos, and oculogyric crisis, occur rarely. Tardive dyskinesia, characterized by tongue protrusion, puffing of the cheeks, and chewing or puckering of the mouth, occurs rarely but may be irreversible. Elderly female patients have a greater risk of developing this reaction. Grand mal seizures may occur in epileptic patients, especially those receiving the drug by IM administration. Neuroleptic malignant syndrome occurs rarely.

DENTAL CONSIDERATIONS

General:

- Monitor vital signs at every appointment because of cardiovascular side effects.
- Patients on chronic drug therapy may rarely have symptoms of blood dyscrasias, which can include infection, bleeding, and poor healing.
- After supine positioning, have patient sit upright for at least 2 min before standing to avoid orthostatic hypotension.
- Assess salivary flow as a factor in caries, periodontal disease, and candidiasis.
- Assess for presence of extrapyramidal motor symptoms, such as tardive dyskinesia and akathisia. Extrapyramidal motor activity may complicate dental treatment.
- Use vasoconstrictors with caution, in low doses, and with careful aspiration.
- Avoid dental light in patient's eyes; offer dark glasses for patient comfort.

- Geriatric patients are more susceptible to drug effects; use lower dose.

Consultations:

- In a patient with symptoms of blood dyscrasias, request a medical consultation for blood studies and postpone dental treatment until normal values are reestablished.
- Take precautions if dental surgery is anticipated and anesthesia is required.
- If signs of tardive dyskinesia or akathisia are present, refer to physician.

Teach Patient/Family to:

- Encourage effective oral hygiene to prevent soft tissue inflammation.
- Use caution to prevent injury when using oral hygiene aids.
- Use powered tooth brush if patient has difficulty holding conventional devices.
- When chronic dry mouth occurs, advise patient to:
  - Avoid mouth rinses with high alcohol content because of drying effects.
  - Use daily home fluoride products to prevent caries.
  - Use sugarless gum, frequent sips of water, or saliva substitutes.

thrombin, topical (thrombinar, thrombin-JMI, thrombostat, etc.)

throm′-bin

CATEGORY AND SCHEDULE

Pregnancy Risk Category: C

Drug Class: Homostatic

MECHANISM OF ACTION

A protein substance produced through a conversion reaction in which prothrombin of bovine origin is activated by tissue thromboplastin in the presence of calcium chloride. It directly clots fibrinogen in the blood.

Therapeutic Effect: Controls bleeding.

USES

Hemostasis

PHARMACOKINETICS

The speed with which thrombin clots blood is dependent upon the concentration of both thrombin and fibrinogen.

INDICATIONS AND DOSAGES

▸ **Hemorrhage, Mild**

Topical

Adults. Apply 100 units/ml as needed.

▸ **Hemorrhage, Severe**

Topical

Adults. Apply 1000 units/ml as needed.

SIDE EFFECTS/ADVERSE REACTIONS

Occasional

Allergic reaction

PRECAUTIONS AND CONTRAINDICATIONS

Sensitivity to thrombin, any of its components and/or to material of bovine origin

DRUG INTERACTIONS OF CONCERN TO DENTISTRY

- None reported

SERIOUS REACTIONS

! Because of its action in the clotting mechanism, thrombin must not be injected or otherwise allowed to enter large blood vessels. Extensive intravascular clotting and even death may result.

DENTAL CONSIDERATIONS

General:

- Solutions (approximately 100 U/ml) are prepared with sterile normal saline or sterile distilled water.
- Can be used with absorbable gelatin sponge but not microfibrillar collagen.

Teach Patient/Family to:

- Report oral lesions, soreness, or bleeding to dentist.

thyroid

thye′-roid

(Armour Thyroid, Nature-Throid NT, Westhroid)

CATEGORY AND SCHEDULE

Pregnancy Risk Category: A

Drug Class: Thyroid hormone

MECHANISM OF ACTION

A natural hormone derived from animal sources, usually beef or pork, that is involved in normal metabolism, growth, and development, especially the CNS of infants. Possesses catabolic and anabolic effects. Provides both levothyroxine and liothyronine hormones.

Therapeutic Effect: Increases basal metabolic rate, enhances gluconeogenesis, stimulates protein synthesis.

USES

Treatment of hypothyroidism, cretinism, myxedema

PHARMACOKINETICS

Partially absorbed from the GI tract. Protein binding: 99%. Widely distributed. Metabolized in liver to active liothyronine (T3), and inactive reverse triiodothyronine (rT3), metabolites. Eliminated by biliary excretion. ***Half-life:*** 2–7 days.

INDICATIONS AND DOSAGES

▸ Hypothyroidism

PO

Adults, Elderly. Initially, 15–30 mg. May increase by 15 mg increments q2–4wk. Maintenance: 60–120 mcg/day. Use 15 mg in patients with cardiovascular disease or myxedema.

Children 12 yr and older. 90 mg/day.

Children 6–12 yr. 60–90 mg/day.

Children older than 1 yr–5 yr. 45–60 mg/day.

Children older than 6–12 mo. 30–45 mg/day.

Children 3 mo and younger. 15–30 mg/day.

SIDE EFFECTS/ADVERSE REACTIONS

Rare

Dry skin, GI intolerance, skin rash, hives, severe headache

PRECAUTIONS AND CONTRAINDICATIONS

Uncontrolled adrenal cortical insufficiency, untreated thyrotoxicosis, treatment of obesity, uncontrolled angina, uncontrolled hypertension, uncontrolled MI, and hypersensitivity to any component of the formulations

Caution:

Lactation, seizure disorders, hypertension, hepatic disease

DRUG INTERACTIONS OF CONCERN TO DENTISTRY

• Increased effects of sympathomimetics when thyroid doses are not carefully monitored or with coronary artery disease

SERIOUS REACTIONS

! Excessive dosage produces signs and symptoms of hyperthyroidism including weight loss, palpitations, increased appetite, tremors, nervousness, tachycardia, hypertension, headache, insomnia, and menstrual irregularities. Cardiac arrhythmias occur rarely.

DENTAL CONSIDERATIONS

General:

• Increased nervousness, excitability, sweating, or tachycardia may indicate uncontrolled hyperthyroidism or a dose of medication that is too high. Uncontrolled patients should be referred for medical treatment.

• Use vasoconstrictors with caution and at low doses.

Consultations:

• Medical consultation may be required to assess disease control.

tiagabine

tye-**ag**′-a-been
(Gabitril)

CATEGORY AND SCHEDULE

Pregnancy Risk Category: C

Drug Class: Anticonvulsant

MECHANISM OF ACTION

An anticonvulsant that enhances the activity of gamma-aminobutyric acid, the major inhibitory neurotransmitter in the CNS.

Therapeutic Effect: Inhibits seizures.

USES

Adjunctive therapy for partial seizures

PHARMACOKINETICS

PO: Rapid absorption, peak plasma levels 0.5–1 hr; highly plasma protein bound (95%), hepatic metabolism (CYP3A isoenzymes), some enterohepatic circulation

INDICATIONS AND DOSAGES

▸ Adjunctive Treatment of Partial Seizures

PO

Adults, Elderly. Initially, 4 mg once a day. May increase by 4–8 mg/day at weekly intervals. Maximum: 56 mg/day.

Children 12–18 yr. Initially, 4 mg once a day. May increase by 4 mg at wk 2 and by 4–8 mg at weekly intervals thereafter. Maximum: 32 mg/day.

SIDE EFFECTS/ADVERSE REACTIONS

Frequent

Dizziness, asthenia, somnolence, nervousness, confusion, headache, infection, tremor

Occasional

Nausea, diarrhea, abdominal pain, impaired concentration

PRECAUTIONS AND CONTRAINDICATIONS

Hepatic disease, Alzheimer's disease, dementia, organic brain disease, stroke

DRUG INTERACTIONS OF CONCERN TO DENTISTRY

• Increased tiagabine clearance: carbamazepine, phenobarbital

• Use CNS depressants with caution because of possible additional effects

SERIOUS REACTIONS

! Overdose is characterized by agitation, confusion, hostility, and weakness. Full recovery occurs within 24 hr.

DENTAL CONSIDERATIONS

General:

• Monitor vital signs at every appointment because of cardiovascular and respiratory side effects.

• Consider semisupine chair position for patient comfort when GI side effects occur.

• Short appointments and a stress-reduction protocol may be required for anxious patients.

• Determine type of epilepsy, seizure frequency, and quality of seizure control.

• Assess salivary flow as factor in caries, periodontal disease, and candidiasis.

• Place on frequent recall if oral side effects occur.

Consultations:

• Consultation with physician may be necessary if sedation or general anesthesia is required.

Teach Patient/Family to:

• Use caution to prevent trauma when using oral hygiene aids.

• Use powered tooth brush if patient has difficulty holding conventional devices.

• Encourage effective oral hygiene to prevent soft tissue inflammation.

• Update health and drug history if physician makes any changes in evaluation or drug regimens; include OTC, herbal, and nonherbal drugs in the update.

• Be aware of oral side effects and potential sequelae.

• When chronic dry mouth occurs, advise patient to:

  • Avoid mouth rinses with high alcohol content because of drying effects.
  • Use daily home fluoride products for anticaries effect.
  • Use sugarless gum, frequent sips of water, or saliva substitutes.

ticagrelor

tye-**ka′**-grel-or

(Brilinta)

CATEGORY AND SCHEDULE

Pregnancy Risk Category: C

Drug Class: Antiplatelet agent

MECHANISM OF ACTION

Inhibits binding of the enzyme adenosine phosphate (ADP) to its platelet receptor and subsequent ADP-mediated activation of a glycoprotein complex, thereby reducing platelet aggregation.

Therapeutic Effect: Inhibits platelet aggregation.

USES

Used in conjunction with aspirin for secondary prevention of thrombotic events in patients with unstable angina (UA), non-ST-elevation myocardial infarction (NSTEMI), or ST-elevation myocardial infarction (STEMI) managed medically or with percutaneous coronary intervention (PCI) and/or coronary artery bypass graft (CABG)

PHARMACOKINETICS

Rapid absorption after oral administration. 99% plasma protein bound. Hepatic metabolism via CYP3A4/5 to an active metabolite. Excreted via the feces (58%) and urine (26%). ***Half-life:*** 7–9 hr.

INDICATIONS AND DOSAGES

▸ Acute Coronary Syndrome: Unstable Angina, Non-ST-Segment Elevation Myocardial Infarction (NSTEMI), ST-Segment Elevation Myocardial Infarction (STEMI)

PO

Adults. Initial: 180-mg loading dose (with a loading dose of aspirin if not already receiving).
Maintenance: 90 mg twice daily; initiated 12 hr after initial loading dose (with low-dose aspirin 75–100 mg/day or 81 mg/day) in patients with UA/NSTEMI.

SIDE EFFECTS/ADVERSE REACTIONS

Frequent

Dyspnea

Occasional

Headache , dizziness, fatigue, bruising, hypokalemia, diarrhea, nausea, back pain, epistaxis, nasopharyngitis

PRECAUTIONS AND CONTRAINDICATIONS

Active pathologic bleeding (e.g., peptic ulcer or intracranial hemorrhage); history of intracranial hemorrhage; hepatic impairment. Use with caution in patients with a history of hyperuricemia or gouty arthritis, respiratory disease.

DRUG INTERACTIONS OF CONCERN TO DENTISTRY

• NSAIDs, aspirin, aspirin-containing products: increased risk of bleeding
• Epinephrine: reduce dose or avoid epinephrine in local anesthetic due to coexisting cardiovascular disease
• CYP3A4 inhibitors (e.g., macrolide antibiotics, azole antifungals): increased blood levels and toxicity of ticagrelor
• CYP3A4 inducers (e.g., carbamazepine, barbiturates): reduced blood levels and efficacy of ticagrelor

SERIOUS REACTIONS

! Ticagrelor increases the risk of bleeding including significant and sometimes fatal bleeding.

DENTAL CONSIDERATIONS

General:

• Monitor vital signs at every appointment due to presence of cardiovascular disease.
• Plan for excessive intraoperative and postoperative bleeding.
• Avoid or limit doses of epinephrine in local anesthetic.
• Short appointments and a stress-reduction protocol may be required for anxious patients.
• Do not modify low-dose aspirin regimen that is used with ticagrelor.

Consultations:

• Consult physician to determine disease status and patient's ability to tolerate dental procedures.

Teach Patient/Family to:

• Report changes in disease status and drug regimen.

ticarcillin

tye-kar-**sill′**-in
(Ticar)

CATEGORY AND SCHEDULE

Pregnancy Risk Category: B

Drug Class: Antibiotic, penicillin

MECHANISM OF ACTION

Binds to bacterial cell wall, inhibiting bacterial cell wall synthesis.
Therapeutic Effect: Bactericidal.

USES

Treatment of infections caused by bacteria

PHARMACOKINETICS

Well absorbed. Widely distributed. Protein binding: 45%–60%. Minimal metabolism in liver. Primarily excreted unchanged in urine. Moderately dialyzable. ***Half-life:*** 1.2 hr (half-life is increased in those with impaired renal function).

INDICATIONS AND DOSAGES

▸ Septicemia; Skin and Skin-Structure, Bone, Joint, and Lower Respiratory Tract Infections; and Endometriosis

IV

Adults, Elderly, Children over 40 kg. 200–300 mg/kg/day q4–6h or 3 g q4h or 4 g q6h. Maximum: 18 g/day.
Children and infants under 40 kg. 200–300 mg/kg/day q4–6h. Maximum: 18 g/day.
Neonates over 2000 g. 75 mg/kg IV q8h under 7 days old; 100 mg/kg IV q8h over 7 old.
Neonates under 2000 g. 75 mg/kg IV q12h under 7 days old; 75 mg/kg q8h over 7 days old.

▸ UTI, Complicated

IV

Adults, Elderly, Children over 40 kg. 150–200 mg/kg/day divided q4–6h or 3 g q6h.
Children under 40 kg. 150–200 mg/kg/day in divided doses q6–8h.

▸ UTI, Uncomplicated

IV/IM

Adults, Elderly, Children over 40 kg. 1 g q6h.
Children under 40 kg. 50–100 mg/kg/day in divided doses q6–8h.

Dosage in Renal Impairment

Creatinine Clearance	Dosage Interval
30–60 ml/min	2 g q4h
10–30 ml/min	2 g q8h
Less than 10 ml/min	2 g q12h

SIDE EFFECTS/ADVERSE REACTIONS

Frequent

Phlebitis, thrombophlebitis with IV dose, rash, urticaria, pruritus, smell or taste disturbances

Occasional

Nausea, diarrhea, vomiting

Rare

Headache, fatigue, hallucinations, bleeding or bruising

PRECAUTIONS AND CONTRAINDICATIONS

Hypersensitivity to any penicillin

DRUG INTERACTIONS OF CONCERN TO DENTISTRY

- Possible increase in bleeding: anticoagulants, thrombolytic drugs, diflunisal (high doses), platelet aggregation inhibitors
- Decreased antimicrobial effectiveness: erythromycins, sulfonamides, tetracyclines
- Possible increase in methotrexate toxicity
- Increased or prolonged plasma levels: probenecid

SERIOUS REACTIONS

! Overdosage may produce seizures and neurologic reactions.
Superinfections including potentially fatal antibiotic-associated colitis; may result from bacterial imbalance.
Severe hypersensitivity reactions, including anaphylaxis, occur rarely.

DENTAL CONSIDERATIONS

General:

- For selected infections in the hospital setting; provide emergency dental treatment only.
- Caution regarding allergy to medication.
- Examine for oral manifestation of opportunistic infection.
- Determine why patient is taking the drug.

Consultations:

- Medical consultation may be required to assess disease control.

Teach Patient/Family to:

- Encourage effective oral hygiene to prevent soft tissue inflammation.
- Report oral lesions, soreness, or bleeding to dentist.
- Prevent trauma when using oral hygiene aids.

ticarcillin disodium/ clavulanate potassium

tie-car-**sill**′-in dye-**soe**′-dee-um/ klah-view-**lan**′-ate poh-**tass**′-ee-um
(Timentin)

CATEGORY AND SCHEDULE

Pregnancy Risk Category: B

Drug Class: Antibiotics, penicillin

MECHANISM OF ACTION

Ticarcillin binds to bacterial cell walls, inhibiting cell wall synthesis. Clavulanate inhibits the action of bacterial β-lactamase.
Therapeutic Effect: Bactericidal.

USES

Treatment of infections caused by bacteria

PHARMACOKINETICS

Widely distributed. Protein binding: ticarcillin 45%–60%, clavulanate 9%–30%. Minimally metabolized in the liver. Primarily excreted unchanged in urine. Removed by hemodialysis. ***Half-life:*** 1–1.2 hr (increased in impaired renal function).

INDICATIONS AND DOSAGES

▸ **Skin and Skin-Structure, Bone, Joint, and Lower Respiratory Tract Infections; Septicemia; Endometriosis**

IV

Adults, Elderly. 3.1 g (3 g ticarcillin) q4–6h. Maximum: 18–24 g/day.
Children 3 mo and older. 200–300 mg (as ticarcillin) q4–6h.

▸ **UTIs**

IV

Adults, Elderly. 3.1 g q6–8h.

▸ **Dosage in Renal Impairment**

Dosage interval is modified on the basis of creatinine clearance.

Creatinine Clearance	Dosage Interval
10–30 ml/min	Usual dose q8h
Less than 10 ml/min	Usual dose q12h

SIDE EFFECTS/ADVERSE REACTIONS

Frequent

Phlebitis or thrombophlebitis (with IV dose), rash, urticaria, pruritus, altered smell or taste

Occasional

Nausea, diarrhea, vomiting

Rare

Headache, fatigue, hallucinations, bleeding, or ecchymosis

PRECAUTIONS AND CONTRAINDICATIONS
Hypersensitivity to any penicillin

DRUG INTERACTIONS OF CONCERN TO DENTISTRY
• Possible increase in bleeding: anticoagulants, thrombolytic drugs, diflunisal (high doses), platelet aggregation inhibitors
• Decreased antimicrobial effectiveness: erythromycins, sulfonamides, tetracyclines
• Possible increase in methotrexate toxicity
• Increased or prolonged plasma levels: probenecid

SERIOUS REACTIONS
! Overdosage may produce seizures and other neurologic reactions. Antibiotic-associated colitis and other superinfections may result from bacterial imbalance. Severe hypersensitivity reactions including anaphylaxis occur rarely.

DENTAL CONSIDERATIONS
General:
• For selected infections in the hospital setting; provide emergency dental treatment only.
• Caution regarding allergy to medication.
• Examine for oral manifestation of opportunistic infection.
• Determine why patient is taking the drug.

Consultations:
• Medical consultation may be required to assess disease control.

Teach Patient/Family to:
• Encourage effective oral hygiene to prevent soft tissue inflammation.
• Report oral lesions, soreness, or bleeding to dentist.
• Prevent trauma when using oral hygiene aids.

T

ticlopidine hydrochloride
tye-**klo′**-pa-deen
high-droh-**klor′**-ide
(Apo-Ticlopidine[CAN], Ticlid, Tilodene[AUS])

CATEGORY AND SCHEDULE
Pregnancy Risk Category: B

Drug Class: Platelet aggregation inhibitor

MECHANISM OF ACTION
An aggregation inhibitor that inhibits the release of adenosine diphosphate from activated platelets, which prevents fibrinogen from binding to glycoprotein IIb/IIIa receptors on the surface of activated platelets.
Therapeutic Effect: Inhibits platelet aggregation and thrombus formation.

USES
Reduction of the risk of stroke in high-risk patients

PHARMACOKINETICS
Peak 1–3 hr, half-life increases with repeated dosing; metabolized by the liver; excreted in urine, feces.

INDICATIONS AND DOSAGES
▸ **Prevention of Stroke**
PO
Adults, Elderly. 250 mg twice a day.

SIDE EFFECTS/ADVERSE REACTIONS
Frequent
Diarrhea, nausea, dyspepsia including heartburn, indigestion GI discomfort, and bloating
Rare
Vomiting, flatulence, pruritus, dizziness

PRECAUTIONS AND CONTRAINDICATIONS

Active pathologic bleeding, such as bleeding peptic ulcer and intracranial bleeding, hematopoietic disorders including neutropenia and thrombocytopenia; presence of hemostatic disorder; severe hepatic impairment

Caution:

Past liver disease, renal disease, elderly, lactation, children; increased bleeding risk requires hematologic monitoring every 2 wk for the first 3 mo of therapy

DRUG INTERACTIONS OF CONCERN TO DENTISTRY

- Increased bleeding tendencies: aspirin, NSAIDs

SERIOUS REACTIONS

! Neutropenia occurs in approximately 2% of patients. Thrombotic thrombocytopenia purpura, agranulocytosis, hepatitis, cholestatic jaundice, and tinnitus occur rarely.

DENTAL CONSIDERATIONS

General:

- Patients on chronic drug therapy may rarely have symptoms of blood dyscrasias, which can include infection, bleeding, and poor healing.
- Consider local hemostatic measures to prevent excessive bleeding.
- Do not discontinue for routine dental procedures.

Consultations:

- Medical consultation may be required to assess disease control and patient's ability to tolerate stress. Consultation should include data on hematologic profile.

Teach Patient/Family to:

- Prevent injury when using oral hygiene aids.

tiludronate

ti-**loo**′-dro-nate
(Skelid)

CATEGORY AND SCHEDULE

Pregnancy Risk Category: C

Drug Class: Bisphosphonate derivative

MECHANISM OF ACTION

A calcium regulator that inhibits functioning osteoclasts through disruption of cytoskeletal ring structure and inhibition of osteoclastic proton pump.
Therapeutic Effect: Inhibits bone resorption.

USES

Treatment of Paget's disease of bone in patients with twice normal upper limit values for serum alkaline phosphatase (SAP) and who are symptomatic and at risk for future complications

PHARMACOKINETICS

PO: Rapid but incomplete absorption, bioavailability 6% (fasted), peak plasma levels 2 hr, little or no metabolism, excreted in urine.

INDICATIONS AND DOSAGES

▸ **Paget's Disease**

PO

Adults, Elderly. 400 mg once a day for 3 mo. Must take with 6–8 oz plain water. Do not give within 2 hr of food intake. Avoid giving aspirin, calcium supplements, mineral supplements, or antacids within 2 hr of tiludronate administration.

SIDE EFFECTS/ADVERSE REACTIONS

Frequent

Nausea, diarrhea, generalized body pain, back pain, headache

Occasional

Rash, dyspepsia, vomiting, rhinitis, sinusitis, dizziness

PRECAUTIONS AND CONTRAINDICATIONS

GI disease, such as dysphagia and gastric ulcer, impaired renal function

Caution:

Lactation, safety in children younger than 18 yr not established

DRUG INTERACTIONS OF CONCERN TO DENTISTRY

- Bioavailability decreased by calcium, food, aluminum or magnesium antacids.
- Do not take indomethacin, aspirin, or calcium supplements 2 hr before or after tiludronate.

SERIOUS REACTIONS

! Acute renal failure associated with hypocalcemia

DENTAL CONSIDERATIONS

General:

- Potential for osteonecrosis of the jaw (emphasize preventive care and avoid invasive procedures).
- Be aware of oral manifestations of Paget's disease (macrognathia, alveolar pain).
- Consider semisupine chair position for patient comfort when GI side effects occur.
- Consider short appointments for patient comfort.
- Assess salivary flow as a factor in caries, periodontal disease, and candidiasis.

Consultations:

- Medical consultation may be required to assess disease control.

Teach Patient/Family to:

- Use caution to prevent trauma when using oral hygiene aids.
- Encourage effective oral hygiene to prevent soft tissue inflammation.
- Update health and drug history if physician makes any changes in evaluation or drug regimens; include OTC, herbal, and nonherbal drugs in the update.
- When chronic dry mouth occurs, advise patient to:
  - Avoid mouth rinses with high alcohol content because of drying effects.
  - Use daily home fluoride products for anticaries effect.
  - Use sugarless gum, frequent sips of water, or saliva substitutes.

timolol maleate

tim′-oh-lole **mal′**-ee-ate

(Apo-Timol[CAN], Apo-Timop[CAN], Betimol, Blocadren, Gen-Timolol[CAN], Istalol, Optimol[AUS], PMS-Timolol[CAN], Tenopt[AUS], Timoptic, Timoptic Ocudose, Timoptic XE, Timoptol[AUS], Timoptol XE[AUS])

Do not confuse timolol with atenolol, or Timoptic with Viroptic.

CATEGORY AND SCHEDULE

Pregnancy Risk Category: C (D if used in second or third trimester)

Drug Class: Nonselective β-adrenergic blocker

MECHANISM OF ACTION

An antihypertensive, antimigraine, and antiglaucoma agent that blocks β_1- and β_2-adrenergic receptors. ***Therapeutic Effect:*** Reduces intraocular pressure (IOP) by reducing aqueous humor production, lowers B/P, slows the heart rate, and decreases myocardial contractility.

USES

Treatment of mild-to-moderate hypertension, reduction of mortality risk after MI, migraine prophylaxis; unapproved uses: essential tremors, angina, cardiac dysrhythmias, anxiety, mild-to-moderate heart failure

PHARMACOKINETICS

Route	Onset	Peak	Duration
PO	15–45 min	0.5–2.5 hr	4 hr
Ophthalmic	30 min	1–2 hr	12–24 hr

Well absorbed from the GI tract. Protein binding: 60%. Minimal absorption after ophthalmic administration. Metabolized in the liver. Primarily excreted in urine. Not removed by hemodialysis. ***Half-life:*** 4 hr. Systemic absorption may occur with ophthalmic administration.

INDICATIONS AND DOSAGES

▸ Mild-to-Moderate Hypertension

PO

Adults, Elderly. Initially, 10 mg twice a day, alone or in combination with other therapy. Gradually increase at intervals of not less than 1 wk. Maintenance: 20–60 mg/day in 2 divided doses.

▸ Reduction of Cardiovascular Mortality in Definite or Suspected Acute MI

PO

Adults, Elderly. 10 mg twice a day, beginning 1–4 wk after infarction.

▸ Migraine Prevention

PO

Adults, Elderly. Initially, 10 mg twice a day. Range: 10–30 mg/day.

▸ Reduction of IOP in Open-Angle Glaucoma, Aphakic Glaucoma, Ocular Hypertension, and Secondary Glaucoma

Ophthalmic

Adults, Elderly, Children. 1 drop of 0.25% solution in affected eye(s) twice a day. May be increased to 1 drop of 0.5% solution in affected eye(s) twice a day. When IOP is controlled, dosage may be reduced to 1 drop once a day. If patient is switched to timolol from another antiglaucoma agent, administer concurrently for 1 day. Discontinue other agent on following day.

Ophthalmic (Timoptic XE)

Adults, Elderly. 1 drop/day.

Ophthalmic (Istalol)

Adults, Elderly. Apply once a day.

SIDE EFFECTS/ADVERSE REACTIONS

Frequent

Diminished sexual function, drowsiness, difficulty sleeping, unusual tiredness or weakness

Ophthalmic: Eye irritation, visual disturbances

Occasional

Depression, cold hands or feet, diarrhea, constipation, anxiety, nasal congestion, nausea, vomiting

Rare

Altered taste, dry eyes, itching, numbness of fingers, toes, or scalp

PRECAUTIONS AND CONTRAINDICATIONS

Bronchial asthma, cardiogenic shock, CHF unless secondary to tachyarrhythmias, COPD, patients receiving MAOI therapy, second- or third-degree heart block, sinus bradycardia, uncontrolled cardiac failure

Caution:

Major surgery, lactation, diabetes mellitus, renal disease, thyroid disease, COPD, well-compensated heart failure, CAD, nonallergic bronchospasm

DRUG INTERACTIONS OF CONCERN TO DENTISTRY

• Increased B/P, bradycardia: anticholinergics, sympathomimetics (epinephrine)
• Decreased antihypertensive effects: indomethacin and other NSAIDs
• Suspected increase in plasma levels: diphenhydramine
• May slow metabolism of lidocaine

Optic

• Avoid use of anticholinergic drugs, atropine-like drugs, propantheline, and diazepam (benzodiazepines)

SERIOUS REACTIONS

! Overdose may produce profound bradycardia, hypotension, and bronchospasm.
! Abrupt withdrawal may result in diaphoresis, palpitations, headache, and tremors.
! Timolol administration may precipitate CHF and MI in patients with cardiac disease, thyroid storm in those with thyrotoxicosis, and peripheral ischemia in those with existing peripheral vascular disease. Hypoglycemia may occur in patients with previously controlled diabetes.
! Ophthalmic overdose may produce bradycardia, hypotension, bronchospasm, and acute cardiac failure.

T

DENTAL CONSIDERATIONS

General:

• Potentially reduced effectiveness of epinephrine administered for anaphylaxis.
• Monitor vital signs at every appointment because of cardiovascular side effects.
• Patients on chronic drug therapy may rarely have symptoms of blood dyscrasias, which can include infection, bleeding, and poor healing.
• Assess salivary flow as a factor in caries, periodontal disease, and candidiasis.
• Limit use of sodium-containing products, such as saline IV fluids, for patients with a dietary salt restriction.
• After supine positioning, have patient sit upright for at least 2 min before standing to avoid orthostatic hypotension.
• Stress from dental procedures may compromise cardiovascular function; determine patient risk.
• Short appointments and a stress-reduction protocol may be required for anxious patients.
• Consider semisupine chair position for patients with nausea or respiratory distress.

Consultations:

• In a patient with symptoms of blood dyscrasias, request a medical consultation for blood studies and postpone dental treatment until normal values are reestablished.
• Medical consultation may be required to assess disease control and patient's ability to tolerate stress.

Teach Patient/Family to:

• Encourage effective oral hygiene to prevent soft tissue inflammation.
• Use caution to prevent injury when using oral hygiene aids.
• When chronic dry mouth occurs, advise patient to:
  • Avoid mouth rinses with high alcohol content because of drying effects.
  • Use daily home fluoride products to prevent caries.
  • Use sugarless gum, frequent sips of water, or saliva substitutes.

Optic

General:

- Check compliance of patient with prescribed drug regimen for glaucoma.
- Avoid dental light in patient's eyes; offer dark glasses for patient comfort.

Consultations:

- Consultation with physician may be necessary if sedation or anesthesia is required.

tinzaparin sodium

tin-**za'**-pair-in **soe'**-dee-um
(Innohep)

CATEGORY AND SCHEDULE

Pregnancy Risk Category: B

Drug Class: Anticoagulant

MECHANISM OF ACTION

A low-molecular-weight heparin that inhibits factor Xa. Causes less inactivation of thrombin, inhibition of platelets, and bleeding than standard heparin. Does not significantly influence bleeding time, PT, aPTT.
Therapeutic Effect: Anticoagulant.

USES

Prevention and/or treatment of deep venous thrombosis (DVT), a condition in which harmful blood clots form in the blood vessels of the legs

PHARMACOKINETICS

Well absorbed after subcutaneous administration. Primarily eliminated in urine. ***Half-life:*** 3–4 hr.

INDICATIONS AND DOSAGES

▸ **DVT**

Subcutaneous

Adults, Elderly. 175 anti-Xa international units/kg once a day. Continue for at least 6 days and until patient is sufficiently anticoagulated with warfarin (INR of 2 or more for 2 consecutive days).

SIDE EFFECTS/ADVERSE REACTIONS

Frequent

Injection site reaction, such as inflammation, oozing, nodules, and skin necrosis

Rare

Nausea, asthenia, constipation, epistaxis

PRECAUTIONS AND CONTRAINDICATIONS

Active major bleeding, concurrent heparin therapy, hypersensitivity to heparin or pork products, thrombocytopenia associated with positive in vitro test for antiplatelet antibody

DRUG INTERACTIONS OF CONCERN TO DENTISTRY

- Increased risk of bleeding: drugs that interfere with coagulation or platelet function, such as NSAIDs and aspirin

SERIOUS REACTIONS

! Overdose may lead to bleeding complications ranging from local ecchymoses to major hemorrhage. Antidote: Dose of protamine sulfate (1% solution) should be equal to dose of tinzaparin injected. 1 mg protamine sulfate neutralizes 100 units of tinzaparin. A second dose of 0.5 mg tinzaparin per 1 mg protamine sulfate may be given if aPTT tested 2–4 hr after the initial infusion remains prolonged.

DENTAL CONSIDERATIONS

General:

- Do not discontinue for routine dental procedures.
- Determine why patient is taking the drug.
- Consider local hemostasis measures to prevent excessive bleeding.
- Avoid products that affect platelet function, such as aspirin and NSAIDs.
- Antibiotic prophylaxis prior to dental treatment may be required for joint prosthesis.
- Patient may need assistance in getting into and out of dental chair. Adjust chair position for patient comfort.
- Product may be used in outpatient therapy. Delay elective dental treatment until patient completes tinzaparin therapy.

Consultations:

- Medical consultation should include routine blood counts including platelet counts and bleeding time.

Teach Patient/Family to:

- Prevent trauma when using oral hygiene aids.
- Report oral lesions, soreness, or bleeding to dentist.
- Encourage effective oral hygiene to prevent soft tissue inflammation.

T

tioconazole

tyo-**con′**-ah-zole
(Gynecure[CAN], Monistat-1, Trosyd[CAN], Vagistat)

CATEGORY AND SCHEDULE

Pregnancy Risk Category: C

Drug Class: Antifungals, topical, dermatologics

MECHANISM OF ACTION

An imidazole derivative that inhibits synthesis of ergosterol (vital component of fungal cell formation). ***Therapeutic Effect:*** Fungistatic.

USES

Treatment of infections caused by a fungus or yeast

PHARMACOKINETICS

Negligible absorption from vaginal application.

INDICATIONS AND DOSAGES

▸ Vulvovaginal Candidiasis

Intravaginal

Adults, Elderly. 1 applicatorful just before bedtime as a single dose.

SIDE EFFECTS/ADVERSE REACTIONS

Frequent

Headache

Occasional

Burning, itching

Rare

Irritation, vaginal pain, dysuria, dryness of vaginal secretions, vulvar edema/swelling

PRECAUTIONS AND CONTRAINDICATIONS

Hypersensitivity to tioconazole or other imidazole antifungal agents

DRUG INTERACTIONS OF CONCERN TO DENTISTRY

- None reported

SERIOUS REACTIONS

! None reported

DENTAL CONSIDERATIONS

General:

- Be aware that broad-spectrum antibiotics can exacerbate vaginal candidiasis.

tiotropium bromide

tee-oh-**trow′**-pea-um **broe′**-mide
(Spiriva)

CATEGORY AND SCHEDULE

Pregnancy Risk Category: C

Drug Class: Anticholinergics, bronchodilators

MECHANISM OF ACTION

An anticholinergic that binds to recombinant human muscarinic receptors at the smooth muscle, resulting in long-acting bronchial smooth-muscle relaxation. ***Therapeutic Effect:*** Relieves bronchospasm.

USES

Treatment of bronchospasm (wheezing or difficulty in breathing) that is associated with chronic obstructive pulmonary disease (COPD)

PHARMACOKINETICS

Route	Onset	Peak	Duration
Inhalation	N/A	N/A	24–36 hr

Binds extensively to tissue. Protein binding: 72%. Metabolized by oxidation. Excreted in urine. ***Half-life:*** 5–6 days.

INDICATIONS AND DOSAGES

▸ COPD

Inhalation

Adults, Elderly. 18 mcg (1 capsule)/day via HandiHaler inhalation device.

SIDE EFFECTS/ADVERSE REACTIONS

Frequent

Dry mouth, sinusitis, pharyngitis, dyspepsia, UTI, rhinitis

Occasional

Abdominal pain, peripheral edema, constipation, epistaxis, vomiting, myalgia, rash, oral candidiasis

PRECAUTIONS AND CONTRAINDICATIONS

History of hypersensitivity to atropine or its derivatives, including ipratropium

DRUG INTERACTIONS OF CONCERN TO DENTISTRY

• Dental drug interactions have not been studied.

SERIOUS REACTIONS

! Angina pectoris, depression, and flu-like symptoms occur rarely.

DENTAL CONSIDERATIONS

General:

• Monitor vital signs, especially respiration.
• Ask patient about exercise and activity tolerance.
• Caution: Not for acute episodes or emergency use.
• Assess salivary flow as a factor in caries, periodontal disease, and candidiasis.
• Place on frequent recall due to oral side effects.
• Acute asthmatic episodes may be precipitated in the dental office. A rapid-acting sympathomimetic inhalant (rescue inhaler) should be available for emergency use. Many patients may already have a prescribed rescue inhaler they normally use for acute asthmatic events.
• Consider semisupine chair position for patients with respiratory disease.

Consultations:

• Medical consultation may be required to assess disease control and patient's ability to tolerate stress.

Teach Patient/Family to:
• Gargle, rinse mouth with water, and expectorate after each aerosol dose.
• When chronic dry mouth occurs, advise patient to:
  • Avoid mouth rinses with high alcohol content due to drying effects.
  • Use daily home fluoride products for anticaries effect.
  • Use sugarless gum, frequent sips of water, or saliva substitutes.

tirofiban

tye-roe-**fye**′-ban
(Aggrastat)
Do not confuse Aggrastat with Aggrenox.

CATEGORY AND SCHEDULE

Pregnancy Risk Category: B

Drug Class: Platelet inhibitor

MECHANISM OF ACTION

An antiplatelet and antithrombotic agent that binds to platelet receptor glycoprotein IIb/IIIa, preventing binding of fibrinogen.
Therapeutic Effect: Inhibits platelet aggregation and thrombus formation.

T

USES

An antiplatelet in combination with heparin, treatment of acute coronary syndrome, including those to be managed medically and those undergoing percutaneous transluminal coronary angioplasty (PTCA) or atherectomy

PHARMACOKINETICS

Poorly bound to plasma proteins; unbound fraction in plasma: 35%. Limited metabolism. Primarily eliminated in the urine (65%) and, to a lesser amount, in the feces. Removed by hemodialysis. ***Half-life:*** 2 hr. Clearance is significantly decreased in severe renal impairment (creatinine clearance less than 30 ml/min).

INDICATIONS AND DOSAGES

▸ **Inhibition of Platelet Aggregation**
IV
Adults, Elderly. Initially, 0.4 mcg/kg/min for 30 min; then continue at 0.1 mcg/kg/min through procedure and for 12–24 hr after procedure.
▸ **Severe Renal Insufficiency (Creatinine Clearance Less Than 30 ml/min)**
Adults, Elderly. Half the usual rate of IV infusion.

SIDE EFFECTS/ADVERSE REACTIONS

Occasional
Pelvis pain, bradycardia, dizziness, leg pain
Rare
Edema and swelling, vasovagal reaction, diaphoresis, nausea, fever, headache

PRECAUTIONS AND CONTRAINDICATIONS

Active internal bleeding or a history of bleeding diathesis within previous 30 days, arteriovenous malformation or aneurysm, history of intracranial hemorrhage, history of thrombocytopenia after prior exposure to tirofiban, intracranial neoplasm, major surgical procedure within previous 30 days, severe hypertension, stroke

DRUG INTERACTIONS OF CONCERN TO DENTISTRY

• Increased risk of bleeding: drugs that interfere with coagulation or platelet function, such as NSAIDs and aspirin

SERIOUS REACTIONS

! Signs and symptoms of overdose include generally minor mucocutaneous bleeding and bleeding at the femoral artery access site. Thrombocytopenia occurs rarely.

DENTAL CONSIDERATIONS

General:

• An acute-use drug for use in hospitals or emergency departments. If a patient should report this drug in his/her medical history, question about cardiovascular disease and drugs he or she may be taking.

• Patients are at risk for bleeding while receiving this drug; provide palliative dental care for dental emergencies only.

• Avoid products that affect platelet function, such as aspirin and NSAIDs.

Consultations:

• Medical consultation should include routine blood counts, including platelet counts and bleeding time.

• Medical consultation may be required to assess disease control and patient's ability to tolerate stress.

Teach Patient/Family:

• To inform dentist of unusual bleeding episodes following dental treatment.

tobramycin

toe-bra-**mye′**-sin

(Nebcin, Nebcin Pediatric, TOBI)

CATEGORY AND SCHEDULE

Pregnancy Risk Category: C

Drug Class: Antiinfective

MECHANISM OF ACTION

An aminoglycoside antibiotic that irreversibly binds to protein on bacterial ribosomes reduces protein synthesis of susceptible microorganisms.

Therapeutic Effect: Bacteriostatic.

USES

Treatment of serious bacterial infections

PHARMACOKINETICS

Rapid, complete absorption after IM administration. Protein binding: less than 30%. Widely distributed but does not cross the blood-brain barrier and is in low concentrations in CSF. Excreted unchanged in urine. Removed by hemodialysis. ***Half-life:*** 2 hr. Half-life is increased with impaired renal function and in neonates. Half-life is decreased in cystic fibrosis, febrile, or burn patients.

INDICATIONS AND DOSAGES

▸ **Skin/Skin-Structure, Bone, Joint, Respiratory Tract, Postoperative, Burn, Intraabdominal Infections; Complicated UTI; Septicemia; Meningitis**

IM/IV

Adults, Elderly. 3 mg/kg/day in 3 divided doses. May use up to 5 mg/kg/day in 3 to 4 equal doses.

▸ **Cystic Fibrosis**

Inhalation

Adult, Elderly, Children 6 yr and older. 1 ampule (300 mg) via nebulizer twice daily (28 days on, 28 days off). Consider starting elderly patients at 3 mg/kg IV q8h.

▸ **Dosage in Renal Impairment**

Dosage and frequency are modified on the basis of degree of renal impairment and the serum concentration of the drug. After a loading dose of 1–2 mg/kg, the

T

maintenance dose and frequency are based on serum creatinine levels and creatinine clearance. Dosage should be reduced to 3 mg/kg/day as soon as clinically indicated. Dosage should not exceed 5 mg/kg/day.

SIDE EFFECTS/ADVERSE REACTIONS

Occasional

IM: Pain, induration at IM injection site

IV: Phlebitis, thrombophlebitis

Rare

Hypotension, nausea, vomiting

PRECAUTIONS AND CONTRAINDICATIONS

Hypersensitivity to aminoglycosides (cross-sensitivity)

DRUG INTERACTIONS OF CONCERN TO DENTISTRY

- Increased risk of nephrotoxicity: cephalosporins, enflurane, vancomycin
- Increased neuromuscular blocking effects: neuromuscular blockers

SERIOUS REACTIONS

! Nephrotoxicity, as evidenced by increased BUN and serum creatinine and decreased creatinine clearance, may be reversible if the drug is stopped at the first sign of nephrotoxic symptoms.

! Irreversible ototoxicity, manifested as tinnitus, dizziness, ringing or roaring in ears, impaired hearing and neurotoxicity, as evidenced by headache, dizziness, lethargy, tremors, and visual disturbances, occur occasionally. The risk of irreversible neurotoxicity and ototoxicity is greater with higher dosages, prolonged therapy, or if the solution is applied directly to the mucosa.

! Superinfections, particularly with fungi, may result from bacterial imbalance with any route of administration. Anaphylaxis may occur.

DENTAL CONSIDERATIONS

General:

- For selected infections in the hospital setting; provide emergency dental treatment only.
- Caution regarding allergy to medication.
- Examine for oral manifestation of opportunistic infection.
- Determine why patient is taking the drug.

Consultations:

- Medical consultation may be required to assess disease control in the patient.

Teach Patient/Family to:

- Encourage effective oral hygiene to prevent soft tissue inflammation.
- Report oral lesions, soreness, or bleeding to dentist.
- Prevent trauma when using oral hygiene aids.

tobramycin sulfate

tow-bra-**my′**-sin **sull′**-fate

(AK-Tob, Apo-Tobramycin[CAN], Nebcin, PMS-Tobramycin, TOBI, Tobrex)

CATEGORY AND SCHEDULE

Pregnancy Risk Category: C (B, ophthalmic form)

Drug Class: Antiinfective

MECHANISM OF ACTION

An aminoglycoside antibiotic that irreversibly binds to protein on bacterial ribosomes; interferes with

T

protein synthesis of susceptible microorganisms.
Therapeutic Effect: Bacteriostatic.

USES

Treatment of serious bacterial infections

PHARMACOKINETICS

Rapid, complete absorption after IM administration. Protein binding: less than 30%. Widely distributed (doesn't cross the blood-brain barrier; low concentrations in CSF). Excreted unchanged in urine. Removed by hemodialysis. ***Half-life:*** 2–4 hr (increased in impaired renal function and neonates; decreased in cystic fibrosis and febrile or burn patients).

INDICATIONS AND DOSAGES

▸ Skin and Skin-Structure, Bone, Joint, Respiratory Tract, Postoperative, Intraabdominal, and Burn Wound Infections; Complicated UTIs; Septicemia; Meningitis

IV, IM
Adults, Elderly. 3–6 mg/kg/day in 3 divided doses or 4–6.6 mg/kg once a day.

▸ Superficial Eye Infections Including Blepharitis, Conjunctivitis, Keratitis, and Corneal Ulcers

Ophthalmic Ointment
Adults, Elderly. Usual dosage, apply a thin strip to conjunctiva q8–12h (q3–4h for severe infections).
Ophthalmic Solution
Adults, Elderly. Usual dosage, 1–2 drops in affected eye q4h (2 drops/hr for severe infections).

▸ Bronchopulmonary Infections in Patients with Cystic Fibrosis

Inhalation Solution
Adults. Usual dosage, 60–80 mg twice a day for 28 days, then off for 28 days.
Children. 40–80 mg 2–3 times a day.

▸ Dosage in Renal Impairment

Dosage and frequency are modified on the basis of the degree of renal impairment and the serum drug concentration. After a loading dose of 1–2 mg/kg, the maintenance dose and frequency are based on serum creatinine levels and creatinine clearance.

SIDE EFFECTS/ADVERSE REACTIONS

Occasional
IM: Pain, induration
IV: Phlebitis, thrombophlebitis
Topical: Hypersensitivity reaction (fever, pruritus, rash, urticaria)
Ophthalmic: Tearing, itching, redness, eyelid swelling
Rare
Hypotension, nausea, vomiting

PRECAUTIONS AND CONTRAINDICATIONS

Hypersensitivity to tobramycin, other aminoglycosides (cross-sensitivity), and their components

DRUG INTERACTIONS OF CONCERN TO DENTISTRY

• Antibiotics: potentially reduced effectiveness

SERIOUS REACTIONS

! Nephrotoxicity (as evidenced by increased BUN and serum creatinine levels and decreased creatinine clearance) may be reversible if the drug is stopped at the first sign of nephrotoxic symptoms. Irreversible ototoxicity (manifested as tinnitus, dizziness, ringing or roaring in ears, and hearing loss) and neurotoxicity (manifested as headache, dizziness, lethargy, tremor, and visual disturbances) occur occasionally. The risk of these reactions increases with higher dosages or prolonged therapy and when the solution is applied directly to the mucosa. Superinfections, particularly fungal infections, may result from bacterial imbalance with any administration route.

! Anaphylaxis may occur.

DENTAL CONSIDERATIONS

General:

- Avoid directing dental light into patient's eyes; provide dark glasses during treatment to avoid irritation.
- Protect patient's eyes from accidental spatter during dental treatment.

tocainide hydrochloride

toe'-kay-nide high-droh-**klor'**-ide
(Tonocard)

CATEGORY AND SCHEDULE

Pregnancy Risk Category: C

Drug Class: Antidysrhythmic (class IB), lidocaine analogue

MECHANISM OF ACTION

An amide-type local anesthetic that shortens the action potential duration and decreases the effective refractory period and automaticity in the His-Purkinje system of the myocardium by blocking sodium transport across myocardial cell membranes.

Therapeutic Effect: Suppresses ventricular dysrhythmias.

USES

Treatment of documented life-threatening ventricular dysrhythmias

PHARMACOKINETICS

PO: Peak 0.5–3 hr. ***Half-life:*** 10–17 hr; metabolized by liver; excreted in urine.

INDICATIONS AND DOSAGES

▸ Suppression and Prevention of Ventricular Arrhythmias

PO

Adults, Elderly. Initially, 400 mg q8h. Maintenance: 1.2–1.8 g/day in divided doses q8h. Maximum: 2400 mg/day.

SIDE EFFECTS/ADVERSE REACTIONS

Tocainide is generally well tolerated.

Frequent

Minor, transient light-headedness, dizziness, nausea, paresthesia, rash, tremor

Occasional

Clammy skin, night sweats, myalgia

Rare

Restlessness, nervousness, disorientation, mood changes, ataxia (muscular incoordination), visual disturbances

PRECAUTIONS AND CONTRAINDICATIONS

Hypersensitivity to local anesthetics, second- or third-degree AV block

Caution:

Lactation, children, renal disease, liver disease, CHF, respiratory depression, myasthenia gravis, blood dyscrasias

DRUG INTERACTIONS OF CONCERN TO DENTISTRY

- No specific interactions are reported with dental drugs; however, any drug that could affect the cardiac action of tocainide (local anesthetics, vasoconstrictors, and anticholinergics) should be used in the least effective dose.

SERIOUS REACTIONS

! High dosage may produce bradycardia or tachycardia, hypotension, palpitations, increased ventricular arrhythmias, premature ventricular contractions (PVCs), chest pain, and exacerbation of CHF.

DENTAL CONSIDERATIONS

General:

- Monitor vital signs at every appointment because of cardiovascular and respiratory side effects.
- After supine positioning, have patient sit upright for at least 2 min before standing to avoid orthostatic hypotension.
- Patients on chronic drug therapy may rarely have symptoms of blood dyscrasias, which can include infection, bleeding, and poor healing.
- Assess salivary flow as a factor in caries, periodontal disease, and candidiasis.
- Stress from dental procedures may compromise cardiovascular function; determine patient risk.

Consultations:

- In a patient with symptoms of blood dyscrasias, request a medical consultation for blood studies and postpone dental treatment until normal values are reestablished.
- Medical consultation may be required to assess disease control and patient's ability to tolerate stress.

Teach Patient/Family to:

- Encourage effective oral hygiene to prevent soft tissue inflammation.
- Use caution to prevent injury when using oral hygiene aids.
- When chronic dry mouth occurs, advise patient to:
  - Avoid mouth rinses with high alcohol content because of drying effects.
  - Use daily home fluoride products to prevent caries.
  - Use sugarless gum, frequent sips of water, or saliva substitutes.

tolazamide

tole-**az**′-ah-mide
(Tolinase)
Do not confuse with tolbutamide, tocainide, or tolazine.

CATEGORY AND SCHEDULE

Pregnancy Risk Category: D

Drug Class: Sulfonylurea (first-generation) oral antidiabetic

MECHANISM OF ACTION

A first-generation sulfonylurea that promotes release of insulin from beta cells of pancreas.
Therapeutic Effect: Lowers blood glucose concentration.

USES

Treatment of type 2 diabetes mellitus

PHARMACOKINETICS

Well absorbed from the GI tract. Extensively metabolized in liver to five metabolites, three of which are active. Primarily excreted in urine. Unknown if removed by hemodialysis. ***Half-life:*** 7 hr.

INDICATIONS AND DOSAGES

▸ Diabetes Mellitus

PO

Adults, Elderly. Initially, 100–250 mg once a day, with breakfast or first main meal. Maintenance: 100–1000 mg once a day. May increase by increments of 100–250 mg weekly on the basis of blood glucose response. May increase by 100–250 mg/day at weekly intervals. Maximum: 1000 mg/day. Doses more than 500 mg/day should be given in 2 divided doses with meals.

SIDE EFFECTS/ADVERSE REACTIONS

Frequent

Altered taste sensation, dizziness, drowsiness, weight gain, constipation, diarrhea, heartburn, nausea, vomiting, stomach fullness, headache

Occasional

Increased sensitivity of skin to sunlight, peeling of skin, itching, rash

PRECAUTIONS AND CONTRAINDICATIONS

Diabetic complications, such as ketosis, acidosis, and diabetic coma, sole therapy for type 1 diabetes mellitus, hypersensitivity to tolazamide or its components

Caution:

Elderly, cardiac disease, thyroid disease, severe hypoglycemic reactions, renal disease, hepatic disease

DRUG INTERACTIONS OF CONCERN TO DENTISTRY

- Increased hypoglycemic reaction: NSAIDs, salicylates, ketoconazole, miconazole
- Decreased action of tolazamide: corticosteroids, sympathomimetics (epinephrine)

SERIOUS REACTIONS

! Severe hypoglycemia may occur due to overdosage and insufficient food intake, especially with increased glucose demands.

! GI hemorrhage, cholestatic hepatic jaundice, leukopenia, thrombocytopenia, pancytopenia, agranulocytosis, and aplastic or hemolytic anemia occur rarely.

DENTAL CONSIDERATIONS

General:

- Patients on chronic drug therapy may rarely have symptoms of blood dyscrasias, which can include infection, bleeding, and poor healing.
- Be prepared to manage hypoglycemia.
- Place on frequent recall to evaluate healing response.
- Short appointments and a stress-reduction protocol may be required for anxious patients.
- Diabetics may be more susceptible to infection and have delayed wound healing.
- Anticipate possible hypoglycemic episodes.
- Ensure that patient is following prescribed diet and regularly takes medication.
- Question patient about self-monitoring of drug's antidiabetic effect.
- Avoid prescribing aspirin-containing products.

Consultations:

- In a patient with symptoms of blood dyscrasias, request a medical consultation for blood studies and postpone dental treatment until normal values are reestablished.
- Medical consultation may be required to assess disease control.

Teach Patient/Family to:

- Encourage effective oral hygiene to prevent soft tissue inflammation.
- Avoid mouth rinses with high alcohol content because of drying effects.

tolbutamide

tole-**byoo**′-ta-mide
(Apo-Tolbutamide[CAN], Orinase, Orinase Diagnostic, Rastinon[AUS], Tol-Tab)
Do not confuse with tolazamide, tocainide, or tolazine.

CATEGORY AND SCHEDULE

Pregnancy Risk Category: C

Drug Class: Sulfonylurea (first-generation) oral antidiabetic

MECHANISM OF ACTION

A first-generation sulfonylurea that promotes the release of insulin from β cells of pancreas.
Therapeutic Effect: Lowers blood glucose concentration.

USES

Treatment of type 2 diabetes mellitus

PHARMACOKINETICS

Route	Onset	Peak	Duration
PO	1 hr	5–8 hr	12–24 hr
IV	N/A	30–45 min	90–180 min

Well absorbed from the GI tract. Protein binding: 80%–99%. Extensively metabolized in liver to two inactive metabolites, primarily via oxidation. Excreted in urine. Removed by hemodialysis. ***Half-life:*** 4.5–6.5 hr.

INDICATIONS AND DOSAGES

▸ **Diabetes Mellitus**

PO

Adults. Initially, 1 g daily, with breakfast or first main meal, or in divided doses. Maintenance: 0.25–3 g once a day. After dose of 2 g is reached, dosage should be increased in increments of up to 2 mg q1–2wk, based on blood glucose response. Maximum: 3 g/day.

▸ **Endocrine Tumor Diagnosis**

IV

Adults. 1 g infused over 2–3 min.

SIDE EFFECTS/ADVERSE REACTIONS

Frequent

Increased sensitivity of skin to sunlight, peeling of skin, itching, rash, dizziness, drowsiness, weight gain, constipation, diarrhea, heartburn, nausea, headache, pain at injection site, oral lichenoid reaction

Occasional

Altered taste sensation, constipation, vomiting, stomach fullness

PRECAUTIONS AND CONTRAINDICATIONS

Diabetic ketoacidosis with or without coma, sole therapy for type 1 diabetes mellitus, use in children, hypersensitivity to tolbutamide or any component of its formulation

Caution:

Elderly, cardiac disease, thyroid disease, severe hypoglycemic reactions, renal disease, hepatic disease

DRUG INTERACTIONS OF CONCERN TO DENTISTRY

- Increased hypoglycemic reactions: NSAIDs, salicylates, ketoconazole, miconazole
- Decreased effects: corticosteroids, sympathomimetics

SERIOUS REACTIONS

! Severe hypoglycemia may occur because of overdosage or insufficient food intake, especially with increased glucose demands.
Cardiovascular mortality has been reported higher in patients treated

with tolbutamide. GI hemorrhage, cholestatic hepatic jaundice, leukopenia, thrombocytopenia, pancytopenia, agranulocytosis, and aplastic or hemolytic anemia occur rarely.

DENTAL CONSIDERATIONS

General:

- Patients on chronic drug therapy may rarely have symptoms of blood dyscrasias, which can include infection, bleeding, and poor healing.
- Ensure that patient is following prescribed diet and regularly takes medication.
- Question patient about self-monitoring of drug's antidiabetic effect including blood glucose values or finger-stick records.
- Anticipate possible hypoglycemic episodes.
- Place on frequent recall to evaluate healing response.
- Short appointments and a stress-reduction protocol may be required for anxious patients.
- Diabetics may be more susceptible to infection and have delayed wound healing.
- Avoid prescribing aspirin-containing products.

Consultations:

- In a patient with symptoms of blood dyscrasias, request a medical consultation for blood studies and postpone dental treatment until normal values are reestablished.
- Medical consultation may be required to assess disease control.
- Medical consultation may include data from patient's blood glucose monitoring including glycosylated hemoglobin or HbA_{1c} testing.

Teach Patient/Family to:

- Encourage effective oral hygiene to prevent soft tissue inflammation.
- Avoid mouth rinses with high alcohol content because of drying effects.

tolcapone

toll′-ka-pone
(Tasmar)

CATEGORY AND SCHEDULE

Pregnancy Risk Category: C

Drug Class: Antiparkinsonian

MECHANISM OF ACTION

An antiparkinson agent that inhibits the enzyme catechol-O-methyltransferase (COMT), potentiating dopamine activity and increasing the duration of action of levodopa.

Therapeutic Effect: Relieves signs and symptoms of Parkinson's disease.

USES

An adjunct to levodopa and carbidopa in the treatment of Parkinson's disease

PHARMACOKINETICS

Rapidly absorbed after PO administration. Protein binding: 99%. Metabolized in the liver. Eliminated primarily in urine (60%) and, to a lesser extent, in feces (40%). Unknown if removed by hemodialysis. ***Half-life:*** 2–3 hr.

INDICATIONS AND DOSAGES

▸ Adjunctive Treatment of Parkinson's Disease

PO

Adults, Elderly. Initially, 100–200 mg 3 times a day concomitantly with each dose of carbidopa and levodopa. Maximum: 600 mg/day.

▸ **Dosage in Hepatic Impairment**

Patients with moderate to severe cirrhosis should not receive more than 200 mg tolcapone 3 times a day.

SIDE EFFECTS/ADVERSE REACTIONS

Alert

Frequency of side effects increases with dosage. The following effects are based on a 200-mg dose.

Frequent

Nausea, insomnia, somnolence, anorexia, diarrhea, muscle cramps, orthostatic hypotension, excessive dreaming, dry mouth

Occasional

Headache, vomiting, confusion, hallucinations, constipation, diaphoresis, bright yellow urine, dry eyes, abdominal pain, dizziness, flatulence

Rare

Dyspepsia, neck pain, hypotension, fatigue, chest discomfort

PRECAUTIONS AND CONTRAINDICATIONS

Hypersensitivity, patients with SGPT/ALT and SGOT/AST exceeding upper limit of normal or other signs of hepatic impairment; informed consent required; history of nontraumatic rhabdomyolysis, hyperpyrexia, and confusion related to medication

Caution:

Discontinue drug with signs of hepatocellular injury, MAOIs, hypotension, dyskinesia, lactation

DRUG INTERACTIONS OF CONCERN TO DENTISTRY

- Increased sedation: alcohol and all CNS depressants
- No other data for dental drugs reported

SERIOUS REACTIONS

! Upper respiratory tract infection and UTI occur in 5%–7% of patients. Too-rapid withdrawal from therapy may produce withdrawal-emergent hyperpyrexia, characterized by fever, muscular rigidity, and altered LOC.

Dyskinesia and dystonia occur frequently.

DENTAL CONSIDERATIONS

General:

- Notify physician immediately if symptoms of liver failure are observed (bleeding, jaundice, etc.).
- Assess salivary flow as a factor in caries, periodontal disease, and candidiasis.
- After supine positioning, have patient sit upright for at least 2 min before standing to avoid orthostatic hypotension.
- Consider semisupine chair position for patient comfort because of GI side effects of drug.

Consultations:

- Medical consultation may be required to assess disease control.
- Take precaution if dental surgery is anticipated and general anesthesia is required.

Teach Patient/Family to:

- Use powered tooth brush if patient has difficulty holding conventional devices.
- When chronic dry mouth occurs, advise patient to:
  - Avoid mouth rinses with high alcohol content because of drying effects.
  - Use daily home fluoride products for anticaries effect.
  - Use sugarless gum, frequent sips of water, or saliva substitutes.

tolmetin

tole′-met-in
(Novo-Tolmetin[CAN], Tolectin, Tolectin DS)

CATEGORY AND SCHEDULE

Pregnancy Risk Category: C (D if used in third trimester or near delivery)

Drug Class: Nonsteroidal antiinflammatory

MECHANISM OF ACTION

A nonsteroidal antiinflammatory that produces analgesic and antiinflammatory effects by inhibiting prostaglandin synthesis. ***Therapeutic Effect:*** Reduces inflammatory response and intensity of pain stimulus reaching sensory nerve endings.

USES

Treatment of osteoarthritis, rheumatoid arthritis, juvenile rheumatoid arthritis

PHARMACOKINETICS

Rapidly absorbed from the GI tract. Metabolized in liver. Excreted in urine. Minimally removed by hemodialysis. ***Half-life:*** 5 hr.

T

INDICATIONS AND DOSAGES

▸ **Rheumatoid Arthritis, Osteoarthritis**

PO

Adults, Elderly. Initially, 400 mg 3 times a day (including 1 dose upon arising, 1 dose at bedtime). Adjust dose at 1- to 2-wk intervals. Maintenance: 600–1800 mg/day in 3–4 divided doses.

▸ **Juvenile Rheumatoid Arthritis**

PO

Children more than 2 yr. Initially, 20 mg/kg/day in 3–4 divided doses. Maintenance: 15–30 mg/kg/day in 3–4 divided doses.

SIDE EFFECTS/ADVERSE REACTIONS

Occasional

Nausea, vomiting, diarrhea, abdominal cramping, dyspepsia (heartburn, indigestion, epigastric pain), flatulence, dizziness, headache, weight decrease or increase

Rare

Constipation, anorexia, rash, pruritus

PRECAUTIONS AND CONTRAINDICATIONS

Severely incapacitated, bedridden, wheelchair bound, hypersensitivity to aspirin or other NSAIDs

Caution:

Lactation, children, bleeding disorders, GI disorders, cardiac disorders, hypersensitivity to aspirin, NSAIDs, peptic ulcer disease, geriatric patients

DRUG INTERACTIONS OF CONCERN TO DENTISTRY

- Increased risk of GI side effects: ASA, NSAIDs, ethanol (alcohol)
- Nephrotoxicity: acetaminophen (prolonged use and high doses)
- Possible risk of decreased renal function: cyclosporine
- Decreased antihypertensive effect of diuretics, α-adrenergic blockers, and ACE inhibitors
- SSRIs: increased risk of GI side effects

SERIOUS REACTIONS

! Peptic ulcer, GI bleeding, gastritis, and severe hepatic reaction (cholestasis, jaundice) occur rarely. Nephrotoxicity (dysuria, hematuria, proteinuria, nephrotic syndrome) and severe hypersensitivity reaction (fever, chills, bronchospasm) occur rarely.

DENTAL CONSIDERATIONS

General:

- Patients on chronic drug therapy may rarely have symptoms of blood dyscrasias, which can include infection, bleeding, and poor healing.
- Monitor vital signs at every appointment because of cardiovascular side effects.
- Assess salivary flow as a factor in caries, periodontal disease, and candidiasis.
- Avoid prescribing in last trimester of pregnancy.
- Possibility of cross-allergenicity when patient is allergic to aspirin.

Consultations:

- Medical consultation may be required to assess disease control.
- In a patient with symptoms of blood dyscrasias, request a medical consultation for blood studies and postpone dental treatment until normal values are reestablished.

Teach Patient/Family to:

- Encourage effective oral hygiene to prevent soft tissue inflammation.
- Use caution to prevent injury when using oral hygiene aids.
- When chronic dry mouth occurs, advise patient to:
  - Avoid mouth rinses with high alcohol content because of drying effects.
  - Use daily home fluoride products to prevent caries.
  - Use sugarless gum, frequent sips of water, or saliva substitutes.

tolterodine tartrate

tol-**tare**′-oh-deen **tar**′-trate
(Detrol, Detrol LA)

CATEGORY AND SCHEDULE

Pregnancy Risk Category: C

Drug Class: Antispasmodic

MECHANISM OF ACTION

An antispasmodic that exhibits potent antimuscarinic activity by interceding via cholinergic muscarinic receptors, thereby inhibiting urinary bladder contraction.
Therapeutic Effect: Decreases urinary frequency, urgency.

USES

Treatment of overactive bladder with symptoms of urinary frequency or incontinence

PHARMACOKINETICS

Rapidly and well absorbed after PO administration. Protein binding: 96%. Extensively metabolized in the liver to active metabolite. Primarily excreted in urine. Unknown if removed by hemodialysis. ***Half-life:*** 1.9–3.7 hr.

INDICATIONS AND DOSAGES

▸ **Overactive Bladder**

PO

Adults, Elderly. 1–2 mg twice a day.

▸ **Dosage in Severe Renal or Hepatic Impairment**

PO

Adults, Elderly. 1 mg twice a day.

PO (Extended-Release)

Adults, Elderly. 2–4 mg once a day.

SIDE EFFECTS/ADVERSE REACTIONS

Frequent
Dry mouth
Occasional
Headache, dizziness, fatigue, constipation, dyspepsia (heartburn, indigestion, epigastric discomfort), upper respiratory tract infection, UTI, dry eyes, abnormal vision (accommodation problems), nausea, diarrhea
Rare
Somnolence, chest or back pain, arthralgia, rash, weight gain, dry skin

PRECAUTIONS AND CONTRAINDICATIONS

Uncontrolled angle-closure glaucoma, urine retention
Caution:
Bladder obstruction, pyloric stenosis, GI obstructive disorders, treated narrow-angle glaucoma, significant hepatic dysfunction, renal impairment, lactation, pediatric use

DRUG INTERACTIONS OF CONCERN TO DENTISTRY

• Studies not available; however, drugs that inhibit cytochrome P-450 3A4 enzymes, such as erythromycin, clarithromycin, ketoconazole, itraconazole, and fluoxetine, require a dose reduction to 1 mg twice daily
• Increased anticholinergic effects: possibly with other anticholinergic drugs

SERIOUS REACTIONS

! Overdose can result in severe anticholinergic effects including abdominal cramps, facial warmth, excessive salivation or lacrimation, diaphoresis, pallor, urinary urgency, blurred vision, and prolonged QT interval.

DENTAL CONSIDERATIONS

General:
• Assess salivary flow as a factor in caries, periodontal disease, and candidiasis.
• Consider semisupine chair position for patient comfort because of GI side effects of drug.
• Avoid dental light in patient's eyes; offer dark glasses for patient comfort.
• Avoid drugs with anticholinergic activity, such as antihistamines, opioids, benzodiazepines, propantheline, atropine, and scopolamine.
Consultations:
• Physician should be informed if significant xerostomic side effects occur (e.g., increased caries, sore tongue, problems eating or swallowing, difficulty wearing prosthesis) so that a medication change can be considered.
Teach Patient/Family to:
• Encourage effective oral hygiene to prevent soft tissue inflammation.
• When chronic dry mouth occurs, advise patient to:
  • Avoid mouth rinses with high alcohol content because of drying effects.
  • Use daily home fluoride products for anticaries effect.
  • Use sugarless gum, frequent sips of water, or saliva substitutes.

tolvaptan

tol-**vap**′-tan
(Samsca)

CATEGORY AND SCHEDULE

Pregnancy Risk Category: C

Drug Class: Vasopressin receptor antagonist

T

MECHANISM OF ACTION

A non-peptide vasopressin V(2)-receptor antagonist that blocks the effect of vasopressin.
Therapeutic Effect: Increases urine water excretion; results in aquaresis (free water clearance), decrease in urine osmolality, increase in serum sodium concentrations.

USES

Hyponatremia (serum sodium <125 mEq/L or less marked hyponatremia that is symptomatic and resistant to fluid restriction)

PHARMACOKINETICS

Well absorbed after PO administration. Bioavailability: ~40%. Protein binding: 99%. Metabolized in liver, primarily by CYP3A; substrate and inhibitor of P-glycoprotein. Eliminated via nonrenal routes. ***Half-life:*** 12 hr.

INDICATIONS AND DOSAGES

▸ Hyponatremia

PO

Adults. 15 mg a day, without regard to meals. Increase dose to 30 mg a day, after at least 24 hr, to a maximum of 60 mg a day, as needed to achieve the desired level of serum sodium.

SIDE EFFECTS/ADVERSE REACTIONS

Frequent

Nausea, xerostomia, pollakiuria or polyuria, thirst

Occasional

Asthenia, constipation, anorexia, hyperglycemia, pyrexia, dehydration

Rare

Deep vein thrombosis, disseminated intravascular coagulation, intracardiac thrombus, ventricular fibrillation, respiratory failure, cerebrovascular accident, ischemic colitis, vaginal hemorrhage, diabetic ketoacidosis, rhabdomyolysis, pulmonary embolism, prolonged prothrombin time, urethral hemorrhage

PRECAUTIONS AND CONTRAINDICATIONS

Hypersensitivity to tolvaptan or its components
Alcoholism—Black Box Warning
Malnutrition—Black Box Warning
Hepatic disease—Black Box Warning
Anuria
Urgent need to raise serum sodium acutely
Inability of the patient to sense or appropriately respond to thirst
Hypovolemic hyponatremia
Concurrent use with strong CYP3A inhibitors (e.g., atazanavir, ritonavir, nelfinavir, indinavir, saquinavir, itraconazole, ketoconazole, clarithromycin, telithromycin, nefazodone)

Caution:

Renal or hepatic impairment
Chronic alcoholics, SIADH (increase risk for overly rapid correction of hyponatremia)

DRUG INTERACTIONS OF CONCERN TO DENTISTRY

- CYP3A inducers: May reduce the effectiveness of tolvaptan
- CYP3A inhibitors: May increase tolvaptan concentrations; avoid concurrent use
- Drugs that increase potassium: May increase the risk of hyperkalemia
- Hypertonic solutions: not recommended
- P-glycoprotein inhibitors: May increase tolvaptan exposure; consider dose reduction

SERIOUS REACTIONS

! Dehydration and hypovolemia can occur, especially in potentially volume-depleted patients receiving diuretic or those on fluid restrictions.
! Rapid correction of hyponatremia may cause osmotic demyelination resulting in dysarthria, mutism, dysphagia, lethargy, affective changes, spastic quadriparesis, seizures, coma, and death.

DENTAL CONSIDERATIONS

General:

• Monitor vital signs at every appointment.
• Patients taking this medication are treated on an inpatient basis.
• Assess salivary flow as a factor in caries, periodontal disease, and candidiasis.

Consultations:

• Consult physician to determine disease control and ability of patient to tolerate dental procedures, if needed while receiving drug.

Teach Patient/Family to:

• Report signs and symptoms of dry mouth.

topiramate

toe-**peer**′-ah-mate
(Topamax)
Do not confuse topiramate or Topamax with Toprol XL.

CATEGORY AND SCHEDULE

Pregnancy Risk Category: C

Drug Class: Anticonvulsant

MECHANISM OF ACTION

An anticonvulsant that blocks repetitive, sustained firing of neurons by enhancing the ability of gamma-aminobutyric acid to induce an influx of chloride ions into the neurons; may also block sodium channels.
Therapeutic Effect: Decreases seizure activity.

USES

Adjunctive therapy for adult patients with partial-onset seizures or for primary generalized tonic-clonic seizures; Lennox-Gastaut syndrome

PHARMACOKINETICS

Rapidly absorbed after PO administration. Protein binding: 13%–17%. Not extensively metabolized. Primarily excreted unchanged in urine. Removed by hemodialysis. ***Half-life:*** 21 hr.

INDICATIONS AND DOSAGES

▸ **Adjunctive Treatment of Partial Seizures, Lennox-Gastaut Syndrome**

PO

Adults, Elderly, Children older than 17 yr. Initially, 25–50 mg for 1 wk. May increase by 25–50 mg/day at weekly intervals. Maximum: 1600 mg/day.
Children 2–16 yr. Initially, 1–3 mg/kg/day to maximum of 25 mg. May increase by 1–3 mg/kg/day at weekly intervals. Maintenance: 5–9 mg/kg/day in 2 divided doses.

▸ **Tonic-Clonic Seizures**

PO

Adults, Elderly, Children. Dosage is individualized and titrated.

▸ **Migraine Prevention**

PO

Adults, Elderly. 100 mg/day in 2 divided doses.

▸ **Dosage in Renal Impairment**

Expect to reduce drug dosage by 50% in patients with tonic-clonic seizures who have a creatinine clearance of less than 70 ml/min.

SIDE EFFECTS/ADVERSE REACTIONS

Frequent

Somnolence, dizziness, ataxia, nervousness, nystagmus, diplopia, paresthesia, nausea, tremor

Occasional

Confusion, breast pain, dysmenorrhea, dyspepsia, depression, asthenia, pharyngitis, weight loss, anorexia, rash, musculoskeletal pain, abdominal pain, difficulty with coordination, sinusitis, agitation, flu-like symptoms

Rare

Mood disturbances, such as irritability and depression; dry mouth; aggressive behavior

PRECAUTIONS AND CONTRAINDICATIONS

Renal impairment, hepatic impairment, rapid drug withdrawal, kidney stones, lactation, children

Caution:

Renal impairment, hepatic impairment, rapid drug withdrawal, kidney stones, lactation, children

DRUG INTERACTIONS OF CONCERN TO DENTISTRY

- Increased CNS depression: opioids, sedatives, ethanol, and other CNS depressants
- Decreased serum levels: carbamazepine

SERIOUS REACTIONS

! Psychomotor slowing, impaired concentration, language problems (such as word-finding difficulties), and memory disturbances occur occasionally. These reactions are generally mild to moderate but may be severe enough to require discontinuation of drug therapy.

DENTAL CONSIDERATIONS

General:

- Patients on chronic drug therapy may rarely have symptoms of blood dyscrasias, which can include infection, bleeding, and poor healing.
- Short appointments and a stress-reduction protocol may be required for anxious patients.
- Assess salivary flow as factor in caries, periodontal disease, and candidiasis.
- Avoid dental light in patient's eyes; offer dark glasses for patient comfort.
- Determine type of epilepsy, seizure frequency, and quality of seizure control. A stress-reduction protocol may be required.

Consultations:

- In a patient with symptoms of blood dyscrasias, request a medical consultation for blood studies and postpone dental treatment until normal values are reestablished.
- Medical consultation may be required to assess disease control.

Teach Patient/Family to:

- Encourage effective oral hygiene to prevent soft tissue inflammation.
- Use caution to prevent trauma when using oral hygiene aids.
- Use powered tooth brush if patient has difficulty holding conventional devices.
- Update health and drug history if physician makes any changes in evaluation or drug regimens; include OTC, herbal, and nonherbal drugs in the update.
- When chronic dry mouth occurs, advise patient to:
    - Avoid mouth rinses with high alcohol content because of drying effects.
    - Use daily home fluoride products for anticaries effect.
    - Use sugarless gum, frequent sips of water, or saliva substitutes.

topotecan

toe-**poh′**-teh-can
(Hycamtin)

CATEGORY AND SCHEDULE

Pregnancy Risk Category: D

Drug Class: Antineoplastic

MECHANISM OF ACTION

A DNA topoisomerase inhibitor that interacts with topoisomerase I, an enzyme that allows DNA replication by producing reversible single-strand breaks in DNA that relieve torsional strain. Topotecan prevents relegation of the DNA strand, resulting in damage to double-strand DNA and cell death.
Therapeutic Effect: Kills cancer cells.

USES

Treatment of breast cancer that has spread to other parts of the body

PHARMACOKINETICS

Hydrolyzed to active form after IV administration. Protein binding: 35%. Excreted in urine. ***Half-life:*** 2–3 hr (increased in impaired renal function).

INDICATIONS AND DOSAGES

▸ **Ovarian Carcinoma, Small-Cell Lung Cancer**

IV

Adults, Elderly. 1.5 mg/m^2/day over 30 min for 5 consecutive days, beginning on day 1 of a 21-day course. Minimum of 4 courses recommended. If severe neutropenia (neutrophil count less than 1500/mm^2) occurs during treatment, reduce dose for subsequent courses by 0.25 mg/m^2 or administer filgrastim (G-CSF) no sooner than 24 hr after the last dose of topotecan.

▸ **Dosage in Renal Impairment**

No dosage adjustment is necessary in patients with mild renal impairment (creatinine clearance of 40–60 ml/min). For moderate renal impairment (creatinine clearance of 20–39 ml/min), give 0.75 mg/m^2.

SIDE EFFECTS/ADVERSE REACTIONS

Frequent

Nausea, vomiting, diarrhea, total alopecia, headache, dyspnea

Occasional

Paresthesia, constipation, abdominal pain

Rare

Anorexia, malaise, arthralgia, asthenia, myalgia

PRECAUTIONS AND CONTRAINDICATIONS

Baseline neutrophil count less than 1500 cells/mm^3, breast-feeding, pregnancy, severe myelosuppression

DRUG INTERACTIONS OF CONCERN TO DENTISTRY

- None reported

SERIOUS REACTIONS

! Severe neutropenia (neutrophil count less than 500 cells/mm^3) occurs in 60% of patients, usually during the first course of therapy. The neutrophil nadir usually occurs at a median of 11 days after starting therapy. Thrombocytopenia (platelet count less than 25,000/mm^3) occurs in 26% of patients, and severe anemia (RBC count less than 8 g/dl) occurs in 40% of patients. The platelet and RBC nadirs usually occur at a median of 15 days after starting the first course of therapy.

DENTAL CONSIDERATIONS

General:

• If additional analgesia is required for dental pain, consider alternative analgesics (NSAIDs) in patients taking opioids for acute or chronic pain.
• Examine for oral manifestations of opportunistic infection.
• This drug may be used in the hospital or on an outpatient basis. Confirm the patient's disease and treatment status.
• Chlorhexidine mouth rinse prior to and during chemotherapy may reduce severity of mucositis.
• Patient on chronic drug therapy may rarely present with symptoms of blood dyscrasias, which can include infection, bleeding, and poor healing. If dyscrasia is present, caution patient to prevent oral tissue trauma when using oral hygiene aids.
• Palliative medication may be required for management of oral side effects.
• Short appointments and a stress-reduction protocol may be required for anxious patients.
• Consider semisupine chair position for patient comfort if GI side effects occur.
• Caution: patients may be at high risk for infection.
• Patients may have received other chemotherapy or radiation; confirm medical and drug history.
• Oral infections should be eliminated and/or treated aggressively.

Consultations:

• Medical consultation should include routine blood counts including platelet counts and bleeding time.
• Consult physician; prophylactic or therapeutic antiinfectives may be indicated if surgery or periodontal treatment is required.
• Medical consultation may be required to assess immunologic status during cancer chemotherapy and determine safety risk, if any, posed by the required dental treatment.
• Medical consultation may be required to assess disease control and patient's ability to tolerate stress.
• In a patient with symptoms of blood dyscrasias, request a medical consultation for blood studies and postpone treatment until normal values are reestablished.

Teach Patient/Family to:

• See dentist immediately if secondary oral infection occurs.
• Be aware of oral side effects.
• Encourage effective oral hygiene to prevent soft tissue inflammation.
• Report oral lesions, soreness, or bleeding to dentist.
• Prevent trauma when using oral hygiene aids.
• Update health and medication history if physician makes any changes in evaluation or drug regimens; include OTC, herbal, and nonherbal remedies in the update.
• Use soft tooth brush to reduce risk of bleeding.

toremifene citrate

tor-**eh**′-mih-feen **sih**′-trate
(Fareston)

CATEGORY AND SCHEDULE

Pregnancy Risk Category: D

Drug Class: Antineoplastic, antiestrogen agent

MECHANISM OF ACTION
A nonsteroidal antiestrogen and antineoplastic agent that binds to estrogen receptors on tumors, producing a complex that decreases DNA synthesis and inhibits estrogen effects.
Therapeutic Effect: Blocks growth-stimulating effects of estrogen in breast cancer.

USES
Treatment of metastatic breast cancer in postmenopausal women with estrogen receptor-positive or unknown tumors

PHARMACOKINETICS
Well absorbed after PO administration. Metabolized in the liver. Eliminated in feces. ***Half-life:*** Approximately 5 days.

INDICATIONS AND DOSAGES
▸ **Breast Cancer**
PO
Adults. 60 mg/day until disease progression is observed.

SIDE EFFECTS/ADVERSE REACTIONS
Frequent
Hot flashes, diaphoresis, nausea, vaginal discharge, dizziness, dry eyes
Occasional
Edema, vomiting, vaginal bleeding
Rare
Fatigue, depression, lethargy, anorexia

PRECAUTIONS AND CONTRAINDICATIONS
History of thromboembolic disease
Caution:
Thromboembolic diseases, endometrial hyperplasia, hypercalcemia with bone metastases, monitor leukocyte and platelet counts, tumor flare

DRUG INTERACTIONS OF CONCERN TO DENTISTRY
• None reported

SERIOUS REACTIONS
! Ocular toxicity (cataracts, glaucoma, decreased visual acuity) and hypercalcemia may occur.

DENTAL CONSIDERATIONS
General:
• Patients on chronic drug therapy may rarely have symptoms of blood dyscrasias, which can include infection, bleeding, and poor healing.
• Consider semisupine chair position for patient comfort because of GI side effects of drug.
Consultations:
• Medical consultation may be required to assess disease control.
Teach Patient/Family to:
• Encourage effective oral hygiene to prevent soft tissue inflammation.

torsemide
tor′-se-mide
(Demadex)
Do not confuse torsemide with furosemide.

CATEGORY AND SCHEDULE
Pregnancy Risk Category: B

Drug Class: Loop diuretic

MECHANISM OF ACTION
A loop diuretic that enhances excretion of sodium, chloride, potassium, and water at the ascending limb of the loop of Henle; also reduces plasma and extracellular fluid volume.

T

Therapeutic Effect: Produces diuresis; lowers B/P.

USES

Treatment of hypertension and edema associated with CHF, liver disease, chronic renal failure

PHARMACOKINETICS

Route	Onset	Peak	Duration
PO	1 hr	1–2 hr	6–8 hr
IV	10 min	1 hr	6–8 hr

Rapidly and well absorbed from the GI tract. Protein binding: 97%–99%. Metabolized in the liver. Primarily excreted in urine. Not removed by hemodialysis. ***Half-life:*** 3.3 hr.

INDICATIONS AND DOSAGES

▸ **Hypertension**

PO

Adults, Elderly. Initially, 5 mg/day. May increase to 10 mg/day if no response in 4–6 wk. If no response, additional antihypertensive added.

▸ **CHF**

PO, IV

Adults, Elderly. Initially, 10–20 mg/day. May increase by approximately doubling dose until desired therapeutic effect is attained. Doses greater than 200 mg have not been adequately studied.

▸ **Chronic Renal Failure**

PO, IV

Adults, Elderly. Initially, 20 mg/day. May increase by approximately doubling dose until desired therapeutic effect is attained. Doses greater than 200 mg have not been adequately studied.

▸ **Hepatic Cirrhosis**

PO, IV

Adults, Elderly. Initially, 5 mg/day given with aldosterone antagonist or potassium-sparing diuretic. May increase by approximately doubling dose until desired therapeutic effect is attained. Doses greater than 40 mg have not been adequately studied.

SIDE EFFECTS/ADVERSE REACTIONS

Frequent

Headache, dizziness, rhinitis

Occasional

Asthenia, insomnia, nervousness, diarrhea, constipation, nausea, dyspepsia, edema, ECG changes, pharyngitis, cough, arthralgia, myalgia

Rare

Syncope, hypotension, arrhythmias

PRECAUTIONS AND CONTRAINDICATIONS

Anuria, hepatic coma, severe electrolyte depletion

Caution:

Lactation, children younger than 18 yr, dehydration, systemic lupus erythematosus, ototoxicity, electrolyte imbalance

DRUG INTERACTIONS OF CONCERN TO DENTISTRY

- Increased electrolyte imbalance: systemic corticosteroids
- Masked ototoxicity: phenothiazines
- Decreased antihypertensive effects: NSAIDs
- Increased sweating, hot flashes, weakness, cardiovascular symptoms: chloral hydrate (rare)

SERIOUS REACTIONS

! Ototoxicity may occur with high doses or a too-rapid IV administration. Overdose produces acute, profound water loss; volume and electrolyte depletion; dehydration; decreased blood volume; and circulatory collapse.

DENTAL CONSIDERATIONS

General:

• Monitor vital signs at every appointment because of cardiovascular side effects.
• After supine positioning, have patient sit upright for at least 2 min before standing to avoid orthostatic hypotension.
• Patients on high-potency loop diuretics should be questioned about serum potassium levels or potassium supplement use.
• Short appointments and a stress-reduction protocol may be required for anxious patients.
• Consider semisupine chair position for patient comfort if GI side effects occur.

Consultations:

• Medical consultation may be required to assess disease control and patient's ability to tolerate stress.

Teach Patient/Family to:

• Update health history/drug record if physician makes any changes in evaluation or drug regimens; include OTC, herbal, and nonherbal drugs in the update.

T

tramadol hydrochloride

tram′-ah-dole high-droh-**klor′**-ide
(Tramal[AUS], Tramal SR[AUS], Ultram, Zydol[AUS])
Do not confuse tramadol with Toradol, or Ultram with Ultane.

CATEGORY AND SCHEDULE

Pregnancy Risk Category: C

Drug Class: Synthetic opioid analgesic

MECHANISM OF ACTION

An analgesic that binds to μ-opioid receptors and inhibits reuptake of norepinephrine and serotonin. Reduces the intensity of pain stimuli reaching sensory nerve endings. ***Therapeutic Effect:*** Alters the perception of and emotional response to pain.

USES

Treatment of moderate-to-severe pain

PHARMACOKINETICS

Route	Onset	Peak	Duration
PO	Less than 1 hr	2–3 hr	4–6 hr

Rapidly and almost completely absorbed after PO administration. Protein binding: 20%. Extensively metabolized in the liver to active metabolite (reduced in patients with advanced cirrhosis). Primarily excreted in urine. Minimally removed by hemodialysis. ***Half-life:*** 6–7 hr.

INDICATIONS AND DOSAGES

▸ **Moderate to Moderately Severe Pain**

PO

Adults, Elderly. 50–100 mg q4–6h. Maximum: 400 mg/day for patients 75 yr and younger; 300 mg/day for patients older than 75 yr.

▸ **Dosage in Renal Impairment**

For patients with creatinine clearance of less than 30 ml/min, increase dosing interval to q12h. Maximum: 200 mg/day.

▸ **Dosage in Hepatic Impairment**

Dosage is decreased to 50 mg q12h.

SIDE EFFECTS/ADVERSE REACTIONS

Frequent

Dizziness or vertigo, nausea, constipation, headache, somnolence

Occasional

Vomiting, pruritus, CNS stimulation (such as nervousness, anxiety, agitation, tremor, euphoria, mood swings, and hallucinations), asthenia, diaphoresis, dyspepsia, dry mouth, diarrhea

Rare

Malaise, vasodilation, anorexia, flatulence, rash, blurred vision, urine retention or urinary frequency, menopausal symptoms

PRECAUTIONS AND CONTRAINDICATIONS

Acute alcohol intoxication; concurrent use of centrally acting analgesics, hypnotics, opioids, or psychotropic drugs

Caution:

Not a controlled substance, but dependence and abuse are possible

DRUG INTERACTIONS OF CONCERN TO DENTISTRY

- Increased risk of respiratory depression: anesthetics, alcohol
- Significant increase in metabolism: carbamazepine
- Increased serum concentrations: quinidine
- Increased risk of seizures: MAOIs, tricyclic antidepressants, selective serotonin reuptake inhibitors
- Increased risk of sedation: other CNS depressant drugs, alcohol

SERIOUS REACTIONS

! Overdose results in respiratory depression and seizures. Tramadol may have a prolonged duration of action and cumulative effect in patients with hepatic or renal impairment.

DENTAL CONSIDERATIONS

General:

- Determine why the patient is taking the drug.
- Patients taking opioids for acute or chronic pain should be given alternative analgesics for dental pain.
- Geriatric patients are more susceptible to drug effects; use lower dose.
- Assess salivary flow as a factor in caries, periodontal disease, and candidiasis.
- Take precautions if dental surgery is anticipated and general anesthesia is required.
- Risk of cross-hypersensitivity to other opioid analgesics.

Teach Patient/Family to:

- Use caution to prevent trauma when using oral hygiene aids.
- Use caution when driving or operating complex equipment.
- When chronic dry mouth occurs, advise patient to:
  - Avoid mouth rinses with high alcohol content because of drying effects.
  - Use daily home fluoride products for anticaries effect.
  - Use sugarless gum, frequent sips of water, or saliva substitutes.

trandolapril

tran-**doe′**-la-pril

(Gopten[AUS], Mavik, Odrik[AUS])

Do not confuse trandolapril with tramadol.

CATEGORY AND SCHEDULE

Pregnancy Risk Category: C (D if used in second or third trimester)

Drug Class: Angiotensin-converting enzyme (ACE) inhibitor

MECHANISM OF ACTION

An ACE inhibitor that suppresses the renin-angiotensin-aldosterone system and prevents the conversion of angiotensin I to angiotensin II, a potent vasoconstrictor; may also inhibit angiotensin II at local vascular and renal sites. Decreases plasma angiotensin II, increases plasma renin activity, and decreases aldosterone secretion.

Therapeutic Effect: Reduces peripheral arterial resistance and pulmonary capillary wedge pressure; improves cardiac output and exercise tolerance.

USES

Treatment of hypertension alone or in combination with other antihypertensive medications; maintenance therapy to prevent CHF after MI; ventricular dysfunction after MI

PHARMACOKINETICS

Slowly absorbed from the GI tract. Protein binding: 80%. Metabolized in the liver and GI mucosa to active metabolite. Primarily excreted in urine. Removed by hemodialysis. ***Half-life:*** 24 hr.

INDICATIONS AND DOSAGES

▸ **Hypertension (Without Diuretic)**

PO

Adults, Elderly. Initially, 1 mg once a day in nonblack patients, 2 mg once a day in African-American patients. Adjust dosage at least at 7-day intervals. Maintenance: 2–4 mg/day. Maximum: 8 mg/day.

▸ **CHF**

PO

Adults, Elderly. Initially, 0.5–1 mg, titrated to target dose of 4 mg/day.

SIDE EFFECTS/ADVERSE REACTIONS

Frequent

Dizziness, cough

Occasional

Hypotension, dyspepsia (heartburn, epigastric pain, indigestion), syncope, asthenia (loss of strength), tinnitus

Rare

Palpitations, insomnia, drowsiness, nausea, vomiting, constipation, flushed skin

PRECAUTIONS AND CONTRAINDICATIONS

History of angioedema from previous treatment with ACE inhibitors

Caution:

Angioedema (higher rate in African-American patients), CHF, ischemic heart disease, aortic stenosis, cerebrovascular disease, monitor WBC count in SLE or scleroderma, impaired renal function, hyperkalemia, pediatric patients, potassium-sparing diuretics

DRUG INTERACTIONS OF CONCERN TO DENTISTRY

- Decreased absorption of tetracycline
- Drugs that lower B/P could possibly exaggerate hypotensive effects

SERIOUS REACTIONS

! Excessive hypotension ("first-dose syncope") may occur in patients with CHF and in those who are severely salt or volume depleted.

! Angioedema and hyperkalemia occur rarely.

! Agranulocytosis and neutropenia may be noted in those with collagen vascular disease including scleroderma and systemic lupus erythematosus and impaired renal function.

! Nephrotic syndrome may be noted in those with history of renal disease.

DENTAL CONSIDERATIONS

General:

• Monitor vital signs at every appointment because of cardiovascular disease.
• Limit use of sodium-containing products, such as saline IV fluids, for patients with a dietary salt restriction.
• Stress from dental procedures may compromise cardiovascular function; determine patient risk.
• Short appointments and a stress-reduction protocol may be required for anxious patients.
• Use precaution if sedation or general anesthesia is required; risk of hypotensive episode.
• After supine positioning, have patient sit upright for at least 2 min before standing to avoid orthostatic hypotension.
• Consider semisupine chair position for patient comfort because of respiratory side effects of drug.
• Patients on chronic drug therapy may rarely have symptoms of blood dyscrasias, which can include infection, bleeding, and poor healing.

Consultations:

• Medical consultation may be required to assess disease control and patient's ability to tolerate stress.

Teach Patient/Family to:

• Encourage effective oral hygiene to prevent soft tissue inflammation.
• Use caution to prevent trauma when using oral hygiene aids.
• Update health and drug history if physician makes any changes in evaluation or drug regimens; include OTC, herbal, and nonherbal drugs in the update.

tranexamic acid

tran-ex-**am′**-ik ass-id
(Cyklokapron, Lysteda)

CATEGORY AND SCHEDULE

Pregnancy Risk Category: B

Drug Class: Hemostatic, antithrombolytic

MECHANISM OF ACTION

A competitive inhibitor of plasminogen activation and, at much higher concentrations, a noncompetitive inhibitor of plasmin (i.e., actions similar to aminocaproic acid), which exerts its antifibrinolytic effects primarily by forming a reversible complex with a modified plasminogen.
Therapeutic Effect: Inhibits fibrinolysis, hemostatic.

USES

Prophylaxis and treatment of hemophilia patients to reduce or prevent hemorrhage during and after extractions; unapproved uses: in hyperfibrinolysis-induced hemorrhage, angioedema; oral rinse (with systemic therapy) to reduce bleeding in oral surgery patients who are also taking anticoagulants

PHARMACOKINETICS

Absorption after PO administration represents 30%–50% of the ingested dose, and bioavailability is not affected by food intake. Protein binding: 3%. Site of metabolism is not established. Excreted in urine.
Half-life: Unknown.

INDICATIONS AND DOSAGES

▸ **Hemorrhage Prophylaxis, Tooth Extraction**

IV/PO

Adults, Children. 10 mg/kg body weight immediately before dental extraction. Following surgery, a dose of 25 mg/kg body weight can be given orally 3 or 4 times daily for 2–8 days. Alternatively, tranexamic acid can be administered entirely orally, 25 mg/kg body weight 3–4 times per day beginning 1 day before surgery.

Dosage in Renal Impairment

Serum Creatinine	IV Dosage	Tablets
120–250 μmol/L (1.36–2.83 mg/dl)	10 mg/kg twice daily	15 mg/kg twice daily
250–500 μmol/L (2.83–5.66 mg/dl)	10 mg/kg daily	15 mg/kg daily
More than 500 μmol/L (2–5.66 mg/dl)	10 mg/kg q48h or 5 mg/kg q24h	15 mg/kg q48h or 7.5 mg/kg q24h

SIDE EFFECTS/ADVERSE REACTIONS

Occasional

Hypotension, diarrhea, nausea, vomiting, dizziness

PRECAUTIONS AND CONTRAINDICATIONS

Acquired defective color vision, subarachnoid hemorrhage, active intravascular clotting process, hypersensitivity to tranexamic acid or any component of the formulation

Caution:

Lactation, reduce dose in renal impairment, limited use experience in children

DRUG INTERACTIONS OF CONCERN TO DENTISTRY

- Increased risk of bleeding: drugs that affect coagulation
- Factor IX complex: increased risk of thrombotic complications when used concurrently

SERIOUS REACTIONS

! Thromboembolic events (e.g., deep vein thrombosis, pulmonary embolism, cerebral thrombosis, acute renal cortical necrosis, central retinal artery and vein obstruction) have been reported.

DENTAL CONSIDERATIONS

General:

- Used as an antifibrinolytic mouthwash following oral surgery to prevent hemorrhage in patients taking oral anticoagulants.

Consultations:

- Hematologist consultation is strongly recommended.

Teach Patient/Family to:

- Update health and drug history if physician makes any changes in evaluation or drug regimens; include OTC, herbal, and nonherbal drugs in the update.
- Report hemorrhage or bleeding not responding to postsurgical hemostasis.
- Use caution to prevent trauma when using oral hygiene aids.

tranylcypromine sulfate

tran-ill-**sip**′-roe-meen **sull**′-fate

(Parnate)

CATEGORY AND SCHEDULE

Pregnancy Risk Category: C

Drug Class: Antidepressant, MAOI

MECHANISM OF ACTION

An MAOI that inhibits the activity of the enzyme monoamine oxidase at CNS storage sites, leading to increased levels of the neurotransmitters epinephrine, norepinephrine, serotonin, and dopamine at neuronal receptor sites. ***Therapeutic Effect:*** Relieves depression.

USES

Treatment of depression (when uncontrolled by other means)

PHARMACOKINETICS

Well absorbed from GI tract. Metabolized in the liver. Primarily excreted in urine. Removed by hemodialysis. ***Half-life:*** 1.5–3.5 hr.

INDICATIONS AND DOSAGES

▸ Depression Refractory to or Intolerant of Other Therapy

PO

Adults, Elderly. Initially, 10 mg twice a day. May increase by 10 mg/day at 1- to 3-wk intervals up to 60 mg/day in divided doses.

SIDE EFFECTS/ADVERSE REACTIONS

Frequent

Orthostatic hypotension, restlessness, GI upset, insomnia, dizziness, lethargy, weakness, dry mouth, peripheral edema

Occasional

Flushing, diaphoresis, rash, urinary frequency, increased appetite, transient impotence

Rare

Visual disturbances

PRECAUTIONS AND CONTRAINDICATIONS

CHF, children younger than 16 yr, pheochromocytoma, severe hepatic or renal impairment, uncontrolled hypertension

Caution:

Suicidal patients, convulsive disorders, severe depression, schizophrenia, hyperactivity, diabetes mellitus

DRUG INTERACTIONS OF CONCERN TO DENTISTRY

- Increased pressor effects: indirect-acting sympathomimetics (ephedrine)
- Hyperpyretic crisis, convulsions, hypertensive episode, and death: carbamazepine, meperidine, and possibly other opioids
- Increased anticholinergic effects: anticholinergics and antihistamines
- Increased effects of alcohol, barbiturates, benzodiazepines, CNS depressants, fluoxetine, tricyclic antidepressants

SERIOUS REACTIONS

! Hypertensive crisis occurs rarely and is marked by severe hypertension, occipital headache radiating frontally, neck stiffness or soreness, nausea, vomiting, diaphoresis, fever or chills, clammy skin, dilated pupils, palpitations, tachycardia or bradycardia, and constricting chest pain.

! Intracranial bleeding has been reported in association with severe hypertension.

DENTAL CONSIDERATIONS

General:

- After supine positioning, have patient sit upright for at least 2 min before standing to avoid orthostatic hypotension.
- Monitor vital signs at every appointment because of cardiovascular side effects.

• Assess salivary flow as a factor in caries, periodontal disease, and candidiasis.
• Hypertensive episodes are possible even though there are no specific contraindications to vasoconstrictor use in local anesthetics.

Consultations:
• Medical consultation may be required to assess patient's ability to tolerate stress.

Teach Patient/Family to:
• Use powered tooth brush if patient has difficulty holding conventional devices.
• When chronic dry mouth occurs, advise patient to:
  • Avoid mouth rinses with high alcohol content because of drying effects.
  • Use daily home fluoride products to prevent caries.
  • Use sugarless gum, frequent sips of water, or saliva substitutes.

trastuzumab

traz-**two**′-zoo-mab
(Herceptin)

CATEGORY AND SCHEDULE

Pregnancy Risk Category: B

Drug Class: Antineoplastic, monoclonal antibody

T

MECHANISM OF ACTION

Binds to the HER-2 protein, which is overexpressed in 25%–30% of primary breast cancers, thereby inhibiting proliferation of tumor cells.

Therapeutic Effect: Inhibits the growth of tumor cells and mediates antibody-dependent cellular cytotoxicity.

USES

Treatment of breast cancer that has spread to other parts of the body

PHARMACOKINETICS

Half-life: 5.8 days (range: 1–32 days).

INDICATIONS AND DOSAGES

▸ **Breast Cancer**

IV

Adults, Elderly. Initially, 4 mg/kg as a 30- to 90-min infusion, then 2 mg/kg weekly as a 30-min infusion.

SIDE EFFECTS/ADVERSE REACTIONS

Frequent

Pain, asthenia, fever, chills, headache, abdominal pain, back pain, infection, nausea, diarrhea, vomiting, cough, dyspnea

Occasional

Tachycardia, CHF, flu-like symptoms, anorexia, edema, bone pain, arthralgia, insomnia, dizziness, paresthesia, depression, rhinitis, pharyngitis, sinusitis

Rare

Allergic reaction, anemia, leukopenia, neuropathy, herpes simplex

PRECAUTIONS AND CONTRAINDICATIONS

Preexisting cardiac disease

DRUG INTERACTIONS OF CONCERN TO DENTISTRY

• Dental drug interactions have not been studied.

SERIOUS REACTIONS

! Cardiomyopathy, ventricular dysfunction, and CHF occur rarely.
! Pancytopenia may occur.

DENTAL CONSIDERATIONS

General:

- If additional analgesia is required for dental pain, consider alternative analgesics (NSAIDs) in patients taking narcotics for acute or chronic pain.
- Monitor and record vital signs.
- Avoid products that affect platelet function, such as aspirin and NSAIDs.
- This drug may be used in the hospital or on an outpatient basis. Confirm the patient's disease and treatment status.
- Patient on chronic drug therapy may rarely present with symptoms of blood dyscrasias, which can include infection, bleeding, and poor healing. If dyscrasia is present, caution patient to prevent oral tissue trauma when using oral hygiene aids.
- Consider semisupine chair position for patient comfort if GI side effects occur.
- Caution: patients may be at high risk for infection.
- Patients may be at risk for bleeding; check oral signs.
- Oral infections should be eliminated and/or treated aggressively.

Consultations:

- Medical consultation should include routine blood counts including platelet counts and bleeding time.
- In a patient with symptoms of blood dyscrasias, request a medical consultation for blood studies and postpone treatment until normal values are reestablished.
- Consult physician; prophylactic or therapeutic antiinfectives may be indicated if surgery or periodontal treatment is required.
- Medical consultation may be required to assess immunologic status during cancer chemotherapy and determine safety risk, if any, posed by the required dental treatment.
- Medical consultation may be required to assess disease control and patient's ability to tolerate stress.

Teach Patient/Family to:

- Inform dentist of unusual bleeding episodes following dental treatment.
- See dentist immediately if secondary oral infection occurs.
- Encourage effective oral hygiene to prevent soft tissue inflammation.
- Report oral lesions, soreness, or bleeding to dentist.
- Prevent trauma when using oral hygiene aids.
- Update health and medication history if physician makes any changes in evaluation or drug regimens; include OTC, herbal, and nonherbal remedies in the update.

travoprost

tra′-voe-prost

(Apo-Timop[CAN], Gen-Timolol[CAN], Optimol[AUS], Tenopt[AUS], Travatan)

CATEGORY AND SCHEDULE

Pregnancy Risk Category: C

Drug Class: Synthetic prostaglandin F_2-α analogue

T

MECHANISM OF ACTION

An ophthalmic agent that is a prostanoid-selective FP receptor agonist.

Therapeutic Effect: Reduces intraocular pressure (IOP) by reducing aqueous humor production.

USES

Reduction of elevated IOP in patients with open-angle glaucoma or ocular hypertension in patients intolerant to, or who show insufficient response to, other IOP-reducing drugs

PHARMACOKINETICS

Absorbed through the cornea and hydrolyzed to the active free acid form. Metabolized in cornea and liver. Metabolites are inactive. Excreted in urine. ***Half-life:*** 17–86 min.

INDICATIONS AND DOSAGES

▸ Open-Angle Glaucoma, Ocular Hypertension

Ophthalmic

Adults, Elderly. 1 drop in affected eye(s) once daily, in the evening.

SIDE EFFECTS/ADVERSE REACTIONS

Frequent

Ocular hyperemia

Occasional

Ocular pain, pruritus, eye discomfort, decreased visual acuity, foreign body sensation

Rare

Abnormal vision, cataract, conjunctivitis, dry eye, eye disorder, flare, iris discoloration, keratitis, lid margin crusting, photophobia, subconjunctival hemorrhage, and tearing

PRECAUTIONS AND CONTRAINDICATIONS

Hypersensitivity to travoprost or benzalkonium chloride, or any other component of the formulation

Caution:

May cause changes in pigmented tissues (iris, eyelid) and growth of eyelashes (length, thickness, color); do not administer with contact lens in place; renal or hepatic impairment, lactation, pediatric use, macular edema

DRUG INTERACTIONS OF CONCERN TO DENTISTRY

• None reported

SERIOUS REACTIONS

! Ocular adverse events including accidental injury, angina pectoris, anxiety, arthritis, back pain, bradycardia, bronchitis, chest pain, cold syndrome, depression, dyspepsia, gastrointestinal disorder, headache, hypercholesterolemia, hypertension, hypotension, infection, pain, prostate disorder, sinusitis, urinary incontinence, and UTI, occur rarely.

DENTAL CONSIDERATIONS

General:

• Monitor vital signs at every appointment because of cardiovascular and respiratory side effects and question patient about occurrence of cardiovascular side effects.

• Avoid drugs with anticholinergic activity, such as antihistamines, opioids, benzodiazepines, propantheline, atropine, and scopolamine.

• Avoid dental light in patient's eyes; offer dark glasses for patient comfort.

Consultations:

• Medical consultation may be required to assess disease control.

Teach Patient/Family to:

• Update health and drug history if physician makes any changes in evaluation or drug regimens.

trazodone hydrochloride

trah′-zoe-doan
high-droh-**klor**′-ide
(Apo-Trazodone [CAN], Desyrel, Oleptro, Novo-Trazodone [CAN], PMS-Trazodone [CAN])
Do not confuse Desyrel with Delsym or Zestril.

CATEGORY AND SCHEDULE

Pregnancy Risk Category: C

Drug Class: Antidepressant

MECHANISM OF ACTION

An antidepressant that blocks the reuptake of serotonin at neuronal synaptic membranes, increasing its availability at postsynaptic receptor sites.
Therapeutic Effect: Relieves depression.

USES

Treatment of depression

PHARMACOKINETICS

Well absorbed from the GI tract. Protein binding: 85%–95%. Metabolized in the liver. Primarily excreted in urine. Unknown if removed by hemodialysis. ***Half-life:*** 5–9 hr.

INDICATIONS AND DOSAGES

▸ **Depression**

PO

Adults. Initially, 150 mg/day in equally divided doses. Increase by 50 mg/day at 3- to 4-day intervals until therapeutic response is achieved. Maximum: 600 mg/day.
Elderly. Initially, 25–50 mg at bedtime. May increase by 25–50 mg every 3–7 days. Range: 75–150 mg/day.
Children 6–18 yr. Initially, 1.5–2 mg/kg/day in divided doses. May increase gradually to 6 mg/kg/day in 3 divided doses.

SIDE EFFECTS/ADVERSE REACTIONS

Frequent
Somnolence, dry mouth, lightheadedness, dizziness, headache, blurred vision, nausea, vomiting
Occasional
Nervousness, fatigue, constipation, generalized aches and pains, mild hypotension
Rare
Photosensitivity reaction

PRECAUTIONS AND CONTRAINDICATIONS

Hypersensitivity to tricyclic antidepressants, recovery phase of MI, convulsive disorders, prostatic hypertrophy
Caution:
Suicidal patients, severe depression, increased intraocular pressure, narrow-angle glaucoma, urinary retention, cardiac disease, hepatic disease, hyperthyroidism, electroshock therapy, elective surgery

DRUG INTERACTIONS OF CONCERN TO DENTISTRY

- Increased risk of CNS depression: all CNS depressants, alcohol. May potentiate mental impairment and somnolence.
- Increased effects of anticholinergic drugs (e.g., atropine, glycopyrrolate).

DENTAL CONSIDERATIONS

General:

- Monitor vital signs at every appointment because of adverse cardiovascular effects.

• Patients on chronic drug therapy may rarely have symptoms of blood dyscrasias, which can include bleeding, infection, and poor healing.
• Assess salivary flow as a factor in caries, periodontal disease, and candidiasis.
• After supine positioning, have patient sit upright for at least 2 min before standing to avoid orthostatic hypotension.

Consultations:

• In a patient with symptoms of blood dyscrasias, request a medical consultation for blood studies and postpone dental treatment until normal values are reestablished.
• Medical consultation may be required to assess disease control and ability of patient to tolerate dental procedures.
• Physician should be informed if significant salivary flow reduction occurs (e.g., increased caries, sore tongue, difficulty wearing prosthesis) so that a medication change can be considered.

Teach Patient/Family to:

• Report oral lesions, soreness, or bleeding to dentist.
• When chronic dry mouth occurs, advise patient to:
  • Avoid mouth rinses with high alcohol content because of drying effect.
  • Use daily home fluoride products to prevent caries.
  • Use sugarless/xylitol gum, frequent sips of water, or saliva substitutes.

treprostinil sodium

treh-**prost**′-in-ill **soe**′-dee-um
(Remodulin)

CATEGORY AND SCHEDULE

Pregnancy Risk Category: B

Drug Class: Antihypertensive (pulmonary), vasodilator

MECHANISM OF ACTION

An antiplatelet that directly dilates pulmonary and systemic arterial vascular beds, inhibiting platelet aggregation.
Therapeutic Effect: Reduces symptoms of pulmonary arterial hypertension associated with exercise.

USES

Treatment of the symptoms of primary pulmonary hypertension or high B/P

PHARMACOKINETICS

Rapidly, completely absorbed after subcutaneous infusion; 91% bound to plasma protein. Metabolized by the liver. Excreted mainly in the urine with a lesser amount eliminated in the feces. ***Half-life:*** 2–4 hr.

INDICATIONS AND DOSAGES

▸ **Pulmonary Arterial Hypertension**

Continuous Subcutaneous Infusion

Adults, Elderly. Initially, 1.25 ng/kg/min. Reduce infusion rate to 0.625 ng/kg/min if initial dose cannot be tolerated. Increase infusion rate in increments of no more than 1.25 ng/kg/min per week for the first 4 wk and then no more than 2.5 ng/kg/min per wk for the duration of infusion.

▸ Hepatic Impairment (Mild to Moderate)
Adults, Elderly. Decrease the initial dose to 0.625 ng/kg/min on the basis of ideal body weight and increase cautiously.

SIDE EFFECTS/ADVERSE REACTIONS

Frequent
Infusion site pain, erythema, induration, rash
Occasional
Headache, diarrhea, jaw pain, vasodilation, nausea
Rare
Dizziness, hypotension, pruritus, edema

PRECAUTIONS AND CONTRAINDICATIONS

None known

DRUG INTERACTIONS OF CONCERN TO DENTISTRY

• Increased risk of bleeding: drugs that interfere with coagulation or platelet function, such as NSAIDs and aspirin

SERIOUS REACTIONS

! Abrupt withdrawal or sudden large reductions in dosage may result in worsening of pulmonary arterial hypertension symptoms.

DENTAL CONSIDERATIONS

General:
• An acute use drug for use in hospitals or emergency departments.
• If a patient reports this drug in his or her medical history, question about cardiovascular disease and drugs he or she may be taking.
• Patients are at risk for bleeding while receiving this drug; provide palliative dental care for dental emergencies only.
• Avoid products that affect platelet function, such as aspirin and NSAIDs.
Consultations:
• Medical consultation should include routine blood counts including platelet counts and bleeding time.
• Medical consultation may be required to assess disease control and patient's ability to tolerate stress.
Teach Patient/Family to:
• Inform dentist of unusual bleeding episodes following dental treatment.

tretinoin

tret′-ih-noyn
(Altinac, Avita, Renova, Retin-A, Retin-A Micro, Vesanoid)

CATEGORY AND SCHEDULE

Pregnancy Risk Category: D (oral), C (topical)

Drug Class: Vitamin A acid

MECHANISM OF ACTION

A retinoid that decreases cohesiveness of follicular epithelial cells. Increases turnover of follicular epithelial cells. Bacterial skin counts are not altered. Transdermal: Exerts its effects on growth and differentiation of epithelial cells. Antineoplastic: Induces maturation, decreases proliferation of acute promyelocytic leukemia (APL) cells.
Therapeutic Effect: Causes expulsion of blackheads; alleviates fine wrinkles, hyperpigmentation; causes repopulation of bone marrow and blood by normal hematopoietic cells.

USES

Treatment of acne vulgaris, reducing fine facial wrinkles associated with

T

sun exposure and aging; unlabeled uses: skin cancer, lichen planus (Renova: not for use in acne)

PHARMACOKINETICS

Topical: Minimally absorbed. Oral: Well absorbed following oral administration. Protein binding: 95%. Metabolized in liver. Primarily excreted in urine, minimal excretion in feces. ***Half-life:*** 0.5–2 hr.

INDICATIONS AND DOSAGES

▸ Acne

Topical
Adults. Apply once daily at bedtime.
Transdermal
Adults. Apply to face once daily at bedtime.

▸ Acute Promyelocytic Leukemia

PO
Adults. 45 mg/m^2/day given as two evenly divided doses until complete remission is documented. Discontinue therapy 30 days after complete remission or after 90 days of treatment, whichever comes first.

SIDE EFFECTS/ADVERSE REACTIONS

Expected
Topical: Temporary change in pigmentation, photosensitivity. Local inflammatory reactions (peeling, dry skin, stinging, erythema, pruritus) are to be expected and are reversible with discontinuation of tretinoin

Frequent
PO: Headache, fever, dry skin/oral mucosa, bone pain, nausea, vomiting, rash

Occasional
PO: Mucositis, earache or feeling of fullness in ears, flushing, pruritus, increased sweating, visual disturbances, hypo-/hypertension, dizziness, anxiety, insomnia, alopecia, skin changes

Rare
PO: Change in visual acuity, temporary hearing loss

PRECAUTIONS AND CONTRAINDICATIONS

Sensitivity to parabens (used as preservative in gelatin capsule)
Caution:
Pregnancy category C, lactation, eczema, sunburn

DRUG INTERACTIONS OF CONCERN TO DENTISTRY

- Increased peeling: medication-containing agents, such as alcohol or astringents
- Avoid concurrent use with photosensitizing drugs: tetracycline, fluoroquinolones, sulfonamides

SERIOUS REACTIONS

PO
! Retinoic acid syndrome (fever, dyspnea, weight gain, abnormal chest auscultatory findings, episodic hypotension) occurs commonly, as does leukocytosis. Syndrome generally occurs during first month of therapy (sometimes occurs following first dose).
! Pseudotumor cerebri may be noted, especially in children (headache, nausea, vomiting, visual disturbances).
! Possible tumorigenic potential when combined with ultraviolet radiation.

Topical
! Possible tumorigenic potential when combined with ultraviolet radiation.

DENTAL CONSIDERATIONS

General:
- May cause dry, peeling skin if used around lips; provide lip lubricant for patient comfort during dental treatment.

• Advise patient if dental drugs prescribed have a potential for photosensitivity.

Teach Patient/Family to:

• Avoid application on normal skin or getting cream in eyes, mouth, or other mucous membranes.

triamcinolone/ triamcinolone acetonide/ triamcinolone diacetate/ triamcinolone hexacetonide

trye-am-**sin**′-oh-lone/trye-am-**sin**′-oh-lone ah-**set**′-oh-nide/ trye-am-**sin**′-oh-lone dye-**ass**′-ih-tate/trye-am-**sin**′-oh-lone hex-ah-**set**′-oh-nide

triamcinolone (Aristocort) triamcinolone acetonide: (Aristocort, Azmacort, Kenacort A[AUS], Kenalog, Kenalog in Orabase[AUS], Nasacort AQ, Triaderm[CAN]) triamcinolone diacetate: (Amcort, Aristocort Intralesional) triamcinolone hexacetonide: (Aristospan)

Do not confuse triamcinolone with Triaminicin or Triaminicol.

CATEGORY AND SCHEDULE

Pregnancy Risk Category: C (D if used in first trimester)

Drug Class: Glucocorticoid, intermediate-acting

MECHANISM OF ACTION

An adrenocortical steroid that inhibits accumulation of inflammatory cells at inflammation sites, phagocytosis, lysosomal enzyme release and synthesis, and release of mediators of inflammation.

Therapeutic Effect: Prevents or suppresses cell-mediated immune reactions. Decreases or prevents tissue response to inflammatory process.

USES

Maintenance treatment of chronic asthma

PHARMACOKINETICS

PO/IM: Peak 1–2 hr. ***Half-life:*** 2–5 hr.

INDICATIONS AND DOSAGES

▸ **Immunosuppression, Relief of Acute Inflammation**

PO

Adults, Elderly. 4–60 mg/day.

IM (Triamcinolone Acetonide)

Adults, Elderly. Initially, 2.5–60 mg/day.

IM (Triamcinolone Diacetate)

Adults, Elderly. 40 mg/wk.

IM (Triamcinolone Hexacetonide)

Adults, Elderly. Initially, 2.5–40 mg up to 100 mg; 2–20 mg.

Intraarticular, Intralesional

Adults, Elderly. 5–40 mg.

▸ **Control of Bronchial Asthma**

Inhalation

Adults, Elderly. 2 inhalations 3–4 times a day.

Children 6–12 yr. 1–2 inhalations 3–4 times a day. Maximum: 12 inhalations/day.

▸ **Rhinitis**

Intranasal

Adults, Children 6 yr and older. 2 sprays each nostril each day.

▸ **Relief of Inflammation or Pruritus Associated with Corticoid-Responsive Dermatoses**

Topical

Adults, Elderly. 2–4 times a day. May give 1–2 times a day or as intermittent therapy.

SIDE EFFECTS/ADVERSE REACTIONS

Frequent

Insomnia, dry mouth, heartburn, nervousness, abdominal distention, diaphoresis, acne, mood swings, increased appetite, facial flushing, delayed wound healing, increased susceptibility to infection, diarrhea or constipation

Occasional

Headache, edema, change in skin color, frequent urination

Rare

Tachycardia, allergic reaction (including rash and hives), mental changes, hallucinations, depression

Topical: Allergic contact dermatitis

PRECAUTIONS AND CONTRAINDICATIONS

Administration of live-virus vaccines, especially smallpox vaccine; hypersensitivity to corticosteroids or tartrazine; IM injection or oral inhalation in children younger than 6 yr; peptic ulcer disease (except life-threatening situations); systemic fungal infection

Topical: Marked circulation impairment

Caution:

Tuberculosis; untreated fungal, bacterial or viral infections of respiratory tract; lactation, children younger than 6 yr; different doses may be required for patients on systemic glucocorticoids or patients with chickenpox, measles; transfer from systemic glucocorticoid therapy to inhalation must be done cautiously to avoid adrenal insufficiency response

T

DRUG INTERACTIONS OF CONCERN TO DENTISTRY

Triamcinolone/Triamcinolone Acetonide/Triamcinolone Hexacetonide

- Decreased action: barbiturates, rifampin, rifabutin
- Increased GI side effects: alcohol, salicylates, NSAIDs
- Increased action: ketoconazole, macrolide antibiotics

SERIOUS REACTIONS

! Long-term therapy may cause muscle wasting in the arms or legs, osteoporosis, spontaneous fractures, amenorrhea, cataracts, glaucoma, peptic ulcer disease, and CHF.

! Abruptly withdrawing the drug following long-term therapy may cause anorexia, nausea, fever, headache, arthralgia, rebound inflammation, fatigue, weakness, lethargy, dizziness, and orthostatic hypotension.

! Anaphylaxis occurs rarely with parenteral administration.

! Suddenly discontinuing triamcinolone may be fatal.

! Blindness has occurred rarely after intralesional injection around face and head.

DENTAL CONSIDERATIONS

General:

- Place on frequent recall because of oral side effects.
- Evaluate respiration characteristics and rate.
- Midday appointments and a stress-reduction protocol may be required for anxious patients.
- Acute asthmatic episodes may be precipitated in the dental office. Rapid-acting sympathomimetic inhalants should be available for emergency use. Triamcinolone is not a rapid-acting drug and is not

intended for use in acute asthmatic attacks.

- Be aware that aspirin or sulfite preservatives in vasoconstrictor-containing products can exacerbate asthma.
- Examine for oral manifestation of opportunistic infection.

Consultations:

- Medical consultation may be required to assess disease control.

Teach Patient/Family to:

- Encourage effective oral hygiene to prevent soft tissue inflammation.
- Gargle, rinse mouth with water, and expectorate after each aerosol dose.

DENTAL CONSIDERATIONS

Triamcinolone/Triamcinolone Acetonide/Triamcinolone Diacetate/Triamcinolone Hexacetonide

General:

- Symptoms of oral infections may be masked.
- Examine for oral manifestation of opportunistic infections.
- Oral side effects may be more common with inhalation products; significant steroid side effects are more likely to occur with chronic systemic doses.
- Acute asthmatic episodes may be precipitated in the dental office. Rapid-acting sympathomimetic inhalants should be available for emergency use. A stress-reduction protocol may be required.
- Monitor vital signs at every appointment because of cardiovascular side effects.
- Assess salivary flow as a factor in caries, periodontal disease, and candidiasis.
- Place on frequent recall to monitor healing response.
- Determine dose and duration of steroid therapy for each patient to assess risk for stress tolerance and immunosuppression.
- Be aware that aspirin or sulfite preservatives in vasoconstrictor-containing products can exacerbate asthma.
- Patients who have been or are currently on chronic steroid therapy may require supplemental steroids for dental treatment.

Consultations:

- Medical consultation may be required to assess disease control.
- Consultation may be required to confirm steroid dose and duration of use.

Teach Patient/Family to:

- Encourage effective oral hygiene to prevent soft tissue inflammation.
- Report oral lesions, soreness, or bleeding to dentist.
- When chronic dry mouth occurs, advise patient to:
  - Avoid mouth rinses with high alcohol content because of drying effects.
  - Use daily home fluoride products for anticaries effect.
  - Use sugarless gum, frequent sips of water, or saliva substitutes.

Triamcinolone Acetonide (Topical)

General:

- Apply approximately 0.25 inch; measure with cotton-tipped applicator; press on lesion, do not rub. Use after brushing and eating and at bedtime for optimal effect.
- When used for oral lesions, return for oral evaluation if response of oral tissues has not occurred in 7–14 days.

Teach Patient/Family to:
- Avoid sunlight on affected area; burns may occur.
- Not use on herpetic lesions.

triamterene

try-**am**′-ter-een
(Dyrenium)
Do not confuse triamterene with trimipramine.

CATEGORY AND SCHEDULE

Pregnancy Risk Category: C (D if used in pregnancy-induced hypertension)

Drug Class: Potassium-sparing diuretic

MECHANISM OF ACTION

A potassium-sparing diuretic that inhibits sodium-potassium ATPase. Interferes with sodium and potassium exchange in distal tubule, cortical collecting tubule, and collecting duct. Increases sodium and decreases potassium excretion. Also increases magnesium, decreases calcium loss.
Therapeutic Effect: Produces diuresis and lowers B/P.

T

USES

Edema; hypertension; more commonly used in combination with a thiazide diuretic

PHARMACOKINETICS

Route	Onset	Peak	Duration
PO	2–4 hr	N/A	7–9 hr

Incompletely absorbed from the GI tract. Widely distributed. Metabolized in the liver. Primarily eliminated in feces via biliary route.
Half-life: 1.5–2.5 hr (increased in renal impairment).

INDICATIONS AND DOSAGES

▸ **Edema, Hypertension**

PO

Adults, Elderly. 25–100 mg/day as a single dose or in 2 divided doses. Maximum: 300 mg/day.
Children. 2–4 mg/kg/day as a single dose or in 2 divided doses. Maximum: 6 mg/kg/day or 300 mg/day.

SIDE EFFECTS/ADVERSE REACTIONS

Occasional

Fatigue, nausea, diarrhea, abdominal pain, leg cramps, headache

Rare

Anorexia, asthenia, rash, dizziness

PRECAUTIONS AND CONTRAINDICATIONS

Drug-induced or preexisting hyperkalemia, progressive or severe renal disease, severe hepatic disease

Caution:

Dehydration, hepatic disease, lactation, CHF, renal disease, cirrhosis

DRUG INTERACTIONS OF CONCERN TO DENTISTRY

- Nephrotoxicity: possible risk with NSAIDs
- Decreased antihypertensive effect: possible risk with NSAIDs, indomethacin
- Decreased effect of folic acid

SERIOUS REACTIONS

! Triamterene use may result in hyponatremia (somnolence, dry mouth, increased thirst, lack of energy) or severe hyperkalemia (irritability, anxiety, heaviness of legs, paresthesia, hypotension, bradycardia, ECG changes [tented T

waves, widening QRS complex, ST segment depression]).
! Agranulocytosis, nephrolithiasis, and thrombocytopenia occur rarely.

DENTAL CONSIDERATIONS

General:
- Limit use of sodium-containing products, such as saline IV fluids, for patients with a dietary salt restriction.
- Assess salivary flow as a factor in caries, periodontal disease, and candidiasis.
- Monitor vital signs at every appointment because of cardiovascular effects and possible hyperkalemia.
- Patients on chronic drug therapy may rarely have symptoms of blood dyscrasias, which can include infection, bleeding, and poor healing.

Consultations:
- In a patient with symptoms of blood dyscrasias, request a medical consultation for blood studies and postpone dental treatment until normal values are reestablished.
- Medical consultation may be required to assess disease control.

Teach Patient/Family to:
- Encourage effective oral hygiene to prevent soft tissue inflammation.
- Use caution to prevent injury when using oral hygiene aids.
- Report oral lesions, soreness, or bleeding to dentist.
- When chronic dry mouth occurs, advise patient to:
  - Avoid mouth rinses with high alcohol content because of drying effects.
  - Use daily home fluoride products to prevent caries.
  - Use sugarless gum, frequent sips of water, or saliva substitutes.

triazolam

trye-**ay**′-zoe-lam
(Apo-Triazo[CAN], Halcion)
Do not confuse Halcion with Haldol or Healon.

CATEGORY AND SCHEDULE

Pregnancy Risk Category: X
Controlled Substance: Schedule IV

Drug Class: Benzodiazepine, sedative-hypnotic

MECHANISM OF ACTION

A benzodiazepine that enhances the action of the inhibitory neurotransmitter gamma-aminobutyric acid, resulting in CNS depression.
Therapeutic Effect: Induces sleep.

USES

Treatment of insomnia, preoperative sedation (unapproved)

PHARMACOKINETICS

PO: Onset 30–45 min, duration 6–8 hr. ***Half-life:*** 2–3 hr; metabolized by liver (CYP3A4); excreted by kidneys (inactive metabolites); crosses placenta; excreted in breast milk.

INDICATIONS AND DOSAGES

▸ **Insomnia**

PO
Adults, Children 18 yr and older. 0.125–0.5 mg at bedtime.
Elderly. 0.0625–0.125 mg at bedtime.
M.R.D. 0.5 mg

SIDE EFFECTS/ADVERSE REACTIONS

Frequent

Somnolence, sedation, dry mouth, headache, dizziness, nervousness, light-headedness, incoordination, nausea, rebound insomnia (may occur for 1–2 nights after drug is discontinued)

Occasional

Euphoria, tachycardia, abdominal cramps, visual disturbances

Rare

Paradoxic CNS excitement or restlessness (particularly in elderly or debilitated patients)

PRECAUTIONS AND CONTRAINDICATIONS

Angle-closure glaucoma; CNS depression; pregnancy or breast-feeding; severe, uncontrolled pain; sleep apnea

Caution:

Anemia, hepatic disease, renal disease, suicidal individuals, drug abuse, elderly, psychosis, children younger than 15 yr, acute narrow-angle glaucoma, seizure disorders

DRUG INTERACTIONS OF CONCERN TO DENTISTRY

- Increased effects: erythromycin, clarithromycin (CYP3A4 inhibitors)
- Increased sedation: alcohol, CNS depressants, opioid analgesics, diltiazem, anesthetics
- Avoid use with ketoconazole, itraconazole, ritonavir, indinavir, nelfinavir
- Caution if used with fluvoxamine, reduce dose by 50%

SERIOUS REACTIONS

! Abrupt or too-rapid withdrawal may result in pronounced restlessness, irritability, insomnia, hand tremors, abdominal or muscle cramps, vomiting, diaphoresis, and seizures.

! Overdose results in somnolence, confusion, diminished reflexes, respiratory depression, and coma.

DENTAL CONSIDERATIONS

General:

- Assess salivary flow as a factor in caries, periodontal disease, and candidiasis.
- If dizziness occurs, provide assistance when escorting patient to and from dental chair.
- When used for conscious sedation, have someone drive patient to and from dental office.
- Avoid the use of this drug in a patient with a history of drug abuse or alcoholism.
- Geriatric patients are more susceptible to drug effects; use a lower dose.
- Psychological and physical dependence may occur with chronic administration.
- Determine why the patient is taking the drug.
- Patients on chronic drug therapy may rarely have symptoms of blood dyscrasias, which can include infection, bleeding, and poor healing.

Teach Patient/Family:

- When chronic dry mouth occurs, advise patient to:
  - Avoid mouth rinses with high alcohol content because of drying effects.
  - Use daily home fluoride products to prevent caries.
  - Use sugarless gum, frequent sips of water, or saliva substitutes.

trifluoperazine hydrochloride

trye-floo-oh-**per′**-ah-zeen high-droh-**klor′**-ide (Apo-Trifluoperazine[CAN], Nono-Trifluzine[CAN], PMS-Trifluoperazine[CAN], Stelazine)

Do not confuse trifluoperazine with triflupromazine, or Stelazine with selegiline.

CATEGORY AND SCHEDULE

Pregnancy Risk Category: C

Drug Class: Phenothiazine antipsychotic

MECHANISM OF ACTION

A phenothiazine derivative that blocks dopamine at postsynaptic receptor sites. Possesses strong extrapyramidal and antiemetic effects and weak anticholinergic and sedative effects.

Therapeutic Effect: Suppresses behavioral response in psychosis; reduces locomotor activity and aggressiveness.

USES

Treatment of psychotic disorders, nonpsychotic anxiety, schizophrenia

PHARMACOKINETICS

PO: Onset rapid, peak 2–3 hr, duration 12 hr. IM: Onset immediate, peak 1 hr, duration 12 hr. Metabolized by liver, excreted in urine, crosses placenta, excreted in breast milk.

INDICATIONS AND DOSAGES

▸ Psychotic Disorders

PO

Adults, Elderly, Children 12 yr and older. Initially, 2–5 mg once or twice a day. Range: 15–20 mg/day. Maximum: 40 mg/day.

Children 6–11 yr. Initially, 1 mg once or twice a day. Maintenance: Up to 15 mg/day.

IM

Adults. 1–2 mg q4–6h. Maximum: 10 mg/24h.

Elderly. 1 mg q4–6h. Maximum: 6 mg/24h.

Children. 1 mg 2 times a day.

SIDE EFFECTS/ADVERSE REACTIONS

Frequent

Hypotension, dizziness, and syncope (occur frequently after first injection, occasionally after subsequent injections, and rarely with oral form)

Occasional

Drowsiness during early therapy, dry mouth, blurred vision, lethargy, constipation or diarrhea, nasal congestion, peripheral edema, urine retention

Rare

Ocular changes, altered skin pigmentation (in those taking high doses for prolonged periods), photosensitivity

PRECAUTIONS AND CONTRAINDICATIONS

Angle-closure glaucoma, circulatory collapse, myelosuppression, severe cardiac or hepatic disease, severe hypertension or hypotension

Caution:

Breast cancer, seizure disorders, lactation, diabetes mellitus, respiratory conditions, prostatic hypertrophy

DRUG INTERACTIONS OF CONCERN TO DENTISTRY

- Increased sedation: other CNS depressants, alcohol, barbiturate anesthetics, opioid analgesics

• Hypotension, tachycardia: epinephrine
• Increased extrapyramidal effects: phenothiazines and related drugs (haloperidol, droperidol), metoclopramide
• Additive photosensitization: tetracyclines
• Increased anticholinergic effects: anticholinergics

SERIOUS REACTIONS

! Extrapyramidal symptoms appear to be dose related (particularly high doses) and are divided into 3 categories: akathisia (inability to sit still, tapping of feet), parkinsonian symptoms (such as mask-like face, tremors, shuffling gait, and hypersalivation), and acute dystonias (such as torticollis, opisthotonos, and oculogyric crisis). Dystonic reactions may also produce diaphoresis and pallor.
! Tardive dyskinesia, marked by tongue protrusion, puffing of the cheeks, and chewing or puckering of the mouth, occurs rarely but may be irreversible.
! Abrupt withdrawal after long-term therapy may precipitate nausea, vomiting, gastritis, dizziness, and tremors.
! Blood dyscrasias, particularly agranulocytosis, and mild leukopenia may occur.
! Trifluoperazine may lower the seizure threshold.

DENTAL CONSIDERATIONS

General:

• Monitor vital signs at every appointment because of cardiovascular side effects.
• Patients on chronic drug therapy may rarely have symptoms of blood dyscrasias, which can include infection, bleeding, and poor healing.
• After supine positioning, have patient sit upright for at least 2 min before standing to avoid orthostatic hypotension.
• Assess salivary flow as a factor in caries, periodontal disease, and candidiasis.
• Avoid dental light in patient's eyes; offer dark glasses for patient comfort.
• Assess for presence of extrapyramidal motor symptoms, such as tardive dyskinesia and akathisia. Extrapyramidal motor activity may complicate dental treatment.
• Geriatric patients are more susceptible to drug effects; use lower dose.
• Use vasoconstrictors with caution, in low doses, and with careful aspiration.

Consultations:

• In a patient with symptoms of blood dyscrasias, request a medical consultation for blood studies and postpone dental treatment until normal values are reestablished.
• Take precautions if dental surgery is anticipated and anesthesia is required.
• Physician should be informed if significant xerostomic side effects occur (e.g., increased caries, sore tongue, problems eating or swallowing, difficulty wearing prosthesis) so that a medication change can be considered.
• If signs of tardive dyskinesia or akathisia are present, refer to physician.

Teach Patient/Family to:

• Encourage effective oral hygiene to prevent soft tissue inflammation.
• Use caution to prevent injury when using oral hygiene aids.
• Use powered tooth brush if patient has difficulty holding conventional devices.

- When chronic dry mouth occurs, advise patient to:
  - Use daily home fluoride products for anticaries effect.
  - Avoid mouth rinses with high alcohol content because of drying effects.
  - Use sugarless gum, frequent sips of water, or saliva substitutes.

trifluridine

trye-**flure′**-ih-deen
(Viroptic)
Do not confuse with Zostrix.

CATEGORY AND SCHEDULE

Pregnancy Risk Category: C

Drug Class: Antiviral

MECHANISM OF ACTION

An antiviral agent that incorporates into DNA causing increased rate of mutation and errors in protein formation.
Therapeutic Effect: Prevents viral replication.

USES

Treatment of primary keratoconjunctivitis, recurring epithelial keratitis, keratitis associated with human herpes virus types 1 and 2, and vacciniavirus

PHARMACOKINETICS

Intraocular solution is undetectable in serum. ***Half-life:*** 12 min.

INDICATIONS AND DOSAGES

▸ Herpes Simplex Virus Ocular Infections

Ophthalmic
Adults, Elderly, Children older than 6 yr. 1 drop onto cornea q2h while awake. Maximum: 9 drops/day. Continue until corneal ulcer has completely reepithelialized, then 1 drop q4h while awake (minimum: 5 drops/day) for an additional 7 days.

SIDE EFFECTS/ADVERSE REACTIONS

Frequent
Transient stinging or burning with instillation
Occasional
Edema of eyelid
Rare
Hypersensitivity reaction

PRECAUTIONS AND CONTRAINDICATIONS

Hypersensitivity to trifluridine or any component of the formulation
Caution:
Antibiotic hypersensitivity

DRUG INTERACTIONS OF CONCERN TO DENTISTRY

- None reported

SERIOUS REACTIONS

! Ocular toxicity may occur if used longer than 21 days.

DENTAL CONSIDERATIONS

General:

- Avoid dental light in patient's eyes; offer dark glasses for patient comfort.
- Evaluate:
  - Therapeutic response: absence of redness, inflammation, tearing.
  - Allergy: itching, lacrimation, redness, swelling.

trihexyphenidyl

trye-hex-ee-**fen′**-ih-dill
(Artane, Apo-Trihex[CAN])

CATEGORY AND SCHEDULE

Pregnancy Risk Category: C

Drug Class: Antiparkinsonian, anticholinergic

MECHANISM OF ACTION

An anticholinergic agent that blocks central cholinergic receptors (aids in balancing cholinergic and dopaminergic activity).
Therapeutic Effect: Decreases salivation, relaxes smooth muscle.

USES

Treatment of Parkinson symptoms

PHARMACOKINETICS

Well absorbed from GI tract. Primarily excreted in urine.
Half-life: 3.3–4.1 hr.

INDICATIONS AND DOSAGES

▸ Parkinsonism

PO

Adults, Elderly. Initially, 1 mg on first day. May increase by 2 mg/day at 3–5-day intervals up to 6–10 mg/day (12–15 mg/day in patients with postencephalitic parkinsonism).

▸ Drug-Induced Extrapyramidal Symptoms

PO

Adults, Elderly. Initially, 1 mg/day. Range: 5–15 mg/day.

T

SIDE EFFECTS/ADVERSE REACTIONS

Elderly (older than 60 yr) tend to develop mental confusion, disorientation, agitation, psychotic-like symptoms

Frequent
Drowsiness, dry mouth
Occasional
Blurred vision, urinary retention, constipation, dizziness, headache, muscle cramps
Rare
Seizures, depression, rash

PRECAUTIONS AND CONTRAINDICATIONS

Angle closure glaucoma, GI obstruction, paralytic ileus, intestinal atony, severe ulcerative colitis, prostatic hypertrophy, myasthenia gravis, megacolon, hypersensitivity to trihexyphenidyl or any component of the formulation
Caution:
Children, gastric ulcer

DRUG INTERACTIONS OF CONCERN TO DENTISTRY

- Increased anticholinergic effects: scopolamine, atropine, phenothiazines, antihistamines, and other anticholinergics
- Increased CNS depression: alcohol, CNS depressants
- Decreased effects of phenothiazines

SERIOUS REACTIONS

! Hypersensitivity reaction (eczema, pruritus, rash, cardiac disturbances, photosensitivity) may occur.
! Overdosage may vary from CNS depression (sedation, apnea, cardiovascular collapse, death) to severe paradoxic reaction (hallucinations, tremor, seizures).

DENTAL CONSIDERATIONS

General:

- Assess salivary flow as a factor in caries, periodontal disease, and candidiasis.
- Place on frequent recall because of oral side effects.

- After supine positioning, have patient sit upright for at least 2 min before standing to avoid orthostatic hypotension.
- Avoid dental light in patient's eyes; offer dark glasses for patient comfort.

Teach Patient/Family to:

- Encourage effective oral hygiene to prevent soft tissue inflammation.
- Use powered tooth brush if patient has difficulty holding conventional devices.
- When chronic dry mouth occurs, advise patient to:
  - Avoid mouth rinses with high alcohol content because of drying effects.
  - Use daily home fluoride products to prevent caries.
  - Use sugarless gum, frequent sips of water, or saliva substitutes.

trimethobenzamide hydrochloride

trye-meth-oh-**ben′**-za-mide high-droh-**klor′**-ide
(Tigan)

CATEGORY AND SCHEDULE

Pregnancy Risk Category: C

Drug Class: Antiemetic

MECHANISM OF ACTION

An anticholinergic that acts at the chemoreceptor trigger zone in the medulla oblongata.
Therapeutic Effect: Relieves nausea and vomiting.

USES

Treatment of nausea, vomiting

PHARMACOKINETICS

Route	Onset	Peak	Duration
PO	10–40 min	N/A	3–4 hr
IM	15–30 min	N/A	2–3 hr

Partially absorbed from the GI tract. Distributed primarily to the liver. Metabolic fate unknown. Excreted in urine. ***Half-life:*** 7–9 hr.

INDICATIONS AND DOSAGES

▸ Nausea and Vomiting

PO
Adults, Elderly. 300 mg 3–4 times a day.
Children weighing 30–100 lb. 100–200 mg 3–4 times a day.
IM
Adults, Elderly. 200 mg 3–4 times a day.
Rectal
Adults, Elderly. 200 mg 3–4 times a day.
Children weighing 30–100 lb. 100–200 mg 3–4 times a day.
Children weighing less than 30 lb. 100 mg 3–4 times a day.

SIDE EFFECTS/ADVERSE REACTIONS

Frequent
Somnolence
Occasional
Blurred vision, diarrhea, dizziness, headache, muscle cramps
Rare
Rash, seizures, depression, opisthotonos, parkinsonian syndrome, Reye's syndrome (marked by vomiting, seizures)

PRECAUTIONS AND CONTRAINDICATIONS

Hypersensitivity to benzocaine or similar local anesthetics; use of parenteral form in children or suppositories in premature infants or neonates

Caution:
Children, cardiac dysrhythmias, elderly, asthma, prostatic hypertrophy, bladder neck obstruction, narrow-angle glaucoma, stenosing peptic ulcer, pyloroduodenal obstruction

DRUG INTERACTIONS OF CONCERN TO DENTISTRY

• Increased effect: CNS depressants
• May mask ototoxic symptoms associated with antibiotics or large doses of salicylates

SERIOUS REACTIONS

! A hypersensitivity reaction, manifested as extrapyramidal symptoms such as muscle rigidity and allergic skin reactions, occurs rarely.
! Children may experience paradoxic reactions, marked by restlessness, insomnia, euphoria, nervousness, and tremor.
! Overdose may produce CNS depression (manifested as sedation, apnea, cardiovascular collapse, and death) or severe paradoxic reactions (such as hallucinations, tremor, and seizures).

DENTAL CONSIDERATIONS

T

General:
• Nausea and vomiting may be accompanied by dehydration and electrolyte imbalance and should be corrected as part of treatment.
• Postpone elective dental treatment when symptoms are present.

trimetrexate

try-meh-**trex′**-ate
(NeuTrexin)
Do not confuse with Amicar.

CATEGORY AND SCHEDULE

Pregnancy Risk Category: D

Drug Class: Folate antagonist

MECHANISM OF ACTION

A folate antagonist that inhibits the enzyme dihydrofolate reductase (DHFR).
Therapeutic Effect: Disrupts purine, DNA, RNA, protein synthesis, with consequent cell death.

USES

Alternative therapy for *P. carinii* pneumonia (PCP) in immunocompromised patients, including patients with AIDS; unapproved uses: treatment of lung, prostate, colon cancer

PHARMACOKINETICS

Following IV administration, distributed readily into ascitic fluid. Metabolized in liver. Eliminated in urine. ***Half-life:*** 11–20 hr.

INDICATIONS AND DOSAGES

▸ **PCP**

IV Infusion
Adults. Trimetrexate: 45 mg/m^2 once daily over 60–90 min. Leucovorin: 20 mg/m^2 over 5–10 min q6h for total daily dose of 80 mg/m^2, or orally as 4 doses of 20 mg/m^2 spaced equally throughout the day. Round up the oral dose to the next higher 25-mg increment. Recommended course of therapy: 21 days trimetrexate, 24 days leucovorin.

SIDE EFFECTS/ADVERSE REACTIONS

Occasional
Fever, rash, pruritus, nausea, vomiting, confusion
Rare
Fatigue

PRECAUTIONS AND CONTRAINDICATIONS

Clinically significant hypersensitivity to trimetrexate, leucovorin, or methotrexate
Caution:
Lactation, children younger than 18 yr; impaired hematologic, renal, or hepatic function; serious bone marrow depression can occur if leucovorin is not used concurrently

DRUG INTERACTIONS OF CONCERN TO DENTISTRY

• Alteration of plasma levels: concurrent use with erythromycin, ketoconazole, and fluconazole
• Alteration in trimetrexate metabolites: acetaminophen
• Caution with use of drugs that are strong inhibitors of CYP3A4 isoenzymes

SERIOUS REACTIONS

! Trimetrexate given without concurrent leucovorin may result in serious or fatal hematologic, hepatic, and/or renal complications, including bone marrow suppression, oral and GI mucosal ulceration, and renal and hepatic dysfunction.
! In event of overdose, stop trimetrexate and give leucovorin 40 mg/m^2 q6h for 3 days.
! Anaphylaxis occurs rarely.

DENTAL CONSIDERATIONS

General:
• Examine for evidence of oral manifestations of blood dyscrasia (infection, bleeding, poor healing).
• Place on frequent recall because of oral side effects.
• Determine why the patient is taking the drug.
• Examine for oral manifestations of opportunistic infections.
• Consider local hemostasis measures to prevent excessive bleeding.
• Palliative treatment may be required for stomatitis.
• Refer to physician if oral ulcerative lesions occur.
• Consider semisupine chair position for patient comfort because of GI effects of disease.
Consultations:
• Obtain a medical consultation for blood studies (CBC) because leukopenic or thrombocytopenic side effects may result in infection, delayed healing, and excessive bleeding. Postpone elective dental treatment until normal values are maintained.
• Medical consultation may be required to assess disease control.
Teach Patient/Family to:
• Encourage effective oral hygiene to prevent soft tissue inflammation.
• Use caution to prevent injury when using oral hygiene aids.
• See dentist immediately if secondary oral infection occurs.

trimipramine

trye-**mih′**-pra-meen
(Apo-Trimip[CAN], Novo-Tripramine[CAN], Nu-Trimipramine[CAN], Rhotrimine[CAN], Surmontil)
Do not confuse with desipramine.

CATEGORY AND SCHEDULE

Pregnancy Risk Category: C

Drug Class:
Antidepressant-tricyclic

MECHANISM OF ACTION

A tricyclic antibulimic, anticataplectic, antidepressant, antinarcoleptic, antineuralgic, antineuritic, and antipanic agent that blocks the reuptake of neurotransmitters, such as norepinephrine and serotonin, at presynaptic membranes, increasing their concentration at postsynaptic receptor sites. May demonstrate less autonomic toxicity than other tricyclic antidepressants.

Therapeutic Effect: Results in antidepressant effect. Anticholinergic effect controls nocturnal enuresis.

USES

Treatment of depression

PHARMACOKINETICS

Rapidly, completely absorbed after PO administration, and not affected by food. Protein binding: 95%. Metabolized in liver (significant first-pass effect). Primarily excreted in urine. Not removed by hemodialysis. ***Half-life:*** 16–40 hr.

INDICATIONS AND DOSAGES

▸ Depression

PO

Adults. 50–150 mg/day at bedtime. Maximum: 200 mg/day for outpatients, 300 mg/day for inpatients.

Elderly. Initially, 25 mg/day at bedtime. May increase by 25 mg q3–7days. Maximum: 100 mg/day.

SIDE EFFECTS/ADVERSE REACTIONS

Frequent

Drowsiness, fatigue, dry mouth, blurred vision, constipation, delayed micturition, postural hypotension, diaphoresis, disturbed concentration, increased appetite, urinary retention, photosensitivity

Occasional

GI disturbances, such as nausea, and a metallic taste sensation

Rare

Paradoxic reaction marked by agitation and restlessness, nightmares, insomnia, and extrapyramidal symptoms, particularly fine hand tremors

PRECAUTIONS AND CONTRAINDICATIONS

Acute recovery period after MI, within 14 days of MAOI ingestion, hypersensitivity to trimipramine or any component of the formulation

Caution:

Suicidal patients, severe depression, increased intraocular pressure, narrow-angle glaucoma, urinary retention, cardiac disease, hepatic disease, hyperthyroidism, electroshock therapy, elective surgery, MAOIs

DRUG INTERACTIONS OF CONCERN TO DENTISTRY

- Increased anticholinergic effects: muscarinic blockers, antihistamines, phenothiazines
- Increased effects of direct-acting sympathomimetics (epinephrine, levonordefrin)
- Possible risk of increased CNS depression: alcohol, barbiturates, benzodiazepines, and other CNS depressants
- Decreased antihypertensive effects: clonidine, guanadrel, guanethidine

SERIOUS REACTIONS

! High dosage may produce cardiovascular effects, such as severe postural hypotension, dizziness, tachycardia, palpitations, arrhythmias and seizures. High dosage may also result in altered temperature regulation, including hyperpyrexia or hypothermia.

! Abrupt withdrawal from prolonged therapy may produce headache, malaise, nausea, vomiting, and vivid dreams.

DENTAL CONSIDERATIONS

General:

- Monitor vital signs at every appointment because of cardiovascular side effects.
- Assess salivary flow as a factor in caries, periodontal disease, and candidiasis.
- Patients on chronic drug therapy may rarely have symptoms of blood dyscrasias, which can include infection, bleeding, and poor healing.
- After supine positioning, have patient sit upright for at least 2 min before standing to avoid orthostatic hypotension.
- Use vasoconstrictors with caution, in low doses, and with careful aspiration. Avoid use of gingival retraction cord with epinephrine.
- Place on frequent recall because of oral side effects.

Consultations:

- In a patient with symptoms of blood dyscrasias, request a medical consultation for blood studies and postpone dental treatment until normal values are reestablished.
- Medical consultation may be required to assess disease control.
- Physician should be informed if significant xerostomic side effects occur (e.g., increased caries, sore tongue, problems eating or swallowing, difficulty wearing prosthesis) so that a medication change can be considered.

Teach Patient/Family:

- Importance of good oral hygiene to prevent soft tissue inflammation.
- To use caution to prevent injury when using oral hygiene aids.
- When chronic dry mouth occurs, advise patient:
  - To avoid mouth rinses with high alcohol content because of drying effects.
  - To use daily home fluoride products to prevent caries.
  - To use sugarless gum, frequent sips of water, or saliva substitutes.

triptorelin pamoate

trip-toe-**ree′**-linn **pam′**-oh-ate
(Trelstar Depot, Trelstar LA)

CATEGORY AND SCHEDULE

Pregnancy Risk Category: X

Drug Class: Antineoplastic

MECHANISM OF ACTION

A gonadotropin-releasing hormone (GnRH) analogue and antineoplastic agent that inhibits gonadotropin hormone secretion through a negative feedback mechanism. Circulating levels of luteinizing hormone, follicle-stimulating hormone, testosterone, and estradiol rise initially, then subside with continued therapy.

Therapeutic Effect: Suppresses growth of abnormal prostate tissue.

USES

Decreasing testosterone levels

PHARMACOKINETICS

Metabolism may be by CYP450, eliminated by liver, kidneys; terminal half-life is 3 hr in healthy males.

INDICATIONS AND DOSAGES

▸ **Prostate Cancer**

IM (Trelstar Depot)

Adults, Elderly. 3.75 mg once q28 days.

IM (Trelstar LA)

Adults, Elderly. 11.25 mg q84 days.

SIDE EFFECTS/ADVERSE REACTIONS

Frequent

Hot flashes, skeletal pain, headache, impotence

Occasional

Insomnia, vomiting, leg pain, fatigue

Rare

Dizziness, emotional lability, diarrhea, urine retention, UTIs, anemia, pruritus

PRECAUTIONS AND CONTRAINDICATIONS

Hypersensitivity to luteinizing hormone-releasing hormone (LHRH) or LHRH agonists

DRUG INTERACTIONS OF CONCERN TO DENTISTRY

• Dental drug interactions have not been studied.

SERIOUS REACTIONS

! Bladder outlet obstruction, skeletal pain, hematuria, and spinal cord compression (with weakness or paralysis of the lower extremities) may occur.

T

DENTAL CONSIDERATIONS

General:

• If additional analgesia is required for dental pain, consider alternative analgesics (NSAIDs) in patients taking opioids for acute or chronic pain.

• This drug may be used in the hospital or on an outpatient basis. Confirm the patient's disease and treatment status.

• Patients may have received other chemotherapy or radiation; confirm medical and drug history.

• When urinary retention is a problem, use anticholinergic drugs with care.

Consultations:

• Consult patient's physician if an acute dental infection occurs and another antiinfective is required.

• Medical consultation may be required to assess disease control and patient's ability to tolerate stress.

Teach Patient/Family to:

• Encourage effective oral hygiene to prevent soft tissue inflammation.

• Prevent trauma when using oral hygiene aids.

• Update health and medication history if physician makes any changes in evaluation or drug regimens; include OTC, herbal, and nonherbal remedies in the update.

tropicamide

troe-**pik**′-ah-mide

(Diotrope[CAN], Mydriacyl, Opticyl, Tropicacyl)

CATEGORY AND SCHEDULE

Pregnancy Risk Category: C

Drug Class: Mydriatic, cycloplegic

MECHANISM OF ACTION

An antimuscarinic agent that produces competitive antagonism of the actions of acetylcholine.

Therapeutic Effect: Produces dilation of pupil (mydriasis); produces paralysis of accommodation (cycloplegia).

USES
Dilation of the pupil

PHARMACOKINETICS
Onset of action occurs within 20–40 min. The duration is about 6 hr.

INDICATIONS AND DOSAGES
▸ Ocular Diagnostic Procedure, Examination of Fundus

Ophthalmic

Adults, Elderly, Children. 1–2 drops in the eye(s) 15–20 min prior to exam.

▸ Ocular Diagnostic Procedure, Refractive Procedures

Ophthalmic

Adults, Elderly, Children. 1–2 drops in the eye(s). May be repeated in 5 min.

SIDE EFFECTS/ADVERSE REACTIONS
Occasional

Blurred vision, ocular irritation, headache

Rare

Photophobia, increased intraocular pressure

PRECAUTIONS AND CONTRAINDICATIONS
Primary glaucoma or tendency toward glaucoma, hypersensitivity to tropicamide or any component of the formulation

DRUG INTERACTIONS OF CONCERN TO DENTISTRY
• None reported

SERIOUS REACTIONS
! Cardiorespiratory collapse has been reported.

! Systemic absorption, including behavioral disturbances, confusion, dry mouth, fast heartbeat, and psychotic reactions, occurs rarely.

DENTAL CONSIDERATIONS
General:

• An acute use drug for diagnostic purposes.

• Protect patient's eyes from accidental spatter during dental treatment.

• Avoid dental light in patient's eyes; offer dark glasses for patient comfort.

trovafloxacin mesylate/ alatrofloxacin mesylate
troe-va-**flox**′-ah-sin **meh**′-sil-ate/ ala-troe-**flox**′-ah-sin **meh**′-sil-ate

Trovafloxacin mesylate oral: (Trovan) Alatrofloxacin mesylate injection: (Trovan I.V.)

CATEGORY AND SCHEDULE
Pregnancy Risk Category: C

Drug Class: Antibiotic fluoronaphthyridone antiinfective (related to the fluoroquinolones)

MECHANISM OF ACTION
A broad-spectrum anti-bacterial agent that inhibits the enzymes topoisomerase II (DNA gyrase) and topoisomerase IV required for bacterial DNA replication, transcription repair, and recombination.

Therapeutic Effect: Bactericidal.

USES
Treatment of infections caused by susceptible microorganisms in nosocomial pneumonia, community-acquired pneumonia, acute bacterial exacerbated chronic bronchitis, acute sinusitis, abdominal infections, gynecologic infections, UTI, bacterial prostatitis, skin and

T

skin-structure infections, and selected STDs

PHARMACOKINETICS

PO: Good oral absorption, bioavailability 88%, can be administered with food, peak serum levels 1.7 hr, plasma protein binding 76%, wide tissue distribution, excreted in breast milk, hepatic metabolism, excretion in feces and urine, 50% of dose is excreted unchanged in feces. IV: Alatrofloxacin is a prodrug converted to trovafloxacin.

INDICATIONS AND DOSAGES

PO: Skin Infections
Adults older than 18 yr. Dose depends on type of infection; 200 mg daily for 1–14 days.
IV: Nosocomial Pneumonia
Adults older than 18 yr. IV dose depends on type of infection; range 300 mg daily; single IV doses can be followed by appropriate oral doses for 10–14 days.

SIDE EFFECTS/ADVERSE REACTIONS

Oral: Dry mouth, stomatitis, angular cheilitis
CNS: Dizziness, headache, light-headedness, confusion, anxiety, hallucinations
CV: Hypotension, palpitation, flushing, peripheral edema, chest pain
GI: Vomiting, nausea, diarrhea, abdominal pain, flatulence, antibiotic-associated pseudomembranous colitis, hepatic toxicity
Resp: Dyspnea, bronchospasm, coughing
Hema: Anemia, leukopenia, thrombocytopenia
GU: Vaginitis, frequency of urination, abnormal renal function
EENT: Rhinitis, sinusitis
Integ: Pruritus, rash, photosensitization
Meta: Increased liver enzymes
MS: Arthralgia, myalgia, muscle cramps
Misc: Pain on injection, increased sweating, fatigue, fever, anaphylaxis

PRECAUTIONS AND CONTRAINDICATIONS

Hypersensitivity and allergy to the fluoroquinolones
Serious liver injury
Caution:
Children younger than 18 yr, mild to moderate cirrhosis, potential for liver damage, exposure to sunlight, visible or ultraviolet radiation, seizure disorders, cerebral atherosclerosis, lactation, warning associated with possible serious hepatic injury leading to death or transplant

DRUG INTERACTIONS OF CONCERN TO DENTISTRY

- Reduction in absorption: magnesium or aluminum antacid products, iron salts, sucralfate, and morphine within 30 min of oral trovafloxacin; separate doses by at least 2 hr
- Increases serum levels of caffeine

SERIOUS REACTIONS

! Serious liver injury

DENTAL CONSIDERATIONS

General:
- Determine why patient is taking the drug; specific infection.
- Do not use ingestible sodium bicarbonate products, such as the air polishing system Prophy-Jet, within 2 hr of drug use.
- Examine for oral manifestation of opportunistic infection.

• Avoid dental light in patient's eyes; offer dark glasses for patient comfort.
• Use caution in prescribing caffeine-containing analgesics.

Consultations:

• Medical consultation may be required to assess disease control in the patient.
• Consult with patient's physician if an acute dental infection occurs and another antiinfective is required.

Teach Patient/Family to:

• Prevent trauma when using oral hygiene aids.
• Encourage effective oral hygiene to prevent soft tissue inflammation.
• Avoid mouth rinses with high alcohol content because of drying effects.

ulipristal

ue-li-pris-tal
(Ella)
Do not confuse ulipristal with ursodiol.

CATEGORY AND SCHEDULE

Pregnancy Risk Category: X

Drug Class: Contraceptive; progestin receptor modulator

MECHANISM OF ACTION

Postpones follicular rupture when administered prior to ovulation, thereby inhibiting or delaying ovulation. May also alter the normal endometrium, impairing implantation.
Therapeutic Effect: Reduces chance of unintended pregnancy.

USES

Emergency contraception following unprotected intercourse or possible contraceptive failure

PHARMACOKINETICS

Rapidly absorbed after oral administration. 94% plasma protein bound. Hepatic metabolism via CYP3A4 to active and inactive metabolites. ***Half-life:*** 32 hr.

INDICATIONS AND DOSAGES

▸ **Emergency Contraception**

PO

Adults (females). 1 tablet (30 mg) as soon as possible, but within 120 hr (5 days) of unprotected intercourse or contraceptive failure.

SIDE EFFECTS/ADVERSE REACTIONS

Frequent

Headache, abdominal pain, nausea

Occasional

Fatigue, dizziness

PRECAUTIONS AND CONTRAINDICATIONS

Known or suspected pregnancy

DRUG INTERACTIONS OF CONCERN TO DENTISTRY

- CYP3A4 inducers (e.g., carbamazepine, barbiturates, St. John's wort): decreased effectiveness of ulipristal

SERIOUS REACTIONS

! None known

DENTAL CONSIDERATIONS

General:

- Take precaution when seating and dismissing patient due to dizziness.
- Increased risk of nausea and vomiting (e.g., during sedation and impressions).

Teach Patient/Family to:

- Inform dentist when drug has been taken.

unoprostone isopropyl

yoo-noh-**prost′**-ohn eye-seh-**pro′**-pel
(Rescula)

CATEGORY AND SCHEDULE

Pregnancy Risk Category: C

Drug Class: Prostaglandin agonist

MECHANISM OF ACTION

An ophthalmic agent that increases the outflow of aqueous humor.
Therapeutic Effect: Decreases intraocular pressure.

USES

Indicated for lowering intraocular pressure (IOP) in patients with open-angle glaucoma or ocular hypertension who are intolerant to other medications or who failed to achieve a targeted IOP

PHARMACOKINETICS

Peak response occurs in 4–8 wk. The duration of a single dose is about 10 hr. Hydrolyzed to unoprostone free acid form in the cornea. Rapidly eliminated from plasma. Excreted as metabolites in urine. ***Half-life:*** 14 min.

INDICATIONS AND DOSAGES

▸ **Glaucoma, Ocular Hypertension**

Ophthalmic

Adults, Elderly. Instill 1 drop in affected eye(s) 2 times a day.

SIDE EFFECTS/ADVERSE REACTIONS

Frequent

Burning, stinging, dry eyes, itching, increased eyelash length and redness

Occasional

Abnormal vision, eyelid disorder, foreign body sensation

PRECAUTIONS AND CONTRAINDICATIONS

Hypersensitivity to unoprostone isopropyl, benzalkonium chloride, or any other component of the formulation

Caution:

Permanent changes in pigmented tissues of eye, bacterial keratitis, do not use while wearing contact lens, no data on use in renal or hepatic failure or pediatric patients

DRUG INTERACTIONS OF CONCERN TO DENTISTRY

• None reported; avoid use of anticholinergic drugs: atropine-like drugs, propantheline, diazepam, other benzodiazepines.

SERIOUS REACTIONS

! Elevated IOP occurs rarely.

DENTAL CONSIDERATIONS

General:

• Check compliance of patient with prescribed drug regimen for glaucoma.
• Avoid dental light in patient's eyes; offer dark glasses for patient comfort.

Consultations:

• Medical consultation may be required to assess disease control.

ursodiol

your-**soo**′-dee-ol
(Actigall, Urso)

CATEGORY AND SCHEDULE

Pregnancy Risk Category: B

Drug Class: Gallstone solubilizing agent

MECHANISM OF ACTION

A gallstone solubilizing agent that suppresses hepatic synthesis and secretion of cholesterol; inhibits intestinal absorption of cholesterol. ***Therapeutic Effect:*** Changes the bile of patients with gallstones from precipitating (capable of forming crystals) to cholesterol solubilizing (capable of being dissolved).

USES

Dissolution of radiolucent, noncalcified gallbladder stones (<20 mm in diameter) in which surgery is not indicated; prevent gallstones in obese patients experiencing rapid weight loss

INDICATIONS AND DOSAGES

▸ Dissolution of Radiolucent, Noncalcified Gallstones When Cholecystectomy Is Not Recommended; Treatment of Biliary Cirrhosis

PO

Adults, Elderly. 8–10 mg/kg/day in 2–3 divided doses. Treatment may require months. Obtain ultrasound image of gallbladder at 6-mo intervals for first yr. If gallstones have dissolved, continue therapy and repeat ultrasound within 1–3 mo.

▸ Prevention of Gallstones

PO

Adults, Elderly. 300 mg twice a day.

SIDE EFFECTS/ADVERSE REACTIONS

Occasional

Diarrhea

PRECAUTIONS AND CONTRAINDICATIONS

Allergy to bile acids, calcified cholesterol stones, chronic hepatic disease, radiolucent bile pigment stones, radiopaque stones

Caution:

Lactation, children

DRUG INTERACTIONS OF CONCERN TO DENTISTRY

• Reduced action: aluminum-based antacids

SERIOUS REACTIONS

! None significant

DENTAL CONSIDERATIONS

General:

• Consider semisupine chair position for patient comfort because of GI effects of disease.

• Some opioids can cause spasm of bile duct leading to epigastric distress. Use caution in use for sedation or pain control. NSAIDs or acetaminophen may be better choice for pain control.

• Consider drug as a factor in the diagnosis of altered taste.

valacyclovir

val-ah-**sye′**-kloe-ver
(Valtrex)

CATEGORY AND SCHEDULE

Pregnancy Risk Category: B

Drug Class: Antiviral

MECHANISM OF ACTION

A virustatic antiviral that is converted to acyclovir triphosphate, becoming part of the viral DNA chain.
Therapeutic Effect: Interferes with DNA synthesis and replication of herpes simplex virus and varicella-zoster virus, antiviral.

USES

Treatment of herpes zoster in immunocompetent patients, genital herpes, recurrent genital herpes; treatment of herpes labialis

PHARMACOKINETICS

Rapidly absorbed after PO administration. Protein binding: 13%–18%. Rapidly converted by hydrolysis to the active compound acyclovir. Widely distributed to tissues and body fluids (including CSF). Primarily eliminated in urine. Removed by hemodialysis. ***Half-life:*** 2.5–3.3 hr (increased in impaired renal function).

INDICATIONS AND DOSAGES

▸ Herpes Zoster (shingles)
PO
Adults, Elderly. 1 g 3 times a day for 7 days.
▸ Herpes Simplex (cold sores)
PO
Adults, Elderly. 2 g twice a day for 1 day.
▸ Initial Episode of Genital Herpes
PO
Adults, Elderly. 1 g twice a day for 10 days.
▸ Recurrent Episodes of Genital Herpes
PO
Adults, Elderly. 500 mg twice a day for 3 days.
▸ Prevention of Genital Herpes
PO
Adults, Elderly. 500–1000 mg/day.
▸ Dosage in Renal Impairment
Dosage and frequency are modified on the basis of creatinine clearance.

Creatinine Clearance	Herpes Zoster	Genital Herpes
50 ml/min or higher	1 g q8h	500 mg q12h
30–49 ml/min	1 g q12h	500 mg q12h
10–29 ml/min	1 g q24h	500 mg q24h
Less than 10 ml/min	500 mg q24h	500 mg q24h

SIDE EFFECTS/ADVERSE REACTIONS

Frequent
Herpes zoster: Nausea, headache
Genital herpes: Headache
Occasional
Herpes zoster: Vomiting, diarrhea, constipation (50 yr and older), asthenia, dizziness (50 yr and older)
Genital herpes: Nausea, diarrhea, dizziness
Rare
Herpes zoster: Abdominal pain, anorexia
Genital herpes: Asthenia, abdominal pain

PRECAUTIONS AND CONTRAINDICATIONS

Hypersensitivity to or intolerance of acyclovir, valacyclovir, or their components

Caution:
Renal impairment, lactation, children; reduce dose in renal impairment

DRUG INTERACTIONS OF CONCERN TO DENTISTRY
• None reported in otherwise uncompromised patients

SERIOUS REACTIONS
! None known

DENTAL CONSIDERATIONS
General:
• Determine why the patient is taking the drug.
• Be aware of general discomfort associated with shingles; acute symptoms may preclude patient's routine dental visit or mandate short appointments.
• Patients on chronic drug therapy may rarely have symptoms of blood dyscrasias, which can include infection, bleeding, and poor healing.
Consultations:
• Medical consultation may be required to assess disease control.
• In a patient with symptoms of blood dyscrasias, request a medical consultation for blood studies and postpone dental treatment until normal values are reestablished.
Teach Patient/Family to:
• Encourage effective oral hygiene to prevent soft tissue inflammation.
• Use caution to prevent trauma when using oral hygiene aids.

valganciclovir hydrochloride
val-gan-**sye′**-kloh-veer
high-droh-**klor′**-ide
(Valcyte)

CATEGORY AND SCHEDULE
Pregnancy Risk Category: C

Drug Class: Antiviral

MECHANISM OF ACTION
A synthetic nucleoside that competes with viral DNA esterases and is incorporated directly into growing viral DNA chains.
Therapeutic Effect: Interferes with DNA synthesis and viral replication.

USES
Treatment of cytomegalovirus (CMV) retinitis in patients with AIDS

PHARMACOKINETICS
Well absorbed and rapidly converted to ganciclovir by intestinal and hepatic enzymes. Widely distributed. Slowly metabolized intracellularly. Primarily excreted unchanged in urine. Removed by hemodialysis.
Half-life: 18 hr (increased in impaired renal function).

INDICATIONS AND DOSAGES
▸ **CMV Retinitis in Patients with Normal Renal Function**
PO
Adults. Initially, 900 mg (two 450-mg tablets) twice a day for 21 days. Maintenance: 900 mg once a day.
▸ **Prevention of CMV after Transplant**
PO
Adults, Elderly. 900 mg once a day beginning within 10 days of

transplant and continuing until 100 days posttransplant.

▸ **Dosage in Renal Impairment**

Dosage and frequency are modified on the basis of creatinine clearance.

Creatinine Clearance	Induction Dosage	Maintenance Dosage
60 ml/min or more	900 mg twice a day	900 mg once a day
40–59 ml/min	450 mg twice a day	450 mg once a day
25–36 ml/min	450 mg once a day	450 mg every 2 days
10–24 ml/min	450 mg every 2 days	450 mg twice a wk

PRECAUTIONS AND CONTRAINDICATIONS

Hypersensitivity to acyclovir or ganciclovir

Caution:

Renal impairment (requires dose adjustment), preexisting cytopenias, cannot be substituted for ganciclovir capsules on a one-to-one basis, patients older than 65 yr, pediatric use

DRUG INTERACTIONS OF CONCERN TO DENTISTRY

• Increased risk of blood dyscrasias: dapsone, carbamazepine, phenothiazines

• Increased risk of seizures: imipenem/cilastatin (Primaxin)

• Low platelet counts may prevent the use of aspirin, NSAIDs

SERIOUS REACTIONS

! Hematologic toxicity including severe neutropenia (most common), anemia, and thrombocytopenia may occur.

! Retinal detachment occurs rarely.

! An overdose may result in renal toxicity.

! Valganciclovir may decrease sperm production and fertility.

DENTAL CONSIDERATIONS

General:

• Patients on chronic drug therapy may rarely have symptoms of blood dyscrasias, which can include infection, bleeding, and poor healing.

• Examine for oral manifestation of opportunistic infection.

• Place on frequent recall to evaluate healing response.

• Consider local hemostasis measures to control excessive bleeding.

Consultations:

• Medical consultation for blood studies (CBC); leukopenic or thrombocytopenic side effects may result in infection, delayed healing, and excessive bleeding. Postpone elective dental treatment until normal values are maintained.

• Medical consultation may be required to assess disease control.

Teach Patient/Family to:

• Prevent trauma when using oral hygiene aids.

• See dentist immediately if signs of secondary oral infection occur.

• Encourage effective oral hygiene to prevent soft tissue inflammation.

valproic acid/ valproate sodium/ divalproex sodium

val-**pro**′-ick

valproic acid
(Depakene)
valproate sodium
(Depakene syrup, Epilim[AUS] Valpro[AUS])
divalproex sodium
(Depacon, Depakote, Depakote ER, Depakote Sprinkle)

CATEGORY AND SCHEDULE

Pregnancy Risk Category: D

Drug Class: Anticonvulsant

MECHANISM OF ACTION

An anticonvulsant, antimanic, and antimigraine agent that directly increases concentration of the inhibitory neurotransmitter gamma-aminobutyric acid. ***Therapeutic Effect:*** Reduces seizure activity.

USES

Treatment of simple, complex (petit mal) absence, mixed seizures; divalproex for manic episodes in bipolar disorder, complex partial seizures, migraine prophylaxis; unapproved: tonic-clonic (grand mal) seizures

PHARMACOKINETICS

Well absorbed from the GI tract. Protein binding: 80%–90%. Metabolized in the liver. Primarily excreted in urine. Not removed by hemodialysis. ***Half-life:*** 6–16 hr (may be increased in hepatic impairment, the elderly, and children younger than 18 mo).

INDICATIONS AND DOSAGES

▸ Seizures

PO

Adults, Elderly, Children 10 yr and older. Initially, 10–15 mg/kg/day in 1–3 divided doses. May increase by 5–10 mg/kg/day at weekly intervals up to 30–60 mg/kg/day. Usual adult dosage: 1000–2500 mg/day.

IV

Adults, Elderly, Children. Same as oral dose but given q6h.

▸ Manic Episodes

PO

Adults, Elderly. Initially, 750 mg/day in divided doses. Maximum: 60 mg/kg/day.

▸ Prevention of Migraine Headaches

PO (Extended Release)

Adults, Elderly. Initially, 500 mg/day for 7 days. May increase up to 1000 mg/day.

PO (Delayed Release)

Adults, Elderly. Initially, 250 mg twice a day. May increase up to 1000 mg/day.

SIDE EFFECTS/ADVERSE REACTIONS

Frequent

Epilepsy: Abdominal pain, irregular menses, diarrhea, transient alopecia, indigestion, nausea, vomiting, tremors, weight gain or loss

Mania: Nausea, somnolence

Occasional

Epilepsy: Constipation, dizziness, drowsiness, headache, skin rash, unusual excitement, restlessness

Mania: Asthenia, abdominal pain, dyspepsia (heartburn, indigestion, epigastric distress), rash

Rare

Epilepsy: Mood changes, diplopia, nystagmus, spots before eyes, unusual bleeding or ecchymosis

PRECAUTIONS AND CONTRAINDICATIONS

Active hepatic disease

Caution:

MI (recovery phase), hepatic disease, renal disease, Addison's disease, pancreatitis, lactation, children younger than 2 yr have higher risk for hepatotoxicity, urea cycle disorders, thrombocytopenia, acute head injury

DRUG INTERACTIONS OF CONCERN TO DENTISTRY

- Increased effects: CNS depressants; carbamazepine, phenobarbital levels may be increased; phenothiazines can lower the seizure threshold
- Increased bleeding and toxicity: salicylates, NSAIDs
- Increased blood levels: erythromycin
- Increased serum levels of amitriptyline, nortriptyline (start with low dose and monitor)
- Decreased effects of diazepam

SERIOUS REACTIONS

! Hepatotoxicity may occur, particularly in the first 6 mo of valproic acid therapy. It may be preceded by loss of seizure control, malaise, weakness, lethargy, anorexia, and vomiting rather than abnormal serum liver function test results. Blood dyscrasias may occur.

DENTAL CONSIDERATIONS

General:

- Patients on chronic drug therapy may rarely have symptoms of blood dyscrasias, which can include infection, bleeding, and poor healing.
- Evaluate for clotting ability during gingival instrumentation because inhibition of platelet aggregation may occur.
- Consider semisupine chair position for patient comfort if GI side effects occur.
- Place on frequent recall if gingival overgrowth occurs.
- Ask about type of epilepsy, seizure frequency, and quality of seizure control.

Consultations:

- In a patient with symptoms of blood dyscrasias, request a medical consultation for blood studies and postpone dental treatment until normal values are reestablished.
- Medical consultation may be required to assess disease control.

Teach Patient/Family to:

- Encourage effective oral hygiene to prevent soft tissue inflammation and minimize gingival overgrowth.
- Use caution to prevent injury when using oral hygiene aids.
- Use powered tooth brush if patient has difficulty holding conventional devices.
- Schedule frequent oral prophylaxis if gingival overgrowth occurs.
- Report oral lesions, soreness, or bleeding to dentist.

valrubicin

val-**rue**′-bih-sin

(VaHaxan[CAN], Valstar)

Do not confuse valrubicin with valsartan.

CATEGORY AND SCHEDULE

Pregnancy Risk Category: C

Drug Class: Antineoplastic

MECHANISM OF ACTION

An anthracycline antibiotic that inhibits incorporation of nucleosides into nucleic acids after penetrating cells.

Therapeutic Effect: Causes chromosomal damage, arresting cells in the G_2 phase of cell division, and interferes with DNA synthesis.

USES

Treatment of bladder cancer

PHARMACOKINETICS

Concentrated in bladder wall; not absorbed into circulation. Excreted in urine.

INDICATIONS AND DOSAGES

▸ Bladder Cancer

Intravesical

Adults, Elderly. 800 mg once weekly for 6 wk.

SIDE EFFECTS/ADVERSE REACTIONS

Frequent

Local intravesical reaction: Local bladder symptoms, urinary frequency or urgency, dysuria, hematuria, bladder pain, cystitis, bladder spasms

Systemic: Abdominal pain, nausea, UTI

Occasional

Local intravesical reaction: Nocturia, local burning, urethral pain, pelvic pain, gross hematuria

Systemic: Diarrhea, vomiting, urine retention, microscopic hematuria, asthenia, headache, malaise, back pain, chest pain, dizziness, rash, anemia, fever, vasodilation

Rare

Systemic: Flatus, peripheral edema, hyperglycemia, pneumonia, myalgia

PRECAUTIONS AND CONTRAINDICATIONS

Perforated bladder, sensitivity to valrubicin, severe irritated bladder, small bladder capacity, UTI

DRUG INTERACTIONS OF CONCERN TO DENTISTRY

- None reported

SERIOUS REACTIONS

! Serious systemic toxicity if bladder wall perforated

DENTAL CONSIDERATIONS

General:

- If additional analgesia is required for dental pain, consider alternative analgesics (NSAIDs or acetaminophen) in patients taking opioids for acute or chronic pain.
- This drug may be used in the hospital or on an outpatient basis. Confirm the patient's disease and treatment status.
- Offer patient frequent breaks if urinary frequency is a concern.
- Avoid prescribing drugs that could cause urinary retention, such as drugs with anticholinergic activity.

Consultations:

- Medical consultation may be required to assess disease control and patient's ability to tolerate stress.

Teach Patient/Family to:

- Encourage effective oral hygiene to prevent soft tissue inflammation.
- Update health and medication history if physician makes any changes in evaluation or drug regimens; include OTC, herbal, and nonherbal remedies in the update.

valsartan

val-**sar′**-tan
(Diovan)
Do not confuse valsartan with Valstan.

CATEGORY AND SCHEDULE

Pregnancy Risk Category: C (D if used in second or third trimester)

Drug Class: Angiotensin II receptor (AT1) antagonist

MECHANISM OF ACTION

An angiotensin II receptor, type AT_1, antagonist that blocks vasoconstrictor and aldosterone-secreting effects of angiotensin II, inhibiting the binding of angiotensin II to the AT_1 receptors.
Therapeutic Effect: Causes vasodilation, decreases peripheral resistance, and decreases B/P.

USES

Treatment of hypertension as a single drug or in combination with other antihypertensive medications, heart failure

PHARMACOKINETICS

Poorly absorbed after PO administration. Food decreases peak plasma concentration. Protein binding: 95%. Metabolized in the liver. Recovered primarily in feces and, to a lesser extent, in urine. Unknown if removed by hemodialysis. ***Half-life:*** 6 hr.

INDICATIONS AND DOSAGES

▸ **Hypertension**

PO

Adults, Elderly. Initially, 80–160 mg/day in patients who are not volume depleted. May increase up to a maximum of 320 mg/day.

▸ **CHF**

PO

Adults, Elderly. Initially, 40 mg twice a day. May increase up to 160 mg twice a day. Maximum: 320 mg/day.

SIDE EFFECTS/ADVERSE REACTIONS

Rare

Insomnia, fatigue, heartburn, abdominal pain, dizziness, headache, diarrhea, nausea, vomiting, arthralgia, edema

PRECAUTIONS AND CONTRAINDICATIONS

Bilateral renal artery stenosis, biliary cirrhosis or obstruction, hypoaldosteronism, severe hepatic impairment

Caution:

Volume depletion, less effect in African Americans, liver impairment, lactation, children younger than 18 yr, elevated labs for liver function, BUN, and potassium

DRUG INTERACTIONS OF CONCERN TO DENTISTRY

• Possible reduction in effect: ketoconazole
• NSAIDs: decreased antihypertensive effect

SERIOUS REACTIONS

! Overdosage may manifest as hypotension and tachycardia. Bradycardia occurs less often. Viral infection and upper respiratory tract infection (cough, pharyngitis, sinusitis, rhinitis) occur rarely.

DENTAL CONSIDERATIONS

General:

• Monitor vital signs at every appointment because of cardiovascular side effects.

• Limit use of sodium-containing products, such as saline IV fluids, for patients with a dietary salt restriction.
• Stress from dental procedures may compromise cardiovascular function; determine patient risk.
• Short appointments and a stress-reduction protocol may be required for anxious patients.
• Use precaution if sedation or general anesthesia is required; risk of hypotensive episode.

Consultations:

• Medical consultation may be required to assess disease control and patient's ability to tolerate stress.

vancomycin hydrochloride

van-koe-**mye**′-sin high-droh-**klor**′-ide (Vancocin, Vancocin CP[AUS], Vancocin HCl Pulvules[AUS])

CATEGORY AND SCHEDULE

Pregnancy Risk Category: B

Drug Class: Glycopeptide-type antiinfective

MECHANISM OF ACTION

A tricyclic glycopeptide antibiotic that binds to bacterial cell walls, altering cell membrane permeability and inhibiting RNA synthesis. ***Therapeutic Effect:*** Bactericidal.

USES

Treatment of resistant staphylococcal infections, pseudomembranous colitis, staphylococcal enterocolitis, endocarditis

PHARMACOKINETICS

PO: Poorly absorbed from the GI tract. Primarily eliminated in feces. Parenteral: Widely distributed. Protein binding: 55%. Primarily excreted unchanged in urine. Not removed by hemodialysis. ***Half-life:*** 4–11 hr (increased in impaired renal function).

INDICATIONS AND DOSAGES

▸ Treatment of Bone, Respiratory Tract, Skin, and Soft Tissue Infections; Endocarditis, Peritonitis, and Septicemia; Prevention of Bacterial Endocarditis in Those at Risk (If Penicillin Is Contraindicated) When Undergoing Biliary, Dental, GI, GU, or Respiratory Surgery or Invasive Procedures

IV

Adults, Elderly. 500 mg q6h or 1 g q12h.

Children older than 1 mo. 40 mg/kg/day in divided doses q6–8h. Maximum: 3–4 g/day.

Neonates. Initially, 15 mg/kg, then 10 mg/kg q8–12h.

▸ Staphylococcal Enterocolitis, Antibiotic-Associated Pseudomembranous Colitis Caused by *Clostridium difficile*

PO

Adults, Elderly. 0.5–2 g/day in 3–4 divided doses for 7–10 days.

Children. 40 mg/kg/day in 3–4 divided doses for 7–10 days. Maximum: 2 g/day.

▸ Dosage in Renal Impairment

After a loading dose, subsequent dosages and frequency are modified on the basis of creatinine clearance, the severity of the infection, and the serum concentration of the drug.

SIDE EFFECTS/ADVERSE REACTIONS

Frequent

PO: Bitter or unpleasant taste, nausea, vomiting, mouth irritation (with oral solution)

Rare
Parenteral: Phlebitis, thrombophlebitis, or pain at peripheral IV site; dizziness; vertigo; tinnitus; chills; fever; rash; necrosis with extravasation
PO: Rash

PRECAUTIONS AND CONTRAINDICATIONS
Hypersensitivity, decreased hearing
Caution:
Renal disease, lactation, elderly

DRUG INTERACTIONS OF CONCERN TO DENTISTRY
- Ototoxicity or nephrotoxicity: aminoglycosides and high-dose salicylates
- Increased effects of nondepolarizing muscle relaxants

SERIOUS REACTIONS
! Nephrotoxicity and ototoxicity may occur. "Red-neck" syndrome (redness on face, neck, arms, and back; chills; fever; tachycardia; nausea or vomiting; pruritus; rash; unpleasant taste) may result from too-rapid injection.

DENTAL CONSIDERATIONS
General:
- Monitor vital signs at every appointment because of cardiovascular side effects.
- Administer IV slowly over 1 hr; administration that is too rapid can lead to a fall in B/P (monitor) and a red rash on the face, neck, and chest caused by local histamine release. No specific treatment is required for this reaction; evaluate recovery progress.
- Determine why the patient is taking the drug.

Consultations:
- Medical consultation may be required to assess disease control.

vardenafil
var-**den**′-ah-fill
(Levitra)
Do not confuse Levitra with Lexiva.

CATEGORY AND SCHEDULE
Pregnancy Risk Category: B

Drug Class: Impotence therapy

MECHANISM OF ACTION
An erectile dysfunction agent that inhibits phosphodiesterase type 5, the enzyme responsible for degrading cyclic guanosine monophosphate in the corpus cavernosum of the penis, resulting in smooth muscle relaxation and increased blood flow.
Therapeutic Effect: Facilitates an erection.

USES
Treatment of male erectile dysfunction

PHARMACOKINETICS
Rapidly absorbed after PO administration. Extensive tissue distribution. Protein binding: 95%. Metabolized in the liver. Excreted primarily in feces; a lesser amount eliminated in urine. Drug has no effect on penile blood flow without sexual stimulation. ***Half-life:*** 4–5 hr.

INDICATIONS AND DOSAGES
▸ **Erectile Dysfunction**
PO
Adults. 10 mg approximately 1 hr before sexual activity. Dose may be increased to 20 mg or decreased to 5 mg, based on patient tolerance. Maximum dosing frequency is once daily.
Elderly, older than 65 yr. 5 mg.

▸ **Dosage in Moderate Hepatic Impairment**
PO
For patients with Child-Pugh class B hepatic impairment. 5 mg 60 min before sexual activity.
▸ **Dosage with Concurrent Ritonavir**
PO
Adults. 2.5 mg in a 72-hr period.
▸ **Dosage with Concurrent Ketoconazole or Itraconazole (at 400 mg/day), or Indinavir**
PO
Adults. 2.5 mg in a 24-hr period.
▸ **Dosage with Concurrent Ketoconazole or Itraconazole (at 200 mg/day), or Erythromycin**
PO
Adults. 5 mg in a 24-hr period.

SIDE EFFECTS/ADVERSE REACTIONS

Occasional
Headache, flushing, rhinitis, indigestion
Rare
Dizziness, changes in color vision, blurred vision

PRECAUTIONS AND CONTRAINDICATIONS

Concurrent use of α-adrenergic blockers, sodium nitroprusside, or nitrates in any form
Caution:
Men with cardiovascular disease in whom sexual activity is not recommended, left ventricular outflow destruction, vasodilator effects on B/P, strong inhibitors of CYP3A4, anatomic deformation of penis, not approved for use in women or children

DRUG INTERACTIONS OF CONCERN TO DENTISTRY

• Dose adjustments caused by potential drug interactions—do not exceed the maximum single dose of 2.5 mg in a 72-hr period: ritonavir
• Do not exceed 2.5 mg in a 24-hr period: indinavir, ketoconazole (400 mg), itraconazole (400 mg)
• Do not exceed 5 mg in a 24-hr period: ketoconazole (200 mg), itraconazole (200 mg), erythromycin
• Increased plasma levels: drugs that are potent inhibitors of CYP3A4 (e.g., erythromycin, ketoconazole)
• Avoid nitroglycerin within a 24-hr period

SERIOUS REACTIONS

! Prolonged erections (lasting longer than 4 hr) and priapism (painful erections lasting longer than 6 hr) occur rarely.

DENTAL CONSIDERATIONS

General:
• This is an acute-use drug intended to be taken just before sexual activity. Be sure to include drug use in medical history and avoid use of potentially interacting drugs or warn patient of the interaction when CYP3A4 inhibitors are required (e.g., clarithromycin, azole antifungals).
• If signs of angina pectoris occur during dental treatment, do not use sublingual nitroglycerin.

varenicline

ver-**en**′-e-kleen
(Chantix)
Do not confuse with venlafaxine.

CATEGORY AND SCHEDULE

Pregnancy Risk Category: C

Drug Class: Nicotine receptor agonist

MECHANISM OF ACTION
Binds to neuronal nicotinic acetylcholine receptors and blocks nicotine binding, reducing central effects of smoking

USES
Smoking cessation treatment

PHARMACOKINETICS
Well absorbed following oral administration, peak levels in 3–4 hr. Protein binding: 20%. ***Half-life:*** 24 hr. Excreted primarily unchanged in the urine.

INDICATIONS AND DOSAGES
▸ Aid to Smoking Cessation
Adult. PO 0.5 mg per day on days 1–3, PO 0.5 mg twice daily on days 4–7, PO 1 mg twice daily day 8 until end of treatment (up to 24 weeks).

SIDE EFFECTS/ADVERSE REACTIONS
Frequent
Dry mouth, taste alterations, gingivitis, dizziness, headache, insomnia, sleep disturbances, abnormal dreams, anxiety, depression, disturbance in attention, irritability, restlessness, emotional changes, flushing, hypertension, nausea, vomiting, constipation, gastric reflux, flatulence, abnormal liver function test values
Occasional
Epistaxis, respiratory disorders, rhinorrhea, polyuria, menstrual disorders, pruritus, rash, sweating
Rare
Arthralgia, back pain, muscle cramps, myalgia, increased or decreased appetite, chest pain, flu symptoms, edema, fatigue, lethargy, malaise, thirst, weight gain, allergy

PRECAUTIONS AND CONTRAINDICATIONS
Hypersensitivity, nausea, altered metabolism of some drugs due to smoking cessation

DRUG INTERACTIONS OF CONCERN TO DENTISTRY
- None reported

DENTAL CONSIDERATIONS
General:
- Assess salivary flow as a factor in caries, periodontal disease, and candidiasis.
- Take vital signs at every appointment because of cardiovascular side effects.
- Differentiate taste changes due to drug from those associated with restorative materials or preventive aids (e.g., chlorhexidine).
- Consider semisupine chair position to minimize nausea.
- Avoid or use with caution drugs that provoke nausea (e.g., opioids).

Consultations:
- Consult with individual guiding smoking cessation program to assist with compliance and reinforcement of importance of tobacco cessation.

Teach Patient/Family to:
- Avoid mouth rinses with high alcohol content because of drying effect.
- Use home fluoride products to prevent caries.
- Use sugarless gum, frequent sips of water, or saliva substitutes if dry mouth occurs.

Teach Patient/Family to:
- When used in conjunction with a smoking-cessation program in the dental office, be familiar with all aspects of drug use, including drug package insert ("Information for Patients").
- Stop smoking 1 wk after beginning drug therapy.

vasopressin

vay-soe-**press**′-in
(Pitressin, Pressyn[CAN])
Do not confuse Pitressin with Pitocin.

CATEGORY AND SCHEDULE

Pregnancy Risk Category: B

Drug Class: Antidiuretic

MECHANISM OF ACTION

A posterior pituitary hormone that increases reabsorption of water by the renal tubules. Increases water permeability at the distal tubule and collecting duct. Directly stimulates smooth muscle in the GI tract. ***Therapeutic Effect:*** Peristalsis and vasoconstriction.

USES

Control of frequent urination, increased thirst, and loss of water associated with diabetes insipidus

PHARMACOKINETICS

Route	Onset	Peak	Duration
IV	N/A	N/A	0.5–1 hr
IM, Subcutaneous	1–2 hr	N/A	2–8 hr

Distributed throughout extracellular fluid. Metabolized in the liver and kidney. Primarily excreted in urine. ***Half-life:*** 10–20 min.

V

INDICATIONS AND DOSAGES

▸ **Cardiac Arrest**

IV

Adults, Elderly. 40 units as a one-time bolus.

▸ **Diabetes Insipidus**

IV Infusion

Adults, Children. 0.5 m Units/kg/hr. May double dose q30min. Maximum: 10 m Units/kg/hr.

IM, Subcutaneous

Adults, Elderly. 5–10 units 2–4 times a day. Range: 5–60 unit/day.

Children. 2.5–10 units, 2–4 times a day.

▸ **Abdominal Distention, Intestinal Paresis**

IM

Adults, Elderly. Initially, 5 units. Subsequent doses, 10 units q3–4h.

▸ **GI Hemorrhage**

IV Infusion

Adults, Elderly. Initially, 0.2–0.4 unit/min progressively increased to 0.9 unit/min.

Children. 0.002–0.005 unit/kg/min. Titrate as needed. Maximum: 0.01 unit/kg/min.

▸ **Vasodilatory Shock**

IV

Adults, Elderly. Initially, 0.04–0.1 unit/min. Titrate to desired effect.

SIDE EFFECTS/ADVERSE REACTIONS

Frequent

Pain at injection site (with vasopressin tannate)

Occasional

Abdominal cramps, nausea, vomiting, diarrhea, dizziness, diaphoresis, pale skin, circumoral pallor, tremors, headache, eructation, flatulence

Rare

Chest pain; confusion; allergic reaction, including rash or hives, pruritus, wheezing or difficulty breathing, facial and peripheral edema; sterile abscess (with vasopressin tannate)

PRECAUTIONS AND CONTRAINDICATIONS

Hypersensitivity, patients taking nitrates or β-adrenergic blockers, unstable cardiovascular disease, severe hepatic impairment, ESRD, degenerative retinal disorders
Men with cardiovascular disease in whom sexual activity is not recommended, left ventricular outflow destruction, vasodilator effects on B/P, strong inhibitors of CYP3A4 isoenzymes, anatomic deformation of penis, not approved for use in women or children

DRUG INTERACTIONS OF CONCERN TO DENTISTRY

- Decreased effects: demeclocycline, alcohol
- Increased effects: carbamazepine

SERIOUS REACTIONS

! Anaphylaxis, MI, and water intoxication have occurred. The elderly and very young are at higher risk for water intoxication.

DENTAL CONSIDERATIONS

General:

- Normally for acute use in the hospital or emergency department setting.
- Determine why patient is taking the drug.

Consultations:

- Medical consultation may be required to assess disease control and patient's ability to tolerate stress.

venlafaxine

ven-la-**fax′**-een
(Effexor, Effexor XR)

CATEGORY AND SCHEDULE

Pregnancy Risk Category: C

Drug Class: Bicyclic antidepressant

MECHANISM OF ACTION

A phenethylamine derivative that potentiates CNS neurotransmitter activity by inhibiting the reuptake of serotonin, norepinephrine and, to a lesser degree, dopamine.
Therapeutic Effect: Relieves depression.

USES

Treatment of depression, prevention of major depressive disorder relapse; generalized anxiety disorder (XR product only)

PHARMACOKINETICS

Well absorbed from the GI tract. Protein binding: 25%–30%. Metabolized in the liver to active metabolite. Primarily excreted in urine. Not removed by hemodialysis. ***Half-life:*** 3–7 hr; metabolite, 9–13 hr (increased in hepatic or renal impairment).

INDICATIONS AND DOSAGES

▸ **Depression**

PO

Adults, Elderly. Initially, 75 mg/day in 2–3 divided doses with food. May increase by 75 mg/day at intervals of 4 days or longer. Maximum: 375 mg/day in 3 divided doses.

PO (Extended-Release)

Adults, Elderly. 75 mg/day as a single dose with food. May increase by 75 mg/day at intervals of 4 days or longer. Maximum: 225 mg/day.

▸ **Anxiety Disorder**

PO (Extended-Release)

Adults. 37.5–225 mg/day.

▸ **Dosage in Renal and Hepatic Impairment**

Expect to decrease venlafaxine dosage by 50% in patients with moderate hepatic impairment, 25% in patients with mild to moderate renal impairment, and 50% in patients on dialysis (withhold dose until completion of dialysis).

SIDE EFFECTS/ADVERSE REACTIONS

Frequent

Nausea, somnolence, headache, dry mouth

Occasional

Dizziness, insomnia, constipation, diaphoresis, nervousness, asthenia, ejaculatory disturbance, anorexia

Rare

Anxiety, blurred vision, diarrhea, vomiting, tremor, abnormal dreams, impotence

PRECAUTIONS AND CONTRAINDICATIONS

Use within 14 days of MAOIs

Caution:

Lactation, children younger than 18 yr, sustained hypertension with use, renal or hepatic impairment, elderly, long-term use (longer than 4–6 wk), history of seizures, suicidal patients, mania, hyperthyroidism, impairment of driving, avoid use of alcohol

DRUG INTERACTIONS OF CONCERN TO DENTISTRY

• None reported.
• Increased CNS depression: all CNS depressants
• Risk of serotonin syndrome: St. John's wort (herb)

SERIOUS REACTIONS

! A sustained increase in diastolic B/P of 10–15 mm Hg occurs occasionally.

DENTAL CONSIDERATIONS

General:

• Monitor vital signs at every appointment because of cardiovascular side effects.
• After supine positioning, have patient sit upright for at least 2 min before standing to avoid orthostatic hypotension.
• Assess salivary flow as a factor in caries, periodontal disease, and candidiasis.
• Examine for evidence of oral manifestations of blood dyscrasias (infection, bleeding, poor healing).
• Place on frequent recall to evaluate healing response.
• Consider semisupine chair position for patient comfort because of GI effects of disease.

Consultations:

• Medical consultation may be required to assess disease control.
• Physician should be informed if significant xerostomic side effects occur (e.g., increased caries, sore tongue, problems eating or swallowing, difficulty wearing prosthesis) so that a medication change can be considered.
• Obtain a medical consultation for blood studies (CBC) because leukopenic or thrombocytopenic side effects may result in infection, delayed healing, and excessive bleeding. Postpone elective dental treatment until normal values are maintained.

Teach Patient/Family to:
• Encourage effective oral hygiene to prevent soft tissue inflammation.
• Use caution to prevent injury when using oral hygiene aids.
• When chronic dry mouth occurs, advise patient to:
  • Avoid mouth rinses with high alcohol content because of drying effects.
  • Use home fluoride products daily to prevent caries.
  • Use sugarless gum, frequent sips of water, or saliva substitutes.

verapamil hydrochloride

ver-**ap**′-ah-mill
high-droh-**klor**′-ide
(Anpec[AUS], Apo-Verap[CAN], Calan, Calan SR, Chronovera[CAN], Cordilox SR[AUS], Covera-HS, Isoptin[AUS], Isoptin SR, Novo-Veramil[CAN], Novo-Veramil SR[CAN], Veracaps SR[AUS], Verahexal[AUS], Verelan, Verelan PM)
Do not confuse Isoptin with Intropin, or Verelan with Virilon, Vivarin, or Voltaren.

CATEGORY AND SCHEDULE

Pregnancy Risk Category: C

Drug Class: Calcium channel blocker

MECHANISM OF ACTION

A calcium channel blocker and antianginal, antiarrhythmic, and antihypertensive agent that inhibits calcium ion entry across cardiac and vascular smooth-muscle cell membranes. This action causes the dilation of coronary arteries, peripheral arteries, and arterioles. ***Therapeutic Effect:*** Decreases heart rate and myocardial contractility and slows SA and AV conduction. Decreases total peripheral vascular resistance by vasodilation.

USES

Treatment of chronic stable angina pectoris, vasospastic angina, dysrhythmias (class IV), hypertension; unapproved: migraine headache, cardiomyopathy

PHARMACOKINETICS

Route	Onset	Peak	Duration
PO	30 min	1–2 hr	6–8 hr
PO (extended release)	30 min	N/A	N/A
IV	1–2 min	3–5 min	10–60 min

Well absorbed from the GI tract. Protein binding: 90% (60% in neonates). Undergoes first-pass metabolism in the liver to active metabolite. Primarily excreted in urine. Not removed by hemodialysis. ***Half-life:*** 2–8 hr.

INDICATIONS AND DOSAGES

▸ **Supraventricular Tachyarrhythmias, Temporary Control of Rapid Ventricular Rate with Atrial Fibrillation or Flutter**

IV

Adults, Elderly. Initially, 5–10 mg; repeat in 30 min with 10-mg dose.
Children 1–15 yr. 0.1 mg/kg. May repeat in 30 min up to a maximum second dose of 10 mg. Not recommended in children younger than 1 yr.

▸ **Arrhythmias, Including Prevention of Recurrent Paroxysmal Supraventricular Tachycardia and Control of Ventricular Resting Rate in Chronic Atrial Fibrillation or Flutter (with Digoxin)**
PO
Adults, Elderly. 240–480 mg/day in 3–4 divided doses.

▸ **Vasospastic Angina (Prinzmetal's Variant), Unstable (Crescendo or Preinfarction) Angina, Chronic Stable (Effort-Associated) Angina**
PO
Adults. Initially, 80–120 mg 3 times a day. For elderly patients and those with hepatic dysfunction, 40 mg 3 times a day. Titrate to optimal dose. Maintenance: 240–480 mg/day in 3–4 divided doses.
PO (Covera-HS)
Adults, Elderly. 180–480 mg/day at bedtime.

▸ **Hypertension**
PO
Adults, Elderly. Initially, 40–80 mg 3 times a day. Maintenance: 480 mg or less a day.
PO (Covera-HS)
Adults, Elderly. 180–480 mg/day at bedtime.
PO (Extended-Release)
Adults, Elderly. 120–240 mg/day. May give 480 mg or less a day in 2 divided doses.
PO (Verelan PM)
Adults, Elderly. 100–300 mg/day.

SIDE EFFECTS/ADVERSE REACTIONS

Frequent
Constipation
Occasional
Dizziness, light-headedness, headache, asthenia (loss of strength, energy), nausea, peripheral edema, hypotension, possible gingival enlargement
Rare
Bradycardia, dermatitis, or rash

PRECAUTIONS AND CONTRAINDICATIONS

Atrial fibrillation or flutter and an accessory bypass tract, cardiogenic shock, heart block, sinus bradycardia, ventricular tachycardia
Caution:
CHF, hypotension, hepatic injury, lactation, children, renal disease, concomitant blocker therapy

DRUG INTERACTIONS OF CONCERN TO DENTISTRY

- Decreased effect: NSAIDs, phenobarbital
- Increased effect: parenteral and inhalation general anesthetics or other drugs with hypotensive actions, benzodiazepines
- Increased effects of nondepolarizing muscle relaxants
- Increased effects of carbamazepine
- Caution in use of strong inhibitors of CYP3A4, e.g., itraconazole

SERIOUS REACTIONS

! Rapid ventricular rate in atrial flutter or fibrillation, marked hypotension, extreme bradycardia, CHF, asystole, and second- and third-degree AV block occur rarely.

DENTAL CONSIDERATIONS

General:
- Monitor cardiac status; take vital signs at every appointment because of cardiovascular side effects. Consider a stress-reduction protocol to prevent angina during the dental appointment.

• After supine positioning, have patient sit upright for at least 2 min before standing to avoid orthostatic hypotension.
• Place on frequent recall to monitor gingival condition for possible enlargement.
• Limit use of sodium-containing products, such as saline IV fluids, for patients with a dietary salt restriction.
• Assess salivary flow as a factor in caries, periodontal disease, and candidiasis.
• Use vasoconstrictors with caution, in low doses, and with careful aspiration. Avoid use of gingival retraction cord with epinephrine.

Consultations:

• In a patient with symptoms of blood dyscrasias, request a medical consultation for blood studies and postpone dental treatment until normal values are reestablished.
• Medical consultation may be required to assess disease control and patient's ability to tolerate stress.

Teach Patient/Family to:

• Encourage effective oral hygiene to prevent soft tissue inflammation and minimize gingival enlargement.
• Schedule frequent oral prophylaxis if gingival overgrowth occurs.
• When chronic dry mouth occurs, advise patient to:
  • Avoid mouth rinses with high alcohol content because of drying effects.
  • Use daily home fluoride products to prevent caries.
  • Use sugarless gum, frequent sips of water, or saliva substitutes.

vidarabine

vye-**dare**′-ah-been
(Ara-A, Vira-A)
Do not confuse with Zostrix.

CATEGORY AND SCHEDULE

Pregnancy Risk Category: C

Drug Class: Antiviral

MECHANISM OF ACTION

An antiviral agent that appears to interfere with viral DNS synthesis.
Therapeutic Effect: Regenerates corneal epithelium.

USES

Treatment of keratoconjunctivitis caused by human herpes virus, recurrent epithelial keratitis

PHARMACOKINETICS

None reported

INDICATIONS AND DOSAGES

▸ Treatment of Keratitis, Keratoconjunctivitis Caused by Human Herpes Virus, Types 1 and 2

Ophthalmic

Adults, Elderly. Apply 0.5 inch into lower conjunctival sac 5 times a day at 3-hr intervals. After reepithelialization, treat for additional 7 days at dosage of 2 times a day.

SIDE EFFECTS/ADVERSE REACTIONS

Frequent

Burning, itching, irritation

Occasional

Foreign body sensation, tearing, sensitivity to light, pain, photophobia

PRECAUTIONS AND CONTRAINDICATIONS

Hypersensitivity to vidarabine or any component of the formulation
Caution:
Antibiotic hypersensitivity

DRUG INTERACTIONS OF CONCERN TO DENTISTRY

• None reported

SERIOUS REACTIONS

! None significant

DENTAL CONSIDERATIONS

General:
• Avoid dental light in patient's eyes; offer dark glasses for patient comfort.
Teach Patient/Family to:
• Seek evaluation if healing has not occurred in 7–10 days.

vigabatrin

vig-ah-**bat**-trin
Sabril
Do not confuse with Vigamox.

CATEGORY AND SCHEDULE

Pregnancy Risk Category: C

Drug Class: Anticonvulsant

MECHANISM OF ACTION

An anticonvulsant whose exact mechanism is unknown but may be the result of increased levels of gamma-aminobutyric acid (GABA). Vigabatrin irreversibly inhibits GABA transaminase, the enzyme responsible for GABA inactivation.

USES

Adjunctive therapy of refractory complex partial seizures in adults for whom the potential benefits outweigh the risk of vision loss

PHARMACOKINETICS

Extensively absorbed following oral administration (100%), can be taken with food. Peak plasma concentrations reached in 1 hr, widely distributed. Does not bind to plasma proteins. Undergoes hepatic metabolism (CYP2C19). ***Half-life:*** 7.5 hr. Excreted primarily (65%) by the kidneys as unchanged drug.

INDICATIONS AND DOSAGES

▸ **Partial-Onset Seizures**

Adult. PO 500 mg twice daily initially, may be increased by 500 mg/day, up to 2–4 g/day, based on response and tolerability

SIDE EFFECTS/ADVERSE REACTIONS

Frequent
Permanent vision loss, headache, fatigue, somnolence, nystagmus, tremor, blurred vision, memory loss, weight gain, arthralgia, abnormal coordination, confusion
Occasional
Cough

PRECAUTIONS AND CONTRAINDICATIONS

Progressive and permanent bilateral visual field constriction and reduced visual acuity (30% or more of patients, ranging in severity from mild to severe)
Increased risk of suicidal thoughts and behavior

DRUG INTERACTIONS OF CONCERN TO DENTISTRY

• None reported

SERIOUS REACTIONS

! Hypersensitivity, loss of vision

DENTAL CONSIDERATIONS

General:

- Early-morning appointments and stress-reduction protocol may be needed for anxious patients.
- Be prepared to manage seizures and/or nausea.
- After supine positioning, allow patient to sit upright for 2 min to avoid occurrence of dizziness.
- Do not interrupt drug therapy (requires gradual discontinuation by physician).

Consultations:

- Consult with physician to determine seizure control and ability to tolerate dental procedures.

Teach Patient/Family to:

- Update medical and drug history when physician determines change in disease status or alters drug regimen.
- Report changes in vision.

vilazodone

vil az oh done
(Viibryd)
Do not confuse vilazodone with trazodone.

CATEGORY AND SCHEDULE

Pregnancy Risk Category: C

Drug Class: Antidepressant, selective serotonin reuptake inhibitor

MECHANISM OF ACTION

Vilazodone inhibits CNS neuron serotonin uptake with minimal or no effect on reuptake of norepinephrine or dopamine.
Therapeutic Effect: Relieves depression.

USES

Treatment of major depressive disorder

PHARMACOKINETICS

99% plasma protein bound. Extensively hepatic metabolism via CYP3A4 (major pathway) and 2C19 and 2D6 (minor pathways). Excreted via urine and feces. ***Half-life:*** 25 hr.

INDICATIONS AND DOSAGES

▸ **Depression**

PO

Adults. Initially, 10 mg once daily for 7 days, then increase to 20 mg once daily for 7 days, then to recommended dose of 40 mg once daily.

SIDE EFFECTS/ADVERSE REACTIONS

Frequent

Diarrhea, nausea

Occasional

Palpitation, dizziness, insomnia, fatigue, somnolence, migraine, sedation, xerostomia, vomiting, dyspepsia, erectile dysfunction, arthralgia, blurred vision

PRECAUTIONS AND CONTRAINDICATIONS

Concomitant use with MAO inhibitors or within 2 wk of discontinuing MAO inhibitors. May cause increased bleeding risk, CNS depression, serotonin syndrome (SS)/neuroleptic malignant syndrome (NMS)-like reactions. Use with caution in patients with severe hepatic impairment.
May worsen psychosis in some patients or precipitate a shift to mania or hypomania in patients with bipolar disorder. Use with caution in patients with a previous seizure disorder or condition predisposing to

seizures such as brain damage or alcoholism.

DRUG INTERACTIONS OF CONCERN TO DENTISTRY

- CYP3A4 inhibitors (e.g., macrolide antibiotics, azole antifungals): increased likelihood of adverse effects.
- CYP3A4 inducers (e.g., carbamazepine, barbiturates): reduced efficacy of vilazodone.
- Avoid NSAIDs, aspirin, and aspirin-containing products due to increased risk of bleeding.

SERIOUS REACTIONS

! Antidepressants increase the risk of suicidal thinking and behavior in children, adolescents, and young adults (18–24 yr of age) with major depressive disorder (MDD) and other psychiatric disorders.

DENTAL CONSIDERATIONS

General:

- Increased risk of intraoperative and postoperative bleeding.
- Monitor vital signs for possible cardiovascular adverse effects.
- Increased risk of nausea and vomiting (e.g., during sedation and impressions).
- Increased risk of serotonin syndrome.
- Avoid hypoxia and use conservative doses of local anesthetic due to decreased seizure threshold.

Consultations:

- Consult physician to determine status of disease and ability of patient to tolerate dental procedures.

Teach Patient/Family to:

- Report changes in disease and drug regimen.

V

vinblastine sulfate

vin-**blass**′-teen **sull**′-fate
(Oncovin[AUS], Velban, Velbe[AUS])
Do not confuse vinblastine with vincristine or vinorelbine.

CATEGORY AND SCHEDULE

Pregnancy Risk Category: D

Drug Class: Antineoplastic

MECHANISM OF ACTION

A vinca alkaloid that binds to microtubular protein of mitotic spindle, causing metaphase arrest. ***Therapeutic Effect:*** Inhibits cell division.

USES

Treatment of certain kinds of cancer, including lymphoma and cancer of the breast or testicles

PHARMACOKINETICS

Does not cross the blood-brain barrier. Protein binding: 75%. Metabolized in the liver to active metabolite. Primarily eliminated in feces by biliary system. ***Half-life:*** 24.8 hr.

INDICATIONS AND DOSAGES

▸ **Remission Induction in Advanced Testicular Carcinoma, Advanced Mycosis Fungoides, Breast Carcinoma, Choriocarcinoma, Disseminated Hodgkin's Disease, Non-Hodgkin's Lymphoma, Kaposi's Sarcoma (KS), or Letterer-Siwe Disease**

IV

Adults, Elderly. Initially, 3.7 mg/m^2 as a single dose. Increase dose by about 1.8 mg/m^2 at weekly intervals until desired therapeutic response is attained, WBC count falls below

3000/mm^3, or maximum weekly dose of 18.5 mg/m^2 is reached.
Children. Initially, 2.5 mg/m^2 as a single dose. Increase dose by about 1.25 mg/m^2 at weekly intervals until desired therapeutic response is attained, WBC count falls below 3000/mm^3, or maximum weekly dose of 7.5–12.5 mg/m^2 is reached.

▸ Maintenance Dose for Treatment of Advanced Testicular Carcinoma, Advanced Mycosis Fungoides, Breast Carcinoma, Choriocarcinoma, Disseminated Hodgkin's Disease, Non-Hodgkin's Lymphoma, KS, or Letterer-Siwe Disease

IV

Adults, Elderly, Children. Administer one increment less than dose required to produce WBC count of 3000/mm^3. Each subsequent dose given when WBC count returns to 4000/mm^3 and at least 7 days have elapsed since previous dose.

SIDE EFFECTS/ADVERSE REACTIONS

Frequent

Nausea, vomiting, alopecia

Occasional

Constipation or diarrhea, rectal bleeding, headache, paresthesia (occur 4–6 hr after administration and persist for 2–10 hr); malaise; asthenia; dizziness; pain at tumor site; jaw or face pain; depression; dry mouth

Rare

Dermatitis, stomatitis, phototoxicity, hyperuricemia

PRECAUTIONS AND CONTRAINDICATIONS

Bacterial infection, severe leukopenia, significant granulocytopenia (unless it stems from disease being treated)

DRUG INTERACTIONS OF CONCERN TO DENTISTRY

• Suspected increase in metabolism: strong inhibitors of CYP3A4 isoenzymes (erythromycin, clarithromycin, fluconazole, itraconazole, ketoconazole, metronidazole)

SERIOUS REACTIONS

! Hematologic toxicity is manifested as leukopenia and, less commonly, anemia. The WBC count reaches its nadir 4–10 days after initial therapy and recovers within 7–14 days (21 days with high vinblastine dosages). Thrombocytopenia is usually mild and transient, with recovery occurring in a few days. Hepatic insufficiency may increase the risk of toxic drug effects. Acute shortness of breath or bronchospasm may occur, particularly when vinblastine is administered concurrently with mitomycin.

DENTAL CONSIDERATIONS

General:

• If additional analgesia is required for dental pain, consider alternative analgesics (NSAIDs or acetaminophen) in patients taking opioids for acute or chronic pain.
• This drug may be used in the hospital or on an outpatient basis. Confirm the patient's disease and treatment status.
• Short appointments and a stress-reduction protocol may be required for anxious patients.
• Patient on chronic drug therapy may rarely present with symptoms of blood dyscrasias, which can include infection, bleeding, and poor healing. If dyscrasia is present, caution patient to prevent oral tissue trauma when using oral hygiene aids.

• Examine for oral manifestation of opportunistic infection.
• Palliative medication may be required for management of oral side effects.
• Chlorhexidine mouth rinse prior to and during chemotherapy may reduce severity of mucositis.
• Advise patient if dental drugs prescribed have a potential for photosensitivity.
• Assess salivary flow as a factor in caries, periodontal disease, and candidiasis.
• Patients may have received other chemotherapy and radiation; confirm medical and drug history.
• Patients presenting with KS also may be HIV positive.
• Patients may be at risk for infection.

Consultations:

• Medical consultation may be required to assess immunologic status during cancer chemotherapy and determine safety risk, if any, posed by the required dental treatment.
• Medical consultation may be required to assess disease control and patient's ability to tolerate stress.
• In a patient with symptoms of blood dyscrasias, request a medical consultation for blood studies and postpone treatment until normal values are reestablished.

Teach Patient/Family to:

• Maintain fastidious oral hygiene.
• Encourage effective oral hygiene to prevent soft tissue inflammation.
• Report oral lesions, soreness, or bleeding to dentist.
• Prevent trauma when using oral hygiene aids.
• When chronic dry mouth occurs, advise patient to:
• Avoid mouth rinses with high alcohol content because of drying effects.
• Use daily home fluoride products for anticaries effect.
• Use sugarless gum, frequent sips of water or saliva substitutes.
• Update health and medication history if physician makes any changes in evaluation or drug regimens; include OTC, herbal, and nonherbal remedies in the update.

vincristine sulfate

vin-**cris**′-teen **sull**′-fate
(Oncovin, Vincasar PFS)
Do not confuse vincristine with vinblastine, or Oncovin with Ancobon.

CATEGORY AND SCHEDULE

Pregnancy Risk Category: D

Drug Class: Antineoplastic

MECHANISM OF ACTION

A vinca alkaloid that binds to microtubular protein of mitotic spindle, causing metaphase arrest. ***Therapeutic Effect:*** Inhibits cell division.

USES

Treatment of acute leukemia, advanced non-Hodgkin's lymphoma, disseminated Hodgkin's disease, neuroblastoma, rhabdomyosarcoma, Wilms' tumor

PHARMACOKINETICS

Does not cross the blood-brain barrier. Protein binding: 75%. Metabolized in the liver. Primarily eliminated in feces by biliary system. ***Half-life:*** 10–37 hr.

INDICATIONS AND DOSAGES

▸ Acute Leukemia, Advanced Non-Hodgkin's Lymphoma, Disseminated Hodgkin's Disease, Neuroblastoma, Rhabdomyosarcoma, Wilms' Tumor

IV

Adults, Elderly. 0.4–1.4 mg/m^2 once a wk.

Children. 1–2 mg/m^2 once a wk.

Children weighing less than 10 kg or with a body surface area less than 1 m^2 0.05 mg/kg. Maximum: 2 mg.

▸ Dosage in Hepatic Impairment

Reduce dosage by 50% in patients with a direct serum bilirubin concentration more than 3 mg/dl.

SIDE EFFECTS/ADVERSE REACTIONS

Expected

Peripheral neuropathy (occurs in nearly every patient; first clinical sign is depression of Achilles tendon reflex)

Frequent

Peripheral paresthesia, alopecia, constipation or obstipation (upper colon impaction with empty rectum), abdominal cramps, headache, jaw pain, hoarseness, diplopia, ptosis or drooping of eyelid, urinary tract disturbances

Occasional

Nausea, vomiting, diarrhea, abdominal distention, stomatitis, fever

Rare

Mild leukopenia, mild anemia, thrombocytopenia

PRECAUTIONS AND CONTRAINDICATIONS

Patients receiving radiation therapy through ports that include the liver

DRUG INTERACTIONS OF CONCERN TO DENTISTRY

- None reported

SERIOUS REACTIONS

! Acute shortness of breath and bronchospasm may occur, especially when vincristine is administered concurrently with mitomycin.

Prolonged or high-dose therapy may produce foot or wrist drop, difficulty walking, slapping gait, ataxia, and muscle wasting. Acute uric acid nephropathy may occur.

DENTAL CONSIDERATIONS

General:

- If additional analgesia is required for dental pain, consider alternative analgesics (NSAIDs or acetaminophen) in patients taking opioids for acute or chronic pain.
- This drug may be used in the hospital or on an outpatient basis. Confirm the patient's disease and treatment status.
- Short appointments and a stress-reduction protocol may be required for anxious patients.
- Patient on chronic drug therapy may rarely present with symptoms of blood dyscrasias, which can include infection, bleeding, and poor healing. If dyscrasia is present, caution patient to prevent oral tissue trauma when using oral hygiene aids.
- Examine for oral manifestation of opportunistic infection.
- Assess salivary flow as a factor in caries, periodontal disease, and candidiasis.
- Palliative medication may be required for management of oral side effects.
- Chlorhexidine mouth rinse prior to and during chemotherapy may reduce severity of mucositis.

• Patients may have received other chemotherapy or radiation; confirm medical and drug history.
• Patients may be at risk for infection.

Consultations:

• Medical consultation may be required to assess immunologic status during cancer chemotherapy and determine safety risk, if any, posed by the required dental treatment.
• Medical consultation may be required to assess disease control and patient's ability to tolerate stress.
• In a patient with symptoms of blood dyscrasias, request a medical consultation for blood studies and postpone treatment until normal values are reestablished.
• Refer patients to attending physician if symptoms of peripheral neuropathy are present (numbness, tingling, or pain in hands or feet).

Teach Patient/Family to:

• Encourage effective oral hygiene to prevent soft tissue inflammation.
• Report oral lesions, soreness, or bleeding to dentist.
• Prevent trauma when using oral hygiene aids.
• Update health and medication history if physician makes any changes in evaluation or drug regimens; include OTC, herbal, and nonherbal remedies in the update.
• When chronic dry mouth occurs, advise patient to:
  • Avoid mouth rinses with high alcohol content due to drying effects.
  • Use daily home fluoride products for anticaries effect.
  • Use sugarless gum, frequent sips of water, or saliva substitutes.

V

vinorelbine

vin-oh-**rell′**-bean
(Navelbine)
Do not confuse vinorelbine with vinblastine.

CATEGORY AND SCHEDULE

Pregnancy Risk Category: D

Drug Class: Antineoplastic

MECHANISM OF ACTION

A semisynthetic vinca alkaloid that interferes with mitotic microtubule assembly.

Therapeutic Effect: Prevents cell division.

USES

Treatment of some kinds of lung cancer

PHARMACOKINETICS

Widely distributed after IV administration. Protein binding: 80%–90%. Metabolized in the liver. Primarily eliminated in feces by biliary system. ***Half-life:*** 28–43 hr.

INDICATIONS AND DOSAGES

▸ Unresectable, Advanced Non–Small-Cell Lung Cancer (as Monotherapy or in Combination with Cisplatin)

IV

Adults, Elderly. 30 mg/m^2 administered weekly over 6–10 min.

▸ Dosage Adjustment Guidelines

Dosage adjustments should be based on granulocyte count obtained on the day of treatment, as follows:

Granulocyte Count (cells/mm^3)	Dose on Day of Treatment
More than 1500	30 mg/m^2
1000–1499	15 mg/m^2
Less than 1000	Do not administer

▸ **Combination Therapy (with Cisplatin)**

IV Injection

Adults, Elderly. 25 mg/m^2 every wk or 30 mg/m^2 on days 1 and 29, then q6wk.

SIDE EFFECTS/ADVERSE REACTIONS

Frequent

Asthenia; mild or moderate nausea; constipation; erythema, pain, or vein discoloration at injection site; fatigue; peripheral neuropathy manifested as paresthesia and hyperesthesia; diarrhea; alopecia

Occasional

Phlebitis, dyspnea, loss of deep tendon reflexes

Rare

Chest pain, jaw pain, myalgia, arthralgia, rash

PRECAUTIONS AND CONTRAINDICATIONS

Granulocyte count before treatment of fewer than 1000 cells/mm^3

DRUG INTERACTIONS OF CONCERN TO DENTISTRY

- None reported

SERIOUS REACTIONS

! Bone marrow depression is manifested mainly as granulocytopenia, which may be severe. Other hematologic toxicities, including neutropenia, thrombocytopenia, leukopenia, and anemia, increase the risk of infection and bleeding. Acute shortness of breath and severe bronchospasm occur infrequently, particularly in patients with preexisting pulmonary dysfunction and in those receiving mitomycin concurrently.

DENTAL CONSIDERATIONS

General:

- If additional analgesia is required for dental pain, consider alternative analgesics in patients taking narcotics for acute or chronic pain (e.g., acetaminophen).
- Avoid products that affect platelet function, such as aspirin and NSAIDs.
- This drug may be used in the hospital or on an outpatient basis. Confirm the patient's disease and treatment status.
- Patient on chronic drug therapy may rarely present with symptoms of blood dyscrasias, which can include infection, bleeding, and poor healing. If dyscrasia is present, caution patient to prevent oral tissue trauma when using oral hygiene aids.
- Consider semisupine chair position for patients with respiratory disease.
- Caution: patients may be at high risk for infection.
- Patient may have received other chemotherapy or radiation; confirm medical and drug history.
- Oral infections should be eliminated and/or treated aggressively.

Consultations:

- Medical consultation should include routine blood counts including platelet counts and bleeding time.
- Consult physician; prophylactic or therapeutic antiinfectives may be indicated if surgery or periodontal treatment is required.
- Medical consultation may be required to assess immunologic status during cancer chemotherapy and determine safety risk, if any, posed by the required dental treatment.

• Medical consultation may be required to assess disease control and patient's ability to tolerate stress.

Teach Patient/Family to:

• See dentist immediately if secondary oral infection occurs.

• Encourage effective oral hygiene to prevent soft tissue inflammation.

• Report oral lesions, soreness, or bleeding to dentist.

• Prevent trauma when using oral hygiene aids.

• Update health and medication history if physician makes any changes in evaluation or drug regimens; include OTC, herbal, and nonherbal remedies in the update.

vismodegib

vis-**moe**′-deg-ib

(Erivedge)

Do not confuse vismodegib with vandetanib or vemurafenib.

CATEGORY AND SCHEDULE

Pregnancy Risk Category: D

Drug Class: Antineoplastic agent, hedgehog pathway inhibitor

MECHANISM OF ACTION

Basal cell cancer is associated with mutations in hedgehog pathway components. Vismodegib is a selective hedgehog pathway inhibitor that binds to and inhibits smoothened homologue (SMO), the transmembrane protein involved in hedgehog signal transduction.

Therapeutic Effect: Treats basal cell carcinoma.

USES

Treatment of metastatic basal cell carcinoma, or locally advanced basal cell carcinoma that has recurred following surgery or in patients who are not candidates for surgery, and not candidates for radiation therapy

PHARMACOKINETICS

99% plasma protein bound. Metabolized by oxidation, glucuronidation, and pyridine ring cleavage. Excreted primarily via the feces. ***Half-life:*** Continuous daily dosing: 4 days; single dose: 12 days.

INDICATIONS AND DOSAGES

▸ **Basal Cell Cancer, Metastatic or Locally Advanced**

PO

Adults. 150 mg once daily until disease progression or unacceptable toxicity.

SIDE EFFECTS/ADVERSE REACTIONS

Frequent

Fatigue, alopecia, amenorrhea, abnormal taste, weight loss, nausea, diarrhea, constipation, vomiting, muscle spasms

Occasional

Hypokalemia, hyponatremia

PRECAUTIONS AND CONTRAINDICATIONS

Amenorrhea may occur in women of reproductive potential.

DRUG INTERACTIONS OF CONCERN TO DENTISTRY

• P-glycoprotein inhibitors (e.g., macrolide antibiotics): may increase blood levels and adverse effects of vismodegib

SERIOUS REACTIONS

! May result in severe birth defects or embryo-fetal death

DENTAL CONSIDERATIONS

General:

• Dysgeusia and ageusia occur in over 10% of patients taking vismodegib.
• Increased potential for nausea and vomiting (e.g., during sedation and impressions).
• Prepare for interruptions in treatment due to possible diarrhea.

Consultations:

• Consult physician to determine disease status and ability of patient to tolerate dental procedures.

Teach Patient/Family to:

• Report oral adverse effects of drug.
• Use effective, atraumatic oral hygiene measures to prevent soft tissue inflammation.
• Update health and medication history regularly.

vitamin A

vight′-ah-min A
(Aquasol A, Palmitate A)
Do not confuse Aquasol A with Anusol.

CATEGORY AND SCHEDULE

Pregnancy Risk Category: A (X if used in doses greater than recommended daily allowance)

Drug Class: Fat-soluble vitamin

MECHANISM OF ACTION

A fat-soluble vitamin that may act as a cofactor in biochemical reactions.
Therapeutic Effect: Is essential for normal function of retina, visual adaptation to darkness, bone growth, testicular and ovarian function, and embryonic development; preserves integrity of epithelial cells.

USES

Treatment of vitamin A deficiency

PHARMACOKINETICS

Rapidly absorbed from the GI tract if bile salts, pancreatic lipase, protein, and dietary fat are present. Transported in blood to the liver, where it is metabolized; stored in parenchymal hepatic cells, then transported in plasma as retinol, as needed. Excreted primarily in bile and, to a lesser extent, in urine.

INDICATIONS AND DOSAGES

▸ **Severe Vitamin A Deficiency**

PO

Adults, Elderly, Children 8 yr and older. 500,000 units/day for 3 days; then 50,000 units/day for 14 days, then 10,000–20,000 units/day for 2 mo.
Children 1–7 yr. 5000 units/kg/day for 5 days, then 5000–10,000 units/day for 2 mo.
Children younger than 1 yr. 5000–10,000 units/day for 2 mo.

IM

Adults, Elderly, Children 8 yr and older. 100,000 units/day for 3 days; then 50,000 units/day for 14 days.
Children 1–7 yr. 17,500–35,000 units/day for 10 days.
Children younger than 1 yr. 7500–15,000 units/day.

▸ **Malabsorption Syndrome**

PO

Adults, Elderly, Children 8 yr and older. 10,000–50,000 units/day.

▸ **Dietary Supplement**

PO

Adults, Elderly. 4000–5000 units/day.
Children 7–10 yr. 3300–3500 units/day.
Children 4–6 yr. 2500 units/day.
Children 6 mo–3 yr. 1500–2000 units/day.

Neonates younger than 5 mo. 1500 units/day.

SIDE EFFECTS/ADVERSE REACTIONS

None known

PRECAUTIONS AND CONTRAINDICATIONS

Hypervitaminosis A

Caution:

Impaired renal function; pregnancy category A (RDA doses), otherwise pregnancy category C

DRUG INTERACTIONS OF CONCERN TO DENTISTRY

- None listed

SERIOUS REACTIONS

! Chronic overdose produces malaise, nausea, vomiting, drying or cracking of skin or lips, inflammation of tongue or gums, irritability, alopecia, and night sweats. Bulging fontanelles have occurred in infants.

DENTAL CONSIDERATIONS

General:

- Oral manifestation of side effects could indicate hypervitaminosis.
- May cause dry or peeling skin around lips; provide lip lubricant for patient comfort during dental treatment.

vitamin D

vight′-ah-min D
(Calciferol, Drisdol, Ostoforte[CAN])

CATEGORY AND SCHEDULE

Pregnancy Risk Category: A (D if used in doses above recommended daily allowance)

Drug Class: Fat-soluble vitamin

MECHANISM OF ACTION

A fat-soluble vitamin that stimulates calcium and phosphate absorption from the small intestine, promotes secretion of calcium from bone to blood, and promotes resorption of phosphate in renal tubules; also acts on bone cells to stimulate skeletal growth and on parathyroid gland to suppress hormone synthesis and secretion.

Therapeutic Effect: Essential for absorption and utilization of calcium and phosphate and normal bone calcification. Reduces parathyroid hormone level. Improves phosphorus and calcium homeostasis in chronic renal failure.

USES

Varies with the type of vitamin D selected, but generally includes vitamin D deficiency, rickets, renal osteodystrophy, tetany, hypoparathyroidism, and hypophosphatemia; doxercalciferol is indicated for reduction of elevated intact parathyroid hormone (iPTH) levels for secondary hyperparathyroidism in patients receiving chronic renal dialysis

PHARMACOKINETICS

Readily absorbed from small intestine. Concentrated primarily in liver and fat deposits. Activated in the liver and kidneys. Eliminated by biliary system; excreted in urine. ***Half-life:*** 19–48 hr for ergocalciferol.

INDICATIONS AND DOSAGES

Alert

Oral dosing is preferred. Administer the drug IM only in patients with GI, hepatic, or biliary disease associated with malabsorption of vitamin D.

▸ **Dietary Supplement**

PO

Adults, Elderly, Children. 10 mcg (400 units)/day.

Neonates. 10–20 mcg (400–800 units)/day.

▸ **Renal Failure**

PO

Adults, Elderly. 0.5 mg/day.

Children. 0.1–1 mg/day.

▸ **Hypoparathyroidism**

PO

Adults, Elderly. 625 mcg–5 mg/day (with calcium supplements).

Children. 1.25–5 mg/day (with calcium supplements).

▸ **Nutritional Rickets, Osteomalacia**

PO

Adults, Elderly, Children. 25–125 mcg/day for 8–12 wk.

Adults, Elderly (with malabsorption syndrome). 250–7500 mcg/day.

Children (with malabsorption syndrome). 250–625 mcg/day.

▸ **Vitamin D–Dependent Rickets**

PO

Adults, Elderly. 250 mcg–1.5 mg/day.

Children. 75–125 mcg/day.

Maximum: 1500 mcg/day.

▸ **Vitamin D–Resistant Rickets**

PO

Adults, Elderly. 250–1500 mcg/day (with phosphate supplements).

Children. Initially, 1000–2000 mcg/day (with phosphate supplements). May increase in 250- to 600-mcg increments q3–4mo.

SIDE EFFECTS/ADVERSE REACTIONS

None known

PRECAUTIONS AND CONTRAINDICATIONS

Hypercalcemia, malabsorption syndrome, vitamin D toxicity

Caution:

Cardiovascular disease, renal calculi, hyperphosphatemia

DRUG INTERACTIONS OF CONCERN TO DENTISTRY

• Reduction in calcitriol levels: ketoconazole

SERIOUS REACTIONS

! Early signs and symptoms of overdose are weakness, headache, somnolence, nausea, vomiting, dry mouth, constipation, muscle and bone pain, and metallic taste. Later signs and symptoms of overdose include polyuria, polydipsia, anorexia, weight loss, nocturia, photophobia, rhinorrhea, pruritus, disorientation, hallucinations, hyperthermia, hypertension, and cardiac arrhythmias.

DENTAL CONSIDERATIONS

General:

• Sensitivity of eyes to dental light may indicate late toxicity.

Teach Patient/Family to:

• Be aware that oral side effects are associated with early symptoms of overdose.

vitamin E

vight′-ah-min E
(Aqua Gem E, Aquasol E, E-Gems, Key-E, Key-E Kaps)
Do not confuse Aquasol E with Anusol.

CATEGORY AND SCHEDULE

Pregnancy Risk Category: A (C if used in doses above recommended daily allowance)
OTC

Drug Class: Vitamin E (fat-soluble vitamin)

MECHANISM OF ACTION

An antioxidant that prevents oxidation of vitamins A and C, protects fatty acids from attack by free radicals, and protects RBCs from hemolysis by oxidizing agents.
Therapeutic Effect: Prevents and treats vitamin E deficiency.

USES

Treatment of vitamin E deficiency, hemolytic anemia in premature neonates, prevention of retrolental fibroplasia

PHARMACOKINETICS

Variably absorbed from the GI tract (requires bile salts, dietary fat, and normal pancreatic function). Primarily concentrated in adipose tissue. Metabolized in the liver. Primarily eliminated by biliary system.

INDICATIONS AND DOSAGES

▸ **Vitamin E Deficiency**
PO
Adults, Elderly. 60–75 units/day.
Children. 1 unit/kg/day.

SIDE EFFECTS/ADVERSE REACTIONS

CNS: Headache, fatigue
CV: Increased risk of thrombophlebitis
GI: Nausea, cramps, diarrhea
GU: Gonadal dysfunction
EENT: Blurred vision
Integ: Sterile abscess, contact dermatitis
MS: Weakness
Meta: Altered metabolism of hormones (thyroid, pituitary, adrenal), altered immunity

PRECAUTIONS AND CONTRAINDICATIONS

None significant

DRUG INTERACTIONS OF CONCERN TO DENTISTRY

• With doses greater than 400 international units: increased risk of bleeding, oral anticoagulants, NSAIDs

SERIOUS REACTIONS

! Chronic overdose may produce fatigue, weakness, nausea, headache, blurred vision, flatulence, and diarrhea.

DENTAL CONSIDERATIONS

General:

• Determine why the patient is taking the drug.

warfarin sodium

war′-far-in **soe**′-dee-um
(Apo-Warfarin[CAN], Coumadin, Gen-Warfarin[CAN], Jantoven, Marevan[AUS], Tar-Warfarin[CAN])
Do not confuse Coumadin with Kemadrin.

CATEGORY AND SCHEDULE

Pregnancy Risk Category: D

Drug Class: Oral anticoagulant

MECHANISM OF ACTION

A coumarin derivative that interferes with hepatic synthesis of vitamin K–dependent clotting factors, resulting in depletion of coagulation factors II, VII, IX, and X.
Therapeutic Effect: Prevents further extension of formed existing clot; prevents new clot formation or secondary thromboembolic complications.

USES

Treatment of pulmonary emboli, deep vein thrombosis (DVT), MI, atrial dysrhythmias, to reduce risk of recurrent MI and thromboembolic events.

PHARMACOKINETICS

Route	Onset	Peak	Duration
PO	1.5–3 days	5–7 days	N/A

Well absorbed from the GI tract. Metabolized in the liver. Primarily excreted in urine. Not removed by hemodialysis. ***Half-life:*** 1.5–2.5 days.

INDICATIONS AND DOSAGES

Anticoagulant

PO

Adults, Elderly. Initially, 5–15 mg/day for 2–5 days; then adjust based on INR. Maintenance: 2–10 mg/day.
Children. Initially, 0.1–0.2 mg/kg (maximum 10 mg). Maintenance: 0.05–0.34 mg/kg/day.

Usual Elderly Dosage (Maintenance)

PO, IV

Elderly. 2–5 mg/day.

SIDE EFFECTS/ADVERSE REACTIONS

Occasional

GI distress, such as nausea, anorexia, abdominal cramps, diarrhea

Rare

Hypersensitivity reaction including dermatitis and urticaria, especially in those sensitive to aspirin

PRECAUTIONS AND CONTRAINDICATIONS

Neurosurgical procedures, open wounds, pregnancy, severe hypertension, severe hepatic or renal damage, uncontrolled bleeding, ulcers

Caution:

Alcoholism, elderly

DRUG INTERACTIONS OF CONCERN TO DENTISTRY

- Increased action: diflunisal, salicylates, propoxyphene, metronidazole, erythromycin, clarithromycin, ketoconazole, itraconazole, fluconazole, NSAIDs, indomethacin, chloral hydrate, tetracyclines, fluoroquinolones, acetaminophen, ciprofloxacin, levofloxacin
- Decreased action: barbiturates, carbamazepine acetaminophen (monitor INR levels)

• Herbal products with some anticoagulant activity: feverfew, garlic, ginger, ginkgo, ginseng

SERIOUS REACTIONS

! Bleeding complications ranging from local ecchymoses to major hemorrhage may occur. Drug should be discontinued immediately and vitamin K or phytonadione administered. Mild hemorrhage: 2.5–10 mg PO, IM, or IV. Severe hemorrhage: 10–15 mg IV and repeated q4h as necessary.
! Hepatotoxicity, blood dyscrasias, necrosis, vasculitis, and local thrombosis occur rarely.

DENTAL CONSIDERATIONS

General:
• Reports on concomitant use of acetaminophen and warfarin suggest a possible increase in anticoagulant effects, especially in patients with other diseases or contributing factors (diarrhea, age, debilitation, etc.). Patients taking warfarin should be questioned about recent use of acetaminophen and current INR values. Acetaminophen has been shown to increase the INR, depending on the amount of acetaminophen taken and duration of use. A new INR value may be required if surgical procedures are planned.
• Patients on chronic drug therapy may rarely have symptoms of blood dyscrasias, which can include infection, bleeding, and poor healing.
• Consider local hemostasis measures to prevent excessive bleeding.
• Increased bleeding may occur with IM injections.
Consultations:
• Medical consultation should include current INR value.
• For dental surgical procedures that may result in excessive bleeding, consider requesting physician to make dose reduction before dental treatment so that INR is within appropriate therapeutic range.
• In a patient with symptoms of blood dyscrasias, request a medical consultation for blood studies and postpone dental treatment until normal values are reestablished.
Teach Patient/Family to:
• Encourage effective oral hygiene to prevent soft tissue inflammation.
• Use caution to prevent injury when using oral hygiene aids.
• Report oral lesions, soreness, or bleeding to dentist.

zafirlukast

za-**feer**′-loo-kast
(Accolate)
Do not confuse Accolate with Accupril or Aclovate.

CATEGORY AND SCHEDULE

Pregnancy Risk Category: B

Drug Class: Selective leukotriene receptor antagonist

MECHANISM OF ACTION

An antiasthmatic that binds to leukotriene receptors, inhibiting bronchoconstriction caused by sulfur dioxide, cold air, and specific antigens, such as grass, cat dander, and ragweed.
Therapeutic Effect: Reduces airway edema and smooth muscle constriction; alters cellular activity associated with the inflammatory process.

USES

Prophylaxis and chronic treatment of asthma

PHARMACOKINETICS

Rapidly absorbed after PO administration (food reduces absorption). Protein binding: 99%. Extensively metabolized in the liver. Primarily excreted in feces. Unknown if removed by hemodialysis. ***Half-life:*** 10 hr.

INDICATIONS AND DOSAGES

▸ **Bronchial Asthma**

PO
Adults, Elderly, Children 12 yr and older: 20 mg twice a day.
Children 5–11 yr: 10 mg twice a day.

SIDE EFFECTS/ADVERSE REACTIONS

Frequent
Headache
Occasional
Nausea, diarrhea
Rare
Generalized pain, asthenia, myalgia, fever, dyspepsia, vomiting, dizziness

PRECAUTIONS AND CONTRAINDICATIONS

Hypersensitivity, hepatic dysfunction with prior use of zafirlukast
Caution:
Not for acute bronchospasm, food decreases bioavailability, pregnancy category B, lactation, patients younger than 7 yr, hepatic impairment, liver enzyme elevation, elderly (increased infection); if liver dysfunction suspected, discontinue use and measure liver enzymes, serum ALT (SPGT)

DRUG INTERACTIONS OF CONCERN TO DENTISTRY

- Increased PT with concurrent use of warfarin
- Reduced plasma levels: erythromycin, terfenadine, theophylline
- Increased plasma levels with aspirin
- Inhibits CYP2C9 and CYP3A4: use with caution when drugs metabolized by these enzymes are used

SERIOUS REACTIONS

! Concurrent administration of inhaled corticosteroids increases the risk of upper respiratory tract infection.

DENTAL CONSIDERATIONS

General:

- Midday appointments and a stress-reduction protocol may be required for anxious patients.
- Avoid prescribing aspirin-containing products and NSAIDs.
- Acute asthmatic episodes may be precipitated in the dental office. Sympathomimetic inhalants should be available for emergency use. A stress-reduction protocol may be required.
- Be aware that aspirin or sulfite preservatives in vasoconstrictor-containing products can exacerbate asthma.
- Consider semisupine chair position for patients with respiratory disease or if GI side effects occur.

Consultations:

- Medical consultation may be required to assess disease control.

Teach Patient/Family to:

- Use powered tooth brush if patient has difficulty holding conventional devices.
- Update health and drug history if physician makes any changes in evaluation or drug regimens; include OTC, herbal, and nonherbal remedies in the update.

zalcitabine

zal-**site′**-ah-been
(Hivid)

CATEGORY AND SCHEDULE

Pregnancy Risk Category: C

Drug Class: Synthetic pyrimidine antiviral

MECHANISM OF ACTION

A nucleoside reverse transcriptase inhibitor that inhibits viral DNA synthesis.
Therapeutic Effect: Prevents replication of HIV-1.

USES

Treatment of advanced HIV infection in combination with zidovudine

PHARMACOKINETICS

Readily absorbed from the GI tract (absorption decreased by food). Protein binding: less than 4%. Undergoes phosphorylation intracellularly to the active metabolite. Primarily excreted in urine. Removed by hemodialysis. ***Half-life:*** 1–3 hr; metabolite, 2.6–10 hr (increased in impaired renal function).

INDICATIONS AND DOSAGES

▸ **HIV Infection (in Combination with Other Antiretrovirals)**

PO

Adults, Children 13 yr and older. 0.75 mg q8h.

Children younger than 13 yr. 0.01 mg/kg q8h. Range: 0.005–0.01 mg/kg q8h.

▸ **Dosage in Renal Impairment**

Dosage and frequency are modified on the basis of creatinine clearance.

Creatinine Clearance	Dose
10–40 ml/min	0.75 mg q12h
Less than 10 ml/min	0.75 mg q24h

SIDE EFFECTS/ADVERSE REACTIONS

Frequent

Peripheral neuropathy, fever, fatigue, headache, rash

Occasional
Diarrhea, abdominal pain, oral ulcers, cough, pruritus, myalgia, weight loss, nausea, vomiting
Rare
Nasal discharge, dysphagia, depression, night sweats, confusion

PRECAUTIONS AND CONTRAINDICATIONS

Moderate or severe peripheral neuropathy
Caution:
Lactation, children younger than 13 yr, renal impairment, hepatic impairment, risk of serious peripheral neuropathy, risk of severe hepatic impairment, CHF

DRUG INTERACTIONS OF CONCERN TO DENTISTRY

- Increased peripheral neuropathy: metronidazole, dapsone, or other drugs associated with peripheral neuropathy

SERIOUS REACTIONS

! Peripheral neuropathy (characterized by numbness, tingling, burning, and pain in the lower extremities) occurs in 17% to 31% of patients. These symptoms may be followed by sharp, shooting pain and progress to a severe, continuous, burning pain that may be irreversible if the drug is not discontinued in time.
! Pancreatitis, leukopenia, neutropenia, eosinophilia, and thrombocytopenia occur rarely.

DENTAL CONSIDERATIONS

General:
- Examine oral cavity for side effects if on long-term drug therapy.
- Monitor vital signs at every appointment because of cardiovascular side effects.
- Palliative medication may be required for management of oral side effects.
- Assess salivary flow as a factor in caries, periodontal disease, and candidiasis.
- Prophylactic antibiotics may be indicated to prevent infection if surgery or deep scaling is planned.
- Patients may be more susceptible to infection and have delayed wound healing.

Consultations:
- Medical consultation may be required to assess disease control and patient's ability to tolerate stress.

Teach Patient/Family to:
- Encourage effective oral hygiene to prevent soft tissue inflammation.
- Use caution to prevent injury when using oral hygiene aids.
- See dentist immediately if secondary oral infection occurs.
- When chronic dry mouth occurs, advise patient to:
  - Avoid mouth rinses with high alcohol content because of drying effects.
  - Use daily home fluoride products to prevent caries.
  - Use sugarless gum, frequent sips of water, or saliva substitutes.

zaleplon

zal'-eh-plon
(Sonata, Stamoc[CAN])

CATEGORY AND SCHEDULE

Pregnancy Risk Category: C
Controlled Substance: Schedule IV

Drug Class: Hypnotic

MECHANISM OF ACTION

A nonbenzodiazepine that enhances the action of the inhibitory neurotransmitter gamma-aminobutyric acid.
Therapeutic Effect: Induces sleep.

USES

Short-term treatment of insomnia

PHARMACOKINETICS

PO: Rapid absorption, bioavailability 30%, peak plasma levels 1 hr, wide tissue distribution, rapid hepatic metabolism (CYP3A4 minor pathway), excretion in urine; heavy, high-fat meal significantly delays absorption

INDICATIONS AND DOSAGES

▸ **Insomnia**

PO

Adults. 10 mg at bedtime. Range: 5–20 mg.
Elderly. 5 mg at bedtime.

SIDE EFFECTS/ADVERSE REACTIONS

Expected

Somnolence, sedation, mild rebound insomnia (on first night after drug is discontinued)

Frequent

Nausea, headache, myalgia, dizziness

Occasional

Abdominal pain, asthenia, dyspepsia, eye pain, paresthesia

Rare

Tremors, amnesia, hyperacusis (acute sense of hearing), fever, dysmenorrhea

PRECAUTIONS AND CONTRAINDICATIONS

Severe hepatic impairment

Caution:

Abuse potential similar to benzodiazepines, elderly, debilitated, smaller patients adjust dose downward; lactation, children

DRUG INTERACTIONS OF CONCERN TO DENTISTRY

- Caution when using dental drugs that inhibit or induce cytochrome P-450 enzymes; this drug is a minor substrate for CYP3A4; however, use caution (see Appendix I).
- CNS depression: all CNS depressant drugs.

SERIOUS REACTIONS

! Zaleplon may produce altered concentration, behavior changes, and impaired memory.
! Taking the drug while up and about may result in adverse CNS effects, such as hallucinations, impaired coordination, dizziness, and light-headedness.
! Overdose results in somnolence, confusion, diminished reflexes, and coma.

DENTAL CONSIDERATIONS

General:

- Assess salivary flow as a factor in caries, periodontal disease, and candidiasis.
- Determine why patient is taking the drug.
- Consider semisupine chair position for patient comfort if GI side effects occur.

Consultations:

- Medical consultation may be required to assess disease control and patient's ability to tolerate stress.

Teach Patient/Family to:

- When chronic dry mouth occurs, advise patient to:
  - Avoid mouth rinses with high alcohol content because of drying effects.

• Use daily home fluoride products for anticaries effect.
• Use sugarless gum, frequent sips of water, or saliva substitutes.

zanamivir

za-**na**′-mi-veer
(Relenza)

CATEGORY AND SCHEDULE

Pregnancy Risk Category: B

Drug Class: Antiviral

MECHANISM OF ACTION

An antiviral that appears to inhibit the influenza virus enzyme neuraminidase, which is essential for viral replication.
Therapeutic Effects: Prevents viral release from infected cells.

USES

Treatment of uncomplicated influenza in adults and children older than 7 yr with symptoms of no more than 2 days; more effective against influenza type A virus.

PHARMACOKINETICS

Inhalation: 4%–17% of inhaled dose is absorbed, peak serum levels 1–2 hr, low plasma protein binding (less than 10%), excreted unchanged in urine.

INDICATIONS AND DOSAGES

▸ **Influenza Virus**
Inhalation
Adults, Elderly, Children 7 yr and older. 2 inhalations (one 5-mg blister per inhalation for a total dose of 10 mg) twice a day (about 12 hr apart) for 5 days.

▸ **Prevention of Influenza Virus**
Inhalation
Adults, Elderly. 2 inhalations once a day for the duration of the exposure period.

SIDE EFFECTS/ADVERSE REACTIONS

Occasional
Diarrhea, sinusitis, nausea, bronchitis, cough, dizziness, headache
Rare
Malaise, fatigue, fever, abdominal pain, myalgia, arthralgia, urticaria

PRECAUTIONS AND CONTRAINDICATIONS

Hypersensitivity
Caution:
Teach use of inhaler to patient; chronic obstructive pulmonary disease or asthma does not preclude influenza vaccine, safety in children younger than 12 yr not established

DRUG INTERACTIONS OF CONCERN TO DENTISTRY

• None reported

SERIOUS REACTIONS

! Neutropenia may occur.
Bronchospasm may occur in those with a history of COPD or bronchial asthma.

DENTAL CONSIDERATIONS

General:
• Acute influenza patients are unlikely to be seen in the dental office except for dental emergencies.
• Use precautions to prevent spread of flu virus in office.

ziconotide

zi-**koe**′-no-tide
(Prialt)

CATEGORY AND SCHEDULE

Pregnancy Risk Category: C

Drug Class: Analgesic

MECHANISM OF ACTION

A synthetic peptide that selectively binds to and blocks *N*-type voltage-sensitive calcium channels located on afferent nerves in the spinal cord.
Therapeutic Effect: Blocks excitatory neurotransmitter release, reducing sensitivity to painful stimuli.

USES

Reduction of chronic pain in the body

PHARMACOKINETICS

Elimination Half-life: 4.6 hr after intrathecal administration. 50% bound to plasma proteins; metabolized in multiple organs. Excreted in urine as proteolytic degradation products.

INDICATIONS AND DOSAGES

▸ **Pain Control**

Intrathecal
Adults, Elderly. Initially, 2.4 mcg/day (0.1 mcg/hr). May titrate to maximum of 19.2 mcg/day (0.8 mcg/hr).

SIDE EFFECTS/ADVERSE REACTIONS

Frequent
Dizziness, nausea, somnolence, weakness, diarrhea, confusion, ataxia, headache, vomiting, gait disturbance, memory impairment, hypertonia
Occasional
Anorexia, visual disturbances, anxiety, urinary retention, speech disorder, aphasia, nystagmus, paresthesia, fever, hallucinations, nervousness, vertigo
Rare
Insomnia, dry skin, constipation, arthralgia, myalgia, tremor

PRECAUTIONS AND CONTRAINDICATIONS

History of psychosis, presence of infection at the injection site, uncontrolled bleeding, or spinal canal obstruction that impairs CSF circulation, IV administration

DRUG INTERACTIONS OF CONCERN TO DENTISTRY

• Enhanced CNS depression: all CNS depressants

SERIOUS REACTIONS

! Atrial fibrillation, cerebral vascular accident, seizures, kidney failure (acute), myoclonus, and psychosis occur rarely.

DENTAL CONSIDERATIONS

General:
• Determine why patient is taking the drug.
• For use in the hospital setting.
Consultations:
• Medical consultation may be required to assess disease control and patient's ability to tolerate stress.
Teach Patient/Family to:
• Encourage effective oral hygiene to prevent soft tissue inflammation.
• Update health and medication history if physician makes any changes in evaluation or drug

regimens; include OTC, herbal, and nonherbal remedies in the update.

zidovudine

zyde-**oh**′-vue-deen
(Apo-Zidovudine[CAN], AZT, Novo-AZT[CAN], Retrovir)
Do not confuse Retrovir with ritonavir.

CATEGORY AND SCHEDULE

Pregnancy Risk Category: C

Drug Class: Antiviral thymidine analogue

MECHANISM OF ACTION

A nucleoside reverse transcriptase inhibitor that interferes with viral RNA-dependent DNA polymerase, an enzyme necessary for viral HIV replication.
Therapeutic Effect: Interferes with HIV replication, slowing the progression of HIV infection.

USES

Treatment of symptomatic HIV infections (AIDS, ARC), confirmed *P. carinii* pneumonia (PCP), or absolute CD4 lymphocytes less than 200/mm^3; prevention of maternal-fetal transmission.

PHARMACOKINETICS

Rapidly and completely absorbed from the GI tract. Protein binding: 25%–38%. Undergoes first-pass metabolism in the liver. Crosses the blood-brain barrier and is widely distributed, including to CSF. Primarily excreted in urine. Minimal removal by hemodialysis. ***Half-life:*** 0.8–1.2 hr (increased in impaired renal function).

INDICATIONS AND DOSAGES

▸ **HIV Infection**

PO
Adults, Elderly, Children older than 12 yr. 200 mg q8h or 300 mg q12h.
Children 12 yr and younger. 160 mg/m^2/dose q8h. Range: 90–180 mg/m^2/dose q6–8h.
Neonates. 2 mg/kg/dose q6h.
IV
Adults, Elderly, Children older than 12 yr. 1–2 mg/kg/dose q4h.
Children 12 yr and younger. 120 mg/m^2/dose q6h.
Neonates. 1.5 mg/kg/dose q6h.

SIDE EFFECTS/ADVERSE REACTIONS

Expected
Nausea, headache
Frequent
Abdominal pain, asthenia, rash, fever, acne
Occasional
Diarrhea, anorexia, malaise, myalgia, somnolence
Rare
Dizziness, paresthesia, vomiting, insomnia, dyspnea, altered taste

PRECAUTIONS AND CONTRAINDICATIONS

Life-threatening allergic reactions to zidovudine or its components
Caution:
Granulocyte count less than 1000/mm^3 or Hgb less than 9.5 g/dl, lactation, children, severe renal disease, severe hepatic function, risk of severe neutropenia and anemia

DRUG INTERACTIONS OF CONCERN TO DENTISTRY

- Decreased blood levels: acetaminophen, clarithromycin
- Increased serum levels: fluconazole

SERIOUS REACTIONS

! Serious reactions include anemia, which occurs most commonly after 4–6 wk of therapy, and granulocytopenia; both effects are more likely to occur in patients who have a low Hgb level or granulocyte count before beginning therapy.
! Neurotoxicity (as evidenced by ataxia, fatigue, lethargy, nystagmus, and seizures) may occur.

DENTAL CONSIDERATIONS

General:
• Examine for oral manifestations of opportunistic infections.
• Patients on chronic drug therapy may rarely have symptoms of blood dyscrasias, which can include infection, bleeding, and poor healing.
• Avoid dental light in patient's eyes; offer dark glasses for patient comfort.
• Place on frequent recall because of oral side effects.
Consultations:
• In a patient with symptoms of blood dyscrasias, request a medical consultation for blood studies and postpone dental treatment until normal values are reestablished.
• Medical consultation may be required to assess disease control.
Teach Patient/Family to:
• Encourage effective oral hygiene to prevent soft tissue inflammation.
• Use caution to prevent injury when using oral hygiene aids.
• See dentist immediately if secondary oral infection occurs.

zileuton

zye-**lew**′-ton
(zyelo)
Do not confuse Zyflo with Zyban.

CATEGORY AND SCHEDULE

Pregnancy Risk Category: C

Drug Class: Leukotriene pathway inhibitor

MECHANISM OF ACTION

A leukotriene inhibitor that inhibits the enzyme responsible for producing inflammatory response. Prevents formation of leukotrienes (leukotrienes induce bronchoconstriction response, enhances vascular permeability, stimulates mucus secretion).
Therapeutic Effect: Prevents airway edema, smooth muscle contraction, and the inflammatory process, relieving signs and symptoms of bronchial asthma.

USES

Prophylaxis and chronic treatment of asthma

PHARMACOKINETICS

Rapidly absorbed from GI tract. Protein binding: 93%. Metabolized in liver. Primarily excreted in urine. Unknown if removed by hemodialysis. ***Half-life:*** 2.1–2.5 hr.

INDICATIONS AND DOSAGES

▸ Bronchial Asthma
PO
Adults, Elderly, Children 12 yr and older. 600 mg 4 times a day. Total daily dosage: 2400 mg.

SIDE EFFECTS/ADVERSE REACTIONS

Frequent
Headache
Occasional
Dyspepsia, nausea, abdominal pain, asthenia (loss of strength), myalgia
Rare
Conjunctivitis, constipation, dizziness, flatulence, insomnia

PRECAUTIONS AND CONTRAINDICATIONS

Active liver disease, impaired liver function, hypersensitivity to zileuton or any component of the formulation
Caution:
Not for acute bronchospasm, status asthmaticus; theophylline, warfarin, propranolol; hepatic impairment, lactation, children younger than 12 yr, monitor ALT (SGPT) levels

DRUG INTERACTIONS OF CONCERN TO DENTISTRY

- Increased plasma levels of theophylline, propranolol
- Significant increase in PT when taking warfarin
- Use caution when prescribing dental drugs that are strong inhibitors of CYP1A2 isoenzymes

SERIOUS REACTIONS

! Liver dysfunction occurs rarely and may be manifested as right upper quadrant pain, nausea, fatigue, lethargy, pruritus, jaundice, or flu-like symptoms.

DENTAL CONSIDERATIONS

General:
- Consider semisupine chair position for patient comfort because of GI side effects of disease.
- Acute asthmatic episodes may be precipitated in the dental office.
- Avoid prescribing NSAIDs.
- Sympathomimetic inhalants should be available for emergency use.
- Midday appointments and a stress-reduction protocol may be required for anxious patients.
- Be aware that aspirin or sulfite preservatives in vasoconstrictor-containing products can exacerbate asthma.

Consultations:
- Medical consultation may be required to assess disease control.

Teach Patient/Family to:
- Update health and drug history if physician makes any changes in evaluation or drug regimens; include OTC, herbal, and nonherbal remedies in the update.

zinc oxide/zinc sulfate

zink′ ox′-eyed/**zink′ sul′**-fate
(zinc oxide: Balmex, Desitin; zinc sulfate: Orazinc, Zincaps[AUS])

CATEGORY AND SCHEDULE

Pregnancy Risk Category: C

Drug Class: Mineral

MECHANISM OF ACTION

A mineral that acts as a cofactor for enzymes that are important for protein and carbohydrate metabolism.
Therapeutic Effect: Zinc oxide acts as a mild astringent and skin protectant. Zinc sulfate helps maintain normal growth and tissue repair, as well as skin hydration.

USES

Treatment of zinc deficiency

INDICATIONS AND DOSAGES

▸ Mild Skin Irritations and Abrasions (e.g., Chapped Skin, Diaper Rash)

Topical (Zinc Oxide)

Adults, Elderly, Children. Apply as needed.

▸ Treatment and Prevention of Zinc Deficiency, Wound Healing

PO (Zinc Sulfate)

Adults, Elderly. 220 mg 3 times a day.

SIDE EFFECTS/ADVERSE REACTIONS

None known

PRECAUTIONS AND CONTRAINDICATIONS

None known

DRUG INTERACTIONS OF CONCERN TO DENTISTRY

• Decreased absorption: tetracyclines, fluoroquinolones

SERIOUS REACTIONS

! None known

DENTAL CONSIDERATIONS

General:

• Determine why patient is taking the drug.

ziprasidone

zye-**pray**′-za-done

(Geodon)

CATEGORY AND SCHEDULE

Pregnancy Risk Category: C

Drug Class: Antipsychotic, atypical

MECHANISM OF ACTION

A piperazine derivative that antagonizes adrenergic, dopamine, histamine, and serotonin receptors; also inhibits reuptake of serotonin and norepinephrine.

Therapeutic Effect: Diminishes symptoms of schizophrenia and depression.

USES

Treatment of schizophrenia

PHARMACOKINETICS

Well absorbed after PO administration. Food increases bioavailability. Protein binding: 99%. Extensively metabolized in the liver. Not removed by hemodialysis. ***Half-life:*** 7 hr.

INDICATIONS AND DOSAGES

▸ Schizophrenia

PO

Adults, Elderly. Initially, 20 mg twice a day with food. Titrate at intervals of no less than 2 days. Maximum: 80 mg twice a day.

IM

Adults, Elderly. 10 mg q2h or 20 mg q4h. Maximum: 40 mg/day.

▸ Bipolar Mania

PO

Adults, Elderly. 40 mg 2 times a day.

SIDE EFFECTS/ADVERSE REACTIONS

Frequent

Headache, somnolence, dizziness

Occasional

Rash, orthostatic hypotension, weight gain, restlessness, constipation, dyspepsia

PRECAUTIONS AND CONTRAINDICATIONS

Conditions that prolong the QT interval, such as congenital long QT syndrome

Caution:
May antagonize levodopa, dopamine agonists; QT prolongation and risk of sudden death, bradycardia, hypokalemia, hypomagnesemia, electrolyte depletion caused by diarrhea, diuretics, or vomiting, neuromalignant syndrome, tardive dyskinesia, seizures, suicide, lactation, pediatric use

DRUG INTERACTIONS OF CONCERN TO DENTISTRY

- Avoid use of any drug that prolongs the QT interval
- Caution in use of other CNS depressants: increased risk of CNS depressant effects
- Reduced plasma levels: carbamazepine
- Increased plasma levels: ketoconazole and other strong inhibitors of CYP3A4 (see Appendix I)
- Drugs that lower B/P: increased risk of hypotension
- Increased extrapyramidal effects: phenothiazines and related drugs (haloperidol, droperidol), metoclopramide

SERIOUS REACTIONS

! Prolongation of QT interval may produce torsades de pointes, a form of ventricular tachycardia.
! Patients with bradycardia, hypokalemia, or hypomagnesemia are at increased risk.

DENTAL CONSIDERATIONS

General:

- Monitor vital signs at every appointment because of cardiovascular side effects.
- After supine positioning, have patient sit upright for at least 2 min before standing to avoid orthostatic hypotension.
- Assess salivary flow as a factor in caries, periodontal disease, and candidiasis.
- Consider semisupine chair position for patient comfort if GI side effects occur.
- Assess for presence of extrapyramidal motor symptoms, such as tardive dyskinesia and akathisia. Extrapyramidal motor activity may complicate dental treatment.
- Use vasoconstrictors with caution, in low doses, and with careful aspiration; avoid use of epinephrine-impregnated gingival retraction cord.

Consultations:

- Consultation with physician may be necessary if sedation or general anesthesia is required.
- Physician should be informed if significant xerostomic side effects occur (e.g., increased caries, sore tongue, problems eating or swallowing, difficulty wearing prosthesis) so that a medication change can be considered.
- Medical consultation may be required to assess disease control and patient's ability to tolerate stress.

Teach Patient/Family to:

- Encourage effective oral hygiene to prevent soft tissue inflammation.
- Prevent trauma when using oral hygiene aids.
- Use powered tooth brush if patient has difficulty holding conventional devices.
- When chronic dry mouth occurs, advise patient to:
  - Avoid mouth rinses with high alcohol content because of drying effects.
  - Use daily home fluoride products for anticaries effect.
  - Use sugarless gum, frequent sips of water, or saliva substitutes.

zoledronic acid

zole-eh-**drone**′-ick **ass**′-id
(Zometa, Reclast)

CATEGORY AND SCHEDULE

Pregnancy Risk Category: C

Drug Class: Osteoporosis therapy adjunct, bisphosphonate

MECHANISM OF ACTION

A bisphosphonate that inhibits the resorption of mineralized bone and cartilage; inhibits increased osteoclastic activity and skeletal calcium release induced by stimulatory factors produced by tumors.

Therapeutic Effect: Increases urinary calcium and phosphorus excretion; decreases serum calcium and phosphorus levels.

USES

Treatment of hypercalcemia from malignancy, bone metastases associated with prostate and lung cancer; multiple myeloma, bone metastases from solid tumors

PHARMACOKINETICS

IV Infusion: Shows triphasic half-life; plasma protein binding 22%; little to no metabolism; excreted mainly in urine; a high percentage of the dose remains bound to bone

INDICATIONS AND DOSAGES

▸ **Hypercalcemia**

IV Infusion

Adults, Elderly. 4 mg IV infusion given over no less than 15 min. Retreatment may be considered, but at least 7 days should elapse to allow for full response to initial dose.

▸ **Multiple Myeloma**

IV

Adults, Elderly. 4 mg q3–4wk.

SIDE EFFECTS/ADVERSE REACTIONS

Frequent

Fever, nausea, vomiting, constipation

Occasional

Hypotension, anxiety, insomnia, flu-like symptoms (fever, chills, bone pain, myalgia, and arthralgia)

Rare

Conjunctivitis

PRECAUTIONS AND CONTRAINDICATIONS

Hypersensitivity to other bisphosphonates, including alendronate, etidronate, pamidronate, risedronate, and tiludronate. Dental implants are contraindicated for patients taking this drug.

Caution:

Data for use in children not available, monitor hypercalcemic parameters, ensure good hydration, renal impairment, bronchospasm in aspirin-sensitive asthmatics, hypocalcemia, hypoparathyroidism, lactation

DRUG INTERACTIONS OF CONCERN TO DENTISTRY

- None reported

SERIOUS REACTIONS

! Renal toxicity may occur if IV infusion is administered in less than 15 min.

DENTAL CONSIDERATIONS

General:

- Bisphosphonates may increase the risk of osteonecrosis of the jaw.
- This drug is used only in oncology units or hospitals.

• Examine for oral manifestation of opportunistic infection.
• Consider semisupine chair position for patient comfort if GI side effects occur.
• Short appointments may be required.
• If oral candidiasis occurs, treat with suitable antifungal drug.

Consultations:

• Medical consultation may be required to assess disease control.

Teach Patient/Family to:

• Observe regular recall schedule and practice effective oral hygiene to minimize risk of osteonecrosis of the jaw.

zolmitriptan

zohl-mih-**trip**′-tan
(Zomig, Zomig Rapimelt[CAN], Zomig-ZMT)

CATEGORY AND SCHEDULE

Pregnancy Risk Category: C

Drug Class: Serotonin agonist

MECHANISM OF ACTION

A serotonin receptor agonist that binds selectively to vascular receptors, producing a vasoconstrictive effect on cranial blood vessels.

Therapeutic Effect: Relieves migraine headache.

USES

Acute treatment of migraine with or without aura in adults

PHARMACOKINETICS

Rapidly but incompletely absorbed after PO administration. Protein binding: 15%. Undergoes first-pass metabolism in the liver to active metabolite. Eliminated primarily in urine (60%) and, to a lesser extent, in feces (30%). ***Half-life:*** 3 hr.

INDICATIONS AND DOSAGES

▸ Acute Migraine Attack

PO

Adults, Elderly, Children older than 18 yr. Initially, 2.5 mg or less. If headache returns, may repeat dose in 2 hr. Maximum: 10 mg/24 hr.

Intranasal

Adults, Elderly. 5 mg. May repeat in 2 hr. Maximum: 10 mg/24 hr.

SIDE EFFECTS/ADVERSE REACTIONS

Frequent

Oral: Dizziness; tingling; neck, throat, or jaw pressure; somnolence
Nasal: Altered taste, paresthesia

Occasional

Oral: Warm or hot sensation, asthenia, chest pressure
Nasal: Nausea, somnolence, nasal discomfort, dizziness, asthenia, dry mouth

Rare

Diaphoresis, myalgia, paresthesia

PRECAUTIONS AND CONTRAINDICATIONS

Arrhythmias associated with conduction disorders, basilar or hemiplegic migraine, coronary artery disease, ischemic heart disease (including angina pectoris, history of MI, silent ischemia, and Prinzmetal's angina), uncontrolled hypertension, use within 24 hr of ergotamine-containing preparations or another serotonin receptor agonist, use within 14 days of MAOIs, Wolff-Parkinson-White syndrome

Caution:

Renal impairment, hepatic impairment, may cause coronary

vasospasm, lactation, children, elderly

DRUG INTERACTIONS OF CONCERN TO DENTISTRY

• Potential serotonin crises: selective serotonin reuptake inhibitors, ergot-containing drugs (avoid use within 24 hr of taking this drug)
• Decreased plasma levels: cimetidine

SERIOUS REACTIONS

! Cardiac reactions (including ischemia, coronary artery vasospasm, and MI) and noncardiac vasospasm-related reactions (e.g., hemorrhage and CVA) occur rarely, particularly in patients with hypertension, diabetes, or a strong family history of coronary artery disease; obese patients; smokers; males older than 40 yr; and postmenopausal women.

DENTAL CONSIDERATIONS

General:
• This is an acute-use drug; thus, it is doubtful that patients will come to the office if acute migraine is present.
• Be aware of patient's disease, its severity, and its frequency, when known.
• Advise patient if dental drugs prescribed have potential for photosensitivity.
Consultations:
• If treating chronic orofacial pain, consult with physician of record.
• Medical consultation may be required to assess disease control and patient's ability to tolerate stress.
Teach Patient/Family to:
• Be aware that dryness of the mouth may occur when taking this drug.
• Avoid mouth rinses with high alcohol content because of drying effects.
• Update health and drug history if physician makes any changes in evaluation or drug regimens; include OTC, herbal, and nonherbal remedies in the update.

zolpidem tartrate

zole-**pi**′-dem **tar**′-trate
(Ambien, Stilnox[AUS])
Do not confuse Ambien with Amen.

CATEGORY AND SCHEDULE

Pregnancy Risk Category: B
Controlled Substance: Schedule IV

Drug Class: Nonbarbiturate, nonbenzodiazepine sedative-hypnotic

MECHANISM OF ACTION

A nonbenzodiazepine that enhances the action of the inhibitory neurotransmitter gamma-aminobutyric acid.
Therapeutic Effect: Induces sleep and improves sleep quality.

USES

Treatment of insomnia

PHARMACOKINETICS

Route	Onset	Peak	Duration
PO	30 min	N/A	6–8 hr

Rapidly absorbed from the GI tract. Protein binding: 92%. Metabolized in the liver; excreted in urine. Not removed by hemodialysis. ***Half-life:*** 1.4–4.5 hr (increased in hepatic impairment).

INDICATIONS AND DOSAGES

▸ **Insomnia**

PO

Adults. 10 mg at bedtime.
Elderly, Debilitated. 5 mg at bedtime.

SIDE EFFECTS/ADVERSE REACTIONS

Occasional

Headache

Rare

Dizziness, nausea, diarrhea, muscle pain

PRECAUTIONS AND CONTRAINDICATIONS

Hypersensitivity, ritonavir

Caution:

Discontinue if skin rash occurs, pediatric patients at risk for oligohidrosis, hyperthermia; seizures with abrupt withdrawal; use contraception in women of childbearing age; hepatic or renal dysfunction; lactation, kidney stones

DRUG INTERACTIONS OF CONCERN TO DENTISTRY

- Increased CNS depression: alcohol, all CNS depressants, fluconazole, ketoconazole, itraconazole

SERIOUS REACTIONS

! Overdose may produce severe ataxia, bradycardia, altered vision (e.g., diplopia), severe drowsiness, nausea and vomiting, difficulty breathing, and unconsciousness.

! Abrupt withdrawal of the drug after long-term use may produce asthenia, facial flushing, diaphoresis, vomiting, and tremor.

! Drug tolerance or dependence may occur with prolonged, high-dose therapy.

DENTAL CONSIDERATIONS

General:

- Assess salivary flow as a factor in caries, periodontal disease, and candidiasis.
- Monitor vital signs at every appointment because of cardiovascular side effects.

Consultations:

- Medical consultation may be required to assess disease control.

Teach Patient/Family to:

- When chronic dry mouth occurs, advise patient to:
  - Avoid mouth rinses with high alcohol content because of drying effects.
  - Use daily home fluoride products to prevent caries.
  - Use sugarless gum, frequent sips of water, or saliva substitutes.

zonisamide

zoh-**nis'**-ah-mide
(Zonegran)

CATEGORY AND SCHEDULE

Pregnancy Risk Category: C

Drug Class: Anticonvulsant (sulfonamide derivative)

MECHANISM OF ACTION

A succinimide that may stabilize neuronal membranes and suppress neuronal hypersynchronization by blocking sodium and calcium channels.

Therapeutic Effect: Reduces seizure activity.

USES

Adjunctive therapy in partial seizures in adults with epilepsy

PHARMACOKINETICS

Well absorbed after PO administration. Extensively bound to RBCs. Protein binding: 40%. Primarily excreted in urine.
Half-life: 63 hr (plasma), 105 hr (RBCs).

INDICATIONS AND DOSAGES

▸ **Partial Seizures**

PO

Adults, Elderly, Children older than 16 yr. Initially, 100 mg/day for 2 wk. May increase by 100 mg/day at intervals of 2 wk or longer. Range: 100–600 mg/day.

SIDE EFFECTS/ADVERSE REACTIONS

Frequent

Somnolence, dizziness, anorexia, headache, agitation, irritability, nausea

Occasional

Fatigue, ataxia, confusion, depression, impaired memory or concentration, insomnia, abdominal pain, diplopia, diarrhea, speech difficulty

Rare

Paresthesia, nystagmus, anxiety, rash, dyspepsia, weight loss

PRECAUTIONS AND CONTRAINDICATIONS

Allergy to sulfonamides

Caution:

Discontinue if skin rash occurs, pediatric patients at risk for oligohidrosis, hyperthermia; seizures with abrupt withdrawal; use contraception in women of childbearing age; hepatic or renal dysfunction; lactation, kidney stones

DRUG INTERACTIONS OF CONCERN TO DENTISTRY

• None reported.

• Carbamazepine increases renal clearance.

SERIOUS REACTIONS

! Overdose is characterized by bradycardia, hypotension, respiratory depression, and coma.

! Leukopenia, anemia, and thrombocytopenia occur rarely.

DENTAL CONSIDERATIONS

General:

• Determine type of epilepsy, seizure frequency, and quality of seizure control.

• Patients on chronic drug therapy may rarely have symptoms of blood dyscrasias, which can include infection, bleeding, and poor healing.

• Short appointments and a stress-reduction protocol may be required for anxious patients.

• Place on frequent recall to evaluate gingival condition and self-care.

• Consider semisupine chair position for patient comfort if GI side effects occur.

• Warn patient of increased CNS side effects when sedation is used. Advise not to drive a car to and from dental appointment.

Consultations:

• Consultation with physician may be necessary if sedation or general anesthesia is required.

• In a patient with symptoms of blood dyscrasias, request a medical consultation for blood studies and postpone treatment until normal values are reestablished.

• Medical consultation may be required to assess disease control and patient's ability to tolerate stress.

Teach Patient/Family to:

- Encourage effective oral hygiene to prevent soft tissue inflammation.
- Prevent trauma when using oral hygiene aids.
- Update health and drug history if physician makes any changes in evaluation or drug regimens; include OTC, herbal, and nonherbal remedies in the update.
- See physician immediately if rash develops because of drug.

Generic and Trade Name Index

Page numbers followed by "f" indicate figures, "t" indicate tables, and "b" indicate boxes.

INDEX

INDEX

INDEX

INDEX

INDEX

INDEX

INDEX

INDEX